Williams'
Essentials
of Nutrition
and Diet Therapy

Williams'
Essentials
of Nutrition
and Diet Therapy

12th **EDITION**

Eleanor D. Schlenker, PhD, RDN

Professor and Extension Specialist, Emerita
Department of Human Nutrition, Foods, and Exercise
College of Agriculture and Life Sciences
Virginia Polytechnic Institute and State University
Blacksburg, Virginia

Joyce Gilbert, PhD, RDN

President and CEO
Association of Nutrition and Foodservice Professionals
Saint Charles, Illinois

ELSEVIER

ELSEVIER

3251 Riverport Lane
St. Louis, Missouri 63043

WILLIAMS' ESSENTIALS OF NUTRITION AND DIET THERAPY,
TWELFTH EDITION

ISBN: 978-0-323-52971-6

Notices

Previous editions copyrighted 2015, 2011, 2007, 2003, 1999, 1994, 1990, 1986, 1982, 1978, 1974.

Library of Congress Control Number: 2018946505

Content Strategist: Sandra Clark
Content Development Management: Lisa Newton
Content Development Specialist: Melissa Rawe
Publishing Services Manager: Julie Eddy
Senior Project Manager: Cindy Thoms
Design Direction: Brian Salisbury

Printed in China.

Last digit is the print number: 9 8 7 6 5 4 3 2

Working together
to grow libraries in
developing countries

www.elsevier.com • www.bookaid.org

We continue to be indebted to Sue Rodwell Williams who created the
first eight editions of this text, and set the standard that we strive to follow.

The Authors

To my parents, Harold and Nora, who taught me to appreciate
the opportunity to learn.

Eleanor D. Schlenker

To my mom, Helen, who taught me knowledge is power and to
my many mentors who have taught me how to harness
the power of knowledge.

Joyce Gilbert

CONTRIBUTORS

Adriana Campa, PhD
Associate Professor
Florida International University
Miami, Florida
Chapter 24 Acquired Immunodeficiency Syndrome (AIDS)

Pamela Charney, PhD, RD
Associate Professor
University of North Georgia
Dahlonega, Georgia
Chapter 19 Nutrition Support: Enteral and Parenteral Nutrition

Dorothy Chen-Maynard, PhD, RDN, FAND
DPD Director, Nutrition and Food Sciences
California State University, San Bernardino
San Bernardino, California
Chapter 20 Gastrointestinal Diseases

Kary Woodruff, MS, RD, CSSD
Assistant Professor (lecturer), Department of Nutrition and
    Integrative Physiology
University of Utah
Salt Lake City, Utah
Chapter 11 Nutrition During Pregnancy and Lactation
Chapter 12 Nutrition for Normal Growth and Development
Chapter 14 Nutrition and Physical Fitness

Laura Dana, MSN, RN, LCCE, COS-C
ASN Program Director
Cambridge Institute
Altamonte Springs, Florida

Mary M. Flynn, PhD, RD, LDN
Associate Professor of Medicine (Clinical)
The Miriam Hospital, Brown University
Providence, Rhode Island

Wanda Hayes, DNP, RN
Nursing Program Director
Judson College
Marion, Alabama

Kimberly Head, BA, BS, DC
Director
Collin College
Plano, Texas

Ashanti Starr Johnson, MSN, RN
Nursing Faculty
Cambridge Institute
Altamonte Springs, Florida

Kevin Pierce, MBA, CAPM, CMT
Academic Dean
East West College of Natural Medicine
Sarasota, Florida

PREFACE

Through eleven highly successful editions, this nutrition textbook has presented a sound approach to student learning and clinical practice in the health professions. It provides both a strong research base and a person-centered approach to the study and application of nutrition in human health. We have appreciated the suggestions and positive reception of this text by users in colleges, community colleges, and clinical settings throughout the United States and in other parts of the world.

New discoveries in nutrition science and its application to human health provide the foundation for the rapidly evolving protocols in public health and clinical care. Evidence-based practice rather than dependence on custom or prior learning is the new standard for decision-making. The expanding science base in biology, biotechnology, and health is leading to new arenas of practice such as nanotechnology, nutrigenomics, and functional foods. Recent changes in the U.S. population are creating new challenges for the health professional. Government agencies have noted that for the first time in history, our population cannot be considered to be "healthy," based on the prevalence of obesity and growing chronic disease observed in both youth and adults. Our population is also becoming more diverse in culture and ethnicity. These observations carry implications for future health professionals and their formal preparation for working in public health, community, clinical, or industry settings. The health professionals of the future must deal creatively with the realities of chronic disease. They must develop a framework of understanding of the needs of diverse populations and food patterns that differ from their own. The worldwide epidemic of obesity, diabetes, and related chronic disease, fueling the rise in health care costs, is drawing attention to new methods for delivery of health care and disease prevention strategies and the importance of both appropriate food and physical activity patterns in developing a healthy lifestyle. Public interest and concern for nutrition and health are increasing, although consumers often depend on less reliable sources of information. New technology and the Internet offer unlimited opportunities for meaningful nutrition and health intervention programs, despite the appearance of false advertising and misleading health claims. Nutrition has become prominent in the marketplace promoting functional foods and expanding product lines. Such changes present both opportunities and challenges for the future health professional.

This new edition reflects these far-reaching changes. We continue to be guided by a commitment to sound nutrition principles rooted in basic science and their application to human health and well-being. We have built on previous editions to produce this new book—updated and rewritten, with our new design and format—to meet the changing needs of students, faculty, and practitioners in the health professions.

NEW TO THIS EDITION

To accommodate the demands of a rapidly emerging science and an increasingly diverse society, the entire text has been updated. Changes and additions based on input from many teachers, students, and clinicians have been incorporated to increase its usefulness.

Chapter Changes

With the retirement of Dr. Sue Rodwell Williams, the founder and primary author of the first eight editions of this textbook, we continue to share responsibility for the preparation of this new edition. Part 1, *Introduction to Human Nutrition,* provides the foundation in nutrition science and we apply these principles to human nutrition needs and food selection in Part 2, *Community Nutrition and the Life Cycle.* Part 3, *Introduction to Clinical Nutrition,* describes the nutrition care process for nutritional intervention and the application of medical nutrition therapy in the treatment of both acute and chronic diseases and conditions.

We welcome both new and continuing contributors to this edition. Kary Woodruff prepared Chapter 11, "Nutrition During Pregnancy and Lactation," Chapter 12, "Nutrition for Normal Growth and Development," and Chapter 14, "Nutrition and Physical Fitness." Pamela Charney revised Chapter 19, "Nutrition Support: Enteral and Parenteral Nutrition." Dr. Dorothy Chen-Maynard completed Chapter 20, "Gastrointestinal Diseases," and Dr. Adriana Campa contributed Chapter 24, "Acquired Immunodeficiency Syndrome (AIDS)."

New material has been incorporated throughout this edition, reflecting recent research findings and clinical treatment therapies. Examples include new roles for traditional nutrients such as vitamin D, updates on the transmission and treatment of acquired immunodeficiency syndrome (AIDS), and recent attention to protein needs and effective utilization. Health promotion with strategies for implementation is a recurring theme throughout the text, and students are encouraged to look for the *Health Promotion* heading in each chapter for special information to assist with nutrition education in a variety of settings. New research pointing to the application and effectiveness of text messaging and other technologies in support of nutrition education and medical nutrition therapy is reviewed. Full coverage of the U.S. Department of Agriculture and U.S. Department of Health and Human Services health initiatives including MyPlate, the Dietary Guidelines for Americans, and Healthy People 2020 includes goals, practice standards, and application and usefulness to health promotion. We provide an overview of the New Nutrition Label and its helpfulness to consumers. To support future work with the growing elderly population, the MyPlate for Older Adults, developed by Tufts University and the American Association of Retired Persons Foundation is presented in the chapter on nutritional needs for adults. Simple screening protocols for identifying potential malnutrition in older adults will be helpful for students when entering their clinical practice.

The chapters on energy balance and obesity provide readers with a comprehensive review of this public health problem including proposed contributing factors such as sleep deprivation and the intestinal microbiome. Interventions to stem the advance of the obesity epidemic, including new regulations for school breakfast and lunch that limit kilocalories and emphasize fruit, vegetables and whole grains, and current activity recommendations for children are presented. The chapter on nutrition and physical performance includes emerging research pertaining to protein and fluid needs, dietary supplements, and the benefits of exercise on risk factors for cardiovascular disease and diabetes. A public health approach to nutrition and well-being provides a framework for developing and marketing community nutrition and health intervention programs with attention to needs assessment, implementation, and evaluation. Throughout the text students are reminded of factors that contribute to food insecurity among all age and population groups and government agencies and programs that can help individuals and families meet their food needs.

Feature boxes addressing contemporary issues in nutrition and health have been updated. Each chapter includes an example of *Evidence-Based Practice,* guiding students through the critical thought process and reinforcing this concept for future use in the practice setting. The *Complementary and Alternative Medicine (CAM)* boxes—found in all chapters in Part 3—review and evaluate new therapies relevant to chapter topics. *Focus on Culture* boxes introduce students to the concept of cultural competence and the nutritional deficiencies, health problems, and appropriate interventions pertinent to various cultural, ethnic, racial, and age-groups. *Focus on Food Safety* boxes alert readers to food safety issues pertaining to a particular nutrient, medical condition, or segment of the population. *Perspectives in Practice* boxes provide practical elements for nutrition education that students will find helpful in their future roles. Tools available for download from government or other reputable public sites are noted. "Websites of Interest" connect students with accurate and objective Internet resources, useful in finding answers to patient inquiries. "Further Readings and Resources" from the research and professional literature enable further inquiry into a topic of interest.

PERSONAL APPROACH

The person-centered approach that has been a hallmark of the Williams' text over the years continues in this edition. The authors and contributors write in a personal style using materials and examples from personal research and clinical experience. Scientific knowledge is presented in human terms as a tool to develop practical solutions to individual problems.

Illustrations and Design

Numerous illustrations, anatomic figures, graphic line drawings, and photographs, most in full color, enhance the overall design and help students better understand the concepts and clinical practices presented.

Enhanced Readability and Student Interest

Continuing attention has been given to enhancing readability and enlivening the text stylistically with use of boxes, illustrations, and recurring themes that capture student interest and assist in comprehension. New material has been added, and remaining sections have been rewritten. Recent advances in basic and clinical science are explained and applied. Issues of public and professional controversy pertinent to students' future practice are examined.

Learning Aids Within the Text

This twelfth edition continues to include many aids that assist student learning.

Chapter Openers

To alert students to the content of each chapter and draw them into its study, each chapter opens with a preview of chapter topics and their relevance to professional practice. An outline of the major chapter headings is also included on this page.

Key Terms

Key terms important to the student's understanding and application of the chapter content are presented in two steps. First, they are identified in blue type in the body of the text. Then, these terms are grouped and defined in boxes in the lower corners of the pages close to their mention. This dual-level approach to vocabulary development greatly improves the overall study and usefulness of the text.

Pedagogy Boxes

Perspectives in Practice, Focus on Culture, Evidence-Based Practice, Complementary and Alternative Medicine (CAM), and Focus on Food Safety: These special features throughout the text introduce supplemental material, apply subject matter to evidence-based decision-making,

introduce chapter-related issues or controversies, present a deeper look at chapter topics, or describe a practical application of a nutrition concept. These interesting and motivating studies help the student comprehend the importance of scientific thinking and develop sound judgment and openness to varied points of view.

Case Studies

In Parts 2 and 3 realistic case studies provide opportunities for problem solving, relating the information learned to practical situations in nutrition care. Each chapter contains at least one case with questions for analysis, decision-making, and intervention. These case studies help students apply principles of community nutrition and medical nutrition therapy to individuals and groups they will meet in their clinical assignments.

Chapter Summaries

To assist students in drawing the chapter material together as a whole, each chapter concludes with a summary of the key concepts presented and their significance or application. The student can then return to any part of the chapter for repeated study and clarification as needed.

Review Questions

To help students think critically about key components of the chapter and how they relate to community and patient needs or problems, review questions conclude each chapter. Questions go beyond the simple review of facts, requiring problem-solving and critical thinking. Review questions may require the student to seek information or perspective beyond what is found in the text using the scientific literature, the popular literature, community meal or public health programs, nutrition labeling, or population data from government sources.

Chapter References

A strength of this text is the documentation of the topics presented, drawn from a wide selection of pertinent journals. To provide immediate access to all references cited in the chapter text, a full list is given at the end of each chapter rather than collected at the end of the book. Special attention has been directed toward selection of references published within the last 4 to 7 years.

Further Readings And Resources

In addition to referenced material from the text, an annotated list of suggestions for further reading is provided at the end of each chapter. These selections extend or apply the text material according to student needs or special interests. The annotations improve their usefulness by identifying the pertinent topics of the reference. Also included is a list of reliable websites for further reference and study.

Appendices

The appendices contain reference tools and guidelines in learning and practice. These include extended tables for calculating Body Mass Index and a reference list of foods containing oxalates. A table of common conversions between metric and British measurement systems is included for student review. A summary of federal food assistance programs funded and supervised by the U.S. Department of Agriculture and the Administration on Aging, useful for future patient referral, describes the target audience, guidelines for participation, and food resources provided.

Supplementary Materials Available on Evolve

Our Evolve website is designed to provide supplemental online learning opportunities to complement the material in the book. The Evolve website contains sections for both instructor and student resources.

The PowerPoint presentations, Test Bank, and Review Questions were prepared by experienced nutrition writer, editor, and project coordinator, Gill Robertson, MS, RD.

Instructor Resources

- TEACH for Nurses
- Extensive Test Bank of NCLEX-style multiple-choice examination questions
- Image Collection of images from the text
- PowerPoint presentations for each chapter, each created to help guide classroom lecture

Student Resources

- This food database contains over 5000 foods in 18 different categories: Baby Food, Baked Goods, Beverages, Breads/Grains and Pasta, Breakfast Foods/Cereals, Dairy and Eggs, Fats and Oils, Fruits and Vegetables, Meats and Beans, Nuts and Seeds, Frozen Entrees and Packaged Foods, Restaurant Chains–Fast Foods, Restaurant Chains–Other, Seafood and Fish, Snacks and Sweets, Soups, Supplements, and Toppings and Sauces.
- The profile feature allows users to enter and edit the intake and output of an unlimited number of individuals, and the weight management planner helps outline healthy lifestyles tailored to various personal profiles.
- In addition to foods and activities, features include an ideal body weight (IBW) calculator, a basal metabolic rate calculator to estimate total daily energy needs, and sample diets with nutrition recommendations for a variety of conditions.

ACKNOWLEDGMENTS

A textbook of this size is never the work of just authors and contributors. It develops into the planned product through the committed hands and hearts of a number of persons who bring their specialized skills and expertise to its completion. It would be impossible to name all the individuals involved, but several groups deserve special recognition.

First, the authors are grateful to the reviewers, who gave their valuable time and skills to strengthen the manuscript.

Second, we are indebted to Elsevier and the many persons there who had a part in this extensive project. We especially thank our content strategist, Sandra Clark, whose skills and support have always been invaluable; and our content development specialist, Melissa Rawe, whose creative and energetic talents helped shape the book's pages. We also thank our production project manager, Cindy Thoms, for essential guidance; and our book designer, Brian Salisbury, who helped to bring a new look to this twelfth edition. To our marketing managers and the many fine Elsevier sales representatives throughout the country, we owe great appreciation for their help in ensuring the book's success with users.

Eleanor D. Schlenker
Blacksburg, Virginia
Joyce Gilbert
Saint Charles, Illinois

CONTENTS

APPENDICES

Contents

PART 1

Introduction to Human Nutrition

1

Nutrition and Health

Eleanor D. Schlenker

ⓔ http://evolve.elsevier.com/Williams/essentials/

A mother is told that her 11-year-old son, who is overweight and sedentary, will likely develop type 2 diabetes before he reaches the age of 18. A 23-year-old pregnant woman whose sister delivered a low-birth-weight baby is worried that this may happen to her. A 62-year-old man has been told by his doctor that he has hypertension and is at risk of a stroke. A recent edition of the Dietary Guidelines for Americans (DGA) noted that for the first time in our history, the US population could not be described as healthy. Approximately half of all adults have at least one chronic disease, many related to poor eating patterns and low physical activity. Diet-related chronic diseases are affecting our youth, as even adolescents are being diagnosed with elevated blood lipids and high blood pressure. Statisticians predict that today's youth will be the first generation to have a shorter life expectancy than their parents.

Nutrition is the cornerstone of a healthy lifestyle. A diet higher in fruits, vegetables, and whole grains and lower in kilocalories (kcalories or kcal), sugar, and fat could help the 11-year-old boy lower his body fat and disease risk. Appropriate food choices support a successful pregnancy. A healthy diet with attention to sodium and potassium can lower the need for medications to control cardiovascular risk. Nutrition is an effective intervention strategy for addressing health problems.

OUTLINE

New Challenges for Health Professionals
The Science of Nutrition
Nutrition Policy and National Health Problems
Nutrition Guides for Food Selection

A Safe and Healthy Food Supply
Personal Perceptions of Food
Health Promotion

In this chapter, we begin our study of nutrition and human health and see how these principles apply to the health problems of the US population. Current knowledge in nutrition reflects our growing understanding of the relationship between food, health, and well-being. Government agencies and institutions charged with reducing chronic disease and containing health care costs are directing attention to what people are eating and what improvements are needed. Access to a safe and wholesome food supply for all must be our goal.

NEW CHALLENGES FOR HEALTH PROFESSIONALS

Our society is constantly changing, and that includes health care and how it is delivered. The rising incidence of chronic disease among all age groups points to the need for lifestyle education and the availability of affordable and healthy food. The Internet and smartphones are adding cost-effective opportunities to deliver information and help consumers distinguish between appropriate and problematic resources. The rise in life expectancy is bringing rapid shifts in population and growing cohorts of older individuals with unique needs. These changes as described later will continue to affect your future practice as a health professional.

Rise in Chronic Disease

In most developed countries, classic nutrient deficiencies have been replaced by diseases of affluence, resulting from a lifestyle favoring an overabundance of food and low physical activity. Nearly half of the US population suffers from at least one chronic condition as described next.[1]

Obesity: Obesity is a major health problem across the globe. Even countries previously facing food shortages and underweight are now experiencing increasing overweight.[2] According to current US statistics, 35% of men and 40% of women are obese, and of these nearly 6% of men and 10% of women are classed as severely obese. Over the past decade, obesity rates have stabilized in men but are increasing in women.[3] Twenty-one states have obesity rates of at least 30%, and four states have rates of 35% or higher.[4] Moreover, 39% of men and 26% of women are overweight[5]; less than one-third of US adults are normal weight. Among children and youth ages 2 to 19, 17% are obese.[6]

Diabetes: The rise in obesity has fueled the current diabetes epidemic; 29 million people in the United States have type 2 diabetes and another 86 million are living with prediabetes, putting them at risk of developing diabetes and other chronic conditions.[7] Diabetes and its complications account for 20% of all health care costs. Without intervention, it is estimated that by 2050, one-third of the US population

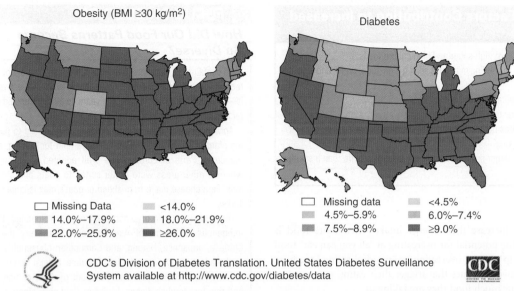

FIG. 1.1 Percentage of US adults who were obese or had diagnosed diabetes in 2015. Notice the relationship between obesity and diabetes; states with a higher prevalence of obesity also had a higher prevalence of diabetes. (Maps from the Behavioral Risk Factor Surveillance System, Centers for Disease Control and Prevention: *PowerPoint Slides on Diabetes,* Maps of Trends in Diabetes and Obesity, Atlanta, GA, US Department of Health and Human Services. https://www.cdc.gov/diabetes/data/center/slides.html.)

will have diabetes. (Note in Fig. 1.1 the pattern of diabetes concentrated in the southern and northeastern regions of the United States.)

Cardiovascular disease (CVD): Heart disease and stroke are among the most widespread and costly health problems and are also among the most preventable. CVD is the cause of one in three deaths, and 20% of these occur in persons under the age of 65. Treatment of CVD accounts for approximately $1 of every $6 spent on health care in the US.[8]

Cancer: Each year more than 1.5 million persons are diagnosed with cancer and more than 500,000 die. In the coming years, cancer is expected to become the leading cause of death as the older population grows in number. On average an individual dying of cancer loses 16.6 years of potential life. More than half of cancer deaths could be prevented through healthy choices, screening, and vaccinations.[9]

Growth of the aging population: Adding to the burden of chronic disease will be the growth of the aging population. Over the past 100 years, life expectancy has risen from approximately 45 years to nearly 80 years, and over the next 50 years the number of persons age 65 and over is expected to double.[10]

Common denominators to the prevention and amelioration of chronic disease, disability, and a deteriorating quality of life is an appropriate diet accompanied by regular physical activity. Recent evaluations of food and nutrient intake and deaths from CVD and diabetes pointed to the protective benefits and detriments to health of particular foods. Fruits, vegetables, legumes, nuts, fish, whole grains, and polyunsaturated fatty acids were protective in preventing these conditions.[11] A greater number of cardiometabolic deaths were associated with higher intakes of sodium, processed meats, and sugar-sweetened beverages and lower use of fruits, vegetables, and fish. Those authors[12] associated dietary intake with 49% of deaths in men and 42% of deaths in women. We will continue to explore the relationships between diet and chronic disease in the following chapters.

Population Diversity and Chronic Disease

As a nation we are becoming increasingly diverse.[13] The numbers of Hispanic Americans, Asian Americans, and Pacific Islander Americans are increasing at rapid rates. Asian Americans are at increased risk of

diabetes, likely fostered by a change from a plant-based diet to the typical American diet high in sugar and fat.[14] African Americans develop heart disease, high blood pressure, and diabetes at younger ages than whites and are twice as likely to die of heart disease before the age of 50.[15] Diabetes screening indicates that Hispanic Americans often develop prediabetes before the age of 40.[16] Obesity is a major risk factor for type 2 diabetes in all race and ethnic groups.

Health disparities: Socioeconomic status, race or ethnic group, and availability of health insurance all contribute to disparities in health care across the US population.[17] Approximately one-third of Americans report skipping dental check-ups or using home remedies for existing ailments rather than seeing a doctor. Even those with health insurance report putting off a recommended examination or treatment. Blacks were more likely to avoid getting a prescription filled or to cut pills in half or to skip medicine doses than were whites or Hispanics,[17] likely related to financial limitations. Postponing treatment for a chronic condition such as type 2 diabetes leads to a worsening situation requiring an even greater level of care, and associated disability or premature death. The Centers for Disease Control and Prevention (CDC) has implemented various programs to address health disparities based on (1) language, (2) isolation, and (3) discrimination.[18] Approximately one in five families in the United States speak a language other than English at home; within this group, more than half speak Spanish.[19]

Lifestyle Intervention and Education

Lifestyle education and management is a necessary adjunct to medication in the prevention and control of chronic disease. Our environment, which promotes the consumption of energy-dense foods, has contributed to the development of obesity and chronic disease. In contrast to earlier times when humans survived as "hunter-gatherers," we now have a plentiful supply of good-tasting, high-calorie food, with little physical activity required to obtain it. The ever-present vending machine, special offers of two hamburgers for the price of one, and accessible food at all sporting and most social events are factors contributing to excessive food intake (Box 1.1). Portions served at fast food restaurants are at least 2 times larger than those offered 20 years

BOX 1.1   Factors Contributing to Increased Food Intake

- Media advertising of high-sugar and high-calorie foods
- Constant access to vending machines selling high-sugar drinks and high-fat snacks
- More meals eaten away from home
- All-you-can-eat restaurant buffets
- Larger portion sizes both at home and in restaurants
- Continuous snacking
- "Supersizing": a larger portion costing only a fraction more than a smaller portion

ago. Most people increase their energy intake when more food is served, adding to the potential for overeating at "all you can eat" food outlets. We can help prevent overeating by "mindful eating," teaching individuals to be aware of cues that trigger their eating and monitor what foods and how much food they are taking in.

As energy intake has risen, energy expenditure has dropped. For many children, television or video games have replaced active outdoor games, and they ride rather than walk to school. Rural localities and new residential developments lack sidewalks, and many neighborhoods are unsafe for walking. Collaborative efforts among schools, community planners, and health professionals will be required to solve these problems.

The Focus on Culture box, "How Did Our Food Patterns Become So Diverse?" introduces factors influencing the food patterns of populations around the world.

KEY TERMS

Overweight
A body weight greater than the average weight for a person of that gender and body height; this measurement does not distinguish between body fat and body muscle.

Type 2 Diabetes
A form of diabetes mellitus usually occurring in middle or older age in which the body no longer produces or uses insulin effectively; type 2 diabetes is often associated with overweight or obesity and a sedentary lifestyle. (Type 2 diabetes differs from type 1 diabetes in which the body can no longer produce any insulin.)

Hypertension
Medical term to describe high blood pressure; dietary and lifestyle interventions can help lower blood pressure and reduce dependence on antihypertensive medications.

Kilocalorie (kcalorie, kcal)
A calorie is the amount of heat energy required to raise the temperature of 1 g of water from 14° C to 15°C. The kilocalorie equals 1000 small calories and is commonly used to describe the energy content of foods and diets.

Obese
An excessive accumulation of body fat.

Energy-Dense
Term used to describe the relative kcalorie content of a food portion; an energy-dense food may also be nutrient dense if it is a good source of essential nutrients.

FOCUS ON CULTURE

How Did Our Food Patterns Become So Diverse?

Food contains the nutrients that sustain life, but for most of us this is not the reason we eat what we do. Food habits—what we eat and when we eat it—have evolved over thousands of years. In all cultures and societies, various factors have influenced food habits.

Agriculture: Available land for crops or animals led to patterns emphasizing plant or animal foods. Cattle require land for grazing, along with water resources. Parts of Europe were well adapted to raising cattle or pigs, whereas other areas were better suited to goats and sheep for meat and milk. Feta cheese made from sheep or goat's milk is common in Greece and Turkey.

The cereal or grain of a particular region influenced daily meals. Rice, indigenous to Southeast Asia, is served at every meal in traditional Chinese, Japanese, Hmong, and Cambodian households, much the same as bread in the American diet. Because animal foods are limited, the Asian pattern combines a small amount of meat or fish with vegetables and rice for stewlike dishes. Maize or field corn along with rice were the traditional cereals in parts of the United States and Central and South America. Corn bread, corn cake, and popcorn were dietary staples among Native Americans, and corn made into tortillas is the basic grain in Mexican meals.

Climate: When people raised all of their own food, the growing season and amount of rainfall defined what they ate. Root vegetables such as potatoes and cold-hardy cabbage, carrots, and apples were common in northern Europe because they could be stored in a root cellar to sustain families over the winter. In contrast, grains and legumes, along with a bountiful supply of fresh produce, provided the plant base of the healthful Mediterranean diet. Olives, olive oil, and dates remain important foods in Mediterranean cultures. The Caribbean region with its extended growing season is known for its tropical fruits and starchy vegetables.

Proximity to water: Populations living near water included fish or seafood in their daily diet. The typical Japanese meal includes fish or shellfish, along with steamed rice. The French-American (Cajun) foods common to southeast Louisiana have a seafood base and are served over rice.

Religion: Religious beliefs define not only what foods are appropriate but also when they may be eaten. The dietary laws of Judaism are defined in the *Rules of Kashruth*, and foods selected and prepared accordingly are called *kosher*, from the Hebrew word meaning *fit* or *proper*. Jewish law governs how animals are slaughtered with the supervision of a rabbi. Many traditional Jewish foods such as matzo, a type of unleavened bread, relate to significant events in Jewish history.

Muslim dietary laws come from the Quran. As in Judaism, pork is forbidden. Certain foods, including figs, olives, dates, honey, milk, and buttermilk, are believed to have special spiritual and physical value. In the ninth month of the Islamic calendar, Muslims celebrate Ramadan, a 30-day period of daylight fasting during which no food or beverages are eaten from dawn to sunset.

Various foods with particular ethnic and cultural origins have joined the mainstream of American foods. Bagels, a traditional Jewish food, sushi from Japan, and olive oil from the Mediterranean are commonly used by many Americans. A balance between the old and the new preserves one's heritage and health.

Bibliography

Goody CM, Drago L, editors: *Cultural food practices*, Chicago, 2010, Diabetes Care and Education Dietetic Practice Group, American Dietetic Association.

Kittler PG, Sucher KP: *Cultural foods: traditions and trends*, Belmont, CA, 2000, Wadsworth/Thomson Learning.

New Directions in Nutrition

New Foods for Health

As nutrition researchers studied the nutrients in food required to prevent deficiency diseases, they also discovered that particular plant foods contain naturally occurring substances in addition to conventional nutrients that positively affect health. These substances, named *phytochemicals* (plant chemicals) and found in fruits, vegetables, and whole grains may play an active role in fighting chronic disease. The foods in which they are found are known as *functional foods*. The finding that certain omega-3 fatty acids found in fish may help prevent CVD has prompted the food industry to develop food sources providing increased amounts of these nutrients. Orange juice has become an alternative source of calcium and vitamin D to prevent bone loss.[20] In contrast, "energy drinks" with added herbs and stimulants and potential deleterious effects on health are being marketed to replace water or other nutritious beverages. Helping consumers make appropriate choices from food in the marketplace is a role for the health professional.

Genes in Nutrition and Health

The Human Genome Project, an international initiative to map the human genetic code, is helping scientists learn how diet interacts with the genetic code and how this affects our nutrient needs and our health. A gene is a DNA sequence that can be translated into a protein, and bioactive components including nutrients, phytochemicals, and functional foods can influence its expression.

Two fields of study have emerged from the Human Genome Project. Nutrigenomics is the study of interactions between the components in our diet and our genome, and how this can change the proteins that control our physiology and metabolism. This may explain why individuals respond differently to nutrient supplementation and have greater or lesser nutrient needs.[21] Evaluations of overweight individuals are providing greater insight into how nutrients affect gene expression. When these individuals modify their diet, their energy metabolism is altered, and these findings may enable clinicians to individualize intervention strategies based on a patient's subtype.[22] Alternatively, nutrigenetics looks at how individual differences in our genetic code affect our nutrient needs, health status, or risk of particular diseases.[21] Phenylketonuria, the inability of an individual to metabolize the amino acid phenylalanine, results from the lack of the required enzyme and is an example of nutrigenetics. Reviewing family history to determine the risk of chronic disease is another application of nutrigenetics. The presence of certain genes in an individual or family member has been associated with cardiovascular risk, and women with a particular genotype are highly susceptible to breast cancer.[23] Genetic testing carried out by reputable health professionals can provide patients with information that will enable them to implement prevention strategies or follow a more aggressive screening protocol.

In the future, it is likely that health professionals will have the required information to generate personalized dietary advice based on an individual's genetic code; however, we still have much to learn before this becomes a reality. Currently, we can make general recommendations regarding disease prevention for individuals whose family history or medical diagnoses put them at risk, and medical research centers are able to offer genetic counseling in respect to various conditions. However, consumers need to be wary of commercial enterprises offering home DNA kits and mail-order sales of supplements meant to supply the nutrient needs of a particular genotype. Genetic screening and intervention should be obtained through a legitimate health care facility.

Disseminating Nutrition Information

Advances in technology, such as Facebook and smartphones, have revolutionized the way individuals communicate with each other and the outside world. Seventy-seven percent of Americans own smartphones. This includes not only individuals ages 18 to 29 (92% own smartphones) but also 42% of those over age 65.[24] Nearly half of smartphone owners have used this technology to seek health information. Approximately three-fourths of Americans have broadband access at home,[24] and the availability of the Internet at any hour of the day or night has made this a source of ready information. Almost 60% of US adults say they have looked online for health information in the past year; 35% say they have gone online to try to figure out what medical condition they or someone else might have.[25] Caregivers of family members with serious health problems are heavy users of technology on health-related topics. Unfortunately, the accuracy or reliability of the information presented on Internet sites is often suspect. An evaluation of 100 health-related websites conducted by the US Office of Disease Prevention and Health Promotion revealed serious problems in both the credibility of the information presented and the transparency as to who owns the site.[26] Only 30 sites clearly disclosed their identity, and only 15% offered credibility and updating of content. Other shortcomings included failure to disclose authorship of the material presented and clearly differentiating between advertisements and factual content.

Internet sites marketing herbs, drugs, and supplements are not monitored by government regulatory agencies and often contain misleading information. Reputable food companies usually provide helpful facts about the nutrient content of their products, but commercial sites devoted to sales often post misleading claims. Internet sites maintained by government agencies, universities, state extension services, and medical facilities offer evidence-based information and should be the first source for guidance on foods, nutrition, and health. At the close of each chapter in this text is a list of recommended websites for consumers or health professionals seeking additional information.

THE SCIENCE OF NUTRITION

Nutrition builds on two branches of science. The life sciences of biochemistry and physiology tell us how nutrition relates to our physical health and body function. The behavioral sciences help us understand how nutrition is interwoven with our psychosocial needs. Both aspects are at work in our lives.

Human organisms are highly complex groupings of chemical compounds constantly at work in an array of reactions that sustain life. Nutrients participate in and help control these chemical reactions. Various physiologic systems integrate the activities of millions of functioning cells, uniting them into a functioning whole. This highly sensitive internal control is called homeostasis.

We also have social and emotional qualities rooted in our earliest awareness. Eating patterns and attitudes toward food develop over a lifetime based on the influences of our primary family and friends, ethnic or cultural group, community, nation, and world. How we perceive food, what we choose to eat, why we eat what we do, and the ways in which we eat are all integral to human nutrition.

Working Definitions

Nutrition means *to nourish* and encompasses the food people eat and how it enriches their lives physically, socially, and personally. From the moment of conception until death, an appropriate supply of food supports optimal growth and maturation and mental and physical well-being. Good nutrition promotes health and reduces the risk of adverse conditions ranging from low birth weight to obesity to CVD. Food supplies the energy to carry out body functions, such as inhaling and exhaling, maintaining body temperature, and engaging in physical activity. Food also nourishes the human spirit. We all have our particular "soul foods," comfort foods that connect us to our family and provide a sense of psychological and emotional well-being.

To study nutrition, we need to define the terms that describe this body of knowledge and the health professionals who work within it. *Nutrition* refers to the food people eat and how it nourishes their bodies, whereas nutrition science defines the nutrient requirements for body maintenance, growth, activity, and reproduction. Dietetics is the health profession tasked with the practical application of nutrition science throughout the life cycle in health and disease. The registered dietitian nutritionist (RDN) is the nutrition expert on the health care team and, in collaboration with the physician and nurse, carries the major responsibility for a patient's nutritional care. Public health nutritionists focus on disease prevention and oversee programs that serve high-risk groups in the community, such as pregnant teens or frail older adults, assessing needs and applying interventions. RDNs cooperate with school nurses to teach weight management classes for children and parents, assist day care providers in planning menus and snacks, or help clients at fitness centers improve their body composition or athletic performance.

Functions of Food and Nutrients

Food serves as the vehicle for bringing nutrients into the body; however, the specific chemical compounds and elements in food—the nutrients—are the substances the body needs. No one particular food or food combination is required to ensure health. The human race has survived for centuries on a wide variety of foods, depending on what was available and what the culture designated as appropriate. Approximately 50 nutrients are known to be essential to human life and health, although countless other elements and molecules are being studied and may be found to be essential. The identification of essential nutrients (nutrients that the body cannot synthesize) is especially important when developing liquid formulas for feeding critically ill patients.

The macronutrients (carbohydrates, fats, and proteins), the micronutrients (vitamins and minerals), and water all have important roles in growth and health. The macronutrients supply energy and build tissue, whereas the micronutrients, needed in much smaller amounts, form specialized structures and regulate body processes. Water is the additional and often-forgotten nutrient that sustains all life systems. The sum of all the chemical reactions occurring in the body that use nutrients is referred to as metabolism. The first section of this text defines the essential nutrients; later chapters describe how they participate in growth, maturation, aging, and dietary interventions in health and disease.

Nutrients have three general functions, as follows:
1. To provide energy
2. To build and repair body tissues and structures
3. To regulate the metabolic processes that maintain homeostasis.

Energy

All three of the macronutrients—carbohydrate, fat, and protein—can be used for energy, although carbohydrate and fat are the preferred energy sources.

Carbohydrates. Dietary carbohydrates—starch and sugars—are the primary sources of fuel for heat and energy. Glucose, the breakdown product of dietary carbohydrate, is the energy currency of the body. *Glycogen* is the storage form of carbohydrate available for quick energy when glucose is needed. Each gram of carbohydrate when metabolized in the body yields 4 kilocalories (kcalories or kcal), known as its fuel factor. In a well-balanced diet for a healthy person, 45% to 65% of total kcalories come from carbohydrate.[27]

The majority of these kcalories should be obtained from complex carbohydrates (starch), with a smaller amount from simple carbohydrates (sugars). Another form of complex carbohydrate, known as *fiber*, does not yield energy but has other important body functions. Although the general public uses the word *calorie* to refer to the energy value of food, nutritionists use the technical term *kilocalorie*. As noted later in this chapter, MyPlate (http://www.choosemyplate.gov), the food guidance system developed for the general public,[28] and the DGA[1,29] use the term *calorie* when indicating the energy value of foods or meals.

KEY TERMS

Nutrigenomics
The study of the effects of nutrients and other bioactive substances found in food on genes, body proteins, and metabolites.

Nutrigenetics
The study of the effect of an individual's particular genetic makeup on metabolic and physiologic functions, including nutrient requirements and risk of certain diseases.

Homeostasis
State of dynamic equilibrium within the body's internal environment, a balance achieved through the control of many interrelated physiologic mechanisms.

Nutrition
The sum of the processes involved in taking in food, releasing the nutrients it contains, and assimilating and using these nutrients to provide energy, maintain body tissue, and regulate body metabolism.

Nutrition Science
The body of scientific knowledge developed through controlled research that relates to all aspects of nutrition and its role in the body; areas of study include national, international, community, and clinical nutrition.

Dietetics
The science related to the application of nutrition principles to the selection and preparation of foods and the development of healthy eating patterns for various ages, physiologic situations, health conditions, and diseases.

Registered Dietitian Nutritionist (RDN)
A health professional who has completed an accredited academic program and a minimum of 1200 hours of postbaccalaureate, supervised practice and has passed the National Registration Examination for Dietitians administered by the Commission on Dietetic Registration of the Academy of Nutrition and Dietetics.

Public Health Nutritionist
A health professional who has completed an academic program in nutrition and a graduate degree (MPH or DrPH) in a school of public health accredited by the Council on Education for Public Health, and supervises the nutrition component of public health programs in county, state, national, or international community settings.

Nutrients
Substances in food that are essential for energy, growth, normal body function, and maintenance of life.

KEY TERMS—cont'd

Essential Nutrients

Substances that cannot be made by the body and must be supplied in food. These include essential fatty acids, vitamins, minerals, and essential amino acids for making proteins.

Macronutrients

The three energy-yielding nutrients: carbohydrate, fat, and protein.

Micronutrients

The two classes of non–energy-yielding elements and compounds—minerals and vitamins; these nutrients control and regulate cell metabolism and are components of specialized body structures.

Metabolism

The sum of all the biochemical and physiologic processes by which the body grows and maintains itself (anabolism), breaks down and reshapes tissue (catabolism), and transforms energy to do its work. Products of these reactions are called metabolites.

Carbohydrate

Nutrient class that includes starch, sugar, and fiber; starch should be the major energy source in the diet; sugar and starch have a fuel factor of 4 kcal/g; fiber is an indigestible form of carbohydrate.

Fuel Factors

The number of kcalories that 1 g of a macronutrient yields when completely oxidized; the fuel factor is 4 for carbohydrate and protein, 9 for fat, and 7 for alcohol. Fuel factors are used in computing the energy values of foods and diets (e.g., 10 g of fat yields 90 kcal).

Note: alcohol also adds kcalories to the diet but contains no nutrients. Its fuel factor is 7 kcal/g.

Fat

Nutrient class providing a concentrated form of energy (yields 9 kcal/g); is stored as adipose tissue as an energy reserve; supplies essential fatty acids in the diet.

Protein

Nutrient class that contains nitrogen and essential amino acids; amino acids serve as building blocks for forming body tissues, enzymes, and hormones; fuel factor is 4 kcal/g.

Fats. Dietary fats from either animal or plant sources provide an alternate or storage form of energy. Fat is a more concentrated fuel than carbohydrate, with a fuel factor of 9, yielding 9 kcal/g. Nutrition experts recommend that fats supply no more than 20% to 35% of total kcalories.[27] Fats contain the essential fatty acids required for life and health. Saturated fats are a less healthy form of fat; therefore the majority of our dietary fat should be unsaturated.

Proteins. The primary function of protein is tissue building, although it can be used for energy if needed. The body draws on dietary or tissue protein for energy when the fuel supply from carbohydrates and fats is not sufficient to meet body needs. Protein yields 4 kcal/g, making its fuel factor 4. Protein can provide 10% to 35% of total kcalories in a well-balanced diet for healthy people.[27]

Tissue Building and Repair

Protein is the primary nutrient for building and maintaining body tissues. Vitamins and minerals are used in smaller amounts in the structure of specialized tissues.

Protein. The basic units of proteins are amino acids, the building blocks for body growth and repair. Body tissues are constantly being broken down and rebuilt to ensure growth and maintenance of body structure. Proteins also form vital substances such as enzymes and hormones that regulate body systems.

Minerals. Minerals help build tissues with very specific functions. Two major minerals—calcium and phosphorus—give strength to bones and teeth. The trace element iron is a component of hemoglobin and binds oxygen for transport to cells and carbon dioxide for return to the lungs.

Vitamins. Vitamins are complex molecules needed in very minute amounts but are essential in certain tissues. Vitamin C produces the intercellular ground substance that cements tissues together and prevents tissue bleeding. Vitamin A in the rods and cones of the eye is needed for vision in dim light.

Metabolic Regulation

Specific vitamins and minerals are necessary for enzyme activities responsible for a host of chemical reactions. Water provides the appropriate environment for these reactions to occur.

Minerals. Minerals serve as cofactors in controlling cell metabolism. One example is iron, which controls the enzyme actions in the cell mitochondria that produce and store high-energy compounds.

Vitamins. Many vitamins are components of cell enzyme systems. They govern reactions that produce energy and synthesize important molecules. For instance, thiamin controls the release of energy for cell work, and vitamin B_{12} is needed for the synthesis and maturation of red blood cells.

Water. Water forms the blood, lymph, and intercellular fluids that transport nutrients to cells and remove waste. Water also functions as a regulatory agent, providing the fluid environment in which all metabolic reactions take place.

Nutrient Interrelationships

An important principle in nutrition is *nutrient interaction*. It has the following two parts:

1. Individual nutrients participate in many different metabolic functions; for some functions a nutrient has a primary role, and for others it has a supporting role.
2. No nutrient ever works alone.

Intimate and ongoing metabolic relationships exist among all the nutrients and their metabolites. Although we look at each nutrient individually to simplify our study, they do not exist that way in the body. Nutrients are always working together within an integrated whole, providing energy, building and rebuilding tissue, and regulating metabolic activities. This synergy and interaction among nutrients is important in carrying out body functions and is sometimes overlooked when we examine the effects of one nutrient at a time.

Nutritional Status

The nutritional health of an individual is known as his or her *nutritional status* and describes how well nutrient needs are being met. Nutritional status is influenced by living situation, social and economic factors, available food, food choices, and state of health. *Nutritional status* differs from *dietary status*. Evaluating nutritional status requires a combination of dietary, biochemical, anthropometric, and clinical measurements (Box 1.2), whereas dietary status addresses only what foods are being consumed and their nutrient content. It is important to know not only what an individual is eating, but also whether the body is absorbing and making use of those nutrients. Blood nutrient levels can help identify a nutrient deficiency or a nutrient excess brought about by overuse of highly fortified foods or dietary supplements. Used together, dietary and biochemical measurements can help us distinguish between a *primary nutrient deficiency* and a *secondary nutrient deficiency*. A primary nutrient deficiency is caused by insufficient dietary intake of a particular nutrient or nutrients. A secondary nutrient deficiency is the result of poor absorption or metabolism of a nutrient caused by an interfering substance, a disease or condition, or an elevated requirement. Body weight for height (body mass index [BMI]) and other anthropometric measurements provide estimates of the proportion of body fat versus lean body mass. An evaluation of nutritional status sometimes includes related clinical conditions associated with food and nutrient intake, such as osteoporosis and calcium. Clinical and biochemical parameters included in a nutritional assessment are discussed in detail in Chapter 16; however, when discussing the individual nutrients, we will often refer to the current status of the US population based on the methods listed in Box 1.2.

KEY TERMS

Amino Acid
An acid containing the essential element nitrogen in the chemical group NH2. Amino acids are the structural units of protein and the building blocks of body tissue.

Synthesize
The action of forming new compounds in the body for use in building tissues or carrying out metabolic or physiologic functions.

Metabolites
Any substance produced by metabolism or by a metabolic process.

Anthropometric
Measurement of the human body to determine height, weight, skinfold thickness, or other dimensions that help estimate the relative proportions of body fat and body muscle; these measurements are used to evaluate health status and risk of chronic disease.

Optimal Nutrition

Individuals with optimal nutritional status have neither a deficiency nor an excess of nutrients. Nutrient stores are at the upper end of the normal range. Evidence of optimal nutrition includes appropriate weight for height and good muscle development and tone. Appetite, digestion, and elimination are normal. Well-nourished persons are more likely to be alert, both mentally and physically. They are not only meeting their day-to-day needs but also maintaining appropriate nutrient stores to resist disease and support body function in times of stress.

Undernutrition

Undernutrition takes various forms ranging from marginal nutritional status to the emaciated famine victim. Persons with *marginal nutritional status* are meeting their minimum day-to-day nutritional needs but lack the nutrient stores to cope with any added physiologic or metabolic demand arising from injury or illness, pregnancy, or growth spurt. Marginal nutritional status results from poor choices from the food available, stressful environments, or insufficient resources to obtain appropriate types or amounts of food.

Current US food trends add to the risk of marginal nutritional status and undernutrition among all age groups. Money spent for food away from home has increased and now equals approximately half of total food expenditures.[30] Men between the ages of 20 and 50 consume nearly 40% of their kcalories, fat, saturated fat, and sodium in food away from home but lower proportions of fiber, vitamin A, vitamin D, and calcium.[31] Mixed dishes such as sandwiches, burgers, tacos, pizza, and pasta supply 29% of the total caloric intake of persons age 2 and older; snacks and sweets, including candy, desserts, cake, cookies, and granola bars, make up an additional 16%, and sugar-sweetened soft drinks and fruit drinks add another 12%.[29] Added sugars account for 270 kcal in the average US diet, well above the recommendation that added sugar contribute less than 10% of daily energy intake. Despite an abundance of kcalories, most Americans have less than recommended intakes of fruit, vegetables, whole grains, and dairy items low in fat and added sugar.[29]

Public health nutritionists describe the American diet as energy rich but nutrient poor. Although persons with less-than-optimal intakes of micronutrients may not suffer from overt malnutrition, they are at greater risk of physical illness than those who are well nourished. The body can adapt to marginal nutrient intake but any added physiologic stress that calls on nutrient stores will result in overt malnutrition.

Overt Malnutrition

When nutrient intake is insufficient to meet day-to-day needs and nutrient stores are depleted, signs of malnutrition begin to appear. Limited-resource individuals and families often have diets lacking in food quantity or quality. When asked about their food supply, approximately 12.7% of US households (15.8 million) reported some level of food insecurity during the preceding 12 months, meaning they were uncertain of having or being able to acquire a sufficient amount of food for all members of their family.[32] Single-parent families, families with incomes below the poverty line, and minority families are most at risk.

Hunger influences the health of all ages and genders, but the most vulnerable are infants, children, pregnant women, and older adults. Toddlers from families that are food insecure are more likely to have poorer health and experience deficits in cognitive development and academic performance that can extend through adolescence.[33] Children with chronically inadequate diets often develop iron-deficiency anemia, with low energy and lessened resistance to infection. Women who are poorly nourished in pregnancy are more likely to give birth to a low-birth-weight infant. Homeless and limited-resource families have low intakes of fruits and vegetables that contain important micronutrients,[34] and these foods are in short supply at many food pantries.[35]

Malnutrition also exists among hospitalized patients and residents of long-term care facilities. Both prescription and over-the-counter medications can diminish appetite or interfere with the absorption of nutrients. Metabolic tests or surgery requiring a prior period of fasting interfere with meals and food intake. Hypermetabolic diseases such as congestive heart failure or cancer increase energy requirements and lead to nutrient depletion and weight loss. Cytokines, secreted by the immune system in response to infection and chronic disease, interfere with the efficient use of nutrients with loss of body protein. In the elderly, even aggressive nutrition intervention cannot always reverse these negative effects.[36]

Overnutrition

Overnutrition takes various forms. Excessive energy intake coupled with low physical activity leads to unwanted weight gain and elevated health risks for chronic conditions such as CVD and diabetes. Overnutrition also occurs with excessive intakes of micronutrients from overuse of dietary supplements. Inappropriate amounts of particular vitamins or minerals damage tissues and interfere with the absorption and metabolism of other essential nutrients. Herbal preparations, growing in popularity, carry the potential for harmful interactions with nutrients or medications.

Nutrient Density

A major factor in nutritional health is the *nutrient density* of the diet. This term refers to the relative nutrient content of a food in relation to its energy content. Nutrition experts[29] define **nutrient-dense** foods as those that provide vitamins, minerals, and other substances that contribute to adequate nutrient intakes or have positive health effects but contain little or no solid fats, added sugars, refined starches, and sodium. A nutrient-dense food contributes vitamins, minerals, essential fatty acids, and/or protein to the diet in addition to kcalories. A food that is not nutrient dense adds kcalories but is lacking in other nutrients. As described in Table 1.1, a hamburger made from lean ground beef, containing only a limited amount of fat, also supplies protein and many vitamins and minerals. Fruits and vegetables high in vitamins and minerals and low in kcalories are nutrient dense. In contrast, a doughnut with high amounts of added sugar and fat and sugar-sweetened soft drinks add only kcalories. These foods we consider to be "**empty calories**" because they contribute no essential nutrients.[37] Americans who consume adequate kcalories may still exhibit undernutrition because the foods they consume are not nutrient dense.

NUTRITION POLICY AND NATIONAL HEALTH PROBLEMS

Diet, Health, and Public Policy

Public policy refers to the laws, regulations, and government programs surrounding a certain topic. Nutrition policies are concerned with food guidance for the public, nutrition standards for government food programs, and the health and well-being of the population. Recently, nutrition policy has focused on obesity and related chronic disease. Food safety regulations and nutrition labeling are other examples of public policy.

Prior to 1950, government policies and programs were intended to eradicate hunger and malnutrition. Nutrient deficiency diseases such as rickets and pellagra still existed in various regions of the United States. A law passed in the 1930s mandated the addition of vitamin D to milk as a measure against rickets, and the enrichment of grains with thiamin, riboflavin, niacin, and iron began sometime later to address the problems of pellagra and anemia. The development of the School Nutrition Program with policies for free and reduced-cost lunches was a response to existing hunger among children and adolescents. However, by the 1980s the focus had shifted to overnutrition as new research linked dietary habits to the growing prevalence of CVD.

TABLE 1.1 Nutrient Density of Selected Foods

	Orange Juice (1 cup)	Glazed Doughnut 3-in Diameter (1)	Beef Patty Pan Broiled (3 oz)	Baked Beans Canned, (1 cup)	Sweet Potato, Canned, Mashed (½ cup)	Milk—1% Fat (1 cup)
Kcalories	117	192	197	266	124	118
Fat (g)	—	10	12	1	<1	3
Protein	—	—	◆	◆	—	◆
Fiber	—	—	—	◆	◆	—
Vitamin A	—	—	—	—	◆	◆
Vitamin C	◆	—	—	—	◆	—
Folate	◆	—	—	◆	—	—
Vitamin B₆	◆	—	◆	◆	◆	◆
Calcium	◆ (if fortified)ᵃ	—	—	◆	—	◆
Iron	—	—	◆	◆	◆	—

ᵃOrange juice is not a good source of calcium unless this nutrient has been added.
NOTE: Blue diamonds indicate at least 10% of the Dietary Reference Intakes (DRI); calculations based on DRI values for men ages 19–50. Red diamonds equal 50% or more of the DRI; foods supplying at least 10% of the DRI are considered a good source of that nutrient.
US Department of Agriculture, Agricultural Research Service: *USDA national nutrient database for standard reference*, Release 26, 2013. Nutrient Data Laboratory home page: http://www.ars.usda.gov/nutrientdata.

- Increase the contribution of total vegetables to the diets of individuals aged 2 and older from 0.8 cups equivalent per 1000 calories to 1.2 cups equivalent per 1000 calories.
- Increase the proportion of schools that do not sell or offer calorically sweetened beverages to students from 9% to 21%.
- Increase the proportion of infants who are breast-fed at 6 months from 43.5% to 60.6%.
- Reduce the proportion of US households reporting food insecurity from 14.6% to 6.0%.
- Reduce the proportion of adults aged 18 years and older with hypertension from 29.9% to 26.9% (10% reduction).

Data from US Department of Health and Human Services: *Healthy People 2020: 2020 Topics and Objectives*, Washington, DC, Office of Disease Prevention and Health Promotion, last updated May 2017. https://www.healthypeople.gov/2020/topics-objectives.

Congressional committees and government agencies began to discuss the role of government in setting dietary guidelines to improve health.

The *Surgeon General's Report on Nutrition and Health*[38] released in 1988 established the connection between the typical American diet high in fat and salt and morbidity and early death from CVD. In 1989 the Food and Nutrition Board of the National Academy of Medicine (formerly the Institute of Medicine) issued another extensive report, *Diet and Health: Implications for Reducing Chronic Disease Risk*.[39] Their conclusions agreed with the Surgeon General and people were advised to (1) reduce total fat to 30% or less of total kcalories, (2) reduce saturated fat and cholesterol, (3) increase fiber and complex carbohydrates, (4) avoid excessive sodium and protein, and (5) maintain appropriate levels of calcium.

Healthy People 2020

In 1990 the US Department of Health and Human Services (USDHHS) introduced the public health initiative Healthy People 2000 that established science-based, national objectives for promoting health. These objectives are updated every 10 years and build on the progress made in the decade prior.[40] Healthy People 2020 includes many nutrition-related goals pertaining to dietary intake, maternal and child health, food safety, and management of chronic disease (see examples in Box 1.3). The Healthy People 2020 website presents ideas for related community programs for each objective.

NUTRITION GUIDES FOR FOOD SELECTION

For the past 100 years, government agencies have been issuing food guides to help Americans meet their nutritional needs. The underlying assumptions have been influenced by emerging nutrition science as well as social, political, and economic events, including wars and national emergencies. Their focus also shifted from preventing undernutrition to controlling chronic diseases related to overnutrition. These guides are of three types: (1) nutrition standards, (2) dietary guidelines, and (3) food guides. Each has a different intention and target audience.

Nutrition Standards
Dietary Reference Intakes

Most countries set standards for nutrient intakes of healthy people according to age and sex. Health professionals use these standards in making decisions about the nutritional health of individuals and groups. In the United States these nutrient and energy standards are called the Dietary Reference Intakes (DRIs) and include several categories of

recommendations.[27] Each category within the DRIs has a different purpose and use for the health professional. Each category is described next:

- *Dietary Reference Intakes (DRIs):* The framework of nutrient standards that provide reference values for use in planning and evaluating diets for healthy people. The DRIs include the Recommended Dietary Allowance (RDA), the Adequate Intake (AI), the Tolerable Upper Intake Level (UL), and the Estimated Average Requirement (EAR).
- *Recommended Dietary Allowance (RDA):* The daily intake of a nutrient that will meet the requirement of 97% to 98% (or two standard deviations of the mean) of healthy people of a given age and sex. The RDAs were established and are reviewed periodically by an expert panel of nutrition scientists; they are amended as needed based on new research findings. RDAs have been set for carbohydrate, protein, essential fatty acids, and most vitamins and minerals. When planning diets the RDA serves as an intake goal.
- *Adequate Intake (AI):* A suggested daily intake of a nutrient to meet body needs and support health. The AI is used when there is insufficient research available to develop an RDA but the nutrient appears to have a strong health benefit. The AI serves as a guide for intake when planning diets.
- *Tolerable Upper Intake Level (UL):* The highest amount of a nutrient that can be consumed safely with no risk of toxicity or adverse effects. The UL is used to evaluate the nutrient content of dietary supplements or review total nutrient intake from food and supplements. Intakes exceeding the UL usually result from concentrated supplements, not food.
- *Estimated Average Requirement (EAR):* The daily intake of a nutrient that will meet the requirement of 50% of healthy people of a given age and sex. The EAR is used to plan and evaluate the nutrient intakes of groups rather than individuals.
- *Acceptable Macronutrient Distribution Range (AMDR):* The AMDR guides the division of kcalories among carbohydrate, fat, and protein in ranges supportive of health; carbohydrate should provide 45% to 65% of total kcalories, fat should provide 20% to 35% of total kcalories, and protein should provide 10% to 35% of total kcalories.

The DRIs for vitamins and minerals are broken into two age categories for persons over age 50, directing our attention to the changes in nutrient requirements as we age. These two categories are ages 51 to 70 and 71 and older.[27]

The first set of DRIs, replacing earlier RDAs, was released in 1997. They provided new standards for calcium, phosphorus, magnesium, and vitamin D and emphasized their role in bone health. Since then, DRIs have been established for the B-complex vitamins, antioxidant nutrients and carotenoids, vitamins A and K and the trace minerals, energy, the energy-yielding macronutrients and fiber, and electrolytes and water. The DRIs for calcium and vitamin D were revised again in 2010, based on bone health. (These original publications can be found on the website of the National Academy of Medicine (formerly the Institute of Medicine) of the National Academies of Science at https://www.nal.usda.gov/fnic/dietary-reference-intakes.) The Institute of Medicine has recently been renamed the National Academy of Medicine.

The nutrient standards of Canada and Great Britain are similar to those of the United States. Developing countries use standards set by the United Nations Food and Agriculture Organization (FAO).

Dietary Guidelines
Origin of the Dietary Guidelines

Dietary guidelines are the second type of nutrition guide. First published in 1980, the DGA expressed the growing concerns of government agencies about the health of the American people. The *Dietary Guidelines are designed for health professionals who are assisting individuals and managing food and nutrition programs that support a healthy and nutritionally adequate diet. The guidelines (1) give direction to government policies and the development of programs relating to nutrition and health, (2) help set standards for food-related programs, such as school meals, and (3) form the basis of nutrition education materials produced and distributed by government agencies.*[59]

By law the guidelines are updated every 5 years and represent a cooperative effort between the USDHHS, the federal agency concerned with health, and the US Department of Agriculture (USDA), the federal agency concerned with food. For each update an advisory panel of experts is charged with the responsibility of reviewing the current guidelines, assessing the nutrition and health status of the general population to identify emerging needs and problems, and reviewing new research findings that impact on public health. When complete, the advisory committee's report is submitted for public comment before the specific guidelines are finalized by government experts.[1,29] (See the Evidence-Based Practice box, "How Do I Use It?" to learn more about this method of decision-making.)

Current Dietary Status of the US Population

The current dietary patterns of most Americans include excessive amounts of sodium and added sugar but inadequate amounts of calcium, potassium, vitamin D, and fiber. All age groups, beginning with toddlers ages 1 to 3 years, consume greater than their recommended limits for sodium. Less than one in five Americans meets their recommended servings of vegetables, and barely one in four takes in their recommended servings of fruit. Although most people meet or exceed the number of daily grain servings recommended for their age and kcalories, they are choosing refined grains rather than whole grains. Only approximately 20% of the US population older than age 4 consumes their needed servings of dairy or calcium-fortified foods, putting them at risk of poor bone growth and/or excessive bone loss. Most persons eat more than their recommended amount of protein, with greater amounts from meat, poultry, and eggs and lesser amounts from fish and vegetable sources. Solid fats still exceed oils in the diets of most Americans.[29]

Dietary Guidelines for 2015–2020

The 2015 Dietary Guidelines Advisory Committee took a somewhat different approach than previous committees. Earlier *Dietary Guidelines* emphasized individual dietary components—the food groups and the nutrients. But as noted by the 2015 Advisory Committee,[29] people do not eat nutrients in isolation, but rather as part of an overall eating pattern. It is this eating pattern with its food and nutrition characteristics that over time influences our health and risk of chronic disease. Accordingly, the 2015 guidelines provide three suggested eating patterns to assist individuals in choosing more healthy foods. Each eating pattern is provided at 12 different energy levels, ranging from 1000 to 3200 kcal, and to the extent possible meets the RDA for each nutrient without exceeding kcalorie limits. The three patterns include the following[1,29]:

- *Healthy US-Style Eating Pattern.* This pattern is based on the types and amounts of food that Americans are generally accustomed to eating but suggests nutrient-dense forms and appropriate amounts. It also stays within the recommended limits of overconsumed nutrients such as fat, sodium, and added sugars.
- *Healthy Mediterranean-Style Eating Pattern.* This pattern was adapted from the Healthy US-Style Pattern while adjusting the amounts of certain foods to more closely align with the Mediterranean diet that has been associated with improved health outcomes. This pattern contains more fruits and seafood and less dairy than the Healthy US-Style Pattern.
- *Healthy Vegetarian Eating Pattern.* In this pattern, soy foods such as tofu, legumes, nuts, seeds, and whole grains are increased, and meat, poultry, and seafood are eliminated. Dairy foods and eggs were included as protein sources because recent surveys indicate that a majority of vegetarians use these foods, although the pattern includes suggestions for substitutions if all animal foods are eliminated.[1,29]

These patterns can be viewed in Appendices 3, 4, and 5 of the 2015 DGA, accessible at https://health.gov/dietaryguidelines/2015/guidelines/. To obtain a copy of the 2015 Guidelines publication visit https://health.gov/dietaryguidelines/2015/.

The 2015–2020 Guidelines use five overarching principles to build a framework for healthy eating, yet allow individuals to enjoy foods that meet their personal, cultural, and traditional food patterns (Fig. 1.2).[1] Most people will need to make some changes or *shifts* in

EVIDENCE-BASED PRACTICE

How Do I Use It?

How will you, as a practicing professional, seek out information when developing a nutrition care plan for a patient or client or establishing a nutrition education program? Over time, new evidence becomes available and new interventions are developed. How do you stay up to date on new findings?

The new paradigm in health care is evidence-based practice: using current research and published findings to make appropriate decisions. Successful evidence-based practice requires that you keep current on new standards of practice, carry out planned protocols to evaluate new methods or programs, and share your outcomes with others.

Evidence-based practice is a three-step process, as follows:

- *Identify the problem:* What is the question that you need to answer? Are you developing a new treatment protocol and need some guidance? Do you need some new ideas on how to motivate pregnant teens to consume a healthy diet?
- *Review the evidence:* Search for studies in your professional journals that address this question and critically evaluate what you find. How many patients or clients participated in the evaluation? What was the time period of the study? Were the research participants and circumstances similar to yours? Based on the outcomes of the studies you find, are there some things that you will try to do differently to achieve a better outcome?
- *Implement the findings:* Following your review of the existing information, develop and implement a plan for your patients or group. Be sure to include an evaluation component so you can rate the outcome and success of your

plan. When you have compiled your results, share them with other professionals at your facility and at local or state professional meetings.

Nutrition and health experts have developed formal systems for evaluating research evidence. Evidence may be rated as good or strong, fair, limited, or supported only by opinion. These rating scales are used in review articles published in professional journals and on reputable websites maintained by government agencies and professional societies. Make use of these systems in your decision-making process.

Examples of evidence-based approaches to nutrition and health issues follow:
National Institutes of Health, Office of Dietary Supplements: *Herbs at a glance*, November 2016. https://nccih.nih.gov/health/herbsataglance.htm.
US Department of Health and Human Services, US Department of Agriculture: *Scientific report of the 2015 Advisory Committee on the dietary guidelines*, Washington, DC, 2015. https://health.gov/dietaryguidelines/2015-scientific-report/.

Bibliography

Laramee SH: Evidence-based practice: a core competency for dietetics, *J Am Diet Assoc* 105:333, 2005.
Vaughan LA, Manning CK: Meeting the challenges of dietetic practice with evidence-based decisions, *J Am Diet Assoc* 104:282, 2004.
Zoellner J, Van Horn L, Gleason PM, et al: What is translational research? Concepts and applications in nutrition and dietetics, *J Acad Nutr Diet* 115:1057, 2015.

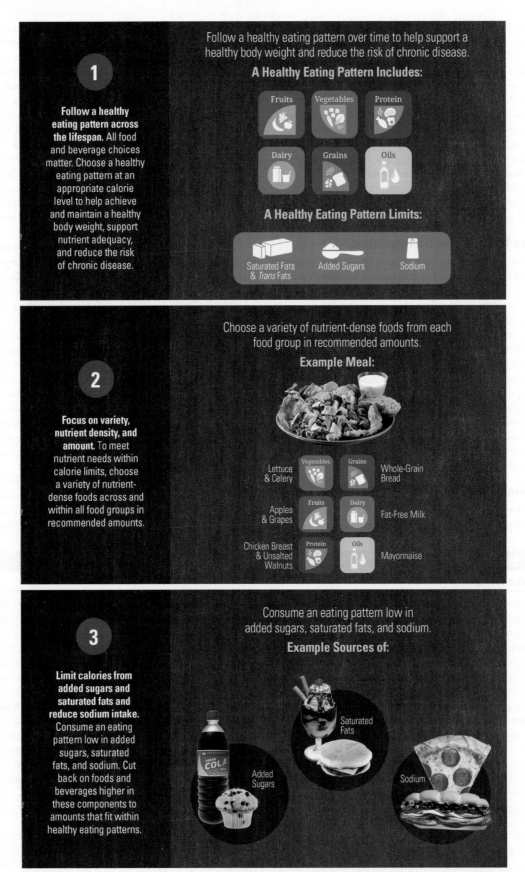

FIG. 1.2 The 2015–2020 Dietary Guidelines proposes five recommendations for choosing a healthy diet for yourself and others. Make shifts in your eating pattern to accommodate more nutrient-dense foods. Support programs that provide healthy food for all age groups. (US Department of Health and Human Services, US Department of Agriculture: Dietary Guidelines for Americans, 2015–2020, ed 8, 2015.)

4

Shift to healthier food and beverage choices. Choose nutrient-dense foods and beverages across and within all food groups in place of less healthy choices. Consider cultural and personal preferences to make these shifts easier to accomplish and maintain.

Replace typical food and beverages choices with more nutrient-dense options. Be sure to consider personal preferences to maintain shifts over time.

Example:

Meal A   *Shift*   Meal B

5

Support healthy eating patterns for all. Everyone has a role in helping to create and support healthy eating patterns in multiple settings nationwide, from home to school to work to communities.

Everyone has a role in helping to create and support healthy eating patterns in places where we learn, work, live, and play.

FIG. 1.2, cont'd

their food choices to accommodate the new guidelines, such as choosing foods higher in nutrient density, eating a wider variety of foods, limiting fat, saturated fat, added sugar, and sodium, and shifting to more healthy beverages. The 2015 guidelines, along with the 2008 *Physical Activity Guidelines for Americans*, emphasize daily physical activity in balance with a kcalorie-appropriate diet to maintain a healthy weight.[1] (See Box 1.4 for further details on the 2015 Dietary Guidelines Recommendations.)

Strategies for Implementation

Adoption of healthy shifts in food practices by the American public will require a change in the food environment at home, at school, at the workplace, and in the community. Consumers need access to fresh produce and healthy choices when eating away from home. Food processors must review the kcalorie, sugar, solid fat, and sodium content of their packaged foods. Nutrition programs for children and older adults must incorporate the dietary guidelines in the meals they serve. Snacks offered at community gatherings, sports events, and religious functions must include healthy options. Community leaders must consider the locations of sidewalks, trails, and

parks that provide accommodations for walking and other physical activity. All individuals and families must have access to healthy food, regardless of their income. We must develop a plan to enable all Americans to eat well, be physically active, and maintain good health and function.

Food Guides

Food guides are developed for use by the general public. They are intended to help individuals with day-to-day food selection and meal planning and provide a practical interpretation of nutrition standards and dietary guidelines. Food guides group foods based on their nutrient content and recommend a certain number of servings from each group. Commonly used food guides are the MyPlate[28] developed by USDA which accompanies the DGA, and *Choose Your Foods: Food Lists for Diabetes* from the American Diabetes Association and the Academy of Nutrition and Dietetics.[41] These guides classify foods differently and serve different purposes.

Food Guides

The USDA issued its first food guide in the 1940s, and food guides evolved over time into various formats and shapes. Variations of the Food Guide Pyramid was the graphic used from 1992 through 2009. The need for a new icon that was simple and easy to put into action led to the development of MyPlate, released in 2010.

MyPlate

MyPlate (Fig. 1.3) illustrates the five major food groups using a familiar mealtime visual—a place setting. Food groups join foods with similar nutrient content, and to include more foods similar in nutrients, several food groups were renamed. The traditional meat and beans group was renamed the protein group and the milk group was renamed the dairy group; the fruit, vegetable, and grains groups remained the same. (Table 1.2 describes the nutrients supplied by each food group.)

> ### BOX 1.4   Dietary Guidelines for Americans 2015–2020—Key Recommendations
>
> Consume a healthy eating pattern that accounts for all foods and beverages within an appropriate calorie level.
>
> A healthy eating pattern includes:
> - A variety of vegetables from all of the subgroups—dark green, red and orange, legumes (beans and peas), starchy, and other
> - Fruits, especially whole fruits
> - Grains, at least half of which are whole grains
> - Fat-free or low-fat dairy, including milk, yogurt, cheese, and/or fortified soy beverages
> - A variety of protein foods including seafood, lean meats and poultry, eggs, legumes (beans and peas), and nuts
> - Oils
>
> A healthy eating pattern limits:
> - Saturated fats and *trans* fats, added sugars, and sodium
>
> Key recommendations that are quantitative are provided for several components of the diet that should be limited. These components are of special public health concern in the United States, and the specified limits can help individuals achieve healthy eating patterns within calorie limits.
> - Consume less than 10% of calories per day from added sugars
> - Consume less than 10% of calories per day from saturated fats
> - Consume less than 2300 mg per day of sodium
> - If alcohol is consumed, it should be consumed in moderation—up to one drink per day for women and up to two drinks per day for men—and only by adults of legal drinking age
>
> In tandem with the previous recommendations, Americans of all ages—children, adolescents, adults, and older adults—should meet the *Physical Activity Guidelines for Americans* to help promote health and reduce the risk of chronic disease. Americans should aim to achieve and maintain a healthy body weight. The relationship between diet and physical activity contributes to calorie balance and managing body weight. People can engage in regular physical activity in a variety of ways throughout the day and by choosing activities they enjoy. (See specific recommendations for various age groups at https://health.gov/dietaryguidelines/2015/guidelines/table-of-contents/).

Taken from US Department of Health and Human Services, US Department of Agriculture: *2015–2020 Dietary Guidelines for Americans*, ed 8, 2015.

FIG. 1.3 MyPlate: The MyPlate food icon was developed by the United States Department of Agriculture as part of a communication initiative to help consumers make better food choices. MyPlate uses a familiar mealtime setting to remind us to eat healthfully and include appropriate amounts of each of the five food groups. (From US Department of Agriculture, Center for Nutrition Policy and Promotion: *MyPlate* [http://www.choosemyplate.gov], Washington, DC; last update October 2016.)

TABLE 1.2 Major Nutrients Supplied by Each MyPlate Food Group

Food Group	Major Nutrients[a]	Serving Equivalents
Fruits (color code red)	Vitamin C Folate Potassium Fiber	1 cup raw or cooked fruit or 1 cup 100% fruit juice or ½ cup dried fruit equals 1 cup from the fruit group
Vegetables (color code green)	Vitamin A Vitamin C Vitamin E Vitamin B_6 Folate Potassium Fiber	1 cup raw or cooked vegetables or 1 cup vegetable juice or 2 cups raw leafy greens equal 1 cup from the vegetable group
Grains (color code deep orange) Enriched grains	Thiamin Riboflavin Niacin Folate Iron	1 slice of bread, 1 oz ready-to-eat cereal (approximately 1 cup cereal flakes), ½ cup cooked rice, pasta, or cooked cereal, 1 tortilla (6-inch diameter) or 1 pancake (5-inch diameter) equals 1 oz from the grains group
Whole grains	Zinc, magnesium, and fiber in addition to the nutrients in enriched grains	
Protein foods (color code purple)	Protein Thiamin Riboflavin Niacin Vitamin B_6 Vitamin B_{12}[b] Iron Zinc Vitamin E (nuts)	1 oz lean meat, poultry, or seafood, 1 egg, 1 Tbsp peanut butter, ¼ cup cooked dry beans or peas, or ½ oz nuts or seeds equals 1 oz from the protein foods group
Dairy (color code blue)	Protein Vitamin A Riboflavin Vitamin B_{12} Calcium Phosphorus Magnesium	1 cup milk, 1 cup yogurt, 1 cup fortified soy or rice beverage, 1½ oz natural cheese (e.g., cheddar) or 2 oz processed cheese (e.g., American) equals 1 cup from the dairy group
Other important food components		
Oils (Not a food group but oils supply essential nutrients)	Vitamin E Linoleic acid[c] Alpha-linolenic acid[c]	Includes vegetable, nut, and fish oils and soft vegetable oil table spreads that have no trans fats (Equivalents differ according to source)

[a]Each of the food groups is a major source of the nutrients listed but also adds smaller amounts of other nutrients to the daily diet.
[b]Vitamin B_{12} is found only in animal foods.
[c]Linoleic acid and alpha-linolenic acid are the essential fatty acids.
Data from Dietary Guidelines Advisory Committee, 2005: *Report of the Dietary Guidelines Advisory Committee on the Dietary Guidelines for Americans 2005*, Beltsville, MD, 2004, US Department of Agriculture, Agricultural Research Service, and US Department of Agriculture and US Department of Health and Human Services: *Dietary Guidelines for Americans, 2010* (Policy Document), ed 7, Washington, DC, 2010, US Government Printing Office.

MyPlate translates the dietary guidelines into action messages for consumers providing menus, recipes, food preparation videos, and best buys at the grocery store that address the barriers to healthy eating—time, money, and cooking skills. Easy-to-read fact sheets supply basic information about foods and their content and ways to reduce your kcalorie intake. The interactive feature, MyPlate Plan, enables consumers to develop individualized daily food plans based on their age, gender, and level of physical activity and generate a daily check list to monitor their personal goals (Fig. 1.4). National surveys indicate that users of the MyPlate website make better food choices than nonusers.[42] Both the dietary guidelines and MyPlate build on current food patterns to encourage Americans to make one small shift and then another to develop a healthy eating style that they can maintain long term.[43]

Successful implementation of any food plan requires an understanding of serving size and related kcalories, but this concept is poorly understood by the general public. Consumers tend to think of a serving size as what they choose to eat or "what I have on my plate," and this confusion contributes to overeating. The MyPlate Daily Checklist describes serving sizes in household measures (Fig. 1.4), and a helpful illustration of cup and ounce equivalents of various foods can be found in Fig. 1.5. Consumers might be encouraged to measure their food servings for several weeks to establish what standard serving sizes look like. Each food plan developed using the MyPlate Plan feature defines the number of kcalories that can be used for solid fats and added sugars, but note that empty calories are quite limited. The 2000-kcal Daily Check List (see Fig. 1.4) allows only 50 g or 200 kcal of added sugar. MyPlate

materials also offer suggestions for measuring your minutes of physical activity.

Food Lists for Meal Planning

Choose Your Food: Food Lists for Diabetes (formerly called the *Exchange Lists*) was introduced in 1950 by the American Diabetes Association and the American Dietetic Association as a meal-planning tool for people with diabetes.[41] The *Food Lists* group foods based on macronutrient content and equivalent energy values, making this tool useful for planning any diet in which control of carbohydrate, fat, protein, and total kcalories is the goal. Because the foods in each list are equal to one another when eaten in the portions indicated, items can be freely interchanged within each list, and food values and kcalories remain constant. The freedom of choice to exchange within groups promotes increased variety and satisfaction with meals and snacks.

United States Department of Agriculture

MyPlate Plan
Find your Healthy Eating Style

Everything you eat and drink matters. Find your healthy eating style that reflects your preferences, culture, traditions, and budget—and maintain it for a lifetime! The right mix can help you be healthier now and into the future. The key is choosing a variety of foods and beverages from each food group—*and making sure that each choice is limited in saturated fat, sodium, and added sugars.* Start with small changes—**"MyWins"**—to make healthier choices you can enjoy.

Food Group Amounts for 2,000 Calories a Day

Fruits	Vegetables	Grains	Protein	Dairy
2 cups	**2 1/2 cups**	**6 ounces**	**5 1/2 ounces**	**3 cups**
Focus on whole fruits	Vary your veggies	Make half your grains whole grains	Vary your protein routine	Move to low-fat or fat-free milk or yogurt
Focus on whole fruits that are fresh, frozen, canned, or dried.	Choose a variety of colorful fresh, frozen, and canned vegetables—make sure to include dark green, red, and orange choices.	Find whole-grain foods by reading the Nutrition Facts label and ingredients list.	Mix up your protein foods to include seafood, beans and peas, unsalted nuts and seeds, soy products, eggs, and lean meats and poultry.	Choose fat-free milk, yogurt, and soy beverages (soy milk) to cut back on your saturated fat.

Limit Drink and eat less sodium, saturated fat, and added sugars. Limit:
- Sodium to **2,300 milligrams** a day.
- Saturated fat to **22 grams** a day.
- Added sugars to **50 grams** a day.

Be active your way: Children 6 to 17 years old should move **60 minutes** every day. Adults should be physically active at least **2 1/2 hours** per week.

FIG. 1.4 The MyPlate Plan is an easy way to track what you had to eat for the day and if you are meeting your goals. The MyPlate Plan indicates the food amounts for a 2000 kcalorie plan. Consumers can access a daily food plan based on their age, gender, body weight, and level of physical activity at https://www.choosemyplate.gov/MyPlatePlan. (From US Department of Agriculture, Center for Nutrition Policy and Promotion: *MyPlate Plan, 2000-calorie daily food plan*, last updated in June 2018; Washington, DC.)

MyPlate Daily Checklist

Write down the foods you ate today and track your daily MyPlate, MyWins!

Food group targets for a 2,000 calorie* pattern are:

Food group		Write your food choices for each food group	Did you reach your target?
Fruits	**2 cups** 1 cup of fruits counts as • 1 cup raw or cooked fruit; or • 1/2 cup dried fruit; or • 1 cup 100% fruit juice.	_____ _____	Y N
Vegetables	**2 1/2 cups** 1 cup vegetables counts as • 1 cup raw or cooked vegetables; or • 2 cups leafy salad greens; or • 1 cup 100% vegetable juice.	_____ _____	Y N
Grains	**6 ounce equivalents** 1 ounce of grains counts as • 1 slice bread; or • 1 ounce ready-to-eat cereal; or • 1/2 cup cooked rice, pasta, or cereal.	_____ _____	Y N
Protein	**5 1/2 ounce equivalents** 1 ounce of protein counts as • 1 ounce lean meat, poultry, or seafood; or • 1 egg; or • 1 Tbsp peanut butter; or • 1/4 cup cooked beans or peas; or • 1/2 ounce nuts or seeds.	_____ _____	Y N
Dairy	**3 cups** 1 cup of dairy counts as • 1 cup milk; or • 1 cup yogurt; or • 1 cup fortified soy beverage; or • 1 1/2 ounces natural cheese or 2 ounces processed cheese.	_____ _____	Y N

Limit:
• Sodium to **2,300 milligrams** a day.
• Saturated fat to **22 grams** a day.
• Added sugars to **50 grams** a day.

Y   N

Be active your way:
Adults:
• Be physically active at least **2 1/2 hours** per week.

Children 6 to 17 years old:
• Move at least **60 minutes** every day.

Y   N

* This 2,000 calorie pattern is only an estimate of your needs. Monitor your body weight and adjust your calories if needed.

MyWins **Track your MyPlate, MyWins**
_____
_____
_____

Center for Nutrition Policy and Promotion
January 2016
USDA is an equal opportunity provider and employer.

FIG. 1.4, cont'd

Choose Your Food: Food Lists for Diabetes[41] arranges foods into the following three groups:

1. *Carbohydrates:* includes starches (grains, starchy vegetables, crackers, snacks, and legumes), fruits, milk, sweets, and nonstarchy vegetables.
2. *Proteins:* includes animal protein foods arranged by fat content (lean, medium fat, and high fat) and plant-based proteins.
3. *Fats:* includes both animal and plant fats arranged by degree of saturation—unsaturated (monounsaturated and polyunsaturated) and saturated.

Serving sizes and macronutrient content for combination foods, fast foods, and free foods are also provided. Use of the *Food Lists* in helping people with diabetes control their carbohydrate intake is discussed in Chapter 22.

A SAFE AND HEALTHY FOOD SUPPLY

Food safety is an important public health priority and included in the Healthy People 2020 initiatives.[40] Foodborne illness arising from microbial contamination, and sometimes incorrectly referred to as "*food poisoning,*" is common and costly, yet preventable.[44] The CDC estimates that each year approximately 1 in 6 Americans (48 million people) gets sick; 128,000 are hospitalized; and 3000 die of foodborne illness. The actual number of individuals who get sick from contaminated food is likely higher because many cases go unreported when people attribute their symptoms to a "stomach virus" or the flu and do not seek medical care. Symptoms of foodborne illness include diarrhea, nausea, and stomach upset and cramping. In most cases, victims feel better in 1 or 2 days; however, in young children, older adults, and patients with compromised immune systems, foodborne pathogens result in severe dehydration, fever, hospitalization, and even death. Careful washing of fresh produce, especially leafy vegetables; thorough cooking of poultry and raw meat; avoiding raw eggs (including not tasting batters containing raw eggs); and always washing your hands before eating and cooking help prevent foodborne illness. Proper food handling should be included in any comprehensive nutrition education program. In Chapter 9 we explore these topics in greater depth.

PERSONAL PERCEPTIONS OF FOOD

What Do I Usually Eat

Each of us develops ways of eating based on our ethnic or cultural background, religious beliefs, family habits, socioeconomic status,

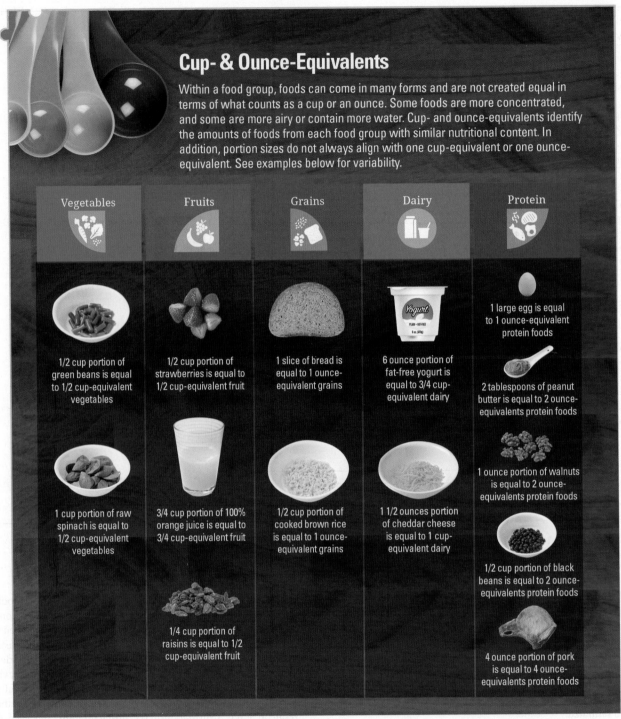

Cup- & Ounce-Equivalents

Within a food group, foods can come in many forms and are not created equal in terms of what counts as a cup or an ounce. Some foods are more concentrated, and some are more airy or contain more water. Cup- and ounce-equivalents identify the amounts of foods from each food group with similar nutritional content. In addition, portion sizes do not always align with one cup-equivalent or one ounce-equivalent. See examples below for variability.

Vegetables	Fruits	Grains	Dairy	Protein

Vegetables

1/2 cup portion of green beans is equal to 1/2 cup-equivalent vegetables

1 cup portion of raw spinach is equal to 1/2 cup-equivalent vegetables

Fruits

1/2 cup portion of strawberries is equal to 1/2 cup-equivalent fruit

3/4 cup portion of 100% orange juice is equal to 3/4 cup-equivalent fruit

1/4 cup portion of raisins is equal to 1/2 cup-equivalent fruit

Grains

1 slice of bread is equal to 1 ounce-equivalent grains

1/2 cup portion of cooked brown rice is equal to 1 ounce-equivalent grains

Dairy

6 ounce portion of fat-free yogurt is equal to 3/4 cup-equivalent dairy

1 1/2 ounces portion of cheddar cheese is equal to 1 cup-equivalent dairy

Protein

1 large egg is equal to 1 ounce-equivalent protein foods

2 tablespoons of peanut butter is equal to 2 ounce-equivalents protein foods

1 ounce portion of walnuts is equal to 2 ounce-equivalents protein foods

1/2 cup portion of black beans is equal to 2 ounce-equivalents protein foods

4 ounce portion of pork is equal to 4 ounce-equivalents protein foods

FIG. 1.5 Serving sizes for various foods. Increasing portion sizes have helped to fuel the growth in overweight and obesity. The 2015–2020 Dietary Guidelines for Americans has provided illustrations of cup and ounce equivalents that can help control your kcalorie intake. (From US Department of Healthand Human Services, US Department of Agriculture: Dietary Guidelines for Americans, 2015–2020, ed 8, 2015.)

health status, geographic location, and personal likes and dislikes. However, the growing ethnic and cultural diversity in our society has brought about a greater intermingling of foods and ideas about food. How people perceive themselves in relation to food and food patterns plays a role in their attitudes toward food and personal eating behavior.

A simple way to get an idea of your own food pattern and beliefs is to look at what you actually eat. See the Perspectives in Practice box,

"My Personal Food Patterns: Do They Need Improvement?" for directions on keeping a food diary. Keeping a record of everything you eat and drink for a day, noting the time, place, any related activity, and people with you provides insight to your true relationship with food. Most of us eat by habit, according to where we are and what is available, rather than by serious thought or plan. Using MyPlate to approximate kcalorie needs and required food servings is a means of rapid dietary assessment.

My Personal Food Patterns: Do They Need Improvement?

Before we can help others make healthy food choices, we need to help our-selves. What do you usually eat? Do you eat regular meals or snack most of the time? Do you make an effort to choose nutritious foods or eat whatever is around? This activity provides an opportunity to evaluate your personal food and nutrient intake.

- To get started, keep a detailed record of everything you eat and drink for 3 days: 2 weekdays and 1 weekend day. List the type and amount of food in household measures (e.g., cups, tablespoons, or dimensions), how it was prepared, and brand name, if applicable. Be specific: was your milk nonfat, 1% fat, 2% fat, or whole? Include butter, margarine, salad dressings, condi-ments, and additions to coffee or tea. When you have completed your record, consider the following:
- What social or emotional factors influenced your food choices? Where and when did you eat? Were you alone or with someone? How did you feel at the time?

- Using MyPlate, compare your intake with the number of servings and serving sizes recommended for your age, gender, and level of physical activity. Did you have too many or too few servings from any of the food groups?
- Using the Nutritrac software available on the Evolve website, evaluate your intakes of macronutrients and micronutrients. Are your kcalories partitioned appropriately? How do your intakes compare with the DRIs for your age and gender?
- Now that you have thought about it, how do you view your diet? Do you have food behaviors that you should modify to promote good health? Do you feel good about certain nutrient categories for which you are meeting current recommendations? If improvements are needed, develop a plan for making changes over time that are consistent with your lifestyle and resources and can be sustained.

Nutritional Analysis by Nutrients and Energy Values

A comprehensive nutritional analysis of food intake is accom-plished using a computer-assisted nutrient analysis program, as found on the Evolve website that accompanies your text. A computer-assisted program enables you to evaluate individual intakes of vitamins and minerals, protein, specific fats, fiber, and energy as compared with the DRIs. Government agencies use such analyses to evaluate dietary information obtained in national surveys and to identify nutrition problems among various age, gender, or ethnic groups.

HEALTH PROMOTION

Healthy People 2020,[40] the National Institutes of Health,[45] and non-profit health groups such as the American Heart Association[46] are encouraging population approaches to health promotion to reach more people with important health messages. Such approaches in-clude the use of media including public service announcements and newspapers, package labeling, school programs, worksite programs, and community programs sponsored by local coalitions, health facili-ties, and other health organizations. The most effective community programs involve several activities that reach a broad base of consum-ers and reinforce the messages in various ways. Several of the Healthy People 2020 objectives pertain to childhood obesity, and schools are well positioned to reach children and families with in-school and after-school activities.

A comprehensive school program could include the school nutri-tion program, school nurse, teachers, parents, parent-teacher associa-tion, and local health care professionals as follows:
- School food service: Review menus to conform to current guidelines limiting fat, sodium, and sugar and emphasizing fruits, vegetables, and whole grains; offer fruit or cereal-based treats for dessert; pro-vide fresh fruit as a snack.
- School art department: Sponsor a student contest for posters or displays that "advertise" healthy cafeteria options or encourage students to drink water rather than sugar-sweetened beverages.
- School health/physical education curriculum: Discuss healthy eating and ways to limit kcalorie intake if you are gaining unwanted weight; support physical activities that are feasible for students of all body weights; set up an after-school walking club.

- Parent/teacher organization: Have a local health professional speak about childhood overweight and intervention strategies; review fundraising policies and determine whether sale items or vending machine contents are in balance with child obesity prevention.
- Engage the local hospital or a health group in sponsoring a walking event for the community at large with emphasis on "getting in the game" rather than how far or how fast a participant can walk. Make step counters available to encourage continued walking.

Health promotion must be ongoing and advance a consistent mes-sage across the community. Programs are most successful if they stress specific goals relating to food or activity rather than overall healthy living.[46] Just as poor eating and activity patterns develop over time, so must intervention be a continuing process. As a health professional, look for other programs and individuals with similar goals with whom you can partner to maximize your impact on community health.[47] (We will learn more about organizing community interven-tions in Chapter 10.)

TO SUM UP

The role of nutrition in human health continues to evolve in response to our changing society and food supply. As available food increased and the physical activity required to obtain it decreased, inappropriate weight gain, diabetes, and CVD have emerged as major health prob-lems worldwide. Discovery of new substances in plant foods that are beneficial to health led to the definition of functional foods and recommendations for their use. Despite the accessibility of nutrient-dense foods, many American diets are high in sugar, fat, and sodium, compromising nutritional status. Children and adults who are chron-ically undernourished as a result of illness, disease, or inadequate food resources are more vulnerable to poor growth, infection, and nutrition-related diseases. Resources developed by government agen-cies are helpful in planning and evaluating the nutrient intakes of all population groups. The DRIs and the DGA, intended for use by health professionals, provide the foundation for MyPlate, which offers practical guidance for family meal planning. Together, these materials build a framework for public policy that directs state and federal nutrition programs and develops health messages reaching people of all ages.

QUESTIONS FOR REVIEW

1. Visit the Maps of Trends in Diagnosed Diabetes and Obesity, produced by the Centers for Disease Control and Prevention at https://www.cdc.gov/diabetes/statistics/slides/maps_diabetesobesity_trends.pdf and scroll down to the state maps and diabetes and obesity statistics. What is the prevalence of obesity and diabetes in your state as compared with national trends? How have they changed over the past 20 years? Note how the growth in diabetes prevalence has paralleled the rise in obesity prevalence.

2. What are the two major fields of science that provide the foundation for the study of nutrition? What does each contribute to our understanding of human nutrition needs?

3. Compare the four levels of nutritional status: optimal nutrition, marginal nutrition, undernutrition, and overnutrition. In what community or clinical situations might you expect to find individuals representing each of these conditions and what physical or clinical signs would you use to identify them?

4. What are the six major nutrient groups? What is the primary function of each?

5. What are the various categories within the DRIs? What is the purpose of each?

6. Compare nutrient standards, dietary guidelines, and food guides: (a) list an example of each, (b) the intended audience (professional or consumer), (c) the type of information included, and (d) a professional situation in which you would use it.

7. Visit the Healthy People 2020 website at https://www.healthypeople.gov and look for a nutrition or health objective of interest. Review the target goals and suggested community-based interventions for that objective. Choose a target audience in your community and develop an intervention that would address this health issue.

8. Research the food patterns of a cultural or ethnic group different from your own. Using MyPlate, develop a 1-day menu for a child or adult in that group using foods common to their daily pattern.

REFERENCES

1. US Department of Health and Human Services, US Department of Agriculture: *Dietary Guidelines for Americans, 2015-2020*, ed 8, December 2015. https://health.gov/dietaryguidelines/2015/guidelines/.

2. Jaacks LM, Kavle J, Perry A, et al: Programming maternal and child overweight and obesity in the context of undernutrition: Current evidence and key considerations for low- and middle-income countries, *Public Health Nutr* 20(7):1286, 2017.

3. Flegal KM, Kruszon-Moran D, Carroll MD, et al: Trends in obesity among adults in the United States, 2005 to 2014, *JAMA* 315(21):2284, 2016.

4. Center for Disease Control and Prevention: *Overweight and Obesity: Adult Obesity Prevalence Maps*, April 1, 2017. https://www.cdc.gov/obesity/data/prevalence-maps.html.

5. US Department of Health and Human Services: *Health, United States, 2015 with Special Feature on Racial and Ethnic Health Disparities, Table 53*, Bethesda, MD, 2016, National Center for Health Statistics.

6. Ogden CL, Carroll MD, Lawman HG, et al: Trends in obesity prevalence among children and adolescents in the United States, 1988-1994 through 2013-2014, *JAMA* 315(21):2292, 2016.

7. Centers for Disease Control and Prevention, Chronic Disease Prevention and Health Promotion: *At a Glance 2016: Diabetes*, July 25, 2016. https://www.cdc.gov/chronicdisease/resources/publications/aag/diabetes.htm.

8. Centers for Disease Control and Prevention, Chronic Disease Prevention and Health Promotion: *Preventing the Nation's Leading Killers. At a Glance 2016 - Heart Disease and Stroke*, March 21, 2017. https://www.cdc.gov/chronicdisease/resources/publications/aag/heart-disease-stroke.htm.

9. Centers for Disease Control and Prevention, Chronic Disease Prevention and Health Promotion: *At a Glance 2016: Cancer*, October 17, 2016. https://www.cdc.gov/chronicdisease/resources/publications/aag/dcpc.htm.

10. Federal Interagency Forum on Aging-Related Statistics: *Older Americans 2016: Key indicators of well-being*, Washington, DC, 2016, US Government Printing Office.

11. Micha R, Shulkin ML, Peñalvo JL, et al: Etiologic effects and optimal intakes of foods and nutrients for risk of cardiovascular diseases and diabetes: Systematic reviews and meta-analyses from the Nutrition and Chronic Diseases Expert Group (NutriCoDE), *PLoS One* 12(4): e0175149, 2017.

12. Micha R, Peñalvo JL, Cudhea F, et al: Association between dietary factors and mortality from heart disease, stroke, and type 2 diabetes in the United States, *JAMA* 317(9):912, 2017.

13. Colby SL, Ortman JM: Projections of the size and composition of the US population: 2014 to 2060: population estimates and projections, *Current Population Reports* pp 25–1143, 2015.

14. Goody CM, Drago L: *Cultural Food Practices, American Dietetic Association (now the Academy of Nutrition and Dietetics)*, Chicago, Ill, 2010, Diabetes Care and Education Dietetic Practice Group.

15. Centers for Disease Control and Prevention: *CDC Vital Signs – African American Health*, May 2017. https://www.cdc.gov/vitalsigns/aahealth/index.html.

16. Valenzuela I, Hosig K, Schlenker ED: *Community-based Lifestyle Intervention for Underserved Hispanics with Type 2 Diabetes in Southwest Virginia*, 2017, Submitted for publication to Hispanic Health International.

17. DiJulio B, Kirzinger A, Wu B, et al: *Data Note: Americans' Challenges with Health Care Costs*, Washington, DC, 20005, March 2, 2017, H J Kaiser Family Foundation. http://kff.org/health-costs/poll-finding/data-note-americans-challenges-with-health-care-costs/.

18. Penman-Aguilar A, Bouye K, Liburd L: Strategies for Reducing Health Disparities — Selected CDC-Sponsored Interventions, United States, 2016, *MMWR* 65(Suppl 1), 2–3, 2016, pp 1–69.

19. US Bureau of Census: *Selected social characteristics in the United States, American Community Survey 5-Year Estimates, 2011-2015*, 2015, American Fact Finder, DP02. https://factfinder.census.gov/faces/tableservices/jsf/pages/productview.xhtml?pid=ACS_15_5YR_DP02&src=pt.

20. Crowe KM, Francis C, Academy of Nutrition and Dietetics: Position paper of the Academy of Nutrition and Dietetics: Functional foods, *J Acad Nutr Diet* 113(8):1096, 2013.

21. Schwartz B: New criteria for supplementation of selected micronutrients in the era of nutrigenetics and nutrigenomics, *Int J Food Sci Nutr* 65(5):529, 2014.

22. Camp KM, Trujillo E, Academy of Nutrition and Dietetics: Position of the Academy of Nutrition and Dietetics: Nutritional genomics, *J Acad Nutr Diet* 114:299, 2014.

23. Rodriguez JL, Thomas CC, Massetti GM, et al: CDC Grand Rounds: Family history and genomics as tools for cancer prevention and control, *MMWR Morb Mortal Wkly Rep* 65(46):1291, November 25, 2016.

24. Smith A: *Record shares of Americans now own smartphones, have home broadband*, Philadephia, PA, 19103, January 12, 2017, Pew Charitable Trust, Pew Research Center. http://www.pewresearch.org/fact-tank/2017/01/12/evolution-of-technology/.

25. Fox S: *Health and Technology in the US Pew Charitable Trust*, Philadephia, PA, 19103, December 4, 2013, Pew Research Center. http://www.pewinternet.org/2013/12/04/health-and-technology-in-the-u-s/.

26. Devine T, Broderick J, Harris LM, et al: Making quality health websites a national public health priority: Toward quality standards, *J Med Internet Res* 18(8):e211, 2016.

27. Institute of Medicine, Otten JJ, Hellwig JP, Meyers LD, et al, editors: *Dietary Reference Intakes [DRI]. The essential guide to nutrient requirements*, Washington, DC, 2006, National Academies Press.

28. US Department of Agriculture, Center for Nutrition Policy and Promotion: *MyPlate,* https://www.choosemyplate.gov.

29. US Department of Health and Human Services, United States Department of Agriculture: *Scientific Report of the 2015 Advisory Committee on the Dietary Guidelines, submitted to the Secretary of the Department of Health and Human Services and the Secretary of the Department of Agriculture,* Washington, DC, 2015, US Department of Agriculture, Agricultural Research Service.

30. Elitzak H, Okrent A: *Food Expenditures,* Economic Research Service, US Department of Agriculture, January 2016. https://www.ers.usda.gov/data-products/food-expenditures.aspx.

31. US Department of Agriculture, Agricultural Research Service: *Table 9. Away From Home: Percentages of Selected Nutrients Contributed by Food and Beverages Consumed Away From Home by Gender and Age, What We Eat in America, NHANES 2013-2014,* 2016. https://www.ars.usda.gov/ARSUserFiles/80400530/pdf/1314/Table_9_AWY_GEN_13.pdf.

32. Coleman-Jensen A, Rabbitt MP, Gregory CA, et al: *Household Food Security in the United States in 2015,* Economic Research Report No. (ERR-215), Washington DC, September 2016, US Department of Agriculture.

33. Shankar P, Chung R, Frank DA: Association of food insecurity with children's behavioral, emotional, and academic outcomes: A systematic review, *J Dev Behav Pediatr* 38(2):135, 2017.

34. Robaina KA, Martin KS: Food insecurity, poor diet quality and obesity among food pantry participants in Hartford, CT, *J Nutr Educ Behav* 45(2):159, 2013.

35. Gany F, Bari S, Crist M, et al: Food insecurity: limitations of emergency food resources for our patients, *J Urban Health* 90(3):552, 2013.

36. Anker SD, Morley JE: Cachexia: A nutritional syndrome? *J Cachexia Sarcopenia Muscle* 6(4):269, 2015.

37. Hingle MD, Kandiah J, Maggi A: Practice Paper of the Academy of Nutrition and Dietetics: Selecting Nutrient-Dense Foods for Good Health, *J Acad Nutr Diet* 116(9):1473, 2016.

38. US Department of Health and Human Services, Public Health Service: *The Surgeon General's report on nutrition and health,* PHS Publication No. 88-50210, Washington, DC, 1988, US Government Printing Office.

39. Food and Nutrition Board, Institute of Medicine: *Diet and health: implications for reducing chronic disease risk,* Washington, DC, 1989, National Academies Press.

40. US Department of Health and Human Services: *Healthy People 2020: 2020 Topics and Objectives,* Washington, DC, 2017, US Department of Health and Human Services. http://www.healthypeople.gov/2020/default.aspx.

41. Academy of Nutrition and Dietetics, American Diabetes Association: *Choose your foods: food lists for diabetes,* ed 7, New York, 2014, Academy of Nutrition and Dietetics, American Diabetes Association.

42. Tagtow A, Raghavan R: Assessing the reach of MyPlate using National Health and Nutrition Examination Survey data, *J Acad Nutr Diet* 117(2):181, 2017.

43. Herring D, Chang S, Bard S, et al: Five years of MyPlate—Looking back and what's ahead, *J Acad Nutr Diet* 116(7):1069, 2016.

44. Centers for Disease Control and Prevention: *Burden of foodborne illness: Overview,* Atlanta, GA, July 2016. https://www.cdc.gov/foodborneburden/estimates-overview.html.

45. US Department of Health and Human Services: *We Can!, Ways to Enhance Children's Activity & Nutrition in Your Community,* Bethesda, MD, 2013, National Heart, Lung and Blood Institute, US Department of Health and Human Services. https://www.nhlbi.nih.gov/health/educational/wecan/community/index.htm.

46. Mozaffarian D, Afshin A, Benowitz NL, et al: Population approaches to improve diet, physical activity, and smoking habits: a scientific statement from the American Heart Association, *Circulation* 126:1514, 2012.

47. Jain A, Langwith C: Collaborative school-based obesity interventions: Lessons learned from 6 southern districts, *J Sch Health* 83:213, 2013.

FURTHER READINGS AND RESOURCES

Readings

Academy of Nutrition and Dietetics: Position of the Academy of Nutrition and Dietetics: total diet approach to healthy eating, *J Acad Nutr Diet* 113:307, 2013.

Slavin J: The challenges of dietary guidance, *Nutr Today* 50(4):169, 2015.

[These articles help us understand the importance of the overall food pattern to health outcomes, and they present ideas on how we can assist others.]

US Department of Agriculture, Center for Nutrition Policy and Promotion: *The Food Environment, Eating Out, and Body Weight: A Review of the Evidence, Nutrition Insight 49,* Alexandria, VA, 2012, US Government Printing Office. Available from: http://www.cnpp.usda.gov/Publications/NutritionInsights/Insight49.pdf.

[This review cites evidence from the Nutrition Evidence Library (NEL) linking frequency of meals away from home and risk of overweight and helps us understand why this occurs.]

Fung TT, Long MW, Hung P, et al: An expanded model for mindful eating for health promotion and sustainability: Issues and challenges for dietetics practice, *J Acad Nutr Diet* 116(7):1081, 2016.

[Dr. Fung and her coworkers help us understand the importance of giving thought to when and what we eat and reduce impulse eating.]

Herring D, Tagtow A: MyPlate, MyState - Personalizing Your Plate with Your Local Flavors, Foods, and Recipes, *J Acad Nutr Diet* 116(8):1239, 2016.

[This article presents some ideas on fitting MyPlate to your local food favorites.]

St-Onge M-P, Ard J, Baskin ML, et al: Meal timing and frequency: Implications for cardiovascular disease prevention: A scientific statement from the American Heart Association, *Circulation* 135:e96, 2017.

[These clinicians offer practical advice about meal planning that can help prevent cardiovascular disease.]

Websites of Interest

• US Department of Agriculture: Nutrition Evidence Library. This website provided the scientific evidence reviewed by the 2015 Dietary Guidelines Advisory Committee in preparation of their report. http://www.cnpp.usda.gov/NEL.htm.

• US Department of Health and Human Services, *2008 Physical Activity Guidelines for Americans.* This site presents science-based physical activity guidelines for both youth and adults along with educational materials for health professionals and consumers. http://www.health.gov/paguidelines/guidelines/default.aspx.

• US Department of Agriculture, Food Surveys Research Group: *What We Eat in America: Data from the National Health and Nutrition Examination Survey.* This site describes the food and nutrient intakes of Americans according to age, gender, race, ethnicity, and economic status. https://www.ars.usda.gov/northeast-area/beltsville-md/beltsville-human-nutrition-research-center/food-surveys-research-group/docs/wweia-data-tables/

• US Department of Health and Human Services, National Heart, Lung and Blood Institute: *Keep an Eye on Portion Distortion.* This site describes portion sizes and how they have changed over the years; includes a downloadable serving size card that can be carried in a wallet or backpack to help with serving size. https://www.nhlbi.nih.gov/health/educational/wecan/eat-right/portion-distortion.htm

• US Department of Agriculture, Center for Nutrition Policy and Promotion. The MyPlate website offers materials for health professionals and practical tips for consumers to use in meal planning. http://www.choosemyplate.gov.

• US Department of Health and Human Services, US Department of Agriculture. 2015 Dietary Guidelines for Americans, Tools and Resources. This site offers brochures and other materials for use by health professionals to assist consumers in choosing healthier meal patterns. https://health.gov/dietary-guidelines/2015/resources.asp

2

Digestion, Absorption, and Metabolism

Eleanor D. Schlenker

ⓔ http://evolve.elsevier.com/Williams/essentials/

We continue our study of nutrition by looking at what happens to food as it follows its path through the digestive system to be broken down into forms the body can use. We see how the tuna sandwich we had for lunch is transformed into the energy-yielding and tissue-building nutrients—glucose, amino acids, and fatty acids. These physiologic and biochemical actions include three parts: digestion, absorption, and metabolism. Although we give little thought to these activities when all are working well, functional changes in the gastrointestinal tract can lead to nutrient deficiency and deteriorating health, loss of pleasure in eating, and poor quality of life. Through the actions of its abundant species of bacteria, the intestine may also help regulate immune function, inflammation, and obesity.

OUTLINE

Human Body: The Role of Nutrition
 Food: Change and Transformation
 Importance for Health and Nutrition
 Gastrointestinal Tract
 Principles of Digestion
Movement of Food Through the Digestive Tract
 Mouth and Esophagus: Preparation and Delivery

Stomach: Storage and Initial Digestion
Small Intestine: Major Digestion, Absorption, and Transport
Colon (Large Intestine): Final Absorption and Waste Elimination
Gastrointestinal Function and Clinical Applications
Health Promotion
 Metabolism

HUMAN BODY: THE ROLE OF NUTRITION

FOOD: CHANGE AND TRANSFORMATION

The food we eat contains the nutrients necessary for our survival, but these nutrients must first be released from other food components and transformed into units the body can use. Through a sequential and interrelated system, foods are broken down into increasingly simple substances that can enter the metabolic pathways in cells. Each section of the gastrointestinal tract has a unique function, but together they form a continuous *whole*. A problem in one segment has clinical consequences for the entire system.

IMPORTANCE FOR HEALTH AND NUTRITION

Gastrointestinal function impacts nutritional well-being. Food, as it occurs in nature and as we eat it, is not a single substance, but a mixture of nutrients and other chemical matter. These substances must be separated so the body can handle each one as an individual unit. Nutrients released from food remain unavailable to the body until they cross the intestinal wall and enter the circulatory system for transport to tissues. Diseases affecting the organs of the gastrointestinal tract or the absorbing surface of the intestinal wall have adverse effects on nutritional status because nutrients are not taken into the body in the amounts needed. At the same time, moderate to severe malnutrition lowers secretion of digestive enzymes and blunts the absorbing structures,

further limiting digestion and nutrient passage. This vicious cycle results in rapid and progressive deterioration in nutritional health.

The output of the gastrointestinal tract is also essential for the chemical work that occurs in tissues and cells. This integrated physiochemical system is fundamental to human nutrition in both health and disease. The internal control responsible for maintaining a constant chemical environment and coordinating the activities of the body's many functional systems is called homeostasis.

> **KEY TERM**
>
> **Homeostasis**
> State of dynamic equilibrium within the body's internal environment; this balance is achieved through the operation of many interrelated physiologic mechanisms.

GASTROINTESTINAL TRACT

Component Parts

The gastrointestinal tract, also called the *alimentary canal*, is a long hollow tube that begins at the mouth and ends at the anus. The specific parts that make up the tract are the mouth, esophagus, stomach, small intestine, large intestine or colon, and rectum. Other organs that lie outside the tract but support its work by secretion of important

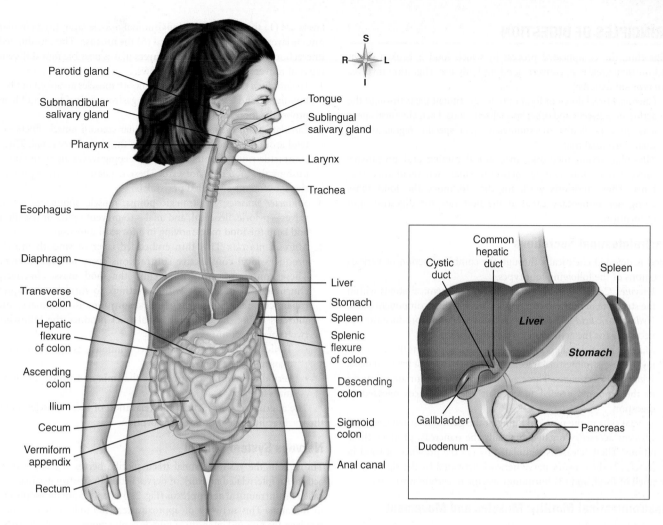

FIG. 2.1 The gastrointestinal system. The successive parts of the gastrointestinal system carry out multiple activities of digestion that liberate and reform food nutrients for our use. (From Thibodeau GA, Patton KT: *Anatomy and physiology,* ed 7, St. Louis, 2010, Mosby.)

enzymes and digestive fluids are the pancreas, gallbladder, and liver. Fig. 2.1 presents the respective components of the gastrointestinal tract and their relative position to one another. These organs, working as a team, can break down and/or absorb several kilograms of carbohydrate, one-half kilogram of fat, one-half kilogram of protein, and 20 or more liters of water daily.[1] We will follow these food components as they travel together through the successive parts of the tract.

General Functions

The gastrointestinal tract has the following four major functions:
1. *Receives food:* The mouth is the entrance to the gastrointestinal tract. From here the food moves to the stomach and other organs for digestion and absorption.
2. *Releases nutrients from food:* Digestion and the separation of nutrients from other food components take place in the stomach and small intestine.
3. *Delivers nutrients into the blood:* Absorbing structures called *microvilli* located in the small intestine transfer the nutrients into the portal blood (glucose and amino acids) or lymph (fatty acids). Water is absorbed later in the colon.
4. *Excretes nondigestible waste:* The fecal mass moves from the colon into the rectum, where it is stored until excreted.
Physical and chemical actions accomplish these tasks.

Sensory Stimulation and Gastrointestinal Function

Both physiologic and psychological stimuli influence the gastrointestinal tract. The physical presence of food in the mouth, stomach, or small intestine initiates a variety of responses that coordinate the muscular movements and chemical secretions necessary for digestion and absorption. Sensory stimuli, such as seeing, smelling, or being close to food, prompt the secretion of digestive juices and muscle motility. Smelling cookies baking, hearing foods sizzle on an outdoor grill, or picking a fresh berry can evoke the physiologic process of digestion. Seeing a sign that advertises your favorite food (or even thinking about food) stimulates the gastrointestinal tract. At the other extreme, dreading an unpleasant-tasting medication or recalling the nausea brought on by chemotherapy can repress the desire for food.

The neural responses resulting from the presence or thoughts of food have an important role in food intake and the digestive process. Neural responses prepare the gastrointestinal tract to receive food by initiating the secretion of enzymes and digestive fluids and promoting gastrointestinal motility. They also control the secretion of hormones that influence appetite, food intake, and satiety.[2] Inappropriate changes in neural regulation that result in feelings of satiety early in the meal limit food intake in some older adults, leading to unwanted weight loss. Maintaining positive associations with food and mealtime supports efficient digestion and absorption of nutrients.

PRINCIPLES OF DIGESTION

Digestion, the complicated process by which food is broken down and nutrients released, converts food for body use. Digestion involves two types of actions:

- Chemical breakdown of food into its constituent parts through the action of enzymes and other specialized fluids. Each chemical agent acts on a particular macronutrient in a specific region of the gastrointestinal tract.
- Muscular action including mechanical mixing and propulsive movements controlled by neuromuscular, self-regulating systems. These motions work together to move the food mass along the alimentary canal at the best rate for digestion and absorption.

Gastrointestinal Secretions

Food is digested chemically through the combined action of various secretions of the following four types.

1. *Enzymes:* Certain enzymes attack designated chemical bonds within the structure of nutrient compounds, freeing their component parts.
2. *Hydrochloric acid and buffer ions:* These secretions produce the pH necessary for the activity of certain enzymes.
3. *Mucus:* This sticky, slippery fluid lubricates and protects the inner lining of the gastrointestinal tract and eases the passage of the food mass.
4. *Water and electrolytes:* These agents provide appropriate solutions in the amounts needed to circulate the substances released in digestion.

Special cells in the mucosal lining of the gastrointestinal tract and in adjacent accessory organs, especially the pancreas, produce these secretions. Their release is stimulated by (1) the presence of food in the tract; (2) the sensory nerve network activated by the sight, taste, or smell of food; and (3) hormones specific to certain nutrients.

Gastrointestinal Motility: Muscles and Movement
Types of Muscles

Organized muscle layers in the gastrointestinal wall provide the motility needed for digestion (Fig. 2.2). From the outer surface inward, the layers are (1) the serosa, (2) a longitudinal muscle layer, (3) a circular muscle layer, (4) the submucosa, and (5) the mucosa. The coordinated interaction of four smooth muscle layers makes possible four different types of movement (Fig. 2.3), as follows:

1. *Longitudinal muscles:* These long, smooth muscles arranged in fiber bundles extend lengthwise along the gastrointestinal tract and help propel the food mass forward.
2. *Circular contractile muscles:* The circular smooth muscle fibers extend around the hollow tube forming the alimentary canal. These contractile rings initiate rhythmic sweeping waves along the tract, pushing the food mass forward. These regularly occurring propulsive movements are called peristalsis.
3. *Sphincter muscles:* At strategic points, muscle sphincters act as valves—pyloric, ileocecal, and anal—to prevent reflux or backflow and keep the food mass moving in a forward direction.
4. *Mucosal muscles:* This thin embedded layer of smooth muscle produces local constrictive contractions every few centimeters. These contractions mix and chop the food mass, effectively churning and mixing it with secretions to form a semiliquid called chyme that is ready for absorption. In summary, the muscles lining the gastrointestinal tract produce the following two types of action:
   - Tonic contractions that ensure continuous passage of the food mass and valve control
   - Periodic rhythmic contractions that mix and propel the food mass forward

The alternating contraction and relaxation of these muscles along the tract facilitate digestion and absorption.

Nervous System Control

Throughout the gastrointestinal tract, specific nerves regulate muscle action. An interrelated network of nerves within the gastrointestinal wall called the intramural nerve plexus (Fig. 2.4) extends from the esophagus to the anus. This network of approximately 100-million nerve fibers regulates the rate and intensity of muscle contractions, controls the speed at which the food mass moves along the tract, and coordinates the digestive process, including the secretion of enzymes and digestive juices.[3]

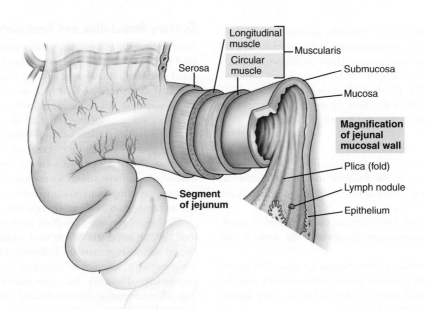

Longitudinal muscle
Circular muscle
Muscularis
Serosa
Submucosa
Mucosa
Segment of jejunum
Magnification of jejunal mucosal wall
Plica (fold)
Lymph nodule
Epithelium

FIG. 2.2 Muscle layers of the intestinal wall. Notice the five layers of muscle that produce the movements necessary for digestion and moving the food mass forward. (Modified from Thibodeau GA, Patton KT: *Anatomy and physiology,* ed 7, St. Louis, 2010, Mosby.)

Stimulus by stretching of intestinal wall

Ring contraction

Contraction travels ——▶ 2 to 25 cm/sec

Peristalsis

Pendular movements

Inactive state

Alternating contractions

Segmentation contractions

FIG. 2.3 Types of movement produced by muscles of the intestine: peristaltic waves from contraction of deep circular muscle, pendular movements from small local muscles, and segmentation rings formed by alternate contraction and relaxation of circular muscle.

KEY TERMS

Digestion
The process of breaking down food to release its nutrients for absorption and transport to the cells; both the chemical action of numerous enzymes and fluids and the mixing and churning action of the embedded musculature accomplish this task.

Serosa
Outer surface layer of the intestines interfacing with the blood vessels of the portal system that go to the liver.

Mucosa
The mucous membrane forming the inner surface of the gastrointestinal tract that has extensive nutrient absorption and transport functions.

Peristalsis
A wavelike progression of alternating contraction and relaxation of the muscle fibers of the gastrointestinal tract that keeps the food mass moving forward.

Chyme
Semifluid food mass resulting from gastric digestion.

Tonic
Ongoing low-level muscle contraction and relaxation

Intramural Nerve Plexus
Network of nerves in the walls of the intestine that control muscle action and secretions for digestion and absorption.

FIG. 2.4 Innervation of the intestine by the intramural nerve plexus. A network of nerves controls and coordinates the movements of the intestinal muscles. (Courtesy Medical and Scientific Illustration.)

MOVEMENT OF FOOD THROUGH THE DIGESTIVE TRACT

We have reviewed the integrated muscular and secretory functions that govern the overall operation of the gastrointestinal tract; now we will follow this process through its successive stages to see what happens to the food we eat.

MOUTH AND ESOPHAGUS: PREPARATION AND DELIVERY

Eating begins the process by which food is broken down into individual nutrients. The first steps in digestion occur in the mouth, where salivary enzymes act on carbohydrate and all foods are broken down into smaller particles to facilitate the later action of digestive juices. The esophagus delivers the food mass to the stomach.

Taste and Smell

Much of our enjoyment of food comes from its unique flavors and aromas. Taste buds located on the tongue, roof of the mouth, and throat contain chemical receptors that produce the four sensations of taste: salty, sweet, sour, and bitter. Recently, a fifth taste has been identified, called *umami,* the taste of amino acids and proteins. Some individuals have a stronger perception of one taste over another, and certain medications produce a bitter taste or loss of taste. Genetically related differences in taste affect our preferences for certain foods.[4] Individuals with enhanced sensitivity to bitter taste might avoid certain fruits and vegetables or prefer sweet or high-fat foods. Such taste preferences that influence what we eat also affect our risk for obesity or particular chronic diseases or conditions.[5] Patients on chemotherapy often have distorted taste (dysgeusia). Smoking also results in changes in taste. Zinc deficiency causes a loss of taste (hypogeusia).

Foods contain volatile components that move from the back of the mouth up into the nasal cavity, where they act on olfactory receptors to produce the pleasant odors we associate with particular foods. In fact, much of what we perceive as a taste may actually be an odor. Radiation therapy of the head or neck, Parkinson disease, and Alzheimer disease often lead to olfactory losses and less interest in eating.

Mastication

Food is broken into smaller particles by biting and chewing.[1] Digestive enzymes act only on the surface of food particles; therefore chewing, which enlarges the surface area available for enzyme action, is an important step in preparing food for digestion. Chewing also produces finer particles, easing the passage of the food mass down the esophagus and into the stomach. Chewing prepares fiber-containing foods such as fruits, vegetables, and whole grains for digestion. Decayed or missing teeth or poorly fitting dentures make eating difficult. Gingivitis and other diseases of the gums and supporting structures of the teeth can result in mouth pain, infection, or further tooth loss, thereby limiting food intake and contributing to malnutrition.

Chemical Digestion

In the mouth, three pairs of salivary glands—parotid, submaxillary, and sublingual—produce a watery fluid containing salivary amylase. This enzyme is specific for starch. The salivary glands also secrete mucus to lubricate and bind the food particles together. The gastrointestinal tract secretes large amounts of digestive fluids (Table 2.1). Saliva secretion alone ranges from 800 to 1500 mL a day. Food remains in the mouth for only a short time; thus starch digestion here

TABLE 2.1 Comparative pH Values and Approximate Daily Volumes of Gastrointestinal Secretions

Secretion	pH	Daily Volume (mL)
Salivary	6.0–7.4	1000
Gastric	1.0–3.5	1500
Pancreatic	8.0–8.3	1000
Small intestinal	7.5–8.0	1800
Brunner gland (bicarbonate)	8.0–8.9	200
Bile	7.5–7.8	1000
Large intestinal	7.5–8.0	200
Total		6700

Modified from Guyton AC, Hall JE: *Textbook of medical physiology,* ed 10, Philadelphia, 2000, WB Saunders.

is brief. However, when salivary amylase binds to starch molecules, it becomes resistant to inactivation by gastric acid, thereby allowing the breakdown of starch to continue in the stomach.[3] A second digestive enzyme released in saliva is lingual lipase, which begins the digestion of fat.

Salivary secretions have other important functions in addition to initiating digestion. They moisten the food particles so they bind together to form a bolus that moves easily down the esophagus, and they lubricate and cleanse the teeth and tissues of the mouth, destroying harmful bacteria and neutralizing any toxic substances entering the mouth. Inadequate secretion leads to the condition known as *dry mouth.* Everyone experiences occasional dry mouth when nervous, upset, or under stress. However, prolonged drastic reduction in the production of saliva leads to swallowing problems as individual particles of food get separated in the esophagus. Infections and ulcers in the mouth, along with tooth decay, are other outcomes of extreme dry mouth, usually referred to as *xerostomia.* Radiation therapy that damages the salivary glands and conditions such as diabetes, Parkinson disease, and autoimmune deficiency diseases can lead to xerostomia. Various medications for management of cardiac failure, hypertension, depression, or chronic pain contribute to dry mouth.[6]

Swallowing

Swallowing involves both the mouth and the pharynx. It is intricately controlled by the swallowing center in the brainstem, and damage to these nerves through radiation therapy, aging, or disease makes swallowing difficult. As illustrated in Fig. 2.5, the tongue initiates a swallow by pressing the food upward and backward against the palate. From this point on, swallowing goes forward as an involuntary reflex and, once begun, cannot be interrupted. Swallowing occurs rapidly, taking less than 1 second, but in that time the larynx must close to prevent food from entering the trachea and moving into the lungs and the soft palate must rise to prevent food from entering the nasal cavity. Patients must never be fed in a supine position because it increases the risk of food aspiration into the lungs.

Esophagus

The esophagus is a muscular tube that connects the mouth and throat with the stomach and serves as a channel to carry the food mass into the body. Functionally, it has the following three parts[1]:

1. *Upper esophageal sphincter (UES):* The UES controls the entry of the food bolus into the esophagus. Between swallows the UES muscle is closed. Within 0.2 to 0.3 seconds after a swallow, nerve stimuli open the sphincter to receive the food mass.

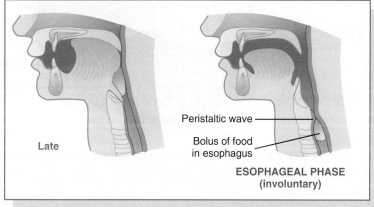

FIG. 2.5 Swallowing is a highly coordinated task directed by a special nerve center in the hypothalamus. (From Mahan KL, Escott-Stump S, editors: *Krause's food, nutrition, and diet therapy,* ed 12, Philadelphia, 2008, Saunders.)

2. *Esophageal body:* The mixed bolus of food immediately passes down the esophagus, moved along by peristaltic waves controlled by nerve reflexes. Degenerative changes in the muscles or nerves lower the intensity and frequency of the peristaltic waves, slowing passage down the channel. Diabetic neuropathy is one cause of such problems. Associated pain and discomfort can lower food intake, resulting in unwanted weight loss. Gravity aids the passage of food down the esophagus when the person eats in an upright position.

3. *Lower esophageal sphincter (LES):* The LES controls the movement of the food bolus into the stomach. When the LES muscles maintain excessively high muscle tone, they fail to open after a swallow, preventing the passage of food into the stomach. This condition is called *achalasia,* meaning "unrelaxed muscle." (See Chapter 20 for a discussion of this condition.)

KEY TERMS

Gingivitis
Red, swollen, bleeding gums, often caused by accumulation of bacterial plaque on the teeth.

Pharynx
Throat.

Bolus
Rounded mass of food formed in the mouth and ready to be swallowed.

Entry Into the Stomach

At the point of entry into the stomach, the gastroesophageal constrictor muscle relaxes to allow the food to pass and then contracts quickly to prevent regurgitation of the acidic stomach contents back into the esophagus. When this mechanism fails and regurgitation occurs, the resulting discomfort is called *heartburn.* The medical name for this condition is gastroesophageal reflux disease (GERD). GERD damages the tissues of the esophagus, which are unprotected from the destructive effects of gastric acid. Mucus secreted by cells in the stomach wall protects those tissues from the harsh effects of this acid. Obesity, overeating, physical inactivity, smoking, and certain medications contribute to GERD. According to national health care data, 7 million Americans per year are diagnosed with GERD and this condition was responsible for more than 300,000 visits to an emergency room.[7] The increasing prevalence of obesity likely contributes to these statistics.

STOMACH: STORAGE AND INITIAL DIGESTION

Motility

The major parts of the stomach are described in Fig. 2.6. Muscles in the stomach wall have three motor functions: (1) storage, (2) mixing, and (3) controlled emptying. As the food mass enters the stomach it rests against the stomach walls, which stretch to store as much as 1 L of food and fluid. Local tonic muscle waves increase their kneading and mixing actions to move the mass of food and secretions toward the pyloric valve at the **distal** end of the stomach. Over time, waves of peristaltic contractions reduce the

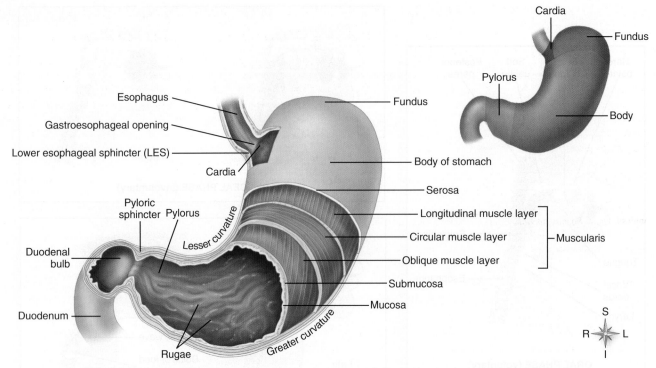

FIG. 2.6 Stomach. The pyloric sphincter controls passage of the food mass from the stomach into the duodenum, the upper section of the small intestine. See also the five layers of muscle found in the stomach wall. (From Thibodeau GA, Patton KT: *Anatomy & physiology,* ed 7, St. Louis, 2010, Mosby.)

food mass to the semifluid chyme. Finally, with each wave, small amounts of chyme pass through the pyloric sphincter into the duodenum. The pyloric sphincter periodically constricts and relaxes to control the rate of emptying. The highly acid chyme must be released slowly enough to allow it to be buffered by the alkaline secretions of the small intestine. The caloric density of a meal, along with its volume and composition, influences the rate of stomach emptying. The speed at which food moves from the gastroesophageal sphincter to the distal end of the stomach and into the small intestine influences food intake, as messages to the brain signaling the arrival of food in the small intestine bring about the release of gastrointestinal hormones that induce feelings of satiety.

Chemical Digestion
Types of Secretions
Secretions produced in the stomach include acid, mucus, and enzymes, as follows:

- *Acid:* Hydrochloric acid creates the acidic environment necessary for certain digestive enzymes to work. For example, a pH of 1.8 to 3.5 is needed for the enzyme pepsin to act on protein; at a pH of 5.0 or greater, there is little or no pepsin activity.
- *Mucus:* This viscous secretion protects the stomach lining from the eroding effect of the acid. Mucus also binds and mixes the food mass and helps move it along.
- *Enzymes:* The major enzyme in the stomach is pepsin, which begins the breakdown of protein. Pepsin is secreted in the form of pepsinogen and activated by hydrochloric acid. The stomach also produces a small amount of gastric lipase (tributyrinase) that acts only on butterfat and has a relatively minor role in

overall digestion. Children have a gastric enzyme called *rennin* (not to be confused with the renal enzyme renin) that aids in the coagulation of milk. Coagulation of milk proteins, changing them from a liquid to a semisolid (as occurs when egg white is heated), slows the rate of stomach emptying, ensuring gradual passage of material to the small intestine. Rennin is absent in adults.

Control of Secretions
Stimuli for the release of gastric secretions come from two sources:
1. *Nerve stimuli* are produced in response to the visual and chemical senses, the presence of food in the gastrointestinal tract, and emotional distress. Anger and hostility increase gastric secretions; fear and depression lower secretions and inhibit blood flow to the region and gastric motility.
2. *Hormonal stimuli* are produced when food enters the stomach. Certain food components, especially caffeine, alcohol, and meat extracts, cause the mucosal cells of the antrum to release the local gastrointestinal hormone gastrin. Gastrin, in turn, stimulates the secretion of hydrochloric acid. When the pH falls to less than three, a feedback mechanism halts the release of gastrin, preventing accumulation of excess acid.[3] A second gastrointestinal hormone, enterogastrone, produced in the mucosa of the duodenum, also prevents excessive gastric response by inhibiting secretion of hydrochloric acid and pepsin and slowing gastric motility. (The Evidence-Based Practice box, "Why Do Some Older Adults With Recommended Intakes of Vitamin B_{12}–Containing Foods Become Deficient: Low Secretion of Gastric Acid" describes a problem that occurs when secretion of gastric acid is inadequate.)

EVIDENCE-BASED PRACTICE

Why Do Some Older Adults With Recommended Intakes of Vitamin B$_{12}$–Containing Foods Become Deficient: Low Secretion of Gastric Acid

Identify the problem: Poor vitamin B$_{12}$ status is observed among many older adults despite their liberal intakes of meat and other animal foods supplying this vitamin.

Review the evidence: Older adults could develop a vitamin B$_{12}$ deficiency because they no longer produce intrinsic factor, the protein carrier secreted by the gastric mucosa and required for vitamin B$_{12}$ absorption. To confirm this hypothesis, older adults who were vitamin B$_{12}$ deficient were given labeled doses of crystalline vitamin B$_{12}$, one dose with intrinsic factor and one without intrinsic factor. Absorption was evaluated by the later appearance of labeled vitamin B$_{12}$ in the urine. It was expected that the dose given without intrinsic factor would remain unabsorbed. Much to the surprise of the researchers, many of these older adults absorbed the vitamin-only test dose—so why were they deficient? Further studies revealed it was not a lack of intrinsic factor, but rather a lack of gastric acid. It is estimated that 50% of older adults secrete very low amounts of hydrochloric acid, and a strongly acid environment is required in the stomach to activate pepsinogen to pepsin, the enzyme needed to break down dietary protein. When animal proteins are not broken down completely, their vitamin B$_{12}$ is not released for absorption and is lost in the feces.

Implement the findings: Crystalline vitamin B$_{12}$ added to fortified breads, cereals, juices, and vitamin supplements is not bound to protein and is not dependent on an acid environment for absorption. Older adults should be encouraged to include a vitamin B$_{12}$–fortified food in their meal pattern several times a week to ensure an adequate body supply. In addition, we have learned that vitamin B$_{12}$ in milk and dairy products is fairly well absorbed, even if gastric acid secretion is limited, because these proteins are more easily digested than those found in meat, poultry, and fish. For older individuals with adequate acid secretion, meat is an excellent source of vitamin B$_{12}$.

Bibliography

Allen LH: Bioavailability of vitamin B$_{12}$, *Int J Vitam Nutr Res* 80(4–5):330, 2010.

Britton E, McLaughlin JT: Ageing and the gut, *Proc Nutr Soc* 72(1):173, 2013.

Brouwer-Brolsma EM, Dhonukshe-Rutten RAM, van Wijngaarden JP, et al: Dietary sources of vitamin B-12 and their association with vitamin B-12 status markers in healthy older adults in the B-Proof Study, *Nutrients* 7:7781, 2015.

Russell RM, Baik H, Kehayias JJ: Older men and women efficiently absorb vitamin B$_{12}$ from milk and fortified bread, *J Nutr* 131:291, 2001.

KEY TERMS

Distal
Away from the point of origin.

Duodenum
The first section of the small intestine entered by food passing through the pyloric valve from the stomach.

Viscous
Sticky.

Antrum
Lower section of the stomach.

Gastrin
Hormone secreted by mucosal cells in the antrum of the stomach that stimulates the parietal cells to produce hydrochloric acid.

Enterogastrone
Hormone produced in the mucous membrane of the duodenum that inhibits gastric acid secretion and motility.

SMALL INTESTINE: MAJOR DIGESTION, ABSORPTION, AND TRANSPORT

Motility

Intestinal Muscle Layers

Review the complex structure of the intestinal wall pictured in Fig. 2.2. Coordination of intestinal motility is accomplished by three layers of muscle: (1) the thin layer of smooth muscle embedded in the mucosa with fibers extending up into the villi, (2) the circular muscle layer, and (3) the longitudinal muscle lying next to the outer serosa.

Types of Intestinal Muscle Action

Under the control of the intramural nerve plexus, wall-stretch pressure from food or hormonal stimuli produces muscle action of the following two types:

1. *Propulsive movements:* Peristaltic waves from contractions of the deep circular muscles propel the food mass slowly forward. Fiber and other indigestible materials from plant foods aid this process, providing bulk for the action of these muscles. The presence of food or irritants brings about long sweeping waves over the entire intestine.
2. *Mixing movements:* Local constrictive contractions occurring every few centimeters mix and chop the food particles in the semiliquid chyme. General tonic contractions ensure continuous passage and valve control, and periodic, rhythmic contractions mix and propel the food mass forward, facilitating ongoing digestion and future absorption.

Chemical Digestion

Major Role of the Small Intestine

In comparison to other sections of the gastrointestinal tract, the small intestine carries the major burden of chemical digestion. It secretes several enzymes, each specific for carbohydrate, fat, or protein, and is assisted by other enzymes entering from the pancreas. The small intestine acts as a regulatory center sensing the nutrient content, pH, and osmolarity of its contents and controls enzyme secretion accordingly.[3]

Types of Secretions

The following four types of secretions complete this final stage of chemical digestion:

1. *Enzymes:* Specific enzymes act on specific macronutrients to bring about their final breakdown to forms the body can absorb and use (Table 2.2).
2. *Mucus:* Glands located at the entrance to the duodenum secrete large amounts of mucus. As in the stomach, mucus protects the

TABLE 2.2 Summary of Macronutrient Digestion

Nutrient	Mouth	Stomach	Small Intestine
Carbohydrate	Salivary amylase breaks down starch to dextrins		Pancreatic amylase breaks down starch to disaccharides: lactose, sucrose, and maltose.
			Disaccharides are broken down to monosaccharides.
			Lactase breaks down lactose to glucose and galactose.
			Sucrase breaks down sucrose to glucose and fructose.
			Maltase breaks down maltose to glucose and glucose.
Protein		Pepsin and HCl break down protein to polypeptides	Trypsin breaks down proteins and polypeptides to dipeptides.
			Chymotrypsin breaks down proteins and polypeptides to dipeptides.
			Carboxypeptidase breaks down polypeptides and dipeptides to amino acids.
			Aminopeptidase breaks down polypeptides and dipeptides to amino acids.
			Dipeptidase breaks down dipeptides to amino acids.
Fat	Lingual lipase has a minor role in beginning fat digestion	Tributyrinase breaks down tributyrin (butterfat) to glycerol and fatty acids	Bile emulsifies fat.
			Pancreatic lipase breaks down fat to glycerol, diglycerides, monoglycerides, and fatty acids.

intestinal mucosa from irritation and digestion by the entering highly acidic chyme. Other cells along the inner intestinal wall, when touched by the moving food mass, secrete mucus to protect the mucosal tissues from abrasion.

3. *Hormones:* When signaled by the presence of acid in the food mass entering from the stomach, mucosal cells in the upper part of the small intestine produce the local gastrointestinal hormone secretin. Secretin, in turn, stimulates the pancreas to send alkaline pancreatic juices into the duodenum to buffer the acidic chyme. The intestinal mucosa in the upper duodenum could not withstand the high acid of the entering chyme without the neutralizing action of the bicarbonate-containing pancreatic juice.

4. *Bile:* Bile emulsifies fat and facilitates its digestion. Bile is produced in the liver as a dilute watery solution and is then concentrated and stored by the gallbladder. When fat enters the duodenum, the local gastrointestinal hormone cholecystokinin (CCK) is secreted by glands in the intestinal mucosa and stimulates the gallbladder to contract and release bile. By means of the *enterohepatic circulation* (Fig. 2.7), molecules of bile are reabsorbed and returned to the liver and gallbladder to be used over and over again. CCK also acts on

the pancreas to stimulate the release of enzymes that break down fats, proteins, and carbohydrates.

End Products of Digestion

When digestion of the macronutrients is complete, the simplified end products (Table 2.3) are ready for absorption. At times, undigested nutrients remain in the small intestine,[8] causing discomfort or distress. When individuals lack the digestive enzyme lactase, the disaccharide lactose remains in the small intestine and attracts large amounts of fluid, resulting in abdominal pain and diarrhea, nausea, and flatulence. (This condition and its clinical management are discussed later in this chapter.)

Absorption
Surface Structures

Viewed from the outside, the small intestine appears smooth, but the inner surface is quite different. As in Fig. 2.8 the following three types of convolutions and projections greatly expand the absorbing surface:

1. *Mucosal folds:* Large folds similar to hills and valleys in a mountain range are easily seen with the naked eye.
2. *Villi:* Fingerlike projections on these folds called villi can be seen through a simple compound microscope.
3. *Microvilli:* These extremely small projections on each villus can be seen only with an electron microscope. The array of microvilli covering the edge of each villus is called the *brush border* because it resembles bristles on a brush. Each villus has an ample network of blood capillaries for the absorption of monosaccharides and amino acids, and a central lymph vessel called a *lacteal* for the absorption of fatty acids.

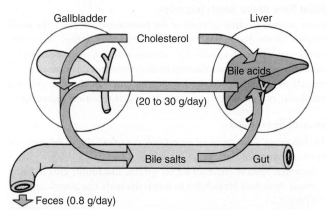

FIG. 2.7 Enterohepatic circulation of bile salts. Bile salts are reabsorbed from the small intestine and returned to the liver and then the gallbladder to be used again and again.

TABLE 2.3 End Products of Digestion

Macronutrient	End Products
Carbohydrate	Glucose, fructose, and galactose (monosaccharides)
Fat	Fatty acids, monoglycerides, diglycerides, and glycerol
Protein	Amino acids, dipeptides

FIG. 2.8 Absorbing structures of the intestine. Note the structures of the intestinal mucosa that increase the surface area for absorption: mucosal folds, villi, and microvilli. (Courtesy Medical and Scientific Illustration.)

The mucosal folds, villi, and microvilli together increase the inner surface area of the small intestine approximately 1000 times over that of the outside covering.[1] These specialized structures, plus the contracted length of the small intestine—630 to 660 cm (21 to 22 feet)—produce a tremendously large surface area to capture and absorb nutrients. This absorbing surface, if stretched out flat, would be as large as a tennis or basketball court. The small intestine is one of the most highly developed organs in the body, making possible its tremendous absorptive capacity for food and fluid (Table 2.4).

Mechanisms of Absorption

Absorption of the nutrients dispersed in the water-based solution entering the small intestine involves several transport mechanisms. The particular transport mechanism used depends on the nutrient and the prevailing electrochemical fluid pressure gradient; these are described as follows:

- *Passive diffusion and osmosis:* When there is no opposing fluid pressure, molecules small enough to pass through the capillary membranes diffuse easily into the villi (Fig. 2.9). High concentrations of nutrients waiting to move into the capillaries where nutrient

---

KEY TERMS

Osmolarity
Number of millimoles of liquid or solid in a liter of solution; used to describe the concentration of body fluids.

Mucus
Viscous fluid secreted by mucous membranes and glands, containing mucin (a glycoprotein), inorganic salts, and water.

Secretin
Hormone produced in the mucous membrane of the duodenum in response to the entrance of acid contents from the stomach; stimulates the flow of pancreatic juices containing digestive enzymes and bicarbonate to neutralize the acid.

Cholecystokinin (CCK)
A hormone secreted by the mucosa of the duodenum in response to the presence of fat; causes the gallbladder to contract and propel bile into the duodenum where needed to emulsify the fat.

Absorption
Transport of nutrients from the lumen of the intestine across the intestinal wall into the blood (glucose and amino acids) or the lymph (fatty acids).

Villi
Fingerlike projections covering the mucosal surface of the small intestine.

Microvilli
Minute vascular structures protruding from the villi that form a "brush border" and facilitate absorption of nutrients.

TABLE 2.4   Volume of Fluid Absorbed Daily by the Gastrointestinal System

Substance	Intake (L)	Intestinal Absorption (L)	Elimination (L)
Food ingested	1.5		
Gastrointestinal secretions	8.5		
TOTAL	10.0		
Fluid absorbed in small intestine		9.5	
Fluid absorbed in large intestine (colon)		0.4	
TOTAL		9.9	
Feces			0.1

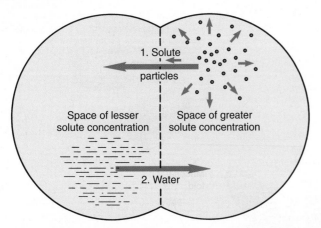

FIG. 2.9 Movement of molecules, water, and solutes through osmosis and diffusion.

concentrations are low create an electrochemical gradient and osmotic pressure that promote absorption.[1]

- *Facilitated diffusion:* Even when the pressure gradient supports absorption, some molecules may be too large to pass easily through the membrane pores and need assistance. Specific proteins located in the membrane facilitate passage by carrying the nutrient across the membrane.
- *Energy-dependent active transport:* Nutrients must cross the intestinal membrane to reach hungry cells even when the flow pressures are against them. Such active work requires extra energy along with a pumping action. A special membrane protein carrier, coupled with the active transport of sodium, assists in the process. The energy-requiring, sodium-coupled transport of glucose is an example of this action. The enzyme sodium/potassium-dependent adenosine triphosphatase (Na^+/K^+-ATPase) in the cell membrane supplies the energy for the pump.
- *Engulfing pinocytosis:* At times, fluid and nutrient molecules are absorbed by pinocytosis. When the nutrient particle touches the absorbing cell membrane, the membrane dips inward around the nutrient, surrounds it to form a vacuole, and then engulfs it. The nutrient is then conveyed through the cell cytoplasm and discharged into the circulation. Smaller whole proteins and fat droplets are absorbed through pinocytosis (Fig. 2.10).

Routes of Absorption

After crossing the intestinal wall, the water-soluble monosaccharides and amino acids enter the portal blood and travel to the liver and other tissues. Fat, which is not water soluble, follows a different route. Fats packaged in a bile complex called a *micelle* (described in detail in Chapter 4) move into the cells of the intestinal wall, where they are processed into human lipid compounds and joined with a carrier protein. These **lipoproteins**, called *chylomicrons,* flow into the lymph, empty into the cisterna chyli (the central abdominal collecting vessel of the lymphatic system), travel upward into the chest through the thoracic duct, and finally flow into the venous blood at the left subclavian vein. The chylomicrons are rapidly cleared from the blood by a special fat enzyme called *lipoprotein lipase.*

Exceptions to this route of fat absorption are the shorter-chain fatty acids with 10 or fewer carbons. Because these short-chain fatty acids are water soluble, they can be absorbed directly into the blood along with the carbohydrate and protein breakdown products. However, most dietary fats are made of long-chain fatty acids that are not water soluble and must take the lymphatic route.

KEY TERMS

Pinocytosis
Means of nutrient absorption by which the molecule is engulfed by the cytoplasm of the receiving cell.

Lipoproteins
Complexes of fat with protein that transport lipids in the blood.

COLON (LARGE INTESTINE): FINAL ABSORPTION AND WASTE ELIMINATION

Role in Absorption

Within a 24-hour period, approximately 1500 mL of remaining food mass leaves the **ileum**, the last section of the small intestine, and enters the *cecum,* the pouch at the entrance to the **colon.** Passage is controlled by the ileocecal valve. Normally the valve remains closed, but each peristaltic wave relaxes the valve muscle, squirting a small amount of remaining chyme into the cecum. This action holds the food mass in the small intestine long enough to ensure maximal digestion and absorption. Nutrients and other materials, including electrolytes, minerals, vitamins, intestinal bacteria, and nondigestible residue, remain in the chyme delivered to the large intestine.

Water Absorption

The main task remaining for the colon is the absorption of water. The capacity of the colon to absorb water is vast, with a net daily maximum

FIG. 2.10 Pinocytosis, the engulfing of large molecules by the cell. (From Nix S: *Williams' basic nutrition and diet therapy,* ed 13, St. Louis, 2009, Mosby.)

of 5 to 8 L.[1] Normally, from 1.0 to 1.5 L is received from the ileum, and 95% of that is absorbed (review Table 2.4).

Much of the water in the chyme (350 to 400 mL) is absorbed in the first half of the colon. Only 100 to 150 mL remains to form the feces.[1] Absorption of water in the colon is important in the regulation of water balance and the elimination of fecal waste. When the chyme first enters the colon, it is a semiliquid, but water absorption during passage changes it to the semisolid nature of normal feces.

The amount of water absorbed in the colon depends on motility and rate of passage. Poor motility and a slow passage rate, often associated with low dietary fiber and low fecal mass, allow greater absorption of water, resulting in hard stools that are difficult to pass, and constipation. Excess motility and too-rapid passage limit the absorption of water and important electrolytes, producing a high volume of loose, watery stool (diarrhea). Diarrhea can result from disease; microbial infection as in foodborne illness; or large amounts of undigested sugar, such as lactose, that exert osmotic pressure and hold vast amounts of fluid. Severe or extended diarrhea leads to dehydration and serious loss of electrolytes.

Mineral Absorption

Sodium and other electrolytes are absorbed from the colon. Intestinal absorption exerts major control on body content of many minerals, and much of our dietary intake is unabsorbed and excreted in the feces. Up to 90% of the calcium and iron in the food we eat is not absorbed. The proportion of a mineral intake that is generally absorbed is an important aspect of nutrient balance and must be considered in dietary evaluation.

Vitamin Absorption

Conditions in the gastrointestinal tract influence the absorption of vitamins. When gastric acid secretion is lower than normal, vitamin B_{12} is less efficiently released from animal tissues and is lost in the feces. Conversely, colonic bacteria synthesize vitamin K and biotin, which are actively absorbed and serve as a major source of the body's supply.

Role of Colon Microflora

At birth the colon is sterile, but intestinal bacteria acquired through passage down the birth canal and infant feeding promote the growth and diversity of particular species. More than 1500 species of bacteria have been identified in the human intestine, and adult composition is usually established by 3 years of age. The microbial population of the gastrointestinal tract is approximately 10 times the total number of cells in the human body.[9] Individuals differ in type and number of bacteria based on genetics, diet, and physical environment. A plant-based diet supports species associated with positive health; use of antibiotics can bring about permanent changes in the microbial community. Differing bacteria acquired through vaginal versus cesarean delivery and breast versus formula feeding may influence health status throughout life.[10] Many bacteria ingested with food do not survive the extreme acid environment in the stomach.

Bacteria from the colon make up approximately one-third of fecal weight[1] and influence the color and odor of the stool. Colonic bacteria acting on bilirubin produce bile pigments, giving the stool its characteristic brown color; thus, when bile flow is hindered, the feces become clay colored or white. The characteristic odor of the stool comes from amines, especially indole and skatole, formed by the action of bacterial enzymes on amino acids.

Gastrointestinal microflora have many roles. Particular microorganisms produce bothersome gas or increase the risk of gastrointestinal disease. Other species make important and positive contributions to health. (We discuss these relationships in the following sections.)

Excessive Gas Production

Colonic bacteria are major contributors to gas production, including carbon dioxide (CO_2), molecular hydrogen (H_2), methane, and sometimes hydrogen sulfide. Gas formation is a normal occurrence in the gastrointestinal tract and, though harmless, is distressing when it causes pain or embarrassment. Intestinal gas, or flatus, can be exaggerated by specific foods or physiologic circumstances in the person eating them.

Usually, gas is produced by the bacterial fermentation of undigested or incompletely absorbed carbohydrate. Humans lack the enzymes necessary to digest the oligosaccharides raffinose and stachyose found in legumes and cause the intestinal gas associated with these foods. Certain starches and fibrous materials in whole grains, fruits, and vegetables are resistant to pancreatic amylase and cannot be broken down and absorbed. Individuals should increase their intakes of fiber gradually to allow a more comfortable adjustment and prevent gastrointestinal distress.

Excessive gas has social implications. Methane, CO_2, and H_2 are odorless, but hydrogen sulfide carries a striking odor. Hydrogen sulfide most often arises from cruciferous vegetables (cabbage, cauliflower, or broccoli) or large amounts of beer, all high in sulfur. Various over-the-counter products claim to reduce the formation of gas or eliminate gaseous odors, but all have limitations. Individuals should check with their physician before using such preparations.[11] (See the Complementary and Alternative Medicine [CAM] box, "Bismuth and Certain Herbs: A Dangerous Combination," for cautions.)

Waste Elimination

Fully formed and ready for elimination, normal feces are approximately 75% water and 25% solids.[1] Solids include fiber, bacteria, inorganic matter such as minerals, a small amount of fat and its derivatives, some mucus, and sloughed-off mucosal cells.

The mass of food residue now slows its passage. Approximately 4 hours after a meal is eaten, food enters the cecum, having traveled the entire length of the small intestine (630 to 660 cm [21 to 22 ft]).

KEY TERMS

Ileum
The distal section of the small intestine that connects with the colon.

Colon
The large intestine extending from the cecum to the rectum.

Bilirubin
A reddish bile pigment resulting from the degradation of heme by reticuloendothelial cells in the liver; a high level in the blood produces the yellow skin symptomatic of jaundice.

 COMPLEMENTARY AND ALTERNATIVE MEDICINE (CAM)

Bismuth and Certain Herbs: A Dangerous Combination

Bismuth-containing medications such as Pepto-Bismol are used to ease gas and bloating. Bismuth also binds with the odor-causing sulfur compounds found in intestinal gas and helps to reduce odor and embarrassment. However, when combined with gingko, garlic, ginger, or ginseng, bismuth and these herbs act as anticoagulants. Individuals should consult their physician before using such a combination.

Bonci L: *American Dietetic Association guide to better digestion,* Hoboken, NJ, 2003, John Wiley & Sons.

Approximately 8 hours later, it reaches the sigmoid colon, having traveled an additional 90 cm (3 ft) through the large intestine. In the sigmoid colon, the residue descends still more slowly toward its final destination, the rectum (review Fig. 2.1 to follow its passage).

The rectum begins at the end of the large intestine immediately past the descending colon and ends at the anus. Feces are usually stored in the descending colon; however, when it becomes full, feces pass into the rectum, presenting the urge to defecate. Anal sphincters under voluntary control regulate the elimination of feces from the body. As much as 25% of a meal may remain in the rectum for up to 72 hours.

GASTROINTESTINAL FUNCTION AND CLINICAL APPLICATIONS

Chronic Gastrointestinal Distress

Most of the time the gastrointestinal tract is a smoothly working system that allows us to enjoy the food we eat while effectively handling digestion, absorption, and the elimination of waste. However, abdominal pain or bloating, early satiety, post-meal discomfort, nausea, or vomiting are regular occurrences for some individuals, and for more than half, diagnostic tests fail to identify a disease or structural explanation.[12] This situation, referred to as *functional dyspepsia*, adds significantly to health care costs and loss of productivity at the workplace and impacts on vitality and quality of life.[13] Anxiety, depression, emotional stress, various prescription medications, certain foods, and chronic disease influence gastrointestinal function and may contribute to symptoms in particular individuals.

We need to listen carefully when people tell us about gastrointestinal problems that limit their enjoyment of food or food selection. Health literacy should include perspectives on over-the-counter drugs or remedies claiming to enhance digestion, inappropriate laxatives, or procedures such as colonic irrigation. Chronic digestive problems demand medical assessment and intervention. (See the Perspectives in Practice box, "Help Your Digestive System Work for You," for practices that support optimal digestive function.)

Lactose Intolerance

Lactose intolerance is a digestive problem related to the inability to digest and absorb lactose. It stems from a deficiency of lactase, the digestive enzyme in the microvilli of the small intestine that breaks lactose into the simple sugars glucose and galactose, necessary for absorption. When undigested lactose remains in the small intestine and colon, it attracts large amounts of water and is fermented by resident bacteria, producing pain, diarrhea, bloating, and gas. Congenital intolerance to lactose is rare; infants usually produce enough lactase to digest the large amounts of lactose in mother's milk. However, adult-onset lactase deficiency is the normal physiologic pattern. It is estimated that at least 80% of Blacks, Asians, and individuals of Mediterranean or Middle Eastern descent are lactase deficient as compared with 20% of whites.[14] In many parts of the world lactose was not present in the diet after weaning; therefore this enzyme was no longer needed. A dairy-based culture in various regions of Europe likely contributed to higher lactase activity among whites.[15]

Individuals with lactose intolerance vary in their ability to digest lactose, although most can tolerate 6 g, equal to ½ cup of milk. Individuals who experience symptoms when ingesting one or two tablespoons of milk likely have another existing condition that is the root cause of the problem.[16] In general, symptoms will not occur with doses of 12 g of lactose (the amount of lactose found in 1 cup of milk), especially if consumed with a meal. Clinical protocols to establish lactose maldigestion have often directed the patient to consume one quart of milk at a single sitting, leading to an overdiagnosis of intolerance.[16] Maldigestion of lactose does not mean that an individual is allergic to milk or dairy foods, although both conditions are sometimes present in the same person. A true milk allergy is caused by the protein in milk, not the lactose.[14]

Other conditions can cause or worsen symptoms after eating foods that contain lactose. Irritable bowel syndrome, celiac disease, cystic fibrosis, or other disorders that damage the intestinal mucosa can interfere with secretion of lactase, and medical diagnosis is often needed to confirm the basis of the malabsorption. Viral infections with prescription of antibiotics can cause temporary lactose intolerance. The identification of genes associated with continuing lactase secretion has enabled genetic testing to confirm true lactose intolerance.[17]

> ### KEY TERMS
>
> **Dyspepsia**
> Gastric distress or indigestion involving nausea, pain, burning sensations, or excessive gas.

PERSPECTIVES IN PRACTICE

Help Your Digestive System Work for You

Our way of eating can either support or stress the normal function of the digestive tract. Positive practices maximize our enjoyment of food and help regulate our food intake.

- Chew your food slowly; allow time for the vapors to enter your sinus cavity and contribute to your sensation of taste.
- Take small bites; eating in a hurry and washing down large mouthfuls with liquid often lead to swallowing an excessive amount of air, causing bloating and belching.
- Wait 15 to 20 min before taking second helpings; when food moves from your stomach into your small intestine, it initiates feelings of satiety and you may find that you do not need that extra spoonful.
- Try to concentrate on pleasant thoughts or conversation while eating; emotional distress such as fear, anger, or worry often depresses the secretion of digestive enzymes and slows peristalsis, leading to gastrointestinal discomfort or upset.
- Focus on your food; try not to combine eating with watching television, completing a homework assignment, or driving to work or class.

- Enjoy the sight, smells, and anticipation of food as you prepare or serve your meal; these responses promote enzyme secretion and digestive function.
- Divide your food across the day; do not consume the majority of your kcalories at one meal; the cells lining the gastrointestinal tract derive most of their energy from the food passing through, and they require a constant supply of nutrients to meet their high metabolic demands.
- Try to eat approximately the same amount of food every day, rather than gorging 1 day and fasting the next; this supports not only efficient gastrointestinal function but also effective body weight management.

Bibliography

Bonci L: *American Dietetic Association guide to better digestion*, Hoboken, NJ, 2003, John Wiley & Sons.

Harvard Medical School: *The sensitive gut. A Harvard Medical School special health report*, Boston, 2012, Harvard Medical School.

Rolls B, Hermann M: *The ultimate volumetrics diet*, New York, 2013, William Morrow, Publishers.

BOX 2.1   Food Sources of Lactose

0 to 2 g Lactose

1 to 2 oz Swiss or cheddar cheese
1 oz American cheese
½ cup cottage cheese
½ cup lactase-treated milk

5 to 8 g Lactose

½ cup regular milk
½ cup white sauce
½ cup yogurt
1 cup ice cream or ice milk
2 tbsp powdered milk

Data from Bonci L: *American Dietetic Association guide to better digestion,* Hoboken, NJ, 2003, John Wiley & Sons. Images copyright 2006 JupiterImages Corporation.

Many people with lactose malabsorption do not need to follow a lactose-free diet but may include milk or other low-lactose dairy foods that will increase their intakes of calcium but avoid the digestive upset associated with lactose intolerance. These individuals may benefit from the action of species of bacteria in the small intestine and colon that produce the lactase enzyme and break down the lactose entering the large bowel. Consuming increasing amounts of lactose in the form of milk or other dairy foods can over the period of several weeks support the growth of bacterial colonies that assist in lactose digestion.[14,16] Yogurt containing active cultures also provides helpful bacteria. (Yogurt as a probiotic will be discussed later in this chapter.)

Following are suggestions on how lactose maldigesters might begin to include dairy foods in their diet[11,16]:

- *Add dairy foods gradually:* Begin with a small amount of one dairy food each day, one-quarter to one-half cup of milk or one-half ounce of cheese; include only one lactose-containing food per meal. (See Box 2.1 for food lactose content.)
- *Include lactose-containing foods with a meal or snack:* This combination slows the movement of lactose into the intestine and may reduce discomfort.
- *Choose dairy foods lower in lactose:* Use lactose-free or lactose-reduced milk. Add lactase drops such as Lactaid or Dairy Ease to milk to break down the lactose. (Acidophilus milk is not lactose free.) Aged cheeses such as cheddar or Swiss are lower in lactose than cheese spreads or other processed cheese. Lactase tablets taken right before eating can reduce gastrointestinal distress.

Lactose is also found in nondairy foods that have milk as an ingredient. Breads and other baked products, some ready-to-eat breakfast cereals, pancake and cookie mixes, instant potatoes, cream soups, hot dogs, and luncheon meats may contain lactose. Read the Nutrition Facts label, and look for the word *milk* or *whey*. (See Chapter 7 for food sources of calcium for persons who cannot tolerate any dairy foods.)

Prebiotics and Probiotics

Elie Metchnikoff, a Russian microbiologist who lived in the 19th century, speculated that fermented milk supplying microbes beneficial to colon health contributed to the long life of many peasants in his country.[18] Since then, we learned that many of the microbes populating the gastrointestinal tract promote human health and provide new tools for improving gastrointestinal and immune function and treating gastrointestinal disorders (Box 2.2). These microbes and their related food

BOX 2.2   Colonic Bacteria Support Health in Various Ways

- Produce short-chain fatty acids that nourish the cells of the intestinal mucosa
- Deactivate carcinogens that enter the gastrointestinal tract through food
- Assist in breaking down binding substances and enabling absorption of minerals
- Prevent harmful bacteria from growing and forming colonies
- Support immune cells that attack harmful body invaders
- Synthesize biotin and vitamin K
- Assist with the regulation of hormones that control appetite and energy balance

components are called *prebiotics* or *probiotics* based on their use and intestinal effects. Prebiotics are indigestible components found in food that selectively stimulate the growth of one or more species of bacteria in the colon. Probiotics are live microorganisms that bring a health benefit to the host.[18]

Prebiotics

Prebiotics are indigestible carbohydrates, often oligosaccharides such as cellulose, hemicellulose, and pectin, found in plants. These fibers are resistant to the digestive secretions of the stomach and small intestine and reach the colon generally intact. Here they are fermented by the existing microflora and stimulate the growth and activity of various healthy bacteria such as *Lactobacillus* and *Bifidobacterium*. This action of prebiotics lowers the existing pH in the colon, reducing the proliferation of pathogenic bacteria such as *Clostridia* and *Helicobacter*.[19,20] All prebiotics are fibers, although not all fibers are prebiotics. Fermentation by colonic bacteria also produces short-chain fatty acids such as butyrate, that serve as preferred energy sources of the mucosal cells. Naturally occurring prebiotics include fibers found in wheat, onions, bananas, garlic, soybeans, artichokes, and asparagus, whereas other fiber derivatives are commercially produced.[21]

Health-promoting bacteria produced by prebiotics bring about various favorable actions, as follows:

- *Immune function:* Prebiotics exert a profound effect on the immune system by way of their action on microbial populations and the protective cells lining the colon. Prebiotics influence the secretion of antibodies and other agents of the immune system to combat pathogens and potential carcinogens entering the lower gastrointestinal tract. Prebiotics support the integrity of the mucosal cells and prevent the binding of pathogens to the intestinal wall and their passage into the body.[19,21] This translation of harmful microbes across the mucosal wall has been termed *"leaky gut"* [22] and will be described further in Chapter 20.

- *Mineral absorption:* Most minerals are absorbed in the small intestine; however, the lower pH of the colon resulting from bacterial fermentation enhances the bioavailability and absorption of calcium, magnesium, and likely other minerals still remaining in the food residue.[21]
- *Normal laxation:* The fermenting action of bacteria can add to stool weight and relieve constipation, helping avoid dependence on laxatives. Prebiotics reduce the prevalence and duration of infectious and antibiotic-induced diarrhea.[19,21]

Probiotics

Probiotics can be obtained in food and dietary supplements. The most commonly used strains are *Lactobacillus*, *Bifidobacterium*, and the yeast *Saccharomyces boulardii*.[18] Lactic acid–producing bacteria have been used over the centuries to acidify and preserve foods such as cultured milk and yogurt, cheese, distilled mash, pickled cabbages, and tempeh. Probiotic cultures are available from pharmaceutical companies for clinical use, although products may not be the same even if they contain the same species. In addition, it is difficult to predict how a particular dose of living bacteria will interact with the microflora already existing in a particular individual. Moreover, clinical benefits depend on the strain, dose, duration of administration, or combination of probiotics; no single probiotic can be effective in all situations.[9] An individual's stress level may influence the composition of the microflora, whether through change in food patterns or digestive or intestinal upset.[22] Despite these uncertainties, probiotics have been used successfully to ameliorate symptoms in such gastrointestinal conditions as follows:

- Inflammatory bowel disease/Crohn disease
- Irritable bowel syndrome
- Traveler's diarrhea and
- *Clostridium difficile* infection.[20]

Two major health conditions in the United States that may benefit from intervention with probiotics are gastric cancer and obesity. A major risk factor for gastric cancer is infestation of the pathogenic bacterium *Helicobacter pylori*.[23] Probiotics seem to inhibit its growth and prevent it from burrowing into the stomach lining. (See the Focus on Culture box, "*Helicobacter pylori*: Risk Factor for African Americans and Hispanics," for more information on the prevalence of this bacterium.)

Evidence suggests that colonic microflora may have a role in the development and prevention of obesity. Obese individuals have been found to have a different population of colonic bacteria than individuals who are not obese.[24,25] Certain bacteria harvest energy by breaking down undigested carbohydrates to sugars and starches that can be absorbed and metabolized and thereby increase energy intake. Gut microflora also influence neural responses and hormones that control satiety and energy metabolism and could lead to weight gain or loss.

Although healthy bacteria have been used successfully in experimental and therapeutic interventions, safety is still a concern. Individuals with compromised immune function should not use probiotics without medical supervision, and clinicians have raised concerns about their use with critically ill patients. Contamination or the passage of a probiotic microorganism across the intestinal mucosa and into the

FOCUS ON CULTURE

Helicobacter Pylori: Risk Factor for African Americans and Hispanics

The bacterium *H. pylori* resides in the stomach lining of nearly half of the world's population. In contrast to *Lactobacillus* and *Bifidobacterium*, which carry out functions in the human colon that contribute to good health, *H. pylori* is a known risk factor for dyspepsia, peptic ulcer, and chronic gastritis and is considered a major risk factor for some types of gastric cancer. *H. pylori* infection burrows into the cells of the mucosa and so is able to interfere with immune function and yet escape the action of gastric acid. Although a national survey reported that 31% of the US population tested positive for *H. pylori*, prevalence among African Americans and Mexican Americans was nearly twice this number. This infection may contribute to the higher incidence of gastric cancer and ulcer disease among African Americans. This bacterium also has a deleterious effect on nutrition status. Individuals who test positive for *H. pylori* have lower serum levels of retinol (vitamin A), beta carotene, and folate, despite dietary intakes equivalent to those with higher serum levels who are free of *H. pylori* infection. Among *H. pylori*–infected patients, low blood levels of ascorbic acid and vitamin B_{12} were restored to normal when their infection was eradicated. *H. pylori* status is related to socioeconomic variables, with higher rates of infection among those with less education, lower income, and poorer living conditions.

Bibliography

Epplein M, Cohen SS, Zheng W, et al: Neighborhood socio-economic characteristics, African ancestry, and Helicobacter pylori sero-prevalence, *Cancer Causes Control* 23(6):897, 2012.

Epplein M, Signorello LB, Zheng W, et al: Helicobacter pylori prevalence and circulating micronutrient levels in a low-income United States population, *Cancer Prev Res (Phila)* 4(6):871, 2011.

Grad YH, Lipsitch M, Aiello AE: Secular trends in Helicobacter pylori seroprevalence in adults in the United States: evidence for sustained race/ethnic disparities, *Am J Epidemiol* 175(1):54, 2012.

Lahner E, Persechino S, Annibale B: Micronutrients (other than iron) and Helicobacter pylori infection: a systematic review, *Helicobacter* 17(1):1, 2012.

Nguyen T, Ramsey D, Graham D, et al: The prevalence of Helicobacter pylori remains high in African American and Hispanic veterans, *Helicobacter* 20:305, 2015.

blood could lead to sepsis in an adult who lacks normal immune response.[20]

At present no legal definitions have been formulated for the terms *prebiotic* or *probiotic*, but as dietary supplements their product labels must comply with applicable US Food and Drug Administration regulations. Accurate information relating to the exact strain or species of bacteria, dosage required for effective intervention, safety of a particular product, or product shelf life can be difficult to obtain.

HEALTH PROMOTION

Choosing Foods That Contain Prebiotics and Probiotics

Individuals can increase their intakes of prebiotics and probiotics by thoughtful food selection. Fruits and vegetables such as bananas, leeks, and asparagus and whole-grain oatmeal and wheat products are good sources of prebiotics.[21] Yogurt, cheese, and kefir (fermented milk prepared by adding kefir grains to cow's milk or goat's milk) all contain potentially live bacteria, but they may not be present in sufficient numbers to be effective. Some yogurts contain not only starter cultures of bacteria but also added *Lactobacillus* or *Bifidobacterium* that produce a probiotic effect. Fermented milk and yogurt marketed as functional foods and containing known strains of bacteria at probiotic levels are entering the marketplace.

METABOLISM

Following absorption, nutrients are transported to cells to provide energy or produce substances and tissues needed to sustain body functions. Metabolic activities within cells describe the total spectrum of chemical reactions associated with use of the individual macronutrients.

Carbohydrate Metabolism

Glucose is an immediate energy source for all body cells but is the preferred energy source for the brain and nervous system. Because glucose is so critical to life, its level in the blood is carefully regulated.

Sources of Blood Glucose

Both carbohydrate and noncarbohydrate molecules are sources of blood glucose, as follows:

- *Carbohydrate sources:* Three carbohydrate substances can be converted to glucose: (1) dietary starches and sugars, (2) glycogen stored in the liver and muscle, and (3) products of carbohydrate metabolism such as lactic acid and pyruvic acid.
- *Noncarbohydrate sources:* Both protein and fat are indirect sources of glucose. Certain amino acids are called *glucogenic amino acids* because they can form glucose after their amino group (NH_2^+) is removed. Approximately 58% of the protein in a mixed diet is made of glucogenic amino acids. Thus more than half of dietary protein might ultimately be used for energy if sufficient carbohydrate and fat are not available. After fats are broken down into fatty acids and glycerol, the glycerol portion (approximately 10% of the fat) can be converted to glycogen in the liver and then to glucose as needed. The formation of glucose from protein, glycerol, and carbohydrate metabolites is called **gluconeogenesis.**

Uses of Blood Glucose

Blood glucose is held within a normal range of 70 to 140 mg/dL (3.9 to 7.8 mmol/L) but is in constant flux as absorbed glucose is transported to cells for immediate use or removed from the circulation and stored as glycogen or fat. Blood glucose is used in three different ways:

- *Energy production:* The primary function of glucose is to supply energy to meet the body's constant demand. An array of metabolic pathways requiring specific and successive enzymes accomplishes this task.
- *Energy storage:* Glucose is stored in two forms: (1) glycogen, which is held in limited amounts in liver and muscle, and (2) fat (adipose tissue), which is the storage form for all excess glucose after energy demands have been met. Only a small supply of glycogen exists at any one time, and it turns over rapidly. In contrast, fat can be stored in unlimited amounts in adipose tissue and provides long-term energy stores.
- *Glucose products:* Small amounts of glucose are used to produce various carbohydrate compounds with important roles in body metabolism. Examples include deoxyribonucleic acid (DNA) and ribonucleic acid (RNA), galactose, and certain amino acids.

These sources and uses of glucose act as checks and balances to maintain normal blood levels, adding or removing glucose as needed.

Hormonal Controls

Several hormones influence glucose metabolism and regulate blood glucose levels.

- *Blood glucose–lowering hormone:* Only one hormone—insulin—lowers blood glucose. Insulin is produced by the beta cells in the pancreas. These cells are scattered in clusters, forming "islands" in the pancreas, which gives rise to the name *islets of Langerhans* after the German scientist who first discovered them.

Insulin lowers blood glucose by the following actions:
- *Glycogenesis* stimulates the conversion of glucose to glycogen in the liver for energy reserve.
- *Lipogenesis* stimulates the conversion of glucose to fat for storage in adipose tissue.
- *Cell permeability* increases, allowing more glucose to enter the cell and be oxidized for energy.
- *Blood glucose–raising hormones:* The following hormones effectively raise blood glucose levels:
- *Glucagon* produced by the alpha cells in the pancreas acts in opposition to insulin, increasing the breakdown of liver glycogen to glucose and maintaining blood glucose levels during fasting or sleep hours. (The hydrolysis of liver glycogen to yield glucose is called **glycogenolysis.**)
- *Steroid hormones,* secreted by the adrenal cortex, release glucose-forming carbon units from protein and oppose the actions of insulin.
- *Epinephrine,* originating from the adrenal medulla, stimulates the breakdown of liver glycogen and quick release of glucose.
- *Somatostatin,* produced in the delta cells of the pancreas and in the hypothalamus, suppresses insulin and glucagon and acts as a general modulator of related metabolic activities.
- *Growth hormone (GH)* and *adrenocorticotropic hormone (ACTH),* released from the anterior pituitary gland, oppose the actions of insulin.
- *Thyroxine,* originating in the thyroid gland, increases the rate of insulin breakdown, increases glucose absorption from the small intestine, and liberates epinephrine.

Lipid Metabolism
Lipid Synthesis and Breakdown

Two organ tissues—liver and adipose tissue—participate in lipid synthesis and breakdown as partners in lipid metabolism. The fatty acids released from lipids supply body cells with concentrated fuel for energy.

Lipoproteins

Lipid-protein complexes are the transport form of lipids in the blood. An excess of blood lipoproteins produces a clinical condition called *hyperlipoproteinemia.* Lipoproteins are produced (1) in the intestinal wall after the initial absorption of dietary lipids and (2) in the liver for constant recirculation to and from cells. Because lipids and carbohydrates work together to supply the body's need for energy, they involve many of the same hormones, as follows:

- *GH, ACTH,* and *thyroid-stimulating hormone (TSH),* all coming from the pituitary gland, increase the release of free fatty acids from stored lipids when energy demands are imposed.
- *Cortisol* and *corticosterone* from the adrenal gland cause the release of free fatty acids.
- *Epinephrine* and *norepinephrine* stimulate the breakdown of lipids and release of free fatty acids.
- *Insulin* promotes lipid synthesis and storage, whereas *glucagon* has the opposite effect of breaking down lipid stores to release free fatty acids.
- *Thyroxine* stimulates release of free fatty acids and lowers blood cholesterol levels.

When fatty acids absorbed from the gastrointestinal tract are delivered to the liver and muscle in larger amounts than needed for immediate energy or synthesis of important molecules, the hormone insulin promotes the formation of triglycerides for storage in the adipose tissue. In situations of prolonged physical activity, starvation, physical stress, or other circumstances that require energy beyond what can be supplied by available glycogen, these triglycerides are broken down and their fatty acids released. Free fatty acids are delivered to the liver to be packaged in lipoproteins for transport to cells for meeting energy needs or redeposition in adipose tissue. Muscle cells, including the heart muscle, depend on free fatty acids for their ongoing energy needs.

Protein Metabolism

Anabolism (Tissue Building)

Protein metabolism centers on the critical balance between anabolism (tissue building) and catabolism (tissue breakdown). The process of anabolism builds tissue through the synthesis of new protein, governed by a definite pattern or "blueprint" provided by DNA in the cell nucleus and calling for specific amino acids. Explicit enzymes and coenzymes along with certain hormones—GH, gonadotropins, and thyroxine—control and stimulate the building of tissue protein.

Catabolism (Tissue Breakdown)

Amino acids released from tissue breakdown are reused for making new proteins or, if not needed for protein synthesis, are broken down further and used for other purposes. The breakdown of amino acids yields two parts: (1) the nitrogen-containing group and (2) the remaining nonnitrogen residue, as follows:

1. *Nitrogen group:* The nitrogen portion is split off first, a process called deamination. This nitrogen can be converted to ammonia and excreted in the urine or retained for use in making other nitrogen compounds.
2. *Nonnitrogen residue:* The nonnitrogen residues are called keto acids. They can be used to form either carbohydrates or fats or, with the addition of a nitrogen group, can form a new amino acid. In health a dynamic equilibrium exists between anabolism and catabolism that sustains growth and maintains sound tissue.

Metabolic Interrelationships

Every chemical reaction occurring in the body is purposeful, and all are interdependent. They have two essential roles: (1) to produce energy and (2) to support the growth and maintenance of healthy tissue. The controlling agents necessary for these reactions to proceed in an orderly manner are the cell enzymes, their coenzymes (often a vitamin or mineral), and special hormones. Overall, human metabolism is an exciting biochemical process designed to develop, sustain, and protect life.

KEY TERMS

Gluconeogenesis
Production of glucose from keto acid carbon skeletons from deaminated amino acids, from the glycerol portion of triglycerides, or from certain carbohydrate metabolites.

Glycogenolysis
Specific term for the conversion of glycogen into glucose in the liver.

Deamination
Removal of an amino group (NH_2) from an amino acid.

Keto Acid
Amino acid residue after deamination; the glycogenic keto acids can be converted to glucose.

TO SUM UP

Digestion breaks down the food we eat to release and convert nutrients to simple forms that the body can use. Digestion involves two types of activities: mechanical and chemical. Muscle action breaks down food through mixing and churning motions and moves the food mass along the gastrointestinal tract. The chemical activity of gastrointestinal secretions breaks food molecules into smaller and more simple components for absorption. Monosaccharides (simple sugars) and amino acids are water soluble and pass from the mucosal cells of the small intestine into the portal blood. Long-chain fatty acids must be packaged in lipid-protein complexes that enter the lymph and then pass through the thoracic duct into the general circulation. The enormous population of bacteria found in the colon participates in immune function and the synthesis and absorption of important nutrients. The day-to-day function of the gastrointestinal tract, often taken for granted, represents a highly coordinated and efficient body system. The breakdown products released through digestion—glucose, amino acids, and fatty acids—participate in multiple metabolic pathways under hormonal and enzymatic control, producing energy, control agents, and tissues necessary for life and health.

QUESTIONS FOR REVIEW

1. You have just eaten a lunch that included a hamburger on a whole wheat bun, a glass of low-fat milk, and a bunch of grapes. Trace the digestion and final use of each of the macronutrients present in your lunch. What are (a) the enzymes, locations, and breakdown products formed in the complete digestion of these foods; (b) the routes taken by the breakdown products after absorption; and (c) one possible body use?

2. It is said that "food does not really enter the body until it is absorbed." What does this mean? What mechanisms support the absorption of nutrients against a concentration gradient?

3. How might long-term antibiotic use affect the overall function of the gastrointestinal tract? What might be the consequences for nutritional status and health?

4. Discuss the roles of muscle movements and motions in digestion. What are the physiologic or pathologic consequences when

(a) movement is absent or too slow and (b) when movement is too rapid?

5. You are working with an older adult who suffered a stroke, resulting in damage to the nerves in his head and throat. What are the implications for his food intake and nutritional well-being?

6. You are working with a young woman who has indicated that she is lactose intolerant and has deleted all dairy products from her diet: (a) What do you need to know about her symptoms and when they occurred? (b) Develop a daily protocol for gradually adding lactose-containing foods to her diet. (c) Prepare a list of calcium-containing foods that will meet her Dietary Reference Intake (DRI) for calcium if consumption of dairy products is not an option.

7. Visit a local supermarket or drug store and examine three over-the-counter medications that claim to (a) reduce stomach acid or (b) alleviate abdominal discomfort or intestinal gas. Make a table

that includes each product and list the active ingredients on the product label. Visit the National Library of Medicine/National Institutes of Health MedlinePlus website at http://www.nlm.nih.gov/medlineplus/druginformation.html or consult another drug index to identify the specific actions of each ingredient. What is the mechanism by which each active ingredient is believed to bring about the desired effect? What is the relative safety of this drug based on the possible side effects or contraindications?

8. Describe the complementary roles of insulin and glucagon in regulating blood glucose levels. What are the effects of these hormones over the course of a day for an individual who eats breakfast at 7:00 a.m., lunch at 12:00 p.m., and dinner at 6:00 p.m., with no snacks?

REFERENCES

1. Guyton AC, Hall JE: *Textbook of medical physiology*, ed 10, Philadelphia, 2000, Saunders.
2. Smeets PAM, Charbonnier L, van Meer F, et al: Food-induced brain responses and eating behavior, *Proc Nutr Soc* 71:511, 2012.
3. Klein S, Cohn SM, Alpers DH: The alimentary tract in nutrition. In Shils MA, Olson JA, Shike M, editors: *Modern nutrition in health and disease*, ed 10, Baltimore, MD, 2006, Lippincott Williams & Wilkins.
4. Loper HB, La Sala M, Dotson C, et al: Taste perception, associated hormonal modulation, and nutrient intake, *Nutr Rev* 73(2):83, 2015.
5. Lampuré A, Castetbon K, Deglaire A, et al: Associations between liking for fat, sweet or salt and obesity risk in French adults: A prospective cohort study, *Int J Behav Nutr Phys Act* 13:74, 2016.
6. Miranda-Rius J, Brunet-Llobet L, Lahor-Soler E, et al: Salivary secretory disorders, inducing drugs, and clinical management, *Int J Med Sci* 12(10):811, 2015.
7. Peery AF, Crockett SD, Barritt AS, et al: Burden of gastrointestinal, liver, and pancreatic diseases in the United States, *Gastroenterology* 149:1731, 2015.
8. Avunduk C: *Manual of gastroenterology: diagnosis and therapy*, ed 4, Philadelphia, 2008, Lippincott Williams & Wilkins.
9. Goulet O: Potential role of the intestinal microbiota in programming health and disease, *Nutr Rev* 73(Suppl 1):32, 2015.
10. Cresci GA, Bawden E: Gut microbiome: What we do and don't know, *Nutr Clin Pract* 30:734, 2015.
11. Bonci L: *American Dietetic Association guide to better digestion*, Hoboken, NJ, 2003, John Wiley & Sons.
12. Holtmann G, Talley NJ: Functional dyspepsia, *Curr Opin Gastroenterol* 31(6):492, 2015.
13. Talley NJ, Ford AC: Functional dyspepsia, *N Eng J Med* 373(19):1853, 2015.
14. Joneja JV: Lactose intolerance. In *The health professional's guide to food allergies and intolerances*, Chicago, 2013, Academy of Nutrition and Dietetics.
15. Misselwitz B: Lactose intolerance: New insights due to blinded testing, *Digestion* 90:72, 2014.
16. Heaney RP: Dairy intake, dietary adequacy, and lactose intolerance, *Adv Nutr* 4:151, 2013.
17. Mattar R, de Campos Mazo DF, Carrilho FJ: Lactose intolerance: diagnosis, genetic, and clinical factors, *Clin Exp Gastroenterol* 5:113, 2012.
18. Marcason W: Probiotics: Where do we stand? *J Acad Nutr Diet* 113:1424, 2013.
19. Verspreet J, Damen B, Broekaert WF, et al: A critical look at prebiotics within the dietary fiber concept, *Annu Rev Food Sci Technol* 7:167, 2016.
20. Mullin GE: Probiotics. In Matarese LE, Mullin GE, Raymond JL, editors: *The health professional's guide to gastrointestinal nutrition*, Chicago, 2015, Academy of Nutrition and Dietetics.
21. Slavin J: Fiber and prebiotics: Mechanisms and health benefits, *Nutrients* 5:1417, 2013.
22. Peregrin T: The inside tract: What RDs need to know about the gut microbiome, *J Acad Nutr Diet* 113(8):1019, 2013.
23. Vipperla K, O'Keefe SJ: The microbiota and its metabolites in colonic mucosal health and cancer risk, *Nutr Clin Pract* 27(5):624, 2012.
24. Duffy LC, Raiten DJ, Hubbard VS, et al: Progress and challenges in developing metabolic footprints from diet in human gut microbial cometabolism, *J Nutr* 145:1123S, 2015.
25. Nova E, Pérez de Heredia F, Gómez-Martínez S, et al: The role of probiotics on the microbiota: effect on obesity, *Nutr Clin Pract* 31:387, 2016.

FURTHER READINGS AND RESOURCES

Readings

O'Connor LE, Eaton TK, Savaiano DA: Improving milk intake in milk-averse lactose digesters and maldigesters, *J Nutr Educ Behav* 47(4):325, 2015.
[These researchers describe interventions to improve milk consumption among individuals who dislike milk or may have problems with lactose digestion.]
Cao Q, Kolasa KM: Gut check: finding the effective dietary approach, *Nutr Today* 46(4):171, 2011.
Carlson MJ, Moore CE, Tsai CM, et al: Child and parent perceived food-induced gastrointestinal symptoms and quality of life in children with functional gastrointestinal disorders, *J Acad Nutr Diet* 114(3):403, 2014.
Marx W, Kiss N, McCarthy AL, et al: Chemotherapy-induced nausea and vomiting: A narrative review to inform dietetics practice, *J Acad Nutr Diet* 116(5):819, 2016.
[These authors provide insight to dietary approaches for treating digestive disorders encountered in the clinical setting.]

Websites of Interest

- National Institutes of Health, National Center for Alternative and Complementary Medicine. This site offers information on herbs sometimes recommended for digestive disorders such as chamomile, ginger, peppermint oil, and turmeric, noting usefulness and risk, if any. https://medlineplus.gov/druginfo/herb_All.html.
- National Institutes of Health, National Center for Complementary and Integrative Health; Probiotics: In Depth. This site discusses the effectiveness, safety, and side effects of probiotics. https://nccih.nih.gov/health/probiotics/introduction.htm.
- National Institutes of Health, National Institute of Diabetes and Digestive and Kidney Diseases; Lactose Intolerance. This site describes causes, diagnosis, and useful interventions for lactose maldigesters. http://digestive.niddk.nih.gov/ddiseases/pubs/lactoseintolerance/index.aspx.

3

Carbohydrates

Eleanor D. Schlenker

ⓔ http://evolve.elsevier.com/Williams/essentials/

With this chapter we begin our study of the macronutrients—carbohydrates, fats, and proteins. These three nutrients share a unique characteristic: the ability to supply energy. Carbohydrates are of prime importance in the human diet as the major source of energy for work and growth. In recent years researchers have looked at digestible and indigestible carbohydrates and their various effects on health. Indigestible carbohydrates, usually referred to as fiber, have specific functions in maintaining gastrointestinal health. Plant foods identified as functional foods have distinct characteristics that positively influence health. Unfortunately, added sugars are making up a greater proportion of the typical American diet at the expense of complex carbohydrates and fiber. We will review the different types of carbohydrate and then examine their functions.

OUTLINE

THE NATURE OF CARBOHYDRATE

Basic Fuels: Sugars and Starch

Two forms of digestible **carbohydrate** occur naturally in plant foods: (1) sugars and (2) starch. Energy on planet Earth comes ultimately from the sun and its action on plants. Using their internal process of **photosynthesis**, plants transform the sun's energy into the stored fuel of carbohydrate (Fig. 3.1). Plants use carbon dioxide (CO_2) from the air and water from the soil—with the plant pigment chlorophyll as a chemical catalyst—to manufacture sugars and starch. The carbohydrates that plants store for their own energy needs become a source of fuel for humans who eat those plants. Because our bodies can rapidly break down starch and sugars, carbohydrates are often referred to as *quick energy foods*. They are our primary source of energy.

Dietary Importance

Carbohydrates make up a major portion of the food of people all over the world. Fruits, vegetables, cereals, grains, and dairy foods supply carbohydrate. Rice is one of the world's most important sources of carbohydrate, feeding an estimated 3.5 billion people worldwide.[1] In the typical American diet, about one half of total kilocalories (kcalories or kcal) come from carbohydrates.[2] Carbohydrate foods are readily available, relatively low in cost, and easily stored. Compared with food items that require refrigeration or have a short shelf life, many carbohydrate foods can be held in dry storage for fairly long periods without spoiling. Modern processing and packaging methods have extended the shelf life of carbohydrate products almost indefinitely.

CLASSIFICATION OF CARBOHYDRATES

The term *carbohydrate* comes from its chemical nature. Carbohydrates contain the elements carbon, hydrogen, and oxygen, with the hydrogen/oxygen ratio usually that of water (CH_2O). Carbohydrates are classified according to the number of basic sugar or saccharide units that make up their structure. The monosaccharides and disaccharides are referred to as *simple carbohydrates* because of their relatively small size and structure. The polysaccharides, including starch and certain fibers, are called *complex carbohydrates* based on their larger size and more complicated structure.

Monosaccharides

The simplest form of carbohydrate is the **monosaccharide**, or single sugar. The three monosaccharides important in human nutrition are (1) glucose, (2) fructose, and (3) galactose.

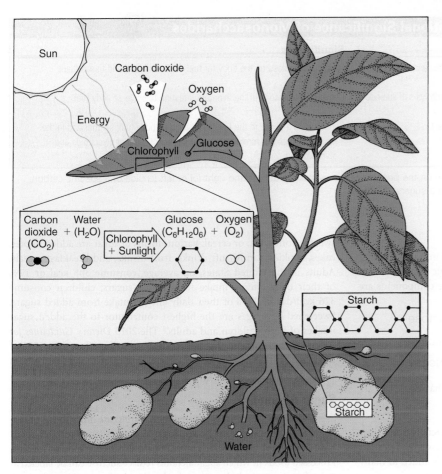

FIG. 3.1 Photosynthesis. In the presence of sunlight and the green leaf pigment chlorophyll, plants use water and carbon dioxide (CO_2) to produce glucose and starch by capturing the sun's energy and transforming it into chemical energy in the food products stored in their roots, stems, and leaves; through this process oxygen is returned to the atmosphere. (Courtesy Medical and Scientific Illustration.)

KEY TERMS

Carbohydrate
Compound made up of carbon, hydrogen, and oxygen; includes starches, sugars, and dietary fiber made and stored in plants; digestible carbohydrates yield 4 kcal/g.

Photosynthesis
Process by which plants containing chlorophyll are able to manufacture carbohydrate by combining CO_2 from the air and water from the soil with sunlight providing energy and chlorophyll as a catalyst.

Monosaccharide
Simple sugar; a carbohydrate containing a single saccharide (sugar) unit. The most common monosaccharides are glucose, galactose, and fructose.

Glucose

Glucose is a moderately sweet sugar found naturally in only a few foods—one being corn syrup. Glucose is the common body fuel oxidized by cells. It is supplied to the body directly from the digestion of starch but is also obtained through conversion of other simple sugars. Glucose (referred to by its older name *dextrose* in hospital intravenous solutions) is the form in which carbohydrates circulate in the blood.

Fructose

Fructose, the sweetest of the simple sugars, is found naturally in fruits and honey. Fructose intake has escalated dramatically since high-fructose corn syrup (HFCS) was introduced for use in processed food.

HFCS is the sweetener in many soft drinks, fruit drinks, commercial baked products, and dessert mixes. In humans, fructose is converted to glucose and burned for energy. Fructose is absorbed less efficiently than glucose, and amounts of 25 to 50 g or more can cause gastrointestinal distress.[3] (An 8-oz container of apple juice may contain 16 g of fructose, whereas a 12-oz can of a sweetened soft drink may supply 22 g or more.[3]) (See the Focus on Food Safety box, "Honey," for cautions relating to infant feeding.)

🍯 FOCUS ON FOOD SAFETY

Honey

Honey is a natural sweetener but in fact contains no vitamins or minerals and has about the same number of kcalories as table syrups. Honey should never be given to infants younger than 1 year because it may contain small amounts of the bacteria spores that produce botulism, a form of food poisoning that is often fatal.

Galactose

The simple sugar galactose is never found free in foods but is released in the digestion of lactose (milk sugar) and then converted to glucose in the liver. This reaction is reversible; in lactation, glucose is reconverted to galactose for use in milk production.

The physiologic and nutritional roles of the monosaccharides (sometimes referred to as *hexoses* because of their six-carbon structure) are summarized in Table 3.1.

TABLE 3.1	**Physiologic and Nutritional Significance of Monosaccharides**	
Monosaccharide	**Source**	**Significance**
D-Glucose[a]	Fruit juices; hydrolysis of starch, cane sugar, maltose, and lactose	Form of sugar used by the body for fuel; found in blood and tissue fluids
D-Fructose	Fruit and fruit juices; honey; hydrolysis of sucrose from cane sugar	Converted to glucose in the liver and intestine to serve as body fuel
D-Galactose	Hydrolysis of lactose (milk sugar)	Converted to glucose in the liver to be used as body fuel; synthesized in the mammary gland to form lactose for milk; constituent of glycolipids and glycoproteins

[a]Monosaccharides can exist in D or L forms depending on the position of the hydroxyl group on the right (D) or left (L) side of a specific carbon. Digestive enzymes are stereospecific and act only on D sugars.

Disaccharides

The disaccharides are double sugars made up of two monosaccharides linked together. The three disaccharides of physiologic importance are sucrose, lactose, and maltose. Their monosaccharide components are as follows:

Sucrose = one glucose + one fructose

Lactose = one glucose + one galactose

Maltose = one glucose + one glucose

Notice that glucose is found in each of the disaccharides.

Sucrose

Sucrose is common "table sugar" and is made commercially from sugar cane and sugar beets. It is found naturally in molasses and certain fruits and vegetables (e.g., peaches and carrots) and is added to many processed foods.

Lactose

Lactose is the sugar found in milk and is the least sweet of the disaccharides, only about one-sixth as sweet as sucrose. Although milk is relatively high in lactose, cheese, one of milk's products, may contain little or no lactose, depending on how the cheese is made. When milk sours in the initial stage of cheese making, the liquid whey separates from the solid curd. The lactose from the milk dissolves into the whey, which is drained away and discarded. The remaining curd is processed into cheese, making it possible for many lactose-intolerant individuals to digest cheese, although cheeses vary in lactose content. (See Chapter 2 for a review of lactose intolerance.)

Maltose

Maltose occurs naturally in relatively few foods but is formed in the body as an intermediate product in starch digestion. It is found in commercial malt products and germinating cereal grains. The physiologic and nutritional significance of disaccharides is summarized in Table 3.2.

Although sugars occur naturally in fruit and milk, the major portion of sugar in the US diet is added in food preparation or processing. We add sugar when we pour syrup on pancakes or use table sugar to sweeten coffee, tea, or cereal. Various forms of sugar are added to pies, cakes, cookies, candy, soft drinks, fruit drinks, and breakfast cereals. Adults in the United States, on average, consume 308 kcal or 17% of their daily energy intake from added sugars; children consume 326 kcal/day or 14% of their daily energy intake from added sugars. Sweetened beverages are the highest contributor to the added sugar intakes of both children and adults.[4] The 2015 *Dietary Guidelines for Americans* recommend that added sugar contribute less than 10% of total energy intake.[5] (See Box 3.1 for examples of foods that contain added or naturally occurring sugars.)

Sugar Alcohols

Sugar alcohols (sometimes referred to as *polyols*) are other forms of carbohydrate with sweetening power. Sugar alcohols, such as sorbitol, mannitol, and xylitol, are found in nature but are also used in food processing. Processed foods in which sugar alcohols replace sucrose can be labeled as *sugar free*. Sugar alcohols are poorly absorbed in the small intestine and, if absorbed, are poorly metabolized. Sugar alcohols commonly used as sugar replacers add only 0.2 to 3.0 kcal/g, compared with other sugars, which add 4 kcal/g.[6] These sweeteners are used in candy, ice cream and other frozen desserts, and baked goods advertised as being artificially sweetened and lower in kcalories. They often replace sugar in products developed to meet the demand for low-carbohydrate foods. Sugar alcohols are also attractive to consumers because the bacteria in the mouth that initiate dental caries do not attack them. These sweeteners offer an alternative for those with diabetes because they do not require insulin for their metabolism; however, they do add kcalories. At high intakes, sugar alcohols can cause abdominal distress or exert a laxative effect; hence foods with these sweeteners are best used in moderation.

Polysaccharides

Complex carbohydrates are called *polysaccharides* because they are made up of many (*poly*) single glucose (saccharide) units. Starch is the most important digestible polysaccharide; others are glycogen and dextrin. Nondigestible polysaccharides, such as cellulose, add important bulk to the diet and are categorized as dietary fiber. Box 3.2 displays some common food sources of complex carbohydrates.

TABLE 3.2	**Physiologic and Nutritional Significance of Disaccharides**	
Disaccharide	**Source**	**Significance**
Sucrose	Cane and beet sugar, sorghum cane, carrots, pineapple	Hydrolyzed to glucose and fructose; fuel for cells
Lactose	Milk	Hydrolyzed to glucose and galactose; fuel for cells; milk production in lactation
Maltose	Starch digestion by amylase or commercial hydrolysis; malt and germinating cereals	Hydrolyzed to yield two molecules of glucose; fuel for cells; can be fermented

BOX 3.1 Food Sources of Sugar

Sources of Naturally Occurring Sugars[a]

Orange juice
Grape juice
Peaches
Apples
Strawberries
Grapes
Bananas
Fluid milk
Powdered milk
Some cheeses (cheeses vary in the amount of lactose they contain, depending on method of manufacture)

Sources of Added Sugars

Pancake syrup
Candy
Fruit drinks
Sports drinks
Soft drinks
Cookies
Cake
Ice cream
Frozen desserts

[a]Fruit, fruit juices, and milk containing naturally occurring sugars also supply other important nutrients; added sugars supply kcalories only.
Images copyright 2006 JupiterImages Corporation.

KEY TERMS

Disaccharides
Class of sugars composed of two molecules of monosaccharides. The three most common disaccharides are sucrose, lactose, and maltose.

Sugar Alcohols
Alcohol formed from a simple sugar; sugar alcohols do not react with bacteria in the mouth to form dental caries; most sugar alcohols are poorly digested and absorbed, and yield less than 4 kcal/g.

Metabolism
Sum of all the various biochemical and physiologic processes by which the body grows and maintains itself (anabolism), breaks down and reshapes tissue (catabolism), and transforms energy to do its work. Products of these various reactions are called *metabolites*.

Glycogen
A polysaccharide made up of many saccharide (glucose) units. Glycogen is the body storage form of carbohydrate (glucose) found mostly in the liver, with lesser amounts in the muscle.

Dextrin
Intermediate breakdown product in the digestion of starch.

Dietary fiber
Nondigestible carbohydrates and lignin found in plants; dietary fiber is eaten as an intact part of the plant in which it is found.

BOX 3.2 Food Sources of Complex Carbohydrates

Hamburger buns
Whole-wheat bread
Corn flakes
Baked potato with skin
Sweet potatoes
Corn
Peas
Oatmeal

Rice
Beans
- Grain foods including bread, cereal, rice, and pasta; legumes; and certain vegetables such as potatoes contain large amounts of starch.
- Whole-grain breads and cereals, legumes, vegetables, and whole fruits supply both digestible carbohydrates and fiber.

Images copyright 2006 JupiterImages Corporation.

Starch

Starch consists of many coiled and branching chains of single glucose units and yields only glucose on complete digestion. Cooking not only improves the flavor of starch but also softens and ruptures the starch cells, making digestion easier. Starch mixtures thicken when cooked, because the substance encasing the starch granules has a gel-like quality that thickens mixtures in the same way as pectin causes jelly to set.

Resistant Starch

At one time it was thought that starch was completely digested and absorbed in the small intestine. Now we know that some starch in certain foods, such as whole grains, potatoes, bananas, and legumes, escapes digestion and enters the colon generally intact. This starch, called *resistant starch*, can make up as much as 15% of the starch in a high starch food.[7]

Undigested starch that moves into the colon is important to health. Microbial fermentation of resistant starch produces short-chain fatty acids, such as butyric acid, the preferred energy source of cells lining the colon. Available butyric acid helps protect against colonic diseases, such as colon cancer.[7] Also, resistant starch has many of the same health benefits as dietary fiber. Based on its health-related properties, food researchers are looking for new plant varieties and processing methods to maximize the resistant starch content of available foods.

Glycogen

Glycogen is the storage form of carbohydrate in animals, whereas starch is the storage form of carbohydrate in plants. Glycogen is synthesized in liver cells and stored in small amounts in liver and muscle. Liver glycogen helps sustain normal blood glucose levels during fasting periods such as sleep hours, and muscle glycogen provides immediate fuel for muscle action. Athletes sometimes practice pregame "glycogen loading" to add fuel stores for athletic competition (see Chapter 14). Dietary carbohydrate is required to maintain normal glycogen stores and prevent the stress symptoms of low-carbohydrate intake—fatigue, dehydration, weakness, and light-headedness. When carbohydrate is not available in sufficient amounts, the body breaks down protein and converts the released amino acids to an energy form. A severe lack of carbohydrate leads to undesirable metabolic effects, such as ketoacidosis, a complication of diabetes (see Chapter 22).

Dextrins

Dextrins are polysaccharide compounds formed as intermediate products in the breakdown of starch (Box 3.3).

Oligosaccharides

Oligosaccharides are small fragments of partially digested starch ranging in size from 3 to 10 glucose units. They are formed in digestion and produced commercially by acid hydrolysis. These small starch molecules are used in special formulas for infants and others with gastrointestinal problems because they are easy to digest. Oligosaccharides are also common in sports drinks, in which they often contribute almost half of the total glucose.

> ### KEY TERM
>
> **Oligosaccharides**
> Intermediate products of polysaccharide digestion that contain from 3 to 10 glucose units.

> ### BOX 3.3 **Breakdown of Starch in Digestion**
>
> Starch + Water ⇒ Soluble starch ⇒ Dextrins
> ⇒ Maltose ⇒ Glucose

Some naturally occurring oligosaccharides are formed with bonds that cannot be broken by human enzymes and therefore remain undigested. Two of these—stachyose and raffinose—are found in legumes such as beans, peas, and soybeans, and provide a feast for colonic bacteria. This produces gas that result in discomfort and embarrassment. The FODMAP diet, proposed for the treatment of irritable bowel syndrome, recommends the avoidance of oligosaccharide-containing foods, along with similar carbohydrates that are fermented by bacteria in the lower intestine.[8] (See Chapter 20 for further discussion of the FODMAP diet.)

Glycemic Index

Carbohydrate foods are digested and absorbed at different rates. Refined carbohydrates, such as white bread or corn flakes, are broken down quickly and rapidly absorbed into the blood. Less refined carbohydrate foods, such as brown rice, beans, or apples, also contain fiber and are digested and absorbed more slowly. These differences have implications for blood glucose control. Rapid entry of large amounts of glucose puts stress on the beta cells of the pancreas to secrete larger amounts of insulin to move glucose into body tissues and lower blood glucose levels. The glycemic index (GI) compares the effect of different carbohydrate-containing foods on blood glucose levels. A food with a high GI will raise blood glucose to a greater extent than a food with a low GI. In clinical practice, GI is measured by comparing blood glucose levels over a 2-hour period following ingestion of 50 g of glucose and after a 50-g carbohydrate portion of the test food. Based on its major effect on blood glucose, the glucose dose is generally assigned the rating of 100, and individual foods are rated accordingly. (See Table 3.3 comparing the GI of various foods.)

Many factors, including the type of digestible carbohydrate, prior cooking, particle size, and presence of fiber, influence the GI of a given food.[9] For example, fruits increase in sugar and decrease in starch as they ripen; as a result, ripe bananas have a higher GI than green bananas. Starches also differ in rate of digestion. Starch exists in two forms: amylose, a long straight chain; and amylopectin, a highly branched chain. Because the starch-digesting enzyme amylase attacks

TABLE 3.3 **Glycemic Index of Common Carbohydrate Foods**[a]

Food	Glycemic Index
Glucose test dose (50 g)	100
Baked potato (without skin)	98
Corn flakes	80
Jelly beans	80
Bread, white	77
Cupcake, frosted	73
Spaghetti, cooked	65
Banana	62
Bread, whole wheat	59
Orange juice	54
Green peas	51
Apple	39
White rice, long grain, cooked	38
All-bran cereal	38
Milk, nonfat	37
Kidney beans, canned	36
Fructose	15

[a]The test dose of 50 g glucose is usually assigned the value of 100 and serves as the standard to evaluate other foods.
Data from Atkinson FS, Foster-Powell K, Brand-Miller JC: International tables of glycemic index and glycemic load values. *Diab Care* 31(12):2281, 2008. (Supplementary Table A1; available online.)

only the molecule at the end of the chain, the straight chain amylose is broken down more slowly than amylopectin, which has many branch chains available for enzyme action. For this reason, potato and wheat, which contain more amylopectin, have a higher GI than does barley, which contains more amylose.[9]

Particle size and indigestible fiber influence the speed of digestion and absorption. Finely milled particles have a higher GI than larger particles because of the greater surface area available to enzyme action. Removal of the bran and fiber from whole grains raises the GI. Hard, compact kernels such as nuts and legumes resist penetration of digestive enzymes and are slow to be broken down as compared with porous white bread or high-carbohydrate liquids.

Other macronutrients or foods in the meal influence the GI of the total meal, although not the GI of individual foods.[10] Fat slows gastric emptying and interferes with the action of digestive enzymes so that high-fat items such as ice cream have a low GI, despite their high sugar content. Protein stimulates the secretion of insulin and hastens removal of glucose from the blood, effectively lowering the GI of the meal. Fiber, particularly viscous fiber, thickens the food mass, slowing the digestive process.[9] Biological differences including age, body mass index, and serum glucose levels influence the GI of particular foods, even in healthy individuals.[11]

Many nutrient-dense foods such as fruits, vegetables, and dairy have relatively low GIs, and whole-grain breads and cereals have moderate GIs when compared with white bread, soda, and fruit drinks. Diets relatively low in overall GI are more likely to meet nutrient requirements.[12]

IMPORTANCE OF CARBOHYDRATES

The complex carbohydrate found in vegetables, legumes, and grains should be the major dietary source of energy. On digestion, starch yields glucose, the favorite energy source of body cells. Fruit and dairy products supply carbohydrate in the form of naturally occurring sugars (fruit contains fructose, and milk contains lactose). Vegetables, legumes, fruits, and grains (especially whole grains) supply other important nutrients, including vitamins, minerals, and fiber. Dairy products are good sources of calcium, magnesium, and protein. Currently major food sources of starch in the American diet are refined grains, such as white bread, ready-to-eat cereals, white potatoes, pasta, and rice, which are often highly processed and limited in micronutrients. Whole grains include the germ and the bran covering of the grain kernel, both rich in nutrients, whereas refined grains have had these components removed (Fig. 3.2). Refined grains are enriched with several B vitamins, iron, and folate but provide less fiber and other trace minerals. Carbohydrate foods high in added sugar supply kcalories but little else. Based on the connection between added sugar and cardiovascular risk factors, including obesity, the American Heart Association recommends that added sugars not exceed 100 to 150 kcal/day, depending on overall energy intake.[13] The Perspectives in Practice box, "Cutting Down on Sugar," offers suggestions on how to lower your intake of added sugar.

Whole grain kernel

Bran
"Outer shell" protects seed
Fiber, B vitamins, trace minerals

Endosperm
Provides energy
Carbohydrates, protein

Germ
Nourishment for the seed
Antioxidants, vitamin E, B vitamins

FIG. 3.2 Nutrients in the bran and germ of whole grains are lost when grains are refined and the bran and germ are discarded. Current laws require that refined grains be enriched with thiamin, riboflavin, niacin, iron, and folate; however, other important nutrients such as zinc and vitamin E, also lost in processing, are not replaced. (From US Department of Agriculture: *Get on the grain train: putting the guidelines into practice.* Home and Garden Bulletin No 267-2, Washington, DC, 2002, US Department of Agriculture.)

FUNCTIONS OF CARBOHYDRATES

Energy

The primary function of starch and sugars is to supply energy to cells, especially brain cells that depend on glucose. When carbohydrate is lacking, fats can be used as an energy source by most organ systems; however, body tissues require a constant supply of glucose to function most efficiently.

Body stores of carbohydrate are relatively small but still serve as an important energy reserve. An adult man has about 300 to 350 g of carbohydrate stored in his liver and muscle in the form of glycogen, and another 10 g of glucose circulates in his blood (Table 3.4). Together this glycogen and glucose will supply the energy for only a half day of moderate activity. To meet the body's constant demand, carbohydrate foods must be eaten regularly and at reasonably frequent intervals.

PERSPECTIVES IN PRACTICE

Cutting Down on Sugar

The Healthy US-Style Eating Pattern included in the 2015 Dietary Guidelines for Americans recommends that empty calories including added sugar not exceed 270 kcal on a 2000-kcal diet. Consider the following substitutions in your meal plans to lower your intake of added sugar:

- Use fresh fruit, such as berries or sliced bananas or no-sugar-added applesauce, in place of syrup to sweeten pancakes or waffles.
- Drink water, low-fat or nonfat milk, or fruit juice in place of soft drinks, fruit drinks, or sports drinks with added sugar.

- Choose fruit canned in water or juice in place of fruit canned in heavy syrup.
- Purchase unflavored yogurt and add fruit or no-sugar-added applesauce for flavor or select flavored yogurt, lower in added sugar, than yogurt with fruit preserves.
- Look for cake and cookie recipes that use fruit purees as sweeteners in place of sugar.
- Read the food labels on salad dressings, catsup, and other condiments and avoid those with added sugar.

TABLE 3.4 Carbohydrate Storage in an Adult Man (70 kg [154 lb])

	Glycogen (g)	Glucose (g)
Liver	72	
Muscles	245	
Extracellular fluids		10
Component totals	317	10
TOTAL STORAGE	327	

Special Functions

Carbohydrates have other specialized roles in overall body metabolism.

Glycogen–Carbohydrate Storage

Liver and muscle glycogen are in constant interchange with the body's overall energy system. These energy reserves protect cells, especially brain cells, from depressed metabolic function and injury and support urgent muscle responses.

Protein-Sparing Action

Carbohydrates help regulate protein metabolism. An adequate supply of carbohydrate to satisfy ongoing energy demands prevents the channeling of protein for energy. This protein-sparing action of carbohydrate allows protein to be reserved for tissue building and repair.

Antiketogenic Effect

Carbohydrates influence fat metabolism. The supply of carbohydrate determines how much fat must be broken down to meet energy needs, thereby controlling the formation of *ketones*. Ketones are intermediate products of fat metabolism that normally are produced in very small amounts. However, when carbohydrate is inadequate to meet cell energy needs, as in starvation or uncontrolled diabetes or very low-carbohydrate diets, fat is oxidized at extreme rates. Sufficient amounts of dietary carbohydrates prevent any damaging excess of ketones.

Heart Action

Heart action is a life-sustaining muscle activity. Although fatty acids are the preferred fuel for the heart, the glycogen stored in cardiac muscle is an important emergency source of contractile energy.

Central Nervous System

The brain and central nervous system (CNS) depend on carbohydrate for energy but have very low carbohydrate reserves—enough to last only 10 to 15 minutes. This makes them especially dependent on a minute-to-minute supply of glucose from the blood. Sustained *hypoglycemic* shock causes irreversible brain damage. Providing an adequate morning supply of glucose for brain function may help explain why individuals who eat breakfast do better in school than those who skip breakfast.[14]

RECOMMENDED INTAKE OF CARBOHYDRATE

Dietary Reference Intakes

The Recommended Dietary Allowance (RDA) for carbohydrate is the same for all persons older than 1 year. Children, adolescents, and adults need a minimum of 130 g/day, the amount required to supply the energy demands of the CNS for 1 day.[15] Most people consume more than this minimum amount to meet their overall energy requirement and keep fat and protein intakes at acceptable levels.

Acceptable Macronutrient Distribution Range

A diet rich in plant-based foods supplies important nutrients and fiber, but it is unwise to take in excessive amounts of carbohydrate, just as it is not prudent to severely limit carbohydrate. To provide guidance for developing dietary patterns, nutrition experts established the Acceptable Macronutrient Distribution Ranges (AMDRs) (Box 3.4) for allocating macronutrient intakes in proportion to total kcalories. The adult AMDR for carbohydrate is 45% to 65% of total energy intake.[15] The AMDRs enable us to individualize diets to meet specific health situations and personal food preferences yet encourage sound nutrition habits.

Nonnutritive Sweeteners

Most of us have an inborn desire for foods that are sweet; however, we are faced with the dilemma of moderating our energy intakes to maintain a healthy weight. Nonnutritive sweeteners (NNSs) allow us to indulge our taste for sweets while limiting kcalorie intake. Sweeteners are grouped as *nutritive* or *nonnutritive*, depending on the kcalories they add to a food. Sucrose (table sugar) and other natural sugars yield 4 kcal/g. In contrast, NNSs, sometimes referred to as *noncaloric sweeteners,* contribute no kcalories or an insignificant number of kcalories. This is because NNSs have a higher intensity of sweetness when compared with nutritive sweeteners, such as corn syrup or sucrose; thus very small amounts are needed to produce the desired level of sweetness.[6]

The Food and Drug Administration (FDA) has approved five NNSs or their derivatives for use in the United States. They sweeten beverages, baked products, soft drinks, fruit drinks, and candy marketed as low or reduced calorie, and some are available for home preparation or baking. The NNS aspartame contains the amino acid phenylalanine, and aspartame-containing products must carry a label indicating that phenylalanine is present.[6] This protects individuals with phenylketonuria, who lack the enzyme needed to metabolize phenylalanine and so must eliminate it from their diets. The NNS most recently approved is a purified derivative extracted from the leaves of the stevia plant, common to South America.[6] An example of the intense sweetening power of NNSs is the fact that a 12-oz can of soda may be sweetened with 17 mg of the stevia derivative compared with 35 g of sugar (140 kcal). Table 3.5 compares the properties of FDA-approved NNSs. (NOTE: Although the FDA has approved the

KEY TERM

Nonnutritive Sweeteners
Substances with sweetening power that cannot be efficiently absorbed or metabolized to provide energy or can be used in very minute amounts based on their intense sweetness.

BOX 3.4 Acceptable Macronutrient Distribution Ranges

Carbohydrate: 45%–65% of total kcalories
Fat: 20%–35% of total kcalories
Protein: 10%–35% of total kcalories

Data from Institute of Medicine, National Academy of Sciences: *Dietary (DRI) reference intakes. The essential guide to nutrient requirements,* Washington, DC, 2006, National Academies Press.

TABLE 3.5 **Properties and Applications of Common Nonnutritive Sweeteners**

Name	Sweetening Power (Compared With Sucrose)	Effect of Heat	Trade Names	Applications
Aspartame	160–220 times sweeter	Degrades during heating and loses sweetening power	NutraSweet, Equal, Sugar Twin (blue box)	Beverages, table sweetener, gelatin, pudding, chewing gum, cold breakfast cereal
Acesulfame-K	200 times sweeter	Stable at baking temperatures	Sweet One, Sweet & Safe	Beverages, table sweetener, baked goods, all-purpose sweetener; excluded for use in meat and poultry
Saccharin[a]	300 times sweeter	Not affected by heat	Sweet and Low, Sweet Twin, Necta Sweet, Sweet 'N Low Brown	Beverages, table sweetener, chewing gum, baked goods, pudding
Sucralose	600 times sweeter	Not affected by heat in cooking and baking	Splenda	Beverages, desserts, baked goods, candy, table sweetener, all-purpose sweetener
Stevia (steviol glycosides-rebaudioside A extracted from stevia plant leaves)	250 times sweeter	Shelf-stable in dry forms or liquids	Truvia, Rebiana, PureVia, SweetLeaf	Beverages, cereals, energy bars, table sweetener

[a]Limited to <12 mg/fl oz in beverages; 20 mg/serving in individual packages; or 30 mg/serving in processed foods.
Data from Academy of Nutrition and Dietetics: Position of the Academy of Nutrition and Dietetics: use of nutritive and nonnutritive sweeteners. *J Acad Nutr Diet* 117:739, 2012; and Gardner C, Wylie-Rosett J, Gidding SS, et al: On behalf of the American Heart Association Nutrition Committee: nonnutritive sweeteners: current use and health perspectives. A scientific statement from the American Heart Association and the American Diabetes Association, *Diabetes Care* 35:1798, 2012.

stevia derivative for use in food and beverages, the actual stevia leaf has not received FDA-approval for use in foods at this time. It is being sold as a dietary supplement, which is not regulated by FDA rules. We will discuss current legislation relating to dietary supplements in Chapter 9.)

Over the past decade, use of NNS-sweetened beverages increased from 18% to 24% of adults and doubled from 6% to 12% of children,[16] likely fueled by increased concerns about body weight. Evidence-based evaluations have concluded that both nutritive sweeteners and NNSs can be used within the context of a balanced diet; however, current evidence is only fair to good that use of NNSs will bring about a loss in body weight.[6] (See the Evidence-Based Practice box, "Do Nonnutritive Sweeteners Help You Lose Weight?," for more discussion.)

EVIDENCE-BASED PRACTICE

Do Nonnutritive Sweeteners Help You Lose Weight?

Identify the problem: Obesity continues to be a major public health problem in the United States and beyond. Consumers attempting to lose unwanted weight, or avoid unwanted weight gain, have turned to nonnutritive sweeteners (NNSs) as a way to decrease their kcalorie intake yet enjoy their favorite foods, especially sweet foods. Use of NNSs that satisfy the palate and add few if any kcalories is rising in both commercial food processing and home food preparation.

Review the evidence: It is logical to conclude that replacing sugar-sweetened food items with NNSs would lead to reduced kcalorie intake with less weight gain or modest weight loss, but research evidence is varied. Those who gain weight or have a higher body mass index are more likely to use NNSs in an effort to address their weight problem, but weight loss does not always follow. At one time it was suggested that NNSs created metabolic effects that actually increased food intake, but this has not been found to be true. The 2015 Dietary Guidelines Advisory Committee concluded that replacing sugar-containing items with NNSs reduced kcalorie intake, body weight, and body fat. However, NNSs are not a weight management tool in and of themselves—they will influence energy intake and assist in weight management *only* if they replace higher-kcalorie foods and beverages.

Implement the findings: For individuals drinking sugar-sweetened beverages regularly, substituting two calorie-free beverages for two 12-oz cans of a sugar-sweetened beverage would save 300 kcal (150 kcal/can) per day. But, the kcalories "saved" by use of reduced-calorie or calorie-free items cannot be used to add other foods to the diet or enjoy larger portions if weight loss is the goal. Use food labels to evaluate the content of added sugars, naturally occurring sugars, and NNSs in foods and beverages.

Bibliography

Fitch C, Keim KS, Academy of Nutrition and Dietetics: Position of the Academy of Nutrition and Dietetics: use of nutritive and nonnutritive sweeteners, *J Acad Nutr Diet* 112:739, 2012.

Miller PE, Perez V: Low-calorie sweeteners and body weight and composition: a meta-analysis of randomized controlled trials and prospective cohort studies, *Am J Clin Nutr* 100:765, 2014.

Roberts JR: The paradox of artificial sweeteners in managing obesity, *Curr Gastroenterol Rep* 17:423, 2015.

US Department of Health and Human Services, US Department of Agriculture: *Scientific Report of the 2015 Dietary Guidelines Advisory Committee*, Washington, DC, 2015, Center for Nutrition Policy and Promotion, US Department of Agriculture. https://www.health.gov/dietaryguidelines/2015-scientific-report/PDFs/Scientific-Report-of-the-2015-Dietary-Guidelines-Advisory-Committee.pdf.

CARBOHYDRATES AND ORAL HEALTH

Nutrient intake and oral health have a synergy that acts in two directions. Malnutrition and nutrition-related diseases lead to deterioration of the teeth and supporting tissues of the mouth and gums, such that eating becomes difficult and nutrient intake is further compromised. Conversely, untreated and progressive periodontal disease results in systemic infections, increases inflammatory responses, and worsens blood glucose control in diabetes.

Dental caries is one of the most frequently occurring and preventable infectious diseases of the oral cavity and a major cause of tooth loss. Oral hygiene, diet, and specific nutrients have been related to dental caries. Normal salivary flow and exposure to fluoride, either systemically through fluoridated water or topically with use of fluoridated toothpaste or dental treatments, help protect against dental caries.

The amounts and types of dietary carbohydrate and the conditions under which they are eaten influence dental caries. All carbohydrates can be cariogenic, although fructose and lactose are less cariogenic than sucrose (Fig. 3.3). Individuals who consume higher amounts of added sugar have increased incidence of dental caries. Although naturally occurring sugars can cause tooth decay, citrus fruits with a high proportion of water and fruits containing citric acid, which stimulates salivary secretion, rinse the teeth and help remove sugars from the enamel's surface. The period of exposure to a sweet solution affects its **cariogenic** potential. Continuous sipping of a sugar-sweetened beverage throughout the day increases the risk of tooth decay. Sticky foods such as raisins, crackers, or potato chips are cariogenic, and soft drinks and sport drinks with an acid pH contribute to erosion of the dental enamel and subsequent caries.

Prevention of dental caries may be yet another reason to choose whole-grain breads and cereals over highly processed grains and grain foods with added sugar. Unprocessed starch as a large molecule cannot pass through the dental plaque to attack the enamel, whereas shorter-chain oligosaccharides are easily broken down by salivary amylase to yield maltose, a choice substrate for plaque bacteria. Grain-sugar mixtures, such as sweetened breakfast cereals or cakes, are especially cariogenic.[17]

Chronic disease can compromise oral health. Age-related loss of calcium from the bones (or the drastic bone loss occurring in osteoporosis) affects the alveolar bone, resulting in tooth loss. Reduced salivary secretion (dry mouth) associated with diabetes and use of particular medications accelerates both tooth decay and damage to oral tissues.[17]

IMBALANCES IN CARBOHYDRATE INTAKE

High-Carbohydrate Diets

Although the AMDR recommends that carbohydrate provide 45% to 65% of total energy,[15] diets containing 75% carbohydrate have been adopted in an effort to lower intakes of fat and kcalories or normalize blood lipoproteins. When carbohydrate intake exceeds 65% of total kcalories, fat intake may be disproportionately low, jeopardizing the supply of essential fatty acids and vitamins and minerals found in higher-fat foods. Such an increase in dietary carbohydrate can trigger a rise in plasma triglycerides and **low-density lipoprotein (LDL)-cholesterol**, and a drop in **high-density lipoprotein (HDL)-cholesterol**, thereby increasing cardiovascular risk.[15] Excessive carbohydrate intake, high in simple carbohydrates or added sugars, brings about rapid elevations in blood glucose, putting heavy demands on the pancreas for insulin production and release. Whole-grain foods, legumes, or fruits and vegetables high in fiber and other complex carbohydrates are better choices when increasing carbohydrate intake.

Low-Carbohydrate Diets

Diets very low in carbohydrate have been popularized as efficient ways to lose weight. Such diets may restrict daily carbohydrate intake to 40 g or less,[18] or 10% or less,[19,20] of total kcalories. These regimens bring about weight loss over the short term *if* energy intake is also reduced, and have a favorable effect on metabolic parameters, including blood LDL-cholesterol, HDL-cholesterol, and triglycerides. Nevertheless, questions remain as to their appropriateness when followed for weeks or months.[19,20] It is important that all dietary patterns include the minimum daily servings of fruits, vegetables, and whole grains as recommended in the 2015 *Dietary Guidelines for Americans*.[5] Limiting these healthy carbohydrate foods lowers dietary fiber as well as important vitamins and minerals. Low-carbohydrate diets that replace carbohydrate foods with items high in saturated fat add to cardiovascular risk. Low-carbohydrate diets that replace carbohydrate with protein and exceed the AMDR for protein increase the burden on the kidneys. The best approach to reducing carbohydrate is eliminating foods high in added sugar that contribute little to nutrient intake.

Low-carbohydrate diets falling below the AMDR change the energy currency of cells from glucose to fatty acids, although the CNS remains

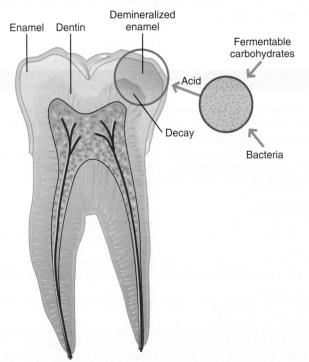

Enamel   Dentin   Demineralized enamel

Fermentable carbohydrates

Acid

Decay

Bacteria

FIG. 3.3 Dental caries can result from poor dental hygiene and continuous snacking and drinking of items high in added sugar or other refined carbohydrates. (From Mahan LK, Escott-Stump S: *Krause's food and nutrition therapy,* ed 12, St. Louis, 2008, Saunders.)

KEY TERMS

Cariogenic
Promotes the development of dental caries or tooth decay.

Low-density Lipoprotein (LDL)-Cholesterol
A lipoprotein produced in the liver that transports fatty acids and cholesterol to the cells and tissues; this lipoprotein contains large amounts of cholesterol.

High-density Lipoprotein (HDL)-Cholesterol
A lipoprotein produced in the liver that carries cholesterol from the tissues back to the liver for degradation and elimination.

dependent on glucose. Low-carbohydrate diets have been effective in lowering blood glucose levels in some people with diabetes, although watchful medical supervision is required.[19] The accelerated breakdown of fat for energy, producing ketones, has an anticonvulsant effect and has been used to treat pediatric epilepsy. The ketosis resulting from low-carbohydrate diets can assist in the management of nonalcoholic fatty liver disease, certain cancers, and neurodegenerative conditions, such as Alzheimer and Parkinson diseases.[20] However, even moderate ketosis increases water loss, demanding attention to water intake. Moreover, when glucose is in short supply, amino acids are broken down to provide carbon skeletons for glucose synthesis, yielding amino groups that must be disposed of via the urine. Calcium and potassium are also lost in this process, so intakes meeting recommended levels are critical.[20] (Note that ketosis as discussed here differs significantly from ketoacidosis, a potentially fatal condition arising in uncontrolled diabetes.)

Clinical trials comparing weight loss patterns among individuals following popular diets, either low or moderate in carbohydrate and low in fat, have revealed no major differences in pounds lost or cardiovascular parameters—*as long as kcalorie intake was reduced*.[21] The apparent safety and effectiveness of low-carbohydrate diets with appropriate medical supervision supports the need for more than one dietary approach to weight control, adapted to individual preferences and metabolic needs. Regardless, establishing a kcalorie deficit between energy intake and energy expenditure using a combination of foods that support nutritional well-being is the cornerstone of long-term weight management and health.

FIBER: THE NONDIGESTIBLE CARBOHYDRATE

Fiber is the nondigestible material found in whole-grain cereals, fruits, vegetables, and legumes that our grandmothers referred to as *roughage*. Because humans lack the enzymes necessary to break down these complex carbohydrates into forms that can be absorbed, they travel the length of the gastrointestinal tract and are eliminated in the feces. Fiber's ability to promote regular bowel function has been recognized for generations. All types of fiber are beneficial to health, but different fibers have different physiologic effects; therefore we need a variety of foods that supply various types. Although most foods contain more than one type of fiber, they likely have more of one than another.

Types of Fiber

In the past, fibers were classified as soluble or insoluble, based on their chemical properties in the laboratory. It was believed that these properties influenced their actions in the body as well. We have since learned that the health benefits of fiber are dependent on two characteristics: viscosity and fermentability. Viscous fibers, formerly referred to as *soluble* fibers, influence blood glucose levels and lower LDL-cholesterol levels. Fibers that are fermented by the microflora in the gastrointestinal tract and provide bulk to the stool were referred to as *insoluble* fibers; however, not all viscous fibers are soluble, and not all fibers that influence laxation are insoluble. Accordingly, these terms are no longer used to describe health benefits, although they still appear on food labels.[15]

For our purposes, fiber is divided into two categories: dietary fiber and **functional fiber**.

Dietary Fiber

Dietary fiber includes the nondigestible carbohydrates and lignin found intact in plant foods. Several dietary fibers important in human nutrition are described as follows:

- *Cellulose:* Cellulose is the material in plant cell walls that provides structure. We find it in the stems and leaves of vegetables, in the coverings of seeds and grains, and in skins and hulls. Because humans are unable to break down cellulose, it remains in the digestive tract and contributes bulk to the food mass.
- *Hemicellulose:* This polysaccharide is found in plant cell walls and often surrounds cellulose. Some hemicelluloses help regulate colon pressure by providing bulk for normal muscle action, whereas others are fermented by colonic bacteria.
- *Lignin:* Lignin is the only dietary fiber that is not a carbohydrate. It is a large molecule that forms the woody part of plants and in the intestine combines with bile acids and prevents their reabsorption. Lignin contributes the sandy texture to pears and lima beans.
- *Pectin:* This fiber is found in plant cell walls. It forms a viscous, sticky gel that binds cholesterol and prevents its absorption. Pectin also helps slow gastric emptying and extend feelings of satiety.
- *Gums:* Plants secrete gums in response to plant injury. In the intestine gums bind cholesterol and prevent its absorption. Bacteria in the colon ferment gums to form short-chain fatty acids that nourish colonic cells (this also occurs with resistant starch).
- *β-Glucans:* These water-soluble fibers are found in oats and oat bran, foods that carry a health claim on the label indicating they can reduce the risk of heart disease. (β-glucans interfere with the absorption of cholesterol.)

Box 3.5 gives examples of foods that provide specific varieties of fiber.

BOX 3.5 Sources of Dietary Fiber

Pectin, β-Glucans, Gums

Oatmeal
Oranges
Kidney beans
Carrots
Apples

Cellulose, Hemicellulose, Lignin

Whole-wheat bread
Popcorn
Baked beans
Bananas
Pears

Functional Fiber

Functional fibers are nondigestible polysaccharides that have been added to a food to increase its fiber content.[15] The term *functional fiber* is used to distinguish those fibers that are added to foods from those that are intact in plants and eaten in that form. Functional fibers can be isolated from plant foods or manufactured, and they are used as dietary supplements or added to processed foods. A particular fiber can be either a dietary fiber or a functional fiber, depending on how it is eaten or used. The pectin in the apple you ate at lunch is considered a dietary fiber. On the other hand, pectin that was isolated from fruit sources and added to homemade or commercial jellies or used as a fiber ingredient in patient tube feedings is classified as a functional fiber. Functional fibers added in food processing must be listed on the food label. Flaxseed and psyllium are two common functional fibers. Flaxseed is added to many breads and cereals marketed as high fiber. Psyllium, an ingredient in bulk laxatives, is also available as a dietary supplement.

A person's total fiber intake includes both dietary and functional fiber. Selected food sources of dietary fiber and their energy content are listed in Table 3.6. Note that foods high in fiber tend to be low to moderate in kcalories.

TABLE 3.6 Dietary Fiber and Energy Content of Selected Foods

Food Group	Serving Size	Dietary Fiber (g)	Energy (kcal)
Grains Group			
All Bran (wheat flakes)	¾ cup	5.0	95
Wheaties	1 cup	3.6	127
Shredded wheat (plain)	2 biscuits	5.8	158
Instant oatmeal, cooked	1 package	4.0	150
Cheerios	1 cup	2.6	105
Air-popped popcorn	1 cup	1.2	31
Whole-wheat bread	1 slice	1.9	81
Vegetable Group			
Kidney beans, canned	½ cup	5.5	108
Green peas, frozen, cooked	½ cup	3.6	62
Corn, frozen, cooked	½ cup	2.3	78
Potato, baked, with skin	1 medium	3.8	161
Carrots, raw	1 medium	1.7	25
Broccoli, chopped, frozen, cooked	½ cup	2.8	26
Spinach, frozen, cooked	1 cup	7.0	65
Fruit Group			
Apple, with skin	1 medium	4.4	95
Strawberries, sliced	1 cup	3.3	53
Orange	1 medium	3.1	62
Banana	1 medium	3.1	105

Data from US Department of Agriculture, Agricultural Research Service: USDA National Nutrient Database for Standard Reference, Release 28, September 2015 (slightly revised, May 2016). Nutrient Data Laboratory Home Page. http://www.ars.usda.gov/ba/bhnrc/ndl.

HEALTH PROMOTION

Health Benefits of Fiber

Dietary fiber influences the food mix in the gastrointestinal tract and associated gastrointestinal function. Individuals who follow dietary patterns that include recommended amounts of fiber are less likely to develop chronic conditions such as type 2 diabetes, cardiovascular disease, or metabolic syndrome.[22] Fiber influences various risk factors associated with chronic conditions, outlined as follows:

- *Increases fecal mass and promotes laxation:* The capacity of dietary fiber to hold water and bacteria creates its bulk-forming and laxative effects. The added mass helps the food bolus move more rapidly through the small intestine, promoting normal bowel action and preventing or alleviating constipation. A larger food mass in the colon averts the development of diverticula, small pouches that protrude outward through the lining of the colon. When the food residue entering the colon is low in bulk, the muscles must contract more forcefully to move it forward, which over time contributes to the formation of diverticula with risk of inflammation and infection. Dietary fiber has been effective in treating diarrhea and may be useful in treating other gastrointestinal conditions.[22]

- *Promotes growth of beneficial colonic microflora:* Bacteria living in the colon ferment dietary fiber along with resistant starch. This action produces short-chain fatty acids that nourish the cells lining the colon and stimulate their growth. Fiber encourages the proliferation of health-promoting bacteria and has been used to treat irritable bowel syndrome (see discussion of prebiotic agents in Chapter 2).[22]

- *Binds bile acids and cholesterol:* Fiber binds cholesterol and bile acids in the lower section of the small intestine and prevents their absorption. Bound to fiber, cholesterol and bile acids are eliminated in the feces.[22] When bile acids are lost, cholesterol must be removed from circulating blood lipoproteins to synthesize their replacements, with a resulting decrease in blood cholesterol.

- *Slows rise in blood glucose and insulin levels:* Foods rich in fiber have a low GI, with their glucose content released slowly into the blood. This slow release prevents a rapid spike in blood glucose after eating and lessens the amount of insulin needed to move glucose into muscle and fat cells, thereby reducing the work of the pancreas. Fiber intake at recommended levels may assist in the prevention and management of diabetes.[22]

- *Assists in weight management:* Fiber lowers the energy density of the diet by displacing carbohydrate, fat, or protein in a food, thereby reducing its energy content. A diet containing recommended levels of fiber requires more chewing and promotes satiety, helping lower food intake. Diets lower in energy density include more fruits, vegetables, whole grains, and legumes, and fewer kcalories from fat, baked desserts, and fried foods, supporting weight loss and weight maintenance.[23]

- *Protects against colorectal and gastric cancer:* Fiber reduces the risk of colorectal and gastric cancer, although it seems to have a lesser effect on other types of cancer, including breast cancer. Cereal fibers appear to play a special role, as cancer risk was found to decrease by 10% for every 10 g of cereal fiber consumed daily.[22] It may be that other dietary components associated with fiber—particular nutrients or phytochemicals—rather than the fiber itself, confer this resistance to chronic disease (see our later discussion on "Functional Foods").

Recommended Fiber Intake

The Adequate Intake (AI) for total fiber is based on the amount expected to lower the risk of coronary heart disease and type 2 diabetes. Men age 50 and younger should consume 38 g/day; those age 51 and older need 30 g/day. The AIs for younger and older women are 25 g/day and 21 g/day, respectively.[15] Unfortunately, consumer directives are inconsistent, as the current nutrition label recommends a fiber intake of 25 g in a 2000-kcal diet, considerably lower than the AI for men.

Fiber intake in the United States is barely half the amount recommended. Mean daily intake is 18.8 g/day for men and 15.4 g/day for women.[24] Women consume more fiber than men based on energy intake

🌐 FOCUS ON CULTURE

Who Eats More Fiber?

The food we choose affects our intake of fiber; thus we see differences in dietary fiber intake across various racial, ethnic, and income groups with differing food patterns. Hispanic Americans have the highest daily intakes of fiber (20 g) influenced by the fiber-rich beans in their usual meal pattern, followed by Asian Americans who take in 19 g, likely based on their frequent use of rice; whites average 17 g. African Americans take in the least fiber, only 15 g each day.[1] Family income influences fiber intake.[2] Among limited resource mothers and children participating in the Special Supplemental Nutrition Program for Women, Infants and Children (WIC), only 15% of Hispanic American mothers and 5.5% of African American mothers met the recommended intake of fiber. The children in these families were even less likely to meet their fiber recommendations (4.4% of Hispanic American children and 2% of African American children had their suggested intake).[2] Body weight is associated with fiber intake, as obese adults tend to have lower intakes of dietary fiber than overweight or normal weight adults.[3] Nutrition education focusing on appropriate fiber-rich foods that fit into customary and acceptable meal patterns, and the inclusion of high-fiber foods in food distribution programs could lower health risk in these groups.

NOTE: See Appendix E for more information on WIC.

Bibliography

1. US Department of Agriculture, Agricultural Research Service: Nutrient intakes from food and beverages. Mean amounts consumed per individual by race/ethnicity and age in the United States. *In What we eat in America,* NHANES 2013–2014, 2016, Table 2. http://www.ars.usda.gov/ba/bhnrc/fsrg.
2. Kong A, Odoms-Young AM, Schiffer LA, et al: Racial-ethnic differences in dietary intake among WIC families prior to food package revisions, *J Nutr Educ Behav* 45(1):39, 2013.
3. King DE, Mainous AG, Lambourne CA: Trends in dietary fiber intake in the United States, 1999-2008, *J Acad Nutr Diet* 112:642, 2012.

(8.8 g/1000 kcal vs. 7.9 g/1000 kcal). Whole grains account for nearly half of fiber intake (44%) among US adults, followed by vegetables (21%), fruit (13%), and legumes (10%).[25] The MyPlate (http://www.choosemyplate.gov) goal of 4½ cups of fruits and vegetables and three whole-grain servings per day within a 2000-kcal diet provides about 30 g of fiber.[5] (See the Focus on Culture box "Who Eats More Fiber?" to compare intakes among various racial, ethnic, and income groups.)

FUNCTIONAL FOODS: SPECIAL CARBOHYDRATE FOODS

Functional foods are foods believed to have a beneficial effect on health and well-being beyond basic nutrition and may reduce the risk of certain diseases or conditions. All foods are functional at some physiologic level, providing nutrients that furnish energy, build or repair tissues, or support metabolic processes. But functional foods move beyond these necessary roles to provide additional health benefits. In the United States there is no legal definition for "functional foods," so this term serves as a marketing rather than a regulatory term.[26] Nutrition experts hold differing views on the definition applied to functional foods. Some agencies include only those foods containing a naturally occurring bioactive substance that promotes health, whereas others apply this term to foods containing an added substance such as a vitamin or fiber.

The first foods designated as functional foods were carbohydrate foods. Fruits, vegetables, legumes, and grains contain tens of thousands of phytochemicals (from the Greek word *phyton*, meaning plant). Plants produce phytochemicals to protect themselves against bacteria and viruses, and when the plants are eaten, these substances are absorbed and act as protective factors for humans. Tomatoes were identified early on as a functional food because the lycopene they contain has been associated with reduced risk of prostate cancer.[27] (Lycopene is a carotenoid, which we will discuss in Chapter 6.) The concept of functional foods or ingredients also includes new roles for familiar nutrients. Certain polyunsaturated fatty acids appear to reduce cardiovascular risk in addition to their well-known roles in maintaining skin integrity and providing energy.

In our study of nutrition we will consider three categories of functional foods.[26]

1. Conventional or intact foods that contain biologically active food components, such as the probiotics in yogurt or the flavonoids in apples, oranges, red wine, and tea (See Table 3.7 for some examples of functional foods and their bioactive component.)
2. Modified foods to which a biologically active substance has been added, such as the addition of calcium to orange juice or polyunsaturated fatty acids to special margarines
3. Food ingredients that are synthesized, such as oligosaccharides and other indigestible carbohydrates that can act as prebiotics

At this time in the United States there is no specific regulation regarding the labeling or advertising associated with functional foods and their bioactive ingredients, although the FDA does allow health claims for foods for which there is an established body of evidence. We will learn more about label Health Claims in Chapter 9.

Currently there is ongoing discussion about the need for a dietary framework for phytochemicals, similar to the currently existing DRIs for known nutrients.[28] Unfortunately, the content of bioactive substances in particular foods is just being established, and the particular biochemical and physiological effects of these substances in the human body are not well-defined. Based on public interest in these plant substances, many are marketed as dietary supplements, apart from their original food source. Although population studies have associated

TABLE 3.7   Selected Functional Foods and Their Proposed Health Benefits

Functional Food	Active Component or Ingredient	Proposed Health Benefit
Whole-grain oats, barley, and psyllium	β-glucans, soluble fiber	Reduces risk of heart disease[a]
Salmon and other fatty fish	Omega-3 fatty acids	Beneficial effect on blood lipids; helps prevent unwanted blood clotting
Tomatoes	Lycopene	May lower risk of certain cancers
Fortified margarine	Plant sterols (added ingredient)	Beneficial effect on blood lipids; lowers risk of cardiovascular disease[a]
Fortified orange juice	Calcium and vitamin D	Helps meet daily requirement for calcium and vitamin D and lower risk of osteoporosis[a]
Bananas, oatmeal beans	Prebiotics	Promote health and function of the colon
Yogurt	Probiotics	Promote health and function of the colon
Apples, oranges, strawberries, tea, cocoa	Flavonoids (a family of phytochemicals)	Appears to lower risk of diabetes and cardiovascular disease

[a]Health claims approved by the Food and Drug Administration for addition to the food label.

intakes of phytochemicals with lower incidence of type 2 diabetes,[29] heart disease, and stroke,[30] it is difficult to separate a specific phytochemical from the foods in the diet that supply those compounds, suggesting that phytochemicals—like nutrients—work best in combination with one another. Accordingly, eating foods that contain a mixture of these components offers the best protection against chronic disease. Also, phytochemicals are found in foods in minute amounts, and not much is known about the safety of concentrated amounts as found in supplements. Phytochemicals and plant fibers are lost in food processing, so try to choose whole-grain breads and cereals, and eat fruits and vegetables with their skins or peel. For nutrients such as calcium or vitamin D, which can be difficult to obtain from conventional foods, the use of available fortified foods can help meet body needs.

DIGESTION-ABSORPTION-METABOLISM REVIEW

The digestion, absorption, and metabolism of carbohydrates were discussed in Chapter 2. The outline below provides a brief review.

Digestion

The conversion of starch and sugars to glucose begins in the mouth where salivary amylase (ptyalin) from the parotid gland acts on starch to begin its breakdown into dextrins and maltose. No specific enzyme in the stomach acts on carbohydrate; however, by the time the food mass is completely mixed with gastric acid, as much as 20% to 30% of the starch has been broken down to maltose. Enzymes that complete the chemical digestion of carbohydrate come from two sources, the pancreas and the small intestine, as follows:

• *Pancreatic secretions:* Pancreatic amylase entering the duodenum through the common bile duct completes the breakdown of starch to maltose.

• *Intestinal secretions:* Cells within the brush border of the small intestine secrete three disaccharidases, sucrase, lactase, and maltase, which act on their respective disaccharides to release the monosaccharides, glucose, galactose, and fructose (see Table 2.2).

Absorption and Metabolism

Glucose is absorbed by an active pumping system using sodium as a carrier. Of the total carbohydrate absorbed, 80% is in the form of glucose, and the remaining 20% is galactose and fructose.[31] Via the capillaries in the villi, the products of carbohydrate digestion enter the portal blood circulation en route to the liver. Here, fructose and galactose are converted to glucose. Glucose not needed for immediate energy is converted to glycogen or adipose tissue for storage.

KEY TERMS

Amylase
A digestive enzyme that breaks down starch; salivary amylase begins the digestion of starch in the mouth; pancreatic amylase enters the small intestine as part of the pancreatic secretions to continue starch breakdown in the duodenum.

Sucrase
Enzyme that splits the disaccharide sucrose, releasing the monosaccharides glucose and fructose.

Lactase
Enzyme that splits the disaccharide lactose, releasing the monosaccharides glucose and galactose.

Maltase
Enzyme that splits the disaccharide maltose, releasing two units of the monosaccharide glucose.

Portal
An entryway, usually referring to the portal circulation of blood that delivers absorbed nutrients from the small intestine to the liver.

TO SUM UP

Carbohydrates produced by plant photosynthesis supply most of the world's population with its primary source of energy. Fruits, vegetables, grains, legumes, and most milk products provide dietary carbohydrate. Simple carbohydrates—monosaccharides and disaccharides—are easily digested and provide quick energy. Starch, a digestible complex carbohydrate, requires increased breakdown to become available for use, but the final product in the digestion and conversion of both starches and sugars is glucose. Carbohydrates serve special functions through their ability to spare protein, prevent the buildup of ketones, and supply energy for the CNS. Fiber, the nondigestible carbohydrate found in the structural walls, hulls, seeds, leaves, and skins of fruits, vegetables, and whole grains, affects the digestion and absorption of food in ways that are beneficial to health. Carbohydrates should provide 45% to 65% of total kcalories. A healthy diet should emphasize foods containing complex carbohydrates and fiber, with a minimum of added sugar. Plant foods rich in phytochemicals or specific nutrients are referred to as *functional foods* if they contribute to health in ways beyond the actions of the known nutrients they contain.

QUESTIONS FOR REVIEW

1. For breakfast you had a piece of whole-grain bread with jelly, a banana, and a glass of low-fat milk. List both the digestible and the nondigestible forms of carbohydrate in this meal.

2. Based on the special roles of carbohydrate in the body, explain the mechanisms causing the physiologic and metabolic aberrations that result when the body is deprived of carbohydrate.

3. What is resistant starch and why is it called resistant? What are its health benefits?

4. Why would a glass of orange juice raise an individual's blood glucose more rapidly than a whole orange?

5. A mother tells you that her toddler seems to have chronic diarrhea. The mother has been giving her apple juice as an afternoon snack. What might be contributing to the gastrointestinal upset? What might be a better snack choice?

6. Using the materials on the MyPlate website (http://www.choose-myplate.gov) and the Nutritrac software found on the Evolve website, determine the daily energy need of a 25-year-old woman who is 5 ft 6 in tall, weighs 125 lb, and is relatively sedentary. How many grams of carbohydrate should be included in her diet, and how many kcalories should it supply? What is her upper limit for grams of added sugar? How much fiber does she need? Develop a 2-day menu that provides the appropriate amounts of carbohydrate and dietary fiber and does not exceed the limit for sugar.

7. Visit your local grocery store and find two fruit juices, two fruit drinks, and two sports drinks available in single-serving, easy-to-carry containers. Use the nutrition label to construct a table indicating the kcalories, total carbohydrate (g), and total sugar (g), per 8-oz. serving. Check the list of ingredients and indicate which products have added sugar. Do any of these items contain added ingredients to qualify as functional foods? Which are most appropriate for regular use? Which should be limited? Why?

8. Define *functional food*. Research one of the functional foods listed at the end of this question and determine the following: (a) What are the important phytochemicals or functional components? (b) What effects do these components have on the body? (c) What is an appropriate portion size? Choose one: tree nuts, blueberries, apples, rolled oats.

REFERENCES

1. Muthayya S, Sugimoto JD, Montgomery S, et al: An overview of global rice production, supply, trade, and consumption, *Ann NY Acad Sci* 1324:7, 2014.

2. US Department of Agriculture, Agricultural Research Service: *Nutrient Intakes from Food and Beverages: Energy Intakes: Percentages of Energy from Protein, Carbohydrate, Fat, and Alcohol, by Gender and Age in the United States. What We Eat in America, NHANES 2013-2014*, 2016. http://www.ars.usda.gov/nea/bhnrc/fsrg.

3. Latulippe ME, Skoog SM: Fructose malabsorption and intolerance: effects of fructose with and without simultaneous glucose ingestion, *Crit Rev Food Sci Nutr* 51(7):583, 2011.

4. Powell ES, Smith-Taillie LP, Popkin BM: Added sugars intake across the distribution of US children and adult consumers: 1977-2012, *J Acad Nutr Diet* 116:1543, 2016.

5. US Department of Health, Human Services and US Department of Agriculture: *2015-2020 Dietary Guidelines for Americans*, ed 8, December 2015.

6. Fitch C, Keim KS, Academy of Nutrition and Dietetics: Position of the Academy of Nutrition and Dietetics: use of nutritive and nonnutritive sweeteners, *J Acad Nutr Diet* 112:739, 2012.

7. Birt DF, Boylston T, Hendrich S, et al: Resistant starch: Promise for improving human health, *Adv Nutr* 4:587, 2013.

8. Marcason W: What is the FODMAP diet? *J Acad Nutr Diet* 112:1696, 2012.

9. Jones JM: Glycemic index. The state of the science, Part 1—The measure and its variability, *Nutr Today* 47(5):207, 2012.

10. Wolever TMS: Glycemic index. The measure and its variability—the true state of the science, *Nutr Today* 47(5):214, 2012.

11. Matthan NR, Ausman LM, Meng H, et al: Estimating the reliability of glycemic index values and potential sources of methodological and biological variability, *Am J Clin Nutr* 104:1004, 2016.

12. Chiu CJ, Liu S, Willett WC, et al: Informing food choices and health outcomes by use of the dietary glycemic index, *Nutr Rev* 69(4):231, 2011.

13. Van Horn L, Carson JA, Appel LJ, et al: Recommended dietary pattern to achieve adherence to the American Heart Association/American College of Cardiology (AHA/ACC) guidelines: A scientific statement from the American Heart Association, *Circulation* 134(22):e505, 2016.

14. Adolphus K, Lawton CL, Champ CL, et al: The effects of breakfast and breakfast composition on cognition in children and adolescents: A systematic review, *Adv Nutr* 7(3):S590, 2016.

15. Food and Nutrition Board, Institute of Medicine: *Dietary Reference Intakes for energy, carbohydrate, fiber, fat, fatty acids, cholesterol, protein, and amino acids, (macronutrients)*, Washington, DC, 2002, National Academies Press.

16. Sylvetsky AC, Rother KI: Trends in the consumption of low-calorie sweeteners, *Physiol Behav* 164(Pt B):446, 2016.

17. Academy of Nutrition and Dietetics: Practice Paper of the Academy of Nutrition and Dietetics: Oral health and nutrition, *J Acad Nutr Diet* 114(6):958, 2014. (Abstract); Full text available at http://www.eatrightpro.org.

18. Bazzano LA, Hu T, Reynolds K, et al: Effects of low-carbohydrate and low-fat diets: A randomized trial, *Ann Intern Med* 161(5):309, 2014.

19. Matarese LE, Pories WJ: Adult weight loss diets: Metabolic effects and outcomes, *Nutr Clin Pract* 29:759, 2014.

20. Frigolet ME, Ramos Barragán VE, Tamez González M: Low-carbohydrate diets: a matter of love or hate, *Ann Nutr Metab* 58:320, 2011.

21. Johnston BC, Kanters S, Bandayrel K, et al: Comparison of weight loss among named diet programs in overweight and obese adults. A meta-analysis, *JAMA* 312(9):923, 2014.

22. Dahl WJ, Stewart ML, Academy of Nutrition and Dietetics: Position of the Academy of Nutrition and Dietetics: Health implications of dietary fiber, *J Acad Nutr Diet* 115:1861, 2015.

23. Raynor HA, Looney SM, Steeves EA, et al: The effects of an energy density prescription on diet quality and weight loss: a pilot randomized controlled trial, *J Acad Nutr Diet* 112:1397, 2012.

24. US Department of Agriculture, Agricultural Research Service: Nutrient intakes from food and beverages: mean amounts consumed per individual by gender and age in the United States, *What We Eat in America*, NHANES 2013-2014, 2016. http://www.ars.usda.gov/nea/bhnrc/fsrg.

25. King DE, Mainous AG, Lambourne CA: Trends in dietary fiber intake in the United States, 1999-2008, *J Acad Nutr Diet* 112:642, 2012.

26. Crowe KM, Francis C, Academy of Nutrition and Dietetics: Position of the Academy of Nutrition and Dietetics: Functional foods, *J Acad Nutr Diet* 113:1096, 2013.

27. Wang Y, Jacobs EJ, Newton CC, et al: Lycopene, tomato products and prostate cancer-specific mortality among men diagnosed with nonmetastatic prostate cancer in the Cancer Prevention Study II Nutrition Cohort, *Int J Cancer* 138(12):2846, 2016.

28. Gaine PC, Balentine DA, Erdman JW Jr, et al: Are dietary bioactives ready for recommended intakes, *Adv Nutr* 4(5):539, 2013.

29. Jacques PF, Cassidy A, Rogers G, et al: Higher dietary flavonol intake is associated with lower incidence of type 2 diabetes, *J Nutr* 143(9):1474, 2013.

30. Jacques PF, Cassidy A, Rogers G, et al: Dietary flavonoid intakes and CVD incidence in the Framingham Offspring Cohort, *Br J Nutr* 114(9):1496, 2015.

31. Marsh MN, Riley SA: Digestion and absorption of nutrients and vitamins. In Feldman M, Scharschmidt BF, Sleisenger MH, editors: *Gastrointestinal and liver disease*, vol 2, ed 6, Philadelphia, 1998, Saunders.

FURTHER READINGS AND RESOURCES

Readings

Hauge DA, Melroe S, Maschoff B, et al: Whole grains in schools: A supply chain approach, *Nutr Today* 50(3):135, May/June 2015.

Hornick B, Birkett A, Liska DA: The fiber deficit, Part 3. Beyond traditional fiber sources: The role of adding fiber to food in improving fiber intakes, *Nutr Today* 48(4):168, 2013.

[These investigators offer suggestions on ways to increase the fiber intake in various age groups.]

Gardner C, Wylie-Rosett J, Gidding SS, et al, on behalf of the American Heart Association Nutrition Committee: Nonnutritive sweeteners: current use and health perspectives. A scientific statement from the American Heart Association and the American Diabetes Association, *Diabetes Care* 35:1798, 2012.

Hill JO: What do you say when your patients ask whether low-calorie sweeteners help with weight management? *Am J Clin Nutr* 100:739, 2014.

Park S, Thompson FE, McGuire LC, et al: Sociodemographic and behavioral factors associated with added sugars intake among US adults, *J Acad Nutr Diet* 116:1589, 2016.

[These papers address various issues related to excessive sugar consumption and how consumers might lower their sugar intakes.]

Websites of Interest

- American Heart Association: *Sugar 101.* This site describes the different types of carbohydrates, including food sources, suggested intakes, lesser-known whole grains, and label terms for added sugars. http://www.heart.org/HEARTORG/HealthyLiving/HealthyEating/Nutrition/Sugar-101_UCM_306024_Article.jsp#.WQeeWMeG-kg.

- International Food Information Council Foundation. This site provides information for both consumers and health professionals describing functional foods. http://www.ific.org/.

- Medline Plus: *US National Library of Medicine.* Provides guidance in many areas of health: source of patient handouts on fiber. https://medlineplus.gov/dietaryfiber.html.

- Produce for Better Health Foundation. This website promoting the Fruits & Veggies More Matters campaign offers games for children, recipes, and information on portion size, selection, safe handling, and cooking of fruits and vegetables. http://www.fruitsandveggies-morematters.org/.

- US Department of Agriculture, Center for Nutrition Policy and Promotion: *MyPlate.* This site offers information on meal planning, nutritional needs, and menus for different ages, genders, and activity levels that will supply the recommended amounts of fruits, vegetables, and whole grains. http://www.choosemyplate.gov/.

- US Department of Health and Human Services, US Department of Agriculture: *Dietary Guidelines for Americans 2015.* The *Dietary Guidelines* give guidance on increasing intakes of complex carbohydrates and decreasing intakes of sugar. http://www.cnpp.usda.gov/dietaryguidelines.htm.

4

Lipids

Eleanor D. Schlenker

Ⓔ http://evolve.elsevier.com/Williams/essentials/

Lipids or fats, as they are commonly called, are the second of the energy-yielding macronutrients and carry mixed messages for consumers. Although we hear that a high-fat diet promotes chronic disease, we also read about the health benefits of the Mediterranean diet, which is moderately high in fat. Fats add taste and a pleasant mouth feel to our food and contribute to our "feeling full." Fat is an essential nutrient for the fatty acids it contains and has an important role in absorption of the fat-soluble vitamins. Fat is energy-dense and in past years provided the needed kilocalories (kcalories or kcal) for strenuous physical labor. Today we must assess not only how much fat we consume but also what type, because different fats have different effects on our health. Fat is an important component of the total diet, and a low-fat diet is not necessarily nutritionally adequate. In our study of lipids we will learn why we need fat and how to include it in meal planning.

OUTLINE

LIPIDS IN NUTRITION AND HEALTH

Health Issues and Lipids

Lipids perform many essential functions in the body, but discussion continues as to the types and the amounts of fat that we should eat.[1-3] You need what you need, but more is not better. Health concerns related to dietary fat focus on two issues: (1) the high energy content of fat, and (2) the negative health effects of certain fatty acids. In general, polyunsaturated and monounsaturated fatty acids have positive effects on body function, whereas certain saturated fats and trans fats add to health risk.

Amount of Fat

Fat is energy dense, containing over twice as many kcalories per gram as protein or carbohydrate. Too much fat in the diet supplies more kcalories than may be required for immediate use, with the excess stored as adipose tissue. Over time such increases in body weight—or more precisely body fat—increase risk of chronic disease.

Type of Fat

Excessive amounts of saturated fats raise blood low-density lipoprotein (LDL)-cholesterol levels and promote atherosclerosis, the buildup of fatty deposits on the interior walls of the major arteries that add to risk of heart attack or stroke. Saturated fat is found primarily in animal sources, although some appear in plant oils.

Unsaturated fats, contained mostly in vegetable oils and fatty fish, can modify blood lipids to lower the risk of cardiovascular disease.[2] Trans fats produced in the commercial processing of lipids are injurious to health and best eliminated from the diet. It is important to help consumers recognize the different sources and types of fat as critical to their health.[4]

KEY TERMS

Lipids
Chemical group name for fats and fat-related compounds such as cholesterol, lipoproteins, and phospholipids.

Fatty Acids
The building blocks or structural components of fats.

Saturated
Term used for a substance that is united with the greatest possible number of other atoms or chemical groups. A fatty acid is saturated if all available chemical bonds on its carbon chain are filled with hydrogen. A fat is saturated if the majority of fatty acids making up its structure are saturated.

Adipose
Cells and tissues that store fat.

Functions of Lipids

Food Lipids

Dietary lipids, well chosen, not only support nutrition and health but also add to the joy of eating. The following are descriptions of these important characteristics:

- *Provide energy:* Lipids are a concentrated source of fuel to store and use as needed. Food lipids yield 9 kcal/g when oxidized by the body as compared with carbohydrates and protein, which yield only 4 kcal/g.
- *Supply essential fatty acids:* The essential fatty acids linoleic acid and α-linolenic acid must be obtained in food because they cannot be made by the body or made in the amounts needed.
- *Support absorption of the fat-soluble vitamins:* Lipid must be present in the food mix in the small intestine to provide a vehicle for absorption of the fat-soluble vitamins.
- *Add to food palatability:* Lipids add flavor and a pleasant mouth feel to food. Our food choices are strongly influenced by taste,[4] and textures from lipids enhance our sensory response.
- *Promote satiety:* A meal containing lipids satisfies the appetite for a longer period than a meal containing only carbohydrate and protein. Particular brain cells respond to the mouth feel of fat and influence the region of the brain controlling satiety. Fat contributes texture and body to a food mixture that slows its movements out of the stomach and helps prolong the feeling of fullness.[5]

Body Lipids

Lipids are stored in the body as adipose tissue. This tissue performs many essential tasks, as follows:

- *Storage source of energy:* Lipids are an efficient fuel for all tissues except the brain and central nervous system (CNS). In fact, fatty acids are the preferred fuel of the heart muscle.
- *Thermal insulation:* The layer of lipid deposited directly beneath the skin helps maintain body temperature.
- *Protection of vital organs:* A weblike padding of adipose tissue surrounds vital organs such as the kidneys, protecting them from mechanical shock and providing structural support.
- *Transmission of nerve impulses:* Lipid layers surrounding nerve fibers provide electrical insulation and transmit nerve impulses.
- *Formation of membranes:* Lipids are structural components of cell membranes and help transport nutrients, metabolites, and waste products in and out of cells.
- *Carrier of fat-soluble materials:* Lipids transport the fat-soluble vitamins A, D, E, and K to the cells for metabolic use. **Lipoproteins** carry lipids to and from the liver and on to body tissues.
- *Precursors of other substances:* Lipids supply fatty acids and cholesterol for the synthesis of various structural and metabolic compounds; brain tissue and the retina contain many fatty acids.

PHYSICAL AND CHEMICAL NATURE OF LIPIDS

Physical Characteristics

The chemical term *lipid* includes fats, oils, and related compounds that are insoluble in water and greasy to the touch. Some food lipids—butter, margarine, or cooking oil—are easily recognized as fats. Other foods that appear to be carbohydrates, such as bakery items or potato chips, often contain significant amounts of fat.

Chemical Characteristics

Lipids are **organic** compounds consisting of a carbon chain with hydrogen and oxygen atoms attached. Particular lipids may have other radicals or groups of elements attached. Fatty acids and their related compounds are the lipids important in human nutrition. Lipids have something in common with carbohydrates: the same chemical elements that make up carbohydrates—carbon, hydrogen, and oxygen—also make up fatty acids. However, carbohydrates and lipids have two important structural differences:

1. Lipids are more complex, with more carbon (C) and hydrogen (H) atoms and fewer oxygen (O) atoms.
2. The common structural units of lipids are fatty acids, whereas the common structural units of carbohydrates are simple sugars.

We will look first at the unique characteristics of fatty acids—their saturation, chain length, and essentiality—and then focus on the **triglycerides** built from fatty acids.

KEY TERMS

Lipoproteins
Complexes of fat with protein. The lipoproteins carry lipids in the plasma; this combination of fat surrounded by protein makes possible the transport of fatty substances in a water-based solution such as plasma.

Organic
Carbon compounds found in plants or animals

Triglycerides
Chemical name for fats that indicates the structure of three fatty acids attached to a glycerol base. Triglycerides are synthesized from excess dietary carbohydrate and fat and stored in adipose tissue; they release free fatty acids into the blood when needed for energy.

FATTY ACIDS AND TRIGLYCERIDES

Characteristics of Fatty Acids: Chain Length

A characteristic of fatty acids important in human nutrition is the length of their carbon chain. Fatty acids in foods range from 4 to 22 carbons (Box 4.1). Chain length affects intestinal absorption. Long-chain fatty acids are more difficult to absorb and require a helping carrier to enter the lymph and then the blood. Short- and medium-chain fatty acids are soluble in water and absorbed directly into the blood. When intestinal diseases injure the absorbing surface of the small intestine, a commercial product called *medium-chain triglyceride* (MCT) oil (made of short- and medium-chain fatty acids) can replace ordinary vegetable oil in food preparation.

Characteristics of Fatty Acids: Saturation

The saturation or unsaturation of a lipid governs its physical characteristics. Saturated fats are hard, less-saturated fats are soft, and unsaturated fats are liquid at room temperature (Box 4.2). These physical differences are based on the ratio of hydrogen atoms to carbon atoms in the fatty acids making up the lipid. If a fatty acid has a hydrogen atom attached at every available space, then it is completely saturated. If the fatty acid has some hydrogen spaces unfilled, then it is unsaturated. The following three terms are used to describe saturation in fats.

1. *Saturated:* Lipids composed mostly of saturated fatty acids are called *saturated fats.* Although saturated fatty acids are usually found in animal foods, the most saturated food fats are two oils

---

BOX 4.1   Chain Length of Fatty Acids

- Short-chain fatty acids have 4 to 6 carbon atoms.
- Medium-chain fatty acids have 8, 10, or 12 carbon atoms.
- Long-chain fatty acids have 14, 16, 18, or more carbon atoms.

BOX 4.2 Degrees of Saturation of Food Fats

Highly Saturated Fat (solid at room temperature)

Stick margarine

Butter

Beef fat

Less-Saturated Fat (very soft at room temperature)

Tub margarine

Squeeze margarine

Unsaturated Fat (liquid at room temperature)

Salad oil

Images copyright 2006 JupiterImages Corporation.

from plants: (1) coconut oil, which is 88% saturated, and (2) palm kernel oil, which is 80% saturated.[6] All other saturated fats are of animal origin as found in meat; butter; whole, reduced-fat, and low-fat milk; and other dairy products. (Note the degree of saturation of coconut oil, currently promoted in the popular press.)

2. *Monounsaturated:* Food lipids that have a high proportion of fatty acids with a pair of hydrogen atoms missing, creating one double bond, are called *monounsaturated fats.* These lipids are generally from plant sources. Canola oil (isolated from rapeseed) and olive oil are monounsaturated fats.

3. *Polyunsaturated:* When fatty acids have four or more spaces unfilled with hydrogen atoms, creating two or more double bonds, they are *polyunsaturated fats.* Many of these fats are from plant sources and include commonly used cooking oils such as corn oil and safflower oil. Polyunsaturated fatty acids with two or more double bonds are also classified according to the position in the carbon chain where the

first double bond appears. When the first double bond follows the third carbon atom, counting from the methyl end of the fatty acid, it is referred to as an omega (ω) 3 or *n-3* fatty acid. When the first double bond follows the sixth carbon atom in the chain, it is called an omega (ω) 6 or *n-6* fatty acid. Two important fatty acids in human metabolism are linoleic acid, an n-6 fatty acid, and α-linolenic acid, an n-3 fatty acid. These are referred to as essential fatty acids because the body cannot synthesize an n-3 or n-6 fatty acid. The n-3 fatty acids found in fatty fish have a role in cardiovascular health.[2]

Essential Fatty Acids

Two different fatty acids—linoleic acid (an n-6 fatty acid) and α-linolenic acid (an n-3 fatty acid)—are essential fatty acids for humans. Arachidonic acid, another fatty acid important in human nutrition, can be made from linoleic acid. Two n-3 fatty acids associated with cardiovascular health—(1) eicosapentaenoic acid (EPA) and (2) docosahexaenoic acid (DHA)—can be made from α-linolenic acid (Fig. 4.1), but these conversion rates are extremely slow[6] and influenced by age, gender, genetics, and overall dietary intake. Therefore individuals best obtain these acids from regular servings of fish.

KEY TERMS

Linoleic Acid

An essential fatty acid for humans; an n-6 polyunsaturated fatty acid.

α-Linolenic Acid

An essential fatty acid for humans; an n-3 polyunsaturated fatty acid.

Essential Fatty Acids

Fatty acids that must be supplied in the diet because the body cannot make them.

Eicosapentaenoic Acid (EPA)

An n-3 polyunsaturated fatty acid found in fish oil; it helps lower the risk of heart attack or stroke.

Docosahexaenoic Acid (DHA)

An n-3 polyunsaturated fatty acid found in fish oil; it is necessary for brain and neural development in infants and helps lower the risk of heart attack or stroke in adults.

Dietary Linoleic Acid (18:2n-6) → Arachidonic Acid (20:4n-6)

Dietary α-Linolenic Acid (18:3n-3) → Eicosapentaenoic Acid (20:5n-3) → Docosahexaenoic Acid (22:6n-3)

Prostaglandins
Widespread in many tissues

Control contraction of smooth muscle
Regulate blood pressure
Regulate secretion of gastric acid
Regulate body temperature
Regulate aggregation of blood platelets
Control inflammation and vascular permeability
Regulate immune function and resistance to harmful organisms

FIG. 4.1 Linoleic acid and α-linolenic acid (the essential fatty acids) are the starting points for synthesis of various other fatty acids and prostaglandins. Prostaglandins, a type of eicosanoid, help regulate many important body functions.

Linoleic acid and α-linolenic acid have the following physiologic roles[6,7]:

- *Skin integrity:* The essential fatty acids strengthen cell membranes and prevent a harmful increase in skin permeability. Essential fatty acid deficiency causes breakdown in skin tissue, with characteristic eczema and skin lesions.[7] Essential fatty acid deficiency seldom occurs other than in patients receiving a parenteral nutrition formula that does not include the essential fatty acids.
- *Regulation of lipid metabolism:* Polyunsaturated fatty acids can reduce blood lipid levels, particularly if they are replacing saturated fat in the diet.[8]
- *Growth:* Normal growth requires an adequate supply of the essential fatty acids, and growth is impaired in essential fatty acid deficiency; α-linolenic acid is especially important for the development of brain tissue before and after birth.[7]
- *Gene expression:* The essential fatty acids regulate the production of enzymes needed for synthesis of nonessential fatty acids.
- *Immune function:* Persons with essential fatty acid deficiency have an increased rate of infection.
- *Aggregation of blood platelets:* EPA and DHA, arising from α-linolenic acid, may prevent unwanted aggregations of blood platelets that block the flow of blood in major arteries, causing heart attack or stroke.[2]
- *Synthesis of hormone-like agents:* Essential fatty acids are precursors of a group of physiologically and pharmacologically active compounds known as *eicosanoids* (see Fig. 4.1). Prostaglandins, a type of eicosanoid, were first identified in human semen and thought to originate in the prostate gland. Prostaglandins exist in virtually all body tissues and act as local hormones to direct and coordinate biologic functions. They influence blood pressure, blood clotting, and cardiovascular function.

Dietary Reference Intakes

Adequate intakes (AIs) have been established for both linoleic and α-linolenic acids. (See Chapter 1 to review the various categories of the Dietary Reference Intakes [DRIs].) Between the ages of 19 and 50, the AI for linoleic acid (an n-6 fatty acid) is 17 g/day for men and 12 g/day for women; past the age of 50, these reference intakes decrease to 14 g/day for men and 11 g/day for women. The AI for α-linolenic acid (an n-3 fatty acid) is 1.6 g/day for all adult men and 1.1 g/day for all adult women.[7] These recommendations are based on the current median intakes of US adults who appear to be meeting their requirements for linoleic and α-linolenic fatty acids.[9] There are no specific DRI standards for EPA and DHA.

Increased intakes of polyunsaturated fatty acids with multiple double bonds also increase the need for antioxidants to prevent oxidation at double bond sites. We will study the role of vitamin E in preventing unwanted oxidation in Chapter 6.

Special Needs of Infants

Arachidonic acid and DHA play a critical role in the brain and neural development of infants; both are found in breast milk in liberal amounts. Commercial infant formula sold in the United States is fortified with arachidonic acid and DHA to the levels found in human milk. Clinical studies are continuing to assess the potential benefits of fish intake or DHA supplements during pregnancy on childhood health outcomes such as improved psychomotor development and problem-solving skills.[10] DHA supplements during pregnancy may lessen the occurrence of allergic diseases such as eczema and asthma in the offspring.[11]

Food Sources of Essential Fatty Acids

The best sources of the two essential fatty acids are vegetable oils. Corn oil, safflower oil, soybean oil, cottonseed oil, sunflower oil, and peanut oil are rich in linoleic acid (an n-6 acid). Alpha-linolenic acid (an n-3 acid) is found in flaxseed, soybean oil, and rapeseed oil (canola oil).[7] The *Dietary Guidelines for Americans* recommends that both children and adults consume two servings of fish per week to ensure an adequate supply of EPA and DHA.[12] (Box 4.3 lists food sources of important fatty acids.)

BOX 4.3   Food Sources of Fatty Acids Important to Health

Linoleic Acid: n-6 Fatty Acid (essential)

Safflower oil
Corn oil
Cottonseed oil
Soybean oil
Nuts
Wheat germ

α-Linolenic Acid: n-3 Fatty Acid (essential)

Soybean oil
Flaxseed oil

Canola oil
Walnuts
Wheat germ

Fatty Acids from Fish: n-3 Fatty Acids[a]

Eicosapentaenoic acid and docosahexaenoic acid

- Herring
- Mackerel
- Halibut
- Salmon
- Canned tuna

Images copyright 2006 JupiterImages Corporation.
[a]These fatty acids can be synthesized in only limited amounts so regular servings of fish are recommended.

Use of Fish Oil Supplements

Fish oil supplements, promoted in the popular press as an alternative to eating fish, should be used only with the supervision of a health care professional. Because EPA and DHA can excessively prolong bleeding time, persons taking anticoagulants including warfarin and aspirin should use such supplements with caution.[7]

Structure of Triglycerides

The body stores fatty acids in the form of triglycerides made from three fatty acids attached to a **glycerol** base. When glycerol is combined with one fatty acid, it is called a *monoglyceride;* with two fatty acids, it is a *diglyceride;* and with three fatty acids, it is termed a *triglyceride.* **Glycerides** are found in food and also formed in the body. Most natural lipids from animal or plant sources are triglycerides. Triglycerides serve multiple functions throughout the body. They appear in body cells as oily droplets and circulate in the blood in the form of lipoproteins.

> ## KEY TERMS
>
> **Prostaglandins**
> One of a group of naturally occurring substances called eicosanoids derived from long-chain fatty acids; they have multiple local hormone-like actions including regulation of gastric acid secretion, blood platelet aggregation, body temperature, and tissue inflammation.
>
> **Glycerol**
> An alcohol that is esterified with fatty acids to produce triglycerides and released when fats are hydrolyzed.
>
> **Glycerides**
> Group name for fats formed from glycerol by the replacement of one, two, or three hydroxyl (–OH) groups with a fatty acid. Monoglycerides contain one fatty acid, diglycerides contain two fatty acids, and triglycerides contain three fatty acids. Glycerides are found in animal and plant fats and oils and stored in the adipose tissue.

FOOD LIPIDS AND HEALTH

Degree of Saturation

Food lipids contain a mixture of both saturated and unsaturated fats. Animal sources—meat, milk, and eggs—contain more saturated fats, whereas plant sources, primarily vegetable oils, are more unsaturated. The spectrum of food fats (from highly saturated to unsaturated) is illustrated in Fig. 4.2. In general, saturated fats are solid at room temperature, and the unsaturated plant lipids are free-flowing oils even at

TABLE 4.1 Effects of Fatty Acid Saturation on Blood Lipids

Degree of Saturation	Number of Double Bonds	Physiologic Effects
Saturated fats	None	Raises blood levels of total cholesterol and LDL-cholesterol
Monounsaturated fats	One	Decreases blood levels of total cholesterol and LDL-cholesterol when substituted for saturated fat.
Polyunsaturated fats (includes the essential fatty acids and fish oils)	Two or more	Decreases blood levels of total cholesterol and LDL-cholesterol when substituted for saturated fat. Discourages blood platelet aggregation decreasing risk of unwanted clots
Trans fats	One	Raises blood levels of total cholesterol and LDL-cholesterol Decreases blood levels of HDL-cholesterol

HDL, High-density lipoprotein; *LDL,* low-density lipoprotein.
Data from Holligan SD, Berryman CE, Wang L, et al: Atherosclerotic cardiovascular disease. In Erdman JW Jr, Macdonald IA, Zeisel SH, editors: *Present knowledge in nutrition,* ed 10, Ames, IA, 2012, International Life Sciences Institute/Wiley-Blackwell.

low temperatures; however, the exceptions to this usual pattern are important to human health. Coconut oil and palm kernel oil, highly saturated vegetable fats, are used extensively in nondairy creamers and baked goods because they are relatively inexpensive.

The number of double bonds in a fatty acid influences its actions in the body. Certain saturated fats increase cardiovascular risk if eaten in large amounts, although fats with one double bond or more have the opposite effect (Table 4.1). Monounsaturated fatty acids are associated with the health-promoting effects of the Mediterranean diet, a plant-based eating pattern rich in legumes, grains, seeds, and olive oil. Polyunsaturated fats with two or more double bonds include the essential fatty acids and fish oils. Despite the positive effects of unsaturated fats, moderation should be the key.[2,8,12,13]

Cis versus *Trans* Fatty Acids

To meet the demand for solid fats for use as table fats or food ingredients, the process of **hydrogenation** was developed. When unsaturated oils are surrounded with hydrogen gas, hydrogen ions attach at available sites, producing a more saturated (or solid) fat. This process turns

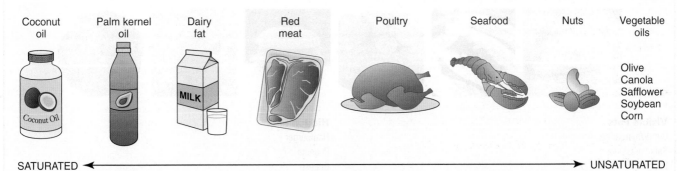

FIG. 4.2 Spectrum of food fats according to degree of saturation. Note that the two food fats with the highest degree of saturation are plant fats, followed by various animal fats in decreasing order of saturation. In general, plant fats are less saturated.

#3

unsaturated vegetable oils into margarine or vegetable shortenings; however, a particular type of unsaturated fatty acid that is formed in this process, a *trans* fatty acid, is extremely detrimental to health.

In Fig. 4.3 we compare the two possible structures of an unsaturated fatty acid. When double bonds occur in nature, the fatty acid chain bends in such a way that both parts are on the same side of the bond. In this case, the fatty acid is called a *cis* fatty acid, meaning same side. Fatty acids

FIG. 4.3 The *cis* and *trans* forms of a fatty acid.

in vegetable oils are in the cis form. However, when oils are partially hydrogenated, the normal bend can change with the two structural parts on opposite sides of the bend. This form is called a trans fatty acid, meaning on the opposite side. Commercially hydrogenated lipids used in soft margarine and other food products often contain trans fatty acids.

Trans fatty acids have been implicated in the development of coronary artery disease, as they raise LDL-cholesterol levels[8] and disrupt essential fatty acid functions in cells (see Table 4.1).[7] In 2006 it became mandatory to add trans fatty acid content to the nutrition label, and since then both food industry and government agencies have worked to reduce the trans fat content in processed food. Prior to the 2006 mandate even young children were consuming significant amounts of trans fats (the goal is 0 g/day). Mean intake in children ages 3 to 5 was 5 g/day, and teenage boys consumed almost 8 g. Men took in 7 g and women about 5 g. Items contributing the greatest proportions of trans fats were cakes, cookies, and pastries, followed by yeast breads, French fries, ethnic dishes, and tortilla chips.[14] In recent years average intake has dropped to 1.3 g/day, although many individuals exceed this level.[15] Based on efforts of public health departments and health professionals, many fast-food restaurants and food manufacturers have voluntarily reduced their use of partially hydrogenated fats containing trans fatty acids. A recent evaluation revealed that fast-food French fries, formerly high in trans fats, now have almost undetectable levels.[16]

The nutrition label guides a consumer's intake of fat. It provides the grams per serving of total fat, saturated fat, and trans fat, although confusion about portion size can add to intake. As for trans fats, it is important to recognize the difference between none or zero trans fats. None means there are no trans fats present. Conversely, a label can list content as zero *if* the amount of trans fat per serving is 0.5 g or less. Eating several servings of such items would add a significant amount of trans fat to the diet. Fats such as coconut oil and palm kernel oil can be found in the list of ingredients on the food label and be identified as sources of saturated fat. Although we should encourage avoidance of trans fats and saturated fats, it is still important to recognize that a food is not necessarily healthy just because it contains no such fats. Such a food may be high in kcalories, total fat, and sugar, and best eaten in limited amounts.

Visible and Hidden Fat

Fat enters the diet in many different forms and foods. Fats are quite visible in butter, margarine, vegetable oil, salad dressing, bacon, and similar added fats; however, less obvious are the fats in milk (unless it is nonfat), egg yolk, cheese, nuts, seeds, and olives, often referred to as *hidden fats*. Other major sources of hidden fats are bakery items, including cake, cookies, crackers, and muffins, or frozen entrees such as baked lasagna (Box 4.4). Meat and

BOX 4.4   Visible and Hidden Fats in Food

Visible Fats	Hidden Fats
Butter/margarine	Hamburger
Salad dressings	Peanuts
Bacon	Cheese
Fat attached to meat	Potato chips
	Chocolate chip cookie

Images copyright 2006 JupiterImages Corporation.

poultry have both visible and hidden fat. Even when visible fat has been trimmed away or the skin removed, the remaining portion still contains some fat. Red meat, especially beef, is marbled with tiny fat deposits within the muscle tissue. When evaluating the nutrient intake of a cultural or ethnic group different from your own, it is important to consider potential sources of hidden fat added in food preparation (see the Focus on Culture box, "Sources of Fat in the Diets of Culturally Diverse Groups").

Acceptable Macronutrient Distribution Range

The Acceptable Macronutrient Distribution Range (AMDR) for fat is 20% to 35% of total kcalories.[7] This range allows appropriate intake of the essential fatty acids and fat-containing foods that are rich sources of other important nutrients, yet controls kcalories. The lower end of the range helps with weight management or weight loss, whereas the upper level will promote weight gain in underweight individuals or ensure sufficient kcalories for an active lifestyle or rapid growth. Fat intakes falling below 10% of total kcalories may not supply needed amounts of essential fatty acids.[7]

Appropriate Intakes of Fat and Carbohydrate

The AMDRs for fat (20% to 35% of total kcalories) and carbohydrate (45% to 65% of total kcalories) set a balance between these two energy sources. Popular low-carbohydrate weight loss regimens often replace carbohydrate with fat and protein to the extent that fat supplies as much as 55% to 65% of total kcalories.[17] It is important that patients with type 2 diabetes not exceed appropriate levels of dietary fat in an effort to lower their intakes of carbohydrates. On the other hand, when fat falls below 20% of total kcalories, carbohydrate and protein levels rise disproportionately.

LIPID-RELATED COMPOUNDS

Cholesterol

Structure

Although cholesterol is not a fat or a triglyceride, it is often associated with dietary lipids. Cholesterol belongs to a family of substances called steroids and travels in the blood attached to long-chain fatty acids. People sometimes confuse cholesterol with saturated fat because both substances are believed to promote atherosclerosis.

Functions

Cholesterol is required for normal body function and synthesized in the liver. If a person obtained no cholesterol whatsoever from food, the body would still have an adequate supply. Cholesterol has broad roles, as follows:

- *Precursor to steroid hormones:* A cholesterol compound in the skin, 7-dehydrocholesterol, is converted to vitamin D when the ultraviolet rays of the sun pass into the skin; cholesterol is also a precursor of estrogen and testosterone.
- *Formation of bile acids:* Cholesterol is used to form bile acids, which emulsify fats and facilitate their digestion; bile acids serve as carriers in fat absorption.
- *Component of brain and neural tissue:* The brain and nerves include cholesterol in their structure.
- *Component of cell membranes:* Cell membranes contain cholesterol.

Food Sources

Cholesterol is found in animal foods but not plant foods. Egg yolk; meat; whole, reduced-fat, and low-fat milk; cheese; and organ meats supply cholesterol. Animal fats (but *not* plant fats) are rich sources.

🌐 FOCUS ON CULTURE

Sources of Fat in the Diets of Culturally Diverse Groups

As our nation becomes increasingly diverse, health professionals need to become familiar with foods that may be different from their own. Traditional foods and dishes can be rich sources of fat, including saturated fat; thus it is important to determine both the content and frequency of use of these ingredients. The following are some strategies to help you get started:

Compile a list of food items common to your target group. The list of typical foods eaten by an East Indian or Chinese or Latino family who recently emigrated to the United States will be very different from a list of foods used by those who have come to adopt more typical American patterns. Even among lifelong residents, racial and ethnic differences may exist as to favorite protein or vegetable choices. Be sure that you can identify each of the foods and the name by which they are recognized. Consult the US Department of Agriculture (USDA) nutrient database to calculate the nutrient content of mixed food dishes or items unfamiliar to you.

Talk with those who do the cooking about the types of food they prepare for their families. Collect recipes to be sure that you understand what grains, fruits, vegetables, meats, and fats are included in each dish. Check to see what ingredients are available in local shops or what substitutions homemakers could possibly make in their native dishes. Be sure to talk with both younger and older homemakers. Older families are more likely to retain traditional food patterns, whereas younger homemakers are more likely to adopt store-bought items used by those around them.

Special problems with fats. Based on the high energy density of fat and its association with chronic disease, we need to obtain good estimates of the types and amounts of fat eaten regularly. Food preparation methods strongly influence fat intake and require particular attention. It is important to determine use of meat, chicken, fish, game meats, or wild birds, if the skin from poultry and birds is eaten, and if these foods are fried or prepared with added fat. An example of the influence of cooking method on fat intake comes from a food survey of Southeast Asian and Chinese families who emigrated to North America. The Southeast Asian families obtained about 40% of their kcalories from fat, with much of it coming from oil-based curry sauces, whereas the Chinese families took in only 34% of their kcalories as fat; yet both added about the same amount of oil to their stir-fry mixtures. When the researchers joined the families for meal preparation, they found their answer. With the stir-fried foods of the Chinese families, much of the fat remained in the pan when the food was served and was later discarded; with the oil-based curry sauces of the Southeast Asian families most of the sauce was eaten along with the other ingredients, adding appreciably to the intake of fat. It may be helpful to visit a family at mealtime to fully appreciate their food habits and sources of added fat.

Bibliography

Bilyk HT: Role of registered dietitian nutritionists in the research and promotion of native and cultural foods, *J Acad Nutr Diet* 115(Suppl 1):S31, 2015.

Kelemen LE, Anand SS, Vuksan V, et al: Development and evaluation of cultural food frequency questionnaires for South Asians, Chinese, and Europeans in North America, *J Am Diet Assoc* 103:1178, 2003.

Suggested Cholesterol Intake

Because the body can synthesize cholesterol as needed, no DRI is necessary. People are encouraged to limit their intake, keeping in mind that eliminating cholesterol entirely would also eliminate meat, eggs, and some dairy products that provide vitamins and minerals important to health. In previous years it was recommended that dietary cholesterol be held to 300 mg/day or less, an intake associated with appropriate blood cholesterol levels. However, the Dietary Guidelines for Americans released in 2015 did not include a goal for cholesterol, noting that an eating pattern consistent with recommended levels of saturated fat would include no more than 100 to 300 mg of cholesterol.[12] In recent years genetic selection has successfully lowered the cholesterol content of eggs and meat; nevertheless, daily intake averages about 348 mg in men and 242 mg in women.[9] Certain plant sterols interfere with the absorption of cholesterol and help lower blood cholesterol levels. (See the Evidence-Based Practice box, "Plant Sterols: Lowering Blood Cholesterol Levels.")

Lipoproteins

Function

The liver is the body's clearinghouse for fatty acids and cholesterol, whether supplied in food or produced in body tissues. When processed by the liver, fatty acids and cholesterol are packaged into lipoproteins and released into the circulation for transport to cells.

Lipid Transport

Lipids are insoluble in water, which poses a problem when they need to be carried in a water-based circulatory system. The body solves this problem by producing lipoproteins, a complex of lipids and lipid-like substances surrounded by water-soluble protein. Special compounds called phospholipids are important in the structure of lipoproteins. Phospholipids are molecules in which one of the three fatty acids attached to a glycerol base is replaced with a phosphate (PO_4^{3-}) group that is water soluble and assists in the transport of lipoproteins. Phospholipids in cell membranes help lipid molecules move from the circulatory system into the cell.

KEY TERMS

Cholesterol
A fat-related compound; a sterol that is normally found in bile and is a principal constituent of gallstones. Cholesterol can be synthesized by the liver and therefore must not be supplied in food; it is a precursor of various steroid hormones and a component of neural tissue and membranes. It is carried in the blood as part of a lipoprotein complex.

Bile
A fluid secreted by the liver and transported to the gallbladder for concentration and storage. It is released into the duodenum on entry of fat and acts as an emulsifier to facilitate fat digestion and assist in fat absorption.

Complex
A chemical compound consisting of several atoms or molecules loosely connected and easily separated. The micelles formed in the lumen of the intestine, which carry fats into the intestinal wall, are bile-lipid complexes.

Phospholipids
A class of fat-related substances that contain a phosphate group and fatty acids. The phospholipids are important components of cell membranes, nerve tissues, and lipoproteins.

EVIDENCE-BASED PRACTICE

Plant Sterols: Lowering Blood Cholesterol Levels

Identify the problem: Plant sterols and stanols, also known as *phytosterols* or *phytostanols,* are found in small amounts in vegetable oils and grains such as corn, rye, and wheat. The chemical structure of plant sterols is much like that of cholesterol; based on this similarity, plant sterols compete with cholesterol for absorption in the small intestine. Nutrition researchers speculated that plant sterols in the digestive food mix would lower the amount of cholesterol absorbed and delivered to the liver. When less cholesterol is available, the liver produces fewer lipoproteins, and blood levels of total cholesterol and LDL-cholesterol decline. Unfortunately, plant sterols occur naturally in food in very small amounts, too small to make a difference in cholesterol absorption. Food technologists have since found ways to incorporate plant sterols into food products to increase dietary intake. Table fats, yogurt, orange juice, grain foods, and cereal bars with added plant sterols are examples of new functional foods.

Review the evidence: Clinical trials with patients having elevated blood cholesterol levels demonstrated the benefits of plant sterols in reducing cardiovascular risk. A daily intake of 2 g of plant sterols/stanols consumed as part of a fortified food or as a dietary supplement lowers LDL-cholesterol levels by 8% to 10%, and long-term studies have not revealed any adverse effects on health.[1] Based on this evidence, the US Food and Drug Administration (FDA) approved a food label health claim for sterol/stanol-containing foods, noting that regular use along with a diet low in saturated fat and cholesterol may reduce the risk of heart disease.[2]

Implement the findings: In order for phytosterols to be effective in helping lower blood LDL-cholesterol levels, they must be eaten regularly. If daily intake is less than the recommended 2 g, the effect will decrease proportionately.

Sterol-fortified foods should be eaten with a meal to effectively stimulate digestive secretions.[3] Importantly, to control kcalorie intake, foods with added sterols must *replace,* not be eaten *in addition to,* the conventional item in the daily meal pattern. An 8-oz serving of orange juice containing 1 g of plant sterols provides 110 kcal but meets the MyPlate (http://www.choose-myplate.gov) equivalent of one serving of fruit. Additional fruit servings, however, are best selected from whole fruits that also supply fiber. Table spreads containing about 0.7 g of plant sterols per tablespoon (1 tbsp being the recommended serving size) add 70 kcal and 8 g of fat per serving. Sterol-containing products advertised as "light" spreads usually contain about 50 kcal/tbsp and 5 g of fat. Overall, it appears that sterol-fortified foods are more effective if delivered in combination with monounsaturated and polyunsaturated fatty acids.[4] Plant sterols can assist in achieving appropriate serum cholesterol levels if used alone or in combination with other lipid-lowering strategies.

References

1. Gylling H, Plat J, Turley S, et al: Plant sterols and plant stanols in the management of dyslipidaemia and prevention of cardiovascular disease, *Atherosclerosis* 232(2):346, 2014.
2. US Food and Drug Administration: *Guidance for industry: A food labeling guide,* Rockville, MD, 2013, US Department of Health and Human Services. http://www.fda.gov/Food/IngredientsPackagingLabeling/LabelingNutrition/default.htm.
3. Rosin S, Ojansivu I, Kopu A, et al: Optimal use of plant stanol ester in the management of hypercholesterolemia, *Cholesterol* 2015:706970, 2015.
4. Cusack LK, Fernandez ML, Volek JS: The food matrix and sterol characteristics affect the plasma cholesterol lowering of phytosterol/phytostanol, *Adv Nutr* 4(6):633, 2013.

Lipoproteins contain fatty acids, triglycerides, cholesterol, phospholipids, and traces of fat-soluble vitamins and steroid hormones. They serve as the major vehicle for lipid transport in the blood.

Classes of Lipoproteins

Lipoproteins are classified according to their density, as determined by their relative content of lipid and protein. The more protein present, the greater the density. The amount of each lipoprotein in the blood is influenced by the time since the last meal and the quantity and type of fat that a person consumes on a regular basis. The five lipoprotein classes are as follows:

1. *Chylomicrons:* These relatively large particles are formed in the intestinal wall after a meal and carry the digested and absorbed fat to the liver for conversion to other lipoproteins.
2. *Very low-density lipoproteins (VLDLs):* The VLDLs are formed in the liver during the fasting interval between meals. When there is no food in the digestive tract and chylomicrons are not entering the circulatory system, VLDLs transport endogenous triglycerides from the liver to tissue cells.
3. *Intermediate-density lipoproteins (IDLs):* IDLs are formed from VLDLs and continue the delivery of endogenous triglycerides to the cells.
4. *Low-density lipoproteins (LDLs):* LDLs are formed from VLDLs and IDLs and carry mainly cholesterol, as most of the triglyceride has already been moved into cells.
5. *High-density lipoproteins (HDLs):* HDLs return cholesterol from the cells to the liver for breakdown and excretion.

Cholesterol, Lipoproteins, and Cardiovascular Risk

The two classes of lipoproteins receiving the most attention in clinical practice are the LDLs and HDLs. Both are primary carriers of cholesterol; thus their levels in the blood have important implications for health. The LDLs transport cholesterol from the liver to the tissues; in fact, about half of the cholesterol circulating in the blood is contained in the LDLs.[18] Conversely, the HDLs return cholesterol from the cells to the liver for excretion. Elevated blood cholesterol in the form of LDL-cholesterol promotes atherosclerosis, the underlying pathologic condition in coronary heart disease. High LDL-cholesterol levels cause a buildup of fatty plaque on the inner walls of the vessels that supply blood to the heart muscle. Over time, these plaques narrow the lumen of the coronary arteries, decreasing delivery of both oxygen and other nutrients. Interruption of blood to the heart, as a result of a blood clot or built-up plaque, causes a heart attack; a similar occurrence in an artery in the brain results in a stroke (cerebral hemorrhage). In contrast to LDLs, high HDLs slow or prevent the progression of atherosclerosis, lowering cardiovascular risk.

Although both the types and amounts of dietary fat affect LDL-cholesterol and HDL-cholesterol levels, it is not that simple. Some people absorb cholesterol more efficiently or synthesize increased

amounts, regardless of dietary intake. Dietary fat rather than dietary cholesterol may play a role in cholesterol synthesis. Genetic factors affect the production of HDL-cholesterol and the rate at which cholesterol is eliminated from the body.[18] In Chapter 21 we will learn about dietary and lifestyle interventions and medications to help control blood lipoprotein levels.

HEALTH PROMOTION

Lowering Fat Intake

Despite public health campaigns directed toward lowering dietary fat, fat intake as a proportion of total energy has remained at 33% to 34% over the past decade,[19] although fat intake is slightly higher among persons above age 60.[20] Fat intake differs according to gender; men consume about 95 g and women consume about 72 g each day, based on differences in total energy intake.[9] Fat intake also differs by race and ethnicity. Hispanics take in more of their kcalories from fat as compared to white and African Americans. Asians consume the least amount of dietary fat based on percentage of kcalories (32%) and total intake (65 g/day compared with 83–86 g/day in other groups).[21,22]

Fast food adds to intakes of both fat and kcalories. Consumers took in an additional 150 to 200 kcalories on days that included a meal at a quick-service restaurant, and that meal provided 40% of their fat kcalories for the day.[23]

Dietary fat can be lowered in various ways. Attempting to eliminate all foods high in fat not only lessens intakes of many important nutrients, such as iron, zinc, vitamin E, and essential fatty acids, but also is unlikely to be sustained over time. Eating a mix of higher-fat and modified-fat or lower-fat foods effectively lowers dietary fat while maintaining appropriate levels of nutrients contained in higher-fat foods. Including one higher-fat food at mealtime adds to satiety and helps curb the urge to overeat. Limiting portion size is another effective way to reduce both fat and kcalories. A balance of both higher-fat and lower-fat foods is the best strategy for overall good health. (See the Perspectives in Practice box, "Lowering Your Fat Intake," for more ideas on moderating your intake of fats.)

Fat Replacers

Fats serve many functions in food recipes and food preparation. In cooking and baking, fats absorb flavors from various ingredients and help blend them throughout the food. Fats also assist in the heat transfer necessary for browning or crispiness; create a velvety mouth feel in foods such as ice cream, pudding, and cheese; and play a critical role in frying. Fat replacers are ingredients that fulfill these functions but are lower in kcalories. Fruit purees made from apples or prunes are often used in home baking as fat replacers in cookies and moist cakes. Other fat replacers used as thickeners and emulsifiers have been developed for use in processed foods.

Most fat replacers are carbohydrates—plant polysaccharides, celluloses, or gums—although protein and fat may provide structure. Several fat replacers have been approved by the FDA for use in the United States. Fat replacers can contribute between 0 and 9 kcal/g, but can be used in smaller amounts than food fats that contain 9 kcal/g.[24] Also, fat replacers are often poorly digested or absorbed, lowering available kcalories. Unfortunately, the general public often assumes that baked goods, frozen desserts, and salad dressings made with fat replacers are lower in kcalories, but this is not always true. In fact, a food containing a fat replacer may contain the same number of kcalories or even more kcalories than its higher-fat counterpart if more

---

KEY TERMS

Chylomicrons
Lipoproteins formed in the intestinal wall after a meal that carry food fats into the lymph and then the general circulation for transport to the liver.

Endogenous
Originating from within the body; an example is endogenous cholesterol, which is produced by cells in the liver.

Lowering Your Fat Intake

Consumers need practical suggestions on how to control their intake of fats, especially unhealthy fats. Encourage small changes that once begun will be continued. Even one change at a time can add up to measurable differences over weeks and months.

The following are some ways to begin:

1. Reduce the fat you add to other foods.
   - Use less butter or margarine on your toast.
   - Be stingy when adding salad dressing.
2. Reduce portion size.
   - Order the small rather than the "super size" portion of French fries.
3. Eat a favorite high-fat food less often.
   - Have ice cream as a snack or dessert on fewer days of the week; choose fresh fruit on other days.
4. Choose a lower-fat version of a food you eat regularly.
   - Use reduced-fat, low-fat, or fat-free milk in place of whole milk. (Gradually reduce the amount of fat until you reach low-fat or fat-free.)
   - Choose a grilled chicken breast without skin rather than a fried chicken breast with skin.
   - Trim all visible fat from meats.
5. Substitute modified foods lower in fat.
   - Look for reduced-fat mayonnaise and salad dressings. (Be sure to check the kcalorie content.)
6. Eliminate fat when preparing foods.
   - Eat raw carrots without added salad dressing or broccoli with nonfat yogurt dip rather than butter or margarine.
   - Season cooked vegetables with lemon juice, orange juice, or low-sodium chicken broth rather than margarine or butter.

sugar has been added to maintain flavor and mouth feel. People who presume they can eat a larger portion of an item made with a fat replacer may be taking in even more kcalories than they would with a smaller portion of the higher-fat item. Better to select snacks from fruit, whole grains, or reduced-fat or fat-free dairy foods, which are not only lower in fat but also rich in nutrients.

DIGESTION-ABSORPTION-METABOLISM REVIEW

Chapter 2 provided an overview of digestion and absorption. A summary of chemical digestion and the absorption process specific to lipids is given here for review.

Digestion

Triglycerides in animal and plant foods must be broken down into individual fatty acids for absorption and body use.

Mouth

Lingual lipase in the salivary secretions begins the process of lipid digestion, although its action is limited.

Stomach

The gastric enzyme specific to lipids is gastric lipase (tributyrinase), which acts on emulsified butterfat. As gastric secretions act on carbohydrates and proteins in the food mix, the lipids begin to separate out, making them more accessible to their own enzymes in the small intestine.

Small Intestine

The major breakdown of lipids begins here. Digestive secretions come from three sources: (1) the biliary tract, (2) the pancreas, and (3) the small intestine, as follows:

1. *Bile from the liver and gallbladder:* The presence of fat in the upper duodenum triggers the release of cholecystokinin (CCK) from the intestinal mucosa, which in turn causes the gallbladder to contract, releasing a flow of bile. Bile acts as an emulsifier, preparing lipids for further digestion by (1) breaking them into smaller particles, thereby increasing the surface area accessible to enzyme action; and (2) lowering the surface tension of the finely dispersed globules, enabling enzymes to penetrate more easily. Bile also provides the alkaline medium needed for the action of pancreatic lipase. If bile secretion is hindered, as much as 40% of dietary fat is lost in the feces.
2. *Enzymes from the pancreas:* Pancreatic lipase breaks off one fatty acid at a time from the glycerol base of triglycerides. The initial action yields one fatty acid plus a diglyceride, and continuing action yields another fatty acid plus a monoglyceride. Each successive step becomes more difficult, with the result that less than one-third of the fat in the food mass is broken down completely. The final products of lipid digestion ready to be absorbed are fatty acids, diglycerides, monoglycerides, and glycerol.
3. *Enzyme from the small intestine:* Lecithinase acts on lecithin, a phospholipid, to prepare it for absorption.

Table 4.2 summarizes lipid digestion.

Absorption

The task of transporting lipids from the small intestine into the bloodstream takes place in three stages.

Stage I: Initial Lipid Absorption

In the small intestine, bile salts combine with the products of lipid digestion to form micelles, a bile-lipid complex. This carrier system (described in Fig. 4.4) moves the lipid molecules from the lumen of the intestine into the intestinal wall.

TABLE 4.2 Summary of Lipid Digestion

Location	Enzyme	Activity
Mouth	Lingual lipase (very limited)	Mechanical, mastication
Stomach	No major enzyme	Mechanical separation of fats as protein and starch are digested and go into solution
	Small amount of gastric lipase (tributyrinase)	Butterfat (tributyrin) to fatty acids and glycerol
Small intestine	Bile salts from gallbladder	Emulsifies fats
	Pancreatic lipase	Triglycerides to diglycerides and monoglycerides in turn; then fatty acids and glycerol
	Lecithinase	Acts on lecithin, a phospholipid, to prepare it for absorption

FIG. 4.4 A micelle complex of fats and bile salts ready for transport into the intestinal wall. The fatty acid in the *2* position of the triglyceride is the most difficult to remove, and some fat is absorbed in this monoglyceride form.

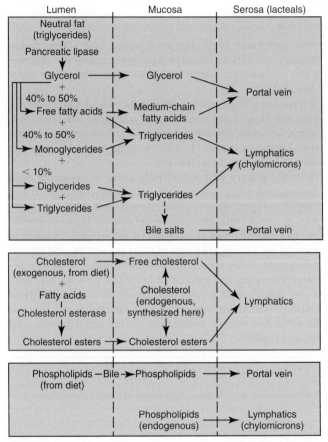

FIG. 4.5 Absorption of fat, cholesterol, and phospholipids. Note that a large proportion of dietary triglycerides are not completely broken down to fatty acids and glycerol before they combine with bile salts to form the micelle; digestion is completed by the lipase enzyme in the lining of the intestine.

Stage II: Absorption Within the Intestinal Wall

Once inside the wall of the small intestine, the bile salts separate from the lipid complex. They are absorbed into the blood and return to the liver via the enterohepatic circulation, ready to carry out their task again. When the lipid products are released from the micellar complex, the following actions take place (Fig. 4.5):

1. *Direct absorption of short- and medium-chain fatty acids:* Fatty acids with a chain length of 12 or fewer carbon atoms are absorbed directly into the **portal** blood. As noted earlier, MCT mixtures are helpful with persons who have problems with fat digestion and absorption.
2. *Enteric lipase digestion:* A lipase within the intestinal wall completes the digestion of the remaining diglycerides and monoglycerides, releasing fatty acids and glycerol.
3. *Triglyceride synthesis:* All longer-chain fatty acids and glycerol form new human triglycerides, ready for absorption and transport via the lymph.

KEY TERMS

Lipase
Group of digestive enzymes that break down triglycerides to fatty acids and glycerol.

Emulsifier
An agent that breaks down large fat globules to smaller, uniformly distributed particles, increasing the surface area available to digestive enzymes and reducing the surface tension. This is the role of bile in the intestine.

Micelles
Complex of bile and fat that carries fat into the wall of the small intestine in preparation for the final stage of absorption into the lymph and general circulation.

Portal
An entryway, usually referring to the portal circulation of blood through the liver. Blood is brought into the liver via the portal vein and moves out via the hepatic vein.

Enteric
Relating to the intestine.

Stage III: Final Absorption and Transport

The newly formed human triglycerides, along with any other lipid materials present, receive a protein covering to form the lipoproteins called *chylomicrons*. These lipid packages cross the cell membrane to enter the lymphatic system and drain into the portal blood. In the liver the lipids are converted into new lipoproteins for transport to body cells. Review Fig. 4.5 to follow lipid absorption through its three stages.

Metabolism

The metabolisms of carbohydrates, proteins, and lipids are closely intertwined to effectively meet the body's constant demand for energy.

TO SUM UP

Lipids are the most energy dense of the macronutrients and a concentrated source of fuel yielding 9 kcal/g. Lipids provide insulation to assist in temperature regulation, protect vital organs from damage, and contribute flavor and texture to foods. They have a role in neural transmission, structure of steroid hormones and cell membranes, and transport of the fat-soluble vitamins. The building blocks of lipids are fatty acids. Fatty acids are classified on the basis of chain length and degree of saturation. Fatty acids from vegetable fats are usually unsaturated, whereas animal fats are more likely to be saturated, although there are exceptions. Linoleic acid, an n-6 fatty acid, and α-linolenic acid, an n-3 fatty acid, are two polyunsaturated fatty acids that are *essential* and must be supplied in food. The essential fatty acids are necessary for skin integrity, growth (especially the prenatal and postnatal development of brain and neural tissue), control of blood lipid metabolism, and immune function. Several n-3 fatty acids in fish discourage platelet aggregation and may lower the risk of heart attack and stroke. Both the type and amount of dietary lipids affect health. Inappropriately high intakes of fat, especially saturated fats and trans fats, increase cardiovascular risk, and excessive levels of kcalories from fat add to the risk of obesity. The AMDR for fat is 20% to 35% of total kcalories. When lipids provide less than 10% of total kcalories, supplies of the essential fatty acids may be inadequate. Consumers should consult the nutrition label and list of ingredients on processed foods to control their intakes of total fat, trans fat, and saturated fat. Nutrition education should reinforce wise selection of higher-fat and lower-fat foods to maintain a prudent intake of healthy fats, control energy intake, and maximize vitamins and minerals.

QUESTIONS FOR REVIEW

1. Describe the roles of fat in the body.
2. Comparing saturated, monounsaturated, polyunsaturated, and trans fatty acids, which are healthy fats and which are unhealthy? What is it about their structures that make them healthy or unhealthy? What fat sources would you recommend to consumers?
3. Name the two essential fatty acids. Why are they considered essential? What happens when they are not available in the amounts needed?
4. You are working with an individual who has been told to reduce his dietary cholesterol. His list of foods indicates that he may have fat-free milk but not reduced-fat or low-fat milk, and he doesn't understand why. What would you tell him?
5. You are counseling a patient who has been told that he should lose 10 to 15 lb. His usual fat intake is about 35% of his total energy intake. He has agreed to lower his intake of fat to 30% in an effort to reduce his daily kcalories. What are some strategies that might help him accomplish this? He and his coworkers eat their lunch at fast-food restaurants. Develop two fast-food lunch menus that limit fat and kcalories.
6. Two persons with strong family histories of cardiovascular disease are concerned about their heart health. Both have lowered their cholesterol intake and avoid eating butter. One person started to use a stick margarine made from corn oil and the other a soft tub corn oil margarine. Which person made the better choice? Why?
7. A consumer tells you that she has begun to read food labels and buys only those items that are made with plant fats rather than animal fats, as she heard that plant fats were healthier. Is this always true? What does she need to look for on the food label to be sure that she is avoiding unhealthy fats?
8. Go to the grocery store and identify a cracker, cookie, or salad dressing that offers both a regular and a reduced-fat or fat-free version. Using the nutrition label, make a chart indicating (a) the serving size, (b) total kcalories per serving, (c) grams of total fat per serving, (d) grams of saturated fat per serving, (e) grams of trans fat per serving, (f) grams of sugar per serving, and (g) cost per serving. What nutritional differences did you observe between the regular and reduced-fat or fat-free versions? Was there a cost difference? If so, was the reduced-fat or fat-free version worth the difference in price? How do the regular and reduced-fat or fat-free versions compare in serving size, kcalories, total fat, and sugar?

REFERENCES

1. Drehmer M, Pereira MA, Schmidt MI, et al: Total and full-fat, but not low-fat, dairy product intakes are inversely associated with metabolic syndrome in adults, *J Nutr* 146:81, 2016.
2. Bowen KJ, Harris WS, Kris-Etherton PM: Omega-3 fatty acids and cardiovascular disease: Are there benefits? *Curr Treat Options Cardio Med* 18:69, 2016.
3. Bloomfield HE, Koeller E, Greer N, et al: Effect on health outcomes of a Mediterranean diet with no restriction on fat intake. A systematic review and meta-analysis, *Ann Intern Med* 165:491, 2016.
4. International Food Information Council Foundation: *2016 Food & Health Survey: Consumer Attitudes Toward Food Safety, Nutrition, and Health*, International Food Information Council Foundation. http://www.foodinsight.org/2016-FHS.
5. Samra RA: Fats and satiety. In Montmayeur JP, le Coutre J, editors: *Fat detection: taste, texture, and post ingestive effects*, Boca Raton, FL, 2010, CRC Press.
6. Jones PJH, Papamandjaris AA: Lipids: cellular metabolism. In Erdman JW Jr, Macdonald IA, Zeisel SH, editors: *Present knowledge in nutrition*, ed 10, Ames, IA, 2012, International Life Sciences Institute/Wiley-Blackwell.
7. Institute of Medicine, Otten JJ, Hellwig JP, Meyers LD, editors: *Dietary reference intakes: the essential guide to nutrient requirements*, Washington, DC, 2006, National Academies Press.
8. Van Horn L, Carson JAS, Appel LJ, et al: Recommended dietary pattern to achieve adherence to the American Heart Association/America College of Cardiology (AHA/ACC) Guidelines. A scientific statement from the American Heart Association, *Circulation* 134(22):e505, 2016.
9. US Department of Agriculture, Agricultural Research Service: Nutrient Intakes from Food and Beverages. Table 1. Mean Amounts Consumed per Individual by Gender and Age in the United States, 2013-2014 *In What We Eat in America*, NHANES 2013-2014, 2016. http://www.ars.usda.gov/nea/bhnrc/fsrg.
10. Gould JF, Makrides M, Columbo J, et al: Randomized control trial of maternal omega-3 long-chain PUFA supplementation during pregnancy and early childhood development of attention, working memory, and inhibitory control, *Am J Clin Nutr* 99(4):851, 2014.
11. Best KP, Gold M, Kennedy D, et al: Omega-3 long-chain PUFA intake during pregnancy and allergic disease outcomes in the offspring: A systematic review and meta-analysis of observational studies and randomized controlled trials, *Am J Clin Nutr* 103(1):128, 2016.
12. US Department of Health and Human Services and US Department of Agriculture: *2015-2020 Dietary Guidelines for Americans*, ed 8, December 2015. https://health.gov/dietaryguidelines/2015.
13. Baum SJ, Kris-Etherton PM, Willett WC, et al: Fatty acids in cardiovascular health and disease, *J Clin Lipidol* 6:216, 2012.
14. Kris-Etherton PM, Lefevre M, Mensink RP, et al: Trans fatty acid intakes and food sources in the US population: NHANES 1999-2002, *Lipids* 47:931, 2012.
15. Doell D, Folmer D, Lee H, et al: Updated estimate of trans fat intake by the US population, *Food Addit Contam Part A Chem Anal Control Expo Risk Assess* 29(6):861, 2012.
16. Urban LE, Roberts SB, Fierstein JL, et al: Sodium, saturated fat, and trans fat content per 1,000 kilocalories: Temporal trends in fast-food restaurants, United States, 2000-2013, *Prev Chronic Dis* 11:E228, December 2014.

17. Bray GA, Siri-Tarino PW: The role of macronutrient content in the diet for weight management, *Endocrinol Metab Clin North Am* 45:581, 2016.

18. Grundy SM: Nutrition in the management of disorders of serum lipids and lipoproteins. In Shils ME, Shike M, Olson J, editors: *Modern nutrition in health and disease*, ed 10, Baltimore, MD, 2006, Lippincott Williams & Wilkins.

19. US Department of Health and Human Services, Centers for Disease Control and Prevention: *Health, United States, 2015: With Special Feature on Racial and Ethnic Health Disparities*, DHHS Publ No 2016-1232, Hyattsville, MD, May 2016.

20. US Department of Agriculture, Agricultural Research Service: Nutrient Intakes from Food and Beverages. Table 5. Percentages of Energy from Protein, Carbohydrate, Fat, and Alcohol, by Gender and Age in the United States, 2013-2014. *In What We Eat in America*, NHANES 2013-2014, 2016. http://www.ars.usda.gov/nea/bhnrc/fsrg.

21. US Department of Agriculture, Agricultural Research Service: Nutrient Intakes from Food and Beverages. Table 6. Percentages of Energy from Protein, Carbohydrate, Fat, and Alcohol, by Race/Ethnicity and Age in the United States, 2013-2014. *In What We Eat in America*, NHANES 2013-2014, 2016. http://www.ars.usda.gov/nea/bhnrc/fsrg.

22. US Department of Agriculture, Agricultural Research Service: Nutrient Intakes from Food and Beverages. Table 2. Mean Amounts Consumed per Individual, by Race/Ethnicity and Age in the United States, 2013-2014. *In What We Eat in America*, NHANES 2013-2014, 2016. http://www.ars.usda.gov/nea/bhnrc/fsrg.

23. US Department of Agriculture, Agricultural Research Service: Nutrient Intakes from Food and Beverages. Table 49. Percent Reporting, Mean Amounts, and Percent of Selected Nutrients From Foods Obtained from Quick Service Restaurants by Gender and Age in the United States, 2013-2014. *In What We Eat in America*, NHANES 2013-2014, 2016. http://www.ars.usda.gov/nea/bhnrc/fsrg.

24. American Dietetic Association: Position of the American Dietetic Association: fat replacers, *J Am Diet Assoc* 105:266, 2005.

FURTHER READINGS AND RESOURCES

Readings

Flores G, Maldonado J, Duran P: Making tortillas without lard: Latino parents' perspectives on healthy eating, physical activity, and weight-management strategies for overweight Latino children, *J Acad Nutr Diet* 112:81, 2012.
[Dr. Flores and his collaborators help us understand the cultural issues in helping families choose healthier foods and ingredients.]
Ludwig DS: Lowering the bar on the low-fat diet: viewpoint, *JAMA* 316(20):2087, 2016.
[Dr. Ludwig reviews the pros and cons of the low-fat diet.]
Van Horn L, Carson, JAS, Appel LJ, et al: Recommended dietary pattern to achieve adherence to the American Heart Association/America College of Cardiology (AHA/ACC) Guidelines. A scientific statement from the American Heart Association, *Circulation* 134(22):e505, 2016.
[This article provides practical advice for helping persons develop a healthier eating pattern with counseling tips, menus, and suggestions for substituting more healthy for less healthy food items.]

Websites of Interest

- International Food Information Council Foundation. This site contains fact sheets and brochures for both consumers and health professionals on food fats and fat replacers. http://www.foodinsight.org/Food_Ingredients_Colors.
- National Heart, Lung and Blood Institute, National Institutes of Health. Information for the Public: This government agency provides tutorials on various aspects of heart disease, recipe books for good eating that include cultural and ethnic food patterns, and health assessment tools, including a menu planner to help monitor fat intake. https://medlineplus.gov/dietaryfats.html.

5

Proteins

Eleanor D. Schlenker

(e) http://evolve.elsevier.com/Williams/essentials/

This chapter describing protein completes our sequence of the macronutrients. Protein is quite different from carbohydrate or fat. First, it is the body's major source of nitrogen, the essential element of all living things. Second, its main task is forming body tissue using its individual building units, the amino acids. Protein is critical to growth and health, and protein deficiency associated with crop failure, poverty, or other food shortages causes widespread malnutrition and death among infants, children, and adults in the developing world. In affluent societies, intakes of protein—especially animal protein—have escalated and for some individuals may be inappropriately high. Protein is critical to the rehabilitation of patients recovering from surgery, trauma, or critical illness. Our growing understanding of the health benefits of plant proteins encourages their use in menu planning for all age groups.

OUTLINE

Physical and Chemical Nature of Proteins
The Building of Proteins
Functions of Protein
Protein and Nitrogen Balance
Protein Quality

Protein Requirements
Protein Intake
Health Promotion
Vegetarian Eating Patterns
Digestion-Absorption-Metabolism Review

PHYSICAL AND CHEMICAL NATURE OF PROTEINS

General Definition

In 1838, when Dutch chemist Johann Mulder first identified protein as a substance in all living things, it is unlikely he realized the importance of his discovery. Proteins shape our lives. Protein enzymes break down our food into nutrients the cells can use. As antibodies, they shield us from disease. Peptide hormones carry messages that coordinate continuous body activity. They guide our growth in childhood and maintain our bodies thereafter; they make us each unique.

Chemical Nature

The structural units of proteins—the amino acids—are the working currency of protein in body cells. Amino acids contain carbon, hydrogen, and oxygen—the same three elements that make up carbohydrates and fats; however, amino acids and their proteins have the additional element nitrogen. Protein is approximately 16% nitrogen. Several amino acids also contain sulfur.

The term *amino acid* tells us they have a dual nature. The word *amino* refers to a base or alkaline substance, so at once we have a contradiction. How can a chemical substance be both a base and an acid, and why is this important? Consider the significance of this fact as we learn more about amino acids and their roles in the body.

General Pattern and Structure

A common structural pattern holds for all amino acids. This pattern is built around a central α-carbon, with several attached chemical groups (Fig. 5.1) as follows:

- *Amino (base, NH₂) group:* The amino group contains the essential element nitrogen and in solution carries a positive charge.
- *Carboxyl (acid, COOH) group:* The carboxyl group is found in all acids, and in solution carries a negative charge.
- *An attached radical (R) group:* The R stands for *radical*, a general term referring to a group of elements attached to a chemical compound. In this case it refers to the attached side chains on amino acids, each one different. The distinctive side chain on an amino acid gives it a unique size, shape, and set of properties. Compare the structure of the two simplest amino acids—glycine and alanine (Fig. 5.2)—with the larger and more complex amino acid arginine (Fig. 5.3), with its extended carbon chain (R) and three additional amino groups.

Twenty different amino acids are used to build body proteins.[1] Each has the same core pattern but a specific and different side group. The dual chemical structure of amino acids, including both acid and base groups, gives them a unique amphoteric nature, meaning that an amino acid can behave as either an acid or a base, depending on the pH of the solution in which it is found. This makes it possible for amino acids to act as buffers, important in clinical care.

FIG. 5.1 Basic structure of an amino acid.

Glycine   **Alanine**

FIG. 5.2 Structure of the amino acids glycine and alanine.

Arginine

FIG. 5.3 Structure of the amino acid arginine.

KEY TERMS

Amino Acids
Acids containing the essential element nitrogen within an amino group—NH_2. Amino acids are the structural units of protein.

Amino Group
The monovalent radical, NH_2, an essential component of all amino acids.

Carboxyl Group
The monovalent radical, COOH, found in organic acids.

Essential Amino Acids

Of the 20 amino acids used to build body proteins, nine cannot be synthesized by the body and must be supplied in food. These nine amino acids are designated as indispensable (essential) amino acids. Another five of the 20 can be synthesized in the amounts needed and are termed dispensable (nonessential) amino acids. The remaining six fall in between and are known as *conditionally indispensable (essential) amino acids* (Box 5.1). Although the body is able to synthesize the conditionally indispensable amino acids, it cannot meet the demand when tissue needs are elevated or the supply of necessary precursors is inadequate. Arginine is such an amino acid. The quantity that can be produced in the liver is not sufficient to meet the needs of the newborn, so additional amounts must be supplied in food. The concept of *dietary* essentiality for the indispensable and conditionally indispensable amino acids is important when assessing protein quality.

BOX 5.1   Categories of Amino Acids

Indispensable (Essential)
- Histidine
- Isoleucine
- Leucine
- Lysine
- Methionine
- Phenylalanine
- Threonine
- Tryptophan
- Valine

Dispensable (Nonessential)
- Alanine
- Aspartic acid

- Asparagine
- Glutamic acid
- Serine

Conditionally Indispensable (Conditionally Essential)
- Arginine
- Cysteine
- Glutamine
- Glycine
- Proline
- Tyrosine

Data from Food and Nutrition Board, Institute of Medicine: *Dietary Reference Intakes for energy, carbohydrate, fiber, fat, fatty acids, cholesterol, protein, and amino acids (macronutrients)*, Washington, DC, 2002, National Academies Press.

KEY TERMS

Amphoteric
Having opposite characteristics; capable of acting either as an acid or a base or combining with an acid or a base.

pH
A scale ranging from 1 to 14 that describes the hydrogen ion concentration of a solution and its relative acidity or alkalinity; 7 is neutral, with lower numbers becoming progressively more acidic and higher numbers becoming progressively more alkaline.

Buffers
Mixtures of acid and alkaline components that, as part of a solution, protect against large changes in pH even if strong acids and bases are added. If an acid is added, then the alkaline partner reacts to counteract the acidic effect. If a base is added, then the acid partner reacts to counteract the alkalizing effect. This process keeps body fluids at the pH levels required for life.

Indispensable (Essential) Amino Acids
Amino acids that the body cannot synthesize or cannot synthesize in sufficient amounts to meet body needs so must be supplied in the diet.

Dispensable (Nonessential) Amino Acids
Amino acids that can be synthesized by the body from available precursors.

Precursor
A substance from which another substance is derived.

THE BUILDING OF PROTEINS

Protein Structure

Peptide Bond

The dual chemical nature of amino acids, with a base group on one end and an acid group on the other, enables them to form the unique chain structure found in all proteins. The end amino group of one amino acid joins with the end carboxyl group of the amino acid next to it. This joining of amino acids is called a peptide bond. Specific amino acids are joined in a particular sequence to form long chains called *polypeptides,* and specific polypeptides come together to form proteins. Polypeptides vary in length from relatively short chains of 3 to 15 amino acids called *oligopeptides* to medium-sized polypeptides with chains of 21 to 30 amino acids, such as insulin. Larger still are complex proteins made up of several hundred amino acids.

To build a compact structure, long polypeptide chains coil or fold back in a spiral shape called a helix. Other proteins form a pleated sheet held together by strengthening cross-links of sulfur and hydrogen bonds. Learning more about the structure of body proteins helps medical researchers develop effective medications and understand how genes influence disease risk.

Types of Proteins

Proteins are a widely diverse group of compounds. They have important roles in body structure and metabolism made possible by their specific content and placement of amino acids. Consider the following examples.

Myosin

This fibrous protein found in muscle (Fig. 5.4) is built from chains of 153 amino acids that coil and unfold as needed. Shaped into long rods, these fibers end in two-headed bundles so they can change shape and bend, making it possible to tighten and contract muscles and then relax them.

Collagen

This structural protein contains three separate polypeptide chains that wind around each other to produce a triple helix (Fig. 5.5). Thus reinforced, collagen is shaped into long rods and bundled into stiff fibers to do its job of strengthening bone, cartilage, and skin to maintain body form.

Hemoglobin

This globular protein (Fig. 5.6) includes four globin polypeptide chains per molecule of hemoglobin. Each chain has several hundred amino acids conjugated with a nonprotein, the iron-containing pigment called *heme.* The globin wraps around the heme and forms

Myosin molecule

Thick filament of muscle

Myosin molecules

FIG. 5.4 Myosin is a globular protein in muscle that combines with actin to form actomyosin, the fundamental contractile unit of muscle.

protective pockets to secure the iron. The iron in heme has a special ability to bind oxygen and, as part of the red blood cell, delivers oxygen to the tissues and returns carbon dioxide for excretion via the lungs.

Albumin

Albumin is the major plasma protein and has a compact globular shape. It consists of a single polypeptide chain of 584 amino acids, twisted and coiled into helix structures held together by disulfide bridges.[2] Albumin serves as a carrier protein for drugs, hormones, enzymes, and trace elements. It helps maintain fluid balance by exerting colloidal pressure in the capillaries that forces the flow of nutrients and fluids into the cells and the return of fluid and waste products out of the cells. (The role of albumin in maintaining fluid balance is described in detail in Chapter 7.) In serious illness, albumin is broken down to supply amino acids for the synthesis of new proteins to meet the body emergency.

KEY TERMS

Peptide Bond
The characteristic joining of amino acids to form proteins. Such a chain of amino acids is termed a peptide.

Helix
A coiled structure found in protein. Some are simple chain coils; others are made of several coils, such as the triple helix.

Synthesis
The making of a substance or compound by the body.

Proteins with Special Roles

Proteins with special structural or metabolic roles include the antibodies of the immune system and the blood protein fibrinogen, important in blood clotting. Hormones, such as insulin and thyroxin, and the enzymes that regulate our day-to-day metabolic activities and produce energy for work are proteins.

FUNCTIONS OF PROTEIN

Growth, Tissue Building, and Maintenance

Dietary protein supplies the amino acid building blocks for the growth and maintenance of body tissues across the life cycle. It must furnish amino acids in the appropriate patterns and amounts for efficient synthesis of specific structural molecules. Although we often consider dietary protein to be most important during growth and development when new tissues are being formed, protein needs are also important for maintenance and well-being after the growth potential has been realized.

Infancy, childhood, and adolescence: Every cell in the human body contains protein, so a constant supply is needed to support the expansion of body tissue as an individual grows from a 7-lb infant to a 160-lb man. Protein is especially important to support the rapid growth occurring in the first years of life when protein deficits can have lifelong effects. Protein needs escalate approaching the adolescent growth spurt as bone matrix and muscle tissues expand rapidly. Good-quality protein is needed to support fetal growth and the production of breast milk.

Adult maintenance: Following the attainment of full growth and maturity, protein requirements reach a steady state based on replacing lost cells and worn-out protein molecules. Loss of cells from the skin and gastrointestinal tract; new cells formed in growth of hair and nails;

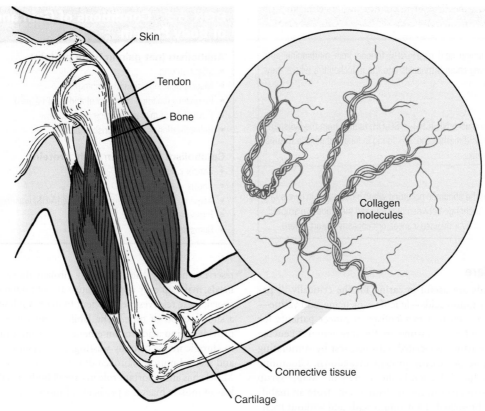

FIG. 5.5 Tissues that contain collagen, a structural protein forming connective tissue.

FIG. 5.6 Hemoglobin is the iron-containing protein in red blood cells that carries oxygen to body cells and tissues and returns carbon dioxide to the lungs for excretion.

and formation of enzymes, hormones, and other control proteins constitute daily protein needs. Individuals who participate in strength training and muscle growth require additional protein. Protein requirements demand special attention following recovery from critical illness when depleted protein stores must be replenished.

Specific Physiologic Roles

All amino acids participate in tissue growth and maintenance. However, some have important metabolic roles of their own, as follows:

- *Form neurotransmitters for brain and nerve function:* Methionine assists in the formation of choline, a precursor of acetylcholine, and tyrosine is used to synthesize the neurotransmitters dopamine and epinephrine; tryptophan is the precursor of the neurotransmitter serotonin. Age-related decreases in the neurotransmitter dopamine are associated with Parkinson disease and related muscle tremors and rigidity.[3]
- *Form other amino acids:* Methionine is the precursor of the conditionally indispensable amino acid cysteine, as well as **carnitine** and **taurine**; carnitine transports long-chain fatty acids into the mitochondria for energy production, and taurine, found in bile salts, also regulates fluid pressure in the eyes.
- *Form hormones:* Tyrosine is needed to make thyroxin and epinephrine.
- *Support immune function:* Protein is needed to make antibodies for the immune system. Protein molecules referred to as cytokines participate in the acute phase response that alters body metabolism to handle the demands resulting from critical illness, burns, or trauma.
- *Maintain fluid balance:* Plasma proteins control the flow of fluids, nutrients, and waste products back and forth between the capillaries and the cells. When protein is lacking in quantity or quality and serum proteins such as albumin are not produced in the amounts needed, body fluids accumulate in the tissues and abdomen, resulting in the edema associated with the protein-deficiency disease kwashiorkor. Low serum albumin complicated by liver disease can lead to **ascites**.
- *Formation of lipoproteins:* Amino acids supply nitrogen for synthesis of the nitrogen-containing lipoproteins that transport fatty acids and triglycerides from the liver to body cells.
- *Formation of genetic materials:* The synthesis of deoxyribonucleic acid (DNA) and ribonucleic acid (RNA) requires various amino acids.
- *Formation of enzymes and control molecules:* All body enzymes are proteins; examples are the digestive enzymes that break down our food to a form the body can use for energy and tissue building.

BOX 5.2 Conditions of Gain and Loss of Body Protein

Anabolism (net gain in body protein)
- Infant growth
- Muscle building (strength training)
- Pregnancy (building of maternal and fetal tissues)
- Production of milk in lactation
- Rehabilitation of a malnourished patient

Catabolism (net loss in body protein)
- Cancer cachexia
- Sepsis
- Acquired immunodeficiency syndrome (AIDS) wasting
- Pressure ulcers
- Burns or trauma

Role in Critical Care

Particular amino acids are useful in caring for the critically ill patient. Branched chain amino acids—leucine, isoleucine, and valine—have positive effects on protein metabolism in cancer patients for whom malnutrition and body wasting are life threatening.[4] Leucine reverses the muscle wasting associated with bed rest by stimulating protein synthesis while decreasing protein breakdown. Glutamine has been shown to reduce infection in the severely ill.[5] Maple syrup urine disease, an inborn error of metabolism, results from an inability to metabolize the branched chain amino acids and without treatment is fatal.

Role as Energy Source

Protein contributes to overall energy metabolism if needed. Protein is seldom used for energy in the fed state when glucose is readily available; however, it may be called upon in the fasting state, or in strenuous aerobic exercise. Before amino acids can be burned for energy, the nitrogen-containing amino group must be removed, and then the remaining carbon skeleton is converted to either glucose or fat. In adults approximately 17 to 25 g of every 100 g of dietary protein is not needed for tissue building or repair and is oxidized for energy.[1] This breakdown of amino acids to a form that can be burned for energy does itself require energy, leading to the popularity of high-protein diets for weight reduction.[6] Adequate carbohydrate spares protein for its primary purpose of tissue growth and repair.

PROTEIN AND NITROGEN BALANCE

Concept of Balance

Interdependent checks and balances keep the body in working order. This is true for protein ebb and flow, with tissues being built and broken down, and body materials being stored and released. These coordinated activities enable the body to respond to any situation disturbing its normal cycles.

Protein Reserves

The average man contains approximately 11 kg of protein.[1] Forty percent is in the skeletal muscle, with the remainder in skin, blood, kidney, liver, brain, and other organs. Body distribution of protein changes with growth and development. The newborn has relatively little skeletal muscle, with proportionately more protein in the brain and visceral organs.

In contrast to the substantial fat reserves held by most people, body protein reserves are quite limited. What we call the labile *protein reserves*, meaning they are easily broken down to meet immediate needs, make up only approximately 1% of total body protein; like glycogen, these reserves are sufficient to maintain body functions for only a short period of time.[1] The labile protein reserves are intended to provide amino acids for an emergency; if the condition continues, as in chronic illness or body wasting, these reserves are rapidly depleted and skeletal muscle is broken down to furnish amino acids as needed. Muscle has an important role in overall body metabolism, and extreme loss of muscle mass is a predictor of mortality.[7]

Protein Balance

The concept of balance as applied to protein balance refers to the steady state between protein synthesis (anabolism) and protein breakdown (catabolism). In periods of growth, such as infancy or childhood, or the increase in muscle as a result of strength training, protein synthesis exceeds breakdown, with a net gain of new tissue (Box 5.2). When food intake is drastically reduced, as in famine or extreme voluntary food restriction, tissue breakdown exceeds synthesis as body protein is broken down to yield energy; this results in a net loss of body protein. Protein catabolism is accelerated during periods of critical illness, as amino acids are needed for the synthesis of new proteins to fight infection, and other responses to metabolic stress cause protein breakdown and loss of nitrogen in the urine. Serious injuries, such as extensive burns, or surgery, or infection, are accompanied by catabolic protein losses that continue despite a high protein intake. When healing has begun or the illness has subsided, rehabilitation can bring about increased protein anabolism and restoration of body tissue.

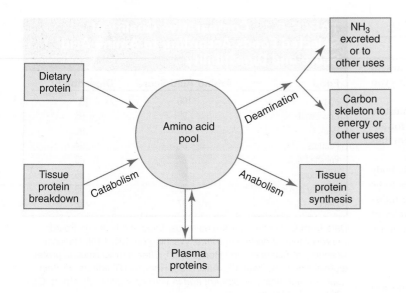

FIG. 5.7 Flow between protein compartments and the amino acid pool. Amino acids are constantly entering and leaving the body's amino acid pool to form new proteins or other nitrogen-containing compounds, to be converted to carbohydrate and used for energy, or to be converted to fat for storage.

Finely tuned mechanisms regulate protein synthesis and breakdown across all body tissues. When less protein is supplied in the diet, protein is conserved and protein losses are minimized. When fighting infection, the body uses available protein reserves to obtain amino acids for making immune cells or other proteins necessary to preserve life. When more protein is available than is needed for body growth or repair and protein reserves are optimum, amino acids are broken down and used for energy or stored as fat. In healthy individuals, adjustments in protein balance on a day-to-day basis manage the daily variations in protein intake or short-term emergencies.

Various processes and protein compartments participate in the control of protein metabolism, as follows:

- *Protein turnover:* Protein turnover is the process by which body proteins are continuously broken down and the released amino acids made into new proteins.[1] New proteins replace worn-out proteins, and different proteins are formed to meet changing needs. When an amino acid labeled with a radioactive carbon atom is incorporated into a protein food and eaten, it can be traced; that is, we can follow its journey through the body. By these studies we learned that amino acids are rapidly incorporated into body proteins. Then, when these proteins are broken down, they are reused to form new proteins. Protein turnover varies among tissues. Turnover rates are higher in the intestinal mucosa, liver, pancreas, kidney, and plasma, tissues that are more metabolically active, and lower in muscle, brain, and skin. Protein turnover is very slow in structural tissues such as collagen. Total body protein turnover is higher in infants and children who are growing rapidly and lower in older adults.
- *Protein compartments:* Body protein is divided between two compartments: (1) tissue protein and (2) plasma protein. Protein from one compartment may be drawn to supply a need in the other. Muscle tissue becomes an important source of amino acids in periods of stress or low-protein intake. Plasma proteins such as prealbumin have rapid turnover and are early indicators of protein catabolism brought on by inflammation, surgery, cancer, or other serious illness. Low plasma albumin is characteristic of children with kwashiorkor, the protein deficiency disease seen in countries with food shortages. Although albumin is not a specific marker of protein deficiency, it can alert the clinician to the need for nutrition intervention.[8] Plasma protein levels are restored to normal when the disease or catabolic stress has abated and protein and kilocalories (kcalories or kcal) become available.

- *Metabolic amino acid pool:* Amino acids derived from tissue breakdown or supplied by dietary protein contribute to a common metabolic "pool." Amino acids from this pool are used to synthesize body proteins as needed. Fig. 5.7 summarizes the many aspects of protein metabolism.

Nitrogen Balance

Protein balance is sometimes described as **nitrogen balance**. Nitrogen balance involves all of the nitrogen in the body—protein nitrogen as well as nonprotein nitrogen in such compounds as urea, uric acid, and ammonia. Nitrogen balance is the net result of nitrogen gain and loss across all body tissues. **Negative nitrogen balance** occurs when body nitrogen loss exceeds the nitrogen taken in from food as occurs in long-term illness, hypermetabolic wasting disease, and inadequate protein intake. **Positive nitrogen balance** occurs during growth, pregnancy, or strength training as more nitrogen is retained. Healthy persons with an adequate protein intake are in **nitrogen equilibrium**, with nitrogen intake and loss approximately equal on a daily basis.

KEY TERMS

Nitrogen Balance
The metabolic balance between nitrogen intake from dietary protein and nitrogen losses in urine, feces, sweat, and cells; dietary protein is 16% nitrogen (6.25 g dietary protein contains 1 g of nitrogen).

Negative Nitrogen Balance
The situation when nitrogen intake from dietary protein does not equal nitrogen losses through urine, feces, sweat, and cells from the skin and gastrointestinal tract; negative nitrogen balance results in a net loss of nitrogen from the body.

Positive Nitrogen Balance
The situation when nitrogen intake from dietary protein exceeds nitrogen losses through the urine, feces, sweat, and cells from the skin or gastrointestinal tract; positive nitrogen balance results in a net increase in body nitrogen.

Nitrogen Equilibrium
The situation that occurs when nitrogen intake from dietary protein equals total nitrogen losses, with no net gain or loss in body nitrogen.

PROTEIN QUALITY

Evaluating Food Proteins

The nutritional quality of a protein is defined by its ability to sustain the growth and repair of body tissues and is based on the following two characteristics[9]:

1. *Protein digestibility:* To be of use to the body, amino acids must be released from other food components and made available for absorption. If nondigestible components in the food prevent this breakdown, then the amino acids are lost in the feces.
2. *Amino acid composition:* All 20 amino acids needed to make body proteins must be available at the same time for new tissues to be formed; therefore food proteins should supply each of the indispensable amino acids in the amount required. Other sources of amino (NH_2) groups in a food protein can be used to synthesize any dispensable amino acids needed.

Comparing Food Proteins

The nutritive value of a food protein is often expressed as its amino acid score, a value based on both its digestibility and amino acid composition. The amino acid reference pattern used to evaluate proteins is quite similar to the pattern of egg white, the reference protein often used in nutrition studies. When evaluating an amino acid score, it is important to identify the limiting amino acid (or acids). A limiting amino acid is any indispensable amino acid falling below the amount recommended in the amino acid reference pattern. For protein synthesis to take place, all indispensable amino acids must be available in the required amount. Thus the limiting amino acid "limits" or hinders the body from effectively using the other amino acids in that protein regardless of their adequacy. When one or two limiting amino acids are identified in a food protein having optimal levels of the other indispensable amino acids, that protein can be combined with another food protein that will supply the amino acid or acids needed. A comparison of the amino acid scores and digestibility of various protein foods is found in Table 5.1. In general, proteins from animal sources have higher scores than those from plant sources.

Amino Acid Content of Plant and Animal Foods

Plant and animal foods differ in their content of indispensable amino acids. Animal foods contain all of the indispensable amino acids in the amounts and ratio needed to support protein synthesis and are referred to as complete proteins. These foods include eggs, milk, cheese, meat, poultry, and fish (Box 5.3). Plant proteins vary in quality but are incomplete proteins; either they supply less than the required amount of one or more indispensable amino acids or they are missing an indispensable amino acid (Box 5.4). However, several plant proteins eaten together or combined with a small amount of animal protein can

TABLE 5.1   Comparative Quality of Selected Foods According to Amino Acid Score and Digestibility

Food	Amino Acid Score	Digestibility
Egg	100	100
Cow's milk	95	95
Beef	89	95
Peanuts	65	94
Polished rice	57	89
Soy flour	47	86
Sesame seeds	42	90
Peas	37	88

Data from Committee on Amino Acids, Food and Nutrition Board: *Improvement of protein nutriture,* Washington, DC, 1974, National Academy of Sciences; and Hopkins, DT: Effects of variation in protein digestibility. In Bodwell CE, Adkins JS, Hopkins DT, editors: *Protein quality in humans: assessment and in vitro estimation,* Westport, CT, 1981, Avi Publishing Company.

supply the amino acids required to support tissue growth and repair.[1,10] This concept of complementary proteins, by which one protein helps meet the amino acid shortage in another, has been at work in the traditional food patterns of families worldwide. See Fig. 5.8 for examples of complementary vegetable proteins. Legumes are among the few plant proteins that are high in lysine, an indispensable amino acid, and thus important to protein nutrition.[11] Soy protein, although lower in methionine than animal protein, meets the amino acid needs of adults. (See the Focus on Culture box, "Soy: A Protein Source Since Ancient Times," to learn more about soy foods.)

KEY TERMS

Limiting Amino Acid
The indispensable amino acid present in a food in the lowest amount as compared with the reference amino acid pattern.

Complete Protein
A protein that contains all indispensable amino acids in the amounts needed for synthesis of body proteins according to the reference amino acid pattern.

Incomplete Protein
A protein with a lower amount of one or more of the indispensable amino acids as compared with the reference amino acid pattern or missing an indispensable amino acid needed to form body proteins.

BOX 5.3   Complete Proteins

- Egg
- Hamburger
- Milk
- Chicken
- Cheese
- Fish fillet

Animal foods are complete proteins and include all the indispensable amino acids in the amounts needed for protein synthesis.

Images copyright 2006 JupiterImages Corporation.

🌐 FOCUS ON CULTURE

Soy: A Protein Source Since Ancient Times

Families throughout Asia have used soybeans for centuries. In China, Japan, Vietnam, Indonesia, the Philippines, Cambodia, and Laos, soybeans in various forms are a dietary staple and a major source of protein. Traditional soy foods such as tofu, tempeh, and soy milk were introduced by newcomers to the United States and have gained broad acceptance by vegetarians and vegans, those who are lactose intolerant, and others looking to expand their food horizons. A growing interest in Asian cooking and the increasing popularity of ethnic restaurants have encouraged more people to eat these foods.

The most important soy-based protein foods are tofu and tempeh, described as follows:

- *Tofu:* In Chinese, *fu* means "riches," so tofu is usually served at New Year's celebrations to bring good luck. Tofu is made by a process similar to cheese making. A coagulating agent such as calcium sulfate, vinegar, or lemon juice is added to pureed soybeans. After the curd has formed, it is placed in molds to form cakes and the liquid whey is discarded. Tofu made with calcium sulfate has higher calcium content. Some types of tofu look much like farmer cheese, but they are very different in flavor. Whereas most cheeses have strong flavors, tofu is bland and absorbs its flavors from other foods. This makes it an excellent addition to cooked mixed dishes with a variety of seasonings or highly spiced ingredients. Tofu is available in two forms: (1) soft and (2) firm. Soft tofu can be mashed and used in recipes in place of ground beef or ricotta cheese; firm tofu can be grilled or stir-fried. Tofu has a limited shelf life, so consumers should check the expiration date on the package and keep it refrigerated.
- *Tempeh:* This soy food originated in Indonesia and is a mixture of soy and grain. When fermented, it becomes a firm mass that can be sliced or made into patties. Tempeh has more flavor than tofu and is a rich source of protein.

Soybeans are mixed with other ingredients to make sauces and seasonings common in Asian cooking.

Several of these mixtures are described as follows:

- *Hoisin sauce:* Used in Chinese cooking, hoisin sauce is a combination of fermented soybeans, water, flour, sugar, and garlic.
- *Miso*: Miso originated in Japan and is a fermented mixture of soybeans and rice or barley. It is a pungent, salty paste used as a seasoning or soup base. Miso is very high in sodium, containing 900 mg of sodium or more per tablespoon.
- *Soy sauce:* This seasoning is a combination of steamed rice, roasted soybeans, and salt that is fermented. Based on its high sodium content, it should be used in moderation. Low-sodium varieties of soy sauce are readily available and can be used as a substitute.

Tofu and tempeh are available in supermarkets and Asian food stores and add variety and nutrition to the meal pattern. If you have not tasted these foods, look for an Asian cookbook in your local library or ask a classmate to share a family recipe.

Bibliography

Diabetes Care and Education Practice Group of the American Dietetic Association, Goody CM, Drago L, editors: *Cultural food practices*, Chicago, 2010, American Dietetic Association.

Kittler PG, Sucher KP: *Cultural foods: traditions and trends*, Belmont, CA, 2000, Wadsworth/Thompson Learning.

Margen S, editor: *The wellness encyclopedia of food and nutrition*, New York, 1992, Health Letter Associates.

PROTEIN REQUIREMENTS

Factors Influencing Protein Requirements

Protein Quality

The quality of dietary protein according to its amino acid composition influences the type and amount needed. Individuals who consume some animal protein along with plant protein will have an adequate supply of all amino acids. Those who eat no animal protein should consume a wide variety of complementary plant proteins to ensure appropriate amounts of the indispensable amino acids.

Protein Digestibility

Food processing and food preparation affect amino acid availability. Heat applied in drying or baking causes chemical bonding between some sugars and amino acids, forming compounds that cannot be digested. Lysine, methionine, and cysteine can be lost in this way.[12] Protein digestion and amino acid absorption are influenced by the time interval between meals, with longer intervals lowering the competition for available enzymes and absorption sites.

Tissue Growth

Protein requirements reflect the growth patterns of infancy, childhood, and adolescence. Pregnancy and lactation increase protein needs.

Energy Content of the Diet

When carbohydrate intake is sufficient to meet energy needs, dietary protein can be used exclusively for tissue building. This is often referred to as the protein-sparing action of carbohydrate. Dietary carbohydrates also support protein use by stimulating the release of insulin, which promotes the use of amino acids for protein synthesis.

Health Status

Conditions and diseases that increase the rate of protein turnover and tissue breakdown raise the protein requirement. After trauma or surgery, amino acids are needed for wound healing and formation of new tissue, as well as the production of infection-fighting immune factors. Serious burns with extensive tissue destruction substantially increase protein needs. In critically ill patients, protein requirements may

BOX 5.4   Incomplete Proteins

- Soy meat analog
- Beans
- Peanuts
- Rice
- Tofu
- Sesame seeds

Plant foods are incomplete proteins, but two or more can be combined to form a complete protein with all indispensable amino acids in the amounts needed for protein synthesis.

Images copyright 2006 JupiterImages Corporation.

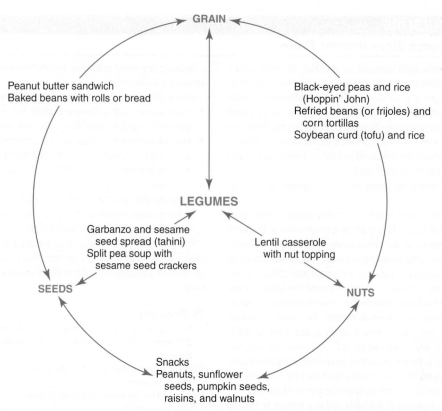

GRAIN

Peanut butter sandwich
Baked beans with rolls or bread

Black-eyed peas and rice
(Hoppin' John)
Refried beans (or frijoles) and
corn tortillas
Soybean curd (tofu) and rice

LEGUMES

Garbanzo and sesame
seed spread (tahini)
Split pea soup with
sesame seed crackers

Lentil casserole
with nut topping

SEEDS

NUTS

Snacks
Peanuts, sunflower
seeds, pumpkin seeds,
raisins, and walnuts

FIG. 5.8 Complementary vegetable proteins. Examples of common plant foods that, when eaten together, supply the amounts of indispensable (essential) amino acids required for protein synthesis. (Redrawn from Stanfield PS, Hui YH: *Nutrition and diet therapy: self-instructional modules,* ed 4, Sudbury, MA, 2003, Jones & Bartlett, with permission.)

reach 1.5 to 2.0 g/kg of body weight or 2 to 2½ times the usual recommendation.[13,14] Supplementation with the amino acid leucine appears to limit the loss of muscle protein that occurs with bed rest or immobilization.[15]

Dietary Reference Intakes
Protein
The Recommended Dietary Allowance (RDA) for protein is 0.8 g/kg body weight or 56 g/day for men and 46 g/day for women.[1] This intake is intended to maintain body tissues and replace daily nitrogen losses via the urine, feces, and sweat. An additional 25 g/day is needed for pregnancy and lactation. Protein requirements of infants and children vary according to age and stage of growth.

There continue to be differences of opinion regarding the current RDAs for protein. New methods of evaluation indicate that protein needs are higher than the current standards for children and pregnant women.[16] Higher protein intakes may help prevent sarcopenia, the loss of muscle contributing to frailty in many persons older than 60 years.[17] These issues will be discussed further in the appropriate chapters.

A Tolerable Upper Intake Level (UL) has not been established for protein; however, the safety of protein intakes well in excess of the RDA is a concern. Protein waste products are excreted via the urine; thus fluid intake must be adjusted accordingly. It is recommended that protein intake, under normal conditions, not exceed 2 times the RDA.[1]

Amino Acids
Individuals meeting the RDA who eat both animal and plant proteins will have an adequate supply of the indispensable amino acids. If no animal foods are consumed, then an intake of mixed plant proteins obtained from legumes (including soy), grains, nuts, seeds, and vegetables can supply amino acids in the pattern needed.[10]

ULs have not been set for individual amino acids because imbalances and toxicity are not usually a hazard when amino acids are supplied in food. However, supplements that exaggerate the intake of one or more amino acids interfere with protein synthesis and can lead to toxicity.[1] Leucine has become popular among both amateur and professional athletes based on its ability to promote protein synthesis. Unsupervised supplementation is a risk to health.[18]

Acceptable Macronutrient Distribution Range
The Acceptable Macronutrient Distribution Range (AMDR) for protein is 10% to 35% of total kcalories.[1] In general, protein needs are met if protein makes up 10% of energy intake; however, if total energy intake is low, as is often the case with older individuals, then it will be necessary to obtain more kcalories from protein to meet the RDA. The suggested kcalorie range for protein provides flexibility to achieve a healthy diet pattern.

PROTEIN INTAKE
Protein-Energy Malnutrition
Protein intake differs widely across population groups, with some getting far more and others far less than they need. Protein-energy malnutrition (PEM) is a major health problem in many developing countries where protein intakes are low in both quantity and quality. Nearly 7 million children under the age of 5 die each year from undernutrition, and an estimated 178 million experience stunted growth.[19] PEM also contributes to the morbidity and mortality associated with infectious diseases such as diarrhea, measles, respiratory tract infections, and gastroenteritis.

Two forms of extreme malnutrition occurring across all age groups when food supplies are insufficient are kwashiorkor and marasmus (Fig. 5.9). Marasmus represents extreme starvation with deficits of energy, protein, and micronutrients. These patients have little or no body fat and exhibit extreme wasting. Rehabilitation must be implemented on a gradual basis to avoid refeeding syndrome, with severe complications or death. Kwashiorkor occurs in children and adults when diets are deficient in protein and likely limiting in energy and micronutrients as well. The word *kwashiorkor* comes from a Ghanaian word meaning "illness striking a child when the second child is born," because it frequently befell a child when a new baby replaced him at the breast, and weaning foods were inadequate to meet his nutritional needs. This form of PEM results in a characteristic edema, hypoalbuminemia, skin lesions, and fatty liver. The primary cause of PEM is most often a lack of food supplying appropriate levels of nutrients; however, impaired digestion or absorption, infection, chronic or acute vomiting, or diarrhea are secondary causes or contributors to this condition.

FIG. 5.9 Protein-energy malnutrition (PEM). (A) Marasmus results from starvation, a diet lacking in both kcalories and protein. (B) Kwashiorkor results from a diet that may be sufficient in kcalories but is deficient in protein. Note the abdominal bloating typical of kwashiorkor. (From Thibodeau GA, Patton KT: *The human body in health & disease*, ed 5, St Louis, 2010, Mosby.)

Population Differences in Protein Intake

Plant researchers are working to improve the amino acid patterns of grains such as rice and maize that are dietary staples for millions of people around the world who take in little or no animal protein. At the other extreme, most people in the United States meet or exceed their RDA for protein, with 42% to 60% of their intake coming from animal sources.[20,21] Average protein intakes of adults are more than 1½ times their Dietary Reference Intake (DRI).[22] Protein intakes are also high among US children who consume more than 2 times their current recommended intakes.

Clinical Applications: Protein Intake
Low-Protein Diets

We usually associate low-protein diets with the severe PEM evident in famine-ravaged countries; however, degrees of malnutrition exist in all areas of the world, including the United States. Children with chronic PEM have poor growth (low weight for height) and stunting (low height for age). Marginal protein status impairs immune function, contributing to the chronic respiratory infections and diarrhea that trouble many poorly nourished children and adults. Low protein intake during pregnancy increases the risk of a low-birth-weight infant. Inappropriately low protein intake as part of a weight reduction regimen promotes loss of lean body mass.

However, in certain clinical situations, protein intake less than the recommended level is warranted. In that case it becomes especially important to choose protein high in biologic value. The following serve as examples of when protein intake may be limited:

- *Parkinson disease:* Protein intake is controlled to prevent the buildup of excessive amino acids that compete with the treatment drug levodopa for passage across the blood-brain barrier.[3]
- *Phenylketonuria (PKU):* Individuals with this inborn error of metabolism lack the enzyme required to metabolize the indispensable amino acid phenylalanine, and accumulation of inappropriately high blood levels of this amino acid results in mental retardation. All infants born in the United States are tested for PKU at birth, and immediate intervention with a protein-restricted diet limiting the intake of phenylalanine prevents harmful changes.
- *Chronic kidney disease (CKD):* When kidney function declines, protein intake is reduced to minimize the burden of excreting urea and other nitrogen-containing waste.
- *Vegan diets:* Individuals who consume no animal foods and must obtain all of their protein from plant sources may have marginal protein intakes based on the added bulk of plant protein foods. Protein may provide only 10% of total kcalories, the minimum AMDR.[1,10]

High-Protein Diets

High-protein diets moved into the spotlight when media attention focused on weight loss regimens that restricted carbohydrate in preference to protein and fat. Protein intakes of 25% to 40% of total kcalories (approximately 1.2 to 1.6 g protein/kg body weight) have been shown to support weight loss and effective energy regulation.[23-25] One benefit of a weight loss diet high in protein is its positive effect on satiety that promotes adherence to the dietary regimen, although this may differ among individuals.[26] Protein also increases energy expenditure as compared with carbohydrate and fat, based on the extra kcalories needed to remove the amino group from amino acids and enable their use as a fuel.[23] Liberal protein intakes protect muscle mass during long-term weight reduction. Retention of muscle mass helps preserve weight loss because these tissues add to basal energy needs and contribute to the overall energy requirement. Genetics may play a role in the macronutrient composition of the diet that is most successful for a given individual. Nevertheless, a reduction in kcalorie intake and/or an increase in energy expenditure are still key to weight loss, regardless of the proportion of specific macronutrients. Personal preferences, cultural food patterns, and metabolic considerations should form the basis for individual interventions, while keeping protein intake within the AMDR upper limit of 35%.

Although high-protein diets have some advantages, their long-term effects on calcium balance[1] and renal function[27] remain under discussion. High intakes of protein, particularly animal protein, can increase urinary calcium; however, protein also stimulates the release of stomach acid and promotes calcium absorption,[1] making this a complicated issue. High-protein diets also require attention to related water needs.

HEALTH PROMOTION

Health Benefits of Plant Proteins

Soy foods and other legumes supply good-quality protein, along with an array of important nutrients, phytochemicals, and fiber with roles in preventing chronic disease.[10] Higher intakes of flavonoids, a class of phytochemicals found in soy, peanuts, and many fruits and vegetables, were associated with lower risk of stroke and mortality in older adults followed for 7 years.[28] Regular use of legumes improved glucose control among patients with type 2 diabetes.[29] Vegetable protein foods also contain healthful fats. One cup of tofu or soybean curd supplies nearly 25%, and one cup of chickpeas supplies 12% of the RDA for linoleic acid.[1,30] Tree nuts and peanuts, often considered snack items rather than alternate sources of protein, are rich in antioxidants, trace minerals, and essential fatty acids[30] and add rich protein to sandwiches and stews. Beans and nuts are important foods in the Mediterranean food

pattern and likely contribute to the healthful benefits attributed to that pattern.[31]

Nutritional Contributions of Animal Proteins

Proteins from animal sources—meat, fish, poultry, eggs, and milk—whether eaten alone or in combination with vegetable proteins, meet the amino acid needs of children and adults. Animal foods supply trace minerals such as iron and zinc that are difficult to obtain in sufficient amounts from plant foods based on their lower content and interfering substances. Dairy foods are rich in calcium and riboflavin and provide preformed vitamin A. Vitamin B_{12} and vitamin D occur naturally in animal foods only. (See the Evidence-Based Practice box, "Dividing Your Protein Across the Day," to learn how your body can best use your dietary protein.)

VEGETARIAN EATING PATTERNS

Vegetarian food patterns existed in ancient times, as described in early Greek culture. People choose to follow a plant-based diet and limit or exclude animal foods for many reasons. Several major world religions, including Hinduism and Buddhism, advocate avoidance of meat for the preservation of animal life. For an urban university group, ethical considerations followed by concerns for health were the overwhelming reasons for selecting a vegetarian or vegan food pattern.[32] Sustainability of the food supply and protection of the environment are growing issues in many parts of the world. In the United States, land requirements for producing a meat-based diet are twice that needed to produce a lacto-ovovegetarian diet; 100 times more water is required to produce 1 kg of animal protein than 1 kg of plant protein.[33] Such reports have led some consumers to plant-based diets to assist in reducing food shortages throughout the world.

EVIDENCE-BASED PRACTICE

Dividing Your Protein Across the Day

Identify the problem: All indispensable amino acids must be present at the same time or become available over the course of a day for protein synthesis to take place; otherwise the amino acids that are available are broken down for energy or other uses. Recent findings indicate that equally dividing your dietary protein across your three meals promotes most efficient use of your amino acid intake.

Review the evidence: The meal pattern most common in the United States consists of a light breakfast, a moderate lunch, but a very heavy dinner. Adults consume 17% to 18% of their daily protein intake at breakfast, 27% to 28% at lunch, and 42% to 43% at dinner. For the average American man, this translates to 16 g of protein at breakfast, 26 g at lunch, and 41 g at dinner. Women, who have a lower intake of protein overall, take in only 12 g at breakfast, 20 g at lunch, and 30 g at dinner. Researchers working with both younger and older adults compared the effects on body protein synthesis and tissue repair when dietary protein was divided equally across the three meals and when intake was skewed with the bulk of daily protein eaten at the dinner meal. Muscle protein synthesis over the succeeding 24-hour period was 25% higher when protein was equally divided as compared with the skewed intake at dinner. This finding is especially pertinent to the physical well-being of older adults, for whom sarcopenia (the loss of muscle mass) leads to disability and loss of independence. Although muscle loss accelerates in later years, it begins in middle age; thus the recommendation to divide protein equally across the day has application for all adult age groups.

Implement the findings: Protein is used most efficiently with an intake of 25 to 30 g at each meal. For men whose daily intake is 98 g, reaching the recommended

level of 30 g at each meal is easily accomplished on their present intake, with some reallocation of protein from dinner to breakfast. However, for women, their average daily intake of 70 g will not supply even 25 g at each meal. Health professionals must stress the importance of optimum daily protein for women, especially older women, for preservation of muscle mass. Both men and women would benefit from nutrition education focusing on protein foods at breakfast. Adding a glass of milk, a high-protein cereal, a cup of yogurt with fruit, a hard-boiled egg, a tuna salad sandwich, a handful of nuts, peanut butter on toast, or melted cheese on toast are various ways to add protein to breakfast.

Bibliography

Mamerow MM, Mettler JA, English KL, et al: Dietary protein distribution positively influences 24-h muscle protein synthesis in healthy adults, *J Nutr* 144:876, 2014.

Paddon-Jones D, Campbell WW, Jacques PF, et al: Protein and healthy aging, *Am J Clin Nutr* 101(Suppl 6):S1339, 2015.

US Department of Agriculture, Agricultural Research Service: *Table 1. Nutrient Intakes from Food and Beverages: Mean Amounts Consumed per Individual by Gender and Age in the United States, 2013–2014; Table 13. Breakfast: Percentages of Selected Nutrients Contributed by Food and Beverages Consumed at Breakfast by Gender and Age in the United States, 2013–2014; Table 17. Lunch: Percentages of Selected Nutrients Contributed by Food and Beverages Consumed at Lunch by Gender and Age in the United States, 2013–2014; Table 21. Dinner: Percentages of Selected Nutrients Contributed by Food and Beverages Consumed at Dinner by Gender and Age in the United States, 2013–2014.* All four tables from *What We Eat in America, NHANES 2013–2014,* 2016. http://www.ars.usda.gov/nea/bhnrc/fsrg.

Although food patterns that emphasize plant foods are generally referred to as *vegetarian diets,* they are exceedingly difficult to quantify. Vegetarian food patterns differ greatly according to the types of animal foods they include or exclude, as follows[10,21]:

- Lacto-ovovegetarian (includes all plant foods, dairy, and eggs)
- Lactovegetarian (includes all plant foods and dairy)
- Ovovegetarian (includes all plant foods and eggs)
- Pescovegetarian (includes all plant foods, dairy, eggs, and fish)
- Vegan (includes plant foods only)
- Raw vegan (includes plant foods only; 75%–100% eaten raw)
- Semivegetarian (includes predominantly plant foods with eggs and dairy, and fish or chicken several times a month)

Approximately 3.3% of the population in the United States describe themselves as vegetarians who never eat meat, fish, or poultry, and approximately half of these are vegans.[10] Food manufacturers have responded to this new interest in vegetarian diets; annual sales of alternative meat products now exceed $553 million. Most fast food restaurants offer a soy burger or meatless option. The availability of these foods in the marketplace assists vegetarians in meal planning and obtaining required nutrients.

Nutritional Implications of Vegetarian Food Patterns

Vegetarian food patterns, including vegan food patterns, will support growth and well-being across the life cycle *if* well planned. Conversely, vegetarian and vegan food patterns, as well as food patterns that include animal foods, will be inadequate if items high in fat and sugar and low in important nutrients are emphasized. In general, the more restrictive the diet, the more planning is required to avoid nutrient deficiencies.

Vegetarians who regularly include eggs and vitamin D–fortified dairy foods and juices in their meal patterns can obtain adequate amounts of protein, vitamin D, and vitamin B_{12}. Vegans need to include a wide variety of plant foods to obtain sufficient amounts of indispensable amino acids with regular use of legumes and soy. A variety of plant proteins eaten over the course of a day should supply sufficient amounts of the indispensable amino acids if energy requirements are met.[11] Vegans must seek out fortified foods or supplements to obtain vitamin D and vitamin B_{12}. Soy milk, rice milk, and orange juice are often fortified with vitamin D and calcium to the amounts found in cow's milk; fortified breakfast cereals and margarine can supply some vitamin D. Vegetarians consuming only limited amounts of milk and/or eggs should also include reliable sources of vitamin B_{12} in their meal patterns. All vegetarians must read labels carefully to determine sources of important nutrients.[10]

Daily intakes of the essential fatty acids (linoleic acid and alpha linolenic acid) are similar in nonvegetarians, pescovegetarians, ovovegetarians or lactovegetarians, and vegans.[21] Linoleic acid (an n-6 fatty acid) is found in various oils, easily accessible in food patterns that do not contain animal foods. For individuals who do not consume fish to supply docosahexaenoic (DHA) and eicosapentaenoic (EPA) acids, appropriate intakes of alpha-linolenic acid (an n-3 fatty) is especially important. As described in Chapter 4, DHA and EPA can be synthesized from alpha-linolenic acid, although this occurs at a rather slow rate. Optimum intakes of alpha-linolenic acid may hasten this conversion.[10] Concentrated sources of the n-3 fatty acids are flax seeds, canola seeds, soy beans, walnuts, and their oils. Low-dose DHA supplements are well absorbed and provide an alternative to those with increased needs.[10]

Minerals require special attention in the vegetarian or vegan food pattern. Calcium intakes of lactovegetarians and ovovegetarians exceed those of nonvegetarians; however, calcium intakes of vegans fall below both groups.[21] Calcium is well absorbed from broccoli, Chinese cabbage, kale, and bok choy (all vegetables low in oxalate). Conversely, spinach and Swiss chard are poor sources of calcium, based on their oxalate content, which interferes with calcium absorption. Beans, almonds, and tahini provide moderate amounts of calcium. Fortified plant foods such as soy milk, rice milk, fruit juices, and breakfast cereals supply calcium.[10]

Iron and zinc are found naturally in many plant foods; however, phytates interfere with their absorption. Including a vitamin C source at the same meal facilitates iron absorption, and soaking beans before cooking makes the iron more available. Fortified grains and cereals add iron in a form that is fairly well absorbed. Based on the presence of substances in plant foods known to interfere with iron absorption, nutrition experts have recommended higher iron intakes for vegetarians than nonvegetarians. Nevertheless, iron intakes are approximately the same in nonvegetarians, vegetarians, and vegans, and their measures of iron status do not differ, suggesting that vegetarians achieve higher levels of iron absorption than would be expected.[10] Based on their plentiful intakes of legumes, nuts, and unrefined grains, vegans are likely to reach their DRI for zinc, although absorption of that nutrient also may be impaired by phytates and fiber. Soaking beans, grains, and seeds and the leavening action in bread improve the availability of zinc. Fruits and vegetables provide many sources of vitamin A and the carotenoids, vitamin K, the B complex vitamins (with the exception of vitamin B_{12}), and potassium.

In general, plant-based diets contain more fiber, antioxidants, carotenoids, and phytochemicals and less saturated fat than the average diet, depending on the animal foods included. Vegetarians eat more fruits and dark green vegetables than do nonvegetarians and twice the whole grains and legumes.[34]

Planning Vegetarian Diets

Vegetarian diets are planned as any diet is planned, to include needed amounts of essential nutrients and sufficient kcalories for energy. The US Department of Agriculture has developed guidelines listing the food groups and amounts needed to supply the essential nutrients in a Healthy Vegetarian Eating Pattern and suggests substitutions for dairy and eggs that will provide a healthy dietary pattern for vegans.[31] Portion sizes of equivalent plant protein foods are described in Box 5.5.

Individuals accustomed to food patterns that include meat may find it difficult to adopt vegetarian meal patterns, even if motivated by health or environmental concerns.[35] This hesitation could relate to the familiar meal triangle including a meat, a starch, and a vegetable, and the need to find a substitute for the meat, fish, or poultry. When asked if they preferred meals that combined ingredients, such as pasta with added ground meat, or meals with separate components such as a chicken leg, baked potato, and vegetable, responses differed by age.[35] Older individuals much preferred the food items arranged separately, whereas younger people were more receptive to mixed dishes. Vegetarian food plans are often based on mixtures that combine beans and nuts to achieve a full set of indispensable amino acids. The 7-day sample menu cycle found on the MyPlate website (http://www.choosemyplate.gov) includes several vegetarian meals. Substitution of soy milk or other soy products could adapt other menus to the vegan food pattern.

Use of complementary proteins to obtain sufficient amounts of the indispensable amino acids is especially important when planning a vegan diet. Review Fig. 5.8 and see the Perspectives in Practice box, "Increase Your Variety: Exploring Complementary Proteins," to consider food combinations for the daily plan.

BOX 5.5 Ounce-Equivalent of Plant Protein Foods

Each of the following servings provides one ounce-equivalent of protein: A plant protein can be combined with a small amount of animal protein to form a complete protein, or two or more different plant proteins can be combined to form a complete protein (see Fig. 5.8).

• Cooked chicken, fish, lean beef, lean ham	1 ounce
• Egg	1
• Nuts (12 almonds, 7 walnut halves)	½ ounce
• Seeds (pumpkin, sunflower, squash – hulled, roasted)	½ ounce
• Peanut butter or almond butter	1 tablespoon
• Cooked beans (black, pinto, pinto, white)	¼ cup
• Cooked peas (chickpeas, lentils, split peas	¼ cup
• Baked beans or refried beans	¼ cup
• Tofu	¼ cup (2 ounces)
• Tempeh (cooked)	1 ounce
• Hummus	2 tablespoons
• Falafel patty	4 ounces
• Soy or bean burger patty	½ patty

Images copyright 2006 JupiterImages Corporation.
Data from US Department of Agriculture: All about the protein foods group. ChooseMyPlate.gov, 2016. https://www.choosemyplate.gov/protein-foods.

Vegetarian Diets and Chronic Disease

Vegetarian diets represent a wide diversity of dietary practices described by what foods are included or excluded. When a vegetarian diet is well planned, it promotes health and lowers the risk of chronic disease. Vegetarians tend to have diets lower in saturated fat and higher in fiber, fruits and vegetables, whole grains, and phytochemicals, foods and substances associated with the prevention of cardiovascular disease, type 2 diabetes, and cancer. Blood levels of low-density lipoprotein (LDL)-cholesterol, body weights, and blood pressures are lower among vegetarians and vegans as compared with nonvegetarians and may help explain their resistance to chronic disease and metabolic syndrome.[10,21,36]

DIGESTION-ABSORPTION-METABOLISM REVIEW

Food proteins must be broken down into their building units—the amino acids—to meet body needs. A brief review of this process is outlined next. (See Chapter 2 for more discussion of digestion, absorption, and metabolism.)

Digestion
Mouth

The only digestive action on proteins in the mouth is the mechanical effect of chewing, breaking food into smaller particles for passage into the stomach.

PERSPECTIVES IN PRACTICE

Increase Your Variety: Exploring Complementary Proteins

Traditional diets the world over are plant based, emphasizing cereals, legumes, and vegetables. In many cultures the main dish is a stew made up of a variety of plant foods; sometimes a small amount of animal protein is added. Exploring complementary proteins is a way to learn more about the foods of different cultural and ethnic groups. Try a new recipe, and calculate the amounts of protein coming from animal and vegetable sources.
Some traditional plant-based meals follow:

• *Mexican:* Corn tortillas combined with beans and vegetables provide a complete protein, as do beans and rice. The addition of cheese to stews or tortillas complements the incomplete proteins of the grain foods. Eggs with beans are a favorite breakfast.

• *East Indian:* A stew containing rice, vegetables, and beans might be served with yogurt, cheese, or peanuts. Bread is made from wheat flour, often combined with flour from ground peas or beans.

• *Hmong (Vietnamese):* Rice mixed with green vegetables and small amounts of fish or peanuts is a typical dish from this region. Rice rather than bread is the basic grain and is included in every meal, including breakfast.

• *Traditional American:* A peanut butter sandwich, ready-to-eat cereal with milk, macaroni and cheese, pinto beans and corn bread, and "Hoppin' John" (black-eyed peas and rice) illustrate complementary proteins.

Bibliography

Diabetes Care and Education Practice Group of the American Dietetic Association, Goody CM, Drago L, editors: *Cultural food practices,* Chicago, 2010, American Dietetic Association.
Kittler PG, Sucher KP: *Cultural foods: traditions and trends,* Belmont, CA, 2000, Wadsworth/Thompson Learning.

Stomach

The enzymatic breakdown of protein begins in the stomach. Three components in the gastric secretions initiate this process: (1) **pepsin**, (2) hydrochloric acid, and (3) rennin.

• *Pepsin:* Pepsin is released by the chief cells in the stomach wall as the inactive proenzyme pepsinogen and requires hydrochloric acid to be transformed into the active enzyme pepsin. Pepsin splits the peptide linkages between amino acids, breaking large polypeptides into successively smaller peptides.

• *Hydrochloric acid:* This provides the acid medium needed to convert pepsinogen to pepsin.

• *Rennin:* This enzyme exists only in infancy and childhood. Rennin acts on casein, the major protein in milk, to produce a curd that slows the passage of food out of the infant's stomach.

Small Intestine

Protein digestion is completed in the small intestine assisted by enzymes secreted by the pancreas and glands in the intestinal wall. These include the following:

• Pancreatic secretions:

1. **Trypsin** is secreted as inactive trypsinogen and activated by the hormone enterokinase produced in the wall of the duodenum. Trypsin acts on proteins and large polypeptides to yield smaller polypeptides and dipeptides.

2. **Chymotrypsin** is secreted as chymotrypsinogen and activated by the trypsin already present in the duodenum. Chymotrypsin continues the same protein-splitting action of trypsin.

3. **Carboxypeptidase** attacks the carboxyl (COOH) end of the peptide chain to produce smaller peptides and some free amino acids.

- Intestinal secretions:
  1. Aminopeptidase releases amino acids one at a time from the amino (NH_2) end of the peptide chain to produce smaller short-chain peptides and free amino acids.
  2. Dipeptidase breaks any remaining dipeptides into two free amino acids.

A summary of the steps in protein digestion can be reviewed in Table 2.2.

KEY TERMS

Pepsin
A gastric enzyme that breaks large protein molecules into shorter-chain polypeptides; gastric hydrochloric acid is required to activate pepsin.

Proenzyme
An inactive precursor converted to the active enzyme by the action of an acid or other enzyme.

Trypsin
A pancreatic enzyme secreted into the small intestine that acts on proteins and polypeptides to yield smaller peptides and dipeptides.

Chymotrypsin
A pancreatic enzyme secreted into the small intestine that breaks peptide linkages forming smaller polypeptides and dipeptides.

Carboxypeptidase
A protein-splitting enzyme secreted by the pancreas into the small intestine that splits the peptide bond at the carboxyl (COOH) end of the chain, producing smaller peptide chains and free amino acids.

Aminopeptidase
A protein-splitting enzyme secreted by the intestinal mucosa that releases amino acids one at a time from the amino (NH_2) end of the peptide chain to produce smaller short-chain peptides and free amino acids.

Dipeptidase
Final enzyme in the protein-splitting series that cleaves dipeptides to yield two free amino acids.

Absorption

Amino acids are absorbed by an energy-requiring, sodium-assisted transport system and enter the portal blood for passage to the liver. A few short-chain peptides and smaller intact proteins escape digestion and are absorbed in that form. Most are broken down as they cross the intestinal wall; however, those protein molecules that pass into the blood intact may play a part in the development of immunity and protein sensitivity. We know that antibodies in the mother's colostrum, the first milk secreted after birth, are passed on to her nursing infant. Inadvertent absorption of intact proteins has been implicated in the development of some food allergies.

Metabolism

The construction sites for building tissue proteins are in the cells. Each cell, depending on its nature and function, requires a unique mix of amino acids to build the specific proteins needed. The metabolic activities of protein are interwoven with those of carbohydrate and fat, which provide the energy to drive ongoing tissue growth and repair.

TO SUM UP

The primary function of dietary protein and its constituent amino acids is to build and repair body tissues and form the regulatory proteins that direct important metabolic tasks. Of the 20 amino acids used to build proteins, 9 cannot be synthesized by the body and are referred to as *indispensable* or *essential amino acids;* another 6 cannot be synthesized in adequate amounts under conditions of stress or accelerated growth and are considered *conditionally indispensable*. The remaining five amino acids can be synthesized by the body and are termed the *dispensable* or *nonessential amino acids*. Both indispensable and conditionally indispensable amino acids must be supplied in the diet. Animal proteins are considered complete proteins because they contain all the indispensable amino acids in the amounts and ratios needed for protein synthesis. Plant proteins or incomplete proteins are missing one or more indispensable amino acids or contain less than the amounts needed to make new proteins. Plant proteins can be mixed with animal proteins or with each other to provide the necessary proportions of all amino acids for body growth and maintenance. Certain amino acids such as leucine and glutamate have application in meeting the escalated needs of patients in critical care. Protein requirements are influenced by growth, food protein quality, health status, and the availability of carbohydrate as an energy source. In many countries protein shortages lead to malnutrition with body wasting, stunted growth, chronic infection, and disease. In the United States, overconsumption rather than underconsumption of protein is becoming a problem. Vegetarian food plans emphasizing plant proteins can meet nutrient needs at all stages of the life cycle if well planned. Vegan food plans excluding all animal foods require supplementation or foods fortified with vitamin D and vitamin B_{12} to meet nutritional needs. Well-planned vegetarian diets are appropriate interventions for the treatment of both type 2 diabetes and obesity.

QUESTIONS FOR REVIEW

1. What is the difference between an indispensable, a dispensable, and a conditionally indispensable amino acid? Indicate appropriate food sources of each.
2. What is meant by protein turnover, and how does it relate to nitrogen balance?
3. Distinguish between protein anabolism and protein catabolism. Describe a clinical situation in which protein anabolism exceeds protein catabolism and one in which the opposite is true.
4. Explain the term *protein-sparing effect*. What happens to protein requirements when weight loss diets are inappropriately low in carbohydrate?
5. Visit your local grocery store and find two liquid protein supplements and two snack bars advertised to provide additional protein. Check the nutrition label and make a table that includes (1) the grams of protein per serving, (2) the grams of sugar per serving, and (3) the total kcalories per serving. What proportion of the adult DRIs for protein do these products provide? Compare the kcalories and protein content of these items with the kcalorie and protein content of 8 oz of nonfat milk, 3 oz of chicken breast, and ½ cup of beans. What is the best choice in terms of cost and nutrition. (The nutrient content of common foods can be found on the Evolve website that accompanies your text.)

6. A pediatrician told a vegan couple that their 2-year-old daughter was falling behind in her growth rate. What dietary factors are likely related to her poor growth? Plan 1 day of meals for this child, indicating food amounts that would meet her protein and energy needs and respect the vegan food pattern. Visit the web site of the Center for Nutrition Policy and Promotion at https://www.cnpp.usda.gov/USDAFoodPatterns for vegetarian/vegan meal patterns and tables of calorie needs. Note that patterns at 1000-, 1200-, and 1400-calorie levels meet the nutritional needs of children ages 2 to 8 years.

7. Protein intakes 2 to 3 times the RDA are not uncommon in the United States. Using the food values found on the Evolve website that accompanies your textbook, calculate the energy value and the number of grams of protein in a fast food meal that includes one double-patty cheeseburger, a large serving of French fries, and a 12-oz milkshake. Compare the total grams of protein and the total kcalories with the protein and energy DRIs for a 16-year-old boy. What proportion of his daily protein and energy needs are provided in this meal?

8. You have a patient who is using calcium-containing antacids to supplement her calcium intake. How might this influence her use of dietary protein?

REFERENCES

1. Institute of Medicine: *Dietary Reference Intakes for energy, carbohydrate, fiber, fat, fatty acids, cholesterol, protein, and amino acids (macronutrients)*, Washington, DC, 2002, National Academies Press.
2. Guyton AC, Hall JE: *Textbook of medical physiology*, ed 10, Philadelphia, 2000, Saunders.
3. Timiras PS: *Physiological basis of aging and geriatrics*, ed 4, New York, 2007, Taylor & Francis.
4. Jonker R, Engelen MPK, Deutz NEP: Role of specific dietary amino acids in clinical conditions, *Br J Nutr* 108(Suppl 2):S139, 2012.
5. Bollhalder L, Pfeil AM, Tomonaga Y, et al: A systematic literature review and meta-analysis of randomized clinical trials of parenteral glutamine supplementation, *Clin Nutr* 32:213, 2013.
6. Bender DA: The metabolism of "surplus" amino acids, *Br J Nutr* 108(Suppl 2):S113, 2012.
7. Weijs PJM, Cynober L, DeLegge M, et al: Proteins and amino acids are fundamental to optimal nutrition support in critically ill patients, *Crit Care* 18:591, 2014.
8. Ferrie S, Allman-Farinelli M: Commonly used "nutrition" indicators do not predict outcome in the critically ill: a systematic review, *Nutr Clin Pract* 28(4):463, 2013.
9. Tome D: Criteria and markers for protein quality assessment – a review, *Br J Nutr* 108(Suppl 2):S222, 2012.
10. Melina V, Craig W, Levin S, Academy of Nutrition and Dietetics: Position of the Academy of Nutrition and Dietetics: vegetarian diets, *J Acad Nutr Diet* 116:1970, 2016.
11. Messina V: Nutritional and health benefits of dried beans, *Am J Clin Nutr* 100(Suppl 1):S437, 2014.
12. Rutherfurd SM, Moughan PJ: Available versus digestible dietary amino acids, *Br J Nutr* 108(Suppl 2):S298, 2012.
13. Hoffer LJ: Protein requirement in critical illness, *Appl Physiol Nutr Metab* 41:573, 2016.
14. McClave SA, Taylor BE, Martindale RG, et al: Guidelines for the provision and assessment of nutrition support therapy in the adult critically ill patient: Society of Critical Care Medicine (SCCM) and American Society for Parenteral and Enteral Nutrition (A.S.P.E.N), *JPEN* 40(2):159, 2016.
15. Galvan E, Arentson-Lantz E, Lamon S, et al: Protecting skeletal muscle with protein and amino acid during periods of disuse, *Nutrients* 8:404, 2016.
16. Arentson-Lantz E, Clairmont S, Paddon-Jones D, et al: Protein: a nutrient in focus, *Appl Physiol Nutr Metab* 40:755, 2015.
17. Paddon-Jones D, Campbell WW, Jacques PF, et al: Protein and healthy aging, *Am J Clin Nutr* 101(Suppl 6):S1339, 2015.
18. Pencharz PB, Elango R, Ball RO: Determination of the tolerable upper intake level of leucine in adult men, *J Nutr* 142:2220S, 2012.
19. Bhutta ZA, Salam RA: Global nutrition epidemiology and trends, *Ann Nutr Metab* 61(Suppl 1):19, 2012.
20. Berner LA, Becker G, Wise M, et al: Characterization of dietary protein among older adults in the United States: amount, animal sources, and meal patterns, *J Acad Nutr Diet* 113:809, 2013.
21. Rizzo NS, Jaceldo-Siegl K, Sabate J, et al: Nutrient profiles of vegetarian and nonvegetarian dietary patterns, *J Acad Nutr Diet* 113:1610, 2013.
22. US Department of Agriculture, Agricultural Research Service: Table 1. Nutrient Intakes from Food and Beverages: Mean Amounts Consumed per Individual by Gender and Age in the United States. *What We Eat in America*, NHANES 2013-2014, 2016. http://www.ars.usda.gov/nea/bhnrc/fsrg.
23. Leidy HJ, Clifton PM, Astrup A, et al: The role of protein in weight loss and maintenance, *Am J Clin Nutr* 101(Suppl 6):1320S, 2015.
24. Astrup A, Raben A, Geiker N: The role of higher protein diets in weight control and obesity-related comorbidities, *Int J Obes* 39:721, 2015.
25. Bray GA, Siri-Tarino PW: The role of macronutrient content in the diet for weight management, *Endocrinol Metab Clin North Am* 45:581, 2016.
26. Dhillon J, Craig BA, Leidy HJ, et al: The effects of increased protein intake on fullness: a meta-analysis and its limitations, *J Acad Nutr Diet* 116:968, 2016.
27. Juraschek SP, Appel LJ, Anderson CAM, et al: Effect of a high-protein diet on kidney function in healthy adults: results from the OmniHeart Trial, *Am J Kidney Dis* 61(4):547, 2013.
28. McCullough ML, Peterson JJ, Patel R, et al: Flavonoid intake and cardiovascular disease mortality in a prospective cohort of US adults, *Am J Clin Nutr* 95:454, 2012.
29. Jenkins DJ, Kendall CW, Augustin LS, et al: Effect of legumes as part of a low glycemic index diet on glycemic control and cardiovascular risk factors in type 2 diabetes mellitus: a randomized controlled trial, *Arch Intern Med* 172(21):1653–1660, 2012.
30. US Department of Agriculture, Agricultural Research Service: September 2015 with slight revision May 2016. USDA National Nutrient Database for Standard Reference, Release 28. Nutrient Data Laboratory Home Page. https://ndb.nal.usda.gov/ndb/.
31. US Department of Health and Human Services and US Department of Agriculture: *2015-2020 Dietary Guidelines for Americans*, ed 8, December 2015.
32. Timko CA, Hormes JM, Chubski J: Will the real vegetarian please stand up? An investigation of dietary restraint and eating disorder symptoms in vegetarians versus non-vegetarians, *Appetite* 58:982, 2012.
33. Nelson ME, Hamm MW, Hu FB, et al: Alignment of healthy dietary patterns and environmental sustainability: a systematic review, *Adv Nutr* 7:1005, 2016.
34. Farmer B, Larson BT, Fulgoni VL, et al: A vegetarian dietary pattern as a nutrient-dense approach to weight management: an analysis of the National Health and Nutrition Examination Survey 1999-2004, *J Am Diet Assoc* 111:819, 2011.
35. Schösler H, de Boer J, Boersema JJ: Can we cut out the meat of the dish? Constructing consumer-oriented pathways towards meat substitution, *Appetite* 58:39, 2012.
36. Le LT, Sabaté J: Beyond meatless, the health effect of vegan diets: findings from the Adventist cohorts, *Nutrients* 6:2131, 2014.

FURTHER READINGS AND RESOURCES

Readings

Academy of Nutrition and Dietetics: Position of the Academy of Nutrition and Dietetics: vegetarian diets, *J Acad Nutr Diet* 116:1970, 2016.

US Department of Health and Human Services, US Department of Agriculture: *2015–2020 Dietary Guidelines for Americans,* ed 8, December 2015. https://health.gov/dietaryguidelines/2015/resources.asp.
[These materials provide a vegetarian food guide that will meet nutritional requirements and describe the adequacy of vegetarian and vegan food plans.]
Beasley JM, Shikany JM, Thomson CA: The role of dietary protein intake in the prevention of sarcopenia of aging, *Nutr Clin Pract* 28(6):684, 2013.
[This article describes the importance of protein in preventing muscle loss in older adults that results in disability and loss of independence.]
Pasiakos SM, Lieberman HR, Fulgoni VL: Higher-protein diets are associated with higher HDL cholesterol and lower BMI and waist circumference in US adults, *J Nutr* 145:605, 2015.
[These researchers discuss a possible connection between dietary protein intake and chronic disease.]

Websites of Interest

- National Institutes of Health, National Library of Medicine: *Medline Plus: Trusted Health Information for You.* This site provides links to many resources on protein needs throughout the life cycle. http://www.nlm.nih.gov/medlineplus/dietaryproteins.html; and information on vegetarianism including planning healthy diets, dangers of inadequate diets, and sources of problem nutrients. http://www.nlm.nih.gov/medlineplus/vegetariandiet.html; information is provided in English and Spanish.
- US Department of Agriculture: *MyPlate.* This site provides many resources on both animal and vegetable proteins. Go to https://www.choosemyplate.gov and search for proteins to obtain a comprehensive list of materials that can be downloaded for nutrition education.

6

Vitamins

Eleanor D. Schlenker

http://evolve.elsevier.com/Williams/essentials/

Here we begin our study of the non–energy-yielding micronutrients: vitamins and minerals. First, we look at the vitamins: why we need them and how we obtain them. No other group of nutritional components has so captured the interest of scientists, health professionals, and the general public as the vitamins. Researchers are discovering new roles for vitamins in preventing chronic disease that exceed their known functions as nutrients. Consumers are being bombarded with opinions about vitamin needs that run the gamut from wise and thoughtful use to wild, flagrant abuse. Health professionals are trying to learn more about functional foods and the vitamin-like substances they contain and how these substances interact with known vitamins. In time we may identify new vitamins essential to human health.

OUTLINE

VITAMINS: ESSENTIAL NUTRIENTS

General Nature

Most of the vitamins we know about nowadays were discovered between 1900 and 1950. The name *vitamin* was adopted when one of the scientists working with a nitrogen-containing substance called an **amine** named his discovery *vitamine* ("vital amine"), thinking this was the common nature of all vitamins. At first, a letter designation was given to each new vitamin; however, as the number grew, this became confusing, and scientific names based on the structure or function of the vitamin were developed. Letter designations have been retained for the fat-soluble vitamins because for each of these vitamins a number of closely related compounds have similar metabolic activities and structures.

KEY TERM

Amine
An organic compound containing nitrogen. Amino acids and pyridoxine (vitamin B_6) are examples of amines.

What Is a Vitamin?

To be classified as a vitamin, a compound has to meet several criteria:
- It must be an organic dietary substance that is not energy producing, as are carbohydrate, fat, and protein.
- It is needed in very small quantities to perform a particular metabolic function and prevent an identified deficiency disease.
- It cannot be synthesized by the body, so it must be supplied in food.

These principles form the basis for establishing that a vitamin is essential. However, for each vitamin we must define the specific requirements for each age and gender and determine how those needs can be met from the available food supply.

Basic Principles

Over the years we have learned more about individual vitamins and how they interact with each other and with other nutrients in carrying out their work. The following principles will guide our study of these nutrients:
- *Individual vitamins are multifunctional:* Most vitamins have multiple roles or actions in the body, sometimes working independently and sometimes working cooperatively with other nutrients. For

example, although we associate vitamin A with its major role of helping us see in dim light, this vitamin also maintains the mucous membranes in the nasal passages that protect against infection.

- *One vitamin cannot substitute for another vitamin:* All vitamins must be available in sufficient amounts for the body to function normally and for tissues to remain healthy. For example, an abundant supply of vitamin C cannot take the place of folate in preventing a neural tube defect (NTD).
- *Vitamins work together in carrying out body functions:* The formation and maturation of red blood cells require the actions of folate, pyridoxine, vitamin B_{12}, and ascorbic acid, along with several important minerals.
- *Vitamins function best when all are present in the appropriate proportions:* High-potency vitamin A supplements interfere with the action of vitamin D, decreasing calcium absorption and increasing the risk of hip fracture.

These functional truths underscore the importance of eating a variety of foods to obtain essential vitamins and the other important substances that contribute to health.

Classification

As the vitamins were discovered, they were grouped according to their solubility in fats or water, and this system has continued (Box 6.1).

Fat-Soluble Vitamins

The fat-soluble vitamins are A, D, E, and K. They are closely associated with body lipids and are easily stored. Their functions are usually related to structural activities with proteins.

Water-Soluble Vitamins

The water-soluble vitamins are vitamin C and the B-complex family. These vitamins are more easily absorbed and transported, but, unlike the fat-soluble vitamins, they cannot be stored except in the general sense of tissue saturation. The B vitamins function mainly as coenzyme factors in cell metabolism. Vitamin C works with enzymes that support tissue building and maintenance.

Current Knowledge and Key Questions

In our study we will answer the following questions for each vitamin:
- *Chemical and physical nature:* What is the general structure of the vitamin?

- *Absorption, transport, and storage:* How does the body handle this particular vitamin?
- *Function:* What does this vitamin do?
- *Related deficiency symptoms or disease:* What happens when this vitamin is absent or not available in sufficient amounts?
- *Clinical role in health:* Does this vitamin prevent or ameliorate a chronic health problem?
- *Recommended intake and possible toxicity:* How much of this vitamin do we need, and how much is too much? What are the consequences of excessive intake? See Chapter 1 to review the Dietary Reference Intakes (DRIs).
- *Food sources:* How do we obtain this vitamin?

In the following sections we discuss the four fat-soluble vitamins and the nine water-soluble vitamins.

FAT-SOLUBLE VITAMINS

VITAMIN A

Chemical and Physical Nature

Vitamin A is the generic name for a group of compounds with similar biologic activity: retinol, retinal, and retinoic acid. The term *retinoids* refers to the natural forms of vitamin A and its synthetic copies. Retinol, an alcohol of high molecular weight ($C_{20}H_{29}OH$), was given its name based on its specific function in the retina of the eye. It is soluble in fat and fat solvents. Because retinol is insoluble in water, it is fairly stable in cooking.

Forms

There are two dietary forms of vitamin A: (1) preformed vitamin A and (2) provitamin A (Box 6.2):
1. *Preformed vitamin A (retinol):* This is the natural form of vitamin A found only in animal foods and usually associated with fat. Vitamin A is stored mostly in the liver but also in small amounts in the kidneys, lungs, and adipose tissue, so organ meats are a rich source. Other dietary sources are the fat portion of dairy foods, egg yolk, and fish.
2. *Provitamin A or β-carotene:* Plants cannot synthesize vitamin A, but instead produce a family of compounds called carotenoids. These substances in plants are eaten by animals and then converted to vitamin A. Thus humans can obtain their vitamin A directly by eating animal foods or by converting carotenoids obtained from plant foods. The carotenoids were so named because β-carotene ($C_{40}H_{56}$) was found in the yellow and orange pigment in carrots and other vegetables and fruits. Examples of other carotenoids found in plant foods include β-cryptoxanthin, lutein, and zeaxanthin, but not all of these can be converted to vitamin A.

   The carotenoids have an important role in human nutrition. β-carotene and other carotenoids converted to vitamin A in the body provide 37% of the total vitamin A intake in the United States.[1] Enzymes found in the mucosal cells of the small intestine and in the liver split the carotenoid molecule to yield retinol. The yellow and red carotenoid pigments in many fruits and vegetables and in red palm oil are the major food sources of vitamin A in most developing countries. Unfortunately, the conversion of carotenoids to retinol is much less efficient than we thought (Table 6.1), raising concerns as to whether plant foods can provide an adequate supply of vitamin A when animal foods are scarce.[2]

BOX 6.1 Classification of Vitamins

Fat-Soluble Vitamins
- A
- D
- E
- K

Water-Soluble Vitamins
- Vitamin C (ascorbic acid)
- Thiamin
- Riboflavin
- Niacin
- Pantothenic acid
- Biotin
- Vitamin B_6 (pyridoxine)
- Folate
- Vitamin B_{12} (cobalamin)

BOX 6.2 Sources of Preformed and Provitamin A

Preformed Vitamin A
Reduced-fat milk
Cheese
Egg yolk
Liver

Provitamin A
Broccoli
Carrots
Spinach
Cantaloupe
Tomato juice
Apricots

Images copyright 2006 JupiterImages Corporation.

TABLE 6.1 Conversion of Carotenoids to Vitamin A

Amount Consumed	Amount Available to the Body
1 mcg retinol	1 mcg retinol
12 mcg β carotene	1 mcg retinol
24 mcg α carotene or β cryptoxanthin	1 mcg retinol

NOTE: Although many carotenoids can be converted to retinol (vitamin A) to help meet body needs, greater amounts of the carotenoids are required to produce one retinol of vitamin A.

Absorption, Transport, and Storage

Substances Needed for Absorption

Whether vitamin A enters the body as preformed vitamin A or as the **precursor** β-carotene, various materials are needed for its absorption, as follows:

- *Bile salts:* Vitamin A joins with fat, other fat-related compounds, and bile salts in the small intestine to form **micelles**, a bile-lipid complex. Bile salts are necessary for carrying fats and fat-soluble materials into the intestinal wall for further breakdown. Clinical conditions affecting the biliary system such as a bile duct obstruction, infectious hepatitis, or liver cirrhosis that interfere with production or release of bile salts hinder vitamin A absorption.
- *Pancreatic lipase:* This fat-splitting enzyme released into the upper small intestine carries out the hydrolysis of fat emulsions containing vitamin A. Water-based preparations of retinol are used when lipase secretion and absorption of fat is curtailed, as in cystic fibrosis or pancreatitis.[3]
- *Dietary fat:* Absorption of vitamin A and provitamin A requires the presence of fat to stimulate the release of bile salts and form micelles. At least 3 to 5 g of fat at the same meal is needed to absorb provitamin A.[3]

Age is a factor in absorption. Newborns, especially premature infants, absorb vitamin A poorly. Persons using mineral oil as a laxative reduce their absorption of vitamin A.

KEY TERMS

Coenzyme
A substance that partners with a cell enzyme in carrying out a chemical reaction; vitamins are important coenzymes in energy, lipid, and protein metabolism.

Retinol
Chemical name for vitamin A derived from its function in the retina of the eye producing light-dark adaptation.

Retinal
The aldehyde form of retinol (vitamin A) derived from the splitting of β-carotene in the intestinal wall. In the retina, retinal combines with opsin to form visual pigments.

Carotenoids
A group of yellow-red-orange pigments widely distributed in plants that act as antioxidants and may have additional health-promoting properties; some carotenoids such as β-carotene can be converted to retinal in the intestinal wall.

Precursor
A substance from which another substance is derived.

Micelles
Complex of bile and fat that carries fat into the intestinal wall in preparation for the final stage of absorption into the lymph and general circulation.

Conversion of Beta Carotene

β-Carotene can be absorbed and used by the body in its original form or be converted to vitamin A. Although at one time we believed that carotenoids were biologically important only as precursors to vitamin A, we have since learned that as members of that broad category of phytochemicals active in functional foods, they have roles in human health over and above the actions of vitamin A. (To learn about the importance of obtaining needed vitamins and phytochemicals from food rather than depending on supplements, see the Evidence-Based Practice box, "Best Sources of Phytochemicals: Food or Supplements?")

EVIDENCE-BASED PRACTICE

Best Sources of Phytochemicals: Food or Supplements?

Identify the problem: The physiologic functions of phytochemicals such as the carotenoids, associated with the colored pigments in fruits and vegetables, are poorly understood. Because the general public is paying closer attention to nutrition and its relation to lifelong health, several of the better-known carotenoids, such as lycopene, have been isolated from their natural sources and are being marketed in supplement form. However, will we receive the same benefit if we shop in the supplement section and forget about eating fruits and vegetables?

Review the evidence: Comparisons of the effects of vitamin and phytochemical supplements or fruit and vegetable intake on chronic disease and mortality found that individuals who ate more daily servings of fruits and vegetables experienced fewer heart attacks or strokes than those with fewer daily servings; supplements were not effective in lowering the incidence of these conditions. Components of the flavonoid family of phytochemicals when consumed in food decreased the risk of stroke in a multiethnic population in the southern United States.

Implement the findings: Scientists have speculated as to why these dietary components are best consumed in their food form to convey their important benefits. One reason could be that fruits, vegetables, and other plant sources contain a mixture of these chemical substances that must work together to bring about their effects on health. To achieve this important **synergy**, they may need to be present in the natural combinations found in a food or in several phytochemical-containing foods eaten at the same time. In contrast to the DRIs developed for the essential vitamins, we have no guidelines as to the amounts of each phytochemical that is required or could lead to toxicity. Studies comparing cardiovascular risk in adults according to their flavonoid intake from fruits and vegetables found the maximum benefit occurred at intakes of 3½ to 5 servings per day. Additional servings, although providing greater amounts of important vitamins and minerals, did not add more months to life. On the other hand, no fruit servings and fewer than three vegetable servings per day reduced the life span by nearly 3 years. This would suggest that just a small amount of these important substances found in fruits and vegetables can make a big difference in life and health, and concentrated amounts contained in supplements may overestimate body needs. Fruits and vegetables also add variety and taste to our meals, features that pills cannot deliver. Encourage your patients to head to the fruit and vegetable sections of their local grocery stores or, better yet, start a garden and grow their own.

Bibliography

Bellavia A, Larsson SC, Bottai M, et al: Fruit and vegetable consumption and all-cause mortality: a dose-response analysis, *Am J Clin Nutr* 98:454, 2013.

Egert S, Rimbach G: Which sources of flavonoids: complex diets or dietary supplements? *Adv Nutr* 2:8, 2011.

Goetz ME, Judd SE, Safford MM, et al: Dietary flavonoid intake and incident coronary heart disease: the reasons for geographic and racial differences in stroke (REGARDS) study, *Am J Clin Nutr* 104:1236, 2016.

Liu RH: Health-promoting components of fruits and vegetables in the diet, *Adv Nutr* 4:S384, 2013.

McCullough ML, Peterson JJ, Patel R, et al: Flavonoid intake and cardiovascular disease mortality in a prospective cohort of US adults, *Am J Clin Nutr* 95:454, 2012.

Transport and Storage

The route of absorption of vitamin A and the carotenoids parallels that of fat. In the intestinal mucosa, retinol—whether from preformed animal sources or converted from carotenes—along with intact plant carotenoids are incorporated into the chylomicrons. In this form, they enter the bloodstream via the lymphatic system and are carried to the liver for storage or distribution to tissues. Vitamin A is transported to body tissues by special retinol-binding proteins.

The liver is an efficient storage organ for vitamin A, containing up to 80% of the body's total supply. Liver stores are usually sufficient to prevent deficiency for 6 to 12 months and in some individuals for as long as 4 years. The capacity of the liver to store substantial amounts of vitamin A has special significance in parts of the world where vitamin A–containing foods are in short supply, because prophylactic doses administered occasionally through government programs can prevent blindness, reduce mortality, and support normal growth in infants and young children.[4]

Functions of Vitamin A

The role of vitamin A in vision is best known, but vitamin A also influences the integrity of body coverings and linings (epithelial tissues), cell division and differentiation, growth, immunity, and reproductive function.

Vitamin A Deficiency and Clinical Applications

Vision

The ability of the eye to adapt to changes in light depends on the light-sensitive pigment, rhodopsin, located in the rods of the retina. Rhodopsin—commonly known as *visual purple*—is made up of the vitamin A molecule retinal and the protein opsin (Fig. 6.1). When vitamin A is lacking, normal rhodopsin cannot be formed and the rods and cones of the retina become increasingly sensitive to changes in light, causing **night blindness**. This condition is reversed with an injection of vitamin A (retinol), which is readily converted to retinal and then rhodopsin.

Cell Differentiation

This vitamin also controls the differentiation of cells, or in other words, the formation of specialized cells from basic stem cells. Vitamin A is needed to develop and maintain healthy epithelial tissue, which provides our primary barrier to infection. The epithelium includes both the outer skin and the mucous membranes that line many body structures. Without vitamin A, the cells formed are dry and flat rather than soft and moist. These dry, flat cells gradually harden to form keratin, a process called **keratinization**. Keratin is a protein that creates dry, scaly tissue, normal for nails and hair but abnormal for skin and mucous membranes. In vitamin A deficiency, such abnormal tissue changes occur in many body systems, as follows:

- *Eye:* The cornea dries and hardens, a condition called *xerophthalmia* (Fig. 6.2). The tear ducts become dry, robbing the eye of its cleansing and lubricating fluid, and infection follows quickly. In extreme deficiency the keratinization progresses to blindness. Blindness caused by vitamin A deficiency is a world public health problem, and mortality is higher among children with even mild xerophthalmia.[4]
- *Respiratory tract:* The epithelium lining the nasal passages becomes dry and the cilia are lost, removing a barrier to infectious organisms.

FIG. 6.1 The vision cycle: light-dark adaptation role of vitamin A.

FIG. 6.2 Xerophthalmia resulting from vitamin A deficiency and a leading cause of blindness in the developing world. (From McLaren DS: *A colour atlas and text of diet-related disorders*, ed 2, London, 1992, Mosby-Year Book Europe Limited.)

FIG. 6.3 Follicular hyperkeratosis resulting from vitamin A deficiency. (From McLaren DS: *A colour atlas and text of diet-related disorders*, ed 2, London, 1992, Mosby-Year Book Europe Limited.)

KEY TERMS

Synergy
Situation when the combined actions of several agents is greater than the sum of their individual actions.

Night Blindness
Inability to see well in dim light because of vitamin A deficiency.

Keratinization
The process of creating the protein keratin, a principal component of skin, hair, nails, and the matrix forming tooth enamel.

Nasal secretions that trap invading particles and remove them from the body are no longer produced.

- *Gastrointestinal tract:* Salivary fluids are no longer secreted, and the mouth becomes dry and cracked, open to invading bacteria. The esophagus becomes red and inflamed. Mucosal secretions decrease throughout the digestive tract, and tissues dry and slough off, lowering the absorption of nutrients that are available.
- *Genitourinary tract:* When epithelial tissue begins to break down, vaginal infections and urinary tract infections ensue.
- *Skin:* As skin becomes dry and scaly, small pustules (hardened, pigmented, papular eruptions) appear around hair follicles, a condition known as *follicular hyperkeratosis* (Fig. 6.3).
- *Tooth formation:* Certain epithelial cells surrounding tooth buds in fetal gum tissue that normally become specialized cup-shaped organs called *ameloblasts* do not develop properly. These little organs form the enamel of the developing tooth.

Growth

Vitamin A is essential for the growth of bones and soft tissues because it controls protein synthesis and cell division and stabilizes cell membranes. The growth and maintenance of bone require constant remodeling, reshaping, and expansion. Vitamin A participates in the important job of tunneling out old bone to make way for new bone. Then the tunnels are filled in to accommodate growth according to the embryonic cartilage model. Although an inadequate supply of vitamin A is detrimental to bone health, so are excessive intakes that cause old bone to be lost more rapidly than new bone can be formed. Intakes of preformed vitamin A exceeding the DRI can result in lower bone mass and increased risk of hip fracture; however, β-carotene and other precursors of vitamin A supplied in fruits and vegetables do not

lead to excessive body levels of vitamin A or bone loss. Based on its role in cell growth and differentiation, vitamin A is an important nutrient in the treatment of protein-energy malnutrition (PEM).

Reproduction

Vitamin A is required for normal sexual maturation and function. It participates in gene expression and plays an important role in fetal growth, including development of the central nervous system (CNS).[3] A sufficient intake is required for successful lactation.

Immunity

Poor vitamin A status lowers resistance to infection in two ways: (1) changes in epithelial and mucosal tissues allow disease organisms to enter the body more easily, and (2) vitamin A has a direct effect on immune function. Both cell-mediated and antibody-mediated immunity are impaired when intake is low, as is the effectiveness of the gastrointestinal mucosal barrier. Measles is more likely to be fatal in vitamin A–deficient children in developing countries. Immune response returns to normal when vitamin A is restored.[4]

Vitamin A Requirement
Influencing Factors

A number of variables modify the vitamin A needs of a given individual, as follows:

- *Liver stores:* High vitamin A stores can supply body needs for an extended period; those with low body stores depend on day-to-day intakes.
- *Intake of preformed versus provitamin A:* Increased amounts of carotenoids are required to meet the DRI for vitamin A.
- *Illness and infection:* Needs increase to support the production of immune cells and body defenses.
- *Gastrointestinal or hepatic defects:* Gallbladder or liver disease interfering with production of bile salts limits fat absorption and in turn the absorption of vitamin A and carotenoids.

Causes of Vitamin A Deficiency

In the United States the primary cause of vitamin A deficiency is inadequate dietary intake, often the result of poor food selection rather than unavailability. Vitamin A deficiency also results from poor absorption, inadequate conversion of β-carotene, or liver or intestinal disease. A high intake of alcohol brings about loss of vitamin A from the liver even if liver function remains normal.[3] Individuals who malabsorb fat can develop vitamin A deficiency.

Dietary Reference Intake

The Recommended Dietary Allowance (RDA) for vitamin A is the amount required to maintain optimal liver stores. It is based on micrograms (mcg) of retinol,[3] and the term retinol activity equivalent (RAE) takes into account the ratios for converting carotenoids to vitamin A. Early on, vitamin A was measured in international units (IU), and some food composition tables still use those units. Many older tables overestimate the amount of vitamin A available from carotenoid-containing foods, such that intakes are calculated to be greater than is true. The RDA for men ages 19 and older is set at 900 mcg RAE and the RDA for women of this age is 700 mcg RAE. To ensure sufficient vitamin A to support a successful pregnancy and appropriate vitamin A content in breast milk, the RDA increases in pregnancy and in lactation.

The Advisory Committee Report accompanying the 2015 Dietary Goals noted that vitamin A was a problem nutrient for the American public because almost half of adults ages 19 and older are taking in less than 67% of their RDA.[1] Fast food meals can influence vitamin A status because meals that include a hamburger or chicken sandwich with fries and a sweetened beverage contain only approximately 25 mcg RAE. Choosing milk as a beverage would add approximately 150 mcg of vitamin A to this meal.[5]

KEY TERM

Retinol Activity Equivalent (RAE)
Unit of measure for dietary sources of vitamin A, including preformed retinol and the provitamins β-carotene, α-carotene, and β-cryptoxanthin.

Vitamin A Toxicity
Hypervitaminosis A

Because the liver can store very large amounts of vitamin A, persons taking high-potency supplements over months or years that exceed the Tolerable Upper Intake Level (UL) can develop toxicity. Impaired vision, gastrointestinal disturbances, and skin abnormalities are evident in both vitamin A deficiency and excess, although expressed in different ways. Daily intakes greater than the UL of 3000 mcg of preformed vitamin A are especially dangerous for pregnant women and can result in congenital malformations, depending on intake.[3] Teens and young adults prescribed acne medications such as isotretinoin (Accutane), which are nonnutritive sources of vitamin A, need to talk with their doctor when contemplating pregnancy. Excessive use of vitamin supplements combined with highly fortified food items can bring children and adults dangerously close to the UL of 3000 mcg.

Food Sources of Vitamin A

Animal sources of preformed vitamin A include liver, milk, cheese, butter, egg yolk, and fish. Reduced-fat, low-fat, and fat-free milk, as well as certain soy and rice milks, are fortified with vitamin A to the level found in whole milk. Nonanimal products such as margarine, ready-to-eat cereals, and cereal bars are often fortified with vitamin A. Dark-yellow, orange, red, and green vegetables and fruits contain a variety of carotenoids and help meet the vitamin A requirement. Cooked vegetables can be better dietary sources of carotenoids than raw vegetables because cooking helps release these substances from their plant component, making them more available for absorption. The vitamin A content of various foods is listed in Box 6.3.

BOX 6.3 Food Sources of Vitamin A

Food Source	Quantity	Vitamin A (mcg RAE)
Grains Group		
Fortified Ready-to-Eat Cereals		
Instant oatmeal (plain)	1 packet	216
Special K	1 cup	155
Cheerios	1 cup	277
Wheaties	¾ cup	199
Vegetable Group		
Sweet potato, baked in skin	1 medium	1096
Pumpkin, canned	½ cup	953
Spinach, leaf, frozen, cooked	½ cup	573
Collard greens, frozen, cooked	½ cup	489
Carrot, raw	1 medium (7½ inches)	601
Chinese cabbage (bok choy), cooked	1 cup	360
Lettuce, dark green	1 cup	205
Peppers, red, sweet, chopped	½ cup	117
Broccoli, frozen, cooked	½ cup	94
Brussels sprouts, frozen, cooked	1 cup	71
Fruit Group		
Cantaloupe	⅛ melon	117
Apricots, canned in juice	½ cup	104
Watermelon	1 wedge (4 × 8 inches)	80

Continued

BOX 6.3   Food Sources of Vitamin A—cont'd

Food Source	Quantity	Vitamin A (mcg RAE)
Meat, Beans, Eggs, and Nuts Group		
Chicken livers, cooked	1	1752
Clams, canned	3 oz	127
Milk Group		
Milk, nonfat, fortified	1 cup	149
Milk, 1% milk fat, fortified	1 cup	142
Milk, whole, 3.5% fat, unfortified	1 cup	112
Soy milk, unfortified	1 cup	00
Cheddar cheese	1 oz	74
Fats, Oils, and Sugar		
Margarine, tub	1 tbsp	116
Butter	1 tbsp	97

Recommended Dietary Allowances for adults: women, 700 mcg RAE; men, 900 mcg RAE. 1 RAE (retinol activity equivalent) = 1 mcg retinol. Images copyright 2006 JupiterImages Corporation. Data from US Department of Agriculture, Agricultural Research Service: *USDA National Nutrient Database for Standard Reference, Release 28*, revised May 2016. Nutrient Data Laboratory Home Page: https://www.ars.usda.gov/northeast-area/beltsville-md/beltsville-human-nutrition-research-center/nutrient-data-laboratory/docs/usda-national-nutrient-database-for-standard-reference/.

🌐 FOCUS ON CULTURE

Acculturation: Does It Affect Food Patterns?

The term *acculturation* refers to the adoption of local customs and practices by families entering a new country. Dietary acculturation can be associated with healthy or unhealthy dietary changes, and such changes influence disease risk. Acculturation is multidimensional and influenced by generation status, favorite language, age at immigration, and years of residence, and these criteria are useful in evaluating degree of acculturation.[1] The diet of many Latinos who take up residence in the United States decreases over time in their use of fruits and vegetables, including beans, lowering their intakes of fiber, provitamin A, ascorbic acid, and the B-complex vitamins. When defined by language preference, both first- and second-generation Mexican-American women who preferred Spanish to English had higher intakes of healthy foods overall.[2] When defined by nativity, low-income Hispanic women born in the United States used fewer orange-colored vegetables as compared to their counterparts born elsewhere.[3]

Changes in food patterns may proceed more slowly when language holds ties to a native culture. Health professionals working with populations new to a host country must recognize the role of language and nativity in the acculturation process.

References

1. Park S, Blanck HM, Dooyema CA, et al: Association between sugar-sweetened beverage intake and proxies of acculturation among US Hispanic and non-Hispanic white adults, *Am J Health Promot* 30(5):357, 2016.
2. Reininger B, Lee M, Jennings R, et al: Healthy eating patterns associated with acculturation, sex and BMI among Mexican Americans, *Public Health Nutr* 20(7):1267–1278, 2017. doi:10.1017/S1368980016003311.
3. Di Noia J, Monica D, Cullen KW, et al: Differences in fruit and vegetable intake by race/ethnicity and by Hispanic origin and nativity among women in the Special Supplemental Nutrition Program for Women, Infants, and Children, 2015, *Prev Chronic Dis* 13:E115, 2016.

(The Focus on Culture box, "Acculturation: How Does It Affect Food Patterns?" points to problems with low intakes of fruits and vegetables among families immigrating to the United States.)

VITAMIN D

Chemical and Physical Nature

When first discovered, vitamin D was classified as a vitamin, although it is now clear that vitamin D is actually a prohormone and in its active form functions as a hormone. Chemically, vitamin D is a sterol and its precursor found in human skin is the lipid molecule 7-dehydrocholesterol. All compounds with vitamin D activity are soluble in fat but not water, and they are heat stable.

Forms

The body uses two forms of vitamin D: (1) ergocalciferol (vitamin D_2) and (2) cholecalciferol (vitamin D_3). Vitamin D_2 is formed by irradiating ergosterol found in ergot (a fungus growing on rye and other cereal grains) and yeast. The more important form is vitamin D_3, made by the action of ultraviolet light from the sun on the 7-dehydrocholesterol in the skin and found naturally in fish liver oils. Vitamin D_3 is also the form used in the fortification of milk and other dairy products, cereals, and juice.

KEY TERMS

Prohormone
A substance that when converted to its active form acts as a hormone; vitamin D obtained from food or synthesized in the skin is a prohormone, and its active hormonal form is called calcitriol.

7-Dehydrocholesterol
A precursor cholesterol compound in the skin that when irradiated by sunlight produces cholecalciferol (D_3).

Absorption, Transport, and Storage

Absorption

Vitamin D is absorbed in the small intestine as part of the micelles, as are all fat-soluble vitamins. Conditions associated with malabsorption, such as celiac disease, cystic fibrosis, Crohn disease, or pancreatic insufficiency, hinder vitamin D absorption.

Active Hormone Synthesis

The active hormone form of vitamin D is 1,25-dihydroxycholecalciferol [1,25$(OH)_2D_3$], with the chemical name calcitriol. Calcitriol is produced by the combined action of the skin, liver, and kidneys, an overall process referred to as the *vitamin D endocrine system*.

We will look at each of the following three steps in this process (Fig. 6.4):

1. *Skin:* When 7-dehydrocholesterol, the vitamin D precursor in the skin, is exposed to the ultraviolet rays of the sun, it is converted into vitamin D_3. The amount produced depends on the length and intensity of sun exposure and skin pigment. For many living in northern climates, sun exposure is not sufficient to supply all

of their vitamin D needs, especially in the winter months. People who are confined indoors and those residing in crowded city areas with high air pollution do not receive adequate ultraviolet exposure to synthesize vitamin D. Dark skin pigment prevents ultraviolet rays from reaching the deep layer in the skin where synthesis of vitamin D_3 occurs. The use of sunscreen lowers vitamin D production; however, staying in the shade and wearing long sleeves may influence blood vitamin D levels to an even greater extent than use of sunscreen.[6] Obesity increases blood vitamin D levels because body vitamin D is sequestered in body fat.[7]

2. *Liver:* Vitamin D, whether produced in the skin or obtained from dietary sources, is transported to the liver, where it is converted to 25-hydroxycholecalciferol [25$(OH)D_3$]. This intermediate metabolite goes on to the kidneys for final activation.

3. *Kidneys:* In the kidneys a special enzyme completes the last step in forming the physiologically active vitamin D hormone 1,25-dihydroxycholecalciferol [1,25$(OH)_2D_3$], referred to as calcitriol. Individuals with kidney disease are often unable to convert vitamin D to its active form.

Functions of Vitamin D

Over the years, vitamin D has been most closely associated with calcium and phosphorus absorption and bone formation, although we are learning of other functions important to health.

Control of Calcium and Phosphorus Levels in Bone and Blood

The vitamin D endocrine system cooperates with parathyroid hormone and calcitonin to (1) stimulate the active absorption of calcium and phosphorus in the small intestine, (2) promote bone mineralization, and (3) maintain blood calcium at normal levels. Each hormone—calcitriol, parathyroid hormone, and calcitonin—has a specific role in controlling bone and blood calcium levels. Vitamin D brings about the synthesis of important proteins that act on the intestine to stimulate calcium and phosphorus absorption and facilitate their deposition in bone tissue. Parathyroid hormone and calcitonin are responsible for keeping blood calcium and phosphorus levels in the normal ranges to support bone deposition.

FIG. 6.4 Formation of the active vitamin D hormone. Vitamin D undergoes a conversion in the liver and then a second conversion in the kidneys to form the vitamin D hormone calcitriol. Notice that vitamin D is handled the same way whether it was synthesized in the skin or obtained from dietary sources.

Vitamin D Deficiency and Clinical Applications

Bone Disease

Without sufficient vitamin D, the body cannot build or maintain normal bone. In children, the vitamin D deficiency disease is called *rickets* and results in a malformed skeleton (Fig. 6.5). Vitamin D–deficient adults develop osteomalacia, in which previously deposited bone mineral is mobilized, resulting in bone pain and weak, brittle bones. Osteomalacia occurs in women of child-bearing age who have little exposure to sunlight, diets low in calcium and vitamin D, and frequent pregnancies followed by periods of lactation. Older adults who use antacids that contain aluminum are at risk of osteomalacia because aluminum binds phosphorus and causes it to be excreted along with calcium. Osteomalacia sometimes accompanies osteoporosis, another bone disease common in older men and women that is treated with vitamin D (see Chapter 7).

The widespread use of vitamin D–fortified milk had nearly eliminated rickets in the United States, but breast-fed infants who do not receive vitamin D supplements are at risk. Breast milk is generally low in vitamin D, and especially so among mothers with poor vitamin D status. It is recommended that breast-fed African-American infants and infants in northern climates be given vitamin D supplements.

Because of its regulatory role in balancing bone mineral absorption and deposition, vitamin D has been used to treat renal osteodystrophy. This condition is secondary to renal failure and results in defective bone formation.

FIG. 6.5 Bowlegs in child with rickets resulting from a lack of vitamin D. (From McLaren DS: *A colour atlas and text of diet-related disorders,* ed 2, London, 1992, Mosby-Year Book Europe Limited.)

Vitamin D Requirement

Influencing Factors

Setting dietary recommendations for vitamin D is complicated by differing degrees of sun exposure and skin synthesis. Those individuals who work indoors must obtain more of their vitamin D from dietary sources than people who work outdoors. Individuals who reside in northern latitudes are more vulnerable to vitamin D deficiency. Older adults are less able to synthesize vitamin D regardless of sun exposure because of aging changes in the skin.[8]

Dietary Reference Intake

The current DRI estimates the amount of dietary vitamin D required to sustain appropriate blood levels when sun exposure is minimal. The RDA for all persons age 1 to 70 is 15 mcg (600 IU). For adults older than 70 years, it increases to 20 mcg (800 IU)[8] based on body changes that occur as people age. Infants pose special problems. Vitamin D–fortified formula and cereal provide the current Adequate Intake (AI) of 10 mcg or 400 IU; breast-fed infants require supplementation.

Vitamin D Toxicity

Vitamin D is stored in the adipose tissue and released slowly, so toxic amounts can accumulate when intake is excessive. Toxicity usually results from inappropriate doses of vitamin D supplements, not fortified foods. Adults exceeding the UL of 100 mcg (4000 IU) may develop hypercalcemia with progressive muscle weakness, bone pain, bone fractures, and falls. Symptoms of toxicity in young children include failure to thrive and calcium deposits in soft tissues such as the kidneys.[8]

HEALTH PROMOTION

Implications of Vitamin D Deficiency

Leaders in nutrition, calling attention to the broad spectrum of individuals who are vitamin D deficient, view the low dietary intakes of vitamin D as a major public health problem.[1] Most adults take in only one-third to one-half of their current RDA,[1] and medical advice for reducing skin cancer encourages people to stay out of the sun or use sunscreen. Poor vitamin D status may not only affect bone health but also impact general health and resistance to chronic disease. It has been established that vitamin D is actively involved in DNA metabolism and has a role in preventing cardiovascular disease, cancer, and other chronic diseases. Although additional vitamin D can be obtained from natural sources or supplements, increased sunlight exposure is recommended. Fifteen minutes in the sun with face, arms, and legs exposed during the months of May through October can help meet annual needs.[9] In contrast, melanoma is associated with tens of thousands of hours of sun exposure and risk of sunburn. Vitamin D also acts as a nerve growth factor, regulating neurotransmitters and producing endorphins that support feelings of well-being.[10]

Food Sources of Vitamin D

Natural sources of vitamin D are few. Vitamin D_2 is found only in yeast and vitamin D_3 mostly in fish liver oils. Fatty fish such as mackerel or salmon provide significant amounts of vitamin D, and egg yolk contains a small amount. Major dietary sources are fortified foods. Milk was selected as a practical carrier more than 50 years ago because it contained calcium and phosphorus and was commonly used by children. The vitamin D added to milk is standardized at 10 mcg (400 IU)/qt, and other dairy foods such as yogurt have added vitamin D. Fortification of milk was credited with eradicating rickets in the United States in the 1930s; however, replacement of milk by soft drinks and fruit drinks has lowered intakes of calcium and vitamin D. Margarine is fortified with 37.5 mcg (1500 IU)/lb to serve as a butter substitute, and various ready-to-eat cereals have vitamin D added. Juices, soy milk, and rice milk fortified with calcium and vitamin D to the level usually found in cow's milk are potential sources for the lactose intolerant and persons avoiding all animal foods. Increasing servings of fish support intakes of both healthy fats and vitamin D. Based on the need to increase intakes, vitamin D is becoming a required nutrient on the nutrition label.[11] Food sources of vitamin D are displayed in Box 6.4.

BOX 6.4 Food Sources of Vitamin D

Vitamin D occurs naturally in eggs and fish. Fortified dairy foods, soy milk, juices, and cereals are other good sources for persons with limited exposure to sunlight.

Food Source	Quantity	Vitamin D (mcg)
Grains Group		
Fortified ready-to-eat cereal (e.g., Total)	¾ to 1 cup	1.0–2.5
Fruit Group		
Orange juice, fortified[a]	1 cup	2.5
Meat, Beans, Eggs, and Nuts Group		
Tuna fish, canned in oil[b]	3 oz	5.7
Tuna fish, canned in water[b]	3 oz	1.0
Egg yolk, large	1	0.9
Milk Group		
Milk, fortified[a] (includes nonfat, 1%, and 2% fat)	1 cup	2.5
Milk, whole (3.5% fat)	1 cup	3.2
Soy milk, fortified[a]	1 cup	2.7

[a]Consumers should check the nutrition label to be sure the product selected is fortified with vitamin D.
[b]Note the difference in vitamin D content between canned tuna fish packed in oil or water.
Recommended Dietary Allowance for adults: ages 19–70, 15 mcg (600 IU); ages ≥71, 20 mcg (800 IU).
Images copyright 2006 JupiterImages Corporation. Data from US Department of Agriculture, Agricultural Research Service: *USDA National Nutrient Database for Standard Reference, Release 28*, revised May 2016. Nutrient Data Laboratory Home Page: https://www.ars.usda.gov/northeast-area/beltsville-md/beltsville-human-nutrition-research-center/nutrient-data-laboratory/docs/usda-national-nutrient-database-for-standard-reference/.

VITAMIN E

Chemical and Physical Nature

Scientists studying reproduction in laboratory animals first discovered vitamin E. Because of its association with birth and its chemical structure as an alcohol, it was named tocopherol, from the Greek word *tokos,* meaning childbirth. Vitamin E came to be known as the *antisterility vitamin,* although this has been demonstrated in animals only, not in humans.

Forms

Vitamin E is the generic name given to a group of eight compounds having to some degree the biologic activity of α-tocopherol. Vitamin E is a pale yellow oil, stable to acids and heat, and insoluble in water. It oxidizes very slowly, which gives it an important role as an antioxidant.

Absorption, Transport, and Storage

Vitamin E is absorbed in the micelles with the aid of bile salts and transported in the chylomicrons. Vitamin E is stored in the liver and adipose tissue, where it is held in bulk liquid droplets. Mobilization of α-tocopherol from these storage sites occurs very slowly.

Functions of Vitamin E
Antioxidant Activity

In our study of the vitamins, we will continue to hear the term *antioxidant* and the role such nutrients play in destroying molecules called *free radicals.* Free radicals have an unpaired electron and are constantly on the lookout for another molecule with an unpaired electron that they can join with. Free radicals are highly active molecules, and the oxidation reactions they initiate are very damaging to body tissues. Free radicals are formed as by-products of normal cell metabolism but also originate in tobacco smoke, car exhaust fumes, and other air pollutants.

Polyunsaturated fatty acids having several double bonds and the tissues where they are found are especially vulnerable to attack. Cell membranes contain a high proportion of polyunsaturated fatty acids, and oxidation by free radicals alters their structure and destroys their ability to recognize harmful substances and prevent them from entering the cell. Brain tissue and nerve fibers are high in unsaturated fatty acids. Deoxyribonucleic acid (DNA) and other proteins in the cell nucleus, if modified by unwanted oxidation reactions, produce molecules that are ineffective in carrying out body functions. Antioxidants such as vitamin E join with the unpaired electron of free radicals and interrupt the chain of oxidation reactions. Vitamin E is nature's most potent antioxidant.

Partnership With Selenium

In addition to vitamin E, a second line of defense against free radical damage is an enzyme containing selenium, a trace mineral. Selenium can spare vitamin E and reduce the vitamin E requirement. In this partnership role, vitamin E can also reduce the selenium requirement.

KEY TERMS

Tocopherol
Chemical name for vitamin E; it functions as an antioxidant to preserve structural membranes and other tissues with a high content of polyunsaturated fatty acids.

Antioxidant
A substance that prevents the formation and destructive actions of free radicals.

Vitamin E Deficiency and Clinical Applications
Premature Infants

Vitamin E deficiency has disastrous effects on red blood cells. When polyunsaturated fatty acids in the lipid membranes of red blood cells are exposed to oxidation, the membranes break, the cell contents are lost, and the cell is destroyed. Continued loss of red blood cells leads to anemia, and this vitamin E deficiency disease is called hemolytic anemia. Premature infants are especially vulnerable to hemolytic anemia because they miss the last month or two of fetal life when vitamin E stores are normally built up. This condition responds positively to vitamin E therapy and is prevented with vitamin E supplementation at birth. Adequate vitamin E during pregnancy can help ensure optimum vitamin E stores in the full-term infant.

Children and Adults

In older children and adults, vitamin E deficiency presents a different set of symptoms associated with the nervous system. Nerves affected are (1) the spinal cord fibers that control physical movement such as walking and (2) the retina of the eye.[12] Vitamin E deficiency also contributes to anemia in both adults and children.[13] These problems were identified in children with cystic fibrosis and pancreatic insufficiency that had defective absorption of fat and fat-soluble vitamins. Vitamin E deficiency disrupts the making of myelin, the protective lipid covering of the nerve cell axons that helps transmit messages along to muscles. The lack of vitamin E also leads to degeneration of the pigment in the rods and cones of the retina that depend on vitamin E to prevent oxidation damage. Optimum intakes of vitamin E and other antioxidants are especially important for cystic fibrosis patients and obese children and adults[13] who have high rates of tissue oxidation. Vitamin E replacement is needed for those with fat malabsorption.

Vitamin E Requirement
Dietary Reference Intake

The RDA for this vitamin is expressed in milligrams of α-tocopherol, the form of vitamin E with the highest biologic activity. Approximately 80% of the vitamin E from dietary sources (including fortified foods) is α-tocopherol, and approximately 20% are other forms. The RDA is 15 mg for both males and females ages 14 and older,[12] but actual intake falls much below this level. In the United States, adult men average 10.4 mg/day of α-tocopherol and adult women average 8.4 mg/day[14]; nevertheless, it is difficult to identify vitamin E deficiency within the general population.[13]

Vitamin E Toxicity

No toxicity syndrome has been identified for vitamin E; however, clinicians warn against self-prescribed supplementation. Despite early

reports in the popular press, current findings have not associated vitamin E with a reduction in cardiovascular risk[15] or prevention of cognitive decline,[16] other than as part of an overall healthful diet. In fact, mortality was higher among individuals supplementing with vitamin E.[17] (The UL for vitamin E is 1000 mg).[12] Intakes greater than recommended levels can interfere with blood platelet aggregation and prevent normal blood clotting. This is important information for persons with low intakes of vitamin K or patients using anticlotting medications.

Food Sources of Vitamin E

Vegetable oils are rich dietary sources of vitamin E. Sunflower, safflower, and canola oils contain the highest amounts, followed by corn oil and olive oil.[5] As might be expected, these oils are also rich sources of polyunsaturated fatty acids, which vitamin E protects from oxidation. Other sources include peanut butter, nuts, and certain vegetables and fruits, especially tomatoes and spinach. Fortified ready-to-eat cereals add to intake. Box 6.5 lists major food sources of vitamin E.

VITAMIN K

Chemical and Physical Nature

The studies of Henrik Dam, a biochemist at the University of Copenhagen working on a hemorrhagic disease in chicks, led to the discovery of vitamin K. Because of its blood-clotting function, he called it the *koagulations vitamin,* or vitamin K. For this discovery he received the Nobel Prize in physiology and medicine.

Chemical Nature

The form of vitamin K found in plants is named phylloquinone for its chemical structure. Phylloquinone is the major dietary form and is widely distributed in both animal and plant foods. Menaquinone is synthesized by intestinal bacteria, but either form can be used by the body. A water-soluble analog of vitamin K, menadione, can be absorbed directly into the portal blood, making it an important source for individuals with fat malabsorption.

Absorption, Transport, and Storage

Both phylloquinone and menaquinone require pancreatic lipase and bile salts for absorption. In the liver, vitamin K is stored in small amounts but excreted rapidly after administration of therapeutic doses.

Functional Roles of Vitamin K
Blood Clotting

The major function of vitamin K is to initiate liver synthesis of four proteins necessary for blood clotting.[12] Each clotting factor is in the form of an inactive precursor that depends on vitamin K for activation. This activation step converts the precursor protein prothrombin to thrombin, which in turn acts on the precursor fibrinogen to form fibrin and complete the clotting process. Both calcium ions and vitamin K are needed for normal clotting. Vitamin K requires a functioning liver to carry out its tasks. When liver damage is the cause of low prothrombin levels and hemorrhage, vitamin K is ineffective as a therapeutic agent. Vitamin K also controls the liver synthesis of other proteins that regulate the speed and duration of coagulation. These regulatory proteins prevent the development of dangerous, unwanted blood clots or thromboses.[3]

Bone Metabolism

Vitamin K has a role in bone health, stimulating the synthesis of osteocalcin and other proteins important to bone. Bone is constantly being

---

KEY TERMS

Anemia
Condition of low blood hemoglobin levels caused by too few red blood cells or red blood cells with a low hemoglobin content.

Hemolytic Anemia
An anemia caused by breakdown of the outer membrane of red blood cells and loss of their hemoglobin; occurs in vitamin E deficiency.

Myelin
Substance made of fat and protein that forms a fatty sheath around the nerve axons to protect and insulate the nerves and facilitate transmission of neuromuscular impulses.

BOX 6.5 Food Sources of Vitamin E

Food Source	Quantity	Vitamin E (mg)
Grains Group		
Fortified ready-to-eat cereal (e.g., Total Whole Grain)	¾ cup	13.5
Rice Krispies	1¼ cup	8.8
Cheerios	1 cup	0.2
Vegetable Group		
Spaghetti sauce, tomato	1 cup	6.3
Spinach, frozen, cooked	½ cup	3.4
Meat, Beans, Eggs, and Nuts Group		
Dry-roasted sunflower seeds	¼ cup	8.4
Peanut butter, smooth	2 tbsp	2.9
Sardines, canned	3 oz	1.7
Red kidney beans, canned	1 cup	0.1
Pinto beans	1 cup	1.6
Fats, Oils, and Sugar		
Corn oil	1 tbsp	1.9
Olive oil	1 tbsp	1.9
Safflower oil	1 tbsp	4.6

Recommended Dietary Allowance for adults: 15 mg.
Images copyright 2006 JupiterImages Corporation. Data from US Department of Agriculture, Agricultural Research Service: *USDA National Nutrient Database for Standard Reference, Release 28,* revised May 2016. Nutrient Data Laboratory Home Page: https://www.ars.usda.gov/northeast-area/beltsville-md/beltsville-human-nutrition-research-center/nutrient-data-laboratory/docs/usda-national-nutrient-database-for-standard-reference/.

remodeled, and vitamin K–dependent proteins are necessary for the formation of bone matrix and mineral deposition. Optimum intakes of vitamin K reduced the incidence of bone fractures and vertebral fractures in older women.[18]

Vitamin K Deficiency and Clinical Applications
Neonatology
The sterile intestinal tract of the newborn cannot supply vitamin K during the first few days of life until normal bacterial flora develop. To prevent hemorrhage during this immediate postnatal period, a prophylactic dose of vitamin K is usually given soon after birth.

Malabsorption
Any defect in fat absorption impairs vitamin K absorption, resulting in slower blood clotting; thus several clinical situations demand supplemental vitamin K. Patients with bile duct obstruction are usually given vitamin K before surgery. Children with cystic fibrosis can become deficient because frequent use of antibiotics interferes with colonic bacterial synthesis of this vitamin.

Drug Therapy
Several drug-nutrient interactions involve vitamin K. Anticlotting drugs such as Coumadin (warfarin), Plavix (clopidogrel), or Aggrenox (dipyridamole and aspirin) act as **antimetabolites**, preventing the synthesis of blood-clotting factors in the liver and so inhibiting the action of vitamin K. When these drugs are used to prevent unwanted clots in the lungs or blood vessels, dietary intake of vitamin K must be closely monitored. Too much vitamin K will oppose the action of the drug and neutralize its effect; too little vitamin K could lead to serious hemorrhage. Dark green leafy vegetables are rich in naturally occurring vitamin K, and vitamin K is added to many multivitamin supplements. With extended use of antibiotics, much of the intestinal bacterial flora is lost, eliminating one of the body's main sources of vitamin K, and supplements may be required.

KEY TERMS

Phylloquinone
A fat-soluble vitamin of the K group found in green plants.

Menaquinone
Form of vitamin K synthesized by intestinal bacteria.

Menadione
A water-soluble analog of vitamin K.

Prothrombin
Blood-clotting factor synthesized in the liver and activated by vitamin K.

Antimetabolite
Substance bearing a close structural resemblance to an essential nutrient or metabolite that interferes with its physiologic function or use.

Vitamin K Requirement

Dietary Reference Intake

It is difficult to set a DRI for vitamin K because at least part of the requirement can be met by intestinal bacterial synthesis. Moreover, reliable information as to the vitamin K content of many foods or its bioavailability is lacking. With this in mind the expert committee established an AI rather than an RDA. For men ages 19 and older the AI is 120 mcg/day, and for women it is 90 mcg/day.[3] These values represent the median intakes of nearly 20,000 men and women who participated in national nutrition and health surveys between 1988 and 1994. This intake is adequate to preserve blood clotting, but it may not be sufficient to support bone health.[18] Toxicity has not been reported.

Food Sources of Vitamin K

Phylloquinone is found in many vegetables but is highest in dark green vegetables and liver. Menaquinones occur in milk, meat, and certain cheeses. Vegetable oils, such as soybean and canola oil, also supply vitamin K.[3,12] A list of good food sources can be found in Box 6.6.

Table 6.2 provides a complete summary of the fat-soluble vitamins.

BOX 6.6   Food Sources of Vitamin K

Spinach	Cabbage
Brussels sprouts	Canned tuna (packed in oil)
Broccoli	Spaghetti sauce
Lettuce	

Adequate intake for adults: women, 90 mcg; men, 120 mcg. Images copyright 2006 JupiterImages Corporation.

TABLE 6.2   Summary of Fat-Soluble Vitamins

Vitamin	Physiologic Functions	Results of Deficiency	Dietary Reference Intake	Food Sources
Vitamin A				
Provitamin: β carotene	Production of rhodopsin and	Poor dark adaptation, night	Males ages ≥19: 900 mcg	Butter; fortified margarine
Preformed vitamin: retinol	other light-receptor pigments	blindness, xerosis, xerophthalmia	retinol activity equivalent[a]	Whole, fortified low-fat, fortified reduced fat, and fortified nonfat cow's milk
	Formation and maintenance of epithelial tissue	Keratinization of epithelial tissue	Females ages ≥19: 700 mcg RAE	
	Immune function		Pregnancy	Fortified soy milk
	Growth	Growth failure	Ages ≤18: 750 mcg RAE	Dark green, deep yellow, and orange vegetables
	Reproduction	Reproductive failure	Ages ≥19: 770 mcg RAE	
	Toxic in large amounts		Lactation	Yellow and orange fruits
			Ages ≤18: 1200 mcg RAE	
			Ages ≥19: 1300 mcg RAE	
Vitamin D				
Provitamins:	Calcium and phosphorus	Defective bone growth, rick-	Adult males/females	Fortified cow's milk
ergosterol (plants);	absorption	ets (in children and youth),	Ages 19–70: 15 mcg (600 IU)	Fortified soy milk
7-dehydrocholesterol (skin)	Calcitriol is major hormone regulator of bone mineral	osteomalacia (in adults)	Ages ≥71: 20 mcg (800 IU)	Fortified orange juice
Vitamins: D_2 (ergocalcif-	metabolism		Pregnancy	Fortified margarine
erol) and D_3 (cholecal-	Possible roles in muscle		All ages: 15 mcg (600 IU)	Fortified cereals
ciferol, used in food	function and control of		Lactation	Oily fish (e.g., salmon, tuna)
fortification)	cell growth		All ages: 15 mcg (600 IU)	Egg yolk
	Toxic in large amounts			Sunlight on the skin
Vitamin E				
Tocopherols	Antioxidant	Anemia in premature infants	Adult males/females	Vegetable oils
Most active form is	Protects cell membranes includ-	Increased risk of oxidative	Ages ≥19: 15 mg	Fortified ready-to-eat cereals
α-tocopherol	ing red blood cell membranes	damage to body tissues	Pregnancy	Nuts
	Partners with selenium in		All ages: 15 mg	Dark green leafy vegetables
	antioxidant function		Lactation	Tomatoes/spaghetti sauce
			All ages: 19 mg	
Vitamin K				
K_1 (phylloquinone)	Activates blood-clotting factors	Hemorrhagic disease of the	Males ages ≥19: 120 mcg	Green leafy vegetables
Found in plant and	(e.g., converts prothrombin to	newborn	Females ages ≥19: 90 mcg	Canned tuna
animal foods	thrombin)	Defective blood clotting	Pregnancy	Spaghetti sauce
K_2 (menaquinone)	Participates in bone formation	Deficiency symptoms	Ages ≤18: 75 mcg	Synthesized by intestinal
Synthesized by intestinal	and remodeling (synthesis of	produced by anticoagulant	Ages ≥19: 90 mcg	bacteria
bacteria	osteocalcin)	and antibiotic therapy	Lactation	
Analog: K_3 (menadione,	Interferes with anticoagulant		Ages ≤18: 75 mcg	
water soluble)	therapy		Ages ≥19: 90 mcg	

WATER-SOLUBLE VITAMINS

VITAMIN C (ASCORBIC ACID)

Chemical and Physical Nature

The discovery of vitamin C is associated with the ancient hemorrhagic disease scurvy. Early observations of British sailors led to the detection of an acid in lemon juice that could prevent or cure this disease. Its chemical name *ascorbic acid* is based on its antiscorbutic properties. The structure of vitamin C is similar to glucose, and most animals can convert glucose to ascorbic acid. However, humans lack this enzyme. Therefore human scurvy could be called a *disease of distant genetic origin*, an inherited metabolic defect. Vitamin C is an unstable, easily oxidized acid. It is destroyed by oxygen, alkali, and heat.

Absorption, Transport, and Storage

Vitamin C is easily absorbed from the small intestine but requires an acid environment. When gastric hydrochloric acid is lacking, absorption is hindered. In contrast to the fat-soluble vitamins that are stored mostly in the liver, vitamin C is generally distributed throughout the body, maintaining limited tissue saturation. Any excess is excreted in the urine. The total body pool in adults varies from approximately 2 g to as little as 0.3 g, depending on intake.[12] Optimum tissue saturation can meet day-to-day needs for as long as 3 months when intake is lacking. This explains why generally healthy people in isolated living situations could survive the winter without eating fresh fruits and vegetables.

Breast milk provides sufficient vitamin C for early infancy if the mother is eating a good diet. Cow's milk contains very little vitamin C because these animals have the enzymes to make their own vitamin C from glucose. Human infant formulas made from cow's milk are supplemented with this vitamin.

Functions of Vitamin C

Antioxidant Capacity

Vitamin C, along with vitamin E, is a powerful antioxidant. Vitamin C joins with free oxygen arising from cell metabolism, making it unavailable to fuel the destructive actions of free radicals. In this role, ascorbic acid may help protect the gastric mucosa from the damaging effect of *Helicobacter pylori* and formation of gastric ulcers.[19] (See Chapter 2 for a review of this pathogen.)

Formation of Intercellular Cement

Vitamin C helps build and maintain many body tissues, including bone matrix, cartilage, dentin, and collagen. Collagen is a protein found in the white fibers of connective tissue. When vitamin C is absent, an important ground substance is not formed and collagen fibers are defective and weak. Blood vessels require this cementing substance to form firm capillary walls. In vitamin C deficiency, capillaries are fragile and easily ruptured by blood pressure or trauma, resulting in small hemorrhages in the skin and other tissues. When vitamin C is restored, the formation of normal collagen follows quickly. Formation of collagen is also important for bone health, providing an appropriate matrix for the deposition of bone minerals. Box 6.7 lists common signs of vitamin C deficiency.

BOX 6.7   Signs of Vitamin C Deficiency

- Easy bruising
- Pinpoint hemorrhages of the skin (petechiae)
- Weak bones that fracture easily
- Poor wound healing
- Bleeding gums (often termed *gingivitis*)
- Anemia

Support of General Body Metabolism

Vitamin C is found in greater amounts in metabolically active tissues such as the adrenal and pituitary glands, brain, eyes, and white blood cells. The multiplying tissues of children contain more vitamin C than the resting tissues of adults. Vitamin C helps in the formation of hemoglobin and the development of red blood cells by promoting iron absorption and assisting in the removal of iron from the protein-iron complex called *ferritin*, in which it is stored.

Vitamin C participates in other functions of metabolic importance, described as follows:

- Assists in the synthesis of carnitine, an amino acid that transports long-chain fatty acids into cell mitochondria where they are burned for energy.
- Assists in the synthesis of neurotransmitters such as norepinephrine and serotonin, and receptors for the neurotransmitter acetylcholine.
- Supports the action of the mixed-function oxidase system that metabolizes drugs and breaks down carcinogens and other foreign molecules; this system also sequesters lead and other heavy metals and neutralizes their effects.
- Controls the conversion of phenylalanine, an indispensable amino acid, to tyrosine, a conditionally indispensable amino acid; this is clinically important in children with phenylketonuria.

Clinical Applications

- *Wound healing:* The role of vitamin C in forming the cement for building supporting tissues creates added demands in traumatic injury or surgery when extensive tissue regeneration is required. Formulas for parenteral feeding generally provide 100 mg/day of vitamin C. Protocols for burn patients with elevated needs for tissue growth and defense against infection call for 1000 mg/day.[20]
- *Fever and infection:* The body's response to infection depletes tissue vitamin C stores. Fever adds to losses because it accompanies infection and produces a catabolic response.
- *Growth:* Additional vitamin C is required during periods of rapid growth in infants and children. An adequate supply is critical in pregnancy to support fetal development and expansion of maternal tissues. Pregnant women who smoke or use drugs may have elevated needs.[12]
- *Stress and body response:* Body stress arising from injury, illness, debilitating disease, or emotional upset calls on vitamin C stores. The adrenal glands, which have a primary role in stress response, contain large amounts of vitamin C.

Vitamin C Requirement

Dietary Reference Intake

The RDA for vitamin C is set at the level required to maintain tissue saturation and provide antioxidant protection of body cells and membranes. For men the RDA is 90 mg. Based on their smaller body size, the RDA for women is 75 mg.[12] Cigarette smokers require an additional 35 mg. Added vitamin is needed in pregnancy, lactation, and periods of growth. Less than half of US adults are meeting the minimum recommended amounts

---

KEY TERMS

Scurvy
A hemorrhagic disease caused by lack of vitamin C.

Collagen
Protein substance of the white fibers of skin, tendon, bone, cartilage, and other connective tissue.

Parenteral
A mode of feeding that does not use the gastrointestinal tract but instead provides nutrition by intravenous delivery of nutrient solutions.

of vitamin C; this would be expected in light of their low use of the fruit and vegetable group that supplies this vitamin.[1] Nevertheless, the occurrence of scurvy in developed nations is usually associated with clinical conditions such as iron overload related to sickle cell anemia, chemotherapy, or treatment for neurologic conditions, not dietary deficiency.[21]

Vitamin C Toxicity

Vitamin C intakes exceeding the recommended level have been promoted for curing the common cold, protecting against degenerative disease, and delaying the signs of aging. Extreme intakes of vitamin C can lead to formation of kidney stones, although they are more likely to occur in men and if intake exceeds 700 mg/day.[22] Kidney stones are usually the result of unwise supplementation, not dietary intake. The UL for ascorbic acid is set at 2000 mg; gastrointestinal symptoms and diarrhea have been observed at these doses.[12]

Food Sources of Vitamin C

The best-known sources of vitamin C are citrus fruits and tomatoes. Broccoli, salad greens, strawberries, watermelon, cabbage, and sweet potatoes are other good sources. Vitamin C is easily oxidized when exposed to the air or heated, so storage, preparation, and cooking methods must be chosen carefully to preserve vitamin content (Box 6.8). Vitamin C is quite stable in acid solutions, so citrus and tomato products remain good sources even if heated. Box 6.9 lists the vitamin C content of various

---

BOX 6.8   Food Preparation Methods to Prevent Vitamin Loss

Vitamins can be destroyed by heat, light, or the action of oxygen from the air. Water-soluble vitamins, especially vitamin C, are particularly vulnerable to such loss. The following storage and preparation practices help retain vitamins in fruits and vegetables:

- Store cut-up fruits and vegetables in the refrigerator in tightly covered containers that protect them from light and oxygen; when preparing fresh fruit or vegetables for salads or cooking, try to minimize the length of time they are exposed to the air.
- Avoid cutting fruits and vegetables into very small pieces; this increases the surface area for nutrient loss.
- Cook vegetables for a *limited* amount of time in a *limited* amount of water in a tightly covered pan to retain nutrients, flavor, color, and texture. (Vegetables should be tender but still retain their shape.)

- Steam vegetables in a steamer basket with the water below to prevent the dissolving of nutrients into the water; vegetables need not be covered with water, as the steam in the covered container will soften the food.
- Use the microwave to reduce the time and amount of water needed for cooking, but avoid overcooking. Remember that foods continue to cook for several minutes after being removed from the microwave.
- Stir-fry vegetables using only a small amount of fat to conserve nutrients and food quality.
- Fruits and vegetables add color and variety to meals, along with important nutrients. Include both raw and cooked vegetables to add interest to menus.

BOX 6.9   Food Sources of Vitamin C

Food Source	Amount	Vitamin C (mg)
Vegetable Group		
Tomato soup, canned, water added	1 cup	16
Vegetable juice cocktail	1 cup	137
Pepper, chili, red	1	65
Peppers, sweet, green, chopped	½ cup	60
Peppers, sweet, red, chopped	½ cup	95
Broccoli, cooked	½ cup	51
Cole slaw	1 cup	48
Sweet potato, canned, vacuumed packed	½ cup	34
Cauliflower, frozen, cooked	½ cup	28
Fruit Group		
Strawberries, sliced	1 cup	98
Orange juice, frozen, reconstituted	1 cup	90
Grape juice, fortified	1 cup	63
Orange	1 medium	70
Cantaloupe	⅛ melon	25
Watermelon	1 wedge (4 × 8 inches)	23
Other		
Fruit punch, fortified	1 cup	73

Recommended Dietary Allowances for adults: women, 75 mg; men, 90 mg.
Images copyright 2006 JupiterImages Corporation. Data from US Department of Agriculture, Agricultural Research Service: *USDA National Nutrient Database for Standard Reference, Release 28,* revised May 2016. Nutrient Data Laboratory Home Page: https://www.ars.usda.gov/northeast-area/beltsville-md/beltsville-human-nutrition-research-center/nutrient-data-laboratory/docs/usda-national-nutrient-database-for-standard-reference/.

TABLE 6.3 Summary of Vitamin C (Ascorbic Acid)

Physiologic Functions	Clinical Applications	Dietary Reference Intake	Food Sources
Antioxidant activity	Wound healing	Males ages ≥19: 90 mg	Citrus fruits and berries
Collagen synthesis	Tissue formation	Females ages ≥19: 75 mg	Vegetables: broccoli, cabbage, chili
General metabolism	Fevers and infections	Cigarette smokers require an additional 35 mg	peppers, potatoes, tomatoes
Makes iron available for	Stress reactions	Pregnancy	
hemoglobin synthesis	Growth	Ages ≤18: 80 mg	
Controls conversion of the amino	Scurvy (classic deficiency	Ages ≥19: 85 mg	
acid phenylalanine to tyrosine	disease)	Lactation	
		Ages ≤18: 115 mg	
		Ages ≥19: 120 mg	

🌐 FOCUS ON FOOD SAFETY

Did You Wash That Orange?

Oranges, apples, pears, grapes, bananas, and raw carrots are healthy snacks and travel well in a backpack or school bag. However, all fresh produce must be washed before you eat or cook it to remove any remaining pesticides, soil particles, and bacteria that accumulated as it was picked, shipped, and handled in the store. Fruits and vegetables to be peeled still need to be washed. After your hands touch the unwashed banana peel, you will transfer those bacteria to the fruit as you peel it. It is also important to wash all "prewashed" vegetables and salad greens to be sure that all soil particles and bacteria have been removed.

foods. A summary of vitamin C functions and requirements is found in Table 6.3. (For tips on the proper handling of fresh fruits and vegetables, see the Focus on Food Safety box, "Did You Wash That Orange?")

B VITAMINS

DEFICIENCY DISEASES AND VITAMIN DISCOVERIES

The discovery of the B vitamins is a story of people dying of a puzzling, age-old disease for which no cure existed. Eventually it was learned that common, everyday food held the answer. The paralyzing disease was beriberi, which plagued East Asia for centuries (Fig. 6.6). It was named by the native words, *I can't, I can't*, which described its crippling effects. The "vitamine" connection was established when an American chemist, R.R. Williams, used extracts of rice polishings to cure the epidemic infantile beriberi. The food factor that brought the cure was labeled *water-soluble B* because it was thought to be a single vitamin. Now we know several vitamins exist in the B group, all water-soluble but with unique metabolic functions. Each of the B vitamins has been given a specific chemical name.

COENZYME ROLE

The B vitamins have important metabolic roles as coenzyme partners with cell enzymes that control energy metabolism and build tissue. Eight vitamins are in this group. First we consider the three associated with classic deficiency diseases—thiamin, riboflavin, and niacin; then the more recently discovered coenzyme factors—pantothenic acid, biotin, and pyridoxine (vitamin B_6); and, finally, the important blood-forming factors—folate and vitamin B_{12} (cobalamin).

FIG. 6.6 Beriberi is the classic thiamin-deficiency disease characterized by impaired neural function, extreme weakness, paralysis, and wasting related to the inability to metabolize glucose for energy. (From McLaren DS: *A colour atlas and text of diet-related disorders,* ed 2, London, 1992, Mosby-Year Book Europe Limited.)

KEY TERMS

Beriberi
A disease of the peripheral nerves caused by thiamin deficiency.

Pantothenic Acid
A member of the B vitamin complex widely distributed in nature and throughout body tissues; it functions as a part of coenzyme A (CoA), important in lipid and carbohydrate metabolism.

THIAMIN

The search for the cause of beriberi was successfully concluded with the identification of thiamin. Its nature and metabolic role were clarified in the early 1930s.

Chemical and Physical Nature

Thiamin is a water-soluble and fairly stable vitamin, although it is destroyed in alkaline solutions. Its name comes from its chemical ringlike structure.

Absorption, Transport, and Storage

Thiamin is absorbed most efficiently in the acid environment of the upper small intestine before the food mass is buffered by the alkaline fluids entering from the pancreas. Thiamin is not stored in large amounts, so a continuous dietary supply is needed.[23] Tissue thiamin responds rapidly to increased metabolic demand as occurs in fever, high muscular activity, pregnancy, and lactation. Tissue stores depend on both thiamin intake and general diet composition. Carbohydrate increases the need for thiamin, whereas fat and protein spare thiamin. Food patterns with a high proportion of simple carbohydrates may elevate the need for thiamin. When the tissues are saturated, unused thiamin is excreted in the urine.

Function of Thiamin

Coenzyme Role

Thiamin functions as a control agent in energy metabolism. When combined with phosphorus to form **thiamin pyrophosphate (TPP)**, it serves as a coenzyme in reactions involving glucose. Approximately 90% of body thiamin is in the coenzyme form.[23] The symptoms of beriberi can be traced to the loss of energy usually provided by glucose metabolism.

Thiamin Deficiency

When thiamin levels are insufficient to support cellular energy metabolism, clinical effects become apparent, as follows:

- *Gastrointestinal system:* Anorexia, constipation, gastric atony, and poor hydrochloric acid secretion progress as the deficiency continues. When the cells of the smooth muscles and the secretory glands do not receive enough energy from glucose, they cannot perform the digestive work needed to supply still more glucose to meet body needs. This vicious cycle accelerates as the deficiency continues.
- *Nervous system:* The CNS depends on glucose to do its work. Without sufficient thiamin to provide this constant fuel, nerve activity is impaired, alertness and reflex responses are diminished, and general apathy and fatigue take over. If the deficiency continues, then lipogenesis is hindered, followed by damage to the myelin sheaths—the lipid tissue covering the nerve fibers. This causes increasing nerve irritation, pain, and prickly or deadening sensations. If unchecked, paralysis will result as in the classic deficiency disease beriberi. Classic symptoms of beriberi include cognitive deficits with reduced levels of glucose metabolism in the brain. Such changes in brain glucose metabolism are also associated with Alzheimer disease.[24]
- *Cardiovascular system:* The heart muscle weakens, leading to cardiac failure and edema of the lower extremities.
- *Musculoskeletal system:* Inadequate TPP in muscle tissue results in widespread chronic pain that responds to thiamin therapy.

Thiamin status is evaluated by the activity of a TPP-dependent enzyme transketolase found in red blood cells. This is a common test to determine whether a clinical observation is related to thiamin deficiency or another cause.

Thiamin Requirement

Dietary Reference Intake

The thiamin requirement is based on energy intake with a minimum of 0.3 mg of thiamin/1000 kcal. To provide a margin of safety, the RDA is set at 1.2 mg for men and 1.1 mg for women.[23] Additional thiamin is needed during pregnancy and lactation. Because the kidneys excrete excess thiamin, there are no reports of toxicity arising from oral doses up to 50 mg. No UL has been established.

Clinical Applications

Several conditions influence thiamin needs:

- *Alcohol abuse:* Thiamin is important when planning nutritional intervention for patients with alcohol problems.[24] Both a primary deficiency (an inadequate diet) and a conditioned deficiency (the effect of alcohol) contribute to thiamin malnutrition and, over time, serious neurologic disorders. Alcohol interferes with the active absorption of thiamin, resulting in rapid depletion of tissue stores.
- *Acute illness or disease:* Fever and infection increase energy requirements and the need for thiamin. Patients on hemodialysis lose thiamin and require supplementation to prevent deficiency.
- *Normal growth and development:* Thiamin needs increase in pregnancy and lactation to meet the demands of rapid fetal growth, the elevated metabolic rate of pregnancy, and milk production. Continuing growth throughout infancy, childhood, and adolescence requires attention to thiamin intake. At any point in the life cycle, the larger the body and its tissue mass, the greater are the cellular energy requirements and need for thiamin.
- *Cardiovascular function:* Various diuretics used to manage heart failure promote urinary loss of thiamin and increase the thiamin requirement.[25] If thiamin intake is low, then these patients can develop a thiamin deficiency that worsens their cardiac symptoms. The B vitamins might work together in supporting cardiac and circulatory function because thiamin, riboflavin, and folate intakes were found to be inversely associated with systolic blood pressure.[26]
- *Gastric bypass surgery:* Thiamin supplementation is likely to be necessary after gastric bypass surgery because energy intake is drastically reduced and absorption less efficient. Thiamin deficiency may play a role in the neurologic and CNS complications that sometimes occur following bariatric surgery.[27]

Food Sources of Thiamin

Thiamin is widespread in plant and animal foods, although the amount found in individual foods is usually small. As a result, intakes can be low when kcalories are curtailed. Major sources in the American diet are whole grain and enriched breads, ready-to-eat cereals, and legumes.[1] Lean pork and beef are also good sources. Thiamin is extremely water soluble and readily lost in cooking water. Box 6.10 lists foods containing thiamin.

RIBOFLAVIN

Discovery

In 1897 a London chemist observed in milk whey a water-soluble pigment with a peculiar yellow-green fluorescence. However, it was not until many years later that researchers in Germany actually discovered riboflavin. This vitamin was given the chemical name *flavin*, from the Latin word for yellow. Later, when it was found to contain a sugar called *ribose*, the name *riboflavin* was officially adopted.

Chemical and Physical Nature

Riboflavin is a yellow-green fluorescent pigment that forms yellowish-brown, needlelike crystals. It is water soluble and relatively heat stable but easily destroyed by light and irradiation.

Absorption, Transport, and Storage

Riboflavin is easily absorbed in the upper small intestine. Bulk fiber supplements such as psyllium, especially when taken with milk or near

---

KEY TERM

Thiamin Pyrophosphate (TPP)
Active coenzyme form of thiamin needed for carbohydrate metabolism.

BOX 6.10 Food Sources of Thiamin

Food Source	Amount	Thiamin (mg)
Grains Group		
Ready-to-Eat Cereals		
All-Bran Complete Wheat Flakes	¾ cup	1.50
Total Raisin Bran	1 cup	1.48
Rice Krispies	1¼ cup	0.58
Wheaties	1 cup	1.01
Corn flakes	1 cup	0.38
Instant oatmeal	1 packet	0.30
Rice, white, long grain, cooked, enriched	1 cup	0.26
Pancake, frozen, ready to eat	3 in	0.28
Bagel, enriched	3½ in	0.57
Macaroni/spaghetti, enriched	1 cup	0.42
Hamburger roll, enriched	1	0.24
Bread, white, enriched	1 slice	0.13
Vegetable Group		
Green peas, frozen, cooked	½ cup	0.23
Potatoes, mashed, prepared from instant flakes	½ cup	0.14
Tomato juice, canned	1 cup	0.24
Fruit Group		
Orange juice, frozen, reconstituted	1 cup	0.17
Grapes (red or green)	1 cup	0.11
Meat, Beans, Eggs, and Nuts Group		
Pork, roasted, lean	3 oz	0.47
Ham, baked, lean	3 oz	0.59
Kidney beans, cooked	1 cup	0.28
Baked beans, canned, plain or vegetarian	1 cup	0.24
Milk Group		
Milk, 3.5% fat, 2% fat, or nonfat (may vary slightly)	1 cup	0.11

Recommended Dietary Allowances for adults: women, 1.1 mg; men, 1.2 mg.
Images copyright 2006 JupiterImages Corporation. Data from US Department of Agriculture, Agricultural Research Service: *USDA National Nutrient Database for Standard Reference, Release 28,* Revised May 2016. Nutrient Data Laboratory Home Page: https://www.ars.usda.gov/ northeast-area/beltsville-md/beltsville-human-nutrition-research-center/nutrient-data-laboratory/docs/usda-national-nutrient-database-for-standard-reference/.

mealtimes, can hinder riboflavin absorption and contribute to deficiency. Body stores are limited, although small amounts are found in the liver and kidney. Day-to-day tissue needs must be supplied in the diet.

Functions of Riboflavin

Coenzyme Role

Riboflavin is a part of the cell enzymes called *flavoproteins*. These enzymes—flavin mononucleotide (FMN) and flavin adenine dinucleotide (FAD)—are integral to both energy metabolism and deamination. Deamination is the removal of a nitrogen-containing amino group from an existing amino acid so that a new amino acid can be formed. Accordingly, riboflavin is active in both energy production and tissue building.

Riboflavin Deficiency and Clinical Applications

Riboflavin deficiency leads to the condition termed ariboflavinosis. This includes a combination of clinical signs that center on tissue inflammation and breakdown and poor healing of even minor injuries (Box 6.11 and Fig. 6.7). Tissues subject to persistent abrasion that require continual replacement, such as the cells in the corners of the mouth, are affected first, followed by changes in the skin, and gastrointestinal tract. Riboflavin deficiency seldom occurs alone, but rather develops in combination with other B vitamin deficits. Because riboflavin is light sensitive, infants with elevated blood levels of bilirubin who are treated with phototherapy may require additional riboflavin.

BOX 6.11   **Signs of Riboflavin Deficiency**

- Lips become swollen and cracked with characteristic cracks at the corners of the mouth (**cheilosis**).
- Nasal angles develop cracks and irritation.
- Tongue becomes swollen and reddened (**glossitis**) (see Fig. 6.7).
- Extra blood vessels develop in the cornea (corneal vascularization).
- Eyes burn, itch, and tear.
- Skin becomes greasy and scaly, especially in skinfolds (**seborrheic dermatitis**).

FIG. 6.7 Glossitis resulting from riboflavin deficiency. (From McLaren DS: *A colour atlas and text of diet-related disorders,* ed 2, London, 1992, Mosby-Year Book Europe Limited.)

KEY TERMS

Ariboflavinosis
Group of clinical manifestations of riboflavin deficiency.

Cheilosis
Cracks and scaly lesions on the lips and mouth resulting from riboflavin deficiency.

Glossitis
Swollen, reddened tongue; symptom of riboflavin deficiency.

Seborrheic Dermatitis
Greasy scales and crusts that appear on the skin and moist folds of the body in riboflavin deficiency.

Riboflavin Requirement

Dietary Reference Intake

The RDA for riboflavin is based on the amount needed to sustain optimal levels of the flavoprotein enzymes. Recommended intakes are 1.3 mg/day for adolescent and adult men and 1.1 mg/day for adolescent and adult women.[23] The higher level for men relates to their higher kcalorie intakes and larger body size. No UL has been set for riboflavin, but supplements exceeding the RDA still carry possible harm.

Populations at Risk

Certain groups have special needs for riboflavin. Patients on hemodialysis must replace the riboflavin lost in the dialysate fluids. Pregnant and lactating women and infants and children are at risk of riboflavin deficiency based on their rapid tissue growth and high energy and protein metabolism. People who engage in vigorous physical activity have a greater need for riboflavin, possibly related to increased energy expenditure and muscle maintenance and repair. Cancer, heart disease, and diabetes

mellitus may add to riboflavin requirements.[12] Individuals who are lactose intolerant and avoid milk or milk products may be low in riboflavin.

Food Sources of Riboflavin

Major sources of riboflavin are milk and cheese. One quart of cow's milk or fortified soy or rice milk contains 2 mg of riboflavin, more than the daily requirement. Because riboflavin is destroyed by exposure to ultraviolet light, milk is usually packaged in cardboard or opaque plastic containers. Nursing mothers who store breast milk need to be reminded of potential riboflavin losses from glass containers. Other good sources of riboflavin are meat, whole or enriched grains and ready-to-eat cereals, and certain vegetables. Riboflavin is stable to heat and not easily destroyed with proper cooking. Box 6.12 describes some food sources of riboflavin.

NIACIN

The age-old disease related to niacin is pellagra. It is characterized by a typical dermatitis and eventually leads to fatal effects on the nervous system.[23] Pellagra was first observed in 18th-century Europe and was common in the southern region of the United States in the early 1900s among families whose diet was largely based on corn. The American physician Joseph Goldberger noticed that children who did not have pellagra had higher intakes of meat and milk. His investigation established that pellagra was related to a food factor, not an infectious pathogen; however, it was not until 1937 that a researcher at the University of Wisconsin associated niacin with pellagra by using it to cure a related disease—black tongue—in dogs.

Chemical and Physical Nature

Niacin exists in two forms: (1) nicotinic acid and (2) nicotinamide. Nicotinic acid is easily converted to nicotinamide, which is water soluble, is stable to acid and heat, and forms a white powder when crystallized.

Niacin also bears a close connection to the essential amino acid tryptophan, as described as follows:

- *Precursor role of tryptophan:* Curious observations by early researchers raised puzzling questions. Why was pellagra rare in some populations whose diets were low in niacin but common in others whose diets were higher in niacin? Why did milk, which is low in niacin, cure or prevent pellagra? Why was pellagra so common in families subsisting on diets high in corn? Then came the key discovery—tryptophan can be used by the body to make niacin. In other words, tryptophan is a precursor of niacin. Milk prevents pellagra because it is high in tryptophan. A corn-based diet results in pellagra because it is low in both tryptophan and niacin, but this depends on how the corn is prepared. In the American South, where corn was eaten as a vegetable or made into corn bread or corn meal, the bound niacin present in corn could not be released and absorbed. In contrast, pellagra was rare in Mexican families who soaked corn in lime (alkali) when preparing tortillas, because the lime treatment released the bound niacin so it was able to be absorbed. Others with diets low in niacin escaped pellagra because they had sufficient intakes of animal protein that supplied tryptophan.
- *Niacin equivalent (NE):* The tryptophan-niacin relation led to the development of the unit of measure called a *niacin equivalent (NE).* In general, 60 mg of tryptophan can produce 1 mg of niacin, the amount designated as the NE. This is the unit used in the DRI for niacin.[23]

KEY TERM

Niacin Equivalent (NE)
A measure of the total dietary sources of niacin; 1 NE equals 1 mg of niacin or 60 mg of tryptophan.

BOX 6.12 Food Sources of Riboflavin

Food Source	Amount	Riboflavin (mg)
Grains Group		
Ready-to-Eat Cereals		
Total Whole Grain	¾ cup	1.70
Wheaties	1 cup	1.12
Rice Krispies	1¼ cup	0.43
Corn flakes	1 cup	0.43
Instant oatmeal	1 packet	0.06
Waffle, frozen, ready to eat	1	0.22
Bagel	3½ in	0.06
Rice, white, long grain, enriched, cooked	1 cup	0.02
Bread, white, enriched	1 slice	0.06
Vegetable Group		
Spinach, frozen, cooked	½ cup	0.17
Broccoli, cooked	½ cup	0.10
Meat, Beans, Eggs, and Nuts Group		
Pork, lean, braised	3 oz	0.23
Egg, hard-cooked	1	0.26
Turkey, dark meat, roasted	3 oz	0.29
Kidney beans, canned	1 cup	0.13
Baked beans, canned, plain or vegetarian	1 cup	0.10
Milk Group		
Yogurt, low fat, with fruit	1 cup	0.40
Milk, 2% fat, 1% fat, nonfat	1 cup	0.45
Pudding, instant, chocolate	½ cup	0.21
Cottage cheese, low fat	½ cup	0.28

Recommended Dietary Allowances for adults: women, 1.1 mg; men, 1.3 mg.

Images copyright 2006 JupiterImages Corporation. Data from US Department of Agriculture, Agricultural Research Service: *USDA National Nutrient Database for Standard Reference, Release 28,* revised May 2016. Nutrient Data Laboratory Home Page: https://www.ars.usda.gov/northeast-area/beltsville-md/beltsville-human-nutrition-research-center/nutrient-data-laboratory/docs/usda-national-nutrient-database-for-standard-reference/.

Functions of Niacin

Coenzyme Role

Niacin has two coenzyme forms: (1) nicotinamide-adenine dinucleotide (NAD) and (2) nicotinamide-adenine dinucleotide phosphate (NADP). In these forms, niacin partners with riboflavin in the cellular enzyme systems that convert amino acids and glycerol to glucose and then oxidize the glucose to release energy. (Recall that glycerol is obtained from the hydrolysis of triglycerides.)

Use as a Drug

Pharmacologic doses of nicotinic acid have been prescribed for cardiovascular patients in an effort to raise blood high-density lipoprotein (HDL)-cholesterol levels and prevent a recurrence of cardiovascular events; however, large-scale evaluations have not reported decreases in heart attacks, stroke, or deaths following use of this therapy.[28] Also, at therapeutic levels of 3- to 100-fold the DRI, nicotinic acid acts as a vasodilator, causing skin flushing and itching.[29] Side effects of this

therapy include gastrointestinal upset, muscle weakness, worsening of existing diabetes mellitus, and liver damage, so patients treated with these doses require constant medical supervision.[28,29]

Niacin Deficiency and Clinical Applications

Niacin deficiency and pellagra result in muscle weakness, anorexia, and indigestion. More specific symptoms involve the skin and nervous system, and skin areas exposed to sunlight develop a dark, scaly dermatitis (Fig. 6.8). If the deficiency continues, then deterioration of the CNS leads to confusion, disorientation, neuritis, and finally death.

Niacin Requirement

Dietary Reference Intake

The current RDAs for niacin are 16 mg NE/day for adult men and 14 mg NE/day for adult women.[23] These recommendations allow for gender differences in energy intake and body size, as well as the availability and relative efficiency of converting tryptophan to niacin. Various medications such as isoniazid interfere with the

FIG. 6.8 Pellagra is caused by niacin deficiency, with damage to the nervous system and a characteristic dermatitis. (From McLaren DS: *A colour atlas and text of diet-related disorders,* ed 2, London, 1992, Mosby-Year Book Europe Limited.)

conversion of tryptophan to niacin and contribute to niacin deficiency.[30] Rapid growth, pregnancy, lactation, physical activity, or the need to replace tissues after surgery or trauma increase the need for niacin.

Food Sources of Niacin

Meat and dairy products are major sources of niacin in the American diet and are also high in tryptophan. Other foods include peanuts, dried beans and peas, and whole grain or enriched breads and ready-to-eat cereals. Corn and rice are relatively poor sources because they are low in tryptophan. Box 6.13 lists some comparative food sources of niacin.

PANTOTHENIC ACID

Discovery

Pantothenic acid is found in all living things and participates in many body functions. Intestinal bacteria synthesize considerable amounts. This source, along with its occurrence in a wide variety of foods, makes pantothenic acid deficiency unlikely.

Chemical and Physical Nature

Pantothenic acid is a white crystalline compound. It is readily absorbed in the small intestine and combines with phosphorus to make the active molecule acetyl coenzyme A (CoA). In this form,

BOX 6.13   Food Sources of Niacin

Food Source	Amount	Niacin (mg NE)[a]
Grains Group		
Ready-to-Eat Cereals		
All-Bran Complete Wheat Flakes	¾ cup	20.0
Wheaties	1 cup	13.3
Rice Krispies	1¼ cup	5.9
Corn flakes	1 cup	5.0
Instant oatmeal	1 packet	0.3
Bagel, enriched	3½ in	4.7
Spaghetti, enriched	1 cup	2.6
Bread, white, enriched	1 slice	1.2
Vegetable Group		
Spaghetti sauce, no meat	1 cup	10.3
Potato, baked, flesh only	1 medium	2.2
Sweet potato, baked	1 medium	1.7
Meat, Beans, Eggs, and Nuts Group		
Chicken breast, roasted	½	11.8
Tuna, light, canned in water	3 oz	8.6
Haddock, baked	3 oz	3.5
Beef, ground meat patty	3 oz	3.9
Peanuts, dry roasted	1 oz (about 28)	4.0

[a] Recommended Dietary Allowances for adults: women, 14 mg NE; men, 16 mg NE. 1NE (niacin equivalent) = 1 mg niacin or 60 mg tryptophan. Images copyright 2006 JupiterImages Corporation. Data from US Department of Agriculture, Agricultural Research Service: *USDA National Nutrient Database for Standard Reference, Release 28,* revised May 2016. Nutrient Data Laboratory Home Page: https://www.ars.usda.gov/northeast-area/beltsville-md/beltsville-human-nutrition-research-center/nutrient-data-laboratory/docs/usda-national-nutrient-database-for-standard-reference/.

pantothenic acid has broad metabolic presence and use throughout the body. No known toxicity or natural deficiency exists.

Functions of Pantothenic Acid

As an essential constituent of CoA, pantothenic acid controls metabolic reactions involving carbohydrate, fat, and protein.

Pantothenic Acid Requirements

The AI of 5 mg/day for all adults will replace the pantothenic acid lost daily in the urine. No UL exists for this nutrient.[23]

Food Sources of Pantothenic Acid

Pantothenic acid is found in both plant and animal foods. Good sources include egg yolk, milk, and broccoli.

BIOTIN

General Nature of Biotin

Biotin is a sulfur-containing vitamin, and the minute traces in the body perform multiple metabolic tasks. Natural deficiency is unknown; however, induced deficiencies have occurred in patients on long-term parenteral nutrition that omitted biotin. The protein avidin found in raw egg white binds biotin and, if consumed regularly, induces biotin deficiency. Cooking denatures this protein and destroys its ability to combine with biotin. (Raw eggs also carry the risk of foodborne illness that can be fatal to young children, older adults, and those with compromised immune function.) No known toxicity exists for biotin.

Functions of Biotin

Biotin functions as a partner with CoA in reactions that transfer carbon dioxide (CO_2) from one molecule to another. Examples of this cofactor at work include (1) the synthesis of fatty acids, (2) the synthesis of amino acids, and (3) CO_2 fixation to form purines for making genetic material.

Biotin Requirement

Because the amount of biotin needed is so small, the AI for this nutrient is 30 mcg/day for all adults.[23] Synthesis by intestinal bacteria adds to the body's supply.

Food Sources of Biotin

Biotin is found in many foods, but its bioavailability varies greatly. The biotin in corn and soy is well absorbed, whereas the biotin in wheat is almost totally unavailable. Excellent food sources include egg yolk, liver, tomatoes, and yeast.

VITAMIN B₆ (PYRIDOXINE)

Chemical and Physical Nature

The chemical structure of vitamin B_6 is a pyridine ring, which accounts for its name. It is water soluble and heat stable but sensitive to light and alkali.

Forms

Vitamin B_6 is the generic term for the three forms of this vitamin found in nature: (1) pyridoxine, (2) pyridoxal, and (3) pyridoxamine. All three forms are equally active as precursors of the coenzyme pyridoxal phosphate (B_6–PO_4), or PLP.[23]

Absorption, Transport, and Storage

Vitamin B_6 is well absorbed in the upper segment of the small intestine. It is stored in muscle but found in tissues throughout the body, evidence of its many metabolic activities involving protein and amino acids.

Functions of Vitamin B₆

Coenzyme in Protein Metabolism

In its active phosphate form (PLP), vitamin B_6 is a coenzyme in more than 100 amino acid reactions involving the synthesis of important proteins. Examples include the following:

- *Neurotransmitters:* PLP is needed to convert the essential amino acid tryptophan to serotonin, which carries messages across the cells in the brain; it helps form γ-aminobutyric acid (GABA) found in the gray matter of the brain.
- *Amino group transfer:* PLP transfers nitrogen-containing amino groups from amino acids to form new amino acids and release carbon residues for energy.
- *Niacin:* PLP is needed to form niacin from tryptophan.
- *Hemoglobin:* PLP incorporates amino acids into heme, the nonprotein core of hemoglobin.
- *Immune function:* PLP participates in the production and release of antibodies and immune cells, making it especially important for patients in critical care.

Coenzyme in Fat Metabolism

PLP converts the essential fatty acid linoleic acid to arachidonic acid.

Vitamin B₆ Deficiency and Clinical Applications

Vitamin B_6 is key in a number of clinical situations:

- *Anemia:* A lack of vitamin B_6 interrupts heme formation, resulting in a hypochromic anemia. This occurs despite a ready supply of iron and is reversed when vitamin B_6 is restored.
- *CNS abnormalities:* Vitamin B_6 controls brain function through its role in the formation of serotonin and GABA. When a batch of commercial infant formula was mistakenly heated to a very high temperature, destroying the vitamin B_6, babies fed this formula experienced increasing irritability progressing to convulsions. Immediate supplementation with vitamin B_6 restored their normal function. Seizures and abnormal neural function can occur with both vitamin B_6 deficiency and excess, demanding close attention to sufficient intake but restraint with supplementation.[31]
- *Physiologic demands in pregnancy:* Vitamin B_6 deficiency has been identified in expectant mothers with preeclampsia (hypertension with edema and proteinuria) and eclampsia (convulsions).[23] Growth of the fetus, along with rising metabolic needs of the mother, increase the need for this vitamin.
- *Chronic disease:* Patients in end-stage renal disease undergoing hemodialysis require vitamin B6 supplements to maintain normal blood levels.[32]
- *Medications:* The drug isoniazid (isonicotinic acid hydrazide [INH]) used to treat tuberculosis is a vitamin B_6 **antagonist**; vitamin B_6 intakes of 50 mg/day appear to be a safe level of supplementation to overcome this effect.[31] Levodopa, a medication for Parkinson disease, lowers blood PLP levels. Oral contraceptive users may require vitamin B_6 supplements to avoid metabolic changes associated with deficiency of this vitamin.[33]

Vitamin B₆ Requirement
Dietary Reference Intake

The RDA is expected to maintain optimum blood PLP levels in most individuals,[23] although relatively high protein intakes increase the need

---

KEY TERM

Antagonist
A substance that acts in opposition to another physiologic substance preventing its normal action; vitamin antagonists prevent the usual action of the vitamin.

for vitamin B_6. Men and women ages 19 to 50 should take in 1.3 mg/day. Older adults require higher amounts, and older men need more than older women. For men older than 50 years, the RDA is 1.7 mg/day; for women of this age, it is 1.5 mg/day.

Vitamin B_6 Toxicity

Vitamin B_6 is one of the two water-soluble vitamins, along with vitamin C, with a demonstrated and physiologically deleterious toxicity. Vitamin B_6 toxicity was first reported in women taking supplements 1000 times the RDA in the belief that such a dose would alleviate premenstrual syndrome. Such intakes result in seborrheic dermatitis, interfere with muscle coordination and brain function, and over time damage the nervous system. In most cases, symptoms gradually disappear after the supplements are discontinued. The UL for vitamin B_6 is 100 mg/day.[23]

Food Sources of Vitamin B_6

Vitamin B_6 is widespread among many foods but usually in rather small amounts. Good sources include whole grains, legumes, meat, poultry, bananas, and potatoes. Fruits, vegetables, and whole grain breads and cereals are the major contributors of vitamin B_6 in the Healthy Meal Patterns developed by the 2015 Dietary Guidelines Advisory Committee.[1] Box 6.14 displays some food sources of this vitamin.

BOX 6.14   Food Sources of Vitamin B_6 (Pyridoxine)

Vitamin B_6 (pyridoxine) is found in both plant and animal foods, although the milk group has low amounts. Ready-to-eat cereals, potatoes, and poultry are especially good sources.

Food Source	Amount	Vitamin B_6 (mg)
Grains Group		
Corn flakes	1 cup	0.50
Instant oatmeal	1 packet	0.05
Vegetable Group		
Potato, baked, flesh only	1 medium	0.47
Spaghetti sauce, tomato, no meat	1 cup	0.46
Fruit Group		
Banana	1	0.43
Meat, Beans, Eggs, and Nuts Group		
Chicken breast, roasted	½	0.52
Tuna, light, canned, packed in water	3 oz	0.27
Beef, ground beef patty	3 oz	0.29
Baked beans, canned, plain or vegetarian	1 cup	0.21

Recommended Dietary Allowances for adults: men and women, ages 19–50, 1.3 mg; women, ages ≥51, 1.5 mg; men, ages ≥51, 1.7 mg. Images copyright 2006 JupiterImages Corporation. Data from US Department of Agriculture, Agricultural Research Service: *USDA National Nutrient Database for Standard Reference, Release 28,* Revised May 2016. Nutrient Data Laboratory Home Page: https://www.ars.usda.gov/northeast-area/beltsville-md/beltsville-human-nutrition-research-center/nutrient-data-laboratory/docs/usda-national-nutrient-database-for-standard-reference/.

FOLATE

Discovery

Folates were first extracted from dark green leafy vegetables and given the name *folic acid* from the Latin word for *leaf.* Studies investigating anemia among poor pregnant East Indian women led to the discovery of this vitamin group.

Chemical and Physical Nature

Folic acid, a yellow crystal, has the chemical name of *pteroylmonoglutamic acid,* based on its structure. Folic acid is seldom found naturally but is the form used in supplements and fortified foods. Naturally occurring folate or food folate is the compound pteroylpolyglutamate, which contains additional glutamic acid molecules.[23] Both forms are well used by the body.

Absorption, Transport, and Storage

The absorption of folate depends on the source. Approximately 50% of the folate occurring naturally in plant foods (food folate) is absorbed, compared with 85% of the folic acid added to fortified foods. Conversion factors have been developed for calculating folate intake (Box 6.15).[34]

Functions of Folate

Coenzyme Role

Folate is the coenzyme that attaches single carbons to metabolic compounds. Several key molecules provide examples, as follows:

- *Purines:* Nitrogen-containing compounds in genetic material that participate in cell division and the transmission of inherited traits.
- *Thymine:* A component of DNA, the material in the cell nucleus that controls and transmits genetic characteristics.
- *Hemoglobin:* Heme is the iron-containing nonprotein portion of hemoglobin that transports oxygen and CO_2 in the blood.
- *Conversion of methionine to cysteine:* If folate is not available, homocysteine, an intermediate metabolite, accumulates in the blood and adds to the risk of cardiovascular and other chronic diseases.

Folate Deficiency and Clinical Applications

Anemia

A nutritional megaloblastic anemia occurs in simple folate deficiency. Because folate needs are high during periods of rapid growth, folate deficiency anemia is most likely to occur in pregnant women, growing infants, and young children. Adolescent girls who severely limit their food intake are also at risk.

BOX 6.15   Calculating Dietary Folate Equivalents

- 1 mcg of food folate (occurring naturally in a food) = 1 mcg dietary folate equivalent (DFE).
- 1 mcg folic acid (added in food fortification) = 1.7 mcg DFE (Folic acid added to a food is absorbed more efficiently than naturally occurring food folate.)

  To estimate the DFEs in foods such as fortified breakfast cereals in which most or all of the folate is added folic acid, use the percentage daily value listed on the food label:

  % Daily value × 400 mcg (the daily value for folic acid) × 1.7 = DFEs per serving

Data from Suitor CW, Bailey LB: Dietary folate equivalents: interpretation and application, *J Am Diet Assoc* 100:88, 2000.

Presence of Gastric Acid

An acid environment is required to release food folate from its food source and enable its absorption. Low gastric secretion of hydrochloric acid, a common problem in older adults, or use of medications that raise the pH in the gastrointestinal tract adversely affect folate status.

Medications

The drug amethopterin (methotrexate) used in cancer treatment is a folate antagonist and prevents the synthesis of DNA and purines, thereby preventing the growth of the cancer. High intakes of folate interfere with the action of the drug phenobarbital used to control seizures.[23]

Folate and Birth Defects

NTDs, a worldwide problem, are congenital malformations occurring when the spinal cord and its coverings fail to develop normally. If part of the brain fails to develop (anencephaly), then the infant is likely to die shortly after birth. The more common NTD is spina bifida, in which the neural tube fails to close during embryonic development and the spinal cord remains on the outside of the body (Fig. 6.9). In less severe cases a child may live a productive life if surgical and medical intervention is effective, but for many a normal life is not achievable.

Folate is essential for the formation and closure of the neural tube in the early weeks of fetal development (between day 21 and day 28 of gestation), before a woman is even aware that she might be pregnant. Therefore it is critical that a mother be in good folate status *before* conception occurs. To improve the folate status of women of childbearing age the US Food and Drug Administration (FDA) in 1998 instituted mandatory fortification of flours and grains to the level of 140 mcg of folic acid per 100 g. In practical terms, one slice of fortified bread and one cup of fortified pasta provide 136 mcg DFE or approximately one-third of the RDA.[12] However, many ready-to-eat cereals provide 400 mcg of folic acid per serving or 100% of the RDA.

Although folate fortification has been declared a public health success based on the significant decline in NTD-related births, it remains controversial. First, not all cases of NTDs are the result of folate deficiency, thus additional folate will not address the genetic or other unknown causes that result in this birth defect.[35] Second, excessive folate intake can be harmful for individuals of all ages. It has been reported that high intakes of folate may promote the growth of existing tumors in the colon whereas too low intakes may also add to cancer risk.[36] Surveys indicate that 75% of adult men are taking in more than 470 µg of folate each day and more than 50% of women are taking in more than 450 µg of folate each day from naturally occurring folates and fortified foods. Five percent to 10% of both men and women are obtaining more than 1000 µg of folate from food alone. If such individuals are also taking a supplement, intakes could well exceed the UL of 1000 µg DFE.[1] In the following section we will also explore the problem that high intakes of folic acid can mask a vitamin B_{12} deficiency with injurious results. A continuing question is how we achieve optimum folate status in women of childbearing age while avoiding negative effects on men and older adults who may eat numerous servings of fortified cereals and grains and also take folate supplements.

Folate Requirement
Dietary Reference Intake

The RDA for folate is expressed as Dietary Folate Equivalents (DFEs), which adjusts for the difference in absorption between naturally occurring folate and folic acid added in fortification or obtained in supplements. The RDA for adults is 400 mcg DFE/day and increases to 600 mcg DFE/day in pregnancy.[23] Women of reproductive age average 155 to 165 mcg DFE of folic acid daily from fortified foods.[37] Folic acid intake from fortification is lowest among African-American women (136 mcg DFE).

Folate Toxicity

The UL for folate is 1000 mcg DFE/day,[23] and supplements exceeding the recommended intake of 400 mcg DFE are best avoided. The basis for concern is the relationship between folate and vitamin B_{12}. If vitamin B_{12} levels are low but folate levels are high, then folate will substitute for vitamin B_{12} in the formation of red blood cells and prevent the development of a megaloblastic anemia. However, vitamin B_{12} also has a critical role in maintaining the myelin sheath surrounding nerve

FIG. 6.9 Neural tube defects (NTDs) include anencephaly and spina bifida. Spina bifida can result from a lack of folate needed to close the neural tube that becomes the spinal cord in the developing fetus. (Redrawn from Centers for Disease Control and Prevention: Facts about anencephaly and Facts: spina bifida, Atlanta, 2013.)

BOX 6.16   Food Sources of Folate

Food Source	Amount	Folate (mcg DFE)
Grains Group		
Fortified Ready-to-Eat Cereals		
All-Bran Complete Wheat Flakes	¾ cup	400
Wheaties	1 cup	449
Corn flakes	1 cup	163
Instant oatmeal	1 packet	9
Rice, white, long grain, cooked, enriched	1 cup	153
Spaghetti, enriched, cooked	1 cup	185
Hamburger roll, enriched	1	58
Bread, white, enriched	1 slice	43
Vegetable Group		
Spinach, frozen, cooked	½ cup	115
Broccoli, cooked	½ cup	84
Lettuce, dark green (romaine or similar)	1 cup	64
Tomato juice, canned	1 cup	49
Fruit Group		
Orange juice, frozen, reconstituted	1 cup	47
Strawberries	1 cup	40
Meat, Beans, Eggs, and Nuts Group		
Kidney beans, canned	1 cup	59

Recommended Dietary Allowance for adults: 400 mcg DFE (women capable of becoming pregnant should take in 400 mcg of folic acid in addition to food folate from a varied diet). 1 mcg DFE (dietary folate equivalent) = 1 mcg food folate = 0.6 mcg of folic acid.
Images copyright 2006 JupiterImages Corporation. Data from US Department of Agriculture, Agricultural Research Service: *USDA National Nutrient Database for Standard Reference, Release 28*, Revised May 2016. Nutrient Data Laboratory Home Page: https://www.ars.usda.gov/northeast-area/beltsville-md/beltsville-human-nutrition-research-center/nutrient-data-laboratory/docs/usda-national-nutrient-database-for-standard-reference/.

tissue, and folate cannot meet that need. The appearance of a megaloblastic anemia is often the first alert to vitamin B$_{12}$ deficiency. If high intakes of folate "mask" this effect, then irreversible damage to the nervous system continues unabated.[38]

Food Sources of Folate

Folate is widely distributed in plant foods. Good sources include dark green leafy vegetables, citrus fruits, tomatoes, cantaloupe, and legumes, as well as fortified grains. Ready-to-eat cereal is a major contributor of folic acid in the US diet.[39] Box 6.16 summarizes food sources of folate.

VITAMIN B$_{12}$ (COBALAMIN)

Discovery

The discovery of vitamin B$_{12}$ coincided with the search for a cure for **pernicious anemia**. In 1948 workers crystallized a red compound from

liver that controlled both the blood-forming defect and the nerve degeneration associated with pernicious anemia. This molecule was numbered *vitamin B$_{12}$* and later named *cobalamin*, based on the single red atom of the trace element cobalt at its center.

Chemical and Physical Nature

Vitamin B$_{12}$ is a complex red crystal of high molecular weight. It occurs as a protein complex in animal foods only. Vitamin B$_{12}$ is synthesized by bacteria in the intestinal tract of herbivorous animals and some bacterial synthesis also occurs in the human intestine.

Absorption, Transport, and Storage

Vitamin B$_{12}$ is split from its protein complex by the hydrochloric acid in the stomach and then bound to a specific protein called *intrinsic factor*, secreted by the gastric mucosa. This vitamin B$_{12}$–intrinsic factor complex then moves into the intestine, where special receptors in the wall of the ileum enable its absorption. The loss of gastric acid or failure of the gastric mucosa to secrete intrinsic factor will prevent absorption and result in deficiency.

Approximately 50% of body vitamin B$_{12}$ is stored in the liver, with the remainder distributed among active tissues. These amounts are minute but held tenaciously and only slowly depleted. Vitamin B$_{12}$ deficiency does not become apparent for 3 to 5 years after a gastrectomy and loss of required secretions.

KEY TERM

Pernicious Anemia

A macrocytic anemia caused by the absence of intrinsic factor necessary for absorption of vitamin B$_{12}$; it is treated with intramuscular injections of vitamin B$_{12}$; if untreated it results in death.

Functions of Vitamin B₁₂
Basic Coenzyme Role
Vitamin B₁₂ participates in amino acid metabolism and formation of the heme portion of hemoglobin. It has a role in the synthesis and maintenance of important lipids and proteins that form the myelin sheath covering the nerves of the brain and spinal cord.

Vitamin B₁₂ Deficiency and Clinical Applications
Vitamin B₁₂ deficiency disrupts blood formation and affects brain and cognitive function:

- *Pernicious anemia:* The megaloblastic anemia arising from vitamin B₁₂ deficiency took on the name *pernicious anemia* because it is fatal if left untreated. When this vitamin is lacking, the production and maturation of red blood cells is halted because the heme portion of the hemoglobin molecule cannot be synthesized, and the activated molecule of folate needed to assist in the process cannot be formed. The root cause of pernicious anemia is a lack of intrinsic factor required for vitamin B₁₂ absorption; thus another way must be found to supply this vitamin to the body. Monthly intramuscular injections or high-dose oral supplements that enable the absorption of small amounts of vitamin by mass action control the blood-forming disorder and prevent the degenerative effects on the nervous system.[40]

- *Brain and cognitive function:* Progressive vitamin B₁₂ deficiency causes fatigue, lassitude, muscle weakness, and tingling sensations in the extremities. As damage to the nervous system continues, there are declines in cognitive and thought processes and often changes in personality. Even in the absence of overt deficiency, long-term studies indicate that older adults with lower blood vitamin B₁₂ levels are more likely to experience cognitive decline and depression than those with normal levels.[41] At the same time it is important to note that supplementation with vitamin B₁₂ will not reverse cognitive changes in older adults that are not associated with their B₁₂ status.[42]

- *Low gastric acid secretion:* Low gastric acid levels as a result of *H. pylori* infection, gastrectomy or bariatric surgery, or age-related changes in secretion results in lower B₁₂ absorption from food. Use of acid-depressing medications can contribute to this problem. It is estimated that 20% of older adults experience problems absorbing vitamin B₁₂ from food.[40] The problem of low gastric acid can be bypassed depending on the source of the B₁₂ included in the diet. The vitamin used in food fortification and vitamin supplements is not bound in a protein complex and does not require gastric acid for effective absorption as does the B₁₂ bound in food. Use of vitamin B₁₂–fortified foods several times each week will help to supply the amount needed.

- *Pregnancy and lactation:* For normal brain development, sufficient vitamin B₁₂ must be available to the growing fetus and the breast-fed infant. Pregnant and breast-feeding mothers who have undergone gastric surgery, are vegans, or consume very few animal foods need special counseling regarding appropriate supplements.[40]

- *Diabetes:* Metformin, frequently prescribed in treatment of type 2 diabetes, has been associated with vitamin B₁₂ deficiency in some long-term patients.[43]

Vitamin B₁₂ Requirement
The amount of vitamin B₁₂ required is minute. The RDA is 2.4 mcg for both younger and older adults.[23]

Food Sources of Vitamin B₁₂
In nature, vitamin B₁₂ is found only in animal foods; rich sources include lean meat, fish, poultry, milk, eggs, and cheese. For individuals who include any animal foods in their diet, the recommended intake is easily obtained. Vegans and individuals with low gastric acid levels can meet their requirement from fortified grains, cereals, juices, soy milk, or vitamin B₁₂ supplements. Box 6.17 lists various sources.

A summary of the water-soluble B vitamins is found in Table 6.4.

BOX 6.17 Food Sources of Vitamin B₁₂ (Cobalamin)

Vitamin B₁₂ (cobalamin) is found naturally in animal foods only, but various grain foods and juices are fortified with this vitamin. Vegans who consume no animal foods and older persons with reduced gastric acid levels should check the nutrition label to identify products with added vitamin B₁₂.

Naturally Occurring Sources of Vitamin B₁₂
Meat patty
Chicken leg
Fish serving
Milk
Cheese

Examples of Nonanimal Foods Sometimes Fortified with Vitamin B₁₂
Ready-to-eat cereal
Bread
Orange juice

Recommended Dietary Allowance for adults: 2.4 mcg.
Images copyright 2006 JupiterImages Corporation.

TABLE 6.4 Summary of B-Complex Vitamins

Vitamin	Coenzyme: Physiologic Functions	Clinical Applications	Dietary Reference Intake	Food Sources

Thiamin	Carbohydrate metabolism
	Thiamin pyrophosphate (TPP): active form
	Production of glucose for energy
		Beriberi (classic deficiency disease)
		Neuropathy
		Wernicke-Korsakoff syndrome (alcoholism)
		Depressed muscular and secretory functions
			Males ages ≥19: 1.2 mg
			Females ages ≥19: 1.1 mg
			Pregnancy
			  All ages: 1.4 mg
			Lactation
			  All ages: 1.4 mg
				Pork, beef, organ meats
				Whole or enriched grains and cereals
				Legumes

Continued

TABLE 6.4   Summary of B-Complex Vitamins—cont'd

Vitamin	Coenzyme: Physiologic Functions	Clinical Applications	Dietary Reference Intake	Food Sources
Riboflavin	General metabolism FMN (flavin mononucleotide) FAD (flavin adenine dinucleotide)	Cheilosis, Glossitis, Seborrheic dermatitis	Males ages ≥19: 1.3 mg Females ages ≥19: 1.1 mg Pregnancy 　All ages: 1.4 mg Lactation 　All ages: 1.6 mg	Milk products Organ meats Enriched grains and cereals
Niacin (nicotinic acid, nicotin-amide)	General metabolism Nicotinamide adenine dinucleotide (NAD) Nicotinamide adenine dinucleotide phosphate (NADP)	Pellagra (classic deficiency disease) Weakness, anorexia Scaly dermatitis Neuritis Death (if untreated)	Males ages ≥19: 16 mg NE[a] Females ages ≥19: 14 mg NE Pregnancy 　All ages: 18 mg NE Lactation 　All ages: 17 mg NE	Meat and dairy foods containing tryptophan Peanuts Enriched grains and cereals
Vitamin B_6 (pyridoxine, pyridoxal, pyridoxamine)	General metabolism Pyridoxal phosphate (PLP): active form Transamination and decarboxylation reactions Active in protein and amino acid metabolism Synthesis of neurotransmitters	Reduced serum levels associated with pregnancy and use of certain oral contraceptives Antagonists include isoniazid and penicillamine, Toxic with excessive supplement intake	Adult males 　Ages 19–50: 1.3 mg 　Ages ≥51: 1.7 mg Adult females 　Ages 19–50: 1.3 mg 　Ages ≥51: 1.5 mg Pregnancy 　All ages: 1.9 mg Lactation 　All ages: 2.0 mg	Meat, organ meats Whole grains and cereals Legumes Bananas, Potatoes
Pantothenic acid	General metabolism Coenzyme A (CoA): active form Metabolism of carbohydrates, fats, and amino acids	Many roles in lipogenesis, amino acid activation, and formation of cholesterol, steroid hormones, and heme	Males/females 　Ages ≥19: 5 mg Pregnancy 　All ages: 6 mg Lactation 　All ages: 7 mg	Egg, milk, liver Widely distributed in food
Biotin	General metabolism CO_2 transfer reactions	Deficiency induced by avidin (a protein in raw egg white) and by antibiotics	Males/females 　Ages ≥19: 30 mcg Pregnancy 　All ages: 30 mcg Lactation 　All ages: 35 mcg	Egg yolk, liver Widely distributed in food Synthesized by intestinal bacteria
Folate – naturally occurring in food Folic acid - used in food fortification and supplements	General metabolism Single carbon transfer reactions (e.g., purine nucleotide, thymine, heme synthesis)	Megaloblastic anemia Conversion of methionine to cysteine Neural tube defect–affected pregnancy Phenobarbital and methotrexate interfere with folate	Males/females 　Ages ≥19: 400 mcg Pregnancy 　All ages: 600 mcg Lactation 　All ages: 500 mcg	Green leafy vegetables Oranges, orange juice, tomatoes Liver and organ meats Fortified breads and cereals
Vitamin B_{12} (cobalamin)	General metabolism Methylation reactions in synthesis of amino acids Production and maturation of red blood cells Synthesis and maintenance of myelin sheath surrounding nerves	Pernicious anemia induced by lack of intrinsic factor for B_{12} absorption Megaloblastic anemia Peripheral neuropathy Changes in cognitive function Vegan diet requires supplementation Low gastric acid secretion hinders absorption	Males/females 　Ages ≥19: 2.4 mcg Pregnancy 　All ages: 2.6 mcg Lactation 　All ages: 2.8 mcg	Meat, milk, cheese, egg, liver (found in all animal foods) Fortified cereals, juices, and soy milk

[a]Niacin equivalent; 1 mg of niacin = 60 mg tryptophan.

PERSPECTIVES IN PRACTICE
Choosing a Vitamin-Mineral Supplement: Do I Need One?

The general public is constantly bombarded by advertisements promoting a vitamin or mineral supplement to prevent or cure real or imagined nutrient deficiencies or chronic health problems. National surveys indicate that 52% of the general public take a nutritional supplement. These include multivitamin-mineral supplements or individual nutrients such as calcium, vitamin D, and fish oils.[1]

The best strategy for obtaining appropriate amounts of vitamins and minerals is to eat a variety of nutrient-dense foods. Fortified foods such as breakfast cereals or juices can add vitamins or minerals that may be difficult to obtain in sufficient amounts. Individuals at particular stages in their life cycle or with elevated needs may require supplements to meet their recommended intakes as follows[2,3]:

- Infants who are breast-fed and children, teenagers, and adults who eat or drink limited amounts of vitamin D–containing foods will need a supplement to meet their Daily Recommended Intake (DRI).
- Women of childbearing age who may become pregnant are encouraged to consume 400 mcg of folic acid daily in addition to food folate obtained from a varied diet to help prevent neural tube defects (NTDs); folic acid added to fortified foods and supplements is better absorbed than naturally occurring folate.
- Older adults with low levels of gastric acid who are less able to absorb vitamin B_{12} from animal sources require vitamin B_{12}–fortified foods or supplements.
- Vegans who consume no animal foods will require additional sources of vitamin B_{12}.
- Individuals with low energy needs, such as sedentary older adults, or others who eat very limited amounts of food or follow unhealthy food patterns will benefit from a multivitamin-mineral supplement.
- Individuals with specific medical conditions, such as cystic fibrosis, that interfere with fat absorption, or who have had bariatric surgery, or who are undergoing hemodialysis will require continuing evaluation of their nutritional status and need for supplements.
- Pregnant women are unlikely to meet their iron requirement of 27 mg from food only, even including fortified foods, and are usually prescribed a supplement.
- Recommendations for the use of vitamin-mineral supplements must be individualized and based on need as evaluated by a health professional. For those individuals who cannot or will not achieve nutritional adequacy with food alone, consider the following when recommending supplements.

Guidelines for Selecting a Vitamin-Mineral Supplement
- Use supplements in addition to, not in place of, real food. A poor diet with added supplements is still a poor diet.
- Avoid multivitamin-mineral supplements or single-nutrient supplements that exceed 100% of the DRI for any nutrient. Individuals using highly fortified foods, such as a cereal that supplies 100% of the DRI for most vitamins, is likely not in need of a supplement.
- If using more than one supplement be sure to add the amounts of any nutrient supplied in each. Total intake should not exceed the DRI for any vitamin or mineral.
- Check with a physician or other health professional who can evaluate the relative benefits and risks before beginning a supplement. Inappropriately high amounts of particular vitamins or minerals can interfere with the action of certain prescription or over-the-counter medications or become toxic.
- Store your vitamin-mineral supplement in a cool, dry place, not the kitchen or bathroom or other area with high heat and humidity. Vitamins that are easily oxidized will absorb moisture when the bottle is opened and deteriorate rapidly.

For vitamins and minerals, "more is not necessarily better." Once you reach your DRI, combining what was provided in your food and any supplement, there is no benefit to taking in an additional amount. Excessive amounts of nutrients, such as vitamin A, vitamin D, or vitamin B_6 consumed in supplements, can lead to toxic conditions. In addition, recent analyses[4] of popular brands revealed that many supplements contain as much as 26% more of a particular nutrient than is stated on the label, noting the importance of prudent use.

References
1. Kantor ED, Rehm CD, Du M, et al: Trends in dietary supplement use among US adults from 1999-2012, *JAMA* 316(14):1464, 2016.
2. Marra MV, Boyar AP, American Dietetic Association: Position of the American Dietetic Association: nutrient supplementation, *J Am Diet Assoc* 109:2073, 2009.
3. Biesalski HK, Tinz J: Multivitamin/mineral supplements: Rationale and safety—a systematic review, *Nutrition* 33:76, 2017.
4. Andrews KW, Roseland JM, Gusev PA, et al: Analytical ingredient content and variability of adult multivitamin/mineral products: National estimates for the Dietary Supplement Ingredient Database, *Am J Clin Nutr* 105(2):526, 2017.

As we conclude our discussion of this important micronutrient group, consider your own vitamin intake and review the Perspectives in Practice box, "Choosing a Vitamin-Mineral Supplement: Do I Need One?"

TO SUM UP

A vitamin is an organic, non–energy-yielding substance that is (1) required in very small amounts; (2) participates in specific metabolic functions, often as a coenzyme; and (3) must be supplied in the diet. The metabolic tasks of the fat-soluble vitamins A, D, E, and K involve the synthesis of important proteins related to vision, blood clotting, and bone health. Vitamin A influences the differentiation of cells and tissues, and vitamin E, a powerful antioxidant, protects polyunsaturated fatty acids in membranes and neural tissue from harmful free radicals. The fat-soluble vitamins are absorbed and transported with lipids and easily stored; thus excessive intake can lead to toxicity.

The water-soluble vitamins including ascorbic acid and the B-complex vitamins are synthesized by plants and, with the exception of vitamin B_{12} (found only in animal sources), are supplied in both plant and animal foods. They function as coenzymes in cell metabolism and protein synthesis and must be consumed regularly as body stores are limited. Excess intake is excreted in the urine. Ascorbic acid functions as an antioxidant and is important for tissue integrity. Folate and vitamins B_6 and B_{12} have important roles in formation of red blood cells and development and function of nerve structures. Vitamin B_6 and ascorbic acid have shown evidence of toxicity with excessive supplement use, and intakes of folate greater than recommended levels can interfere with the body's use of vitamin B_{12}. Water-soluble vitamins, especially vitamin C and folate, are easily oxidized, and appropriate cooking and storage practices are required to prevent losses from food sources.

QUESTIONS FOR REVIEW

1. Explain how the absorption and storage of a vitamin influence the risk of deficiency and toxicity. Provide several examples to illustrate this concept.

2. A young man with cystic fibrosis has just been diagnosed with night blindness although he eats a variety of dark green and deep yellow vegetables and fruits. How would you explain this?

3. What organ systems participate in the formation of the vitamin D hormone calcitriol, and what are their roles? How has the use of sunscreen and choice of soft drinks rather than milk increased the vulnerability of youth to vitamin D deficiency? How does renal failure impact vitamin D function?

4. What is an antioxidant, and how does it protect body tissues? A woman tells you that she is taking 1000 mg of vitamin E daily to prevent signs of aging. How would you advise her?

5. How does the B vitamin complex influence functions of the brain and nervous system? What vitamins are necessary to synthesize neurotransmitters such as serotonin?

6. Name the B vitamins involved in blood formation. Describe their roles and interactions.

7. You are helping a young woman develop an eating pattern that will meet her needs for folate and vitamin D. Develop menus for 2 days that will meet her DRI for these nutrients. What are the problems related to meeting the DRI for vitamin D with food only?

8. Visit a grocery store and choose two ready-to-eat cereals advertised as being "healthy" and two sugar-sweetened cereals advertised for children. Compare the food labels and record the levels or proportion of the Daily Value provided for vitamin A, vitamin D, folic acid, vitamin B_6, and vitamin B_{12}. Did you observe any vitamin differences between the "healthy" cereals and sugar-sweetened cereals? Are any of the vitamins actually provided by the accompanying milk rather than the cereal itself? If a young man had two servings of a "healthy" cereal, would he be in danger of exceeding the UL for any nutrient?

REFERENCES

1. US Department of Health and Human Services, US Department of Agriculture: *Report of the Dietary Guidelines Advisory Committee on the Dietary Guidelines for Americans 2015*, Washington, DC, 2015, Center for Nutrition Policy and Promotion, US Department of Agriculture. https://health.gov/dietaryguidelines/2015-scientific-report/.

2. Tang G, Hu Y, Yin SA, et al: β-carotene in golden rice is as good as β-carotene in oil at providing vitamin A to children, *Am J Clin Nutr* 96:658, 2012.

3. Food and Nutrition Board, Institute of Medicine: *Dietary Reference Intakes for vitamin A, vitamin K, arsenic, boron, chromium, copper, iodine, iron, manganese, molybdenum, nickel, silicon, vanadium, and zinc*, Washington, DC, 2001, National Academies Press.

4. Wiseman EM, Bar-El DS, Reifen R: The vicious cycle of vitamin A deficiency: A review, *Crit Rev Food Sci Nutr* 57(17):3703–3714, 2017.

5. US Department of Agriculture, Agricultural Research Service: *USDA National Nutrient Database for Standard Reference*, Release 28, revised May 2016. https://ndb.nal.usda.gov/ndb/.

6. Linos E, Keiser E, Kanzler M, et al: Sun protective behaviors and vitamin D levels in the US population: NHANES 2003-2006, *Cancer Causes Control* 23:133, 2012.

7. Ganji V, Zhang X, Tangpricha V: Serum 25-hydroxyvitamin D concentrations and prevalence estimates of hypovitaminosis D in the US population based on assay-adjusted data, *J Nutr* 142:498, 2012.

8. Food and Nutrition Board, Institute of Medicine: *DRI, Dietary Reference Intakes: calcium, vitamin D*, Washington, DC, 2011, National Academies Press.

9. Hoel DG, Berwick M, de Gruijl FR, et al: The risks and benefits of sun exposure 2016, *Dermatoendocrinol* 8(1):e1248325, 2016.

10. Holick MF: Vitamin D and brain health: The need for vitamin D supplementation and sensible sun exposure, *J Intern Med* 277(1):90, 2015.

11. US Food and Drug Administration: *Food labeling: Revision of the nutrition and supplement facts labels. A rule by the Food and Drug Administration on 5/27/2016.* 81 FR 33741, 21 CFR 101, 2016-11867, May 2016.

12. Food and Nutrition Board, Institute of Medicine: *Dietary Reference Intakes. The essential guide to nutrient requirements*, Washington, DC, 2006, National Academies Press.

13. Traber MG: Vitamin E inadequacy in humans: Causes and consequences, *Adv Nutr* 5:503, 2014.

14. US Department of Agriculture, Agricultural Research Service: Table 1. Nutrient Intakes from Food and Beverages. Mean Amounts Consumed per Individual by Gender and Age in the United States, 2013-2014. *What We Eat in America*, NHANES 2013-2014, 2016. https://www.ars.usda.gov/northeast-area/beltsville-md/beltsville-human-nutrition-research-center/food-surveys-research-group/docs/wweia-data-tables/.

15. Hosseini B, Saedisomeolia A, Skilton MR: Association between micronutrients intake/status and carotid intima media thickness: A systematic review, *J Acad Nutr Diet* 117(1):69–82, 2017.

16. Tucker KL: Nutrient intake, nutritional status, and cognitive function with aging, *Ann N Y Acad Sci* 1367:38, 2016.

17. Bjelakovic G, Nikolova D, Gluud LL, et al: Antioxidant supplements for prevention of mortality in healthy participants and patients with various diseases (review), *Cochrane Database Syst Rev* (3):CD007176, 2012.

18. Gröber U, Reichrath J, Holick MF, et al: Vitamin K: An old vitamin in a new perspective, *Dermato endocrinol* 6(1):e968490, 2014.

19. Aditi A, Graham DY: Vitamin C, gastritis, and gastric disease: A historical review and update, *Dig Dis Sci* 57(10):2504, 2012. doi:10.1007/s10620-012-2203.

20. Winkler MA, Manchester S: Medical nutrition therapy for metabolic stress, sepsis, trauma, burns, and surgery. In Mahan KL, Escott-Stump S, editors: *Krause's food, nutrition, & diet therapy*, ed 12, Philadelphia, PA, 2008, Saunders.

21. Golriz F, Donnelly LF, Devaraj S, et al: Modern American scurvy—experience with vitamin C deficiency at a large children's hospital, *Pediatr Radiol* 47(2):214, 2017.

22. Ferraro PM, Curhan GC, Gambaro G, et al: Total, dietary, and supplemental vitamin C intake and risk of incident kidney stones, *Am J Kidney Dis* 67(3):400, 2016.

23. Food and Nutrition Board, Institute of Medicine: *Dietary Reference Intakes for thiamin, riboflavin, niacin, vitamin B_6, folate, vitamin B_{12}, pantothenic acid, biotin, and choline*, Washington, DC, 1998, National Academies Press.

24. Gibson GE, Hirsch JA, Fonzetti P, et al: Vitamin B1 (thiamine) and dementia, *Ann N Y Acad Sci* 1367:21, 2016.

25. Ahmed M, Azizi-Namini P, Yan AT, et al: Thiamin deficiency and heart failure: The current knowledge and gaps in literature, *Heart Fail Rev* 20:1, 2015.

26. Tzoulaki I, Patel CJ, Okamura T, et al: A nutrient-wide association study on blood pressure, *Circulation* 126:2456, 2012.

27. Frantz DJ: Neurologic complications of bariatric surgery: involvement of central, peripheral, and enteric nervous systems, *Curr Gastroenterol Rep* 14:367, 2012.

28. Garg A, Sharma A, Krishnamoorthy P, et al: Role of niacin in current clinical practice: A systematic review, *Am J Med* 130(2):173–187, 2017.

29. MacKay D, Hathcock J, Guarneri E: Niacin: chemical forms, bioavailability, and health effects, *Nutr Rev* 70(6):357, 2012.

30. Li R, Yu K, Wang Q, et al: Pellagra secondary to medication and alcoholism: A case report and review of the literature, *Nutr Clin Pract* 31(6):785, 2016.

31. Ghavanini AA, Kimpinski K: Revisiting the evidence for neuropathy caused by pyridoxine deficiency and excess, *J Clin Neuromusc Dis* 16:25, 2014.

32. Clase CM, Ki V, Holden RM: Water-soluble vitamins in people with low glomerular filtration rate or on dialysis: A review, *Semin Dial* 26(5):546, 2013.

33. Rios-Avila L, Coats B, Ralat M, et al: Pyridoxine supplementation does not alter in vivo kinetics of one-carbon metabolism but modifies patterns of one-carbon and tryptophan metabolites in vitamin B-6-insufficient oral contraceptive users, *Am J Clin Nutr* 102:616, 2015.

34. Suitor CW, Bailey LB: Dietary folate equivalents: interpretation and application, *J Am Diet Assoc* 100(1):88, 2000.

35. Osterhues A, Ali NS, Michels KB: The role of folic acid fortification in neural tube defects: A review, *Crit Rev Food Sci Nutr* 53:11, 2013.

36. Mason JB, Tang SY: Folate status and colorectal cancer risk: A 2016 update, *Mol Aspects Med* 53:73, 2017.

37. Bailey RL, Dodd KW, Gahche JJ, et al: Total folate and folic acid intake from foods and dietary supplements in the United States: 2003-2006, *Am J Clin Nutr* 91:231, 2010.

38. Paul L, Selhub J: Interaction between excess folate and low vitamin B12 status, *Mol Aspects Med* 53:43, 2017.

39. US Department of Health and Human Services, US Department of Agriculture: *Report of the Dietary Guidelines Advisory Committee on the Dietary Guidelines for Americans 2010*, Washington, DC, 2010, Center for Nutrition Policy and Promotion, US Department of Agriculture. https://www.cnpp.usda.gov/sites/default/files/dietary_guidelines_for_americans/2010DGACReport-camera-ready-Jan11-11.pdf.

40. Stabler SP: Vitamin B_{12} deficiency, *New Engl J Med* 368:149, 2013.

41. Moorthy D, Peter I, Scott TM, et al: Status of vitamins B-12 and B-6 but not of folate, homocysteine, and the methylenetetrahydrofolate reductase C677T polymorphism are associated with impaired cognition and depression in adults, *J Nutr* 142:1554, 2012.

42. Dangour AD, Allen E, Clarke R, et al: Effects of vitamin B-12 supplementation on neurologic and cognitive function in older people: A randomized controlled trial, *Am J Clin Nutr* 102:639, 2015.

43. Aroda VR, Edelstein SL, Goldberg RB, et al, and the Diabetes Prevention Program Research Group: Long-term metformin use and vitamin B12 deficiency in the Diabetes Prevention Program Outcomes Study, *J Clin Endocrinol Metab* 101(4):1754, 2016.

FURTHER READINGS AND RESOURCES

Readings

Haynes-Maslow L, Parsons SE, Wheeler SB, et al: A qualitative study of perceived barriers to fruit and vegetable consumption among low-income populations, North Carolina, 2011, *Prev Chronic Dis* 10:E34, 2013. http://dx.doi.org/10.5888/pcd10.120206.
[These authors help us understand the many factors influencing fruit and vegetable intake.]

Linos E, Keiser E, Kanzler M, et al: Sun protective behaviors and vitamin D levels in the US population: NHANES 2003-2006, *Cancer Causes Control* 23:133, 2012.
[This article points to a vitamin deficiency that continues to occur in the United States.]

Rautiainen S, Lee IM, Rist PM, et al: Multivitamin use and cardiovascular disease in a prospective study of women, *Am J Clin Nutr* 101(1):144, 2015.
[This study tries to answer the question if high vitamin intakes protect against chronic disease.]

Websites of Interest

- US Department of Agriculture: *Choose My Plate*. This site offers various educational materials on vitamin needs throughout the life cycle, vitamin supplements, and good food sources of individual vitamins. https://search.usa.gov/search?utf8=✓&affiliate=choosemyplate_i14yb&query=vitamins&commit=Search
- US Library of Medicine, National Institutes of Health: *MedlinePlus*. Vitamins. This website is a source of reputable health information for the general public, including specific information on vitamins and their roles in the body, and guidance on use of vitamin supplements. https://medlineplus.gov/vitamins.html.
- US Department of Health and Human Services, Office of Dietary Supplements: *Vitamin and Mineral Supplement Fact Sheets*. Fact sheets for both consumer and professional use provide background information on vitamin functions and guidance on use of supplements. https://ods.od.nih.gov/factsheets/list-VitaminsMinerals/.
- Centers for Disease Control and Prevention: *Spina bifida*. This site presents the types, causes, diagnosis, and treatment for spina bifida. https://www.cdc.gov/ncbddd/spinabifida/facts.html.

7

Minerals and Water

Eleanor D. Schlenker

(e) http://evolve.elsevier.com/Williams/essentials/

This chapter completes the review of the two remaining classes of nutrients: minerals and water. As individual elements, minerals seem simple in comparison to the complex structures of vitamins, but they fulfill equally important roles. New technologies that make it possible to measure extremely small quantities of trace minerals in body tissues have opened new opportunities to study the roles of these nutrients and how they interact with vitamins to maintain body function and prevent disease. In time we may identify additional minerals essential to human health. An equally important but often overlooked nutrient is water. Water is second only to oxygen in that it is vital for survival. Growing interest in sports nutrition and athletic performance has brought new attention to water as a beverage, and bottled water is now the bottled drink with the highest sales volume. As with the vitamins, we will focus on why we need them and how we obtain them.

OUTLINE

MINERALS IN HUMAN NUTRITION

Comparison of Vitamins and Minerals

The two classes of micronutrients, vitamins and minerals, have both similarities and differences (Table 7.1). Vitamins are complex organic molecules that serve primarily as coenzymes or regulators of body metabolism, especially energy metabolism. In contrast, minerals are simple elements with important roles in both structure and function. Minerals also serve as cofactors in many important enzyme systems and, in fact, sometimes partner with vitamins in regulating essential metabolic functions. As was true for vitamins, an excess of one mineral cannot remedy a deficit of another, making it important to eat a wide variety of foods.

Cycle of Minerals

On Earth we live within a vast slow-motion cycle of minerals essential to life. Elements in water find their way into rocks and soil; through plants they find their way to animals and humans. At one time our access to these elements depended on where we happened to live—because people obtained all of their food from nearby farms. However, with expanding knowledge of how these elements are incorporated into foods, plus the fact that much of the food we eat is grown outside of our immediate surroundings, people living in all parts of the world have the potential for adequate mineral nutrition.

TABLE 7.1	**Comparisons of Vitamins and Minerals**	
Characteristic	Minerals	Vitamins
Similarities		
Essentiality	Must be obtained in food	Must be obtained in food
Unique role	One cannot substitute for another	One cannot substitute for another
Interactions	Interferes with other minerals if present in inappropriate amounts	Interferes with other vitamins if present in inappropriate amounts
Impact on chronic disease	May have a role in prevention of chronic disease	May have a role in prevention of chronic disease
Differences		
Structure	Simple organic elements	Complex organic structures
Absorption	Problems in absorption caused by interfering or binding substances	More easily absorbed
Classification	Based on amount needed by the body (major minerals or trace elements)	Based on solubility in water or lipid
Roles in body	Structural and metabolic	Only metabolic
Relative amount needed	Varies among minerals (more needed for structural roles)	Needed in very minute amounts
Stability	Seldom destroyed in cooking	Easily destroyed in cooking

Metabolic Roles

Differing Functions

The roles of minerals in the body are as varied as the elements themselves. They participate in an impressive array of structural and metabolic activities:

- *Structural:* Calcium and phosphorus give strength to bones and body frame. Iron provides the core for the heme in hemoglobin that carries oxygen to the tissues and returns carbon dioxide to the lungs for excretion.
- *Metabolic:* Ionized sodium and potassium exercise control over body water. Iodine is a necessary constituent of the thyroid hormone that sets the rate of metabolism in the cells. Iron is a cofactor in the mitochondrial enzyme system that supplies our body with energy.

Some minerals such as iron contribute to structure and function. Far from being static and inert, minerals are active participants in many systems that support life.

Differing Amounts

Minerals differ from vitamins in the amounts needed. All vitamins are required in very small amounts, but minerals vary depending on their role. A man weighing 150 lb has almost 3 lb of calcium in his body, most of it in the skeleton. This same man contains only approximately 3 g (¹⁄₁₀ oz) of iron, found mainly in the hemoglobin of red blood cells.

Concept of Bioavailability

In general, minerals are absorbed less efficiently than vitamins. The amount of mineral in a food as determined by laboratory analysis may not be the amount that can be absorbed. The term bioavailability refers to the proportion of a food nutrient that can be successfully absorbed and made available for body use. Bioavailability is influenced by the food source and the host, as follows:

- *Binding substances:* In some plants, minerals are bound in chemical complexes and not easily released. Oxalates in green leafy vegetables and phytates in whole grains bind minerals and prevent their absorption.

- *Gastric acidity:* Most minerals are better absorbed in an acid environment.
- *Chemical form:* Iron cannot be absorbed in the ferric form; it must first be reduced to ferrous iron for absorption to take place.
- *Other foods in the meal:* Some foods, such as tea, contain substances that interfere with the absorption of certain minerals.
- *Body need:* Various minerals, such as iron, are absorbed at higher rates in periods of active growth, pregnancy, and lactation.

Bioavailability issues make it difficult to set dietary recommendations for minerals.

> **KEY TERMS**
>
> **Hemoglobin**
> Oxygen-carrying pigment in red blood cells.
>
> **Bioavailability**
> Amount of a nutrient in a food that is absorbed and available to the body for metabolic use.

Classification

The essential minerals are organized into two groups: (1) major minerals and (2) trace elements. Those minerals required in amounts of more than or equal to 100 mg/day are called *major minerals*, not because they are more important, but because there are more of them in the body. Those needed in smaller amounts are called *trace elements*, and a few that are required in only minute amounts are referred to as *ultratrace elements*.

The seven minerals present in the body in large amounts are calcium, phosphorus, magnesium, sodium, potassium, sulfur, and chloride. Nine trace elements that occur in very small amounts are also essential for human health. All required minerals are listed in Box 7.1. We will review five aspects of each: (1) absorption, (2) physiologic function, (3) clinical applications, (4) daily requirement, and (5) food sources.

MAJOR MINERALS

CALCIUM

Of all the minerals in the body, calcium is present in the largest amounts. The adult woman contains approximately 1000 g (2.2 lb) of calcium, and the adult man contains approximately 1200 g (2.6 lb). Total body calcium reflects the constant interchange of calcium supplied in food or supplements, calcium stored in the skeleton, and urinary calcium loss. Calcium balance is applied at three levels: (1) the intake-absorption-excretion balance, (2) the bone-blood balance, and (3) the calcium-phosphorus blood serum balance.

Intake-Absorption-Excretion Balance
Calcium Intake
Calcium has been identified as a nutrient of public health importance in respect to bone health. Except for children ages 1 to 3, 50% to 75% of the population is not meeting their Recommended Dietary Allowances (RDAs).[1] Calcium intake in early life carries lifelong implications for bone health. Females with higher intakes of calcium as adolescents enjoyed higher bone mass as adults,[2] lowering their risk of fractures later in life.

Calcium Absorption
In general, approximately 25% of ingested calcium is absorbed, although absorption can reach 60% in infancy or other periods of high demand. Absorption falls to very low levels in advanced age.[3] Calcium is absorbed in the small intestine, chiefly in the duodenum. Here the gastric acidity is still effective, but as the food mass is buffered by pancreatic juices and becomes more alkaline, absorption is reduced.

Factors increasing calcium absorption. The following factors increase calcium absorption:
- *Vitamin D hormone:* Vitamin D is necessary for the active transport of calcium in the upper small intestine. Calcitriol, the vitamin D hormone, controls the synthesis of a calcium-binding protein that carries the mineral across the mucosal cell and into the blood.[3]
- *Body need:* Physiologic conditions over the life cycle—growth, pregnancy, lactation, and older age—influence the rate of absorption. Absorption is highest in times of greater need, such as pregnancy or the adolescent growth spurt.
- *Amount of calcium in the diet:* Percent absorption increases when intake is limited; at high calcium intakes, a smaller proportion is absorbed, although the net amount may be higher.

- *Acidic environment:* Lower pH or a more acidic environment in the gastrointestinal tract favors the solubility of calcium and enhances absorption.
- *Dietary protein and carbohydrate:* Optimal protein intake supports bone health and increases calcium absorption by promoting gastric acid secretion.[4] Lactose enhances calcium absorption through the action of the intestinal bacterium *Lactobacilli*, which produces lactic acid and lowers intestinal pH.

Factors decreasing calcium absorption. The following factors decrease calcium absorption:
- *Vitamin D deficiency:* A lack of vitamin D or inability to form the active vitamin D hormone calcitriol as a result of liver or kidney disease depresses absorption.
- *Fat malabsorption:* Excessive amounts of fatty acids remaining in the small intestine combine with calcium to form insoluble soaps that cannot be absorbed.
- *Fiber and other binding agents:* Dietary fiber can bind calcium and hinder its absorption. Other binding agents include oxalic acid and phytic acid. Oxalic acid is found in varying amounts in green leafy vegetables; consequently, some vegetables are better sources of calcium than others. The outer hull of many cereal grains, especially wheat, contains phytates.
- *Alkaline environment:* Calcium is insoluble in an alkaline medium (a high pH) and poorly absorbed. Overuse of antacids will lower calcium absorption.

Calcium Excretion

Calcium balance is controlled primarily at the point of absorption, as is true for many minerals. A large proportion of dietary calcium (50%–90%) remains unabsorbed and is eliminated in the feces. A small amount of calcium, usually no more than 200 mg/day, is excreted in the urine to maintain normal levels in body fluids.

Bone-Blood Balance
Calcium in the Bones
The skeleton is the major site of calcium storage. Bones and teeth contain approximately 99% of body calcium, but these stores are not static. Bone is constantly being built and reshaped according to period of growth and hormonal influences (Fig. 7.1). As much as 700 mg of

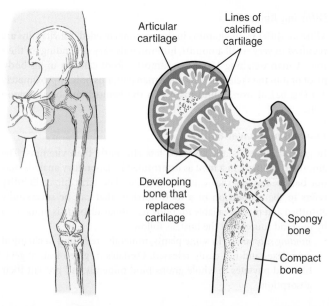

FIG. 7.1 Bone and cartilage development.

calcium enters and leaves the bones each day.[3] Under certain conditions, withdrawals exceed deposits: immobility from a body cast or the bone disease **osteoporosis** results in excessive calcium withdrawal and loss.

Calcium in the Blood

The small amount of body calcium that is not in bone—approximately 1%—circulates in the blood and other body fluids. Blood calcium exists in two forms:

1. *Bound calcium:* In general, 40% of the calcium in the blood is bound to plasma proteins and not *diffusible* (i.e., not able to move into cells or enter into other activities).
2. *Free ionized calcium:* Free calcium carrying an electrical charge moves about unhindered and diffuses through membranes to control body functions. Free calcium accomplishes a great deal of metabolic work because it is in an activated form. Free calcium is critical to ongoing tissue metabolism and so is more closely regulated than bound calcium. When calcium intake is low and blood calcium levels drop, calcium is mobilized from the bones to restore levels to normal.

Calcium-Phosphorus Serum Balance

The final level of calcium balance is the calcium-phosphorus balance in the serum. These two minerals maintain a defined relationship based on their relative solubility. The calcium-phosphorus serum balance is the solubility product of calcium and phosphorus expressed in milligrams per deciliter (mg/dL). Normal calcium serum levels are 10 mg/dL in children and adults. For phosphorus, normal levels are 4 mg/dL in adults and 5 mg/dL in children. Thus the normal serum calcium-phosphorus solubility products are $10 \times 4 = 40$ in adults and $10 \times 5 = 50$ in children. Any situation that increases the serum phosphorus level will decrease the serum calcium level to keep the calcium-phosphorus solubility product constant. A drop in serum calcium interferes with important functions such as muscle contraction, including contraction of the heart muscle.

The three hormones that work together to maintain calcium balance are the parathyroid hormone (PTH), the vitamin D hormone calcitriol, and the hormone **calcitonin**. The cooperative action of these hormones is an example of the synergism among metabolic control agents:

1. *PTH:* The parathyroid glands lying adjacent to the thyroid glands are particularly sensitive to changes in the blood level of free ionized calcium. When ionized calcium levels begin to fall, PTH is released and restores the levels to normal by the following actions:
   - Stimulates the intestinal mucosa to absorb more calcium
   - Rapidly withdraws calcium from bone
   - Increases calcium reabsorption and phosphorus excretion by the kidneys
2. *Vitamin D hormone (calcitriol):* Calcitriol cooperates with PTH to control the absorption of calcium in the small intestine and regulate the deposit of calcium and phosphorus in bone. Calcitriol exerts more control on calcium absorption and its deposit in bone, and PTH exerts more control on calcium withdrawal from bone and kidney excretion of phosphorus.
3. *Calcitonin:* Calcitonin is produced by special C cells in the thyroid gland. It prevents an abnormal rise in serum calcium by modulating the release of bone calcium. Thus its action counterbalances that of PTH to keep serum calcium at normal levels. The overall relationship of the factors involved in calcium balance and regulation is illustrated in Fig. 7.2.

Physiologic Functions of Calcium
Bone Formation

Calcium, along with phosphorus, gives strength and rigidity to the skeleton. Building and maintaining bone mass is accomplished

FIG. 7.2 Calcium metabolism. Note the relative distribution of calcium in body tissues.

through the action of specialized cells that handle the deposit and withdrawal of bone calcium.

Tooth Formation

Special organs in the gums deposit calcium to form teeth, and this mineral exchange continues as in bone. Calcium deposit and withdrawal occur mainly in the dentin and cementum. Very little exchange occurs in the enamel once the tooth is formed.

General Metabolic Functions

The relatively small amount of ionized calcium in blood and body fluids has an amazing number of physiologic roles:

- *Blood clotting:* Serum calcium ions are required for the cross-linking of fibrin, giving stability to the fibrin threads.
- *Nerve transmission:* A current of calcium ions triggers the flow of signals from one nerve cell to another. Calcium ions in cells of the cardiac muscle direct the nerve signals to these fibers.
- *Muscle contraction and relaxation:* Ionized serum calcium initiates the contraction of muscle fibers and controls their return to steady state. Calcium ions released into the cytoplasm of the muscle cell create the attractive forces between actin and myosin that result in the contraction of the muscle fiber. This action of calcium is particularly critical to the constant contraction-relaxation cycle of the heart muscle. Calcium channel blockers slow heart action by preventing this release of calcium.
- *Cell membrane permeability:* Ionized calcium controls the passage of fluids and solutes across cell membranes by its effect on the intercellular membrane cement.
- *Enzyme activation:* Calcium ions activate certain cell enzymes, particularly those that release energy for muscle contraction. They have a similar role with protein-splitting enzymes and the lipase enzyme that digests fat.

KEY TERMS

Osteoporosis
The abnormal loss of bone mineral and matrix leading to porous, fragile bone tissue with enlarged spaces that is prone to fracture or deformity; common disease of aging in both men and women.

Calcitonin
A polypeptide hormone secreted by the C cells in the thyroid gland in response to hypercalcemia, which lowers calcium levels in the blood.

Solutes
Particles of a substance in solution; a solution consists of a solute and a dissolving medium (solvent), usually a liquid.

Clinical Applications

Disruption of the physiologic and metabolic functions of calcium is associated with several clinical problems.

Tetany

A drop in serum ionized calcium causes tetany, marked by severe, intermittent spastic muscle contractions and muscular pain. Seizures and convulsions ensue if the situation is not corrected.

Rickets and Osteomalacia

A deficiency of vitamin D hormone causes rickets in growing children and osteomalacia in adults. When exposure to sunlight is limited and dietary intake of vitamin D is poor, calcium absorption is inadequate

and bone mineral is lost. (See Chapter 6 to review vitamin D and these deficiency diseases.)

Resorptive Hypercalciuria and Renal Calculi

Resorption of bone calcium and its excretion in the urine accelerates during prolonged immobilization. A full body cast, spinal cord injury, or body brace after a back injury decreases the normal muscle tension needed to preserve bone. The subsequent rise in urinary calcium increases the risk of renal stones.

Calcium and Health
Bone Disease

A calcium-related condition increasing in prevalence with the growth of the aging population is osteoporosis. Although a recent national survey indicated that approximately 16% of men and 30% of women 50 years of age and over have osteoporosis, this prevalence rises to 46% and 77%, respectively, by age 80.[5] With advancing age and loss of bone mineral, bones become progressively more fragile, with increasing risk of fractures, physical disability, and mortality. Loss of the steroid hormones estrogen and testosterone bring about alterations in calcium balance such that bone is broken down more rapidly than it can be replaced, with a net loss of bone mass and changes in bone structure (Fig. 7.3).

Metabolic Disease

Low calcium intake or limited use of dairy foods has been put forth as a possible contributor to chronic conditions unrelated to bone health, including obesity,[6,7] hypertension,[6,8] and certain types of cancer.[6] Increased servings of dairy foods, rather than total calcium intake from all sources, appeared to influence these findings. This suggests that other components found in dairy foods, in addition to calcium, factored in these outcomes. Calcium may contribute to weight management by increasing the excretion of fat in the feces through the formation of calcium soaps that prevent fat absorption.[7]

Calcium Requirement
Dietary Reference Intake

Concerns about the amount of calcium required for lifetime maintenance of healthy bones led to the current Dietary Reference Intakes (DRIs).[3] For youths 9 to 18 years of age, the RDA of 1300 mg/day ensures maximum deposition of bone calcium. Men and women ages

Normal bone   Bone with osteoporosis

FIG. 7.3 Comparison of normal and osteoporotic spongy bone. Scanning electron micrograph (SEM) of (A) normal bone and (B) bone with osteoporosis. Note the loss of bone linkages and enlarged pores in the osteoporotic bone. (From Kumar V, Abbas A, Fausto N: *Robbins basic pathology*, ed 7, Philadelphia, 2002, Saunders.)

19 to 50 should take in 1000 mg/day to maintain positive calcium balance. Women ages 51 to 70 require 1200 mg to offset the calcium losses associated with menopause, whereas for men in this age group, the RDA remains at 1000 mg. All persons older than 70 years require 1200 mg to support bone health and prevent bone loss. Intakes greater than the Tolerable Upper Intake Level (UL) of 2500 mg/day for adults younger than 51 years and 2000 mg/day for adults age 51 and older can interfere with the absorption of other important minerals or lead to complications such as kidney insufficiency and milk-alkali syndrome. Milk-alkali syndrome got its name from the condition that arose when patients with peptic ulcers were treated with large amounts of antacids (alkaline) such as calcium carbonate over a long period of time. This shifts the body's acid-base balance to alkaline and results in calcium deposits in the kidneys and other soft tissues.

Sources of Calcium

Calcium is highly available from dairy products, making these foods ideal sources. One quart of cow's milk supplies 1200 mg of calcium, along with 10 mg (400 IU) of vitamin D. Green leafy vegetables such as bok choy, broccoli, and kale are good sources, but spinach, collard greens, sweet potatoes, and beans are high in oxalic acid, which compromises bioavailability. Whole grains and nuts contain phytic acid, making these foods poor sources. Calcium-fortified soy milk, juices, and cereals meet calcium needs for the lactose intolerant. Aged cheeses such as cheddar or Swiss, good sources of calcium, are low in lactose. It is important to emphasize low-calorie, reduced-fat, low-fat, or nonfat dairy foods to young women for whom weight gain is a major concern. Box 7.2 suggests additional food sources of calcium.

BOX 7.2   Food Sources of Calcium

Food Source	Amount	Calcium (mg)
Grains Group		
Fortified Ready-to-Eat Cereals		
Total	¾ cup	1000
All Bran	½ cup	121
Cheerios	1 cup	112
Bread, white, commercially prepared	1 slice	73
Bread, whole wheat, commercially prepared	1 slice	52
Vegetable Group		
Vegetable juice (fortified)	8 fl oz	299
Collard greens (cooked)	1 cup	268
Potato (baked), flesh and skin	1 med	26
Kale (frozen, cooked)	1 cup	179
Broccoli (frozen, cooked)	½ cup	30
Fruit Group		
Orange juice (fortified)	8 fl oz	349
Figs (dried)	2 figs	27
Meat, Beans, Eggs, and Nuts Group		
Soybeans (mature beans, cooked)	1 cup	175
Almonds (roasted)	1 oz (24 nuts)	80
Milk Group		
Yogurt (fruited, low fat)	8 oz container	345
Milk, (nonfat, reduced fat, whole)	1 cup	295
Soy milk (fortified with calcium)	1 cup	299
Soy milk (unfortified)	1 cup	61
Fats, Oils, and Sugar		
These foods do not supply calcium.		

RDA for adults: men ages 19 to 70, 1000 mg; men ages >70, 1200 mg; women ages 19 to 50, 1000 mg; women ages >50, 1200 mg.
Images copyright 2006 JupiterImages Corporation. Data from US Department of Agriculture, Agricultural Research Service: *USDA National Nutrient Database for Standard Reference, Release 28.* Nutrient Data Laboratory Home Page, revised May, 2016. https://www.ndb.nal.usda.gov/ndb/.

TABLE 7.2 Choosing a Calcium Supplement

Characteristic	Recommendation
Amount of elemental calcium present	Calcium compounds contain different amounts of elemental calcium; calcium carbonate is 40% calcium by weight, but calcium citrate is only 21% calcium; you would need twice as much calcium citrate to get the same amount of calcium.
Absorption	Calcium carbonate, calcium citrate, and calcium citrate malate (the form found in fortified juices) are all well absorbed; calcium citrate is better absorbed than calcium carbonate when gastric acid is low.
Purity	Do not use supplements made from bone meal, oyster shell, or dolomite because they may contain lead or other toxic elements; coral calcium may contain lead and mercury; look for a well-known brand of pharmaceuticals or check for the USP (United States Pharmacopeia) symbol or the word "purified."
Dose	Calcium is absorbed best when taken in doses of 500 mg or less; depending on need, take divided doses rather than one massive dose
When best taken	Calcium carbonate is best absorbed with food; calcium citrate can be taken anytime.
Combination products	Some calcium supplements are combined with other nutrients such as phosphorus, magnesium, or vitamin D; phosphorus is readily available in the US diet and not needed in supplements; unless vitamin D is supplied in another supplement, it could be included here.
Potential interactions	Calcium can decrease the absorption of various medications, including phenytoin and tetracycline, and interacts with thiazide and similar diuretics; medications to be taken on an empty stomach should not be taken with a calcium supplement; persons on prescription or over-the-counter medications should check with their physician or pharmacist before adding a calcium supplement.
Form	Calcium supplements are available in tablets, gel capsules, liquids, and chewables; chewables and liquids might be helpful for those with difficulty swallowing.
Ability to dissolve in the stomach	Chewables and liquids are broken down before they enter the stomach; to test a tablet place one in warm water for 30 minutes and stir occasionally; if it has not dissolved in this time it likely will not dissolve in your stomach.

Data from National Institutes of Health: Medline Plus. Trusted Health Information for You. *Calcium supplements: who should take calcium supplements,* Bethesda, MD, 2015, US Department of Health and Human Services. http://www.nlm.nih.gov/medlineplus/ency/article/007477.htm; Office of Dietary Supplements: *Dietary supplement fact sheet: calcium,* Bethesda, MD, 2016, National Institutes of Health, US Department of Health and Human Services. https://ods.od.nih.gov/factsheets/Calcium-HealthProfessional/; Blumberg S: Is coral calcium a safe and effective supplement? *J Am Diet Assoc* 104:1335, 2004.

Calcium Supplements

Many persons cannot or will not consume enough calcium-rich foods to meet their requirement and depend on supplements. Table 7.2 outlines criteria to be considered in selecting and using calcium supplements. To help meet all dietary requirements, it is best to obtain at least half your daily calcium from food that will supply other important nutrients in addition to calcium and will also provide calcium in a highly bioavailable form. (For further reading on calcium and bone health see the Evidence-Based Practice box, "Optimum Calcium and Vitamin D: Can We Lower Fracture Risk?")

EVIDENCE-BASED PRACTICE

Optimum Calcium and Vitamin D: Can We Lower Fracture Risk?

Identify the problem: Age-related bone loss and development of osteoporosis are responsible for more than 2 million fractures each year at great financial and human cost. As the number of older adults continues to grow, bone health has moved into the forefront as a public health problem, but a solution has proven to be elusive.

Review the evidence: Although optimal intakes of calcium along with sufficient vitamin D provided in the form of food or supplements might be expected to slow the loss of bone, research trials have not always reached the same conclusions. Meta-analyses including nearly 31,000 adults middle age and older reported that supplementation with calcium and vitamin D to meet recommended takes reduced the risk of all fractures by 15% and hip fractures by 30%.[1] Other experts point to the side effects associated with excessive calcium supplements, including gastrointestinal upset and renal stones.[2] Although it is agreed that recommended intakes of these nutrients improve bone health, should all older persons take supplements?

Implement the findings: Adults can promote their bone health by following these suggested guidelines:

- Maintain a consistent intake of 1000 to 1200 mg of calcium and 600 to 800 IU of vitamin D each day, depending on the RDA for your age group.[3] Use fortified foods to help supply these nutrients.
- Individuals with insufficient dietary intakes of calcium and vitamin D might rely on supplements to reach the RDA for their age group.
- Avoid intakes of calcium and vitamin D that exceed the RDA; if you have a healthy diet, you may not need a supplement. The Healthy US-Style Food

Pattern included in the 2015 Dietary Guidelines for Americans supplies more than 1200 mg of calcium at an 1800 kcal intake level but supplies less than 300 IU of vitamin D.[4]

- Maintain a healthy lifestyle that includes regular physical activity; weight-bearing exercise and strength training support retention of bone mass.
- Have a bone scan on a regular basis to monitor bone status and possible need for medical intervention.

Meeting current recommendations but not exceeding target intakes of calcium and vitamin D during adulthood minimizes bone loss and risk of bone fracture.

References

1. Weaver CM, Alexander DD, Boushey CJ, et al: Calcium plus vitamin D supplementation and risk of fractures: an updated meta-analysis from the National Osteoporosis Foundation, *Osteoporos Int* 27:367, 2016.
2. Harvey NC, Biver E, Kaufman JM, et al: The role of calcium supplementation in healthy musculoskeletal aging: an expert consensus meeting of the European Society for Clinical and Economic Aspects of Osteoporosis, Osteoarthritis and Musculoskeletal Diseases (ESCEO) and the International Foundation for Osteoporosis (IOF), *Osteoporos Int* 28(2):447, 2017.
3. Food and Nutrition Board, Institute of Medicine: *Dietary Reference Intakes for calcium and vitamin D,* Washington, DC, 2011, National Academies Press.
4. US Department of Health and Human Services, US Department of Agriculture: *Report of the Dietary Guidelines Advisory Committee on the Dietary Guidelines for Americans 2015,* Washington, DC, 2015, Center for Nutrition Policy and Promotion, US Department of Agriculture. https://www.health.gov/dietaryguidelines/2015-scientific-report/.

PHOSPHORUS

Phosphorus is closely associated with body calcium, although it has some unique characteristics and functions of its own. The adult human body on average contains 850 g (1.9 lb) of phosphorus, with 85% in the skeleton, 14% in the soft tissues, and the remaining 1% in extracellular fluids (ECFs) and cell membranes. Phosphorus makes up approximately 1% of body weight.

Absorption-Excretion Balance
Absorption
Free phosphate is absorbed along the entire length of the small intestine. Absorption is regulated by the vitamin D hormone calcitriol and phosphate carrier proteins.[9] Phosphorus exists in food joined with calcium and must be split off as a free mineral to be absorbed. An excess of other minerals such as aluminum or iron or calcium depresses phosphorus absorption. Phytates in whole grains prevent its absorption.

Excretion
Phosphorus is excreted via the kidneys, which help regulate serum phosphorus levels. Usually 85% to 95% of the plasma phosphate filtered by the renal glomeruli is reabsorbed along with calcium under the influence of vitamin D hormone. However, when phosphate must be excreted to preserve the normal serum calcium-phosphorus balance, PTH overrides vitamin D hormone and increases excretion.

Bone-Blood-Cell Balance
Bone
The phosphorus in the skeleton and teeth is combined with calcium. Bone phosphorus is in constant interchange with the phosphorus in blood and other body fluids.

Blood
The normal adult range for serum phosphorus is 3.0 to 4.5 mg/dL; levels less than 2.5 mg/dL or greater than 5.0 mg/dL demand immediate medical attention.[9] High phosphorus intakes leading to elevated serum levels stimulate PTH release and mobilization of bone calcium to restore the normal serum calcium-phosphorus balance. Antacids that contain aluminum bind phosphorus and lower serum levels.

Cells
In its active phosphate form, phosphorus works with proteins, lipids, and carbohydrates to produce energy, build and repair tissues, and act as a buffer to maintain appropriate pH.

Hormonal Controls
Because calcium and phosphorus work closely together, phosphorus balance is under the control of the vitamin D hormone calcitriol and PTH, two hormones that also control calcium balance. Phosphate depletion results from (1) low intake; (2) poor absorption, usually caused by an interfering substance such as phytate or aluminum; or (3) excessive wasting by the kidney.

Physiologic Functions
Bone and Tooth Formation
Phosphorus helps build bones and teeth. As a component of calcium phosphate, it is constantly deposited and resorbed in the continuing process of bone formation and remodeling.

General Metabolic Activities
Phosphorus is found in every living cell where it participates in overall metabolism. Several activities are described next:
- *Absorption of glucose and glycerol:* Phosphorus combines with these molecules to assist their absorption from the intestine. Phosphorus also promotes the reabsorption of glucose in the renal tubules.
- *Transport of fatty acids:* Phospholipids transport fats in the blood.
- *Energy metabolism:* Phosphorus-containing compounds such as adenosine triphosphate (ATP) are high-energy storage molecules that meet instant demands for energy.
- *Buffer system:* The buffer system of phosphoric acid and phosphate helps maintain blood acid-base balance.

Clinical Applications
Changes in the normal serum phosphorus level occur under particular circumstances, as follows:
- *Recovery from diabetic acidosis:* Active carbohydrate absorption and metabolism place a high demand on serum phosphorus, causing temporary hypophosphatemia. Phosphate is combined with glucose to form glycogen.
- *Growth:* Children have higher serum phosphate levels related to their high levels of growth hormone.
- *Hypophosphatemia:* Low serum phosphorus levels occur with intestinal diseases, such as sprue and celiac disease, that hinder phosphorus absorption. Excessive secretion of PTH (primary hyperparathyroidism) causes inappropriate excretion of phosphorus and hypophosphatemia. Low serum phosphorus may accompany the refeeding syndrome often seen in the first days of nutritional repletion of a severely wasted patient when glycogen stores are being rapidly replenished. This can occur in patients suffering from extreme eating disorders.[10] One symptom of hypophosphatemia is muscle weakness, because cells are deprived of the phosphorus needed for energy metabolism. If left untreated, it will lead to metabolic acidosis, heart failure, and sudden death.
- *Hyperphosphatemia:* In renal failure and hypoparathyroidism, excess phosphate accumulates in the serum. This causes the serum calcium level to drop, resulting in tetany. Highly elevated serum phosphate levels, left untreated, lead to cardiac paralysis and sudden death.

Phosphorus Requirement
Dietary Reference Intake
The RDA for phosphorus is 1250 mg/day for individuals 9 to 18 years of age and 700 mg/day for all adults.[3] At one time, the relative intake of calcium to phosphorus was considered important in building and remodeling bone. Phosphorus intakes that were higher than calcium intakes were believed to hinder bone mineral deposition. We have learned since that sufficient amounts of both nutrients are more important than their ratio to each other.[3] Because both minerals are found in many of the same foods, meeting calcium needs will likely provide adequate phosphorus.

Food Sources of Phosphorus

Milk and milk products contain significant amounts of phosphorus. Because phosphorus is important in muscle metabolism, lean meats also are a good source. Phosphorus-containing food additives add phosphorus to the typical American diet. Substitution of soft drinks high in phosphorus for milk-based beverages has led to increased intakes of phosphorus in place of calcium.[3]

SODIUM

Sodium is a plentiful mineral in the body. The average adult contains approximately 100 g (3.5 oz) of sodium. Half circulates in the ECF (extracellular fluid) as free ionized sodium, 40% is found in bone, and 10% resides inside the cell.

Absorption-Excretion Balance

Sodium is easily absorbed in the small intestine; usually no more than 2% remains to be excreted in the feces. The major route of excretion is through the kidneys under the control of **aldosterone**, the sodium-conserving hormone produced in the adrenal cortex. For individuals in temperate climates in a steady state of fluid and sodium balance, urinary sodium excretion is approximately equal to intake. Sodium is lost in sweat during exercise or in hot environments.

> ### KEY TERM
>
> **Aldosterone**
> Hormone secreted from the cortex of the adrenal glands that acts on the distal renal tubule to reabsorb sodium in exchange for potassium; the aldosterone mechanism conserves sodium and also water because water absorption follows sodium reabsorption.

Physiologic Functions of Sodium

Water balance: Ionized sodium is the major guardian of the body water outside the cells. Differences in the sodium concentrations of body fluids largely determine the distribution of water via osmosis from one area to another.

Acid-base balance: In cooperation with chloride and bicarbonate ions, ionized sodium helps regulate acid-base balance.

Cell permeability: The sodium pump located in all cell membranes controls the passage of materials in and out of the cell. Potassium is moved into the cell, and sodium is moved out of the cell. Glucose also moves into the cell via this active transport system.

Muscle action: Sodium ions help transmit electrochemical impulses along nerve and muscle membranes. Potassium and sodium ions work together to balance the response of nerves to stimulation. They control the flow of nerve impulses to muscles and the contraction of muscle fibers.

Sodium Requirement

Dietary Reference Intake

The body can adjust to a wide range of sodium intakes. When intake is low, the body conserves sodium by reducing output in urine and sweat. At high intakes, excretion equals intake. The Adequate Intake (AI) for sodium covers short-term sweat losses from physical activity or exposure to high environmental temperatures. Those with exceptionally high losses, such as endurance runners, will require more sodium.[11] For young adults the AI is 1500 mg of sodium or 3800 mg of table salt. (Sodium chloride or table salt is 40% sodium by weight.) The AI drops to 1300 mg of sodium for those ages 51 to 70, and to 1200 mg for those

ages 71 and older based on their reduced energy intakes. The UL is 2300 mg of sodium or 5800 mg of table salt.[11]

Sodium Intake

Current national surveys indicate that 97% of the American public have sodium intakes exceeding the AI, beginning with children ages 1 to 3. Adult mean intakes are highest among men ages 20 to 29 (4466 mg) but drop to 3424 mg by ages 70 and older. In women, intakes are highest between ages 30 and 39 (3269 mg) and lowest at ages 70 and older (2597 mg).[12]

A matter of growing concern for policy makers is the sodium intake of children and teens and its possible role in the development of hypertension in these age groups.[13] Approximately 96% of boys between ages 9 and 10 exceed the UL for sodium.[1]

HEALTH PROMOTION

Sodium and Blood Pressure

Although it is generally agreed that excessive sodium intake is associated with increased blood pressures, particularly in salt-sensitive individuals, there continue to be differences of opinion as to what the optimum intake should be and who, if any, needs to restrict their sodium intake.[1,14-17] The 2010 Dietary Guidelines for Americans, based on the recommendation of the American Heart Association,[14] proposed that most persons would benefit from lowering their sodium intake to 1500 mg, the current AI. Since then, new evidence[15] and a comprehensive report by the Institute of Medicine (IOM)[16] has advised that such restriction is not only unrealistic for the general population but could be dangerous for individuals with existing diabetes, cardiovascular disease, and chronic kidney disease. Too little sodium can influence insulin action, blood lipids, and hormonal control of body water; thus the IOM recommends intakes no lower than 2300 mg.[16] There may be a range of optimal sodium intakes, as some researchers have found cardiovascular mortality to be lowest on sodium intakes between 2650 mg and 4950 mg.[17]

The 2015 Dietary Guidelines Advisory Committee noting sodium as a nutrient with implications for public health, encourages a sodium intake of less than 2300 mg for adults and lesser amounts for children, commensurate with their lower energy intake.[1] Certain individuals, including African Americans, postmenopausal women, and those with existing hypertension, are salt-sensitive, meaning that they respond differently to increased sodium than the general population; however, experts suggest they may benefit more from increasing their intakes of calcium and potassium and adopting the Dietary Approaches to Stop Hypertension (DASH) food pattern, than restricting their sodium intake.[18] Persons looking to reduce their daily sodium intake to less than 2300 mg should consult a health professional. (To learn more about dietary intervention for hypertension, see the Focus on Culture box, "Low Mineral Intake: Could It Affect Blood Pressure in Blacks?")

Controlling Sodium Intake

Implementing a reduction in sodium intake will require time and substantial adjustments in the food supply.[1] Dietary sodium comes from various sources, but only 12% of the sodium in the US diet occurs naturally in foods and water. Most (77%) is consumed in the form of salt (sodium chloride) added in commercial food preparation or food processing (Fig. 7.4).[19] Forty-four percent of dietary sodium comes from mixed dishes, with burgers, sandwiches, tacos, and pizza contributing the highest amounts in this category.

When individuals are accustomed to liberal use of salt as a seasoning, adjusting to a reduced level can be difficult. The limited number

🌐 FOCUS ON CULTURE

Low Mineral Intake: Could It Affect Blood Pressure in Blacks?

Black adults are at particular risk for elevated blood pressure, with 43% reported to be hypertensive as compared with 29% of whites, 28% of Hispanic Americans, and 26% of Asian Americans.[1] Generous intakes of calcium, potassium, and magnesium, along with a moderate intake of sodium, influence blood pressure and have been the basis for dietary intervention. The DASH Eating Plan of seven to eight grain, four to five vegetable, four to five fruit, and two to three milk servings each day meets or exceeds the DRIs for calcium, potassium, and magnesium and has helped persons lower their blood pressure.[2] Some individuals were even able to reduce or eliminate their antihypertensive medications.

According to national surveys, black adults take in barely half the potassium and magnesium and approximately two-thirds of the calcium, recommended in the DASH diet (see table).[3] On the other hand, sodium intake greatly exceeds the UL of 2300 mg.

Nutrient	Amount in DASH Diet (mg)	Intake of Blacks (mg)
Potassium	4700	2449
Magnesium	500	278
Calcium	1250	821
Sodium	≤2300	3513

Lowering sodium intake is one step, but equally important is helping individuals with hypertension choose more calcium-, potassium-, and magnesium-rich foods. The DASH Eating Plan can be accessed at: https://www.nhlbi.nih.gov/health/health-topics/topics/dash/followdash, National Heart, Lung, and Blood Institute, National Institutes of Health.

References

1. National Center for Health Statistics: *Hypertension among adults aged 20 and over, by sex and race and Hispanic origin: United States, 1999–2000 through 2013–2014.* Health, United States, 2015 With Special Feature on Racial and Ethnic Health Disparities, Hyattsville, MD, 2016. http://www.cdc.gov/nchs/hus/contents2015.htm#fig23.
2. Epstein DE, Sherwood A, Smith PJ, et al: Determinants and consequences of adherence to the Dietary Approaches to Stop Hypertension diet in African-American and white adults with high blood pressure: results from the ENCORE trial, *J Acad Nutr Diet* 112:1763, 2012.
3. US Department of Agriculture, Agricultural Research Service: *Table 2. Nutrient Intakes from Food and Beverages. Mean Amounts Consumed per Individual, by Race/Ethnicity and Age, in the United States, 2013–2014.* What We Eat in America, NHANES 2013–2014, 2016. https://www.ars.usda.gov/ARSUserFiles/80400530/pdf/1314/Table_2_NIN_RAC_13.pdf.

of reduced-sodium convenience products and the high sodium content of fast food is also a barrier; moreover, foods advertised as "no salt added" or "reduced salt" are often higher in cost. Adjusting to a diet within the UL for sodium will require substituting foods lower in sodium for foods higher in sodium, such as preparing a luncheon sandwich with leftover chicken or turkey or no-salt added peanut butter, rather than luncheon meats. Implementing a diet lower in sodium is likely to require home preparation of more fresh foods seasoned with flavorings or herbs, rather than use of heat-and-serve items. Fruits and most vegetables, with the exception of spinach and celery, are low in sodium. Compare the sodium content of highly processed and less processed foods in Box 7.3. (In Chapter 9 we will use the nutrition label to check the sodium content of processed foods.)

POTASSIUM

Potassium is more than twice as plentiful in the body as sodium. An adult contains approximately 270 g (9.5 oz) or 4000 milliequivalents (mEq).

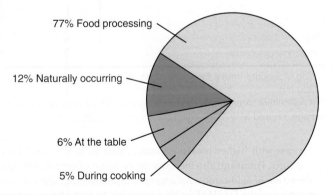

FIG. 7.4 Sources of dietary sodium. Most of our dietary sodium comes from processed food. (Data from Sebastian RS, Enns CW, Steinfeldt LC, et al: *Discontinuation of data processing step: salt adjustment on designated foods likely to be home prepared, what we eat in America,* 2012, NHANES, US Department of Agriculture, Agricultural Research Service.)

Most body potassium is inside cells, where it guards intracellular water; however, the relatively small amount of potassium in ECF is important for muscle activity, especially heart muscle activity. Plasma potassium levels are maintained within very narrow limits of 3.5 to 5.0 mEq/L.

Absorption-Excretion Balance

Dietary potassium is easily absorbed in the small intestine and the potassium circulating in the gastrointestinal secretions is reabsorbed. Prolonged vomiting or diarrhea results in serious losses. The principal route of potassium excretion is the urine. Because plasma potassium is critical to heart muscle action, the kidneys guard potassium carefully, with at least 70% of the potassium filtered by the kidneys being reabsorbed. Aldosterone, the hormone that acts on the kidneys to conserve sodium, also regulates plasma potassium, because potassium is lost in exchange for sodium. Elevated plasma potassium levels stimulate the release of aldosterone. The normal obligatory potassium loss is approximately 160 mg/day, although certain diuretic drugs lead to greater losses.

Physiologic Functions of Potassium

Water balance: The potassium inside the cells balances with the sodium outside the cells to maintain normal osmotic pressures and water distribution.

Muscle activity: Potassium is needed for the action of cardiac and skeletal muscles. Together with sodium and calcium, potassium regulates neuromuscular stimulation, transmission of electrochemical impulses, and contraction of muscle fibers. Low plasma potassium leads to muscle irritability and paralysis. This effect is particularly notable for the heart muscle, which develops a gallop rhythm ending in cardiac arrest. Even small variations in plasma potassium are reflected in electrocardiograms (ECGs).

Carbohydrate metabolism: When glucose is converted to glycogen, 0.36 mmol of potassium is stored in each gram of glycogen. When a patient in diabetic acidosis is treated with insulin and glucose, the ensuing rapid production of glycogen draws potassium from the plasma. Serious **hypokalemia** will result if adequate potassium replacement does not accompany treatment. Even moderate

BOX 7.3   Sodium Content of Foods

Food Source	Amount	Sodium (mg)
Grains Group		
Ready-to-Eat Cereals		
Cheerios	1 cup	139
Total	¾ cup	141
All Bran	½ cup	80
Shredded wheat, no salt added	2 biscuits	1
Bread, white, commercially prepared	1 slice	122
Bread whole wheat, commercially prepared	1 slice	146
Vegetable Group		
Potato (baked), flesh and skin	1 medium	17
Potato salad, homemade	1 cup	1322
Tomato, raw	1 medium	6
Stewed tomatoes (canned)	1 cup	564
Broccoli (frozen), cooked, no salt added	½ cup	10
Broccoli (frozen with cheese sauce)	½ cup	215
Meat, Beans, Eggs, and Nuts Group		
Ham (lean)	3 oz	962
Bacon (broiled/fried)	3 med strips	326
Ground beef, regular (broiled)	3 oz	69
Tuna, light, canned in water	3 oz	210
Halibut, baked	3 oz	70
Peanuts, dry roasted, without salt	1 oz (28 nuts)	2
Peanut butter, creamy (with salt)	1 tbsp	68
Kidney beans, red, cooked, no salt added	1 cup	4
Baked beans, canned, vegetarian	½ cup	436
Milk Group		
Cottage cheese, creamed, low fat	1 cup	764
Cheddar cheese	1 oz	180
Swiss cheese	1 oz	60
American cheese, processed, pasteurized	1 oz	474
Milk, whole, low fat, nonfat	1 cup	116
Fats, Oils, and Sugar		
Margarine, tub, with salt	1 tbsp	93
Butter (salted)	1 tbsp	90
Butter (unsalted)	1 tbsp	0

Sodium is added to food in home food preparation and in food industry processing. Adequate Intake for adults: ages 19 to 50, 1500 mg; ages 51 to 70, 1300 mg; ages ≥71, 1200 mg; Tolerable Upper Intake Level for adults: 2300 mg.
Images copyright 2006 JupiterImages Corporation. Data from US Department of Agriculture, Agricultural Research Service: *USDA National Nutrient Database for Standard Reference, Release 28.* Nutrient Data Laboratory Home Page, revised May, 2016. https://www.ndb.nal.usda.gov/ndb/.

potassium deficiency without overt hypokalemia can aggravate existing glucose intolerance.

Protein synthesis: Potassium is required for the storage of nitrogen as muscle protein or other cell protein. When tissue is broken down, potassium is lost along with nitrogen. Amino acid replacement in rehabilitation includes potassium to ensure nitrogen retention.

Control of blood pressure: Potassium helps control blood pressure by offsetting the pressor effect of sodium that raises blood pressure.

Persons with higher potassium intakes tend to have lower blood pressures. Potassium also increases the excretion of sodium through the action of aldosterone. An appropriate potassium intake is a cornerstone of the DASH (Dietary Approaches to Stop Hypertension) diet, an eating pattern shown to reduce blood pressure in vulnerable individuals.[20] (We will learn more about DASH in Chapter 21.)

Acid-base balance: Potassium helps protect bone mass and reduces the loss of calcium in the urine. Potassium, along with other bicarbonate-yielding compounds in fruits and vegetables, neutralizes sulfur-containing acids produced in the metabolism of meat and other animal protein foods.[4] When potassium and bicarbonate buffers are not available in sufficient amounts, these acids act on bone, releasing bone calcium and lowering bone mass.

Potassium Requirement

Dietary Reference Intake

The AI for potassium is 4700 mg/day for all adults.[11] This intake is expected to offset the blood pressure–raising action of sodium and minimize bone loss, but barely 5% of men and less than 1% of women reach this goal.[1] Median intakes are 3022 mg for men ages 19 and older and 2291 mg for women of this age. Note that these intakes represent approximately two-thirds and less than one-half, respectively, of their DRI,[1] making potassium a nutrient of concern in the 2015 Dietary Goals. Although a sodium-potassium intake ratio of 1500 mg of sodium to 4700 mg of potassium has been recommended, this is met by less than 2% of the adult population.[21] Based on the chronic problems associated with elevated blood pressure and loss of bone that occur across the adult population, increased servings of high-potassium foods would be a cost-effective public health intervention.

Clinical Implications of Excessive Intake

When kidney function is normal, potassium is easily excreted; thus no UL exists for this nutrient. Moreover, potassium toxicity has not been reported as a result of food intake, so dietary sources of potassium should be encouraged; however, potassium supplements can be dangerous, regardless of kidney status. Hyperkalemia with serious cardiac arrhythmias occurs in apparently healthy individuals who accidentally or intentionally take potassium supplements. Salt substitutes that replace sodium with potassium can be unrecognized sources of potassium and should be approved by a health professional. Individuals with diabetes, renal impairment, or heart failure have increased risk of hyperkalemia. Certain medications impair potassium excretion.[11]

Food Sources of Potassium

Potassium as a component of all living cells is found in many foods. Legumes, whole grains, fruits (especially oranges and bananas), leafy green vegetables, broccoli, potatoes, meats, and milk supply considerable amounts (Box 7.4). Persons who eat many servings of fruits and vegetables have potassium intakes of approximately 8 to 11 g/day.[11] It is estimated that three-fourths of the US population does not consume at least five servings of fruits and vegetables daily, a factor contributing to low potassium intake. The two most frequently eaten vegetables are potatoes and tomatoes, accounting for 21% and 18%, respectively, of all vegetable consumption. Fruit juice, high in nutrients but low in fiber, accounts for one-third of all fruit portions.[1] Note that potassium toxicity does not occur from high intakes of potassium-containing foods, but rather from potassium supplements.

Three additional minerals—magnesium, chloride, and sulfur—are assigned to the major minerals group.

BOX 7.4 Food Sources of Potassium

Food Source	Amount	Potassium (mg)
Vegetable Group		
Potato, baked (flesh and skin)	1 medium	926
Potato, baked (flesh only)	1 medium	610
Sweet potato, canned (no syrup)	½ cup	398
Spinach, frozen, cooked	½ cup	287
Fruit Group		
Orange juice, frozen, from concentrate	1 cup	443
Banana	1 medium	422
Meat, Beans, Eggs, and Nuts Group		
Lima beans, baby, frozen, cooked without salt	½ cup	370
Milk Group		
Milk, nonfat (low-fat, reduced-fat, and whole milks vary slightly)	1 cup	382
Cottage cheese, low fat	1 cup	194
Other		
Spaghetti sauce (no meat)	½ cup	422

Adequate Intake for adults: 4700 mg.

Images copyright 2006 JupiterImages Corporation. Data from US Department of Agriculture, Agricultural Research Service: *USDA National Nutrient Database for Standard Reference, Release 28*. Nutrient Data Laboratory Home Page, revised May, 2016. https://www.ndb.nal.usda.gov/ndb/.

MAGNESIUM

An adult body contains approximately 25 g of magnesium, a little less than an ounce. Most is combined with calcium and phosphorus in bone, with the remainder distributed in muscle, other tissues, and fluids. Magnesium activates enzymes for energy production and tissue building and has a role in normal muscle action. As an active nutrient in the enzymatic control of glucose and lipid metabolism, it appears to have a role in lowering the incidence of atherosclerosis, hypertension, type 2 diabetes, and metabolic syndrome.[22,23] The relatively high magnesium content in whole grains may contribute to their positive effect in lowering chronic disease risk. Individuals with gluten-sensitive enteropathy might consider whole grain oat products, labeled gluten free, as a source of magnesium.[24] Excessive intakes of magnesium from nonfood sources such as magnesium salts can lead to metabolic alkalosis, hypokalemia, and paralysis of the ileum.[25]

Magnesium Requirement

The RDA for magnesium is 400 mg for younger men and 310 mg for younger women. To compensate for age-related changes in the kidneys that lead to greater losses, the RDA for persons older than age 30 increases to 420 mg and 320 mg in men and women, respectively.[25]

Food Sources

Magnesium is widespread in nature and unprocessed foods. Whole grains are good sources, but more than 80% of the magnesium is lost when the germ and bran layers of the kernel are removed to produce refined grains. Although milk contains only a modest amount of magnesium, it is a major source in the US diet because it is consumed frequently. Other foods include nuts, soybeans, cocoa, seafood, dried beans and peas, and green leafy vegetables. Except for bananas, fruits are relatively poor sources. Diets rich in vegetables and unrefined grains are higher in magnesium than diets based on highly processed foods and meat. Box 7.5 lists some good sources of magnesium.

CHLORIDE

Chlorine appears in the body as the chloride ion (Cl^-). Chloride accounts for approximately 3% of body mineral, and most is found in the ECF, where it helps control water balance and acid-base balance. Spinal fluid has the highest concentration. A fair amount of ionized chloride is found in the gastrointestinal tract as a component of gastric hydrochloric acid (HCl). Uncontrolled vomiting and diarrhea with continuing loss of gastric fluids can lead to chloride deficiency with muscle cramps and disturbed acid-base balance.

SULFUR

Sulfur is found in all body cells as a constituent of cell protein. Elemental sulfur forms sulfate compounds with sodium, potassium, and magnesium. Other forms of sulfur include: (1) sulfur-containing amino acids such as methionine and cysteine; (2) glycoproteins in cartilage, tendons, and bone matrix; (3) detoxification products formed by intestinal bacteria; (4) organic molecules such as heparin, insulin, coenzyme A (CoA), thiamin, and biotin; and (5) keratin in hair and nails.

The major minerals are summarized in Table 7.3.

BOX 7.5 Food Sources of Magnesium

Food Source	Amount	Magnesium (mg)
Grains Group		
Shredded wheat	2 biscuits	61
Vegetable Group		
Spinach, frozen, cooked	½ cup	78
Meat, Beans, Eggs, and Nuts Group		
Baked beans, canned, vegetarian	1 cup	69
Peanut butter, creamy	2 tbsp	54
Milk Group		
Soy milk	1 cup	60
Milk, reduced fat, low fat, nonfat	1 cup	27

Recommended Dietary Allowance for adults: women ages 19 to 30, 310 mg; women ages ≥31, 320 mg; men ages 19 to 30, 400 mg; men ages ≥31, 420 mg.
Images copyright 2006 JupiterImages Corporation. Data from US Department of Agriculture, Agricultural Research Service: *USDA National Nutrient Database for Standard Reference, Release 28*. Nutrient Data Laboratory Home Page, revised May, 2016. https://www.ndb.nal.usda.gov/ndb/.

TABLE 7.3 Summary of Major Minerals

Mineral	Metabolism	Physiologic Functions	Clinical Applications	Dietary Reference Intake	Food Sources

Calcium (Ca)	Absorption according to body need and requiring Ca-binding protein and vitamin D
	Absorption favored by protein and acidity
	Serum levels regulated by vitamin D, parathyroid hormone, and calcitonin
	Excretion chiefly in feces: 50%–90% of amount ingested
	Deposition and mobilization in bone tissue is regulated by vitamin D and parathyroid hormone
		Constituent of bones and teeth
		Participates in blood clotting, nerve transmission, muscle action, cell membrane permeability, enzyme activation
			Tetany (decrease in serum Ca)
			Rickets, osteomalacia
			Osteoporosis
			Hyperparathyroidism and hypoparathyroidism
				Males Ages 19–70: 1000 mg
				Males Ages ≥71: 1200 mg
				Females Ages 19–50: 1000 mg
				Females Ages ≥51: 1200 mg
				Pregnancy
				  Ages ≤18: 1300 mg
				  Ages ≥19: 1000 mg
				Lactation
				  Ages ≤18: 1300 mg;
				  Ages ≥19: 1000 mg
					Milk, cheese, yogurt
					Green leafy vegetables
					Whole and fortified grains
					Legumes, nuts
					Fortified soy foods
					Fortified fruit juice

Phosphorus (P)	Absorption with Ca aided by vitamin D and parathyroid hormone and hindered by binding agents
	Excretion chiefly by kidney according to serum level as regulated by parathyroid hormone
	Deposition and mobilization in bone compartment is constant
		Constituent of bones and teeth
		Involved in energy metabolism as component of ATP
		Participates in absorption of glucose and glycerol, transport of fatty acids, and buffer system
			Growth
			Recovery from diabetic acidosis
			Hypophosphatemia: bone disease, malabsorption syndromes, primary hyperparathyroidism
			Hyperphosphatemia: renal insufficiency, hypoparathyroidism, tetany
				Male/female adults
				  Ages ≥19: 700 mg
				Pregnancy
				  Ages ≤18: 1250 mg
				  Ages ≥19: 700 mg
				Lactation
				  Ages ≤18: 1250 mg
				  Ages ≥19: 700 mg
					Milk, cheese
					Meat, egg yolk
					Whole grains
					Legumes, nuts
					Soft drinks

TABLE 7.3 Summary of Major Minerals—cont'd

Mineral	Metabolism	Physiologic Functions	Clinical Applications	Dietary Reference Intake	Food Sources

Magnesium (Mg)	Absorption according to intake load; hindered by excessive fat, phosphate, calcium, or phytates
	Excretion (regulated by kidney)
		Constituent of bones and teeth
		Coenzyme in general metabolism, smooth muscle action, neuromuscular irritability
		Cation in intracellular fluid
			Low serum level following gastrointestinal losses
			Tremor, spasm in deficiency
			Alcoholism, certain medications cause losses via the kidney
				Males Ages 19–30: 400 mg
				Males Ages ≥31: 420 mg
				Females Ages 19–30: 310 mg
				Females Ages ≥31: 320 mg
				Pregnancy
				  Ages ≤18: 400 mg
				  Ages 19–30: 350 mg
				  Ages 31–50: 360 mg
				Lactation
				  Ages ≤18: 360 mg
				  Ages 19–30: 310 mg
				  Ages 31–50: 320 mg
					Milk, cheese
					Meat, seafood
					Whole grains
					Legumes, nuts

Sodium (Na)	Readily absorbed
	Excretion chiefly by kidney, controlled by aldosterone
		Major cation in extracellular fluid, water balance, acid-base balance
		Cell membrane permeability
		Energy-requiring absorption of glucose
		Normal muscle irritability
			Losses in gastrointestinal disorders, diarrhea
			Fluid-electrolyte and acid-base balance problems
			Muscle action
			Exerts pressor effect on blood pressure
				Male/female adults
				  Ages 19–50: 1500 mg
				  Ages 51–70: 1300 mg
				  Ages ≥71: 1200 mg
				UL for all adults: 2300 mg
				Pregnancy
				  All ages: 1500 mg
				Lactation
				  All ages: 1500 mg
					Salt (NaCl)
					Sodium compounds used in baking and food processing
					Milk, cheese, carrots, spinach, beets, celery

Potassium (K)	Easily absorbed
	Secreted and reabsorbed in gastrointestinal fluids
	Excretion chiefly by kidney, regulated by aldosterone
		Major cation in intracellular fluid, water balance, acid-base balance
		Normal muscle irritability
		Glycogen formation
		Protein synthesis
			Losses in gastrointestinal disorders, diarrhea
			Fluid-electrolyte, acid-base balance problems
			Muscle action, especially heart muscle; serum level carefully regulated
			Losses in tissue catabolism
			Treatment of diabetic acidosis:
			Losses with diuretic therapy
			Opposes pressor effect of sodium on blood pressure
				Male/female adults
				  All ages: 4700 mg
				Pregnancy
				  All ages: 4700 mg
				Lactation
				  All ages: 5100 mg
					Fruits
					Vegetables
					Legumes, nuts
					Whole grains
					Meat

Chloride (Cl)	Readily absorbed
	Excretion controlled by kidney
		Major anion in extracellular fluid, water balance, acid-base balance
		Gastric hydrochloric acid—digestion
			Losses in gastrointestinal disorders, vomiting, diarrhea, tube drainage
			Hypochloremic alkalosis
				Males/females
				  Ages 19–50: 2300 mg
				  Ages 51–70: 2000 mg
				  Ages ≥71: 1800 mg
				Pregnancy
				  All ages: 2300 mg
				Lactation
				  All ages: 2300 mg
					Salt (NaCl)

Sulfur (S)	Absorbed in elemental form; split from amino acid sources (methionine and cysteine) in digestion and absorbed into portal circulation Excreted by kidney in relation to protein intake and tissue catabolism	Essential component of proteins Detoxification reactions Enzyme activity and energy metabolism	Cystine renal calculi Cystinuria	Adults: No specific recommendation: diets adequate in sulfur-containing amino acids are adequate in sulfur	Meat, eggs Milk, cheese Legumes, nuts

ATP, Adenosine triphosphate.

ESSENTIAL TRACE ELEMENTS

TRACE ELEMENTS: THE CONCEPT OF ESSENTIALITY

By the simplest definition an essential element is one required to sustain life whereas its absence brings death. For major elements found in relatively large amounts in the body, such a determination is fairly easy based on the quantity available for study. It is more difficult to establish the essentiality of the trace elements because we seem to need so little of them. Trace elements have a required intake of less than 100 mg/day, yet some of them exist in fairly large amounts in our diet and our environment.

Trace elements have two major functions: (1) to catalyze chemical reactions and (2) to serve as structural components of larger molecules. They can be separated into two groups: (1) those that are known to be essential and (2) those for which additional research is needed.

Nine trace elements are considered essential for humans based on defined need and function (see Box 7.1). Several other trace elements are thought to be essential for animals, but researchers have yet to demonstrate a role for them in human health.[25] As we develop better techniques of tissue analysis and functional tests appropriate for human studies, we will learn more about these trace elements and if they are required.

IRON

Of all the micronutrients, iron has the longest history, and the body mechanisms regulating its absorption and use are well understood.

Forms of Iron in the Body

The average adult body contains approximately 3 to 4 g of iron. This iron is distributed in the following forms, each with a specific metabolic function:

- *Transport iron:* A trace of iron, 0.05 to 0.18 mg/dL, is found in blood plasma bound to the transport carrier protein transferrin.
- *Hemoglobin and myoglobin:* Most body iron, approximately 70%, resides in the red blood cells as part of the heme portion of the hemoglobin molecule that delivers oxygen to and removes carbon dioxide from body cells. Another 5% helps form myoglobin, the oxygen-carrying molecule found in the heart and skeletal muscles. Skeletal muscles that continue to contract over extended periods of time, as in marathon runners, require an ongoing supply of oxygen from myoglobin.
- *Storage iron:* Approximately 20% of body iron is stored as the protein-iron compound ferritin in the liver, spleen, and bone marrow. Excess iron is held in the body as hemosiderin and exchanges with ferritin as needed.
- *Cellular iron:* The remaining 5% is distributed across all body cells as an enzyme cofactor in oxidative enzyme systems that produce energy.

Absorption-Transport-Storage-Excretion Balance

Iron is regulated differently from most other nutrients. In general, urinary excretion controls plasma and tissue levels by ridding the body of any excess that has accumulated. For iron, control is exerted at the points of absorption, transport, and storage. The body has no system for excreting iron.

Absorption

Major control of iron balance takes place at the site of absorption in the small intestine. Absorption is influenced by two characteristics of iron: its form (heme vs. nonheme) and its chemical state (ferric vs. ferrous).

TABLE 7.4 Characteristics of Heme and Nonheme Dietary Iron

	DIETARY IRON	
	Heme (Smaller Portion)	Nonheme (Larger Portion)
Food sources	None in plant sources; 40% of iron in animal sources	All plant sources; 60% of iron in animal sources
Absorption	Rapid; transported and absorbed intact	Slow; tightly bound in organic molecules; enhanced by acid and presence of heme iron

The two forms of dietary iron are heme iron and nonheme iron (Table 7.4). The larger portion of dietary iron by far is nonheme iron, which includes all plant sources plus 60% of animal sources.[26] Heme iron is absorbed at a much faster rate because it is a smaller molecule than nonheme iron and easily separated from the hemoglobin molecule in meat, fish, and poultry. Nonheme iron is tightly bound to organic components in plants and animal tissues.

The chemical status of dietary iron varies as follows: Nonheme iron found in plant and animal foods is in the chemical form of ferric iron (Fe^{3+}). The gastric acid in the stomach helps separate ferric iron from the organic compounds in which it is bound and reduces it to the more soluble ferrous iron (Fe^{+2}). Ferric iron must be reduced to ferrous iron before it can be absorbed. If not enough gastric acid is available to accomplish this conversion, the ferric iron is lost in the feces. It is expected that approximately 17% of nonheme iron will be absorbed compared with 25% of heme iron,[25] although current researchers suggest that absorption of nonheme iron does not rise to greater than 5%, even in women with high iron needs.[27] Based on the high variability in absorption among individuals and their iron needs, estimating approximate absorption is difficult.

KEY TERMS

Ferritin
Protein-iron compound for storing iron in tissues.

Hemosiderin
Insoluble iron oxide–protein compound for storing iron in the liver when the storage capacity of ferritin is exceeded.

Heme Iron
Form of dietary iron found only in animal sources as part of the heme portion of hemoglobin. Heme iron is more easily absorbed than nonheme iron.

Nonheme Iron
The larger portion of dietary iron that includes all plant food sources and 60% of animal food sources. This form of iron is not part of a heme complex and is less easily absorbed.

Ferric Iron (Fe^{+3})
The oxidized form of iron usually found in food; this form cannot be absorbed and must be reduced to ferrous iron (Fe^{+2}) by the action of gastric acid to be absorbed.

Ferrous Iron (Fe^{+2})
The reduced form of iron that is absorbed in the small intestine.

Iron distribution and transfer within the absorbing cells of the intestinal mucosa involve several carrier substances. Iron never travels unescorted. First, a protein carrier in the mucosal cell binds the ferrous iron. This protein carrier leaves behind enough iron to serve the needs of the energy-producing mitochondria of the absorbing cell and then delivers specific amounts to waiting carriers that control its destination. These carriers are (1) apoferritin, a protein receptor that combines with iron to form the iron-holding compound ferritin for storage in the cell; and (2) apotransferrin, the protein receptor that combines with iron to form the iron-carrier compound serum transferrin, which circulates in the blood.

The proportion of dietary iron that is absorbed or rejected is determined by the amount of ferritin already present in the intestinal mucosal cells. When all available apoferritin has joined with iron to form ferritin, any additional iron arriving at the binding site is rejected and returned to the lumen of the intestine for excretion in the feces. Most absorption takes place in the upper small intestine.

Three factors favor absorption:

1. *Body need:* In iron deficiency or increased demand as in growth, pregnancy, or weight training, more iron is absorbed.[26] When tissue reserves are ample or saturated, iron is rejected and excreted.
2. *Ascorbic acid (vitamin C) or other acids:* An acidic environment increases iron absorption. Acid reduces ferric iron to ferrous iron, the soluble form that is absorbed. Adding ascorbic acid to a meal by including orange juice or similar acid source increases the absorption of nonheme iron.[28] Gastric HCl provides the optimal acid medium to prepare iron for absorption.
3. *Animal tissues:* Heme iron improves the absorption of nonheme iron eaten at the same meal. Peptides released in digestion of meat, fish, and poultry enhance iron absorption from other food sources.

Five factors hinder iron absorption:

1. *Binding agents:* Phosphates, phytates, and oxalates bind iron and prevent its absorption. Certain vegetable proteins, including soy protein, decrease iron absorption independent of their phytate content. Polyphenols in tea and coffee decrease absorption of nonheme iron.[29]
2. *Low gastric acid:* Partial removal of the stomach reduces the number of acid-secreting cells and decreases absorption of both heme and nonheme iron. Iron supplements are necessary after bariatric surgery.[30] Persons who abuse antacids will have trouble absorbing nonheme iron.
3. *Infection:* Severe infection depresses iron absorption because the body attempts to suppress the supply of iron available to the infectious microorganisms.
4. *Gastrointestinal disease:* Malabsorption syndromes such as celiac disease or steatorrhea hinder iron absorption.
5. *Calcium:* Large amounts of calcium can inhibit the absorption of both heme and nonheme iron consumed at the same meal, and this interaction can influence the iron status of those taking concentrated calcium supplements with meals.[31] Adding calcium to meals at the levels normally found in food might be the best approach for optimum absorption of all nutrients.

Transport

After absorption, iron is bound with the protein transferrin for transport to storage sites or body cells. Normally, only 20% to 35% of the iron-binding capacity of transferrin is filled. The remainder serves as a reserve for handling any emergency or variance in iron intake.

Storage

Bound to transferrin, iron is delivered to storage sites in the bone marrow and liver. Here it is recombined with apoferritin to form ferritin, an exchangeable storage form that releases iron as needed. The second less soluble storage form, hemosiderin, provides reserve storage in the liver. From these sites, iron is mobilized for hemoglobin synthesis and production of red blood cells or other body cells. Adults use 20 to 25 mg of iron per day for hemoglobin synthesis, but much of this iron was conserved and recycled when old red blood cells were broken down. The average life span of a red blood cell is approximately 120 days. These interrelationships of body iron absorption-transport-storage are diagrammed in Fig. 7.5.

Excretion

Because iron regulation occurs at the point of absorption, only minute amounts are lost through the kidneys. The body also loses iron by the normal sloughing off of skin cells and gastrointestinal cells, as well as through normal gastrointestinal and menstrual blood loss. Heavy menstrual flow, childbirth, surgery, acute and chronic hemorrhage, gastrointestinal disease, or parasitic infestation causes exceptional iron loss and depletes body stores.

Physiologic Functions of Iron

Oxygen transport: Iron is "pocketed" within the heme molecule, the nonprotein portion of hemoglobin in the red blood cell, and carries oxygen to all body cells for respiration and metabolism. Iron has a similar role in myoglobin, which delivers oxygen within muscle cells.

Cellular oxidation: Iron is a component of cell enzyme systems that oxidize glucose and other energy-yielding nutrients.

Immune function: Iron is needed for the production of immune cells and cytokines that attack foreign bacteria invading the body.

Growth needs: Positive iron balance is imperative for growth. At birth an infant has a 4- to 6-month supply of iron stored in its liver. Breast-fed infants obtain some iron in breast milk, and iron is added to commercial infant formulas. Supplementary iron-rich and iron-fortified foods are introduced to an infant's diet at 4 to 6 months of age to prevent milk anemia. Throughout childhood, iron is needed for continued growth and to build reserves for the physiologic stress of adolescence: muscle development in boys and the onset of menses in girls. Iron needs escalate during pregnancy to produce red blood cells for the mother's expanding blood volume and to build iron reserves in the developing fetal liver. Blood loss in childbirth draws on iron stores.

Brain and cognitive function: Iron is vital for brain development and the synthesis and breakdown of neurotransmitters. Iron deficiency in the critical periods of gestation and early lactation can have long-lasting negative effects on development of motor skills, cognitive and social development, and a child's ability to interact with the environment.[32] Interventions may bring about some improvement; however, many individuals demonstrate long-term alterations in neurobiological processes.

Clinical Applications

Clinical abnormalities result from a deficiency or an excess of iron.

Iron Deficiency Anemia

Iron deficiency is a worldwide public health problem and leads to a hypochromic microcytic anemia. Iron deficiency has various causes, described as follows:

- *Low iron intake or sources with poor bioavailability:* Nutritional anemia develops when iron or other nutrients needed for hemoglobin synthesis

FIG. 7.5 Summary of iron metabolism, showing its absorption, transport, use in hemoglobin synthesis, and storage forms (ferritin and hemosiderin).

and red blood cell production are inadequate. The role of hemoglobin in carrying oxygen to the cells is important in understanding the symptoms of iron deficiency anemia in children and adults (Box 7.6).

- *Blood loss:* Hemorrhagic anemia results from excessive loss of blood and its associated iron. Aspirin leads to blood loss through the gastrointestinal tract, and its long-term use for pain relief can lower body stores. Severe hemorrhoids cause blood loss.
- *Gastrectomy:* Postgastrectomy anemia develops when gastric acid is insufficient to liberate iron for absorption.

BOX 7.6   Signs of Iron Deficiency

Fatigue
Muscle weakness
Pale color
Decreased resistance to infection
Spoon nails
Angular stomatitis

- *Malabsorption:* When the absorbing surface of the small intestine is damaged, iron deficiency anemia often follows.
- *Chronic disease:* Anemia of chronic disease is related to irregularities in the recycling of iron from old red blood cells and the production of new red blood cells, not iron deficiency per se. It is associated with infection, inflammatory disorders, heart disease, renal disease, and connective tissue diseases such as osteoarthritis. Found mostly in older adults, this anemia is highly resistant to treatment.
- *Obesity:* Obese youth and adults can experience changes in iron regulation that lower iron absorption and increase risk of iron deficiency, regardless of iron intake.[33]

Worldwide Problem of Iron Deficiency Anemia

Iron deficiency anemia is second only to protein-energy malnutrition as the most prevalent nutritional deficiency worldwide. It is estimated that 43% of children, 38% of pregnant women, and 29% of nonpregnant women are anemic and approximately half of these are the result of iron deficiency.[34] Iron deficiency anemia respects neither social class nor geographic location; iron balance in developing countries is precarious based on low intakes of bioavailable iron and iron loss through parasitic infections. For more information on how to recognize an iron deficiency anemia, see the Perspectives in Practice box, "Nutritional Anemias: How Are They Identified?"

Iron Requirement
Dietary Reference Intake
The RDAs for iron are 18 mg/day for women ages 19 to 50 and 8 mg/day for men ages 19 and older.[26] When the menses cease, the RDA for women is the same as for men—8 mg/day. Pregnancy has a "high iron cost," and the daily allowance rises to 27 mg/day. Iron needs decrease to 9 mg/day during lactation because the menses are usually absent during this period.[26]

Special Considerations for Vegetarians
Individuals who do not eat meat, fish, or poultry need to give special attention to their iron needs. Not only is the bioavailability of iron lower in plant foods, but also heme iron is unavailable to enhance nonheme iron absorption. As a result, overall iron absorption from plant foods is estimated to be approximately 10%, as compared with 18% for the typical American diet. With this in mind, it is believed that vegetarians have an iron requirement 1.8 times that of individuals consuming heme iron.[25] This would raise the iron requirement of vegetarian premenopausal women to approximately 32 mg/day. This recommendation is nearly twice that for persons of comparable age and gender who consume a mixed diet, so individual counseling regarding iron sources and supplements is warranted.

Iron Toxicity
Hemochromatosis
Iron toxicity was first identified in a population in Southern Africa who cooked their food in iron vessels and also had a genetic tendency to absorb and store abnormally high amounts of dietary iron. In the United States, accidental iron poisoning occurs in children and adults who overuse iron supplements. However, another cause of iron overload is the genetic disease hemochromatosis, in which iron continues to be absorbed at high rates despite elevated

---

KEY TERMS

Anemia
A condition characterized by an abnormally low number of red blood cells or low hemoglobin content.

Hemochromatosis
A genetic-related disorder causing excessive absorption of iron and its deposition in soft tissues such as joints, heart, and liver.

PERSPECTIVES IN PRACTICE

Nutritional Anemias: How Are They Identified?

Nutritional anemias occur when a nutrient required to synthesize hemoglobin or red blood cells is lacking. Two common nutritional anemias are iron deficiency anemia and the megaloblastic anemia related to a lack of vitamin B_{12}.

Various blood parameters can help identify the cause of a nutritional anemia as follows:

Size of the Red Blood Cell
- Microcytic cells are smaller in size than normal red blood cells and are characteristic of iron deficiency anemia.
- Macrocytic cells are very large in size as compared with normal red blood cells and are often associated with a lack of vitamin B_{12}.

Number of Red Blood Cells
- The number of red blood cells is less than normal in both an iron deficiency and a vitamin B_{12}-related anemia; it can alert you to a developing anemia but cannot identify its cause.

Hemoglobin Level
- Women of childbearing age often have lower hemoglobin levels than do men, due to their monthly blood loss; however, hemoglobin levels are reduced in both genders in the case of anemia; for this reason, low hemoglobin is not a sensitive marker for distinguishing between an iron deficiency and a vitamin B_{12}-related anemia.

Other Markers of Iron Status Can Help Identify an Iron Deficiency Anemia.
- Serum iron, which transports iron for metabolic use, falls to low levels as the iron deficiency worsens.
- Serum ferritin carries iron to storage sites; it falls to low levels as less iron is available.
- Transferrin is the protein that binds absorbed iron and delivers it to the bone marrow for production of red blood cells and to body cells for metabolic use; serum transferrin rises as the body attempts to use all available iron.
- Serum transferrin saturation indicates the proportion of available transferrin that is bound with iron; normal transferrin saturation is approximately 20% to 35% but drops to less than 15% in iron deficiency anemia.

Identifying the cause of a nutritional anemia requires a review of various markers providing clues about ongoing red blood cell formation and iron metabolism.

Bibliography

Litchford MD: Assessment: laboratory data. In Mahan LK, Escott-Stump S, editors: *Krause's food and nutrition therapy*, St Louis, 2008, Saunders.

Stopler T: Medical nutrition therapy for anemia. In Mahan LK, Escott-Stump S, editors: *Krause's food and nutrition therapy*, St Louis, 2008, Saunders.

liver stores. It is estimated that 1 in 200 individuals of European descent carry this genetic mutation, but development of this condition is influenced by genetic and environmental factors including gender, alcohol consumption, and blood loss.[35] Excessive body iron is associated with increased tissue oxidation and production of free radicals and, if untreated, is believed to foster cardiac arrhythmias, liver disease, joint disease, and diabetes. Even moderately elevated iron stores, much lower than those associated with hemochromatosis, appear to increase the risk of type 2 diabetes in otherwise healthy persons.[36]

Tolerable Upper Intake Level

Because iron becomes toxic at inappropriately high levels, iron intake should not exceed 45 mg/day.[25] Although it would seem unlikely that one would reach this level from food only, current iron fortification policies developed to meet the iron needs of women in the childbearing years add significant amounts of iron to the diet. Individuals who eat more than one serving of a cereal that contains 15 to 18 mg of iron per serving, along with other iron-containing foods, and possibly a multivitamin-mineral supplement with iron, will approach or exceed

the UL. Men and older women who eat large amounts of meat supplying heme iron, take iron supplements, and use alcoholic beverages on a regular basis, which increases iron absorption, are at risk of iron toxicity. Median intakes of iron from food and beverages among men older than 19 years is 17 mg, more than twice their RDA, whereas women of childbearing age who do not use supplements fall woefully below their RDA of 18 mg with a median intake of barely 13 mg. Men and women of all ages taking supplements containing iron have median intakes approaching 32 mg.[1] Iron supplements should always be approved and supervised by a physician.

Food Sources of Iron

The typical Western diet contains approximately 5 to 7 mg of iron per 1000 kcal. Iron is found in highest amounts in meat, fish, poultry, eggs, dried peas and beans, and whole grain and fortified breads and cereals. Heme iron provides less than 10% of the iron intake of girls and women and less than 12% of the iron intake of boys and men.[26] Fortified grain products such as breakfast cereals are major sources in the American diet. Box 7.7 lists some comparative food sources of iron.

BOX 7.7 Food Sources of Iron

Food Source	Amount	Iron (mg)
Grains Group		
Ready-to-Eat Cereals		
Total	¾ cup	18.00
Cheerios	1 cup	9.29
All Bran	½ cup	5.46
Rice, white, long grain enriched, cooked	1 cup	1.90
Rice, brown, long grain, cooked	1 cup	1.13
Bread, white, commercially prepared	1 slice	0.90
Bread, whole wheat, commercially prepared	1 slice	0.79
Vegetable Group		
Spinach, frozen, cooked	½ cup	1.86
Potato, baked, flesh and skin	1 medium	1.87
Potato, baked, flesh only	1 medium	0.55
Peas, green, canned	½ cup	0.81
Lima beans, frozen, baby, cooked	1 cup	3.53
Broccoli, frozen, cooked	½ cup	0.56
Vegetable juice cocktail, canned	1 cup	0.71
Fruit		
Raisins, seedless	½ cup	1.36
Meat, Beans, Eggs, and Nuts Group		
Ground beef patty, lean	3 oz	2.41
Frankfurter, beef	1	0.55
Ham, canned, lean	3 oz	0.80
Chicken, thigh meat, roasted, without skin	3 oz	0.90
Tuna, light, canned in water	3 oz	1.39
Egg, whole, hard cooked	1 large	0.59

BOX 7.7 Food Sources of Iron—cont'd		
Food Source	**Amount**	**Iron (mg)**
Soybeans, cooked	½ cup	4.42
Refried beans, canned	½ cup	1.71
Soy patty, vegan	3 oz	2.47
Tofu, firm	3 oz	1.80

Recommended Dietary Allowances for adults: men, 8 mg; women ages 19–50, 18 mg; women ages ≥51, 8 mg.
Images copyright 2006 JupiterImages Corporation. Data from US Department of Agriculture, Agricultural Research Service: *USDA National Nutrient Database for Standard Reference, Release 28.* Nutrient Data Laboratory Home Page, revised May, 2016. https://www.ndb.nal.usda.gov/ndb/.

IODINE

Iodine has worldwide interest, based on the occurrence of goiter and other disorders brought about by iodine deficiency. Iodine is a component of the hormone thyroxine produced in the thyroid gland. The body contains only 15 to 20 mg of iodine, and 70% to 80% is in the thyroid gland. This gland has a remarkable ability to concentrate iodine.

Absorption-Excretion Balance
Absorption

Iodine is absorbed in the form of iodides. Iodides are then loosely bound to proteins and carried by the blood to the thyroid gland, which takes up as much as it needs for hormone synthesis. One-third of the available iodide is used to produce active thyroid hormone with the remainder used to form hormone precursors for later use.

Excretion

Absorbed iodide not needed by the thyroid gland is excreted in the urine. More than 90% of the iodine taken into the body appears in the urine.

Hormonal Control

Thyroid-stimulating hormone (TSH) from the anterior lobe of the pituitary gland directs the uptake of iodine by thyroid cells in response to plasma thyroid hormone levels. When plasma levels are high, less thyroid hormone is produced. When plasma levels are low, the thyroid cells are stimulated to take up more iodine and produce more hormone. This feedback mechanism maintains a healthy circular balance between supply and demand and is the characteristic pattern of the endocrine glands controlled by the pituitary gland.

Physiologic Function of Iodine
Thyroid Hormone Synthesis

The major function of iodine is as part of the thyroid hormone, thyroxine. Thyroxine regulates cell oxidation and basal metabolic rate (BMR) by increasing oxygen uptake and the reaction rates of enzyme systems handling glucose. In this role, iodine exerts tremendous control over total body metabolism. Thyroid hormone also regulates protein synthesis and myelin formation in the developing brain. Hyperthyroidism and hypothyroidism affect the rate of thyroxine production and the body's overall metabolic rate.

Plasma Thyroxine

Thyroxine is secreted into the bloodstream bound to plasma protein for transport to cells. After completing its work, the hormone is degraded in the liver and the iodine is excreted in the bile.

Clinical Applications
Iodine Deficiency Disorder: Goiter

Endemic goiter, visible as an enlargement of the thyroid gland, is a problem in geographic areas where water and soil, and in turn locally grown foods, contain little iodine. Up to 2 billion people live in iodine-deficient areas, and 37% are school children.[37] Africa, Southeast Asia, the Eastern Mediterranean, and parts of Europe have had widespread iodine deficiency. When iodine is not available in the amounts needed, the thyroid gland cannot produce a normal quantity of thyroxine. Low plasma thyroxine levels signal the pituitary to release TSH, and, without iodine, the thyroid gland responds by making thyroglobulin (a colloid), which accumulates in the thyroid follicles. Over time the gland becomes increasingly engorged and may attain a size of 500 to 700 g (1 to 1½ lb) or more (Fig. 7.6).

Salt iodization remains the most cost-effective way to deliver iodine to both humans and livestock and is credited with eradicating iodine deficiency in the United States and Canada. Through the use of iodized salt, the number of countries affected by goiter has dropped from 110 to 32.[38] In remote areas where iodization of salt is not practical, iodized rapeseed oil or bouillon cubes, monthly doses of potassium iodide to school children, or slow-release iodide added to drinking water has eradicated severe endemic goiter. Goiter also stems from eating foods containing substances that inhibit the synthesis of thyroxine. Pearl millet, a cereal grain in the Sudan region of Africa, can cause goiter.

Iodine Deficiency Disorder: Cretinism

Iodine deficiency has been referred to as *the most common cause of preventable brain damage in the world,*[38] and for pregnant and lactating women and their infants, the need is critical. When iodine deficiency is severe during fetal and infant periods of critical brain development, the outcome is cretinism, with irreversible mental retardation and disability. Consistent salt fortification programs provide sufficient iodine to support the elevated needs of pregnancy and the production of breast milk with appropriate iodine content.[38]

KEY TERM

Goiter
Enlargement of the thyroid gland caused by lack of available iodine to produce the thyroid hormone thyroxine.

KEY TERM

Cretinism
A congenital disease resulting from a lack of iodine and insufficient thyroxin secretion, characterized by physical deformity, dwarfism, mental retardation, and often goiters.

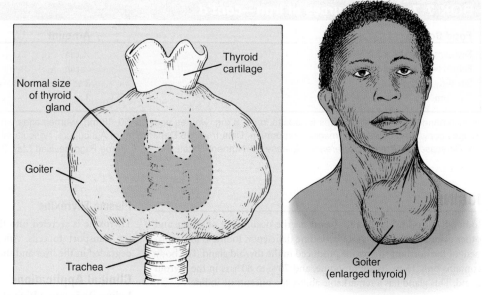

FIG. 7.6 Goiter. The extreme enlargement shown here reflects an extended duration of iodine deficiency.

Iodine Requirement

Dietary Reference Intake

The RDA for iodine in men and women is 150 mcg/day.[26] To meet the needs of mother and developing fetus, the RDA increases to 220 mcg/day in pregnancy and 290 mcg/day throughout lactation. Because of increased demand for iodine during accelerated growth, the allowance for youth ages 14 to 18 is the same as for adults.

Food Sources of Iodine

Seafood is rich in iodine. Plant foods depend on the iodine content of the soil and the iodine compounds used in food processing. Iodized table salt fortified at the level of 1 mg of iodine per 10 g of salt is a major dietary source in the United States, along with calcium and potassium iodates that are common additives in commercially produced bread. Recommended lowering of salt intake will also result in a lowering of iodine intake.

Common food production and processing methods add to iodine intake. Dairy farms use iodophors, iodine-containing chemicals, for sanitizing milking machines and milk tanks. Iodine-containing compounds are used as dough conditioners, and iodine supplements are added to animal feeds. For most people, iodine intake from food and supplements is unlikely to exceed the UL. Toxicity symptoms usually result from intakes of several grams of iodine.

ZINC

Zinc is a component of more than 100 body enzymes and a factor in growth.[26] Total body zinc ranges from 1.5 g in women to 2.5 g in men. It is present in minute quantities in all body organs, tissues, and fluids. Although zinc is vital throughout life, it is especially important in periods of growth. Zinc is intimately involved with DNA and RNA metabolism and protein synthesis and necessary for tissue growth to progress at normal rates.

Absorption-Excretion-Storage

Zinc is absorbed in the midsection of the small intestine, and, as is true for various minerals, individuals in poor status absorb a greater proportion of their dietary zinc than do individuals in good status. Zinc is excreted primarily via the feces, with very small amounts lost in the urine. Zinc absorption is impaired with long-term alcohol consumption, and greater amounts are lost in the urine, putting these persons at risk of poor zinc status. Zinc is stored primarily in the muscle and bone. A very small amount of body zinc circulates in the plasma, but these levels are carefully regulated.

Clinical Applications

Several clinical problems stem from zinc deficiency, as follows:

- *Hypogonadism:* Dwarfism with arrested development and function of the gonads results from pronounced zinc deficiency in childhood and adolescence. Sexual maturation is delayed in male adolescents deprived of zinc.
- *Loss in taste and smell:* Hypogeusia (diminished taste) and hyposmia (diminished smell) are associated with severe zinc deficiency but improve when zinc is restored.
- *Wound healing:* Healing of wounds or tissue injuries from trauma, surgery, or physiologic stress is retarded in those who are zinc deficient. Older adults with pressure sores may benefit from zinc supplementation.
- *Growth, development, and life cycle needs:* Rapid growth in infants, children, and adolescents carries special needs for zinc. When zinc is inadequate, proteins necessary for the linear growth of the long bones are not produced and growth is stunted.[26] Poor zinc intake in pregnancy can result in congenital malformations and low infant birth weight or preterm delivery. Zinc supplements given to very low-birth-weight infants has been shown to lower the incidence of lung disease, gastrointestinal necrosis, sepsis, and mortality.[39] Even subclinical deficiency has adverse effects on brain function in both children and adults.[40]
- *Immune function:* Zinc promotes optimum immune function. Zinc-deficient children in developing countries are more vulnerable to disability and death from diarrhea. Individuals with optimum zinc status have greater resistance to infections.
- *Malabsorption:* Malabsorption diseases such as Crohn disease can lead to zinc deficiency. Dietary restrictions imposed in the treatment of these conditions can further limit zinc availability.

Zinc Requirement

Dietary Reference Intake

The RDA for zinc is 11 mg for men and 8 mg for women.[26] Women's needs are lower because of their generally smaller body size. Beef is a major zinc source in the United States, followed by ready-to-eat cereals, milk, and poultry.[26] Zinc is better absorbed from animal proteins than plant proteins because phytates in plant foods bind to zinc and prevent its absorption.

Concentrated zinc supplements can interfere with iron and copper absorption and can lead to poor copper status. Conversely, there is evidence that iron supplements may interfere with zinc absorption if both are taken without food. This raises a concern about the management of supplement use in pregnancy when both nutrients are vital to growth of maternal and fetal tissues.[25] Excessive zinc intake results in gastrointestinal distress, a decrease in blood high-density lipoprotein (HDL)-cholesterol, and a suppressed immune system. This usually occurs from use of high-potency supplements exceeding the adult UL of 40 mg, not from food.[25] Parents need to be advised regarding the potential hazards of oversupplementation in young children. A national survey indicated that 65% of boys and 56% of girls ages 1 to 3 had zinc intakes greater than their UL of 7 mg.[1]

Food Sources of Zinc

Good sources of dietary zinc are seafood (especially oysters), meat, eggs, and milk. Legumes and whole grains contain zinc, but bioavailability is a problem. Box 7.8 lists some foods containing zinc.

BOX 7.8 Food Sources of Zinc

Food Source	Amount	Zinc (mg)
Grains Group		
Shredded wheat	2 biscuits	1.36
Oat bran muffin	1 (small)	1.21
Vegetable Group		
Peas, green, canned	1 cup	1.07
Meat, Beans, Eggs, and Nuts Group		
Oysters, breaded, fried	3 oz (6 medium)	74.06
Ground beef patty, lean	3 oz	5.47
Baked beans, canned, vegetarian	1 cup	5.79
Peanut butter, creamy	2 tbsp	0.80
Milk Group		
Milk, nonfat (reduced fat, low fat, and whole milk vary slightly)	1 cup	1.03
American cheese, processed, pasteurized	1 oz	0.71

Recommended Dietary Allowance for adults: women, 8 mg; men, 11 mg. Images copyright 2006 JupiterImages Corporation. Data from US Department of Agriculture, Agricultural Research Service: *USDA National Nutrient Database for Standard Reference, Release 28.* Nutrient Data Laboratory Home Page, revised May, 2016. https://www.ndb.nal.usda.gov/ndb/.

Minerals from Cooking Utensils: Safe or Harmful?

Some dishes and containers intended to be decorative are lined with copper or enhanced with glazes that contain lead. Copper and lead are easily dissolved by acid, which includes acids in food. This makes it dangerous to cook or serve foods in unlined copper utensils or ceramic, lead-glazed containers because harmful amounts of these minerals will dissolve and enter one's food, especially at high temperatures. The body requires copper in very minute amounts, but higher levels become toxic. Lead exposure is harmful at all ages but especially for children. The Food Code developed by the US Food and Drug Administration (FDA), which sets standards for safe food handling in restaurants, institutions, and other food service operations, forbids use of such containers. In like manner, very small amounts of iron from cast iron cooking utensils enter food during cooking, especially when cooking acid foods. For most people this is not a problem and may actually be helpful in raising iron intake levels; however, persons with hemochromatosis, who absorb iron in abnormally large amounts, should avoid all cast iron utensils. In general, cookware purchased in reputable retail stores will not pose any health risk, but consumers should avoid cooking or serving food in utensils from international sources or purchased as a craft or collectable.

Data from US Food and Drug Administration: *Food Code: 2005,* Washington, D.C., 2005, US Government Printing Office.
National Library of Medicine, National Institutes of Health: *Medline Plus, Trusted Health Information for You: Cooking utensils and nutrition,* Bethesda, MD, 2015, National Library of Medicine. http://www.nlm.nih.gov/medlineplus/ency/article/002461.htm.

COPPER

Copper and iron have many characteristics in common, as follows:
- Both are components of cell enzymes.
- Both are involved in energy production.
- Both participate in hemoglobin synthesis.

Copper is found in many foods, but deficiency has been reported in patients on total parenteral nutrition (TPN) that excluded copper. Persons using concentrated zinc supplements that interfere with copper absorption can develop copper deficiency. Premature infants fed only cow's milk, which is low in copper, become deficient.[26]

The RDA for copper is 900 mcg/day (0.9 mg/day).[26] Copper, like many trace elements, is lost in food processing. The richest sources are liver, seafood (particularly oysters), nuts, and seeds, with smaller amounts in whole grains and legumes. The Focus on Food Safety box, "Minerals from Cooking Utensils: Safe or Harmful?" describes how copper and other minerals can enter our food in cooking.

MANGANESE

The adult body usually contains 20 mg of manganese distributed in the liver, bones, pancreas, and pituitary gland.[26] Manganese is a part of important cell enzymes. Manganese deficiency has been reported in patients with pancreatic insufficiency and protein-energy malnutrition. Although an essential nutrient, manganese is toxic at prolonged exposure to manganese dust as occurs with miners or industrial workers. Excess manganese accumulates in the liver and central nervous system (CNS), producing psychiatric disturbances and neuromuscular symptoms resembling those of Parkinson disease. Manganese toxicity usually occurs from environmental exposure, not dietary intake.

The AI for manganese is 2.3 mg/day for men and 1.8 mg/day for women.[26] The typical American diet supplies manganese at a level of 1.6 mg/1000 kcal. The best sources are plant foods such as grains, legumes, seeds, nuts, leafy vegetables, tea, and coffee.

CHROMIUM

Chromium is found in minute amounts in liver, soft tissues, and bone, although the precise body total is unknown. Chromium is part of a protein complex that potentiates insulin activity and assists in moving glucose into cells. Through its role with insulin, chromium influences carbohydrate, protein, and fat metabolism. Chromium picolinate is widely advertised as a bodybuilding and weight loss supplement, despite the fact that no research evidence supports these claims.

The AI for chromium is 35 mcg/day for men and 25 mcg/day for women ages 19 to 50. Based on the decline in energy intakes, the AIs decrease to 30 and 20 mcg, respectively, after age 50.[26] Information about the chromium content of common foods is sparse. Brewer's yeast is a rich source. Other food sources include liver, cheddar cheese, wheat germ, and whole grains.

SELENIUM

Selenium is deposited in all body tissues except adipose tissue. Concentrations are highest in liver, kidney, heart, and spleen. Selenium is an integral part of an antioxidant enzyme that protects cells and lipid membranes from oxidative damage. Selenium partners with vitamin E, each sparing the other. Highly bioavailable selenium compounds are found in human milk, with even higher concentrations in colostrum, suggesting an important role for this element in the term and preterm infant.[41] The RDA for all adults is 55 mcg/day.[42] Plant foods vary in selenium based on the content of the soil in which they were grown. In general, good sources include seafood, legumes, whole grains, lean meats, and dairy products; vegetables have the smallest amounts.

MOLYBDENUM

Molybdenum is an enzyme cofactor in reactions that move hydroxyl (OH^-) groups.[26] The RDA is set at 45 mcg/day for all adults. The amount of molybdenum in foods varies according to the soil content. The richest sources generally include legumes, whole grains, and nuts. Animal products, fruit, and most vegetables are poor sources.

FLUORIDE

Fluoride accumulates in the calcified tissues and protects bones and teeth from mineral loss.[43] If fluoride is present when calcium-phosphorus crystals are being formed, then a fluoride ion (F^-) replaces a hydroxyl ion (OH^-) in the crystal, resulting in a material that is more resistant to resorption. Fluoride-containing crystals are also more resistant to the erosion of bacterial acids formed by microorganisms that feed on fermentable carbohydrates adhering to the teeth and initiate tooth decay.[43]

The AI for fluoride is expected to protect against dental caries. Intake is set at 4 mg/day for men and 3 mg/day for women.[25] Fish, fish products, and teas contain the highest amounts. Fluoridated dental products, such as toothpaste and mouthwash, contribute to fluoride intake and may approach the amount ingested from food. Adding fluoride to public water supplies in the amount of 1 part per million (ppm) reduces dental caries in those communities. Cooking with fluoridated water increases the level in many foods. Currently more than 72% of the US population that is served by community water systems has access to fluoridated water.[43]

Excessive fluoride intake leads to pitted and discolored teeth, and this condition was first identified in communities where the natural water source was high in fluoride; however, this condition is unlikely to occur unless fluoride intake exceeds 10 mg a day for a period of 10 years or more. Young children should be monitored to avoid swallowing excessive amounts of fluoride-containing dental products.[25]

The roles of the essential trace elements are summarized in Table 7.5.

TABLE 7.5 Summary of Trace Elements

Element	Metabolism	Physiologic Functions	Clinical Applications	Dietary Reference Intake	Food Sources

Iron (Fe)	Absorption controls body supply; favored by body need, acidity, and reducing agents such as vitamin C; hindered by binding agents, reduced gastric HCl, infection
	Transported as transferrin, stored as ferritin or hemosiderin
	Excreted in sloughed cells, bleeding; no body mechanism for excretion
		Hemoglobin and myoglobin synthesis, oxygen/carbon dioxide carrier
		Cell oxidation; energy metabolism
			Anemia (hypochromic, microcytic)
			Excess: hemosiderosis, hemochromatosis
			Growth and pregnancy needs
				Males ages ≥19: 8 mg
				Females ages 19–50: 18 mg
				Females ages ≥51: 8 mg
				Pregnancy
				  All ages: 27 mg
				Lactation
				  Ages ≤18: 10 mg
				  Ages ≥19: 9 mg
					Meat, eggs, liver
					Whole grain and enriched breads and cereals
					Dark green vegetables
					Legumes, nuts
					Acidic foods cooked in iron utensils

Iodine (I)	Absorbed as iodides, taken up by thyroid gland under control of thyroid-stimulating hormone (TSH)
	Excretion by kidney
		Synthesis of thyroxin, which regulates cell metabolism, basal metabolic rate (BMR)	Endemic colloid goiter
			Cretinism
			Hypothyroidism and hyperthyroidism
				Males/females ages ≥19: 150 mcg
				Pregnancy
				  All ages: 220 mcg
				Lactation
				  All ages: 290 mcg
					Iodized salt
					Seafood

TABLE 7.5 Summary of Trace Elements—cont'd

Element	Metabolism	Physiologic Functions	Clinical Applications	Dietary Reference Intake	Food Sources

Zinc (Zn)	Absorbed in small intestine
	Stored in many tissues
	Excretion mostly intestinal
		Essential coenzyme involved with DNA/RNA metabolism and protein synthesis	Growth: hypogonadism
			Sensory impairment: taste and smell
			Wound healing
			Malabsorption diseases
				Males ages ≥19: 11 mg
				Females ages ≥19: 8 mg
				Pregnancy
				  Ages ≤18: 12 mg
				  Ages ≥19: 11 mg
				Lactation
				  Ages ≤18: 13 mg
				  Ages ≥19: 12 mg
					Beef and other meats, liver
					Oysters, seafood
					Milk, cheese, eggs
					Whole grains
					Widely distributed in food

Copper (Cu)	Absorbed in small intestine
	Stored in many tissues
		Associated with iron in enzyme systems, hemoglobin synthesis
		Metalloprotein enzyme component
			Hypocupremia: nephrosis and malabsorption
			Wilson disease, excess copper storage
				Males/females ages ≥19: 900 mcg
				Pregnancy
				  All ages: 1000 mcg
				Lactation
				  All ages: 1300 mcg
					Meat, liver, seafood
					Whole grains
					Legumes, nuts
					Widely distributed in food

Manganese (Mn)	Absorbed poorly Excretion mainly by intestine	Enzyme component in general metabolism	Low serum levels in protein-energy malnutrition Inhalation toxicity	Males ages ≥19: 2.3 mg Females ages ≥19: 1.8 mg Pregnancy All ages: 2.0 mg Lactation all ages: 2.6 mg	Whole grains and cereals Legumes, soybeans Green leafy vegetables

Chromium (Cr)	Better absorbed in an acid environment
	Excretion mainly by kidney
		Associated with glucose metabolism	Potentiates action of insulin	Males ages 19–50: 35 mcg
				Males ages ≥51: 30 mcg
				Females ages 19–50: 25 mcg
				Females ages ≥51: 20 mcg
				Pregnancy
				  Ages ≤18: 29 mcg
				  Ages ≥19: 30 mcg
				Lactation
				  Ages ≤18: 44 mcg
				  Ages ≥19: 45 mcg
					Whole grains and cereals
					Brewer's yeast
					Animal protein foods

Selenium (Se)	Absorption depends on solubility of compound form
	Excreted mainly by kidney
		Component of enzyme glutathione peroxidase
		Synergistic antioxidant with vitamin E
			Marginal deficiency when soil content is low
			Deficiency secondary to total parenteral nutrition or malnutrition
			Toxicity observed in livestock
				Males/females
				  Ages ≥19: 55 mcg
				Pregnancy
				  All ages: 60 mcg
				Lactation
				  All ages: 70 mcg
					Seafood
					Legumes
					Whole grains
					Vegetables
					Low-fat meats and dairy foods
					Varies with soil content

Molybdenum (Mo)	Readily absorbed
	Excreted rapidly by kidneys
		Component of oxidase enzymes	Deficiency unknown in humans	Males/females ages ≥19: 45 mcg
				Pregnancy
				  All ages: 50 mcg
				Lactation
				  All ages: 50 mcg
					Legumes
					Whole grains
					Milk
					Organ meats
					Leafy vegetables

Fluoride (F)	Absorbed in small intestine; little known of bioavailability
	Excreted by kidneys
		Accumulates in bones and teeth, increases resistance to resorption	Reduces dental caries
			Osteoporosis: may reduce bone loss
			Excess: dental fluorosis
			Toxicity: swallowing fluoridated dental products
				Males ages ≥19: 4 mg
				Females ages ≥19: 3 mg
				Pregnancy
				  All ages: 3 mg
				Lactation
				  All ages: 3 mg
					Fish and fish products
					Tea
					Drinking water (if fluoridated)
					Foods cooked in fluoridated water

OTHER TRACE ELEMENTS

The metabolic functions or need for five other trace elements, arsenic, boron, vanadium, nickel, and silicon, are unclear. Although they appear to have beneficial roles in various animal species, evidence of their nutritional importance, essentiality, or role in human health is lacking.[25] Insufficient research data are available to set an RDA or AI for these minerals. Based on their potential for toxicity, a UL has been established for boron, nickel, and vanadium.[25]

WATER AND ELECTROLYTES

Water, the last nutrient we will review, is essential to the life of every cell. In our discussions of sodium, potassium, and chloride, we noted the roles of these minerals in guarding body water and maintaining its appropriate distribution inside or outside of body cells. Now we will see how this is accomplished.

Hydration status is fundamental to health and a vital part of patient care. Three interdependent factors control fluid balance: (1) the water itself (the solvent base for solutions), (2) the various particles in the water (solutes), and (3) the separating membranes that control flow from one compartment to another.

KEY TERM

Compartment
The collective quantity of material of a given type in the body. The four body compartments are (1) lean body mass (muscle and vital organs), (2) minerals, (3) fat, and (4) water.

BODY WATER

Body Water Distribution

If you are a woman, your body is approximately 50% to 55% water; if you are a man, then it is approximately 55% to 60% water. Men have higher water content because they have proportionately more muscle and less fat. Muscle contains more water than any other tissue except blood. Women have proportionately less muscle and more fat; fat is lower in water content.

Functions of Body Water

Body water serves many purposes (Box 7.9). Much of our body form comes from the turgor water provides for tissues. Cell water furnishes the fluid environment for the vast array of chemical reactions that sustain life. Medications are dissolved in body fluids. The evaporation

BOX 7.9 Functions of Body Water

Gives body form and structure
Provides fluid environment for chemical reactions to take place
Dissolves important substances in tissues and cells
Transports nutrients and waste
Controls body temperature
Dissolves medications

of water from the skin is an important means of regulating body temperature.

Overall Water Balance: Input and Output

The average adult processes 2.5 to 3 L of water each day. Water enters and leaves the body by various routes (Table 7.6), controlled by the thirst mechanism and regulatory hormones.

Water enters the body in three forms:
- As preformed water taken in as water or in other beverages
- As preformed water in food
- As metabolic water produced by cell oxidation

The proportion of fluid intake from water and beverages and from the moisture in food varies according to age. On average, water and other beverages contribute 75% to 84% of total fluid intake and food adds 17% to 25%. Individuals older than 70 years drink the least amount of fluid, obtaining more of their water from food. Plain water, either tap or bottled, contributes at least a third of total fluid intake.[44] Many common foods contain large amounts of water (Table 7.7). Metabolic water contributes the least amount to total water intake. All water, regardless of source, is of equal value in meeting fluid needs.

Water leaves the body via the kidneys, skin, and lungs, as well as through fecal elimination (see Table 7.6). Vomiting and diarrhea bring abnormal fluid losses and serious clinical problems if prolonged. Abnormal loss of body fluid is especially dangerous for infants and children, whose bodies contain a greater proportion of water, and more of their body water is outside the cells and more easily lost. Water retention associated with heart failure or electrolyte disturbances requires immediate medical attention. Intake and output must remain in balance to sustain normal hydration.

KEY TERM

Electrolyte
A chemical element or group of elements that in solution forms ions carrying a positive (e.g., H^+, Na^+, K^+, Ca^{+2}, and Mg^{+2}) or negative (e.g., Cl^-, HCO_3^-, HPO_4^{-2}, and SO_4^{-2}) charge. Electrolytes control fluid concentrations inside and outside the cells.

TABLE 7.6 Daily Adult Water Intake and Output

	Intake (Replacement) (mL/day)		OUTPUT (LOSS) (mL/day)	
			Obligatory (Insensible) (mL/day)	Additional (Based on Need) (mL/day)
Preformed in liquids	1200–1500	Lungs	350	
In foods	700–1000	Skin diffusion	350	
Metabolism (oxidation of food)	200–300	Sweat	100	≈250
		Kidneys	900	≈500
		Feces	150	
TOTAL	2100–2800 (≈2600 mL/day)	TOTAL	1850 (≈2600 mL/day)	750

TABLE 7.7   Water Content of Selected Foods and Beverages

Food	Percent (%)
Coffee, milk, sports drinks, watermelon, broccoli, lettuce	91–100
Soda, fruit drinks, fruit juice, apples, oranges, grapes	80–90
Peas, frozen desserts, bananas, casseroles	70–79
Meat, fish, poultry	60–69
Bread, pasta	30–40
Cereals, nuts	<5

Data from Campbell S: Dietary reference intakes: water, potassium, sodium, chloride, and sulfate, *Nutr MD* 30(6):13, 2004.

WATER REQUIREMENTS

For years we were told to drink eight glasses of water a day, although it is difficult to find documentation as to the origin of this advice. References to hydration in the popular press and advertisements for bottled water promote deliberate water consumption. Nutrition experts note that for most individuals fluid needs are met by drinking when thirsty[11]; however, physiologic changes in older adults diminish the thirst mechanism, with risk of dehydration.[45]

Dietary Reference Intake

The current AIs for fluid (Table 7.8) were developed using the median water intake of participants in recent national surveys[11]; yet, questions remain as to the appropriateness of these recommendations. First, quantifying water intake is difficult,[44,45] and only recently have such questions been added to nutrition surveys.[44] Furthermore, fluids such as sweetened or alcoholic beverages are often consumed for social reasons rather than thirst. Lastly, these guidelines pertain to healthy individuals who are relatively sedentary and live in temperate climates. Older adults with a diminished sense of thirst, athletes engaging in vigorous physical activity of long duration, the critically ill with a high rate of metabolism, persons in very hot environments with high losses of water via sweat, or those doing strenuous physical work require special attention.[11,45]

Fluid intake influences energy intake. Water in replacement of sugar sweetened, nonnutritive beverages can assist in weight loss.[46] Among adults ages 20 to 50, intakes of soda, alcohol, fruit drinks, and energy drinks added 350 kcal to their daily energy intake.[44] Water needs and hydration status appear to be influenced by body weight. Obese persons are more likely to be hypohydrated than normal weight or underweight persons despite meeting or exceeding the DRI for fluid, increasing their risk of kidney stones and changes in physiologic and cognitive function.[47]

TABLE 7.8   Adequate Intakes of Fluid[a]

Age (Years)	Males	Females
1–3	4 cups	4 cups
4–8	5 cups	5 cups
9–13	8 cups	7 cups
14–18	11 cups	8 cups
≥19	13 cups	9 cups

[a]Expressed as cups of beverages/drinking water with additional fluid to be supplied in food.
Data from Food and Nutrition Board, Institute of Medicine: *Dietary Reference Intakes for water, potassium, sodium, chloride, and sulfate,* Washington, DC, 2004, National Academies Press.

Clinical Applications

The following clinical situations influence water needs:

- *Uncontrolled diabetes mellitus:* Patients lose excessive amounts of water through the osmotic effect of high urinary glucose and need additional fluid.
- *Cystic fibrosis:* This disease increases fluid needs.
- *High fiber intake:* As dietary fiber increases, so do fluid requirements. Adequate fluid is needed to replace the water absorbed by the fiber in the gastrointestinal tract.
- *High protein intake:* Protein metabolism produces urea and other nitrogenous wastes that must be excreted via the kidneys. Providing an appropriate level of fluid is important for patients given high-protein supplements.
- *Intense physical activity:* Exercise of high intensity or duration such as marathon runs or strenuous physical work requires consistent fluid intake to replace water lost in sweat, thereby enabling this cooling mechanism to continue. A lack of fluid in such situations can lead to heat stroke and death (see Chapter 14).
- *Impaired thirst in older adults:* Some older persons, especially frail elderly in poor health or who take multiple medications, do not become thirsty when they should, based on aging changes in the thirst center of the hypothalamus.[45] Older adults who suffer from incontinence may voluntarily reduce their fluid intake.
- *Medications:* Diuretics increase fluid output, as do certain analgesics and decongestants.

Water Compartments

Body water is divided into two major compartments: (1) the water outside the cells, known as *ECF*; and (2) the water inside the cells, known as *intracellular fluid (ICF)* (Fig. 7.7). We describe as follows:

- *ECF:* The water outside the cells makes up 20% of total body weight. It is divided into four sections: (1) blood plasma, which accounts for 5% of body weight; (2) interstitial fluid, the water surrounding the cells; (3) secretory fluid, the water circulating in transit; and (4) dense tissue fluid, water in deep connective tissue, cartilage, and bone.
- *ICF:* The water inside the cells makes up 40% to 45% of total body weight. All of the metabolic activity of organs and tissues takes place within cells, so it could be expected that the amount of water inside the cells would be greater than the amount of water outside the cells (intracellular water is approximately double the amount of extracellular water).

> **KEY TERM**
>
> **Interstitial Fluid**
> The fluid between cells or in the interspaces of a tissue.

FORCES CONTROLLING WATER DISTRIBUTION

Two forces control the distribution of body water: (1) the number of solutes or particles in solution and (2) the membranes that separate water compartments. We will look at the properties of each. (Review Fig. 2.9, which illustrates the movement of water across membranes.)

Solutes

A variety of particles are found in body water. Two types control water balance: electrolytes and plasma proteins.

Electrolytes

Several minerals act as major electrolytes in controlling body fluid compartments. In this role, they are called electrolytes because they

FIG. 7.7 Body fluid compartments. Note the relative amounts of water in the intracellular fluid and extracellular fluid compartments. (Data from Gamble JL: *Chemical anatomy, physiology, and pathology of extracellular fluid.* Cambridge, MA, 1964, Harvard University Press.)

are free in solution and carry an electrical charge. Free, charged chemical forms are also called *ions*, a term that refers to atoms, elements, or groups of atoms that in solution carry either a positive or negative electrical charge. An ion carrying a positive charge is called a *cation*: examples are sodium (Na^+), the major cation in extracellular water; potassium (K^+), the major cation in intracellular water; calcium (Ca^{+2}); and magnesium (Mg^{+2}). An ion carrying a negative charge is called an *anion*: examples are chloride (Cl^-), bicarbonate (HCO_3^-), phosphate (HPO_4^{-2}), and sulfate (SO_4^{-2}). By virtue of their small size these ions or electrolytes can diffuse freely across cell membranes and create forces that control the movement of water.

Plasma Proteins

Albumin and globulin, plasma proteins of large molecular size, influence the movement of water in and out of capillaries. In this function these plasma proteins are called *colloids*. Because of their large size, plasma proteins cannot pass through the capillary membrane into the interstitial fluid. Instead they remain in the blood vessels, where they exert **colloidal osmotic pressure (COP)** to maintain vascular blood volume. We will learn about this process a bit later.

Organic Compounds of Small Molecular Size

Other organic compounds small in size, such as glucose, urea, and amino acids, diffuse freely in and out of the various fluid compartments but do not influence movement of water unless they are present in abnormally large concentrations. Such a situation occurs in patients with uncontrolled diabetes mellitus, when large amounts of glucose being excreted in the urine cause an abnormal osmotic diuresis or excess water output.

KEY TERM

Colloidal Osmotic Pressure (COP)

Osmotic pressure produced by the protein molecules in the plasma. Because proteins are large molecules, they do not pass through the separating membranes of the capillary cells, but exert a constant osmotic pull that draws fluid and waste products back into the capillaries for transport to the kidneys for filtration and excretion. Cell proteins exert an osmotic pressure that protects against loss of cell water.

Membranes

Water and solutes move across the separating membranes according to the physiologic mechanisms that handle fluid shifts. These mechanisms include osmosis, diffusion, active transport, and pinocytosis. We learned about these mechanisms in Chapter 2.

INFLUENCE OF ELECTROLYTES ON WATER BALANCE

Measurement of Electrolytes

The concentration of electrolytes or particles in a given solution determines the chemical activity of that solution. It is the number of particles, not the size of the particles, that determines chemical combining power, so electrolytes are measured according to the total number of particles in solution. Each particle contributes chemical combining power according to its **valence**, not its total weight. The unit of measure commonly used is the *equivalent*. Because we are talking about very small amounts, these measurements are expressed in *milliequivalents (mEq)*, or thousandths of an equivalent. This term refers to the number of ions—cations and anions—in solution in a given volume of body fluid. It is expressed as the number of milliequivalents per liter (mEq/L).

Electrolyte Balance

Electrolytes are distributed in body water compartments in a definite pattern. According to biochemical and electrochemical laws, a stable solution must have equal numbers of positive and negative particles. This means it must be electrically neutral. When shifts or losses occur, compensating shifts and gains must follow to maintain this balance of essential electrochemical neutrality.

KEY TERM

Valence

The combining power of an element or group of elements, as indicated by its number of positive or negative charges.

Electrolyte Control of Fluid Movement

Ionized sodium is the chief cation of ECF, and ionized potassium is the chief cation of ICF. These two electrolytes control the amount of water retained in each compartment. Shifts in water from one compartment to the other reflect changes in the ECF concentration of these electrolytes. The terms *hypertonic* and *hypotonic* refer to the electrolyte concentration of the water outside the cell. When surrounded by a hypertonic solution, water flows out of the cell and the cell becomes dehydrated and shrinks in size. When the cell is surrounded by a hypotonic solution, water flows into the cell, causing it to swell and eventually burst if the situation is not corrected.

INFLUENCE OF PLASMA PROTEINS ON WATER BALANCE

COP and Capillary Fluid Shift

Water is constantly circulating through the blood vessels to reach cells; fluid must move out of the vessels to service the tissues and then be drawn back into the vessels to maintain normal transport flow. Two opposing pressures control the movement of water and solute across capillary membranes: (1) the hydrostatic pressure (blood pressure) of the capillary blood flow and (2) the COP from plasma proteins (mainly albumin). The flow of water, nutrients, and waste to and from the cells occurs by the shifting balance of these two pressures. It works as a filtration process driven by the differences in osmotic pressure on either side of the capillary membrane.

When blood first enters the capillary system, the existing blood pressure forces water and small solutes such as glucose out into the tissues to bathe and nourish the cells. However, the plasma proteins are too large to pass through the pores of the capillary membrane and now exert the greater COP that draws fluid and waste materials back into the capillary circulation. This process is called the capillary fluid shift mechanism. It is one of the most important homeostatic mechanisms in the body for maintaining water balance, without which cells would die. Low serum albumin disrupts this process. Low concentrations of serum albumin lower the COP, with the result that less fluid is drawn back into the capillary circulation, leading to fluid retention in the tissues and edema.

Cell Fluid Control

Just as plasma proteins in the capillaries provide COP to maintain the volume of the ECF, cell protein provides the osmotic pressure that maintains the volume of the ICF. Electrolytes also play a role with ionized potassium guarding water within the cell and ionized sodium guarding water outside the cell. This balance supports the sustaining flow of water, nutrients, metabolites, and waste.

INFLUENCE OF HORMONES ON WATER BALANCE

Antidiuretic Hormone

The posterior lobe of the pituitary gland secretes the antidiuretic hormone (ADH), also called *vasopressin*. It controls the reabsorption of water by the kidneys according to body need, acting as a water conservation mechanism. In times of threatened or actual loss of body water, this hormone is released to retain precious fluid.

ADH is secreted in response to (1) an increase in the concentration of particles in the ECF as measured by receptors in the hypothalamus and (2) decreased blood volume and blood pressure as measured by receptors in the major arteries. Secretion of ADH increases water reabsorption in the kidney tubule, thereby decreasing the amount of fluid lost in the urine. When ECF concentration and blood volume have returned to normal, ADH secretion is reduced. ADH levels rise in situations when fluid is lost through heavy sweating, fever, or major blood loss.

Aldosterone

Aldosterone is the sodium-conserving hormone associated with the renin-angiotensin-aldosterone system, but it also exerts secondary control over body water. Renin, an enzyme secreted by the kidney in response to reduced blood volume acts on angiotensin, an enzyme in the plasma, which triggers the release of aldosterone from the adrenal cortex. Aldosterone acts on the kidney to reabsorb sodium, but in the process water is also reabsorbed, restoring normal blood volume. The ADH and aldosterone systems work cooperatively to maintain normal hydration and are continuously present at low levels. Both are activated by injury, surgery, vomiting or diarrhea, or other physiologic stress bringing about losses of body water.

KEY TERMS

Capillary Fluid Shift Mechanism
Process that controls the movement of water, electrolytes, nutrients, and waste between the blood in the capillary and the surrounding interstitial fluid. Shifts in balance between the intracapillary hydrostatic blood pressure and the colloidal osmotic pressure exerted by the plasma proteins accomplish filtration of water and solutes out of the capillary at the arteriole end and reabsorption of waste at the venule end.

Renin-Angiotensin-Aldosterone System
Three-stage system of sodium conservation and control of water loss; in response to diminished blood pressure in the kidney nephrons: (1) the kidneys secrete the enzyme renin, which combines with and activates angiotensinogen in the plasma; (2) active angiotensin stimulates the adjacent adrenal gland to release the hormone aldosterone; and (3) aldosterone causes reabsorption of sodium in the kidney nephrons and water follows.

TO SUM UP

Minerals are inorganic substances widely distributed in nature. They help build body tissues; serve as cofactors for metabolic reactions; participate in muscle contraction and water balance; and assist in transmission of messages along nerve fibers. Minerals are classified as (1) major minerals and (2) trace elements. Major minerals are required in amounts greater than 100 mg/day, whereas trace elements, measured in units as small as a microgram (mcg), are required in lesser amounts. Seven major minerals and nine trace elements are essential in human nutrition; in time others may be found to be essential for humans but their functions and requirements are currently unknown. The major minerals include calcium and phosphorus, with roles in bone health, energy metabolism, and nerve transmission, and magnesium, a participant in many metabolic reactions. Sodium and potassium exert opposing effects on blood pressure, with implications for cardiovascular health. The trace mineral iron (a part of hemoglobin) transports oxygen to the cells and, along with iodine and zinc, regulates growth and body metabolism. Other trace minerals are enzyme partners regulating day-to-day metabolic activities. Sodium, potassium, and chloride particles in body fluids, along with plasma proteins, control the distribution of body water inside (ICF) and outside (ECF) the cells. Maintaining appropriate fluid compartments and hydration status are crucial in clinical care. Loss of trace elements through refinement of grains and food processing negatively impacts the mineral intake and status of many Americans.

QUESTIONS FOR REVIEW

1. List the seven major minerals and describe their (a) physiologic function, (b) problems related to deficiency or excess, and (c) dietary sources.
2. You are working with a teenager who eats no red meat or fish but likes chicken. She is concerned about her weight and limits her food intake to 1600 kcal/day. List the foods with portion sizes that you would select to reach her iron RDA of 18 mg. When making your selections, consider other factors in the diet that will enhance or impede the absorption of the iron provided. (USDA food patterns for various kcalorie levels that conform to the 2015 *Dietary Guidelines for Americans* can be accessed at http://www.cnpp.usda.gov/USDAFoodPatterns.htm.)
3. What causes the edema in protein-energy malnutrition?
4. What minerals are depleted with prolonged diarrhea? What are possible consequences?
5. In the early 1900s the Great Lakes and mountainous regions of the United States suffered from endemic iodine deficiency. What was the cause of this? How has it been eliminated?
6. Go to a nearby grocery store or drug store that sells mineral supplements. Check three multimineral supplements marketed for children or adults or older adults. Prepare a table that lists each brand and include (a) the percentage of the DRI provided for each mineral and (b) the cost of a 1-day supply of the supplement. Did any of the supplements you examined exceed a UL for the intended age group? If so, then what is the danger of toxicity? Based on cost and content, what specific foods might be better choices as nutrient sources?
7. You are working with a 37-year-old man with gradually increasing blood pressure who has been advised to increase his intakes of potassium and calcium and lower his intake of sodium. When his work takes him on the road, he has lunch at a fast food restaurant; on other days he takes a lunch from home to eat at his desk. Develop a menu for a fast food lunch and a packed lunch that will provide 33% of the DRI for potassium and calcium and no more than 33% of the UL for sodium. (He has access to a refrigerator at his worksite for storage of his packed lunch.)
8. You are asked to give a 10-minute talk on water at a meal site for older adults. Prepare an outline of your major points, and justify your choice of content. Develop a handout with suggestions for increasing fluid intake.

REFERENCES

1. US Department of Health and Human Services, US Department of Agriculture: *Report of the Dietary Guidelines Advisory Committee on the Dietary Guidelines for Americans 2015*, Washington, DC, 2015, Center for Nutrition Policy and Promotion, US Department of Agriculture. https://health.gov/dietaryguidelines/2015-scientific-report/.
2. Movassagh EZ, Kontulainen S, Baxter-Jones ADG, et al: Are milk and alternatives and fruit and vegetable intakes during adolescence associated with cortical and trabecular bone structure, density and strength during adulthood, *Osteoporos Int* 28(2):609, 2017.
3. Food and Nutrition Board, Institute of Medicine: *Dietary Reference Intakes for calcium and vitamin D*, Washington, DC, 2011, National Academies Press.
4. Shams-White MM, Chung M, Du M, et al: Dietary protein and bone health: A systematic review and meta-analysis from the National Osteoporosis Foundation, *Am J Clin Nutr* 105(6):1528–1543, 2017. doi:10.3945/ajcn.116.145110.
5. Wright NC, Saag KG, Dawson-Hughes B, et al: The impact of the new National Bone Health Alliance (NBHA) diagnostic criteria on the prevalence of osteoporosis in the USA, *Osteoporos Int* 28(4):1225, 2017.
6. Thorning TK, Raben A, Tholstrup T, et al: Milk and dairy products: good or bad for human health? An assessment of the totality of scientific evidence, *Food Nutr Res* 60:32527, 2016. doi:10.3402/fnr.v60.32527.
7. Soares MJ, Murhadi LL, Kurpad AV, et al: Mechanistic roles for calcium and vitamin D in the regulation of body weight, *Obes Rev* 13:592, 2012.
8. Kim K, Yang YJ, Kim K, et al: Interactions of single nucleotide polymorphisms with dietary calcium intake on the risk of metabolic syndrome, *Am J Clin Nutr* 95:231, 2012.
9. Heaney RP: Phosphorus. In Erdman JW, MacDonald IA, Zeisel SH, editors: *Present knowledge in nutrition*, ed 10, Ames, IA, 2012, International Life Sciences Institute/Wiley-Blackwell.
10. Garber AK, Sawyer SM, Golden NH, et al: A systematic review of approaches to refeeding in patients with anorexia nervosa, *Int J Eat Disord* 49(3):293, 2016.
11. Food and Nutrition Board, Institute of Medicine: *Dietary Reference Intakes for water, potassium, sodium, chloride, and sulfate*, Washington, DC, 2004, National Academies Press.
12. US Department of Agriculture, Agricultural Research Service: Table 1. Nutrient Intakes from Food and Beverages. Mean Amounts Consumed per Individual by Gender and Age in the United States, 2013-2014. *What We Eat in America*, NHANES 2013-2014, 2016. https://www.ars.usda.gov/northeast-area/beltsville-md/beltsville-human-nutrition-research-center/food-surveys-research-group/docs/wweia-data-tables/.
13. Yang Q, Zhang Z, Kuklina EV, et al: Sodium intake and blood pressure among US children and adolescents, *Pediatrics* 130:611, 2012.
14. US Department of Health and Human Services, US Department of Agriculture: *Report of the Dietary Guidelines Advisory Committee on the Dietary Guidelines for Americans 2010*, Washington, DC, 2010, Center for Nutrition Policy and Promotion, US Department of Agriculture. https://www.cnpp.usda.gov/sites/default/files/dietary_guidelines_for_americans/2010DGACReport-camera-ready-Jan11-11.pdf.
15. Kalogeropoulos AP, Georgiopoulou VV, Murphy RA, et al: Dietary sodium content, mortality, and risk for cardiovascular events in older adults: the Health, Aging, and Body Composition (Health ABC) Study, *JAMA Intern Med* 175(3):410, 2015.
16. Strom BL, Anderson CAM, Joachim HI: Sodium reduction in populations. Insights from the Institute of Medicine Committee, *JAMA* 310(1):31, 2015.
17. Alderman MH: Dietary sodium: Where science and policy diverge, *Am J Hypertens* 29(4):424, 2016.
18. Pilic L, Pedlar CR, Mavrommatis Y: Salt-sensitive hypertension: Mechanisms and effects of dietary and other lifestyle factors, *Nutr Rev* 74(10):645, 2016.
19. Sebastian RS, Enns CW, Steinfeldt LC, et al: *Discontinuation of Data Processing Step: Salt Adjustment on Designated Foods Likely To Be Home Prepared*. In What We Eat in America, 2012, NHANES, US Department of Agriculture, Agricultural Research Service. https://www.ars.usda.gov/ARSUserFiles/80400530/pdf/0910/discontinuation%20of%20data%20processig%20step-salt%20adjustment.pdf.
20. Chiu S, Bergeron N, Williams PT, et al: Comparison of the DASH (Dietary Approaches to Stop Hypertension) diet and a higher-fat DASH diet on blood pressure and lipids and lipoproteins: a randomized controlled trial, *Am J Clin Nutr* 103(2):341, 2016.
21. Drewnowski A, Maillot M, Rehm C: Reducing the sodium-potassium ratio in the US diet: a challenge for public health, *Am J Clin Nutr* 96:439, 2012.
22. Nielsen FH: Effects of magnesium depletion on inflammation in chronic disease, *Curr Opin Clin Nutr Metab Care* 17(6):525, 2014.
23. Rosanoff A, Weaver CM, Rude RK: Suboptimal magnesium status in the United States: are the health consequences underestimated? *Nutr Rev* 70(3):153, 2012.

24. Joneja JV: *Celiac disease. (Gluten sensitive enteropathy). The health professional's guide to food allergies and intolerances,* Chicago, 2013, Academy of Nutrition and Dietetics.

25. Institute of Medicine, Otten JJ, Hellwig JP, Meyers LD, editors: *Dietary Reference Intakes (DRI). The essential guide to nutrient requirements,* Washington, DC, 2006, National Academies Press.

26. Food and Nutrition Board, Institute of Medicine: *Dietary Reference Intakes for vitamin A, vitamin K, arsenic, boron, chromium, copper, iodine, iron, manganese, molybdenum, nickel, silicon, vanadium, and zinc,* Washington, DC, 2001, National Academies Press.

27. Armah SM, Carriquiry AL, Reddy MB: Total iron bioavailability from the US diet is lower than the current estimate, *J Nutr* 145(11):2617, 2015.

28. Collings R, Harvey LJ, Hooper L, et al: The absorption of iron from whole diets: a systematic review, *Am J Clin Nutr* 98(1):65, 2013.

29. Hurrell R, Egli I: Iron bioavailability and dietary reference values, *Am J Clin Nutr* 91(Suppl 5):S1461, 2010.

30. Ruz M, Carrasco F, Rojas P, et al: Heme- and nonheme-iron absorption and iron status 12 mo after sleeve gastrectomy and Roux-en-Y gastric bypass in morbidly obese women, *Am J Clin Nutr* 96:810, 2012.

31. Gaitán D, Flores S, Saavedra P, et al: Calcium does not inhibit the absorption of 5 milligrams of nonheme or heme iron at doses less than 800 milligrams in nonpregnant women, *J Nutr* 141:1652, 2011.

32. Lam LF, Lawlis TR: Feeding the brain—The effects of micronutrient interventions on cognitive performance among school-aged children: A systematic review of randomized controlled trials, *Clin Nutr* 36(4):1007, 2017.

33. Tussing-Humphreys L, Pusatcioglu C, Nemeth E, et al: Rethinking iron regulation and assessment in iron deficiency, anemia of chronic disease, and obesity: introducing hepcidin, *J Acad Nutr Diet* 112:391, 2012.

34. Rautiainen S, Manson JE, Lichtenstein AH, et al: Dietary supplements and disease prevention—a global overview, *Nat Rev Endocrinol* 12(7):407, 2016.

35. Powell LW, Seckington RC, Deugnier Y: Haemochromatosis, *Lancet* 388(10045):706, 2016.

36. Zhao Z, Li S, Liu G, et al: Body iron stores and heme-iron intake in relation to risk of type 2 diabetes: a systematic review and meta-analysis, *PLoS One* 7(7):e41641, 2012.

37. Aburto N, Abudou M, Candeias V, et al: *Effect and safety of salt iodization to prevent iodine deficiency disorders: a systematic review with meta-analyses.* WHO eLibrary of Evidence for Nutrition Actions (eLENA), Geneva, 2014, World Health Organization.

38. Zimmerman MB, Andersson M: Assessment of iodine nutrition in populations: past, present, and future, *Nutr Rev* 70(10):553, 2012.

39. Terrin G, Berni Canani R, Di Chiara M, et al: Zinc in early life: A key element in the fetus and preterm neonate, *Nutrients* 7(12):10427, 2015.

40. Sandstead HH: Subclinical zinc deficiency impairs human brain function, *J Trace Elem Med Biol* 26(2–3):70, 2012.

41. Finch CW: Review of trace mineral requirements for preterm infants: what are the current recommendations for clinical practice, *Nutr Clin Pract* 30(1):44, 2015.

42. Food and Nutrition Board, Institute of Medicine: *Dietary Reference Intakes for vitamin C, vitamin E, selenium, and carotenoids,* Washington, DC, 2000, National Academies Press.

43. Palmer CA, Gilbert JA, Academy of Nutrition and Dietetics: Position of the Academy of Nutrition and Dietetics: the impact of fluoride on health, *J Acad Nutr Diet* 112(9):1443, 2012.

44. Drewnowski A, Rehm CD, Constant F: Water and beverage consumption among adults in the United States: cross-sectional study using data from NHANES 2005-2010, *BMC Public Health* 13:1068, 2013.

45. Popkin BM, D'Anci KE, Rosenberg IH: Water, hydration, and health, *Nutr Rev* 68(8):439, 2010.

46. Tate DF, Turner-McGrievy G, Lyons E, et al: Replacing caloric beverages with water or diet beverages for weight loss in adults: main results of the Choose Healthy Options Consciously Everyday (CHOICE) randomized clinical trial, *Am J Clin Nutr* 95:555, 2012.

47. Rosinger AY, Lawman HG, Akinbami LJ, et al: The role of obesity in the relation between total water intake and urine osmolality in US adults, 2009-2012, *Am J Clin Nutr* 104(6):1554, 2016.

FURTHER READINGS AND RESOURCES

Readings

Academy of Nutrition and Dietetics: Position of the Academy of Nutrition and Dietetics: the impact of fluoride on health, *J Acad Nutr Diet* 112:1443, 2012.

[Fluoridation of water is one of the top 10 public health initiatives for this century; this article helps us understand the need for fluoride.]

Kopecky SL, Bauer DC, Gulati M, et al: Lack of evidence linking calcium with or without vitamin D supplementation to cardiovascular disease in generally healthy adults: A clinical guideline from the National Osteoporosis Foundation and the American Society for Preventive Cardiology, *Ann Intern Med* 165:867, 2016.

[These authors help us understand the controversy about calcium supplements and risk of cardiovascular disease.

Hooper L: Why, oh why, are so many older adults not drinking enough fluid? *J Acad Nutr Diet* 116(5):774, 2016.

[This article helps us understand the problem of dehydration in community-living older adults and those in long-term care.]

Centers for Disease Control and Prevention: Vital signs: food categories contributing the most to sodium consumption—United States, 2007-2008, *MMWR* 61(5):92, 2012.

Kolasa KM, Sollid K, Edge MS, et al: Blood pressure management: communicating comprehensive lifestyle strategies beyond sodium, *Nutr Today* 47(4):183, 2012.

[Dr. Kolasa and her colleagues provide us with an intervention strategy for high blood pressure that goes beyond sodium intake but note the MMWR report listing the major contributors to dietary sodium.]

Websites of Interest

Several government sites provide comprehensive information on dietary supplements, what they are or what they contain, guidelines for their use, and their interactions with prescription and over-the-counter medications:

• National Institutes of Health, National Library of Medicine: *Medline Plus, Trusted Health Information for You: Dietary Supplements.* https://www.nlm.nih.gov/medlineplus/dietarysupplements.html; and National Institutes of Health, Office of Dietary Supplements: https://www.ods.od.nih.gov.

• US Food and Drug Administration, Center for Food Safety and Applied Nutrition, Office of Nutritional Products, Labeling, and Dietary Supplements: http://www.fda.gov/food/DietarySupplements/default.htm.

The following sites discuss the role of particular minerals in the prevention of chronic diseases and dietary sources.

• National Institutes of Health: This site provides information on calcium and bone health. http://www.nlm.nih.gov/medlineplus/calcium.html.

• National Institutes of Health: This site provides information on sodium and blood pressure. http://www.nlm.nih.gov/medlineplus/dietarysodium.html.

• US Department of Agriculture. *MyPlate.* This website describes daily food plans and healthy food choices supplying adequate minerals for all age groups. https://www.choosemyplate.gov.

8

Energy Balance

Eleanor D. Schlenker

ⓔ http://evolve.elsevier.com/Williams/essentials/

Thus far we have reviewed the three energy-yielding nutrients (carbohydrate, fat, and protein); the micronutrients (vitamins and minerals) that catalyze the chemical reactions converting food to energy; and water, the medium in which all of these processes occur. Here we look at the relationship between energy intake and energy expenditure and their combined effect on body composition and body weight. A sedentary lifestyle coupled with an abundance of food puts both young people and adults at risk for unwanted weight gain. At the other extreme, an obsession with thinness or food scarcity leads to life-threatening malnutrition. Energy balance is not a simple matter. Energy needs vary under different circumstances and for different body types. Each of us is unique, and our varying body weights and propensity to gain or lose weight reflect this. In this chapter we look at the dynamics of energy metabolism and how these principles apply to a healthy weight.

OUTLINE

THE HUMAN ENERGY SYSTEM

Energy Cycles and Energy Transformation

Forms of Human Energy

In the physical world, energy, like matter, is neither created nor destroyed. When we speak of energy being produced, what we really mean is energy being transformed. Energy constantly changes form as it moves through various systems. In the human body, metabolic reactions convert the stored chemical energy in food to other forms of energy that carry out body work. The ultimate source of energy is the sun, with its vast reservoir of heat and light (Fig. 8.1). By the process of photosynthesis (review Fig. 3.1), plants use water and carbon dioxide (CO_2) to transform the sun's energy into carbohydrate, a storage form of chemical energy. The body converts carbohydrate to glucose, which together with fatty acids is metabolized to release energy and support life. The end products of body energy metabolism are water and CO_2. These end products then become available to plants to produce more carbohydrate for human use.

KEY TERM

Energy
The capacity of a system for doing work, which is manifest in various forms—motion, position, light, heat, and sound. Energy is interchangeable among these various forms and is constantly being transformed and transferred among them.

Transformation of Energy

When food with its stored chemical energy is taken into the body, it undergoes many changes that convert it to different storage forms of chemical energy. This chemical energy is then changed further as work is performed. Our bodies use four forms of energy: (1) chemical, (2) electrical, (3) mechanical, and (4) thermal. In the brain, chemical energy is changed to electrical energy for transmitting nerve impulses and carrying out brain activities. Chemical energy is changed to mechanical energy when muscles contract; it is changed to thermal energy in the regulation of body temperature. Chemical energy is needed to form new tissues and molecules for growth and metabolism. Throughout all of this work, heat is given off to the surrounding atmosphere and larger biosphere.

In the human body, energy is present as either *free energy* or *potential energy*. Free energy is the energy being used at any given moment in the performance of a task. It is unbound and in motion. Potential energy is energy that is stored or bound in a chemical compound and converted to free energy when needed. For example, the energy stored in carbohydrate is potential energy. When we eat carbohydrate and it is metabolized, energy is released for body work. As work is completed, this energy, now in the form of heat or thermal energy, is given off into the air. Measurement of the amount of heat produced over time makes it possible for us to express body energy consumption in kilocalories (kcalories or kcal) or units of heat.

FIG. 8.1 Transformation of energy from its primary source (the sun) to the forms needed for biologic work.

Energy Balance: Input and Output

A constant supply of energy is needed to sustain the activities essential to life. Energy is required to support internal needs along with the added expectations of physical activity. Whether the energy used is electrical, mechanical, thermal, or chemical, the supply of free energy and the reservoir of potential energy decrease as the metabolic and physical work of the body continues. Therefore the system must be constantly refueled from an outside source. For the human energy system, this outside source of fuel is food.

Energy Control in Human Metabolism

If the energy produced in the body through its many chemical reactions was "exploded" all at once, it would damage tissues and systems; therefore mechanisms are needed by which energy release can be controlled to support life, not destroy it. Two means of control make this possible: (1) **chemical bonding** and (2) controlled rates of reaction.

Chemical Bonding

The primary mechanism controlling energy release in the human system is chemical bonding. The chemical bonds that hold elements together in compounds are energy bonds. As long as the compound stays intact, energy is being exerted to maintain it. When the compound is broken into its parts, this energy is released and becomes available for work.

The following three types of chemical bonds transfer energy:

1. *Covalent bonds:* These bonds are based on the relative combining power of the elements that make up a compound. The carbon atoms in organic compounds such as glucose are held together by covalent bonds.

2. *Hydrogen bonds:* Although weaker than covalent bonds, hydrogen bonds are significant because there are so many of them. In addition, the very fact that they are less strong and more easily broken allows them to transfer energy readily from one substance to another. The hydrogen attached to the oxygen molecule in the carboxyl group (COOH) of amino acids and fatty acids is an example of this type of bond.

3. *High-energy phosphate bonds:* The high-energy phosphate bonds in the compound **adenosine triphosphate (ATP)** are the major energy source for carrying out body functions. Working like storage batteries for electrical energy, these bonds are the controlling force of energy metabolism in the human cell.

Controlled Reaction Rates

The chemical reactions making up the body's energy system must have controls to manage the speed at which they occur. For example, some reactions that break down protein, if left alone, occur very slowly. If such reactions were not accelerated by **catalysts**, then getting needed energy from the food in a meal could take years. At the same time, chemical reactions must be prevented from occurring too fast, which would release destructive bursts of energy. **Enzymes, coenzymes,** and hormones regulate energy reactions as follows:

- *Enzymes:* Enzymes are proteins produced in the cell under the direction of individual genes. One gene controls the making of one enzyme, and thousands of enzymes exist in every cell. Each enzyme acts on one particular substance, called its **substrate.** The enzyme and its substrate lock together to produce a new reaction product; however, the enzyme itself remains unchanged, ready to do its work over and over again (Fig. 8.2). Enzymes often act as catalysts.

- *Coenzymes and cofactors:* Many enzymes require partners to assist in completing their work. These coenzyme partners are often vitamins, especially B-complex vitamins. Various minerals also participate in enzyme reactions and in this role are referred to as cofactors. It may

FIG. 8.2 Lock-and-key concept. An enzyme, coenzyme or cofactor, and substrate work together to produce a new substance. Notice that the enzyme is unchanged in the process. *ECS,* Enzyme-coenzyme-substrate.

be helpful to think of coenzymes and cofactors as another substrate, because in receiving the material being transferred they are changed or reduced.

- *Hormones:* In energy metabolism hormones act as messengers to trigger or control enzyme action. The rate of oxidation reactions in the tissues—the body's metabolic rate—is controlled by thyroxine (T_4) from the thyroid gland. Another example is the controlling action of insulin on glucose utilization in the cells.

Types of Metabolic Reactions

Two types of reactions occur in the body: (1) anabolic and (2) catabolic. Each requires energy. The process of anabolism synthesizes new and more complex substances, as in body growth and repair. The process of catabolism breaks down complex substances to more simple ones, as when worn-out proteins are broken down and their released amino acids are used to make new proteins. Both activities release free energy, but the work performed also uses up some free energy. This creates a constant energy deficit that must be met by food.

Sources of Stored Energy

When a person is not taking in food, as in fasting or starvation, the body must draw on its own stores for energy. Sources of stored energy can meet short-term or long-term needs, as described here:

- *Glycogen:* Only a 12- to 36-hour reserve of glycogen exists in liver and muscle; it is quickly depleted.
- *Muscle mass:* Energy stores in the form of muscle protein exist in limited amounts but in greater volume than glycogen stores. Although the body tries to limit the breakdown of protein for energy, the need for glucose to fuel the central nervous system (CNS) results in loss of body protein when the intake of energy and carbohydrate is inadequate. (Review our discussion of deamination of amino acids for glucose production in Chapter 5.) Loss of body protein occurs in rapid weight loss and in body wasting or cachexia. It is a cause for concern and requires prompt intervention.
- *Adipose (fat) tissue:* Although fat stores are generally the largest reserve of stored energy, the supply varies from person to person.

Measurement of Energy Balance
Kilocalorie

Because the release of energy and work performed by the body produces heat, energy expenditure can be measured in heat equivalents. This measure of heat is the calorie. To avoid having to calculate very large numbers, health professionals use the kilocalorie (kcalorie or kcal) to describe energy needs. The kcalorie is equal to 1000 calories; this is the amount of heat required to raise 1 kg of water by 1°C. (Materials prepared for the general public use the term *calorie,* although the actual measurement is the kcalorie.)

Joule

According to the *Système International d'Unités* (SI), the international unit of energy measurement is the joule. It equals the amount of energy expended when 1 kg of a substance is moved 1 m by a force of 1 newton (N). The conversion factor for changing kcalories to kilojoules (kJ) is 4.184 (1 kcal = 4.184 kJ). Some nutrition research

TABLE 8.1   Fuel Factors

Energy Source	kcal/g
Carbohydrate	4
Protein	4
Fat	9
Alcohol	7

journals use kilojoules rather than kcalories to describe energy intake; in clinical practice we use kcalories.

Food Energy Measurement

When helping people develop a food pattern appropriate to their energy needs, it is necessary to know the energy content of each food. There are two methods for determining the energy content of foods: (1) direct calorimetry and (2) calculation of approximate composition.

Calorimetry

The kcalorie values of foods given in food tables were determined by *direct calorimetry*. This method uses a metal container called a *bomb calorimeter*, named for its long tubular shape. A weighed amount of food is placed inside and the bomb calorimeter is then immersed in water. The food is then ignited by an electric spark in the presence of oxygen and burned to ash. The increase in the temperature of the surrounding water indicates the number of kcalories given off by the complete oxidation of the food sample. When you use food tables, remember that these values represent averages from a number of samples of the given food; thus the kcalorie value of a particular serving will vary around that average.

Approximate Composition

An alternative method of estimating the energy value of a food is by calculating the kcalories contributed by the carbohydrate, fat, and protein content as listed in food tables. These calculations are based on the kcalorie value per gram of each of the energy-yielding macronutrients, values known as their fuel factors (Table 8.1). Note that 1 g of fat contains more than twice the number of kcalories as 1 g of carbohydrate or protein. The fuel factor for alcohol (7 kcal/g) falls midway between fat and that of carbohydrate and protein. Using the method of approximate composition, a food containing 12 g of carbohydrate, 8 g of protein, and 5 g of fat would contain 125 kcal.

Calculation:
Carbohydrate: 12 g × 4 kcal/g = 48 kcal
Protein: 8 g × 4 kcal/g = 32 kcal
Fat: 5 g × 9 kcal/g = 45 kcal
Total: 48 + 32 + 45 kcal = 125 kcal

Did you recognize this food as a 1-cup serving of reduced-fat (2%) milk?

TOTAL DAILY ENERGY EXPENDITURE

The total energy expended by an individual stems from three energy needs: (1) basal metabolism, (2) food intake effect, and (3) physical activity. Physical size and body composition, as well as level of physical activity, influence the energy needs of a given individual.

Basal Metabolic Needs

Basal Metabolic Rate

The basal metabolic rate (BMR) is a measure of the energy required to maintain the body at rest. This is the sum of all chemical activities

going on in the body plus the energy needed to fuel the brain, heart, lungs, kidneys, and other organs that must continue to work even when the body rests. Certain small but active tissues—such as the brain, liver, heart, and kidneys—contribute disproportionately to basal needs. For most people, the BMR accounts for 60% to 70% of the total daily energy expenditure.[1] As described in Box 8.1, the feeding status of the patient and the test environment influence the BMR. Consequently the BMR is less common as a clinical measure because of the preparation and details required to determine it. Instead, the resting metabolic rate (RMR) is more generally used because it does not require fasting prior to the test. Recognize, however, that the RMR may be as much as 10% to 20% higher than the BMR because of energy being expended in the processing of food or the delayed effect of recent physical activity.[2]

Measuring Basal Metabolic Rate

The BMR can be measured by direct or indirect methods of calorimetry, as follows:

- *Direct calorimetry:* Using the direct method, a person is placed in an enclosed chamber that has the capacity to measure body heat production while the person is at rest. This instrument is large and costly and usually found only in research facilities.
- *Indirect calorimetry:* Using the indirect method, a portable instrument called a *respirometer* is brought to the side of the bed or chair. This complete apparatus is often referred to as the *metabolic cart*. As the person breathes through a mouthpiece or ventilated hood, the exchange of gases in respiration, called the *respiratory quotient* (CO_2/O_2), is measured. Because more than 95% of the body's energy comes from oxygen-related reactions,[3] the BMR can be calculated from the amount of oxygen consumed in a given period and the CO_2 exhaled. The amount of oxygen used equals the amount of heat released. These numbers can be converted to kcalories using standardized equations.
- *Indirect laboratory tests:* The BMR is regulated by the thyroid hormone T_4; thus thyroid function tests can provide indirect measures of BMR and thyroid activity. These tests include measurements of serum thyroid-stimulating hormone (TSH) from the anterior pituitary gland as well as triiodothyronine (T_3) and T_4. Thyroid hormone levels within the normal range indicate that cell metabolism is occurring at normal rates but cannot be used to calculate BMR.

Factors Influencing Basal Metabolic Rate

Individual characteristics—including gender, body size and composition, genetic makeup, and disease state—influence the BMR of an individual, explained as follows:

- *Body size and body composition:* LBM is the body compartment made up of muscle and vital organs. It is the major factor influencing BMR because of the high metabolic activity of these tissues compared with the less active tissues of fat and bone. Differences in basal energy requirements between men and women of the same

BOX 8.1   Required Conditions for Measuring Basal Metabolic Rate

- Overnight fast (no food for 12–14 h)
- Comfortably resting in a supine position
- Relaxed state (no activity up to 1 h prior)
- Awake but motionless
- Normal body temperature
- Comfortable room temperature (neither hot nor cold)

height and body weight relate to their differences in body composition. Compared with men, women have less muscle and more fat, resulting in a lower BMR. As humans age, the loss of muscle tissue, and to a lesser extent organ tissue, lowers their BMR.

- *Growth:* The increased anabolic work supported by growth hormone adds to the BMR in childhood, adolescence, pregnancy, and lactation.
- *Fever:* With fever, the BMR increases 7% for each 1°F (0.83°C) rise in body temperature.
- *Disease:* Determination of energy expenditure is clinically important in patient care, as disease state can influence energy needs. Diseases that increase cell activity—such as cancer, cardiac failure, and chronic obstructive pulmonary disease—increase BMR and result in loss of body weight and muscle if kcalories are not sufficient to meet body needs.[4] Renal disease and sepsis increase the

metabolic work of the body and raise the BMR. The involuntary muscle tremors of Parkinson disease also increase energy needs.[4] Older adults with pressure ulcers often have increased basal requirements,[5] and untreated human immunodeficiency virus (HIV) infection can raise resting energy expenditure (REE) by 10% or as much as 50% in the presence of opportunistic infections.[6] Inappropriately low energy intake, falling below true energy needs, contributes to growth failure in children with cystic fibrosis.[7] In starvation and protein-energy malnutrition, BMR falls as cell metabolism slows in response to the drop in energy intake and loss of metabolically active tissue.

- *Climate:* BMR rises in response to lower environmental temperatures as the body takes action to increase heat production and minimize heat loss. Opposite reactions that reduce heat production and increase heat loss in a hot environment also raise the BMR. Unless weather conditions are extreme, these changes in BMR are temporary while the individual adapts to the new environmental temperature.
- *Genetics:* Race and ethnicity influence BMR. African American women have a lower RMR per unit of LBM than do Caucasian women, which may make it more difficult for them to lose weight.[8] Energy prediction equations developed with Caucasian youth do not accurately predict REE in obese Hispanic youth.[9] Studies of the human genome indicate that intrafamily differences in RMR may contribute to higher weight gain and the development of metabolic syndrome among particular groups.[10]
- *Age:* Loss of LBM, particularly muscle, results in a drop in REE in frail older adults.[2]

Food Intake Effect (Thermic Effect of Food)

Taking in food stimulates body metabolism as energy is needed to digest, absorb, metabolize, and store nutrients. The amount of kcalories needed to perform these tasks is called the thermic effect of food (TEF). On average, about 10% of the kcalories in a meal or snack are used to process and metabolize that food, although this varies depending on the meal composition. Macronutrients differ in their TEFs. The TEF for fat is 0% to 3%, because fatty acids are easily burned for energy or stored in the form in which they enter the body; therefore few kcalories are needed for processing or storage. For carbohydrate the TEF is 5% to 10% of its kcalories; for protein the TEF is 20% to 30% of its kcalories. The TEF for alcohol is 10% to 30%.[11]

The energy required to metabolize amino acids and synthesize new proteins raises the TEF of this macronutrient, and the TEF effect is especially pronounced with high-quality protein.[11] Removal of the amino group from surplus amino acids, enabling their use as an energy source, is an energy-intensive process and reduces the kcalories available for future use. These factors contribute to the value of a high-protein diet for weight loss or weight management. The very low TEF of fat, along with its high fuel factor (9 kcal/g), can accelerate weight gain on a high-fat diet.

Physical Activity Needs

Physical activity related to employment, personal care, housekeeping, recreation, organized sports, or fitness training produces wide variations

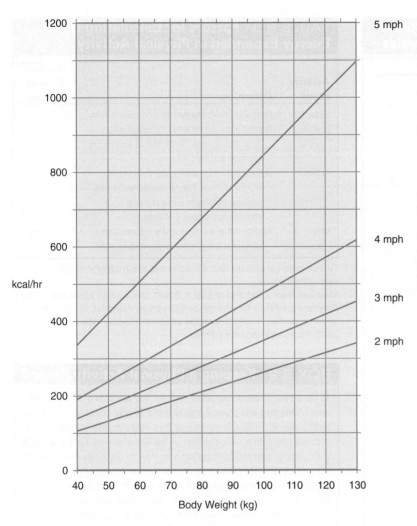

FIG. 8.3 Effect of body weight on the energy required to walk at different speeds. Both body weight and walking speed influence the kcalories burned. Persons with a higher body weight use more kcalories in weight-bearing activities than persons with a lower body weight; the faster they walk, the more kcalories they will use. (Redrawn with permission from Food and Nutrition Board, Institute of Medicine: *Dietary reference intakes for energy, carbohydrate, fiber, fat, fatty acids, cholesterol, protein, and amino acids (macronutrients)*, Washington, DC, 2005, National Academies Press.)

in energy requirements. For sedentary individuals, the kcalories expended in physical activity may be only 15% to 20% of their total energy expenditure, as compared with very active persons whose physical activity kcalories may be 50% to 60% of their total.[1] For weight-bearing activities, energy expenditure is proportional to body weight; accordingly, such an activity will require more kcalories for an individual with a higher body weight and fewer kcalories for one with a lower body weight (Fig. 8.3).[2] Thus an obese child or adult can have the same energy expenditure in physical activity as their nonobese counterparts despite less body movement, based on their higher body weight. Table 8.2 describes the energy cost of common activities per pound of body weight.

The speed at which a person moves also influences the number of kcalories expended. Walking at a speed of 4 mph requires more kcalories than walking at 2 mph, regardless of body weight (see Fig. 8.3).[2] Jogging or running at 5 mph requires more than twice the energy than walking at 3.5 mph (see Table 8.2). The energy cost of movement is also influenced by age-related changes in muscle mass and innervation of muscle cells. Fitness training can benefit older adults and increase their ability to live independently by lowering the energy cost of walking. Such a program enabled older adults over the period of a year to decrease their cost of walking by 5%, while a group of nonparticipants of similar age increased their cost by 5%.[12] The generally slower gait of older individuals may be a compensatory response to offset the greater energy cost of walking brought about by aging and chronic conditions.[13]

Estimating Energy Requirements

Estimating the total energy requirement of a given individual is difficult. An expert panel has defined the estimated energy requirement (EER) as the energy intake that will maintain energy balance in a healthy adult of a certain age, gender, weight, height, and level of physical activity[2] and developed some numerical equivalents to assist in such calculations. Typical ranges for RMR are 0.8 to 1.0 kcal/min for women and 1.1 to 1.3 kcal/min for men (1 kcal/min is about equal to the heat released by a burning candle or 75-watt bulb over the course of a minute).[2] Differences in body dimensions and the proportion of body fat versus muscle influence the RMR and thus the total energy requirement. Individuals with a greater amount of body fat and a lesser proportion of muscle will likely need fewer kcalories.

Your energy expenditure in physical activity can be calculated using a factor that estimates your activity level. Nutrition experts have defined several levels of physical activity and developed factors that estimate the kcalories required (Table 8.3).[2] Consider these definitions and the time span and intensity of activity required. If your only physical activity for the day is the casual walking and routine tasks we all perform as part of our daily living, then your pattern is sedentary. Additional activity in the form of walking at a brisk pace, running, dancing, sports, or use of fitness equipment is needed for the higher categories of activity. Estimate your personal activity level by keeping a daily record; you may be less active than you think you are (Box 8.2).

TABLE 8.2 Energy Expenditure per Pound Body Weight per Hour for Various Activities

Activity	kcal/lb/h[a]
Daily Activities	
Cleaning	1.36
Cooking	0.91
Driving a car	0.91
Gardening	1.81
Reading or writing while sitting	0.70
Sleeping	0.41
Shoveling snow	2.72
Walking	
Moderate: 3 mph (20 min/mile), level	1.50
Moderate: 3 mph (20 min/mile), uphill	2.73
Brisk: 3.5 mph (17 min/mile), level	1.72
Fast: 4.5 mph (13 min/mile), level	2.86
Running	
5 mph (12 min/mile)	3.63
7 mph (8.5 min/mile)	5.22
9 mph (6.5 min/mile)	6.80
Bicycling	
Light (10–11.9 mph)	2.72
Moderate (12–13.9 mph)	3.63
Fast (14–15.9 mph)	4.54
Sports	
Field hockey	3.63
Golf	2.04
Rollerblading	4.42
Soccer	3.85
Swimming, moderate	3.14
Ultimate Frisbee	3.63
Volleyball	1.81
Weight Training	
Light or moderate	1.36
Heavy or vigorous	2.72

[a]Multiply activity factor by weight in pounds by fraction of hour performing activity. Example: a 150-lb person plays soccer for 45 minutes, as follows: 3.85 (factor) × 150 (lb) × 0.75 (hour) = 433 kcalories burned.
Energy expenditure also varies depending on an individual's physical fitness and continuity of exercise.
Data from Nieman DC: *Exercise testing and prescription: a health-related approach*, ed 5, New York, 2003, McGraw-Hill; and Nix S: *Williams' basic nutrition and diet therapy*, ed 13, St Louis, 2009, Mosby-Elsevier.

TABLE 8.3 Factors for Calculating Daily Energy Expended in Physical Activity

Activity Level	Definition	Physical Activity Factor[a]
Sedentary	Normal activities required for independent living	0.2
Low active	Normal activities required for independent living plus at least 30–60 min of moderately intensive activity	0.5
Active	Normal activities required for independent living plus *more* than 60 min of moderately intensive activity or a mix of moderately intensive and vigorous activity	0.7
Very active	Normal activities required for independent living plus 2 h or more of vigorous activity	1.2

[a]These physical activity factors represent the midpoint of the range for each activity level.
Modified from Food and Nutrition Board, Institute of Medicine: *Dietary Reference Intakes for energy, carbohydrate, fiber, fat, fatty acids, cholesterol, protein, and amino acids (macronutrients)*, Washington, DC, 2002, National Academies Press.

BOX 8.2 Keeping a Physical Activity Record

To get a true picture of your activity pattern, you can keep a physical activity record. Recording your physical activity over a 24-hour period is much like recording your food intake. Prepare a chart that allows you to record the time you start and stop each activity and describe the type of activity. Carry a notebook with you and make entries immediately as changes occur. Review the activity expenditure database prior to use, so you are sure to include the appropriate amount of detail when keeping your record. Refer to Table 8.2 for a listing of day to day activities. Using the energy expenditures assigned to your body weight in pounds, calculate your total energy expenditure over a 24-hour period. Keep in mind that databases providing kcalories per activity also account for resting metabolic rate (RMR) per pound of body weight per unit of time; thus you need sum only the time-corrected values to estimate your total energy expenditure for the day. If you are trying to increase your physical activity, keeping a log for several days will help you to identify times through the day or week when you might add or increase an activity. Keeping a record may also alert you to the fact that you need to increase your physical activity.

TABLE 8.4 Estimated Energy Requirements Based on Activity Level and Age

Activity Level	MALE (178 lb, 71 in) (kcalories)[a]		FEMALE (132 lb, 61 in) (kcalories)[a]	
	Age 25	Age 65	Age 25	Age 65
Sedentary	2685	2285	1869	1589
Low active	2934	2534	2072	1792
Active	3250	2850	2325	2045
Very active	3770	3370	2628	2348

[a]An individual of this height and weight has a body mass index (BMI) of approximately 25 kg/m[2], the boundary between normal weight and overweight.
Calculations based on data presented in Food and Nutrition Board, Institute of Medicine: *Dietary Reference Intakes for energy, carbohydrate, fiber, fat, fatty acids, cholesterol, protein, and amino acids (macronutrients)*. Washington, DC, 2002, National Academies Press.

Age influences the RMR and EER. As we age, we lose muscle and organ weight, tissues with high metabolic activity, and gain fat, tissue with low metabolic activity. Table 8.4 illustrates the effect of gender, age, and physical activity on the EER. Within genders individuals are shown to have the same body weight, although the older adults will likely have experienced changes in body composition. Note the significant differences in energy expenditure between sedentary and active adults.

Energy requirements rise during pregnancy, lactation, and other periods of rapid growth and elevated metabolism. (In Chapter 16 we estimate energy requirements using specific equations developed for clinical use that adjust for height, weight, and age.)

New Research Exploring Total Energy Expenditure

As the prevalence of overweight grows worldwide, medical scientists are exploring physiologic and metabolic factors that might influence energy intake and energy expenditure. New areas of research with potential for future intervention include the following:

- *Action of intestinal microflora:* When bacterial fermentation leads to excessive production of fatty acids, the surplus is absorbed into the body, adding to energy intake. Moreover, certain species have an extreme ability to harvest indigestible polysaccharides, thereby increasing carbohydrate absorption. Overweight individuals have been found to have a different profile of intestinal microflora than individuals of normal weight.[14]
- *Brown fat thermogenesis:* Brown fat is a special adipose tissue capable of high-energy metabolism given off as heat. Infants have plentiful amounts of brown fat to assist in their response to cold as they move from the warmth of the womb to the ambient temperature surrounding them. Brown fat is lost as individuals move through childhood and adolescence, although adults retain small amounts. Brown fat affects long-term energy balance by raising the BMR.[15] Capsaicin, a compound found in hot peppers, activates brown fat thermogenesis in some individuals.[16]
- *Sleep deprivation:* It is estimated that 30% of Americans get 6 or fewer hours of sleep per night. Too little sleep influences energy intake and expenditure in several ways: (1) sleep-deprived individuals often experience increases in appetite and crave snack foods high in carbohydrate and fat; (2) lack of sleep reduces one's energy level, so that active pursuits are more likely to be avoided; and (3) hormonal changes set up metabolic patterns that contribute to body weight gain.[17] Night-shift or rotating work shifts can disrupt body metabolism and promote unwanted weight gain. Increasing the hours of sleep may help maintain a healthy weight.

BODY COMPOSITION: FATNESS AND LEANNESS

A person's body composition reflects a lifetime of food intake and energy expenditure. Individuals have different body shapes and sizes depending on their age, gender, genes, body type, and state of health. Ectomorphs have a body type that is generally slender and fragile; mesomorphs have prominent muscle and bone development; and endomorphs have a soft, round physique with some accumulation of body fat (Fig. 8.4). Although each body type has a genetic base, dietary intake and physical activity influence how it is expressed. Some body types are associated with better health, whereas others carry an increased risk of chronic disease. We need to be sensitive to different body types in developing strategies to improve body composition and health.

Body Weight and Body Fat
Overweight Versus Overfat

Because height and weight are easily measured, they are commonly used to assess health status. It is important to know what these measurements do and do not tell us. The terms *overweight* and **obesity** have different meanings as related to body composition, and these distinctions have implications for health. A football player in peak physical condition can be markedly "overweight" according to standard height-weight charts. That is, the player weighs more than the average person of similar height, but that player's body tissues are likely to be very different. A sedentary man above average weight likely has an excess amount of body fat that is adding to his total body weight; an athlete above average weight likely has an exceptionally large amount of muscle. In fact, the overweight athlete may have an even lower proportion of body fat than another individual of average weight. When overweight is the result of excessive body fat rather than enhanced muscle

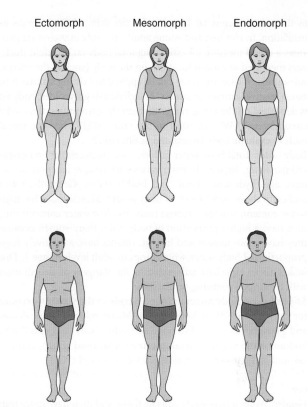

FIG. 8.4 Body types: the ectomorph, the mesomorph, and the endomorph.

or skeletal tissue, *overfat* or *obese* is the appropriate term. The critical element when evaluating body build and health is body composition. What we really need to know is how much of a person's body weight is fat and how much is fat-free mass (FFM). It is more precise to think in terms of *fatness* and *leanness* rather than body weight or overweight.

Body Compartments

Body compartments are defined according to their comparative size and metabolic activity. The relative amounts of specific body tissues sometimes overlap among compartments. The four-compartment model for evaluating body composition includes LBM, body fat, body water, and mineral mass, as follows:

1. *LBM:* This compartment is made up of active cells from muscle and vital organs and largely determines the BMR and related nutrient needs. LBM includes not only cell protein but also a large amount of water (intracellular water) because muscle cells are about 65% water. This compartment also contains very small amounts of fatty acids found in the membranes of muscle and organ cells. In comparison, the term FFM includes cell protein, all body water both inside and outside of cells, and bone mineral mass—all body tissues except for fat. LBM changes in size across the life cycle, with steady growth through childhood and young adulthood and gradual loss in later years. In adults it makes up 30% to 65% of total body weight. Most weight reduction regimens result in a loss of both body fat and LBM.

2. *Body fat:* Total body fat reflects both the number and size of the fat cells (**adipocytes**) that form the adipose tissue. Most adipocytes are white fat cells; rather few are the brown fat cells we referred to earlier. In a man of normal weight, fat comprises 13% to 21% of body weight. In a woman of normal weight, the range of body fat content is 23% to 31%. These amounts vary with age, body type, exercise, and fitness, and many people have body fat levels markedly greater than or less than these ranges. About one half of all body fat is found

in the subcutaneous fat layers under the skin, where it serves as insulation. In children and young adults, the subcutaneous fat provides a useful measure for estimating total body fat. Skinfold thickness measured at various locations on the body (such as the triceps, subscapular region, or waist) can be applied to existing standards to assess relative leanness or fatness. As individuals grow older, body fat is deposited on the trunk rather than on the extremities; thus waist circumference (WC) or waist-to-hip ratio (WHR) become useful tools to evaluate body fatness and health risk.[18]

3. *Body water:* Total body water includes both intracellular and extracellular water. Total body water varies with relative leanness or fatness, age, hydration status, and health status. Generally, water makes up about 50% to 65% of body weight. Muscle tissue has high water content, whereas adipose tissue has low water content; thus men have a higher proportion of body water than women because they have more muscle and less fat. Infants have a relatively high proportion of body water, which drops to adult levels by age 2. This makes them especially vulnerable to the dangers of dehydration with continued vomiting or diarrhea.

4. *Mineral mass:* Body minerals found largely in the skeleton account for only 4% to 6% of body weight. Major minerals are calcium and phosphorus, located in bone and other body cells and fluids. Sodium is the major mineral in extracellular fluid (ECF), and potassium is the major mineral in intracellular fluid (ICF).

The following factors influence the relative sizes of body compartments:

• *Gender:* Women have more adipose tissue and men have more lean tissue, particularly muscle tissue.
• *Age:* Young adults have more LBM and less fat than older adults.
• *Physical activity:* Persons who are physically active tend to have less fat and more LBM than individuals who are sedentary.
• *Race:* Blacks have relatively more bone mineral than whites or Hispanics; white men tend to have more body fat than black men of similar height and weight; Mexican American women tend to have more body fat than black women with similar heights and weights.[19]
• *Climate:* Individuals living in very cold climates develop more subcutaneous fat to insulate against heat loss.

Importance of Body Fat

Although excess body fat is detrimental to health, some body fat is necessary for life. In human starvation, victims die from fat loss, not protein depletion. For mere survival, men require about 3% body fat and women require about 12%; however, for reproductive capacity, women require a level of body fat of about 20%. The initiation of menstruation or menarche occurs when the female body attains a certain size or, more precisely, the critical proportion of body fat. Body fat gained during pregnancy serves as an important energy reserve for lactation. Ill-advised dieting during pregnancy in an attempt to avoid normal weight gain interferes with fetal development and can result in a low-birth-weight infant with associated health risks.

Measuring Body Compartments
Specialized Methods

The classic method for determining body composition is hydrostatic weighing using Archimedes' principle. The individual is first weighed in air and then weighed completely submerged in water. The volume of water displaced is measured, and using standardized equations, the relative amounts of LBM and body fat can be calculated. In a new application of this principle, the individual is weighed in air and then placed in an air-controlled chamber, referred to as a *pod*. The pod can measure the amount of air displaced by the volume of the body (Fig. 8.5). Both air and water displacement methods take advantage of the fact that body fat and lean tissue differ in density, and standard calculations can be applied. The air displacement method offers an opportunity for measuring infants, children, older adults or patients who cannot be weighed under water.[20]

Dual-energy x-ray absorptiometry (DEXA) is an advanced form of radiographic technology that can differentiate between muscle, fat, and bone; this method is used to measure bone mineral density and age-related bone loss. Bioelectrical impedance systems that pass a very small current of electricity through the body can distinguish water, fat, and bone and are easily applied in clinical settings. Body circumferences and skinfold thicknesses are useful and inexpensive methods to estimate body muscle and body fat in a community setting. These procedures are discussed in more detail in Chapter 16.

Development of Height-Weight Tables

The Metropolitan Life Insurance Company, using information obtained from their life insurance policyholders, mostly middle-aged Caucasian men, constructed the first height-weight tables in the 1930s. Desirable weights were based on the body weights of the policyholders who lived the longest. Early height-weight tables presented adult reference weights according to age, based on the assumption that weight gain continued throughout adult life. New concepts have since emerged regarding height-weight tables: (1) Body weight (and body fat) should not increase as individuals move into middle and older ages and (2) body build and body fat patterns differ across racial and ethnic groups, so standard measurements developed using white populations may not be appropriate for blacks, Hispanic Americans, or Asian Americans.

FIG. 8.5 A pod for measuring body composition. The BOD POD uses air-displacement technology to measure body composition. (Courtesy Life Measurement, Inc, Concord, CA.)

KEY TERMS

Obesity
Fatness; an excessive accumulation of body fat.

Adipocyte
A fat cell.

Menarche
The first menstrual period with the onset of puberty.

Reference Tables for Clinical Evaluation

Health and nutrition professionals from the National Academy of Medicine (formally The Institute of Medicine) and the National Heart, Lung, and Blood Institute have developed reference standards to define the terms *overweight* and *obesity*.[2,21,22] Appropriate ranges of body weight for adults of a given height can be of use to health professionals in assessing patients and setting goals for a healthy weight. The body mass index (BMI), which is describe next, provides such a tool.

Body Mass Index

In 1871 Quetelet developed the BMI, which has replaced body weight as the medical standard to define obesity. Although BMI is calculated using body height and weight, it provides a better assessment of appropriate body weight than simple height-weight tables and correlates well with estimates of body fat obtained by underwater weighing. Nevertheless, BMI does not provide a quantitative estimate of body fat and cannot distinguish between excess body fat and increased muscle in persons who weigh more than the standard. Stature influences body composition because taller people have greater bone mass, which adds to their body weight. Thus, individuals with the same BMI may not have the same body composition.[23] Despite these limitations, BMI is useful for relating the increase in health risk with excessive body weight, and providing a base line for intervention when more sophisticated equipment is not available.

The formula for calculating BMI is as follows:

$$BMI = Weight\ (kg) \div Height\ (m)^2$$
Weight: 1 kg = 2.2 lb
Height: 1 m = 39.37 in

The desirable BMI range for adults is 18.5 to 24.9 kg/m². Health risks associated with overweight begin at 25 kg/m² and become apparent at 30 kg/m². Values beyond 35 kg/m² indicate severe obesity (see Tables 8.5 and 8.6 and Appendix A).[2]

Over the past 30 years, the proportion of Americans considered to be of normal weight based on their BMI has declined from 42% to 29%.[24] Data from the recent National Health and Nutrition Examination Survey indicate that 35% of men and about 40% of women are obese; about one-third of US adults are overweight.[24,25] Obesity is more prevalent among women, blacks, and Hispanics, and lowest among Asians. Former smokers are more likely to be obese than current smokers.[25]

BMI is often used to evaluate the effects of overweight and obesity on morbidity and mortality. Age and gender become factors when evaluating the mortality risk associated with a rise in BMI, as older adults and women seem to better tolerate overweight or obesity than younger adults or men.[21] In past years evaluations of BMI and mortality risk have suggested that BMI levels of 25 to 29.9 (overweight) were associated with lower all-cause mortality, and mortality rates of those with grade 1 obesity (BMI = 30 to 34.9) were similar to those of desirable weight (18.5 to 24.9 kg/m²).[26] Two recent evaluations of body weight and mortality among health professionals in the United States and several populations worldwide have challenged those results, reporting that BMI measurements as low as 25 to 27.5 are associated with increases in mortality risk.[27,28]

Various circumstances might contribute to these contrasting findings. First, we noted earlier that BMI is not a true measure of body fat, and individuals of a healthy weight indeed may have a surplus of body fat.[29] Second, some overweight or obese individuals are "metabolically healthy" with limited risk factors for cardiovascular disease, whereas other individuals of healthy weight may have disease risk

TABLE 8.5 Determining Adult Body Mass Index

BMI	19	20	21	22	23	24	25	26	27	28	29	30	31	32	33	34	35[a]
Height								**Body Weight (lb)**									
4 ft 10 in	91	96	100	105	110	115	119	124	129	134	138	143	148	153	158	162	167
4 ft 11 in	94	99	104	109	114	119	124	128	133	138	143	148	153	158	163	168	173
5 ft	97	102	107	112	118	123	128	133	138	143	148	153	158	163	168	174	179
5 ft 1 in	100	106	111	116	122	127	132	137	143	148	153	158	164	169	174	180	185
5 ft 2 in	104	109	115	120	126	131	136	142	147	153	158	164	169	175	180	186	191
5 ft 3 in	107	113	118	124	130	135	141	146	152	158	163	169	175	180	186	191	197
5 ft 4 in	110	116	122	128	134	140	145	151	157	163	169	174	180	186	192	197	204
5 ft 5 in	114	120	126	132	138	144	150	156	162	168	174	180	186	192	198	204	210
5 ft 6 in	118	124	130	136	142	148	155	161	167	173	179	186	192	198	204	210	216
5 ft 7 in	121	127	134	140	146	153	159	166	172	178	185	191	198	204	211	217	223
5 ft 8 in	125	131	138	144	151	158	164	171	177	184	190	197	203	210	216	223	230
5 ft 9 in	128	135	142	149	155	162	169	176	182	189	196	203	209	216	223	230	236
5 ft 10 in	132	139	146	153	160	167	174	181	188	195	202	209	216	222	229	236	243
5 ft 11 in	136	143	150	157	165	172	179	186	193	200	208	215	222	229	236	243	250
6 ft	140	147	154	162	169	177	184	191	199	206	213	221	228	235	242	250	258
6 ft 1 in	144	151	159	166	174	182	189	197	204	212	219	227	235	242	250	257	265
6 ft 2 in	148	155	163	171	179	186	194	202	210	218	225	233	241	249	256	264	272
6 ft 3 in	152	160	168	176	184	192	200	208	216	224	232	240	248	256	264	272	279
6 ft 4 in	156	164	172	180	189	197	205	213	221	230	238	246	254	263	271	279	287
	Healthy Weight						**Overweight**					**Obese**					

[a]Height and weight equivalents for BMI levels above 35 can be found in Appendix A.
To determine BMI, locate the height of interest in the leftmost column and read across the row for that height to the weight of interest. Follow the column of the weight up to the top row that lists the BMI. A BMI of 18.5–24.9 is the range of healthy weight, a BMI of 25–29.9 is the range of overweight, a BMI of 30 to 39.9 is the range of obese, and a BMI of 40 or over is classified as extreme obesity.
BMI, Body mass index.
Data from National Heart, Lung, and Blood Institute: *Aim for a healthy weight: assessing your weight and health risk: body mass index Table 1 and Table 2.* https://www.nhlbi.nih.gov/health/educational/lose_wt/BMI/bmi_tbl.htm.

TABLE 8.6 Body Mass Index and Percent Body Fat

BMI (kg/m²)	Body Weight Status	Body Fat (%): Men	Body Fat (%): Women
<18.5	Underweight	<13	<23
18.5–24.9	Normal	13–21	23–31
25–29.9	Overweight	21–25	31–37
30–34.9	Obese	25–31	37–42
≥35	Severely obese	>31	>42

BMI, Body mass index.
From Food and Nutrition Board, Institute of Medicine: *Dietary Reference Intakes for energy, carbohydrate, fiber, fat, fatty acids, cholesterol, protein, and amino acids (macronutrients)*. Washington, D.C., 2005, National Academies Press.

factors whether or not they have been diagnosed.[26] Finally, it may be important to view an individual's weight history and base the BMI evaluation on his or her maximum weight, as weight loss and a lower BMI later in life may reflect a disease process resulting in the lower body weight.[28] These outcomes have raised questions as to whether all overweight or obese individuals with a BMI of 25 or higher should be approached about weight loss or if identification and intervention for other risk factors is a better approach.[22,29] In any case, appropriate efforts to achieve or maintain a healthy weight should be encouraged. (See the Focus on Culture box, "Evaluating Body Compartments: One Size Does Not Fit All.")

Abdominal Fat/Waist Circumference

Health and disease risk are influenced not only by the amount of body fat but also by where it is positioned. The pear shape, with a smaller waist and larger hip (gynoid shape), is characteristic of younger women and controlled to some extent by the female hormone estrogen. The apple shape, with more fat around the abdomen (android shape), is common in men and postmenopausal women. Because abdominal (**visceral**) fat raises blood lipid levels and increases the risk of cardiovascular disease, extra weight around one's middle is of greater harm than extra weight on the hips or thighs. An appropriate WHR is 0.9 or less for men and 0.8 or less for women. These ratios indicate a smaller waist and a larger hip. Abdominal obesity is defined as a WC greater than or equal to 88 cm (35 in) in women and greater than or equal to 102 cm (40 in) in men.[22] (See the Perspectives in Practice box, "Assessing Energy Expenditure and Body Weight," to estimate your personal energy requirements and evaluate your body weight status.)

⊕ FOCUS ON CULTURE

Evaluating Body Compartments: One Size Does Not Fit All

Body composition differs according to gender, race, and ethnicity. With body mass index (BMI) receiving worldwide attention for estimating body fat and disease risk, researchers have been evaluating differences in body composition among individuals with a similar BMI. Women of all ages have a greater percentage of body fat than men of similar ages and BMIs. Individuals age 70 and over with a BMI of 25 can have 6% to 7% more body fat and significantly less fat free mass as compared with young adults of their comparable race or ethnic group, gender, and BMI.[1]

Differences in body build influence the BMI.[1] Black men have increased skeletal and muscle mass in their lower extremities. Mexican American men tend to be shorter in height, with a greater fat mass on the trunk. At a BMI of 25, young black men have the least body fat (21%) followed by white men (23%), and Mexican American men (25%). Asian American men share some of the characteristics of Mexican American men being shorter in stature, with a larger waist circumference and greater percentage of body fat.[1] Asian Americans and others may be at greater risk of chronic diseases such as diabetes at BMI values considered to be in the healthy range.[2] New prediction standards that accurately assess disease risk among different racial and ethnic groups are urgently needed for targeting early intervention.

References

1. Heymsfield SB, Peterson CM, Thomas DM, et al: Why are there race/ethnic differences in adult body mass index-adiposity relationships? A quantitative critical review, *Obes Rev* 17(3):262, 2016.
2. Jih J, Mukherjea A, Vittinghoff E, et al: Using appropriate body mass index cut points for overweight and obesity among Asian Americans, *Prev Med* 65:1, 2014.

𝒫 PERSPECTIVES IN PRACTICE

Assessing Energy Expenditure and Body Weight

In your professional role you will help clients define their energy needs and assess their body weight and body fat. This exercise provides experience in applying some simple measures.

A. Calculate Your Total Energy Expenditure

Your total energy output per day is the sum of three uses of energy:
1. Resting metabolic rate (RMR).
2. Thermic effect of food (TEF). (The factors we are using to calculate physical activity include the TEF so for this exercise we will not calculate it separately.)
3. Physical activity.

1. Resting Metabolic Rate

Calculate your RMR using one of the following:
    Women: 0.9 kcal/kg per hour[a]
    Men: 1.2 kcal/kg per hour[1]

Convert your body weight from pounds (lb) to kilograms (kg): 1 kg = 2.2 lb
Body weight in pounds _____ ÷ 2.2 = _____ kg
Example: Mr. Frank weighs 176 pounds: 176 ÷ 2.2 = 80 kg
RMR (kcalories) = 0.9 (for women) or 1.2 (for men) × kg body weight × 24 (hours) = _____
Example: Mr. Frank weighs 80 kg and the calculation factor for men is 1.2.
RMR (kcalories) = 1.2 × 80 kg × 24 (hours) = 2304 kcal

2. Physical Activity[1]

Calculate your physical activity expenditure:
Calculate the energy cost of your physical activity using your RMR and the activity factor from Table 8.4 that best fits your current activity level.[1]
    Physical activity kcalories = RMR × physical activity factor = _____
    Example: Mr. Frank's RMR is 2304 kcal, and he is sedentary, so his activity factor is 0.2.
Physical activity kcalories = 2304 × 0.2 = 461 kcal

PERSPECTIVES IN PRACTICE

Assessing Energy Expenditure and Body Weight—cont'd

3. Total Energy Expenditure

To calculate your total energy expenditure (kcalories):

RMR kcalories _____ + physical activity kcalories _____ = _____

Example: Mr. Frank's total energy expenditure: 2304 kcal (RMR) + 461 kcal (physical activity) = 2765 kcal (TEE)

Refer to the dietary intake record that you completed for the Perspectives in Practice box in Chapter 1, and consider the following questions:

a. How does your actual energy intake compare with your estimated total energy expenditure completed above? Are you taking in more kcalories, fewer kcalories, or about the same number of kcalories as you are using each day?

b. What will be the effect on your body weight if you continue this pattern? What will be the effect on your health status?

B. Evaluate Your Body Weight Using the Body Mass Index[2]

Determine your body mass index (BMI) using Table 8.5 or Appendix A.

BMI = _____

Health risks associated with overweight begin at a BMI of 25, and individuals with a BMI of 30 or greater have increasing levels of risk (see Table 8.6).

a. What is your assessment of your weight status using the BMI? Are you underweight, overweight, or in the healthy range?

b. If you are not in the healthy range, how might you begin to improve your status? (Consider underweight to be as needful of attention as overweight.)

C. Evaluate Your Health Status Using Waist Circumference (see text)

Measure your waist circumference (WC) using a nonstretch tape.

WC = _____

If you are a woman, then your WC should not exceed 88 cm (35 in); if you are a man, it should not exceed 102 cm (40 in).

a. What is your assessment of your chronic disease risk based on your WC?

b. If you are not in the healthful range, how might you begin to improve your status?

References

1. Food and Nutrition Board, Institute of Medicine: *Dietary Reference Intakes for energy, carbohydrate, fiber, fat, fatty acids, cholesterol, protein, and amino acids (macronutrients)*. Washington, DC, 2002, National Academies Press.

2. National Heart, Lung, and Blood Institute/National Institute of Diabetes and Digestive and Kidney Diseases: *Aim for a Healthy Weight: Assessing Your Weight and Health Risk: Body Mass Index Table 1 and Table 2*. https://www.nhlbi.nih.gov/health/educational/lose_wt/BMI/bmi_tbl.htm.

[a]These factors represent the midpoint of the suggested range for each gender.

KEY TERM

Visceral
Referring to the organs in the abdominal cavity.

HEALTH PROMOTION

Finding a Healthy Weight

For many people it is difficult to determine what is a normal body weight. In the traditional sense, overweight and excessive body fat represent an energy imbalance arising from a surplus in energy input (fuel from food) over energy output (total energy expenditure). But it is not that simple. Our genetic makeup influences our propensity to gain weight and the amount and position of our body fat. Estrogen and testosterone control the differences in body fat between men and women, but other internal mechanisms also lead to differences in fat accretion. Certain individuals have an exceptionally low RMR and a high metabolic efficiency influenced by an inherited obesity gene,[2] which adds to their risk of unwanted weight. A genetic link has been identified among certain Native Americans that characterizes their lower energy expenditure and higher BMI and contributes to their elevated risk for type 2 diabetes.[30] Fidgeting and ongoing body movement, sometimes referred to as non–exercise activity thermogenesis (NEAT), increases energy expenditure and helps some people resist weight gain even if they are overfed.[31]

Just as weight gain results from a surplus of kcalories, weight loss should follow a kcalorie deficit. Traditionally it was believed that a shortfall of 3500 kcal would bring about the loss of 1 lb of body weight; however, this can be a false promise, and leading clinicians recommend that it not be used.[32] Body mechanisms designed to preserve body mass can decrease spontaneous activity or lower the RMR, making weight loss more difficult. When weight loss is successful, RMR and energy requirements decrease as body tissue is lost. Adding an exercise component assists in weight management *if* energy intake does not increase as a result of the activity. For some individuals the weight loss required to move them into a more appropriate weight range is not possible. Yet, it is critical to interrupt a cycle of continued weight gain. Even small increases in body weight can add to the severity of chronic conditions such as type 2 diabetes or osteoarthritis, adversely affecting the quality of life. Conversely, small losses—even 3% to 5% of body weight—interrupt or slow such changes.[21] So what should be our approach to a healthy weight?

Developing a Healthy Lifestyle

Successful weight management requires a lifelong commitment to positive behaviors that emphasize sustainable and enjoyable eating habits and regular physical activity. A healthy lifestyle is a more appropriate goal than weight loss at any cost. A meal plan low to moderate in fat and rich in fruits, vegetables, whole grains, and fiber at an energy level that prevents further weight gain adds to well-being regardless of weight loss. Regular physical activity such as walking adds to energy expenditure and can assist in moderate weight loss. Weight loss diets celebrated in the popular press often lead to cycles of weight loss followed by even greater weight gain when persons revert to their former eating patterns. Establishing a healthy diet that is acceptable over the long term is the best approach to the control of body weight.[33] (For more discussion on the benefits of walking, see the Evidence-Based Practice box, "Walking, Weight Gain, and Chronic Disease Risk")

Walking, Weight Gain, and Chronic Disease Risk

Identify the problem: Health educators worldwide are encouraging individuals to increase their physical activity. Walking has many advantages as a form of exercise: it requires no special training, no special equipment other than a good pair of walking shoes, does not cost money, and is considered a safe activity for individuals who are overweight or have been sedentary. However, is walking effective in promoting physical well-being?

Review the evidence: When researchers evaluated walking patterns and weight gain among 1155 young adults, a 5-year follow-up indicated that those taking more steps gained less weight.[1] Although both the men and women gained on average 4.4 lb, those who took less than 10,000 steps per day gained 10.1 lb. Other researchers have reported that the number of daily steps of 3388 persons ages 20 and over influenced their cardiovascular risk.[2] Men who walked 9001 steps per day had a BMI of 27.9 and a WC of 99 cm; those walking only 2247 steps per day had a BMI of 29.4 and a WC of 104 cm. Men who accumulated over 12,000 daily steps dropped their WC to 95 cm and their BMI to 26.8, approaching the goal of a healthy weight. Women had fewer steps, ranging from 1755 steps per day to 9824 steps per day, but over this range their WCs varied from 99 cm to 89 cm and their BMIs from 30.0 to 26.4. HDL-cholesterol levels were significantly higher and serum triglyceride levels significantly lower in those taking more steps. Individuals taking more steps also decreased their risk of diabetes, even if walking less than 10,000 steps each day.

Implement the findings: Adults are encouraged to perform at least 30 minutes of moderate-intensity exercise on most days of the week, and walking at a speed of 3 to 4 mph (greater than or equal to 100 steps/min) meets this standard. Daily activities of independent living require about 2500 steps, and 30 minutes of brisk walking will add at least 3000 steps to the daily total.[3] For most people, including older adults or persons with chronic disease, 5500 to 7500 steps per day is an achievable goal. Individuals who stepped in place while television commercials were being aired added 2000 steps to their daily total.[4] Workplace options such as desks for standing rather than sitting are being tested for their effectiveness in increasing energy expenditure.[5]

References

1. Smith KJ, Gall SL, McNaughton SA, et al: Lifestyle behaviours associated with 5-year weight gain in a prospective cohort of Australian adults aged 26-36 years at baseline, *BMC Public Health* 17:54, 2017.
2. Tudor-Locke C, Schuna JM Jr, Han HO, et al: Step-based physical activity metrics and cardiometabolic risk: NHANES 2005-2006, *Med Sci Sports Exerc* 49(2):283, 2017.
3. Tudor-Locke C, Craig CL, Aoyagi Y, et al: How many steps/day are enough? For older adults and special populations, *Int J Behav Nutr Phys Act* 8:80, 2011.
4. Steeves JA, Thompson DL, Bassett DR Jr: Energy cost of stepping in place while watching television commercials, *Med Sci Sports Exerc* 44(2):330, 2012.
5. Tudor-Locke C, Schuna JM Jr, Frensham LJ, et al: Changing the way we work: elevating energy expenditure with workstation alternatives, *Int J Obes (Lond)* 38(6):755, 2014.

FATNESS, THINNESS, AND HEALTH

Obesity and Health

Weight-related health problems can be divided into four categories: (1) metabolic, (2) degenerative, (3) neoplastic, and (4) anatomic.

- *Metabolic:* Type 2 diabetes, hypertension, elevated blood lipids, and the constellation of conditions associated with metabolic syndrome often accompany obesity. Abdominal fat increases the risk of metabolic disorders.
- *Degenerative:* Obesity and physical disability are strongly linked. Osteoarthritis and joint problems, atherosclerotic changes, and pulmonary diseases are more serious in obese persons.
- *Neoplastic:* Many forms of cancer—including colorectal, breast, prostate, esophageal, and ovarian cancer—are more frequent in higher weight categories.
- *Anatomic:* Individuals who exceed a healthy weight have a greater risk of gastroesophageal reflux disease (GERD) and obstructive sleep apnea.

The current prevalence of overweight and obesity will continue to impact health care costs in the years ahead. Among older adults ages 65 to 69, annual Medicare costs of the severely obese (BMI of 35 or higher) were more than twice those of the normal weight (BMI between 18 and 24.9), a difference of $9751 versus $4663.[34]

Obsession with Thinness

An opposite trend to obesity but equally harmful to health is the model of extreme thinness. An image of thinness drives the marketing of clothes, cosmetics, and food. Social pressures have created an abnormally thin and unrealistic ideal that leads to dissatisfaction with the shape of one's body among all age groups. Social discrimination against children and adults who are overweight can intensify the fear of weight gain or result in harmful means of weight loss. Elementary school children have been found to develop restrained eating patterns and dissatisfaction with their bodies in response to social pressures.[35]

If parents restrict food intake, children may react by overeating when those restricted foods are available outside the home. Guilt feelings after eating certain foods and distorted perceptions of body size often form the basis for serious eating disorders that threaten nutritional and physical health.

The family has a role in helping young people develop positive attitudes toward food. Adolescents who reported positive communication and closeness within their family had more frequent meals with family[36] and were less likely to follow inappropriate diets or engage in disordered eating behaviors.[37] Teens participating in weight-related sports are especially vulnerable to unhealthy weight-control practices.

Eating Disorders: A High Price for Thinness

The number of individuals affected by eating disorders is unknown, as these conditions often exist for some time before clinical detection, and based on their secretive nature, they often go unreported. Prevalence differs according to gender and age. Although female adolescents are more vulnerable to a quest for thinness, male adolescents can exhibit disordered eating related to muscle development.[38] Anorexia nervosa and bulimia nervosa are more likely to occur among adolescents, whereas binge eating disorder extends into adulthood.[39] Older adults have been diagnosed with eating disorders. Eating disorders are biologically based mental illnesses that lead to nutritional deficiencies, medical complications, and, in the extreme, disability and death. We associate eating disorders with our society's emphasis on thinness, but physicians in Great Britain and France described anorexia nervosa as far back as the 1800s.

Causes of Eating Disorders

Eating disorders have an emotional/behavioral component and a neurophysiologic/genetic component, although genes appear to play a significant role.[40] Alterations in CNS activity directly affect food behavior and the development of eating disorders. Levels of serotonin and other neurotransmitters are altered, and changes in the hypothalamus affect appetite. Personality traits such as perfectionism and obsessive-compulsive behavior are common among individuals with eating disorders. Family dynamics may be part of the environmental stress that adds to the seriousness of these conditions, but families are not the root cause. Eating disorders often coexist with other psychiatric and anxiety-related disorders, and the longer the nutritional deficits and emotional problems continue, the more severe they become. Individuals do not choose to have eating disorders, and treatment must address both physiologic and emotional components if restoration is to occur.[40]

For every individual who develops an eating disorder, a particular factor may be more or less important. The growing interest in athletics among children and youth can increase risk of eating disorders or assist in prevention. Those participating in activities in which thinness is expected, such as gymnastics or dance, are at greater risk.[39] Students who take part in school or recreational sports that do not require a thin body are at lesser risk. Activities that build self-esteem and help young people feel good about themselves and their accomplishments help protect against eating disorders.

Types of Eating Disorders

The four types of eating disorders recognized by the American Psychiatric Association are (1) anorexia nervosa, (2) bulimia nervosa, (3) binge-eating disorder, and (4) eating disorders not otherwise specified (EDNOS).[39] Each has distinctive diagnostic criteria and symptoms.

Anorexia nervosa means "appetite loss from nervous disease." Anorexia nervosa is a form of starvation with excessive weight loss self-imposed at great physical and psychologic cost. Although these patients may have a body weight only 85% of average or a BMI of less than 17.5, they never see themselves as underweight and emaciated but always as fat.[39] This distorted body image often persists during recovery. Low bone mass is a frequent complication because amenorrhea usually accompanies this condition. Increasing body fat is a major goal in rehabilitation as it triggers resumption of the menses and improved bone health. Body fat in recovering patients for whom menstruation returned was about 28% as compared to 24% in those with continuing amenorrhea.[41]

Bulimia nervosa, meaning "ox hunger," describes the massive amounts of food consumed by these patients. Because this individual is eating, body weight is usually normal or even above normal. Bulimia nervosa is often associated with depression or difficulty in meeting social or role expectations. Patients are consumed with guilt about their food behavior. Eating episodes are followed by purging through self-induced vomiting, use of laxatives or diuretics, enemas, or excessive exercise. Such happenings may occur twice a week or more. Repeated vomiting of the highly acidic stomach contents is harmful to the teeth and tissues of the mouth.[42] This condition is sometimes referred to as the *binge-and-purge syndrome*.

Binge-eating disorder includes binge-eating episodes but without the purging behavior of bulimia nervosa. Binge eating occurs in response to stress or anxiety, or may soothe or relieve painful feelings. Many of these patients are overweight and have the same medical problems as obese individuals who do not binge eat.[42]

EDNOS often include a combination of the conditions described in this section or a frequency of symptoms that differ from established diagnostic criteria. Eating problems such as purging syndrome and night-eating syndrome are included in this category.[42]

Prevention and Treatment

The identification of individuals at risk for eating disorders can prompt early intervention and interrupt the progression of malnutrition. Health professionals, school personnel working with adolescents and athletes, and parents need to be alerted to the characteristics of eating disorders and encouraged to watch for such behaviors (Box 8.3). Staff

---

KEY TERMS

Neoplastic
Describing abnormal growth of tissue, usually associated with the formation of tumors.

Anorexia Nervosa
An eating disorder characterized by (1) an extreme psychophysiologic aversion to food, resulting in life-threatening weight loss, and (2) a distorted body image considered to reflect fat when the body is actually emaciated from self-imposed starvation.

Bulimia Nervosa
An eating disorder in which cycles of gorging on large quantities of food are followed by self-induced vomiting or use of diuretics, laxatives, or extreme levels of exercise to avoid weight gain.

Binge-Eating Disorder
An eating disorder in which individuals consume large amounts of food in a short period of time, but without the purging behavior of bulimia nervosa.

BOX 8.3 Signs Associated With the Development of Eating Disorders in Adolescents[a]

Behavioral Signs
- Obsession with dieting
- Extreme level of exercise
- Dissatisfaction with body size or shape
- Overestimation of kcalorie intake (anorexia nervosa)

Clinical Signs (Anorexia Nervosa)
- Arrested growth and maturation
- Underweight: body mass index <17.5
- Dry and yellowish skin
- Growth of fine hair over the body (e.g., lanugo)
- Drop in internal body temperature; person feels cold
- Severe constipation
- Low blood pressure, slowed breathing and pulse

Clinical Signs (Bulimia Nervosa)
- Chronically inflamed and sore throat
- Swollen glands in the neck and below the jaw
- Worn tooth enamel and decaying teeth
- Intestinal distress and irritation from laxative abuse
- Severe dehydration from purging of fluids

[a]Not all of these signs will be observed in all individuals
Data from Academy of Nutrition and Dietetics: *Practice Paper of the American Dietetic Association: Nutrition Intervention in the Treatment of Eating Disorders*. Published August 2011. Accessible to Academy members at http://www.eatrightpro.org/~/media/eatrightpro%20files/practice/position%20and%20practice%20papers/practice%20papers/practice%20papers/practice_paper_nutrition_intervention.ashx; US Department of Health and Human Services, National Institute of Mental Health: *Eating disorders: about more than food*. NIH Publication No.TR 14-4901, revised 2014. National Institute of Mental Health, Bethesda, MD. https://www.nimh.nih.gov/health/publications/eating-disorders/index.shtml.

need to monitor school-based programs intended to combat obesity,[40] as adolescents with eating disorders may be drawn to such programs.

The treatment of eating disorders requires an experienced team of health professionals including a physician, nurse, dietitian, clinical psychologist or psychiatrist, and dentist. Outpatient services may provide the care needed in less advanced cases, but for life-threatening anorexia nervosa, intense inpatient therapy is essential. An individualized care plan for patients with disordered eating should include nutritional, medical, and behavioral intervention. A framework for meals, snacks, and food choices must be implemented on a gradual basis to address the underweight or overweight. Medical complications arising from severe malnutrition require immediate attention. The psychologist or psychiatrist on the health care team can address the personal and emotional issues contributing to the condition and promote healthy behaviors that will sustain the nutritional and medical recovery. Persons with eating disorders are often resistant to treatment, and progress can be slow.

The Problem of Underweight

We discussed the problem of excessive body weight and body fat, and situations in which individuals deliberately reduce their food intake. Now we consider the causes and effects of underweight caused by lack of food or debilitating illness.

Definition

Underweight, defined as a BMI of less than 18.5 kg/m², is relatively uncommon in the United States. National surveys report that 3.5% of children and youth ages 2 to 19 years are underweight[43] as are 3.3% of community-dwelling older adults.[44] Underweight in older adults is often associated with frailty and health problems, especially in nursing home patients.[45] Low weight for age is a common problem in young children in developing countries where food supplies are limited. Underweight springs from poverty, poor living conditions, long-term illness, or physiologic dysfunction. Infants, young children, and older adults are at greatest risk. Resistance to infection is lower, general health is poorer, and physical strength is decreased in seriously underweight individuals.

General Causes

Malnutrition and underweight can result from decreased food intake, increased energy requirements, or poor utilization of ingested food and nutrients (Box 8.4).

- *Poor food intake:* Lack of sufficient and appropriate food results in failure to thrive in children and older adults. Medications such as digoxin and chemotherapeutic agents, associated with poor appetite and nausea, contribute to the devastating weight loss known as *cachexia* seen in cardiac failure and cancer. Older people in poverty who live alone and lack transportation to a grocery store risk unwanted weight loss. Skilled nursing facilities are required to monitor body weight, as a patient's inability to self-feed can lead to significant weight loss.
- *Increase in energy requirements:* Long-term **hypermetabolic** conditions such as cancer, acquired immunodeficiency syndrome (AIDS),

KEY TERM

Hypermetabolic
Increased rate of body metabolism occurring as a result of infection, trauma, or disease.

advanced heart disease, or infection impose energy demands that drain the body's resources. Hyperthyroidism increases caloric requirements. Extensive physical activity without a sufficient increase in energy intake will over time bring about inappropriate weight loss in the normal weight individual.
- *Poor utilization of available nutrients:* Malabsorption associated with prolonged diarrhea, gastrointestinal disease, or laxative abuse depletes nutrient stores. Cytokines produced by the immune system in response to chronic conditions such as cancer, chronic kidney disease, congestive heart failure, and AIDS accelerate the breakdown of body protein and fat.[46] Cytokines also interfere with the effective utilization of nutritional supplements, making it difficult to reverse the patient's deteriorating condition.

Nutritional Care

Underweight persons require special nutrition intervention to rebuild body tissues and nutrient stores. Food plans must be adapted to the individual's personal preferences, financial situation, and household concerns, and address any existing disease. The dietary recommendation should be (1) high in kcalories (at least 50% beyond standard needs); (2) high in protein to rebuild tissue; (3) high in complex carbohydrates to provide a primary energy source in an easily digested form; (4) moderate in unsaturated fats to add kcalories but not exceed recommended limits; and (5) optimum in vitamins and minerals, including supplements when deficiencies require them. Meals and snacks spread throughout the day that include favorite foods increase interest in eating and promote optimal utilization of nutrients. Liquid nutrition supplements add kcalories and key nutrients. In extreme cases tube feeding or total parenteral nutrition (TPN) may be necessary. (Rehabilitation of undernourished patients will be discussed further in Chapter 19.)

TO SUM UP

Food provides the energy that enables the body to continue its physical and metabolic work. Through a series of ongoing metabolic reactions, the chemical energy in food is converted to thermal, electrical, and mechanical energy. The heat produced by body work, expressed in kcalories, serves as a measure of energy taken in and expended. One's total energy requirement is the sum of (1) basal metabolic needs, (2) the thermic effect of food (TEF), and (3) physical activity. Physical activity is the most variable component, adding relatively few kcalories for sedentary persons but making up half or more of the total energy requirement of highly active people. Both energy intake and physical activity influence the size of the four major body compartments: (1) LBM, (2) body fat, (3) body water, and (4) mineral mass. Both the amount of body fat and its location influence disease risk, with abdominal fat of greatest concern. Conversely, eating disorders with self-imposed food restriction or purging lead to extreme underweight and even death, if prolonged, and treatment prognosis can be poor. Poverty, chronic disease, and medications contribute to underweight through low food intake, poor food utilization, or increased energy requirements. A nutrient- and energy-rich diet can usually restore these malnourished individuals to a healthy weight.

BOX 8.4 Selected Causes of Underweight

- Problems with self-feeding
- Long-term illness and multiple medications
- Cancer
- Cardiac failure (cardiac cachexia)
- Chronic obstructive pulmonary disease
- Acquired immunodeficiency syndrome
- Insufficient resources to obtain adequate food

QUESTIONS FOR REVIEW

1. List the three components contributing to the total energy requirement. What factors influence the BMR and why? What is the most variable component of the total energy requirement and why?

2. What is the difference between the BMR and the RMR? Which is most often used in clinical practice? Why?

3. Name the four body compartments and describe the tissues found in each. How are they measured?

4. You are performing a nutritional assessment of a man who is 6 ft 2 in tall and weighs 248 lb. What is his BMI? Is he overweight, overfat, or do you not know? Explain.

5. You are working with a client who wants to lose weight and has found several diets on the Internet. One is a high-fat diet containing 1800 kcal and the other is a high-protein diet, also containing 1800 kcal. Which diet is most likely to produce long-term weight loss? Why?

6. You are working with a single mother and her 3-year-old daughter who are both underweight. They live in a small apartment in a dilapidated building in the inner city. Their electricity was disconnected, thus they have no working equipment for cooking and no refrigeration. They receive a noon and a supper meal at a nearby food program for the homeless. Plan a breakfast and snacks throughout the day that would increase their kcalorie and nutrient intake. (Remember, all foods you suggest must be safely stored at room temperature.)

7. An adolescent girl with a BMI of 28.6 wants to increase her energy expenditure by 150 kcal a day to encourage weight loss. Develop an activity plan that would mesh with her after-school hours and social time with friends.

8. Visit your local library and review the magazines directed to young adults. Look for an article that suggests a regimen for weight management for either males or females. Evaluate the protocol in terms of (a) nutritional adequacy as compared with the MyPlate recommendations for servings from each food group, (b) suggestions for eating situations such as bag lunches or eating out, (c) reliance on commercial or expensive weight-loss products, and (d) appropriateness for long-term use.

REFERENCES

1. Das SK, Roberts SB: Energy metabolism in fasting, fed, exercise, and re-feeding states. In Erdman JW Jr, Macdonald IA, Zeisel SH, editors: *Present knowledge in nutrition*, ed 10, Ames, IA, 2012, International Life Sciences Institute & Wiley-Blackwell.

2. Food and Nutrition Board, Institute of Medicine: *Dietary Reference Intakes for energy, carbohydrate, fiber, fat, fatty acids, cholesterol, protein, and amino acids (macronutrients)*, Washington, DC, 2002, National Academies Press.

3. Guyton AC, Hall JE: *Textbook of medical physiology*, ed 10, Philadelphia, PA, 2000, Saunders.

4. Psota T, Chen KY: Measuring energy expenditure in clinical populations: rewards and challenges, *Eur J Clin Nutr* 67(5):436, 2013.

5. Little MO: Nutrition and skin ulcers, *Curr Opin Clin Nutr Metab Care* 16(1):39, 2013.

6. van Graan AE: Nutritional management in HIV/AIDS infection, *World Rev Nutr Diet* 111:130, 2015.

7. Kyle UG, Shekerdemian LS, Coss-Bu JA: Growth failure and nutrition considerations in chronic childhood wasting diseases, *Nutr Clin Pract* 30(2):227, 2015.

8. DeLany JP, Jakicic JM, Lowery JB, et al: African American women exhibit similar adherence to intervention but lose less weight due to lower energy requirements, *Int J Obes (Lond)* 38(9):1147, 2014.

9. Klein CJ, Villavicencio SA, Schweitzer A, et al: Energy prediction equations are inadequate for obese Hispanic youth, *J Am Diet Assoc* 111:1204, 2011.

10. Chaput JP, Pérusse L, Després JP, et al: Findings from the Quebec Family Study on the etiology of obesity: Genetics and environmental highlights, *Curr Obes Rep* 3:54, 2014.

11. Westerterp-Plantenga MS, Lemmens SG, Westerterp KR: Dietary protein—its role in satiety, energetics, weight loss and health, *Br J Nutr* 108(Suppl 2):S105, 2012.

12. Valenti G, Bonomi AG, Westerterp KR: Multicomponent fitness training improves walking economy in older adults, *Med Sci Sports Exerc* 48(7):1365, 2016.

13. Schrack JA, Simonsick EM, Chaves PHM, et al: The role of energetic cost in the age-related slowing of gait speed, *J Am Geriatr Soc* 60:1811, 2012.

14. Arora T, Bäckhed F: The gut microbiota and metabolic disease: current understanding and future perspectives, *J Intern Med* 280(4):339, 2016.

15. Feng B, Zhang T, Xu H: Human adipose dynamics and metabolic health, *Ann N Y Acad Sci* 1281:160, 2013.

16. Yoneshiro T, Aita S, Kawai Y, et al: Nonpungent capsaicin analogs (capsinoids) increase energy expenditure through the activation of brown adipose tissue in humans, *Am J Clin Nutr* 95:845, 2012.

17. Shlisky JD, Hartman TJ, Kris-Etherton PM, et al: Partial sleep deprivation and energy balance in adults: an emerging issue for consideration by dietetic practitioners, *J Acad Nutr Diet* 112:1785, 2012.

18. Ashwell M, Gunn P, Gibson S: Waist-to-height ratio is a better screening tool than waist circumference and BMI for adult cardiometabolic risk factors: systematic review and meta-analysis, *Obes Rev* 13:275, 2012.

19. Heo M, Faith MS, Pietrobelli A, et al: Percentage of body fat cutoffs by sex, age, and race-ethnicity in the US adult population from NHANES 1999-2004, *Am J Clin Nutr* 95:594, 2012.

20. Baracos V, Caserotti P, Earthman CP, et al: Advances in the science and application of body composition measurement, *J Parenter Enteral Nutr* 36:96, 2012.

21. US Department of Health and Human Services: *Managing Overweight and Obesity in Adults. Systematic Evidence Review From the Obesity Expert Panel, 2013*, National Heart Lung and Blood Institute, Bethesda, MD, 2013. http://www.nhlbi.nih.gov/files/obesity-evidence-review.pdf.

22. Jensen MD, Ryan DH, Apovian CM, et al: 2013 AHA/ACC/TOS Guideline for the Management of Overweight and Obesity in Adults. A Report of the American College of Cardiology/American Heart Association Task Force on Practice Guidelines and The Obesity Society, *Circulation* 129(25 Suppl 2):S102, 2014.

23. Heymsfield SB, Peterson CM, Thomas DM, et al: Why are there race/ethnic differences in adult body mass index-adiposity relationships? A quantitative critical review, *Obes Rev* 17(3):262, 2016.

24. US Department of Health and Human Services: *Health, United States, 2015: With Special Feature on Racial and Ethnic Health Disparities*. Table 58, Hyattsville, MD, 2016, National Center for Health Statistics.

25. Flegal KM, Kruszon-Moran D, Carroll MD, et al: Trends in obesity among adults in the United States, 2005 to 2014, *JAMA* 315(21):2284, 2016.

26. Loos RJF: The metabolically healthy overweight and obese and their impact on all-cause mortality, *Obesity* 21(9):1750, 2013.

27. The Global BMI Mortality Collaboration, Di Angelantonio E, Bhupathiraju ShN, Wormser D, et al: Body-mass index and all-cause mortality: individual-participant-data meta-analysis of 239 prospective studies in four continents, *Lancet* 388(10046):776, 2016.

28. Yu E, Ley SH, Manson J-AE, et al: Weight history and all-cause and cause-specific mortality in three prospective cohort studies, *Ann Intern Med* 166:613–620, 2017.

29. Heymsfield SB, Cefalu WT: Does body mass index adequately convey a patient's mortality risk? *JAMA* 309(1):87, 2013.

30. Traurig MT, Orczewska JI, Ortiz DJ, et al: Evidence for a role of LPGAT1 in influencing BMI and percent body fat in Native Americans, *Obesity (Silver Spring)* 20(12):2426, 2012.

31. Villablanca PA, Alegria JR, Mookadam F, et al: Nonexercise activity thermogenesis in obesity management, *Mayo Clin Proc* 90(4):509, 2015.

32. Hall KD, Heymsfield SB, Kemnitz JW, et al: Energy balance and its components: implications for body weight regulation, *Am J Clin Nutr* 95:989, 2012.

33. Raynor HA, Champagne CM, Academy of Nutrition and Dietetics: Position of the Academy of Nutrition and Dietetics: Interventions for the treatment of overweight and obesity in adults, *J Acad Nutr Diet* 116:129, 2016.

34. Clark DO, Lane KA, Ambuehl R, et al: Age differences in the association between body mass index class and annualized Medicare expenditures, *J Aging Health* 28(1):165, 2016.

35. Jendrzyca A, Warschburger P: Weight stigma and eating behaviours in elementary school children: A prospective population-based study, *Appetite* 102:51, 2016.

36. Berge JM, Wall M, Larson N, et al: Family functioning: associations with weight status, eating behaviors, and physical activity in adolescents, *J Adolesc Health* 52(3):351, 2013.

37. Berge JM, Wall M, Larson N, et al: The unique and additive associations of family functioning and parenting practices with disordered eating behaviors in diverse adolescents, *J Behav Med* 37:205, 2014.

38. Murray SB, Griffiths S, Mitchison D, et al: The transition from thinness-oriented to muscularity-oriented disordered eating in adolescent males: A clinical observation, *J Adolesc Health* 60(3):353, 2017.

39. Ozier AD, Henry BW, American Dietetic Association: Position of the American Dietetic Association: Nutrition intervention in the treatment of eating disorders, *J Am Diet Assoc* 111:1236, 2011.

40. American Dietetic Association: *Practice paper of the American Dietetic Association: Nutrition intervention in the treatment of eating disorders.* 2011, http://www.eatrightpro.org/resource/practice/position-and-practice-papers/practice-papers/practice-paper-nutrition-intervention-in-the-treatment-of-eating-disorders.

41. El Ghoch M, Calugi S, Chignola E, et al: Body fat and menstrual resumption in adult females with anorexia nervosa: a 1-year longitudinal study, *J Hum Nutr Diet* 29(5):662, 2016.

42. Miller CA, Golden NH: An introduction to eating disorders: clinical presentation, epidemiology, and prognosis, *Nutr Clin Pract* 25:110, 2010.

43. Fryar CD, Ogden CL: *Prevalence of Underweight Among Children and Adolescents Aged 2–19 Years: United States, 1963–1965 Through 2007–2010, Health E-Stats, Center for Disease Control*, Atlanta, GA, 2012. https://www.cdc.gov/nchs/data/hestat/underweight_child_07_10/underweight_child_07_10.htm.

44. Smit E, Winters-Stone KM, Loprinzi PD, et al: Lower nutritional status and higher food insufficiency in frail older US adults, *Br J Nutr* 110(1):172, 2013.

45. Morley JE: Pathophysiology of the anorexia of aging, *Curr Opin Clin Nutr Metab Care* 16:27, 2013.

46. Anker SD, Morley JE: Cachexia: a nutritional syndrome? *J Cachexia Sarcopenia Muscle* 6(4):269, 2015.

FURTHER READINGS AND RESOURCES

Readings

Friend S, Bauer KW, Madden TC, et al: Self-weighing among adolescents: associations with body mass index, body satisfaction, weight control behaviors, and binge eating, *J Acad Nutr Diet* 112(1):99, 2012.
[These authors explore issues relating to eating and body image and how related disorders can be prevented and treated.]

Farley TA: The role of government in preventing excess calorie consumption. The example of New York City, *JAMA* 308(11):1093, 2012.

Shlisky JD, Hartman TJ, Kris-Etherton PM, et al: Partial sleep deprivation and energy balance in adults: an emerging issue for consideration by dietetics practitioners, *J Acad Nutr Diet* 112:1785, 2012.
[These articles address issues of energy intake in our society and potential interventions.]

Websites of Interest

- National Institute of Diabetes and Digestive and Kidney Diseases (NIDDK): *WIN—Weight-Control Information Network.* This site offers up-to-date, science-based information on weight control, obesity, physical activity, and related nutritional issues for health professionals and consumers. https://www.niddk.nih.gov/health-information/health-communication-programs/win/Pages/default.aspx (materials are available in English and Spanish).

- National Institutes of Health and National Library of Medicine: *Weight Control.* This site offers tips on food selection for weight management and links to sites that provide ideas for physical activity. http://www.nlm.nih.gov/medlineplus/weightcontrol.html.

- National Institutes of Health and National Library of Medicine: *Medline Plus; Eating Disorders.* This site offers comprehensive information on eating disorders, including causes, symptoms, treatment, and prevention. http://www.nlm.nih.gov/medlineplus/eatingdisorders.html.

- Nemours Foundation: *TeensHealth: I Think My Friend May Have an Eating Disorder. What Should I Do?* This site assists teens, parents, and teachers who may suspect an eating disorder and need help with intervention. https://kidshealth.org/en/teens/friend-eating-disorder.html.

- US Department of Health and Human Services, Centers for Disease Control and Prevention: *Physical Activity for Everyone.* This site offers physical activity programs and information for all age groups, as well as resources for health professionals, including booklets on airport and mall walking programs. https://www.cdc.gov/physicalactivity/.

PART 2

Community Nutrition and the Life Cycle

9

Food Selection and Food Safety

Eleanor D. Schlenker

Now we begin a two-chapter section in which we apply our knowledge of nutrition science to the food needs and food safety of individuals and families. We look first at the web of factors that influence our personal food choices, including the ever-changing food environment. Health and convenience have joined taste and cost as consumer concerns in the marketplace. Although the expanding food supply offers more choices, it has also created a need for increased food regulation. When families produced their own food, they were responsible for its wholesomeness and safety. As our sphere of food access has broadened to include our region, our nation, and the world, food safety has become a government responsibility. Maintaining a healthy food supply rich in nutrients requires the cooperative efforts of farmers, food processors, and health professionals.

OUTLINE

Personal Food Selection
The Food Environment
Expanding the Food Supply: Biotechnology and the Consumer

Oversight of the Food Supply: Regulation and Information
The Problem of Misinformation: Food and Health
Food Safety and Food Processing

PERSONAL FOOD SELECTION

Food habits, like other human behaviors, do not develop in a vacuum. Rather, they grow out of our cultural, social, and psychological environment and the unique experiences that follow each of us throughout our lives.

Cultural Influences
Cultural Identity
Culture can be defined as the accumulation of a group's learned and shared behaviors in everyday life. Culture reveals the knowledge, values, beliefs, attitudes, and practices accepted by members of a group or community that bring a sense of identity and order to their lives.[1] Often the most significant thing about a culture is what is taken for granted. Culture involves not only the obvious aspects of life—language, religion, family structure, and historical heritage—but also daily patterns such as preparing and serving food and caring for children or elders. Culture defines how an individual describes health, perceives illness, and seeks treatment.[1] These facets of daily life are passed from generation to generation and learned as children grow up within the community.

Food in a Culture
Foodways (food customs or traditions) are among the oldest and most deeply rooted aspects of a culture. They determine what is eaten, when and how it is eaten, and who prepares it.[2] An item considered to be a special treat by families in one part of the world can

be unacceptable somewhere else. The geography of the land, the agriculture in that locality, experiences related to health and food safety, religious beliefs, and local history and traditions influence what we eat. Throughout history, designated foods or meals have commemorated special events of religious or national significance or rites of passage. Many of these customs remain today. (To learn more about food customs, see the Focus on Culture box, "Family Meals: Where Food and Culture Meet.")

Components of a Cultural Food Pattern
All food patterns share several common characteristics, although they differ in the actual foods they contain. These common dietary components are as follows[2]:
- *Core foods:* Core foods, usually complex carbohydrates, are eaten every day and provide the bulk of the energy intake.
- *Complementary foods:* These are items added to improve palatability, such as the vegetables or meat added to a rice or pasta meal.
- *Food flavors and preparation:* How foods are prepared and seasoned is distinctive for every group and is as important as the foods themselves.
- *Frequency and timing of meals:* The number of meals or snacks eaten each day, when they are eaten, and the foods they contain define dietary intake within individuals and cultures.

Maintaining core foods, familiar flavors, and meal sequence serves as a bridge to new meal patterns related to health or other considerations.

FOCUS ON CULTURE

Family Meals: Where Food and Culture Meet

Over the centuries the family meal has been the setting in which children learn about their culture. Common vocabulary, food-related customs, etiquette, food-related holidays, and intergenerational and gender relationships are learned at the family table. In general, celebrations such as weddings, birthdays, religious holidays, or secular holidays involve meals more elaborate in preparation and variety than day-to-day fare and include food items not served at other times. Although Thanksgiving and Christmas mark traditional holiday meals for some groups, Chinese families commemorate the New Year with feasting, and Muslims celebrate the end of Ramadan and its period of fasting with an elaborate meal. In agrarian societies, harvest dinners marked the end of the growing season and the securing of food crops for the coming winter. Sunday dinner was a special meal for many families because this was the day of rest when everyone had time to be together.

Family meals define gender roles and relationships. In East Indian cultures, feeding the family is an important role of the woman of the house. Even if servants or other family members assisted with preparation, the woman of the house delivered the food to the table. Who eats together at mealtime establishes the framework of social standing among family members. In East Asian countries such as China and Japan, and in traditional Native American, Arab, and African cultures, men and guests ate first, and then women and children. In comparison, African-American, Latino, and Asian Indian cultures celebrated the extended family as an important social unit with grandparents, aunts, uncles, and cousins joining in communal meals. In the Hmong community, women prepare the food except for the New Year's celebration, when men do the cooking and eat first.

The blending of families and cultures in the United States has obscured some of these differences in traditional practices. Changes in work patterns of parents and extracurricular activities and sports that occupy children and teens present obstacles to the entire family eating their evening meal together. Eating while watching television also detracts from family interaction. Nevertheless, the research associating better academic performance, lower incidence of disordered eating, and healthier food patterns among youth who eat regular meals with their families reinforces the importance of the learning and social interaction that takes place in this environment. Perhaps the most exceptional outcome of regular family meals is the lower prevalence of obesity among those preschool and school-age children and youth. Nutrition educators should stress to parents the importance of family meals.

Bibliography

Goody CM, Drago L, editors: *Cultural food practices*, Chicago, 2010, Diabetes Care and Education Dietetic Practice Group, American Dietetic Association.

Kittler PG, Sucher KP, Nahikian-Nelms M: *Food and culture*, ed 6, Belmont, CA, 2012, Wadsworth/Cengage Learning.

Martin-Biggers J, Spaccarotella K, Berhaupt-Glickstein A, et al: Come and get it! A discussion of family mealtime literature and factors affecting obesity risk, *Adv Nutr* 5(3): 235, 2014.

Tovar A, Hennessy E, Must A, et al: Feeding styles and evening family meals among recent immigrants, *Int J Behav Nutr Phys Act* 10:84, 2013.

Social Influences

Internal Factors

Food has social roles. Food is a symbol of acceptance, warmth, and friendliness. People are more likely to accept food from those they view as friends or supporters. The offering of food is an expected act of hospitality in many cultures. Strong food patterns develop within the primary family unit, and food practices associated with family celebrations are held tenaciously throughout life (Fig. 9.1). Long into adulthood, certain foods trigger a flood of childhood memories and are valued for reasons totally apart from their nutritional contribution. Nevertheless, income, local availability, and market conditions ultimately influence food choices. People eat foods that are readily available and that they have the money to buy.

External Factors

Peer pressure influences food choices. Foods may be viewed as high-prestige foods or associated with low economic status. Those immigrating to the United States may reject their traditional foods in favor of American foods popular among neighbors or classmates. Children plead for a particular snack item if that is what their friends eat. Adolescents are particularly susceptible to the influence of their peers in selecting healthy or unhealthy foods.[3]

Psychological Influences

People who enjoy a bountiful food supply think less about food because it is always available, whereas those with chronic hunger or food cravings think, talk, and dream about food. For most of us, concerns about food are associated with other needs. Maslow's classic hierarchy describes the five levels of human need, each building on the one before[4]:

1. *Basic physiological needs:* hunger and thirst
2. *Need for safety:* physical comfort, security, and protection
3. *Need to belong:* love, giving and receiving affection
4. *Need for recognition:* self-esteem, sense of self-worth, self-confidence, and capability
5. *Need for self-actualization:* self-fulfillment and creative growth

Although these needs vary with time and circumstance, they help us understand the motivations and actions of others. As summarized in Box 9.1, a complex set of factors influence what a person eats.

FIG. 9.1 A family sharing food. Sharing food with visitors to your home is an established custom among many cultural and ethnic groups. (Reprinted with permission from Food and Nutrition Service, US Department of Agriculture and Food and Nutrition Information Center, National Agricultural Library: *SNAP-Ed Connection: SNAP-Ed photo gallery*, Beltsville, MD, 2005, US Department of Agriculture. https://snaped.fns.usda.gov/photo-gallery?mode=mealtime.)

Data from Sloan AE: The top ten food trends, *Food Technol* 69(4):24, 2015 and Sloan AE: Top ten functional food trends, *Food Technol* 70(4):24, 2016.

BOX 9.1 Factors Influencing Food Choices

Environmental Factors
- Food availability
- Food technology
- Geography, agriculture, food distribution
- Personal economics, income
- Sanitation, housing
- Season, climate
- Storage and cooking facilities

Social Factors
- Advertising
- Culture
- Education, food and nutrition knowledge
- Political and economic policies
- Religion and social customs
- Social class role, peer pressure
- Social problems, poverty, alcoholism
- Distance from food outlets (e.g., grocery stores, restaurants)

Physiologic Factors
- Allergy, food tolerance or intolerance
- Physical disability
- Health-disease status
- Personal food acceptance
- Energy or nutrient needs
- Medical nutrition therapy

BOX 9.2 Current Food Trends

- Gray matters—promoting foods attractive to the growing elderly population
- Rethinking natural—attention to foods that are local, organic, and minimally processed
- Food MD—choosing foods to improve health; seeking healthy convenience foods
- Exclusion diets—adopting diets that are gluten free, lactose free, low in sodium and sugar
- Cook-less meals—looking at one-dish meals; meals prepared in less than 20 min
- Good mornings—healthy starts, taking breakfast with you
- Men in the aisles—men more involved with food shopping and meal preparation

THE FOOD ENVIRONMENT

Food in the Marketplace

Family, ethnic, and regional ties are strong influences in our lives, but new technology and mass media can displace old patterns with new practices. New ethnic flavors are gaining in popularity, and parents or grandparents who took pride in the dishes they prepared can be disheartened if children like the frozen version better. More than 28% of Americans live alone and are a target for single-serving packaging.[5] More than half of at-home meals include at least one semi-prepared item such as precut vegetables, precooked meat loaf, or heat-and-serve mashed potatoes. With the busy lifestyles of parents, children, and singles, 46% of all meals are eaten alone, with family members accessing the kitchen at a time that accommodates their meal preferences and schedules.[5]

According to a national survey, taste, price, and health, in that order, drive the food purchases of the American public. Nevertheless, convenience influences the food purchases of half of the population, and land sustainability was a factor for 40% of the shoppers interviewed. Approximately one-third of consumers indicated they are trying to reduce their food waste by better planning and use of leftovers.[6]

Meal Solutions

The on-the-go lifestyle of the American public has also influenced food shopping and meal preparation (Box 9.2). One food writer described the food goals of the current generation as "gourmet convenience," although a growing number of consumers describe themselves as recreational cooks.[7] Among persons ages 18 to 35, immediate consumption—occasions when food is eaten within one hour of purchase—accounted for 40% of all eating occasions that were not restaurant meals. Consumers are eating more meals at home: families eat dinner at home at least 5 times each week and young adults eat at home at least 4 times each week. Frozen meals are more popular among persons older than 65 years.[7]

Race and ethnicity influence the use of convenience foods and related nutrient intake. The scanning of supermarket items at checkout has enabled the evaluation of items purchased by consumers over time. An evaluation of purchases of more than 157,000 households compared (1) items that required cooking (e.g., sugar, rice, fresh meats); (2) ready-to-heat items (e.g., canned soup, frozen dinners); and (3) ready-to-eat items (e.g., bread, deli items, precut vegetables).[8] Black and Hispanic households had higher purchases of foods requiring cooking and lower purchases of ready-to-eat items than white households. Hispanic households purchased more rice and black households purchased more sugar and fresh meats. Based on records of purchase, black households had higher intakes of saturated fat and sugar than white or Hispanic groups, suggesting that cooking practices influence nutrient intake.[8]

Fresh items can be combined for a quick and healthy meal. A rotisserie chicken from the supermarket or roasted chicken from a fast-food restaurant served with a frozen vegetable and fruit or salad in place of French fries is moderate in kcalories and nutrient dense. A frozen vegetable can be cooked in the microwave in the time it takes to set the table and get the family seated. Packaged salad greens provide a quick addition to a meal. Helping families identify low-fat and nutrient-dense accompaniments to fresh and convenience items improves the nutrition of all family members.

Eating Frequency

The number of eating occasions throughout the day and the time of day that an individual eats influence energy intake and health. Based on a recent National Health and Nutrition Examination Survey (NHANES), 59% of men and 63% of women eat three meals each day, whereas 19% did not eat breakfast and 21% did not eat lunch; only about 8% did not eat dinner.[8] Snacks may take the place of meals, because 90% of those interviewed reported at least one snack for the day and approximately two-thirds had two or more snacks. Both genders obtained nearly one-fourth of their total energy intake from snacks, with after-dinner snacks supplying about 15% of the daily intake.[9] Snacking (defined as any food or beverage other than water taken between meals) is a topic of much discussion among health professionals. Although excessive snacking can contribute to unwanted weight gain, a snack in midmorning or midafternoon can prevent excessive hunger and overeating at the next meal.

Meal frequency has been related to cardiovascular risk and the development of metabolic syndrome.[10] Skipping breakfast alters glucose and insulin metabolism and often leads to overeating later in the day. Such unfavorable alterations in glucose and lipid metabolism increase the risk of diabetes and heart disease and have been associated with excessive night eating. The American Heart Association recommends that health professionals address meal frequency with their patients, in support of healthy lifestyles and reduced cardiometabolic risk.[11]

Smaller meals with snacks (a grazing pattern) rather than one or two very large meals can be a healthy eating pattern *if* the foods being eaten are selected wisely. Individuals who are physically active can benefit from eating more frequently. Older adults who snack are more likely to meet their energy requirement than those who do not snack.[12] Snacking on fruits, vegetables, low-fat dairy foods, low-fat grain products, or protein foods such as peanut butter or hard-cooked eggs adds important nutrients with low to moderate kcalories.

Changing Family Patterns

Extended working hours for parents and increasing sport and club activities for children make it difficult to manage family meals; as a result, the number of middle and high school students eating meals with their families has declined. This is especially true among girls, Asian families, and limited-resource families.[13] Nevertheless, 44% of adolescents still eat at least five meals a week with their parents. Eating together as a family influences nutritional and emotional well-being. The more meals children eat with their parents, the greater their intakes of calcium-rich foods, fruits, and vegetables and the more likely they are to be of normal weight.[14] Moreover, youth who have dinner regularly with their families do better in school and are less likely to use tobacco, alcohol, and drugs.[13] Family meals also influence the food practices of parents, as mothers and fathers eating more meals with their children eat more fruits and vegetables.[15]

Who is responsible for food-related activities in the family is also changing. Food marketing statistics indicate that 43% of men are the primary food shoppers in their families and 46% help with food preparation.[16] Healthy food is an important criterion for male food shoppers. By assuming more responsibility for food shopping and meal preparation, men are providing important role models for children and youth. (See the Perspectives in Practice box, "Returning to Hands-On Food," for ideas on how to get started preparing healthy meals.)

Health Concerns

Americans continue to experience frustration regarding the ever-changing nutrition messages flowing from the mass media. In a recent poll, consumers noted that choosing what they should or should not eat was more difficult than figuring out their taxes.[17] Consumers nowadays tend to identify a "healthy" food on the basis of what it does not contain—components such as additives, salt, saturated fat, or sugar, and approximately half consider a healthy diet to be "the right mix of foods." Nearly three-fourths of responders to a recent poll were making an effort to lose weight, and more than two-thirds were trying to consume smaller portions, choose more whole grains, and cut back on foods with added sugars. Eighty-one percent were attempting to make small changes to eat a more healthy diet such as choosing more fruits and vegetables. Parents appear to worry more about the healthfulness of their children's diets than about their own.[17] Consumers are seeking more information about the food they eat, presenting a challenge for health professionals.

PERSPECTIVES IN PRACTICE

Returning to Hands-On Food

As the pace of life quickens with growing responsibilities of work, school, and child care, preparing meals at home can seem to be a daunting task. Families perceive lack of time as a major barrier to healthful eating; however, lack of confidence in being able to plan a menu or successfully cook a meal that will be acceptable to family members also contributes to limited home preparation. Poor preparation skills add to the time required to prepare meals at home. Involving adolescents in meal preparation has been shown to improve dietary intake in this important age group and other family members as well.

Following are some ways to begin to develop skills for quick and healthy meals:

- *Obtain a family cookbook to help you get started:* The Academy of Nutrition and Dietetics, American Heart Association, and American Diabetes Association offer cookbooks with quick and easy recipes that can be prepared in 30 min and support healthy eating for all ages and chronic diseases.
- *Supplement take-out foods with healthy items prepared at home:* Add a frozen vegetable or salad and oven-browned French fries (made with frozen potato strips) to the chicken or hamburgers purchased on the way home.
- *Try to make foods in advance to keep in your freezer for quick meals:* Instead of making a meat loaf in a loaf pan, make individual meat loaves in a muffin pan. The muffin meat loaves cook in half the time of a regular meat loaf, and leftovers can be frozen individually to thaw and heat as needed. If possible, double a recipe for a stew or casserole to have one meal for now and one meal for another time.
- *Use cut-up chicken parts that can be prepared quickly on the cooktop or in the oven:* Look for recipes that use canned low-sodium chicken broth or low-sodium soups as ready-made sauces.

- *Look for skillet meals or casseroles that mix a protein food with pasta or vegetables:* Consider skillet lasagna, tuna noodle casserole, macaroni and cheese, or chicken and broccoli; one-pot cooking also makes for quick clean-up. Begin to substitute whole grain pasta for refined pasta.
- *Get familiar with legumes:* Lentils and dried green peas can be added directly to a recipe without soaking; make a pot of lentil soup in the evening or on a weekend afternoon to take care of a dinner the following week.
- *Get friendly with vegetables:* When fresh vegetables are out of season and costly, or when time is short, frozen or canned vegetables that are minimally processed are a good option for adding color, texture, and nutrients to your meal; add some cut-up broccoli or carrots to traditional casseroles. Avoid frozen vegetables with added sauces that usually add sodium and fat.

If you have not been cooking, then start by preparing just one or two meals a week. See how quickly you develop your cooking skills and perfect some favorite recipes!

Bibliography

Berge JM, MacLehose RF, Larson N, et al: Family food preparation and its effects on adolescent dietary quality and eating patterns, *J Adolesc Health* 59(5):530, 2016.

Horning ML, Fulkerson JA, Friend SE, et al: Reasons parents buy prepackaged, processed meals: it is more complicated than "I don't have time." *J Nutr Educ Behav* 49(1):60, 2017.

Lavelle F, McGowan L, Spence M, et al: Barriers and facilitators to cooking from 'scratch' using basic or raw ingredients: a qualitative interview study, *Appetite* 107:383, 2016.

Utter J, Denny S: Supporting families to cook at home and eat together: findings from a feasibility study, *J Nutr Educ Behav* 48(10):716, 2016.

EXPANDING THE FOOD SUPPLY: BIOTECHNOLOGY AND THE CONSUMER

Throughout human history, new scientific discoveries have created challenges for society. Biotechnology as it relates to agriculture, food processing, and the environment holds the potential to increase the quantity and quality of our food supply. This field of science allows us to alter the deoxyribonucleic acid (DNA) of a plant or animal species by adding or removing a particular gene, likened to cutting a circle of tape, inserting a different piece, and rejoining both ends to the new piece. This technique has been used to develop new varieties of rice with improved nutrient content and crops with enhanced resistance to disease. However, questions remain about the safety of the food produced using these methods. We will examine some of these issues and the process for biosafety review.

Genetically Modified Plants

Genetically modified (GM) organisms are plants or bacteria in which the natural DNA has been changed in some way to produce a desired trait. Genetic modification can take place through plant breeding methods or through biotechnology. Genetic engineering was first applied in the pharmaceutical industry, and GM bacteria produce human insulin for managing diabetes.

GM food crops were first introduced in the 1990s, and their use has grown dramatically. In the United States the use of GM seeds is regulated by the US Food and Drug Administration (FDA), the Environmental Protection Agency (EPA), and the US Department of Agriculture (USDA).

Goals for Genetic Modification

Since humans first began to cultivate plants, various practices have been used to improve the yield or desirability of particular species. The use of Mendel's principles of inheritance and the development of hybrid plants led to new varieties of wheat and rice with improved yields. Such advances have increased the food supply in the developing world.

Genetic modification of food plants has three goals:

1. *Increased resistance to insects and disease:* If plants carry a protein that acts as a built-in insecticide, farmers can reduce their use of pesticides and herbicides.
2. *Increased tolerance to weather conditions:* Varieties able to survive more extreme environmental conditions are less likely to be destroyed by a late frost.
3. *Increased nutritional value:* Genetic modification increased the monounsaturated fatty acid content of soybean oil. Grains with increased protein and micronutrients have lessened nutrient deficiencies in developing nations.

Corn, soybeans, rapeseed (canola oil), potatoes, tomatoes, and squash are among the genetically altered food crops approved for use in the United States.

Safety of Genetically Modified Crops

Both scientists and consumers have voiced concerns about GM foods as follows:

- *Risk of allergic reaction:* Transfer of a known allergen into a new food, such as adding a peanut allergen to a corn plant, would make the modified plant unsafe for persons with the allergy.
- *Potential toxicity:* Any added DNA must be compared with a protein database to identify any known harmful protein.
- *Danger to the environment:* Transferring insect-resistant genes to weeds or invasive plants could be harmful to helpful insects such as butterflies. Farmers should confine GM plants to specific growing areas so as not to contaminate conventional species.

In response to these concerns, the FDA has implemented strict procedures for the review and testing of food products originating from genetically engineered plants and animals. Petitions must be submitted and all testing completed before such a food can enter the marketplace or be used as feed for animals intended for human food. Both government and professional organizations have declared GM foods as safe. Current US labeling regulations do not require the identification of a food originating from GM sources *unless* the modification has altered its nutrient content.[18] Label identification of all GM foods would provide the information needed for consumers who wish to avoid such foods.

Biotechnology and Animal Foods

Marker-Assisted Breeding

Conventional breeding methods have produced eggs with less cholesterol and beef with reduced fat. Marker-assisted breeding, which combines the skills of classic breeders and molecular geneticists, offers potential for the development of healthy animal foods. When geneticists identify existing DNA patterns that influence traits such as fat composition, breeders can better select for these characteristics.

Bovine Growth Hormone

Growth hormone has an essential role in the growth, development, and health of all animals and humans. Bovine growth hormone (BGH) extracted from the pituitary glands of cattle has long been used to boost milk production. When it became possible to synthesize bovine somatotropin (bST) using recombinant DNA, farmers petitioned the FDA and were granted permission to use recombinant bovine somatotropin (rbST) in their dairy herds. Testing indicated that milk from rbST-treated cows does not differ in bST content from milk obtained from nontreated cows.

When assessing risk as related to a food or biological procedure, answers are seldom clear-cut; no action by either a government agency or an individual is ever completely risk free. Risk is evaluated according to potential benefits versus potential harm and usually involves numerous and often subtle variables. Research evidence must form the basis for judgments that serve the public interest.

OVERSIGHT OF THE FOOD SUPPLY: REGULATION AND INFORMATION

Shared Regulatory System: USDA and FDA

Regulation of the food supply began more than 100 years ago when Congress charged the USDA with safeguarding the nation's food. Early on, the USDA initiated on-site inspection of meatpacking and poultry-processing plants, which continues nowadays. The FDA is responsible for the safety of all foods except meat and poultry. These two agencies work with the EPA to ensure that pesticide residues do not exceed tolerance standards. The USDA, FDA, and Centers for Disease Control and Prevention (CDC) work together to prevent the introduction and spread of such hazards as avian flu or investigate and recall products associated with outbreaks of foodborne illness.

Food and Drug Administration

The FDA enforces all federal regulations intended to keep our food supply safe, pure, and wholesome (Box 9.3). Included in this mandate is the power to seize contaminated and unsafe food, whether grown and processed in the United States or entering from elsewhere. Because it is impossible to inspect all food products before they are sold, the FDA has developed procedures to lower the risk of contamination. These procedures, referred to as *Hazard Analysis and Critical Control Points* (HACCP), identify potential sources of contamination and help food processing plant managers set up ways to control them. The joint

- Ensure that processed foods are free of pathogens and contaminants
- Inspect food-processing facilities (other than meat and poultry plants)
- Approve food additives
- Monitor the content of infant formulas and medical foods
- Oversee nutrition labeling including approval of health claims
- Check shipments of imported foods for purity
- Approve drugs and supplements added to animal feeds

efforts of the FDA and USDA to implement HACCP procedures in poultry processing are credited with reducing by half the number of chickens contaminated with *Salmonella*.

Food Safety Laws

Approval Process for Drugs

The control of drugs by the FDA began in 1938 with the passage of the Federal Food, Drug, and Cosmetic Act (FFDCA). Any new drug, whether developed in the United States or elsewhere, must undergo extensive testing, often extending over a period of years. The manufacturer must present convincing scientific evidence that the product meets the legal standard of "safe and effective." Formal FDA approval is necessary before the drug can be sold.

Regulation of Food Ingredients and Food Additives

Manufacturers of all foods and food additives are legally obligated to assure the public that their products are safe. For conventional foods the FFDCA requires that the food and all ingredients not be "ordinarily injurious." Ingredients with a long history of use are assumed safe, and such food items may be marketed without prior FDA approval. Cookies made with flour, brown sugar, eggs, butter, and baking soda would meet this standard.

In 1960 the FFDCA was expanded to create two legal classes of food additives described as follows:

1. *Generally recognized as safe (GRAS):* The GRAS list includes all food additives and ingredients that were marketed before 1958. The GRAS list includes thousands of additives. One example is the yellow coloring added to margarine that has been in use since the 1930s. Under the law a food is unsafe if an additive "may render injurious" the food product. Food processors are not required to obtain FDA approval to use GRAS list additives; however, the presumed safety of these additives was based on their wide previous use; most were not tested. In 1977 Congress directed the FDA to begin testing the additives on the list, and this is continuing.
2. *Food additives developed since 1958:* For these additives the same legal standard of "may render injurious" applies, but they must undergo rigid testing before approval is obtained. Splenda (sucralose), a nonnutritive sweetener described in Chapter 3, went through the FDA approval process and is now being sold.

Dietary Supplements

Dietary supplements enjoy a very favorable legal status. In 1994 Congress passed the Dietary Supplement Health and Education Act (DSHEA), which effectively deregulated the dietary supplement industry.[19] All substances marketed as supplements prior to 1994 were assumed to be safe, whether or not research evidence supported this claim. The dietary supplement industry markets thousands of products containing vitamins, minerals, amino acids, herbs, botanical compounds, Asian medicinal herbals, and related substances. Under

the law these supplements are classified as neither foods nor drugs. No scientific testing demonstrating either product safety or effectiveness is required. For supplement ingredients developed since 1994, the safety standard is simply that there be no "unreasonable risk." The manufacturer must notify the FDA 75 days before marketing a product containing a new dietary ingredient, but no prior approval is required.

The DSHEA is a controversial law. Dietary supplements are a major industry, with a wide range of products, from single vitamins to complex mixtures. Although a dietary supplement cannot claim to cure a disease, statements about how the human body will respond to the supplement, such as a claim that it will make you burn away unwanted fat, require no substantiating evidence. Supplements containing growth hormone, testosterone, or potentially harmful substances said to restore youthful vitality are often marketed to older adults. Regulations are urgently needed to ensure consumer safety and honest claims describing appropriate use, expected effects, recommended dose, and potential interactions with prescription drugs, herbs, and nutrients.

Agricultural Chemicals

Agricultural chemicals control destructive insects and weeds, improve seed sprouting to increase yield, and prevent plant diseases; however, overuse adds to food pesticide residues and increases farm workers' exposure. Researchers are helping farmers reduce their use of chemical pesticides through integrated pest management, which uses the natural enemies of insect pests to decrease their population. The FDA has the task of assessing health risks and establishing guidelines for the thousands of agricultural chemicals in development and use.

Organically produced foods—grown without the use of chemical pesticides and herbicides—are growing in status as consumers become more concerned about the safety of their food. Organic foods now constitute 4% of all US food sales, with revenues exceeding $35 billion. Fruits and vegetables make up 43% of all organic foods sold.[20] Most organic foods (93%) are sold in conventional and natural food supermarkets, although farmer's markets featuring local sales are growing in number. National standards that govern growing procedures and postharvest handling have been established for producers who wish to label their food as "organic." The USDA must certify farmers before they can use the seal of the National Organic Program (Fig. 9.2).

FIG. 9.2 Seal of the National Organic Program. The US Department of Agriculture has developed a certification program to enable organic farmers to label their produce as *organically grown*. (From National Organic Program, Agricultural Marketing Service, US Department of Agriculture: *The organic seal,* Washington, DC, 2012, US Department of Agriculture. https://www.ams.usda.gov/rules-regulations/organic/organic-seal.)

Water Contamination

Indiscriminate dumping of waste has raised the concentrations of polychlorinated biphenyls (PCBs), heavy metals such as mercury, and other toxic substances in inland and ocean waters. These pollutants are transferred to fish, shellfish, and other wildlife living in or drinking these waters and then to the humans who eat them. State and local health departments post advisories to fishermen regarding the safety of fish caught in local waters, and the FDA monitors the mercury content of ocean and farm-raised fish sold in the United States. Although fish is valued for the protein and omega-3 fatty acids it contains, women who are pregnant or nursing or who may become pregnant should monitor their intake and choose fish low in mercury (Fig. 9.3). This FDA advisory also applies to young children, based on the damaging effect of mercury on the developing nervous system.[21]

Government Agencies Responsible for Food Education

Just as several federal agencies share responsibility for food safety, so several units partner to provide food and health information for consumers. The US Department of Health and Human Services (USDHHS) is the major source of health information. The USDA focuses on food and diet with responsibility for the *Dietary Guidelines for Americans* and MyPlate (http://www.choosemyplate.gov). The FDA oversees consumer food and drug education and reviews food labels, food health claims, and false advertising.

Food Labels

To choose food wisely, consumers must know what nutrients they need, the amounts, and where to find them. Over the past 30 years the FDA, with the advice of experts representing agriculture, foods, nutrition, and health, has developed a framework for food labeling to help individuals monitor their nutrient intake.

Early Efforts at Food Labeling

In the mid-1970s new requirements were set for the food label. All cans and packages had to provide content information including weight, list of ingredients, and the name and address of the manufacturer (Fig. 9.4). The goal at that time was to protect consumers from economic risk—giving true information about food weight and ingredients—not health risk. However, surveys indicated that consumers wanted more nutrition information, including amounts of carbohydrate, fat, and protein, total number of kcalories, and key vitamins and minerals.

Original Nutrition Facts Label

The original nutrition facts label became law under the Nutrition Labeling and Education Act of 1990 and took effect in 1994 (Fig. 9.5). It was required on all prepared or processed foods, including bread, cereal, canned and frozen food, snacks, desserts, and beverages, but was voluntary for fresh fruits, fresh vegetables, and seafood. The nutrition facts label describing the serving size and nutrient content of the contained food as compared with recommended nutrient intakes enabled consumers to compare the nutritional value of one product with another and make an informed choice. Health claims on the food label provided additional information to help consumers lower their risk of chronic disease.

New Nutrition Facts Label

Since the original nutrition facts label was introduced in 1994, our knowledge of nutrition science has expanded and the food patterns and health of the American people have worsened. The prevalence of obesity has escalated across all age groups, and foods high in kcalories

and added sugars but low in nutrient density make up a growing proportion of the American diet. Portion sizes have increased such that the reference servings used in the development of the original nutrition label no longer represent what individuals actually eat. The new nutrition facts label addresses these issues while continuing important information included on the original label.[22] It also portrays a new and refreshed design that draws attention to kcalories and portion size, and other issues important to health. (Compare the original and new nutrition facts labels in Fig. 9.5.)[23]

Kcalories and serving sizes

- *Reference servings.* The food portions consumed by the US population have increased greatly over the past 20 years and so have the kcalories that accompany them. Reference servings on nutrition labels should reflect what individuals actually eat, not what health professionals recommend they eat; thus the reference servings used in labeling have been adjusted to accommodate current eating patterns.
- *Number of servings in a package.* The number of servings in the package as described on the original nutrition facts label was often misunderstood. A food package perceived by the general public to contain a 1-cup single serving, typically eaten in one sitting, might be labeled as two, ½ cup servings; consequently, the portion actually consumed contained twice the kcalories expected. The new nutrition label requires that packages containing between 150% and 200% of the reference serving, such as a 20-oz can of soda or a 15-oz can of soup, must be labeled as containing one serving. Packages containing between 200% and 400% of the reference serving will require dual labeling, listing information both per serving and per package. (See Fig. 9.6 describing this concept.)
- *Number of kcalories contained in one serving and/or per package* now occupies a prominent place on the new nutrition facts label to assist consumers in weight management.

Macronutrient content

- *Carbohydrate:* Total carbohydrate (includes starch, all sugar, and dietary fiber) is listed in grams; dietary fiber and sugars are also listed separately. The 2015 Dietary Guidelines for Americans recommended that consumers limit their intakes of added sugars to no more than 10% of their total kcalorie intake. The original nutrition label indicated the amount of sugar in a food but did not specify how much was added sugar. The new label provides consumers with the amount of added sugar and the total sugar (naturally occurring sugar plus added sugar) in the food portion.
- *Fat:* The new nutrition facts label will continue to note the amounts of total fat, saturated fat, and *trans fats* per portion but will not list the total kcalories coming from fat. This change reflects current thinking that the type of dietary fat is more important to health than the percentage of kcalories obtained from fat. Cholesterol content is listed in milligrams.
- *Protein:* The protein content of a food portion continues to be listed in grams.

Vitamins and minerals

- Sodium and four leader nutrients—vitamin D, calcium, potassium, and iron—are required on the new nutrition label. Sodium is listed in milligrams and as a percentage of the suggested upper limit of 2300 mg.
- Leader nutrients: The original nutrition label drew attention to calcium, iron, vitamin A, and vitamin C, problem nutrients at that time. Recent US dietary surveys have revealed that many population groups are deficient in calcium, iron, vitamin D, and potassium, nutrients with important roles in the prevention of chronic disease, and these nutrients are now mandatory on the new label.

Advice About Eating Fish

What Pregnant Women & Parents Should Know

Fish and other protein-rich foods have nutrients that can help your child's growth and development.

For women of childbearing age (about 16–49 years old), especially pregnant and breastfeeding women, and for parents and caregivers of young children.

- *Eat 2 to 3 servings of fish a week from the "Best Choices" list OR 1 serving from the "Good Choices" list.*
- *Eat a variety of fish.*
- *Serve 1 to 2 servings of fish a week to children, starting at age 2.*
- *If you eat fish caught by family or friends, check for fish advisories. If there is no advisory, eat only one serving and no other fish that week.**

Use this chart!

You can use this chart to help you choose which fish to eat, and how often to eat them, based on their mercury levels. The "Best Choices" have the lowest levels of mercury.

What is a serving?

To find out, use the palm of your hand!

For an adult 4 ounces

For children, ages 4 to 7 2 ounces

Best Choices EAT 2 TO 3 SERVINGS A WEEK

Anchovy	Herring	Scallop
Atlantic croaker	Lobster, American and spiny	Shad
Atlantic mackerel	Mullet	Shrimp
Black sea bass	Oyster	Skate
Butterfish	Pacific chub mackerel	Smelt
Catfish	Perch, freshwater and ocean	Sole
Clam	Pickerel	Squid
Cod	Plaice	Tilapia
Crab	Pollock	Trout, freshwater
Crawfish	Salmon	Tuna, canned light (includes skipjack)
Flounder	Sardine	Whitefish
Haddock		Whiting
Hake		

OR Good Choices EAT 1 SERVING A WEEK

Bluefish	Monkfish
Buffalofish	Rockfish
Carp	Sablefish
Chilean sea bass/ Patagonian toothfish	Sheepshead
Grouper	Snapper
Halibut	Spanish mackerel
Mahi mahi/ dolphinfish	Striped bass (ocean)
	Tilefish (Atlantic Ocean)
	Tuna, albacore/ white tuna, canned and fresh/frozen
	Tuna, yellowfin
	Weakfish/seatrout
	White croaker/ Pacific croaker

Choices to Avoid HIGHEST MERCURY LEVELS

King mackerel	Shark
Marlin	Swordfish
Orange roughy	Tilefish (Gulf of Mexico)
	Tuna, bigeye

www.FDA.gov/fishadvice
www.EPA.gov/fishadvice

EPA United States Environmental Protection Agency   FDA U.S. FOOD & DRUG ADMINISTRATION

*Some fish caught by family and friends, such as larger carp, catfish, trout and perch, are more likely to have fish advisories due to mercury or other contaminants. State advisories will tell you how often you can safely eat those fish.

THIS ADVICE REFERS TO FISH AND SHELLFISH COLLECTIVELY AS "FISH." / ADVICE UPDATED JANUARY 2017

FIG. 9.3 Advice about eating fish: what pregnant women and parents should know. High levels of mercury as found in some ocean fish are harmful to brain development in the fetus and young child. The US Food and Drug Administration provides advice on fish that is safe and fish to be avoided and the relative amounts that can be safely consumed. (This handout can be downloaded for distribution and public information.) (From U.S. Environmental Protection Agency, US Food and Drug Administration, January 2017. https://www.fda.gov/Food/FoodborneIllnessContaminants/Metals/ucm393070.htm.)

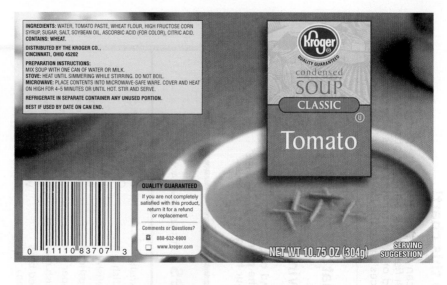

INGREDIENTS: WATER, TOMATO PASTE, WHEAT FLOUR, HIGH FRUCTOSE CORN SYRUP, SUGAR, SALT, SOYBEAN OIL, ASCORBIC ACID (FOR COLOR), CITRIC ACID.
CONTAINS: WHEAT.

DISTRIBUTED BY THE KROGER CO.,
CINCINNATI, OHIO 45202

PREPARATION INSTRUCTIONS:
MIX SOUP WITH ONE CAN OF WATER OR MILK.
STOVE: HEAT UNTIL SIMMERING WHILE STIRRING. DO NOT BOIL.
MICROWAVE: PLACE CONTENTS INTO MICROWAVE-SAFE WARE. COVER AND HEAT ON HIGH FOR 4–5 MINUTES OR UNTIL HOT. STIR AND SERVE.

REFRIGERATE IN SEPARATE CONTAINER ANY UNUSED PORTION.

BEST IF USED BY DATE ON CAN END.

QUALITY GUARANTEED
If you are not completely satisfied with this product, return it for a refund or replacement.

Comments or Questions?
☎ 888-632-6900
🖥 www.kroger.com

0 11110 83707 3

Kroger
QUALITY GUARANTEED
condensed
SOUP
CLASSIC
Ⓤ
Tomato

NET WT 10.75 OZ (304g)   SERVING SUGGESTION

FIG. 9.4 Example of a food label. Notice that this label also informs the consumer that the product contains wheat—one of eight food allergens that must be clearly stated to protect individuals having this allergy. (Courtesy The Kroger Company, Cincinnati, OH.)

FIG. 9.5 The original nutrition facts label as compared with the new nutrition facts label for this fictional product. The new Nutrition Facts label reflects new dietary recommendations and draws attention to calories, serving size, and nutrients lacking in the US diet. The new label also indicates how much of the sugar found in the food is added sugar, as compared to the total sugar present which includes any naturally-occurring sugar. (From US Food and Drug Administration, Silver Spring, MD. http://www.fda.gov/Food/Guidance Regulation/GuidanceDocumentsRegulatoryInformation/LabelingNutrition/ucm385663.htm#images.)

SIDE-BY-SIDE COMPARISON

Original Label

Nutrition Facts
Serving Size 2/3 cup (55g)
Servings Per Container About 8

Amount Per Serving

Calories 230	Calories from Fat 72
	% Daily Value*
Total Fat 8g	**12%**
Saturated Fat 1g	**5%**
Trans Fat 0g	
Cholesterol 0mg	**0%**
Sodium 160mg	**7%**
Total Carbohydrate 37g	**12%**
Dietary Fiber 4g	**16%**
Sugars 1g	
Protein 3g	
Vitamin A	10%
Vitamin C	8%
Calcium	20%
Iron	45%

* Percent Daily Values are based on a 2,000 calorie diet. Your daily value may be higher or lower depending on your calorie needs.

	Calories:	2,000	2,500
Total Fat	Less than	65g	80g
Sat Fat	Less than	20g	25g
Cholesterol	Less than	300mg	300mg
Sodium	Less than	2,400mg	2,400mg
Total Carbohydrate		300g	375g
Dietary Fiber		25g	30g

New Label

Nutrition Facts
8 servings per container
Serving size   2/3 cup (55g)

Amount per serving
Calories   230

	% Daily Value*
Total Fat 8g	**10%**
Saturated Fat 1g	**5%**
Trans Fat 0g	
Cholesterol 0mg	**0%**
Sodium 160mg	**7%**
Total Carbohydrate 37g	**13%**
Dietary Fiber 4g	**14%**
Total Sugars 12g	
Includes 10g Added Sugars	**20%**
Protein 3g	
Vitamin D 2mcg	10%
Calcium 260mg	20%
Iron 8mg	45%
Potassium 235mg	6%

* The % Daily Value (DV) tells you how much a nutrient in a serving of food contributes to a daily diet. 2,000 calories a day is used for general nutrition advice.

Note: The images above are meant for illustrative purposes to show how the new Nutrition Facts label might look compared to the old label. Both labels represent fictional products. When the original hypothetical label was developed in 2014 (the image on the left-hand side), added sugars was not yet proposed so the "original" label shows 1g of sugar as an example. The image created for the "new" label (shown on the right-hand side) lists 12g total sugar and 10g added sugar to give an example of how added sugars would be broken out with a % Daily Value.

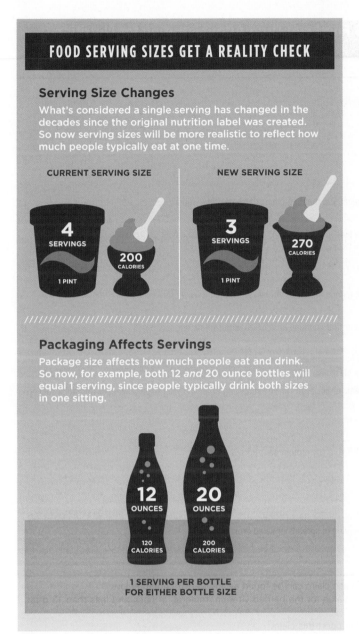

FOOD SERVING SIZES GET A REALITY CHECK

Serving Size Changes

What's considered a single serving has changed in the decades since the original nutrition label was created. So now serving sizes will be more realistic to reflect how much people typically eat at one time.

CURRENT SERVING SIZE | NEW SERVING SIZE

4 SERVINGS — 1 PINT — 200 CALORIES

3 SERVINGS — 1 PINT — 270 CALORIES

Packaging Affects Servings

Package size affects how much people eat and drink. So now, for example, both 12 *and* 20 ounce bottles will equal 1 serving, since people typically drink both sizes in one sitting.

12 OUNCES — 120 CALORIES

20 OUNCES — 200 CALORIES

1 SERVING PER BOTTLE
FOR EITHER BOTTLE SIZE

FIG. 9.6 Changes in Serving Size on the New Nutrition Facts Label. These changes in serving sizes more closely reflect the amount of food that people actually eat at one time. (From US Food and Drug Administration, Silver Spring, MD. https://www.fda.gov/downloads/Food/GuidanceRegulation/GuidanceDocumentsRegulatoryInformation/LabelingNutrition/UCM501663.pdf.)

Vitamin A and vitamin C intakes have become generally adequate in most US population groups and will no longer be mandatory, although they may be added.

Daily values

- *Origin:* The Daily Values (DVs) on the original nutrition label were derived from the 1968 edition of the Recommended Dietary Allowances (RDAs), the standards in use when the original label was developed. The DV represented the highest RDA for that nutrient among the various age and gender groups. For example, the DV for iron is 18 mg, the RDA for women of childbearing age. DVs for sodium, dietary fiber, and vitamin D have been updated on the new

label, based on new evidence from the National Academy of Medicine (formerly the Institute of Medicine) and recommendations of the 2015 Dietary Guidelines Advisory Committee.

- *Usefulness:* The DV serves two purposes: it establishes a maximum intake for a nutrient, such as fat, and it indicates the percentage of the daily requirement of a nutrient, such as calcium, that is contained in a serving. The %DV helps consumers understand the nutrition information in the context of a total daily diet. The new nutrition label includes the %DV for fats, carbohydrates, sodium, vitamin D, calcium, potassium, and iron, based on a reference diet of 2000 kcal. The footnote appearing on the new label has been simplified for consumer understanding: "The % Daily Value tells you how much a nutrient in a serving of food contributes to a daily diet. 2,000 calories a day is used for general nutrition advice." (Review the original and new nutrition facts label in Fig. 9.5.) It will be important to assist consumers in the use and interpretation of the new nutrition label. When consumers were surveyed regarding their understanding of the new nutrition label, 35% did not understand the meaning of Total and Added Sugars.[24] Final date for implementation of the new nutrition facts label is not definite at this time.

Nutrition Labeling for Special Conditions

Since the development of the original nutrition facts label, additional information has been added to the label to assist consumers having special health needs or interests, described as follows:

- *Health claims:* Health claims are label statements that imply a relationship between the consumption of a nutrient or food substance and a disease or health-related condition; however, there can be no suggestion that the nutrient or substance will cure or mitigate the condition.[25] Based on scientific evidence presented for review, the FDA has approved 12 health claims that address such relationships as calcium, vitamin D, and bone health; soluble fiber and heart health; and folate and neural tube defects (Table 9.1).[25]

- *Labels for special needs:* Some nutrition labels include information for the benefit of certain population groups. Animal foods processed under the supervision of a rabbi and meet Jewish dietary standards are labeled as *kosher*.

- *Presence of specific substances:* Foods or beverages containing aspartame must include a warning for the safety of individuals with phenylketonuria, who must avoid the amino acid phenylalanine found in this nonnutritive sweetener. The Food Allergen Labeling and Consumer Protection Act requires that foods containing any amount of a major allergen known to cause anaphylactic shock in allergic individuals must be so labeled. These eight allergens are (1) milk (casein), (2) peanuts, (3) tree nuts, (4) fish, (5) shellfish, (6) wheat, (7) eggs, and (8) soybeans.[25] Casein, eggs, wheat flour, and soy are sometimes added in very small amounts to product formulations to provide texture or stability and would not be apparent to the general consumer if not included on the label. In that very minute amounts of these substances can have lethal consequences in allergic individuals, a label warning must be included. Fig. 9.4 provides such an example, as one might not expect to find a wheat ingredient in tomato soup. With sweet baked items, it is common to see the notation "this product was produced in a plant that also processes peanuts." It is estimated that 1 in 133 persons in the United States has celiac disease, an immune disorder characterized by a response to gluten, a protein found in wheat, rye, barley, and sometimes oats. To prevent resulting damage to the

TABLE 9.1   Health Claims Approved by the US Food and Drug Administration for Nutrition Labels[a]

Claim	Food Requirement
Calcium and osteoporosis and calcium, vitamin D, and osteoporosis	High in calcium[b] High in calcium and vitamin D
Sodium and hypertension	Low in sodium
Dietary fat and cancer	Low fat
Dietary saturated fat and cholesterol and risk of coronary heart disease	Low saturated fat Low cholesterol Low fat
Fiber-containing grain products, fruits, and vegetables, and cancer	A grain product, fruit, or vegetable that is a good source of dietary fiber Low fat
Fruits, vegetables, and grain products that contain fiber, particularly soluble fiber, and risk of coronary heart disease	A fruit, vegetable, or grain product that contains at least 0.6 g soluble fiber per reference serving Low saturated fat Low cholesterol Low fat
Fruits and vegetables and cancer	A fruit or vegetable that is a good source of vitamin A, vitamin C, or dietary fiber Low fat
Folate and neural tube defects	A food or dietary supplement that contains at least 40 μg of folate per serving
Dietary noncariogenic carbohydrate sweeteners and dental caries	Sugar free Contains a Food and Drug Administration–approved sugar alcohol or other nonnutritive sweetener Food must not lower plaque pH to less than 5.7
Soluble fiber from certain foods and risk of coronary heart disease	Food must contain whole oats or barley or Oatrim, supplying at least 0.75 g soluble fiber per reference serving Low saturated fat Low cholesterol Low fat
Soy protein and risk of coronary heart disease[c]	Food must contain at least 6.25 g soy protein per reference serving Low saturated fat Low cholesterol Low fat
Plant sterol/stanol esters and risk of coronary heart disease	Contains at least 0.65 g plant sterol esters per reference serving of spreads/salad dressings *or* at least 1.7 g plant stanol esters per serving of spreads or salad dressings Low saturated fat Low cholesterol

[a]Further details relating to the justification and model label statement for each claim can be found at the website noted below.
[b]Food contains, without fortification, at least 10% of the Daily Reference Value for the named vitamin, mineral, or fiber, and less than 13 g fat, 4 g saturated fat, 60 mg cholesterol, and 480 mg sodium per serving.
[c]The claim for soy protein is now under review as new evidence may not support this claim.
Modified from US Food and Drug Administration: *Guidance for industry. A food labeling guide*, (11. *Appendix C: Health claims*) Rockville, MD, 2013 (updated August 2015), Author. https://www.fda.gov/food/ingredientspackaginglabeling/labelingnutrition/ucm2006876.htm

KEY TERMS

Anaphylactic Shock
A serious and sometimes fatal hypersensitivity reaction to a drug, food, toxin, chemical, or other allergen; the patient experiences weakness, sweating, and shortness of breath or such life-threatening responses as loss of blood pressure and shock, respiratory congestion, or cardiac arrest (see *allergens* next).

Allergens
Substances that cause a hypersensitivity reaction in the body; proteins found in milk, eggs, fish, shellfish, wheat, tree nuts (such as almonds or walnuts), peanuts, and soy can produce serious and sometimes fatal reactions in allergic individuals. The presence of these foods must be indicated on the food label.

lining of the gastrointestinal tract, patients must follow a gluten-free diet. The FDA has defined standards for products carrying the label of "gluten free" to help patients make informed choices.[26]

Public attention to the energy, fat, sodium, and cholesterol content of foods led to legal definitions for terms such as *low* or *reduced* to protect the public from inappropriate or misleading claims. Nevertheless, confusion about serving sizes and differences between the DVs used on the nutrition label and the Dietary Reference Intakes (DRIs) create misperceptions for users.

Food and Botanicals

New foods and beverages with added herbs or stimulants are blurring the distinction between food and supplements. One product receiving increased scrutiny is "energy drinks" that contain high levels of caffeine and may include added B vitamins, taurine (an amino acid), and the botanicals ginseng, ginkgo, or milk thistle.[27] Energy drinks can be marketed as foods or supplements. Those sold as supplements fall under the 1994 DSHEA,[28] enabling manufacturers to bypass label disclosure of ingredients that appear on the GRAS list, such as caffeine. Energy drinks usually contain approximately 80 to 140 mg of caffeine per 8-oz serving, the equivalent of 5 oz of coffee or two cans of caffeinated soft drinks; however, some energy drinks contain as much as 500 mg of caffeine per can—the equivalent of approximately 14 cans of caffeinated soft drinks.[29] A safe intake of caffeine is estimated to be less than 500 mg/day, although individuals with heart disease or liver disease or who take medications that slow the metabolism of caffeine need to consider a lower intake.[27]

Energy drinks and alcohol are a particularly dangerous combination, because the high caffeine content of the energy drink reduces the symptoms of intoxication, encouraging even greater alcohol consumption.[29] Excessive energy drink consumption has been related to caffeine-induced cardiac arrhythmias, which can be fatal.[30] Energy drinks often contain added sugar, adding unwanted kcalories to the diet.

THE PROBLEM OF MISINFORMATION: FOOD AND HEALTH

For centuries people have been anxious about the safety and wholesomeness of their food. Particular foods were believed to possess healing properties or, conversely, cause illness, and certain religious food laws are likely rooted in food safety. Remedies prepared from local plants and herbs were used to cure ailments and sickness. The Internet, Facebook, blogs, and other forms of electronic messaging are currently used to advertise food, drugs, herbs, and other plant botanicals as preventives or cures for common conditions. Some unsubstantiated beliefs about food or plant remedies or bogus drugs are harmless, but others carry serious dangers. False information may be embedded in folklore, built on half-truths, or stem from intentional deception. The FDA supports a vigorous campaign to prevent and prosecute false advertising for particular foods, supplements, or medicines.

False claims usually fall within one of the following categories:
1. The food or product will cure a specific disease or condition.
2. Certain food combinations have special therapeutic effects.
3. Only "natural" foods or plant remedies can meet body needs and prevent disease.

Misleading claims about the healing properties of certain foods or other substances delay appropriate health intervention, with a worsening of the illness and possible death. Patients with difficult-to-treat conditions such as cancer, diabetes, or arthritis are especially vulnerable to fraudulent claims for medicines that promise immediate cures and relief from pain. Diagnostic tests sold online are often the products of illegal pharmaceutical businesses and encourage the purchase of unneeded supplements sold by the same online supplier. Products formulated under unsanitary conditions or that contain harmful substances can lead to further illness or disability. Misleading advertising has a high economic cost. As much as $32 billion per year is spent on more than 85,000 supplement combinations, and many are unnecessary, ineffective, or, at worst, life threatening.[31]

The FDA Division of Consumer Education conducts an active program of public education through its website. A checklist to assist consumers in separating legitimate products and health advice from those that are harmful and waste money is presented in Box 9.4.

> ### BOX 9.4 Checklist for Spotting a Health Scam
>
> - Promises a quick or painless cure
> - Claims to be made from a special, secret, or ancient formula available from only one source
> - Uses testimonials or undocumented case histories from satisfied patients
> - Claims to be effective for a wide range of ailments
> - Claims to cure a disease, such as arthritis, diabetes, or Alzheimer disease, that medical professionals are not able to cure.

Modified from National Institute on Aging, US Department of Health and Human Services: *Age page. Beware of health scams,* Washington, DC, 2014, US Department of Health and Human Services.

FOOD SAFETY AND FOOD PROCESSING

In Chapter 1, we introduced the topic of food safety and the need for vigilance in preparing and handling food. Here we look at the pathogens that cause foodborne illness and how to prevent contamination on the journey from the farm to the market to the kitchen.

Foodborne Illness
Prevalence and Causes of Foodborne Illness
Many disease-producing microorganisms in our environment have the potential to contaminate our food and water, posing a serious threat to public health. New technologies ranging from refrigerated trucks to freeze-drying to food irradiation have brought major improvements in food handling and food safety; yet Americans are still vulnerable to foodborne pathogens. The distribution of food across continents by large corporations presents opportunities for organisms to enter the food chain and be spread regionally and globally. Fruits and vegetables are eaten without being washed. Families eat more precooked foods, seafood salads, and deli meats that are vulnerable to spoilage. Meals picked up at food outlets on the way home are kept warm for extended periods, in contrast to cooked meals eaten immediately after preparation. Those who eat at their desks or in their cars do not take time to wash their hands or use a hand sanitizer.

The CDC is responsible for tracking the incidence of foodborne illness and sharing their findings in an effort to improve food production and handling practices. According to most recent estimates, 1 in 6 Americans (or 48 million people) get sick, 128,000 are hospitalized, and 3000 die from foodborne illness each year.[32] Estimating both the true incidence of foodborne illness and the food responsible is difficult. First, many people experiencing illness assume it is the "flu" or other temporary upset and do not seek medical care. In addition, most of us eat various foods at a meal and are not able to identify the particular cause of any subsequent distress. The food or organism responsible for an outbreak is more likely to be identified if individuals receive medical treatment and provide a bacterial culture or if the outbreak involves an entire family or population who consumed the same food.

Types of Foodborne Illness
Food infection and food poisoning are two different forms of foodborne illness caused by microorganisms.
- *Bacterial food infection* occurs when individuals eat food contaminated with large colonies of bacteria.
- *Bacterial food poisoning* results from toxins produced by bacteria before the food was eaten.

Bacterial food infection. Six common pathogens cause food infection:

1. *Escherichia coli O157:H7:* Most classes of *E. coli* are benign, and some do nutritionally important work, such as fermenting resistant starch. However, *E. coli* O157:H7 produces a toxin that results in severe illness. Found naturally in the intestines of animals and humans, *E. coli* O157:H7 has emerged as a major cause of outbreaks of inflammatory diarrhea with bloody stool and fever. Serious infections can result in renal failure or death. *E. coli* O157:H7 is destroyed by heat, and most outbreaks arise from unpasteurized or undercooked food or contaminated water. Occurrences of *E. coli* O157:H7 infection have resulted from drinking unpasteurized cider made from apples that had fallen to the ground, been contaminated with animal droppings, and not thoroughly washed. These events led to the current emphasis on the pasteurization of juices and beverages. A major outbreak occurred with beef contaminated in processing and then undercooked by restaurants and at home.[33] The restaurant incident reminds us that all parties across the food chain—those who process food *and* those who prepare it—are responsible for food safety. Ground beef must be cooked to a temperature of 165°F to safely destroy *E. coli. E. coli* is also found in salad greens, which reinforces the need to thoroughly wash these foods.

2. *Salmonella: Salmonella* grow quickly in high-protein foods such as milk, custard, egg dishes, and sandwich fillings. Shellfish, such as oysters and clams harvested from polluted waters, are a source of infection. Contamination of eggs with *Salmonella enteritidis* is a worldwide problem. No one should eat raw cookie dough, drink unpasteurized beverages containing milk or egg, or eat undercooked eggs, but these rules are especially important for patients with impaired immune function. *Salmonella* infection is more serious in older adults; 49% of infected persons over age 65 require hospitalization as compared with 26% of younger adults, and death is more frequent.[34] Symptoms develop slowly, usually 12 to 24 hours after ingestion, with mild to bloody diarrhea and fever.

3. *Campylobacter: Campylobacter* is a cause of acute diarrhea in the United States and around the world. It is found in raw and undercooked beef, poultry, and seafood; raw milk; and untreated water. It is destroyed by heating food to 160°F or applying appropriate water purification methods. Cross-contamination, such as using a cutting board for raw poultry and then using it to chop lettuce without appropriate cleansing, is a major cause of infection. *Campylobacter* infection has been associated with Guillain-Barré syndrome and other neuropathies that occur months or years following the initial infection.[35]

4. *Shigella: Shigella* infection is usually confined to the large intestine and varies from simple cramps and diarrhea to fatal **dysentery.** Young children are at particular risk of fatal complications, and treatment with antibiotics may be required. *Shigella* are found in the intestinal tract of animals and in contaminated water. They are spread by insects and unsanitary food handling and grow rapidly in moist or protein foods such as milk, beans, tuna, and turkey. Apple cider or raw fruits and vegetables contaminated by animal droppings are sources of *Shigella.* Foods must be washed and cooked thoroughly and chilled quickly to prevent infection.

5. *Listeria:* This microorganism is a major cause of infection after surgery, but only recently was *Listeria monocytogenes* linked with foodborne illness. In pregnant women, it produces diarrhea and flulike fever and headache that can lead to miscarriage, stillbirth, and life-threatening infection of the newborn; other adults experience fever, muscle aches, confusion, loss of balance, and convulsions.[36] Outbreaks of *Listeria*-related illness have been traced to unpasteurized dairy products, particularly soft Mexican cheeses made with unpasteurized milk. Undercooked poultry and deli foods have been implicated in *Listeria* infections; accordingly, pregnant women are advised to heat to steaming all luncheon meats and processed meats to avoid exposure. Thorough cooking and careful washing of raw fruits and vegetables are other preventive measures (see the Focus on Food Safety box, "Do I Really Need to Wash That Melon?").

6. *Vibrio:* This family of bacteria includes *V. cholerae,* the pathogen causing cholera. The species generally associated with foodborne illness is *V. parahaemolyticus,* found in coastal waters. This is a salt-requiring organism and increases in number in warm weather. Persons who eat raw or undercooked fish, oysters, clams, or other shellfish are at high risk. Cuts or scrapes exposed to infested waters can also cause *Vibrio* infection. *V. parahaemolyticus* causes a watery diarrhea with abdominal cramps, vomiting, fever, and chills that usually last no more than 3 days, and many incidents go unreported. Individuals with compromised immune systems, liver disease, or alcoholism can have serious complications and require medical attention. *V. vulnificus,* a more virulent strain, usually requires hospitalization and can lead to death within a day or two of infection.[37]

Bacterial food poisoning. Foodborne illness arising from toxins already present in the food when it is eaten develops rapidly, with symptoms appearing within 1 to 6 hours. The two most common types of bacterial food poisoning are caused by *Staphylococcus* and *Clostridia* species:

Staphylococcal food poisoning: Staphylococcus aureus is a common cause of food poisoning that affects an estimated 240,000 individuals annually.[38] Symptoms come on suddenly and include severe cramping and abdominal pain with vomiting and diarrhea, sweating, headache, and fever, and in some cases shock and **prostration.** Recovery is fairly

FOCUS ON FOOD SAFETY

Do I Really Need to Wash That Melon?

Unwashed or poorly washed vegetables and fruits are common sources of foodborne illness. Produce can be contaminated with *E. coli* O157:H7, *Salmonella,* or *Cyclospora* through contact with animals, fertilizers containing animal waste, contaminated irrigation water, or poor sanitation practices of workers who pick or sort these crops.

Following are safety tips for preparing fresh fruits and vegetables:

- *Rinse raw produce under running water,* even if you are not going to eat the skin or rind. Any bacteria on the outer surface will be transferred to your hands or to the knife as you peel or cut and then to the food itself. Rub firm-skinned fruits and vegetables or scrub with a small vegetable brush.
- *Remove and discard the outermost leaves* of a head of lettuce or cabbage. Wash each lettuce leaf under running water. Do not dip the entire head of lettuce in a container of water. You may be rinsing in contaminated water.
- *Store fruits and vegetables in the refrigerator within 2 h of peeling or cutting.* Be especially careful with cut melon. Melons are low in acid as compared with oranges, apples, or pineapple, and this allows more rapid growth of bacteria on cut surfaces when the melon stands at room temperature.

KEY TERMS

Dysentery
Disorders marked by inflammation of the intestines, especially the colon, and accompanied by abdominal pain and frequent stools containing blood and mucus; it is caused by chemical irritants, bacteria, protozoa, or parasites.

Prostration
Extreme exhaustion.

rapid, usually within a day, but depends on the amount of toxin ingested and the general health of the victim; consequently, outbreaks in long-term care facilities are especially serious. A frequent source of contamination is an infection on the hand of a food worker, often minor or unnoticed. This bacterium grows rapidly in custard- and cream-filled bakery goods, chicken and ham salads, egg products, and processed meat, cheese, and sauces—all moist foods with a high protein content. There is no change in odor, taste, or appearance, so the consumer has no warning. Although the bacterium is destroyed by heat, the toxin is not, so food stored at an inappropriate temperature will not be safe to eat regardless of further cooking.[38]

Clostridial food poisoning: Clostridium perfringens spores are in soil, water, dust, and refuse—virtually everywhere. It multiplies in cooked meat and meat dishes and develops its toxin in foods held for extended times after cooking. Prevention rests with thorough cooking, prompt serving after cooking, and immediate refrigeration thereafter.

The toxins produced by another *Clostridium, C. botulinum,* cause more serious and often-fatal food poisoning. Depending on the amount of toxin consumed and the individual response, death ensues within 24 hours. The *botulinum* neurotoxin is the most potent substance known, and consuming only a few milligrams of a food that contains this poison can cause illness and death. Initial complaints are vomiting, weakness, and dizziness. Progressively, the toxin irritates motor nerve cells and blocks transmission of neural impulses, causing gradual paralysis ending in respiratory paralysis. *C. botulinum* spores are found in soils throughout the world and carried on harvested food to the canning process. Like all clostridia, this species is anaerobic (i.e., it develops in the absence of air). If spores are not completely destroyed in the canning process, this relatively air-free environment provides ideal conditions for toxin production. The commercial canning industry follows processing standards that eliminate the risk of botulism, but cases still result from foods canned at home using inappropriate methods.

The most recent outbreak of botulism was traced to potato salad served at a community potluck supper that was made with inappropriately processed home-canned potatoes; 28 of the patients were successfully treated, and one patient died.[39] Boiling for 10 minutes destroys the toxin (although not the spore), so all home-canned food, no matter how well preserved, should be boiled at least 10 minutes before eating. Native Alaskan food practices involving uncooked or partially cooked meats have resulted in cases of botulism.[40] Table 9.2 summarizes bacterial sources of foodborne illness.

Viruses. Viruses from the Caliciviridae family, also known as noroviruses, are responsible for more than half of all gastroenteritis cases in the United States. Often referred to as the "stomach bug," norovirus affects as many as 21 million people each year and is responsible for at least 56,000 hospitalizations, often the result of dehydration from prolonged vomiting and diarrhea.[41] There is no vaccine to prevent infection and no drug to cure it. Norovirus infection arises from contaminated and unwashed fruits and vegetables, raw or undercooked shellfish, or touching a contaminated surface. Only 18 viral particles are needed to make you sick. This condition is extremely contagious and also spreads via the fecal-oral route. Health care facilities are subject to outbreaks if health care workers disposing of vomitus, feces, or used dishes or bed linens touch food or serving dishes without washing their hands. In food service facilities, illness can spread from worker to worker and on to food. Vomiting and diarrhea resulting from norovirus contamination usually last no more than 1 to 2 days, but the related dehydration can be serious in young children and older adults.

TABLE 9.2 Selected Examples of Bacterial Foodborne Illness

Foodborne Illness	Causative Organisms (Genus and Species)	Common Food Source	Symptoms and Course
Bacterial Food Infections			
Salmonellosis	*Salmonella* *S. typhi* *S. paratyphi*	Milk, custards, egg dishes, salad dressings, sandwich fillings, polluted shellfish	Mild to severe diarrhea, cramps, vomiting; appears 12–24 h after eating; lasts 1–7 days
Shigellosis	*Shigella* *S. dysenteriae*	Milk and milk products, seafood, salads	Mild diarrhea to fatal dysentery (especially in young children); appears 7–36 h after eating; lasts 3–14 days
Listeriosis	*Listeria* *L. monocytogenes*	Soft cheese made from unpasteurized milk; poultry, seafood, unpasteurized milk, meat products (pâté)	Severe diarrhea, fever, headache, loss of balance, convulsions; can cause miscarriage in pregnant women; symptoms begin after 3–21 days
Vibrio	*Vibrio* *V. parahaemolyticus*	Raw or undercooked oysters, clams, mussels, other shellfish or fin fish;	Watery diarrhea, abdominal cramps, nausea, vomiting, fever, and chills; symptoms occur within 24 h and usually continue for no more than 3 days; severe complications possible with compromised immune systems, liver disease, or alcoholism
Bacterial Food Poisoning			
Staphylococcal	*Staphylococcus* *S. aureus*	Custards, cream fillings, processed meats, ham, cheese, ice cream, potato salad, sauces, casseroles	Severe abdominal pain, cramps, vomiting, diarrhea, perspiration, headache, fever, prostration; appears suddenly 1–6 h after eating; symptoms usually subside within 24 h
Clostridium	*Clostridium* *C. perfringens* (Enteritis)	Cooked meats, meat dishes held at warm or room temperature	Mild diarrhea, vomiting; appears 8–24 h after eating; lasts ≤1 day
	Clostridium *C. botulinum* (Botulism)	Improperly home-canned foods; smoked and salted fish, ham, sausage, shellfish	Severe cases lead to death within 24 h; initial nausea, vomiting, weakness, dizziness, progressing to motor and sometimes fatal respiratory paralysis

Vulnerability to Foodborne Illness

Foodborne illness has health and economic consequences. Microbial foodborne illness results in acute but self-limiting symptoms, and most people require only general supportive care. However, for young children; older adults; and immune-compromised patients with cancer, recent organ or bone marrow transplants, or autoimmune deficiency diseases, foodborne pathogens can lead to septicemia, acute renal failure, or death. In pregnant women, foodborne illness can result in miscarriage. Medical intervention and lost productivity have an annual cost of $1068 per episode, with an estimated total cost of $51 billion.[42]

The increasing use of foods often associated with foodborne illness points to the need for vigilance. In recent years, 46% of reported foodborne illness was attributed to plant foods, with an emphasis on leafy vegetables.[43] Bacteria in the soil cling to growing plants, and failure to properly wash fruits and vegetables prior to eating or processing transfers these pathogens to humans. Poor sanitation on the part of farm workers or irrigation with polluted water elevates the risk from plant foods. Cheeses made with unpasteurized milk, raw milk used as a beverage, or contamination of milk following pasteurization produced 14% of reported foodborne illnesses. Raw or poorly cooked eggs and shellfish are each responsible for 6% of reported outbreaks.[44] Appropriate cooking and holding temperatures for various foods, especially protein foods such as poultry and ground beef, are essential for keeping food safe. See Fig. 9.7 for guidance on recommended cooking and holding temperatures for both in-home and institutional food preparation. Using the information you learned about the importance of family meals, the new nutrition label, and food safety, complete the Case Study box, "Planning the Family Dinner."

Prevention of Foodborne Illness

Protecting food from bacterial contamination begins with appropriate storage. Covered containers or sealable plastic bags for dry, refrigerated, or freezer storage protect food from insects or unwanted contact with other raw foods. Labels on highly perishable foods, such as meat, poultry, and fish, give directions for preventing spoilage and contamination (Fig. 9.8). Raw poultry must be kept separate from other foods and work surfaces. Fight BAC!, a food safety education program, recommends four simple steps[45]:

* CLEAN: Wash hands and surfaces often.
* SEPARATE: Don't cross-contaminate!
* COOK: Cook to proper temperature.
* CHILL: Refrigerate promptly.

The major personal defense against contracting or spreading foodborne illness is hand washing—before touching food and after handling dirty dishes, linens, or trash or using the bathroom. Thorough hand washing with soap and water is superior to use of waterless hand sanitizer.[41] Use of gloves (following hand washing) is required of food handlers and should be the rule for individuals who serve refreshments or present food demonstrations. Those with any infectious diseases or hand injuries, however slight, must not work with food. Fig. 9.9 illustrates proper hand washing.

FIG. 9.7 Chart of food temperatures: avoid the danger zone. 40°F to 140°F It is important to keep hot foods hot and cold foods cold. Foods should be held at temperatures less than 40°F or greater than 140°F to prevent microbial growth. Microorganisms grow rapidly between 40°F and 140°F. Meat and poultry products should be cooked to the internal temperature indicated on the chart. [a]Allow to rest for at least 3 minutes. (From US Department of Agriculture, Food Safety and Inspection Service: "Danger Zone" 40°F to 140°F. https://www.fsis.usda.gov/wps/portal/fsis/topics/food-safety-education/get-answers/food-safety-fact-sheets/safe-food-handling/danger-zone-40-f-140-f/ct_index.)

In the figure:
Minimum Internal Temperature for Safety
165° F — 165° F; Poultry, stuffing, casseroles, reheated leftovers
160° F; Egg dishes and ground meat
Holding temperature for cooked food; **140° F** — 145° F; Beef, pork, lamb, veal[a], roasts, steaks, chops
140° F; Ham, fully cooked (to reheat)
DANGER ZONE
40° F — 40° F; Refrigerator temperature
0° F — 0° F; Freezer temperature

Safe Handling Instructions

This product was prepared from inspected and passed meat and/or poultry. Some food products may contain bacteria that could cause illness if the product is mishandled or cooked improperly. For your protection, follow these safe handling instructions.

 Keep refrigerated or frozen. Thaw in refrigerator or microwave.

 Keep raw meat and poultry separate from other foods. Wash working surfaces (including cutting boards), utensils, and hands after touching raw meat or poultry.

 Cook thoroughly.

 Keep hot foods hot. Refrigerate leftovers immediately or discard.

FIG. 9.8 The safe handling instructions label provides directions for the safe storage and cooking of perishable foods. Labels on fresh and frozen meat, fish, and poultry advise consumers on storing, thawing, and cooking these foods to avoid foodborne illness. (From US Department of Agriculture: *Safe handling instructions label*, Washington, DC, US Department of Agriculture.) https://www.fsis.usda.gov/wps/portal/fsis/topics/food-safety-education/teach-others/download-materials/image-libraries/fsis-images/ct_index.)

CASE STUDY

Planning the Family Dinner

Mrs. G is a single parent with two children: a daughter in third grade and a son in ninth grade. Although they ride different buses to school, both children get home about 3:30 p.m. Mrs. G is employed in a real estate office and usually does not get home until 6:30 p.m. By that time the children have already filled up on snacks and are not really hungry for a meal. Sometimes she calls ahead to tell them that she is stopping at a fast food restaurant and they should wait to eat with her, but most of the time they get something to eat for themselves. Mrs. G's son has been gaining weight at a faster-than-expected rate and has a body mass index (BMI) of 29. At his most recent physical examination, his blood pressure was higher than normal, and the physician recommended that he moderate his weight gain to improve his long-term health.

Questions for Analysis

1. Is it important that the family eat together when Mrs. G gets home? How would you approach this?
2. What are some appropriate snack foods that the children might have when they get home from school that would hold them over until dinner?
3. What are important facts on the new nutrition label that Mrs. G could use in selecting after-school snacks for her children?
4. USDA Food Patterns recommend an energy intake of 2400 kcal for a 14-year-old moderately active boy. What should be the upper level of fat and sodium included in his food for the day? If one-fourth of his daily energy intake is reserved for snacks, then recommend some food combinations that would not exceed the appropriate amounts of kcalories, sodium, and fat.
5. Develop a menu based on foods Mrs. G could bring home and another that the children could begin to prepare for her arrival that are healthy and moderate in cost.
6. Develop five rules for food safety that the children should practice when preparing and eating their after-school snacks and helping with dinner.

FIG. 9.9 Seven-step process for proper hand washing. Failure to wash hands thoroughly before and after preparing and serving food and before eating is a common cause of contamination that leads to foodborne illness. (Courtesy Virginia Cooperative Extension, College of Agriculture and Life Sciences, Virginia Polytechnic Institute and State University, Blacksburg, VA.)

Food Safety Education

Government agencies, food processors, and health organizations have joined forces to develop food safety education programs and certifications to meet the needs of various groups. The initiative of the Partnership for Food Safety Education, called Fight BAC! and described previously, offers website lessons and publicity materials for consumers and professionals (http://www.fightbac.org). Fight BAC! supports food safety messages useful to teachers, public health workers, nutritionists, nurses, or food service managers working with children or adults. The National Restaurant Association Foundation supports a 16-hour national certification program called *ServSafe* for food managers in restaurants, schools, day care centers, hospitals, correctional facilities, and nursing facilities. Most public health departments require all food service managers to have the ServSafe certification or equivalent. *Healthy People 2020* includes goals for reducing foodborne illness and adopting food safety practices.

Food Preservation and Processing

Preservation Methods

As consumers look for shelf-stable convenience foods to feed their families, food scientists are seeking new ways to maintain freshness and flavor and prohibit microbial growth. Many preservation methods used by food processors are similar to those used in the home. Various ways to preserve food are described as follows:

Applying heat: Cooking increases palatability, softens food for chewing, and prepares food for digestion; however, heat is also an important means of ensuring food safety. Most bacteria are killed at temperatures of 180°F to 200°F,[46] and heat also inactivates enzymes that cause spoilage. This is why vegetables are blanched in boiling water to prevent further enzyme activity before being frozen. Pasteurization eliminates pathogens in fluid milk and fruit juices. Factory-canned foods are exposed to temperatures that effectively sterilize the food contents. Foods canned at home at too low a temperature carry the risk of botulism. (To learn more about the importance of pasteurization of milk, see the Evidence-Based Practice box, "Raw Milk—Is it Safe to Drink?")

- *Keeping food cold:* Microbial activity slows at temperatures less than 50°F; thus refrigeration at 45°F or lower will preserve food for a limited period of time.[46] Although freezing prevents microbial growth, bacteria can remain alive, albeit dormant. This is why it is dangerous to refreeze food that has been thawed for some time, because microorganisms have begun to multiply. Cold temperatures will decrease but not eliminate enzyme activity.
- *Removing moisture:* Drying lowers the water activity in a food, and removing available water inhibits the survival and growth of microorganisms. Foods dried at high temperatures, such as ready-to-eat cereals, and foods that are freeze-dried retain more flavor and color. The removal of water from a food also slows enzyme activity and destructive oxidation reactions.
- *Adding acid, sugar, salt, or chemical compounds:* Various natural and chemical additives influence the growth of bacteria and were used to protect food from spoilage before refrigeration and other technologies became available. Acid foods low in pH are resistant to the growth of bacteria, so fermentation with the production of acid was used to turn perishable milk into yogurt or cheese that could be safely stored for a longer time. Adding salt or sugar to a food controls the growth of bacteria by limiting the water available to existing microorganisms. In this way the high sugar content of jams or jellies prevents spoilage. In earlier times, salt curing was a means of preserving meat, and pickling is still used by home and commercial food processors. Chemical compounds such as calcium propionate are added to bread and grain products to retard the growth of mold and bacteria and increase shelf life.
- *Changing the atmosphere:* A new method of food preservation involves changing the atmosphere, that is, removing the oxygen necessary for bacterial growth and enzyme activity and replacing it with carbon dioxide (CO_2) or nitrogen, which slows these activities. Modified atmosphere packaging is used for highly perishable foods such as ready-to-eat chicken pieces and salad mixes.
- *Irradiation:* Irradiation extends shelf life and increases the safety of many foods. Irradiation uses energy sources such as gamma rays, similar to microwaves, that pass through the food and kill harmful bacteria but have little effect on nutrients. Irradiation is used to sterilize rations for space travel and for patients who require completely germ-free food, such as those undergoing bone marrow transplants. Most spices, herbs, and seasonings are irradiated. Irradiation effectively destroys *E. coli* in ground meat and *Salmonella* in fresh eggs and poultry. Although this technology is safe and effective, the sale of irradiated food has been opposed by those who erroneously believe food becomes radioactive or expect that irradiation will mask unsanitary processing or storage. Health care facilities are the primary users of irradiated foods. Irradiation has been endorsed as safe by the Academy of Nutrition and Dietetics, the American Medical Association, and the World Health Organization.
- *High pressure (nonthermal):* An emerging method of food preservation being used for refrigerated foods involves high-pressure treatment in a nonheated environment. Referred to by food processors as a "gentler method" of food processing, it preserves nutrients, taste, and freshness. It is currently used for such products as almond milk, juice drinks, and guacamole.[46]

Chemical Additives

As consumers demand new flavors, improved textures, and increased shelf life, new additives to achieve these goals are being evaluated. Additives serve many functions in processed foods:

- *Provide a smooth and consistent texture:* Emulsifiers in cake mixes and liquid pancake batters prevent ingredients from separating; anticaking agents prevent clumping and allow mixtures to flow freely.
- *Prevent destructive oxidation reactions:* Preservatives prevent rancidity in liquid oils and mixtures containing unsaturated fats; vitamin C or other antioxidants prevent fresh fruit such as sliced apples from turning brown.
- *Prevent microbial growth:* Calcium and sodium propionate prevent the growth of mold in bread and other baked products.
- *Add flavor or color:* Spices add to the flavor and enjoyment of food, and colors provide eye appeal; yellow coloring is added to margarine to take on the appearance of butter.

Table 9.3 lists some examples of food additives and their functions. Vitamins that act as antioxidants are sometimes added to processed foods not to increase their nutrient content but to enhance their shelf life. Other nutrients such as vitamin D and calcium are added to improve dietary intake.

The additives described previously are intentional additives that serve a specific purpose. Unintentional additives are not added on purpose but find their way into the food by some other means. In Chapter 7, we noted the iodine entering the food supply in trace amounts as a result of iodine-containing cleaning agents used in the dairy industry. The FDA is currently evaluating potential residues adsorbed from food packaging materials and containers. A case in point is bisphenol A (BPA), a chemical used in the manufacture of reusable water bottles, food containers, baby bottles, and resin-coated food cans, including those used for infant formula.[47] Trace amounts of BPA can migrate from the container into the food or water and thereby enter the body, although this occurs in very small amounts and absorbed BPA is rapidly metabolized and excreted. The consensus at this time is that BPA in the amounts currently used poses no threat to general health.

TABLE 9.3 Examples of Food Additives and Their Functions

Type	Chemical Compound	Function	Common Food Uses
Anticaking agent	Calcium silicate, calcium stearate	Used to keep food dry and prevent caking if moisture is absorbed from the air; keeps item free-flowing	Table salt, powdered sugar, baking powder
Antimicrobial agent	Calcium propionate, sodium propionate	Prevent growth of mold	Bread
Antioxidants	Butylated hydroxyanisole (BHA) Butylated hydroxytoluene (BHT)	Prevents oxidation reactions and rancidity in unsaturated fatty acids	Vegetable oils, potato chips
Bleaching agent	Chlorine, benzoyl peroxide	Whiten appearance	Freshly milled wheat flour, white flour
Chemical leavening	Sodium bicarbonate	Acts with an acid in a batter to release carbon dioxide for leavening	Double-acting baking powder for quick breads, cakes, cookies
Coloring agent	Annatto (natural) FD&C Red #3 FD&C Yellow #5 (artificial)	Make color of food more appealing	Margarine, candy, carbonated beverages, fruit drinks
Dough conditioners	Ammonium chloride, calcium phosphate	Improves volume	Bread
Emulsifier	Lecithin, monoglycerides and diglycerides	Keeps water-soluble and fat-soluble ingredients evenly distributed throughout a food	Margarine, cake mixes
Humectants	Propylene glycol, sorbitol	Retain moisture, prevent food from becoming hard or stiff	Soft cookies, cake frosting, marshmallow candy
Flavoring agents	Amyl acetate, methyl salicylate, essential oils, monosodium glutamate, sodium chloride (salt)	Enhance flavor or aroma	Most processed foods
Preservative	Sodium nitrate (color) Sodium nitrite (food safety)	Preserves pink color in cured meats; prevents rancidity in meats and botulism	Processed meats, frankfurters, canned foods
Sequestrant	Citric acid	Binds with metals such as iron or copper to prevent changes in flavor, color, or appearance	Wine, juice, mayonnaise
Stabilizers and thickeners	Pectin, locust bean gum, guar gum, carrageenan	Maintain appropriate food texture and mouth feel; thickener	Jelly, ice cream, pudding, yogurt

EVIDENCE-BASED PRACTICE

Raw Milk—Is It Safe to Drink?

Identify the Problem: As consumers reach out to foods that they perceive as "natural" or minimally processed, there is growing attention to "raw milk" or milk that has not undergone pasteurization. Pasteurization is a process by which milk is heated to 161°F for 15 seconds to kill any bacteria or pathogens that may be present, cooled quickly, and stored at 45°F. Raw milk commonly contains *E coli, Campylobacter, Salmonella,* and *Listeria* that can lead to serious illness and even death. Both unpasteurized milk and products such as cheese, yogurt, and ice cream made from unpasteurized milk are a public health hazard.

Review the Evidence: According to the CDC, the number of outbreaks occurring as a result of drinking unpasteurized milk have been increasing. Pregnant women, children, older adults, and individuals with a compromised immune system are most vulnerable to illness related to unpasteurized milk. Fifty-nine percent of recent outbreaks involved at least one child younger than 5 years. (See videos from the CDC regarding foodborne illness in children related to use of unpasteurized milk.)[a]

Misinformation regarding the benefits of unpasteurized milk contribute to the risky use of this food. First, pasteurization does not result in loss of nutrients; unpasteurized milk does not provide nutritional benefits while presenting risk of illness, or even death, in young children. Unpasteurized milk is sometimes thought to carry special health benefits in the prevention or amelioration of such conditions as asthma, allergies, heart disease, and cancer, although these beliefs are unproven. Individuals with lactose malabsorption problems may seek out unpasteurized milk as a possible alternative, although in truth, lactose content is unchanged by pasteurization.

Implement the Findings: Food safety education should emphasize the dangers that accompany the use of unpasteurized milk. Consumers should look for the word "pasteurized" on the labels of both fluid milk and milk products. Soft cheeses made from unpasteurized milk have been associated with miscarriage in pregnant women. Milk labeled as organic can still contain dangerous pathogens if not pasteurized. Organic milk is produced by animals who have not been treated with hormones and have been fed grains grown without the use of pesticides; however, unwanted pathogens and bacteria may still be present. Similarly, milk from healthy cows raised on dairy farms with good safety records cannot be assumed to be safe without undergoing pasteurization. Harmful pathogens usually do not change the look, taste, or smell of milk, so examining, tasting, or smelling a container of raw milk cannot tell you if it is safe to drink. Protect yourself and others by looking for the pasteurized label.

Bibliography

Centers for Disease Control and Prevention: *Food safety and raw milk*, Atlanta, GA, 2015. https://www.cdc.gov/foodsafety/rawmilk/raw-milk-index.html.

Committee on Infectious Diseases, Committee on Nutrition, American Academy of Pediatrics: Consumption of raw or unpasteurized milk and milk products by pregnant women and children, *Pediatrics* 133(1):175, 2014.

Mungai EA, Behravesh CB, Gould LH: Increase in outbreaks associated with nonpasteurized milk, United States, 2007-2012, *Emerg Infect Dis* 21(1):119, 2015.

Silence E, Hardy C, Medeiros LC, et al: Examining trust factors in online food risk information: the case of unpasteurized or 'raw' milk, *Appetite* 99:200, 2016.

[a]Centers for Disease Control and Prevention: *Real stories of the dangers of raw milk,* Atlanta GA, 2014. https://www.cdc.gov/foodsafety/rawmilk/raw-milk-videos.html.

Nutritional Aspects of Food Processing

The effect of food processing on food nutrient content continues to concern both consumers and health advocates. In general, carbohydrates, fats, and proteins are less affected and minerals and vitamins are more affected by food processing. However, both the characteristics of the food and the processing methods used influence the stability or loss of nutrients. Effects on specific nutrients are summarized as follows:

- *Macronutrients:* The major change in carbohydrates and proteins is the Maillard or browning reaction that occurs between sugars and the amino acid lysine. This happens in normal baking and forms new sugar–amino acid compounds that cannot be digested or absorbed; however, in the United States, grain foods are not a major source of lysine. Hydrogenation of liquid vegetable oils to produce solid table fats forms trans fatty acids that have negative effects on health. (See Chapter 4 to review fat hydrogenation.)
- *Minerals:* Major mineral losses result from the refining of cereal grains. When the germ and bran are removed from the kernel to produce a finer-textured flour or cereal, iron, along with zinc, chromium, and magnesium, is lost. Under current food enrichment standards, iron is added back to refined flours and cereals, but the other minerals are not. Mineral content and bioavailability is retained with most other processing methods.
- *Vitamins:* No vitamin is completely stable to food processing, although losses vary from one to another. Vitamins are lost during storage of fruits and vegetables through the action of enzymes and oxidation. Vitamin A is relatively stable to heat, so only small amounts are lost in milk pasteurization. Vitamin E in oils is generally not affected by heat treatment or frying, but freezing rapidly destroys it. Naturally occurring vitamin D is not harmed by heat but must be protected from light and atmospheric oxygen.

Thiamin is sensitive to heat, and losses occur in baking and high-temperature processing of cereals. Light destroys riboflavin, and riboflavin-containing foods must be stored in opaque containers to avoid loss. Riboflavin does withstand the heat treatment of pasteurization, so milk remains a good food source. Folate is destroyed by light, and large amounts are lost in vegetables heated to high temperatures in large amounts of water. Vitamin B_6 is sensitive to light and can be lost in the canning of vegetables. Long exposure to heat or hot storage causes destruction of ascorbic acid.

Food processing as a concept brings forth intense emotions, such that a well-known nutrition expert recently asked if processed food is a four-letter word standing for J-U-N-K food.[48] Health advocates consider processed foods and their content of sugar, fat, and sodium to be a major cause of chronic disease, whereas food companies promote the taste, convenience, and, if applicable, nutritional value of their products. Processed foods are classified as (1) minimally processed (items such as washed and packaged fruits and salad greens that retain most of their inherent properties); (2) processing to enhance preservation, shelf life, or consumer appeal (salad dressing, canned fruit, breakfast cereals, crackers, lunch meat, or cake mix); and (3) prepared foods and ready-to-eat meals packed for freshness and ease of preparation (includes frozen meals and deli items).[48] A recent grocery survey indicated that 68% of family kcalories were contributed by ready-to-eat items. Those authors noted that foods requiring some cooking or preparation are better choices from the standpoint of nutrition.[49] It is important to remember that what a processed food contributes to a healthy diet is based on its nutrient composition, portion size, and frequency of use rather than its degree of processing.

Despite limitations, fortified processed food makes a significant contribution to the American diet. Without fortification, 79% of the US population would not meet even the minimum suggested intake of vitamin A (this fell to 40% with fortification), 50% of the US population would be deficient in thiamin (this fell to 5% with fortification), and 90% would have inadequate intakes of folate (this fell to 10% with fortification). Most women of childbearing age are unable to meet their recommended intake of iron without fortified foods. Among children ages 2 to 18, fortified foods provide between 12% and 20% of their vitamin A, C, B_6, B_{12}, and iron.[48]

Many minimally processed and preserved foods reduce waste and offer convenience, supporting greater use of nutrient-dense items such as fruits and vegetables. At the same time, we must help consumers make prudent choices using the information available to them. A recent study with parents found that snack foods carrying a nutrition claim for an added vitamin or mineral was viewed as a more healthy choice than a similar product not making such a claim, regardless of sugar, fat, or sodium content.[50] A healthy diet can include both minimally processed and ready-to-eat foods if chosen carefully with an emphasis on nutrient density and variety.

TO SUM UP

Food patterns evolve from a social perspective. As our society changes, so does what we eat. Parents are working longer hours, more adults are living alone, and almost half of our food budget is spent on meals away from home. Surveys suggest the American public is becoming more conscious of nutrition and health; however, fast food and convenience meals are the norm in many families. As more of our food comes from farmers and processors across the country and around the globe, the threat of food contamination and risk of widespread outbreaks of food-borne illness escalate. Two government agencies—the FDA and USDA—carry responsibility for maintaining a safe and wholesome food supply. The USDA oversees meat and poultry, and the FDA regulates the processing, labeling, and formulation of all other foods, including GM foods. The nutrition label helps consumers select food to maximize their nutrient intake and avoid inappropriately high levels of kcalories, sugar, sodium, and fat. Under current laws, dietary supplements are largely unregulated, putting undiscerning users at risk. The CDC monitors the incidence of foodborne illness, and several government and private agencies have joined forces to provide public and professional education promoting safe food handling. Public demand for good-tasting food, quickly and easily prepared, and with a long shelf life, has led to growing use of food additives and new processing methods. Consumers and health professionals must continue to monitor the nutrient content of processed food and its implications for nutrition and health.

▉ QUESTIONS FOR REVIEW

1. What are some social and psychological factors that influence your personal food habits? Describe some food customs or special observances in your family that involve food. Do these customs have a positive or negative influence on nutrient intake? Explain.

2. You are preparing a 15-minute lesson on food safety as part of a nutrition education class for young families receiving Supplemental Nutrition Assistance Program benefits. Develop an outline for your presentation, including any visuals you would use. Develop or select a brochure that would be suitable for this audience.

3. A pregnant mother who has been eating more fish to obtain a good supply of omega-3 fatty acids read a newspaper article indicating that all ocean fish are contaminated with mercury. She is concerned

about the safety of her baby. Review the current advisory of the FDA regarding the consumption of fish by pregnant women found in Fig. 9.3 and accessible at (https://www.fda.gov/forconsumers/consumerupdates/ucm397443.htm). How would you advise her? Develop some practical menu suggestions to help her.

4. Find a print or Internet advertisement for a new dietary supplement or health remedy and identify the population to whom it is directed. Using the criteria in Box 9.4, evaluate this product. Does it appear to be helpful or harmful? How would you respond to a consumer seeking your advice on its use?

5. You are helping a day care provider develop a food safety program for her facility. Compile a list of 10 guidelines for the staff that will reduce the risk of foodborne illness among their children. (Visit the Fight BAC! Child Care Training website at http://www.fightbac.org/kidsfoodsafety/young-children-child-care-training/ for some ideas.)

6. Select a type of frozen entree and review the nutrition labels on three examples of that product. Make a table that lists the number of servings; kcalories per serving; grams of protein, fat, fiber, and added sugar; milligrams of sodium; and %DV for vitamin D, iron, potassium, and calcium. Compare the relative merits and disadvantages of each. Which is the best choice based on its contribution of protein, fiber, and vitamin and minerals? Which is the poorest choice in terms of fat, sugar, and sodium?

7. Name five methods of food preservation. Which methods destroy harmful bacteria and which merely retard their growth?

8. Visit the CDC Multistate Foodborne Outbreak Investigations website and review reported outbreaks of foodborne illness that occurred over the past year (https://www.cdc.gov/foodsafety/outbreaks/multistate-outbreaks/outbreaks-list.html). What foods were involved and why/how did the outbreak occur? Which consumer groups were most affected?

REFERENCES

1. Goody CM, Drago L, editors: *Cultural food practices*, Chicago, 2010, Diabetes Care and Education Dietetic Practice Group, American Dietetic Association.
2. Kittler PG, Sucher KP, Nahikian-Nelms M: *Food and culture*, ed 6, Belmont, Calif, 2012, Wadsworth/Cengage Learning.
3. Fitzgerald A, Heary C, Kelly C, et al: Self-efficacy for healthy eating and peer support for unhealthy eating are associated with adolescents' food intake patterns, *Appetite* 63:48, 2013.
4. Maslow AH: *Motivation and personality*, New York, 1954, Harper & Row.
5. Sloan AE: Shoppers shift to fresh, *Food Technol* 71(1):36, 2017.
6. International Food Information Council Foundation: *2016 Food & Health Survey. Food Decision 2016: The impact of a growing national food dialogue*, Washington, DC, 2016, International Food Information Council Foundation. http://www.foodinsight.org/articles/2016-food-and-health-survey-food-decision-2016-impact-growing-national-food-dialogue.
7. Sloan AE: What, when and where America eats, *Food Technol* 70(1):35, 2016.
8. Poti JM, Mendez MA, Ng SW, et al: Highly processed and ready-to-eat packaged food and beverage purchases differ by race/ethnicity among US households, *J Nutr* 146(9):1722, 2016.
9. Kant AK, Graubard BI: 40-year trends in meal and snack eating behaviors of American adults, *J Acad Nutr Diet* 115(1):50, 2015.
10. St-Onge MP, Ard J, Baskin ML, et al: American Heart Association Obesity Committee of the Council on Lifestyle and Cardiometabolic Health; Council on Cardiovascular Disease in the Young; Council on Clinical Cardiology; and Stroke Council: Meal timing and frequency: Implications for cardiovascular disease prevention: A scientific statement from the American Heart Association, *Circulation* 135(9):e96-e121, 2017.
11. Van Horn L, Carson JA, Appel LJ, et al: Recommended Dietary Pattern to Achieve Adherence to the American Heart Association/American College of Cardiology (AHA/ACC) Guidelines: A Scientific Statement From the American Heart Association, *Circulation* 134(22):e505, 2016.
12. Zizza CA: Healthy snacking recommendations: one size does not fit all, *Physiol Behav* 134:32, 2014.
13. Neumark-Sztainer D, Wall M, Fulkerson JA, et al: Changes in the frequency of family meals from 1999 to 2010 in the homes of adolescents: Trends by sociodemographic characteristics, *J Adolesc Health* 52:201, 2013.
14. Fulkerson JA, Larson N, Horning M, et al: A review of associations between family or shared meal frequency and dietary and weight status outcomes across the lifespan, *J Nutr Educ Behav* 46(1):2, 2014.
15. Berge JM, MacLehose RF, Loth KA, et al: Family meals. Associations with weight and eating behaviors among mothers and fathers, *Appetite* 58:1128, 2012.
16. Sloan AE: 10 top functional foods trends, *Food Technol* 70(4), 2016.
17. International Food Information Council Foundation: *Food & Health Survey. Consumer attitudes toward food safety, nutrition, and health*, Washington, DC, 2011, International Food Information Council Foundation.

http://www.foodinsight.org/2011_Food_Health_Survey_Consumer_Attitudes_Toward_Food_Safety_Nutrition_Health.

18. US Food and Drug Administration: *Labeling of Foods Derived From Genetically Engineered Plants*, Silver Spring, MD, January 2017, US Department of Health and Human Services. http://www.fda.gov/Food/IngredientsPackagingLabeling/GEPlants/ucm346858.htm.
19. US Food and Drug Administration: *Dietary Supplements*, Silver Spring, MD, April 2016, US Department of Health and Human Services. http://www.fda.gov/Food/DietarySupplements/default.htm.
20. US Department of Agriculture: *Organic Market Overview*, Washington, DC, October 2016, Economic Research Service. https://www.ers.usda.gov/topics/natural-resources-environment/organic-agriculture/organic-market-overview.aspx.
21. US Food and Drug Administration, US Environmental Protection Agency: *Eating Fish: What Pregnant Women and Parents Should Know*, Silver Spring, MD, January 2017, US Department of Health and Human Services. http://www.fda.gov/Food/FoodborneIllnessContaminants/Metals/ucm393070.htm.
22. US Food and Drug Administration: *Nutrition Facts Label Better Informs Your Food Choices*, Silver Spring, MD, August 2016, US Department of Health and Human Services. http://www.fda.gov/ForConsumers/ConsumerUpdates/ucm387114.htm.
23. US Food and Drug Administration: *Changes to the Nutrition Facts Label*, Silver Spring, MD, January 2017, US Department of Health and Human Services. http://www.fda.gov/Food/GuidanceRegulation/GuidanceDocumentsRegulatoryInformation/LabelingNutrition/ucm385663.htm.
24. Laquatra I, Sollid K, Smith Edge M, et al: Including "Added Sugars" on the Nutrition Facts Panel: How consumers perceive the proposed change, *J Acad Nutr Diet* 115(11):1758, 2015.
25. US Food and Drug Administration: *Guidance for industry: a food labeling guide*, Silver Spring, MD, August 2016, US Department of Health and Human Services. http://www.fda.gov/Food/GuidanceRegulation/GuidanceDocumentsRegulatoryInformation/LabelingNutrition/ucm2006828.htm.
26. US Food and Drug Administration: *Gluten-free labeling of food*, Silver Spring, MD, May 2016, US Department of Health and Human Services. http://www.fda.gov/Food/GuidanceRegulation/GuidanceDocumentsRegulatoryInformation/Allergens/ucm362510.htm.
27. McLellan TM, Lieberman HR: Do energy drinks contain active components other than caffeine? *Nutr Rev* 70(12):730, 2012.
28. US Food and Drug Administration: *Letter to manufacturers regarding botanicals and other novel ingredients in conventional foods*, Silver Spring, MD, September 2001, US Department of Health and Human Services. http://wayback.archive-it.org/7993/20170722024307/https://www.fda.gov/Food/GuidanceRegulation/GuidanceDocumentsRegulatoryInformation/DietarySupplements/ucm103443.htm.
29. Howland J, Rohsenow DJ: Risks of energy drinks mixed with alcohol, *JAMA* 309(3):245, 2013.

30. Sepkowitz KA: Energy drinks and caffeine-related adverse effects, *JAMA* 309(3):243, 2013.

31. Cohen PA: Hazards of hindsight—monitoring the safety of nutritional supplements, *N Engl J Med* 370(14):1277, 2014.

32. Centers for Disease Control and Prevention: *Burden of foodborne illness: Overview*, Atlanta, GA, July 2016, US Department of Health and Human Services. https://www.cdc.gov/foodborneburden/estimates-overview.html.

33. Centers for Disease Control and Prevention: *Multistate Outbreak of Shiga toxin-producing Escherichia coli O157:H7 Infections Linked to Beef Products Produced by Adams Farm (Final Update)*, Atlanta, GA, October 2016, US Department of Health and Human Services. https://www.cdc.gov/ecoli/2016/o157h7-09-16/index.html.

34. Center for Disease Control and Prevention: *Foodborne Diseases Active Surveillance Network (FoodNet). 2015 Preliminary Data: Tables and Figures. Table 12a. Number and Percentage of Hospitalizations by Pathogen and Age Group*, Atlanta, GA, March 2016, US Department of Health and Human Services. https://www.cdc.gov/foodnet/reports/prelim-data-2015.html.

35. Center for Disease Control and Prevention: *Food Safety. Campylobacter*, Atlanta, GA, June 2014, US Department of Health and Human Services. https://www.cdc.gov/foodsafety/diseases/campylobacter/index.html.

36. Center for Disease Control and Prevention: *Listeria (Listeriosis): Symptoms*, Atlanta GA, December 2016, US Department of Health and Human Services. https://www.cdc.gov/listeria/symptoms.html.

37. Center for Disease Control and Prevention: *Vibrio Species Causing Vibriosis. Questions and Answers*, Atlanta, GA, January 2017, US Department of Health and Human Services. https://www.cdc.gov/vibrio/faq.html.

38. Center for Disease Control and Prevention: *Food Safety. Staphylococcal Food Poisoning*, Atlanta, GA, October 2016, US Department of Health and Human Services. https://www.cdc.gov/foodsafety/diseases/staphylococcal.html.

39. McCarty CL, Angelo K, Beer KD, et al: Large Outbreak of Botulism Associated with a Church Potluck Meal–Ohio, 2015, *MMWR (Morb Mortal Wkly Rep)* 64(29):802, 2015. https://www.cdc.gov/mmwr/preview/mmwrhtml/mm6429a6.htm.

40. Center for Disease Control and Prevention: *Botulism*, Atlanta, GA, May 2016, US Department of Health and Human Services. https://www.cdc.gov/botulism/index.html.

41. Center for Disease Control and Prevention: *Norovirus*, Atlanta, GA, August 2016, US Department of Health and Human Services. https://www.cdc.gov/norovirus/index.html.

42. Cody MM, Stretch T, Academy of Nutrition and Dietetics: Position of the Academy of Nutrition and Dietetics: Food and water safety, *J Acad Nutr Diet* 114(11):1819, 2014.

43. Barak JD, Schroeder BK: Interrelationships of food safety and plant pathology: the life cycle of human pathogens on plants, *Annu Rev Phytopathol* 50:241, 2012.

44. Painter JA, Hoekstra RM, Ayers T, et al: Attribution of foodborne illnesses, hospitalizations, and deaths to food commodities by using outbreak data, United States, 1998-2008, *Emerg Infect Dis* 19(3):407, 2013. http://wwwnc.cdc.gov/eid/article/19/3/pdfs/11-1866.pdf.

45. Partnership for Food Safety Education: *The Four Core Practices, Partnership for Food Safety Education*, Arlington, VA, no date given. http://www.fightbac.org/food-safety-basics/the-core-four-practices/.

46. Balasubramaniam VM, Yousef AE, Wan J, et al: Kinder, gentler food processing, *Food Technol* 70(12):20, 2016.

47. US Food and Drug Administration: Bisphenol A (BPA): *Use in food contact application*, Silver Spring, MD, February 2016, US Department of Health and Human Services. http://www.fda.gov/NewsEvents/PublicHealthFocus/ucm064437.htm.

48. Dwyer JT: Trailblazer lecture: Why are processed foods so controversial? *J Acad Nutr Diet* 115(11):1871, 2015.

49. Poti JM, Mendez MA, Ng SW, et al: Is the degree of food processing and convenience linked with the nutritional quality of foods purchased by US households, *Am J Clin Nutr* 101(6):1251, 2015.

50. Verrill L, Wood D, Cates S, et al: Vitamin-fortified snack food may lead consumers to make poor dietary decisions, *J Acad Nutr Diet* 117:376, 2017.

FURTHER READINGS AND RESOURCES

Further Readings

Chaifetz A, Chapman B: Evaluating North Carolina food pantry food safety-related operating procedures. *J Food Prot* 78(11):2033, 2015.

Maughan C, Godwin S, Chambers D, et al: Recipe modification improves food safety practices during cooking of poultry, *J Food Prot* 79(8):1436, 2016.

[These authors describe ways to keep food safe in food pantries and in the home.]

Myers EF: Herbal/botanical medicine: where's the evidence? *Nutr Today* 50(4):194, 2015.

[Dr. Myers provides a framework for evaluating these products.]

Sloan AE: What, when and where America eats, *Food Technol* 70(1):35, 2016.

[Dr. Sloan provides a comprehensive review of food trends among American consumers and the implications for food scientists and nutritionists.]

Websites of Interest

- US Department of Health and Human Services. *FoodSafety.gov is the government gateway to information on appropriate food safety practices, foodborne illness, recalls of unsafe food, and concerns of vulnerable population groups.* http://www.foodsafety.gov (materials available in English and Spanish).

- US Food and Drug Administration. This website includes information on food and drug labeling, recalls of contaminated food and medical supplies, mercury levels in fish, and bogus medical devices along with consumer educational materials. http://www.fda.gov.

- Partnership for Food Safety Education. Fight BAC! Keep Food Safe From Bacteria provides food safety materials for adults, children, and food service workers. http://www.fightbac.org/ (materials available in English and Spanish).

- International Food Information Council: This site provides consumer information on food labeling, food additives, and food ingredients. http://www.ific.org/.

10

Community Nutrition: Promoting Healthy Eating

Eleanor D. Schlenker

http://evolve.elsevier.com/Williams/essentials/

Health and nutrition professionals play active roles in public health programs serving communities across the globe. Despite regional food shortages and famine leading to lost years and poor quality of life, obesity and related chronic diseases continue to rise worldwide. In this chapter, we explore the ecology of malnutrition and food shortages as they exist in the United States and abroad. We describe educational approaches and nutrition intervention programs that help communities and individuals adopt healthy food patterns and lifestyles and look at how nutrition education and intervention programs are developed and marketed. We also consider the use of food resources that can assist individuals and families obtain maximum benefit from their food dollars.

OUTLINE

Nutrition and Public Health
The Ecology of Malnutrition: The Individual and the Environment
Family Food Expenditures

Health Promotion
    Community Education and Program Development
    Food Assistance Programs: Opportunities for Nutrition Education

NUTRITION AND PUBLIC HEALTH

Framework for Health

Our goal for nutrition is optimum health and well-being, but health can be described in various ways. Health for an individual is sometimes defined as soundness of body and mind or as freedom from disease or pain.[1] The National Wellness Institute defines wellness as multidimensional, and this model, adopted by many public health programs, includes physical, emotional, social, occupational, intellectual, and spiritual well-being.[1] The term *public health* focuses on populations rather than individuals, although the size of the population can vary from a healthy-baby clinic to stemming the worldwide invasion of the Ebola virus. Public health programs are directed toward preventing disease rather than curing existing disease, and emphasize positive lifestyle intervention. Public health agencies monitor the health status of the population to determine what services are needed and how they might be implemented. National and international public health agencies investigate outbreaks of disease and existing malnutrition to determine their cause and develop preventive services.

Nutrition is fundamental to public health. In the 20th century, nutrient-deficiency diseases were rampant across the globe and still persist in many low-income regions and developing nations. In this century, nutrient intake is recognized as an environmental factor related to chronic conditions such as cardiovascular disease, diabetes, obesity, and cancer. Although chronic disease is more visible as a public health problem in the developed world, growing nations are coping with the "double burden" of malnutrition: nutrient deficiencies and diseases of affluence.[2] In developing nations, patterns of disease and premature death depend largely on the prevailing social and economic

conditions, and what food is available. In affluent nations, malnutrition is more likely the result of poor choices from the existing food supply rather than a food shortage.

Worldwide Prevalence of Malnutrition

Malnutrition as a worldwide public health problem continues despite progress in managing the food supply. Across the globe, 870 million people suffer from **hunger**, with a kcalorie intake falling below their energy requirement, and 98% live in developing countries.[3] Among children younger than 5 years, 16% are underweight (low weight for age) and 26% are stunted (low height for age), which affects their school performance and future earnings.[3] When food is available, it often consists of a few staple items, mostly grains and cereals. Approximately 25% of the world's population have low intakes of iodine, putting them at risk of goiter or cretinism, and about the same number have anemia resulting from iron or folate deficiency. One in four children in developing countries has poor vitamin A status, adding to the risk of blindness. More than half of child deaths occurring worldwide are preventable and treatable with appropriate access to food, clean water, and sanitation.[3]

Food Insecurity in the United States

Even in the midst of plenty, millions of families in the United States have insufficient supplies of food. Although an estimated 87.3% of US households are **food secure**, with access to adequate food, 12.7% experienced **food insecurity** at least once in the preceding year, meaning they had difficulty providing enough food for all their members.[4] Food-insecure households include more than 42 million people, and 13 million of these are children. These families cope by reducing the variety of their diet or relying on a few basic foods. However, 5% of food-insecure households (including 11 million adults and more than 500,000 children) experience very low food security causing them to reduce their food intake. Household members will not eat even though they are hungry, will skip or reduce the size of a meal, or, in desperate cases, will not eat for an entire day. Parents will sacrifice their own meals to be able to feed their children. Approximately one-fourth of families with very low food security experience an extreme lack of food in only 1 or 2 months of the year, but for one-third of those with low food security, missing meals and reducing portion size is a chronic problem. Food insecurity is more likely to occur in single-parent households, households with children, those living below the poverty line, and in minority households.[4] Box 10.1 provides some screening tools to identify families who are food insecure and require assistance.

Malnutrition and Health

Food shortages affect physical and emotional health. A Gallop World Poll across 147 countries reported that individuals who were food insecure described their daily experience as "struggling" or "suffering" compared with food-secure responders who considered themselves to be "thriving."[5] The worry of not having enough food brings depression, anxiety, and stress; malnutrition in pregnancy results in low birth weight, putting the infant at risk. Malnutrition adds to weakness and disability among older adults, costing years of productive life. At one time, energy and protein deficits were viewed as the major causes of

KEY TERMS

Hunger
A potential consequence of food insecurity resulting from prolonged, involuntary lack of food, and resulting in discomfort, illness, weakness, or pain.

Food Secure
The availability of food adequate in quality and quantity to meet the nutritional needs of all family members at all times throughout the year

Food Insecurity
The limited or uncertain availability of food and the inability or lack of resources to obtain a sufficient supply of nutritionally safe, adequate, and appropriate food through socially acceptable means.

malnutrition in the developing world; however, chronic conditions such as diabetes and hypertension, stemming from overweight, are growing in prevalence in low-income countries.[6] Regions in the Caribbean, Latin America, North Africa, and the Middle East, who in the past suffered from food shortages, now report prevalence rates of overweight/obesity as high as 60% among their urban populations.[7]

Although it is difficult to understand, problems of underweight, stunting, and micronutrient deficiencies exist side by side with growing obesity. Disparities of undernutrition and obesity sometimes exist in the same family. Social norms often reflect differences in food allocation related to age or gender. High-quality foods may be given first to males responsible for the financial support of the family, or parents may indulge their children.[8]

Finally, undernutrition at one stage of the life cycle may hasten the development of obesity at another stage.[8] Children who experienced fetal growth retardation and underfeeding as infants are at risk of rapid and inappropriate weight gain if overfed in childhood, and rapid weight gain among stunted children increases their adult risk of obesity and cardiovascular risk. Parents in food-insecure environments in both low- and high-income countries may encourage children to eat as much as possible when food is available. Nutrition experts in the United States have pointed to the distribution pattern of the Supplemental Nutrition Assistance Program (SNAP) as a contributing factor to the growth of child obesity, as it reinforces a cycle of high kcalorie consumption when benefits are received and lower consumption toward the close of the month when food provisions have been exhausted.[9] This was confirmed among families in Minnesota who spent more than 75% of their food stamp allotment within the first 2 weeks of the month.[10] Food insecurity may lead to binge eating when food is available.

THE ECOLOGY OF MALNUTRITION: THE INDIVIDUAL AND THE ENVIRONMENT

Food Access in Developing Countries

From the biologic standpoint, malnutrition results from an inadequate supply of nutrients to support normal cell growth and function. However, the ecology of malnutrition is the interconnecting set of physical, social, cultural, economic, political, and educational circumstances that impact a person and his need for food (Fig. 10.1). Each component is more or less important at a given time and place for a given individual. If the adverse conditions are only temporary, then the malnutrition is short term and quickly alleviated with no long-standing threat to life and health; however, as nutrient supplies grow short, physiologic changes begin to occur and worsen with time, causing irreparable harm and, in severe conditions, death. Physical characteristics such as infectious or chronic diseases; the needs of growth, pregnancy, or lactation; or heavy physical labor increase the severity of the problem.

To be successful, intervention programs must address both individual and environmental factors. Famine, poverty, war, and unequal distribution of food across a region, all contribute to malnutrition. Lack of clean water, poor sanitation, and depleted soils are common in many parts of the world. Water distribution and pesticide use influence food production. International programs often provide emergency feeding for those who are experiencing crop failure or have been displaced from their homes, but these provide only short-term solutions. Agencies such as the United Nations Food and Agriculture

KEY TERMS

Ecology
The relationship between an individual and his environment.

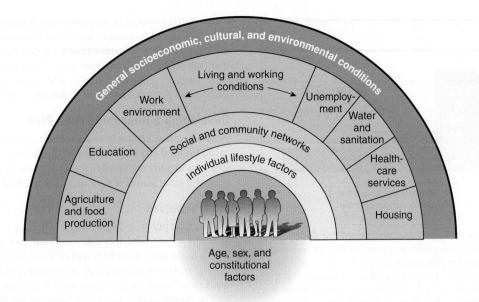

FIG. 10.1 Relationships between the individual, the environment, malnutrition, and disease. The first layer in this figure represents personal behavior and lifestyle including dietary habits that promote or damage health; friendship patterns and community norms also influence personal behavior; the second layer indicates social and community networks that, if available, provide social support; the third layer includes structural factors such as housing, income, and access to services including health care. These three layers represent the interaction between an individual, his or her environment, and the development of malnutrition and disease. (Reprinted with permission from Dahlgren G, Whitehead M: *Policies and strategies to promote social equity in health*, Stockholm, 1991, Institute for Futures Studies.)

Organization (FAO), and the US Agency for International Development (AID) focus on long-term solutions to eliminate hunger, by improving agricultural practices and increasing local food production. Unfortunately, world demand for sugars, oils, and animal foods has lowered the production of staple vegetables and beans in favor of animal feeds and items for export. Cassava, sorghum, and millet—staple foods of Africa's poor—have not benefited from new cultivars or improved technology. As yields of traditional foods are low, prices are high.[11] In many regions, women tend small farms and gardens but are often left out of agricultural extension activities designed to increase local production.[11]

Food Access in the United States

Low-income families in the United States also face what may seem to be an insurmountable task of obtaining enough food. They risk foodborne illness with the purchase of dented cans or foods passed the expiration date. Mothers may try to visit more than one food pantry to adequately feed their families. Shopping strategies reported by mothers of young children who were food insecure included purchasing lower-cost food (83%), taking advantage of sales/discount offers (74%), and purchasing less junk food (73%); 30% reported purchasing fewer fruits and vegetables.[12] Lower-cost food items are often high in carbohydrate, fat, and sugar and may be replacing more nutrient-dense foods.

Among nutrition experts, the question "can low-income Americans afford a healthy diet?" remains controversial. Although cultural and social factors, along with cost, influence nutrient intake, it remains that individuals with higher incomes and more money to spend for food have higher intakes of micronutrients.[13,14] When food budgets shrink, purchases shift toward foods higher in kcalories and lower in cost. Healthy foods such as vegetables are likely to be higher in price per unit weight and so become an expensive source of kcalories as compared with high fat, high sugar items that are energy dense.[15] Grains and

other starches, added sugars, and vegetable fats are a less expensive way to satisfy hunger. An evaluation of food expenditures and nutrient adequacy using the Healthy Eating Index (HEI) reported a direct relationship between money spent and nutrition score. Based on an energy intake of 2000 kcal, persons spending less than $4.21 per day had an HEI score of 44 as compared with those spending at least $7.58 per day, who had a score of 66.[16] Fruits and vegetables, fish, whole grains versus refined grains, and plant proteins were used more frequently in the higher-cost diets. Vitamin C, β-carotene, potassium, and magnesium are the nutrients having the highest cost,[14] whereas foods associated with chronic disease risk have a lower cost. This helps explain why the diets of low-income families deviate from recommended guidelines and why they have higher rates of diet-related chronic diseases.[14]

FAMILY FOOD EXPENDITURES

Family Food Costs

The size and composition of a household influence its food budget. As household size increases, so do food costs, although age and gender make a difference. The weekly food cost of a preschooler is approximately half that of an adult male, and expenditures for women and girls are somewhat lower than for men and boys.[17] As household income rises, the total amount of money spent for food also rises, but not proportionately. Lower-income households are forced to spend significantly more of their income for food as compared with higher-income households (Fig. 10.2).[18] Those with higher incomes may not eat greater amounts of food, but they select more expensive food, buy more pre-prepared items, and eat in restaurants more often.

Family Food Plans

The US Department of Agriculture (USDA) has developed several family food plans that establish the minimum amounts of money required to purchase food for a month that will meet the Dietary

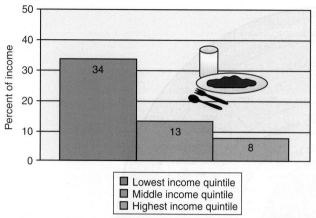

FIG. 10.2 Proportion of family income spent for food. Lower-income families must spend a greater proportion of their income on food than must higher-income families. Lower-income families spend 34% of their income on food compared with higher-income families, who spend only 8%. (Data courtesy of Kuhns A: *Economic Research Service, Food Markets Branch*, Washington, DC, 2017, US Department of Agriculture.)

Reference Intakes (DRIs) and *Dietary Guidelines* for each age and gender group. The plans are categorized as *liberal, moderate, low, and thrifty*, based on the required expenditure (Table 10.1). The thrifty plan is used to calculate the dollar value of SNAP benefits awarded to an individual or family.[19,20]

Each food plan includes a "market basket" of grocery items expected to meet the nutritional needs of the targeted group; however, there are concerns regarding the adequacy of the thrifty food plan (TFP). Food-secure households spend 121% of the TFP to meet their food needs, whereas food-insecure families spend approximately 95%.[4] Even for families spending 100% of the TFP allotment, meeting the recommendation of the 2015 Dietary Guidelines for 2.5 servings of vegetables and 2 servings of fruit per day[21] will be difficult. The TFP allocates 40 cents per edible cup-equivalent for fruits and vegetables. Although many are available at or below this amount, the cup-equivalent cost of dark green, red, and deep yellow vegetables frequently exceeds it. Items such as berries that are rich sources of antioxidants will be available only infrequently on a TFP budget, and vegetable choices can be limited in variety.[22,23]

The USDA food plans now in place were developed several years ago and may not reflect the current American food pattern. In addition, the TFP, for the most part, includes ingredients to be prepared

from scratch, rather than preprepared or convenience items. Nonetheless, a survey of low-income homemakers receiving SNAP benefits indicated that one-third cooked dinner 2 to 5 days per week and more than half cooked 6 to 7 days per week. These families seldom ate away from home.[24] (Suggested menus and market basket items for the USDA food plans can be found in References 19 and 20.)

Developing a Household Food Plan

Each individual or family has a specific amount of money they can spend for food and ideas on how to divide their food dollars. The first step is to identify the family's food resources and preferences because these will enter into how they spend their food dollars.

Food Resources

Food can be purchased with available dollars, produced or preserved at home, or obtained through food assistance programs. Vegetables from a home garden can be frozen or canned for later use, and families in rural areas may raise animals for meat or eggs. Hunters may supplement their family's food supply with fresh meat. SNAP benefits, the Special Supplemental Nutrition Program for Women, Infants, and Children (WIC), free or reduced-cost school meals, meal programs for older adults, or food pantries add to a family's food. Other food-related resources include the following:

- *Access to a well-stocked grocery store* with competitive prices. As supermarkets move from the inner city to suburban areas that offer higher profit margins, people living in downtown urban environments who lack transportation may be forced to food shop at convenience stores with limited selections and higher prices. Older adults may have to shop at the store to which they can get a ride with a neighbor or friend. In rural areas, families must often drive considerable distances to find a store with a broad selection.
- *Time for food shopping and skills in food management.* Working parents and working students may not take the time to read nutrition labels. Busy adults who never learned to cook may rely on preprepared foods regardless of their nutritional value or cost. Retired persons may view store visits as a social experience, although physical limitations can make it difficult to shop and prepare meals.
- *Facilities to store and cook food.* Homeless families and persons who occupy single rooms lack refrigeration and cooking appliances.

Food Preferences

Food is a meaningful part of a family's relationships with one another, their neighbors, and friends. Work and school patterns influence

TABLE 10.1	Examples of USDA Food Plans: Average Cost of Food at Home at Four Levels[a]			
	MONTHLY COST			
Age-Gender Groups	**Thrifty Plan**	**Low-cost Plan**	**Moderate-cost Plan**	**Liberal Plan**
2- to 3-year-old child	$102.20	$130.60	$157.50	$191.80
14- to 18-year-old male	$171.20	$239.00	$303.80	$348.10
19- to 50-year-old female	$162.80	$205.40	$253.30	$323.90
Couple, 51–70 years	$361.30	$466.20	$580.30	$701.30
Couple, 19–50 years and children 6–8 and 9–11 years	$636.70	$836.20	$1044.60	$1268.70

[a]The Food Plans represent food patterns at four different cost levels that meet the nutrient requirements outlined in the 1997 to 2005 *Dietary Reference Intakes*, the 2005 *Dietary Guidelines for Americans*, and the 2005 MyPyramid, and assumes that all meals and snacks are prepared at home. For specific foods and quantities, see *Thrifty Food Plan, 2006* (2007) and *The Low-Cost, Moderate-Cost, and Liberal Food Plans, 2007*; costs given are for individuals in four-person families; data taken from food report for January 2017.
This file may be accessed on the home page of the Center for Nutrition Policy and Promotion at http://www.cnpp.usda.gov/USDAFoodPlans CostofFood.htm.

when and where family members eat. Other characteristics, described as follows, influence family food expenditures.

- *Family traditions:* Cultural, ethnic, and national groups have specific food patterns that they wish to continue. Sometimes it is difficult to obtain certain foods or necessary ingredients or, if available, they are high in price.
- *Special dietary needs:* Family members observing a meal plan related to a chronic condition may need special foods. Food-related conditions such as celiac disease may require home preparation of many foods and unique ingredients.
- *Amount and kind of entertaining:* Families may enjoy sharing meals or joining potluck socials with neighbors, community organizations, or religious affiliations.
- *Meals away from home:* Work or school schedules can require a packed lunch or meals purchased at another location. Families may enjoy eating away from home.
- *Value placed on food and eating:* Food and mealtime may hold high priority in allocation of resources.

Extended discussion with family members about their food resources and preferences provides a framework for developing and implementing a successful food plan.

Food Shopping

Food marketing is a big business, and buying family food is more complex than it may seem. Currently more than 85,000 uniquely formulated food items are available within US supermarkets,[25] and a single food may be marketed in many different ways, each with a different price (Fig. 10.3). To ensure a variety of foods and the number of servings recommended by the 2015 Dietary Guidelines,[21] it is best to plan meals for the week and then compile a shopping list. Avoid shopping

FIG. 10.3 Shoppers are faced with a dazzling array of food choices. (From Food and Nutrition Service, US Department of Agriculture and Food and Nutrition Information Center, National Agricultural Library: *Food stamp nutrition collection: photo gallery*, Beltsville, MD, 2013, US Department of Agriculture. https://www.snaped.fns.usda.gov/woman-looking-can-yams-grocery-store; Reprinted with permission of the Food and Nutrition Service, US Department of Agriculture.)

when you are hungry or rushed because then you will be more likely to buy items that you do not need or cannot afford. Limit shopping to once a week, using frozen or canned items after fresh foods have been exhausted. The Perspectives in Practice box, "Supermarket Skills," will help you sharpen your supermarket skills for teaching others.

PERSPECTIVES IN PRACTICE

Supermarket Skills

As shoppers try to make healthy food choices, developing a "game plan" for smart shopping is a pertinent topic for nutrition education. Supermarket tours help consumers develop more awareness of cost and nutrient quality and also recognize the marketing techniques and triggers for impulse buying. Saving money at the grocery store is not a matter of luck, but rather making smart decisions about what you put in your cart.

Before you shop: Read the weekly sales flyer advertising the specials for the week. They are often released on a Wednesday and can be found in the newspaper, in the store, or on the store's website. Plan your menus for the week, taking advantage of the specials that your family uses regularly and enjoys.

When to shop: Advertised specials available at the beginning of the week are sometimes sold out by the end of the week. In that case, ask for a "rain check" if this is an item you use. This allows you to purchase the item at the sale price when the item is restocked. Weekdays are the best times to shop because stores are less crowded, allowing more time and space for comparison shopping. Avoid Saturdays and dinnertime through the week when stores are congested and checkout lines are long.

Wise use of coupons: Food manufacturers and grocery chains offer coupons in the newspaper, online, and in food packages. There are downsides to coupons: you may have to buy several packages or the largest-size package to use your coupon or be enticed to buy something you do not need because it is "50 cents off." In addition, the store brand at full price may be the equivalent or less than the national brand with a coupon. Limit coupon use to those foods you use regularly.

Shop the inner aisles: The inner aisles of a grocery store contain less expensive staples such as legumes, peanut butter, dried milk, canned tuna fish, bulk cereals, and canned vegetables and fruits. Fresh produce and in-store bakeries are usually located at the front of the store, as these are high-profit items and subject to impulse buying. Displays at the ends of the aisles often represent "sale" items but also are used to draw attention to new or slow-moving items. Check the cost per ounce or unit to discern a true sale.

Placement on the shelf: Stores often place national brands and the most expensive items at eye level; check the prices of the items on the upper and lower shelves as well. Store shelves are usually stocked from back to front, placing the newest items behind the older ones. Reach in the back for the freshest items, especially in the produce, dairy, and meat aisles.

Check for store brands: Many large supermarkets offer their own brands of canned and packaged goods that cost less than national brands and are usually of good quality. National brands and store brands of the same item do not differ in nutrient content.

Unit pricing: Unit pricing is a helpful tool for comparison shopping, but be cautious when comparing a frozen with a canned product. Frozen vegetables contain little or no liquid as compared with canned vegetables that may contain as much as one-third liquid. Even if the canned item costs less per ounce, it may not be a better buy based on the actual amount of food obtained. Measure the liquid in the canned fruits and vegetables that you purchase regularly to calculate the real cost. (See Box 10-2 for an illustration of unit pricing.)

The USDA Cooperative Extension Service found in every state and county is a source of both print and online materials to help consumers develop food shopping skills.

Bibliography

Center for Nutrition Policy and Promotion: *Save More at the Grocery Store. 10 Tips Nutrition Education Series*, DG Tip Sheet No 37, March 2017, US Department of Agriculture. https://www.choosemyplate.gov/ten-tips-save-more-at-the-grocery-store.

US Department of Agriculture: *Healthy Eating on a Budget*. MyPlate. https://www.choosemyplate.gov/budget.

BOX 10.2 Unit Pricing

The unit price is the price per pound, ounce, quart, or serving. Unit price labels are found on the display shelves below canned and packaged foods. Comparing unit prices can help consumers find the brand and size container that costs the least per unit.

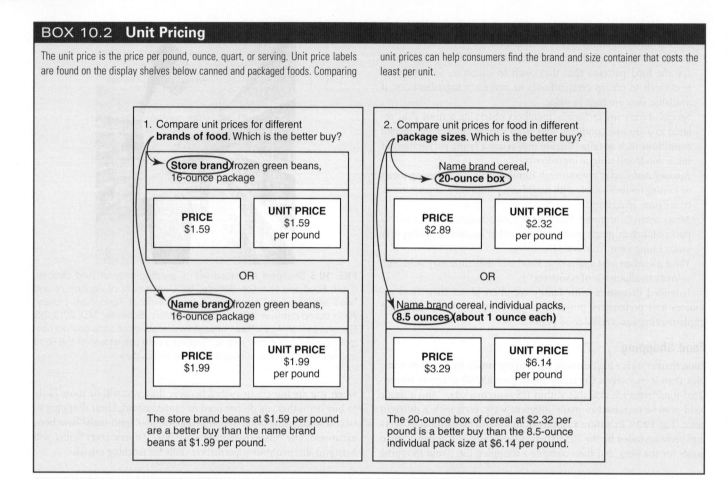

1. Compare unit prices for different **brands of food**. Which is the better buy?

(Store brand) frozen green beans, 16-ounce package

PRICE	UNIT PRICE
$1.59	$1.59 per pound

OR

(Name brand) frozen green beans, 16-ounce package

PRICE	UNIT PRICE
$1.99	$1.99 per pound

The store brand beans at $1.59 per pound are a better buy than the name brand beans at $1.99 per pound.

2. Compare unit prices for food in different **package sizes**. Which is the better buy?

Name brand cereal, (20-ounce box)

PRICE	UNIT PRICE
$2.89	$2.32 per pound

OR

Name brand cereal, individual packs, (8.5 ounces) (about 1 ounce each)

PRICE	UNIT PRICE
$3.29	$6.14 per pound

The 20-ounce box of cereal at $2.32 per pound is a better buy than the 8.5-ounce individual pack size at $6.14 per pound.

Wise Buying

Food labels, as described in Chapter 9, contain important information about food quantity, nutritional quality, and safety and help consumers get the best value for their food dollar. The following information on the food label and store shelf is useful when comparing prices:

- *Unit pricing:* Large packages are sometimes less expensive per unit weight than small packages, but any savings depends on how much is needed and if it can be used before spoiling. If an item has an extended shelf life or is used regularly, then one large box rather than two smaller boxes is a wise choice. The unit pricing label on the store shelf indicates the true price per unit weight and is useful when comparing different brands or package sizes (Box 10.2). Unit pricing tells you if the store brand costs less than the national brand.
- *Open dating:* These dates indicate the freshness of an item or how soon it must be used. Box 10.3 describes the types of dating information used on food labels. Checking the "use by" date is important when considering items reduced for quick sale. Coded dating relates to packing numbers used by the manufacturer to identify dates and lot numbers.
- *Package weight or volume:* The food and nutrition facts labels indicate the weight or volume of food in the package and the number of servings it provides. Deceptive packaging can suggest that the content is greater than it actually is.
- *List of ingredients:* The food label lists by weight the ingredients from the highest to the lowest. As described in Fig. 10.4, fruit drinks contain sugar, water, and flavoring but little or no juice. When purchasing bread or cereal, make certain the first ingredient is a whole grain.
- *Convenience foods:* Use comparison shopping to evaluate the relative cost and time benefit of preprepared items because time saved may not be worth the added cost. Fresh fruits and vegetables peeled and cut into bite-sized pieces and items packaged in single servings are handy when assembling lunches or grabbing snacks but cut into the food budget. Pancake or muffin mixes or precooked meat loaves are helpful to the busy family but add dollars to food costs. Table 10.2 provides examples of added cost according to the form or degree of prepreparation.

BOX 10.3 Types of Open Dating on Food Labels

Sell by	The last date the item can be sold by the store
Best if used by	The date that indicates maximum freshness; after this date, check for signs of spoilage and expect a reduced price
Expiration date or use by	The last date when active ingredients will be good (commonly used with yeast for baking); do not purchase foods after their expiration date, as spoilage may have occurred even if not visible
Pack date	The date the food was packed by the manufacturer; this date is commonly found on canned foods; look for a recent pack date

Ingredient Listing   Ingredients are listed in order from the most to the least amount found in the product.

Grape Juice:

Grape juice, grape juice from concentrate, ascorbic acid (vitamin C). No artificial flavors or colors added

Grape Juice Drink:
(10% Grape Juice)

Water; high fructose corn syrup; sugar; grape juice concentrate; fumaric, citric, and maltic acids (provide tartness); vitamin C; natural flavor; artificial color

Powdered Grape Drink:

Sugar, citric acid (provides tartness), natural and artificial flavor, artificial color, vitamin C

This label tells you:

- Mostly grape juice and juice concentrate
- Vitamin C added

This label tells you:

- Mostly added water, syrup, and sugar
- Some grape juice
- Vitamin C added, plus other things

This label tells you:

- Mostly sugar
- No juice at all
- Vitamin C added, plus other things

FIG. 10.4 Products with similar names can have very different ingredients and nutrient content. Read labels carefully to know what you are receiving for your money. (From US Department of Agriculture: Make your food dollars count, Program Aid No 1345, Washington, DC, 1984)

TABLE 10.2   Cost Comparisons of Food According to Preparation Required

Food[a]	Raw Ingredients	Preprepared	Additional Preparation
Vegetables			
Carrots	Unpeeled and uncut	Small baby carrots peeled and washed	Shredded carrots
	3-oz serving (raw) at 15 cents	3-oz serving (raw) at 27 cents	3-oz serving (raw) at 60 cents
Broccoli	Frozen flowerets in family-size bag	Frozen spears in family-size bag	Frozen spears with cheese sauce
	3-oz serving at 31 cents	3-oz serving at 48 cents	3-oz serving at 90 cents
Potatoes	Fresh potatoes (from 10-lb bag); cooked and mashed with milk	Instant mashed potatoes (milk added)	Refrigerated mashed potatoes (ready to heat)
	½ cup at 17 cents	½ cup at 24 cents	½ cup at 60 cents
Protein Foods			
Chicken	Raw chicken breasts (bone-in) at $2.79 per pound	Raw chicken breasts (boneless, skinless, and thin-sliced) at $4.99 per pound	Chicken breast cutlets (breaded and ready to heat) at $7.84 per pound
Ground beef	Ground chuck hamburger (80% lean)	Ground chuck hamburger preshaped into patties (80% lean)	Meat loaf refrigerated and ready to heat
	3-oz serving (cooked weight) at $0.87	3-oz serving (cooked weight) at $1.12	3-oz serving (heated) at $1.83
Grains			
Oatmeal	Old-fashioned oats (water added)	Quick 1-min oats (water added)	Instant oatmeal, unflavored (water added)
	¾-cup serving at 6 cents	¾-cup serving at 6 cents	¾-cup serving (one packet) at 25 cents
Pancakes	Homemade batter	Dry pancake mix, egg and milk added	Ready-to-pour batter
	One 4-in. pancake at 6 cents	One 4-in. pancake at 11 cents	One 4-in. pancake at 22 cents
Sweets			
Chocolate chip cookie	Homemade cookie batter	Refrigerated cookie dough (preportioned)	Packaged cookie (in-store bakery)
	One 2½-in. cookie at 6 cents	One 2-in. cookie at 12 cents	One 2-in. cookie at 25 cents

[a]Costs based on market prices at the Kroger supermarket in Blacksburg, VA, March 2014. Store brands were used if available for all three food comparisons. Recipes for homemade items taken from Rombauer IS, Rombauer Becker M, Becker E: *Joy of cooking*, ed 75. New York, 2006, Scribner.

Food Preparation

Nutrition education for meal preparers should emphasize preparation methods that maximize nutrient content but also promote the joy of eating. Using herbs and spices to replace salt produces good-tasting food that supports health. Broiling, grilling, or baking rather than frying reduces fat content and kcalories. People eat because they are hungry and because food looks and tastes good. Food demonstrations or hands-on classes with tasting are effective ways to model appropriate food safety and food preparation techniques and to confirm that healthy food is good to eat. (See Box 10.4 for suggestions on planning healthy and attractive menus.)

BOX 10.4 Tips for Menu Planning

- *Strive for balance:* Try to avoid too many high-fat meals in the same week; for every high-fat meal, plan a low-fat meal on another day. If you have a high-fat item as a main dish, serve a low-fat salad or vegetable.
- *Emphasize variety:* Try to mix raw and cooked items within the meal or the menu for the day. Avoid having the same type of food 2 days in a row, such as spaghetti with tomato sauce followed by ravioli with tomato sauce. Look to include different fruits and vegetables throughout the week to avoid monotony and obtain the various nutrients that you need.
- *Add contrast:* Think about how food will look on the plate—avoid all white or all red meals and aim for different sizes and shapes. Mix textures with both soft and crisp foods at the same meal.
- *Consider eye appeal:* Think about color—overcooked vegetables lose color. Try for the most attractive arrangement when placing the food on the plate.

Modified from Office of Superintendent of Public Instruction, Child Nutrition Services: Menu Builder Tool, State of Washington, 2016. http://www.k12.wa.us/ChildNutrition/Programs/NSLBP/pubdocs/MenuBuilderTool.pdf.

Food Shopping Locations

Supermarkets and Supercenters

Large grocery stores and supermarkets carry a wide variety of fresh and processed foods at reasonable prices. When several food outlets are close by, individuals can select where they want to shop or vary their location depending on the particular specials for the week. However, families in low-income urban neighborhoods or rural communities may have limited choices when it comes to food shopping. They may depend on limited-service stores with higher prices and limited selection for their groceries[26] and have no available transportation. A national survey of nearly 9000 stores including supermarkets, grocery stores, and limited-service stores revealed wide disparities in price and selection of fluid milk.[27] Although most supermarkets stocked both whole milk and skim milk, only 78% of limited-service stores sold whole milk and only 35% sold skim milk. Prices per gallon also were proportionately higher in limited-service stores as compared with supermarkets: $4.05 versus $3.33 for whole milk and $3.63 versus $3.26 for skim milk, respectively. The availability of milk at limited-service stores was also influenced by the surrounding population; stores in black or mixed-race neighborhoods were less likely to sell milk than those in white neighborhoods.[27]

Policy makers identify census tracts with high poverty rates and low food access as *food deserts*. When the poverty rate reaches 20% and at least 500 people or one-third of the population live at least 1 mile (if urban) or 10 miles (if rural) from the nearest supermarket or large grocery store, the area is designated a food desert. About two-thirds of food deserts are in urban locations and encompass approximately 24 million persons.[28] Individuals who lack vehicles are dependent on public transportation, and such services are scarce in rural communities. In rural Appalachia, families who could travel the 11 miles to a supermarket were able to save 30% on their food bill as compared with money spent at a nearby limited-service store.[26] Various city governments have partnered with nonprofit organizations and neighborhood groups to improve access to food supplies. Healthy People 2020 recognized the need for government incentives to encourage new food outlets in areas with low food access.[29] (Visit the website of the Philadelphia Food Trust at http://www.thefoodtrust.org to learn more about these accomplishments.[30])

Farmers' Markets

Farmers' markets bring local produce to consumers at prices that can be lower than at supermarkets. Local fruits and vegetables are often considered to be fresher and look and taste better than similar items from a grocery store that may have traveled a long distance. Buying local produce also supports a local sustainable farm system, a priority for a growing number of consumers.[31]

Consumer Cooperatives

Consumer cooperatives offer high-quality foods at the lowest possible price. Food cooperatives usually deal in bulk sales of whole or minimally processed foods and emphasize locally grown foods. Cooperatives usually require volunteer time in addition to or in lieu of a membership fee.

Food Discount Stores

Food stores that stock fresh and processed foods, paper goods, and cleaning supplies at discount prices are growing in popularity. These stores offer few services, and furnishings are sparse. Processed foods sold at food discount stores may be closeouts or excess stock that is nearing its date of expiration or best use. The unit available for purchase often includes multiple cans or packages, so consumers must decide if the quantity being purchased can be used before spoilage occurs.

Food Banks

Food banks are warehouses that collect and store donations of food from supermarkets, food processors, food distributors, growers, and the general public. These foods are made available to soup kitchens or food pantries providing meals or groceries to those in need. Food pantries offer emergency assistance when a family is in need of food and has no resources to purchase food. Feeding America, the nation's largest hunger relief organization, supports a network of more than 200 food banks and 60,000 food pantries across the United States.[32] In the past year, their local partners distributed an estimated 4.8 billion pounds of food, the equivalent of 4 billion meals, to 46 million persons, including 12 million children and 7 million senior citizens. Various local hunger relief organizations obtain food by gleaning or reclaiming wholesome food that would otherwise go to the landfill. It is estimated that 70 billion pounds of food are wasted each year in the United States.[32] The USDA contributes more than $350 million worth of commodity foods for distribution by emergency food providers.[33] (See Appendix D to learn more about commodity foods.)

HEALTH PROMOTION

Eating for Good Nutrition

The USDA Healthy US-Style Eating Pattern, Healthy Mediterranean-Style Eating Pattern, and Healthy Vegetarian Eating Pattern,[21] along with the practical advice found on MyPlate, guide the development of menus that meet nutritional needs. Think first about fruits and vegetables, and aim for a variety over the course of the week. A mix of fresh, frozen, and canned items, depending on season and price, meets financial constraints yet supplies important vitamins and minerals. Home gardening or container gardening increases the availability of vegetables at reduced cost. In urban locations, community gardens offer opportunities for youth and family participation. (The USDA Eating Patterns can be found at https://www.health.gov/dietaryguidelines/2015/guidelines/).

Grain foods are well liked, relatively inexpensive, and offer many varieties for different eating patterns. Whole grains are rich in fiber and especially high in trace minerals. At least three of our daily servings of grains should be whole grains.

Meat, fish, poultry, and eggs are complete proteins and supply B-complex vitamins and trace minerals. Eggs are relatively inexpensive and easy to prepare, and, for most people, one egg a day is acceptable. Fatty fish contributes important omega-3 fatty acids (review Fig. 9.3 for mercury advisories regarding fish consumption). Trimming visible fat and skin from meat and poultry reduces total fat and saturated fat. Dried beans and peas and nuts are good sources of amino acids and, when combined with other plant proteins or small amounts of animal protein, create a complete protein. Legumes are low in fat, high in fiber, versatile in food preparation, and easy to store. Soy protein is found in tofu and added to chips, pasta, trail mix, and other prepared foods.

Dairy foods provide protein, calcium, and magnesium, and most milks and yogurts are fortified with vitamin D. Fat-free, low-fat, and reduced-fat milk and dairy foods are lower in kcalories and total and saturated fat. Soy milk fortified with calcium and vitamin D is an appropriate substitute for milk and yogurt.

Fats and oils supply essential fatty acids and concentrated kcalories for those with high energy needs. Polyunsaturated and monounsaturated oils are the best choices and contain vitamin E. Hydrogenated fats may include trans fatty acids, harmful to health; reviewing the nutrition facts label will help avoid these fats. Butter, containing saturated fat and cholesterol, is best used in limited amounts. (See Table 1.2 to review the nutrient contribution of each food group.) The Case Study box, "Helping with Family Shopping," applies the principles of food shopping and meal planning.)

CASE STUDY

Helping with Family Shopping

Your manager at the local WIC office has asked you to assist a family with their food selection. She is concerned about the nutrient intakes of the mother and children and the family food shopping and food preparation practices. The family consists of three adults: a woman age 26, two men ages 27 and 69, and two children ages 5 and 2. Both children receive WIC food allocations. The mother goes food shopping daily, buying already prepared main dishes and any meat, dairy, and grain foods reduced for quick sale. To save money, she tries to use it all regardless of expiration or "use by" dates. She seldom buys fresh fruits and vegetables because they seem to be expensive, but fruit drinks are a family favorite.

Questions for Analysis

1. Based on the food plans developed by the USDA, what is the minimum amount of money this family must spend on food to meet their nutritional requirements?

2. What questions would you ask this homemaker about her shopping practices?

3. What advice would you give her about food-buying practices to ensure food safety? Which family members are most vulnerable to foodborne illness? (Review food safety principles in Chapter 9 as needed.)

4. What suggestions would you give her about less expensive forms of fruits and vegetables? Are fruit drinks a good use of her food dollars? (See Interactive Chart: *Most expensive and least expensive fruits and vegetables*, 2013, Economic Research Service, US Department of Agriculture. https://www.ers.usda.gov/data-products/fruit-and-vegetable-prices/interactive-chart-most-and-least-expensive-fruits-and-vegetables/.)

5. Develop a 3-day menu for the family observing the MyPlate recommendations for each food group and making use of all WIC foods available to the children. Prepare a shopping list for the purchase of needed foods. (See Appendix D for a list of WIC foods.)

COMMUNITY EDUCATION AND PROGRAM DEVELOPMENT

Community Food and Nutrition Education

Helping individuals and families make positive lifestyle changes to improve their nutrition and well-being is both an art and a science. The DRIs, the USDA Eating Patterns, and the 2015 *Dietary Guidelines for Americans*[21] provide the science—what nutrients and food sources are needed and in what amounts—but adapting those guidelines to individuals and communities with particular food beliefs, incomes, and living situations is an art, requiring patience, sensitivity, and application of behavioral theory.

Nutrition education programs that help people understand the relationship between nutrition and health and assist them in making decisions about their food can take many forms. Community nutrition programs are sponsored by government agencies responsible for the public's health, schools, corporations, faith-based groups, health-related voluntary organizations, health care facilities, and community coalitions. Targeted audiences can include pregnant women, parents, school children, senior citizens, worksite employees, low-income families, or the general public. The SNAP and WIC programs combine food assistance with nutrition education. Other programs may offer only nutrition information, participation in health-related activities, and personal support. These could include classes on healthy eating for mothers with at-risk children, community walking programs, or faith-based programs centered on disease prevention. The Healthy People 2020 objectives[29] emphasize the importance of nutrition and food education beginning in early childhood and continuing through elementary school, high school, and college. Worksites have potential for adult health promotion programs.

Societies shape their own patterns of disease. Dietary, economic, and demographic factors influence health in all age groups.[34,35] Individuals new to the United States may experience difficulties in acculturation to a new food environment.[36] As described in Fig. 10.5, our task is to provide families with the information and tools for decision making that will support positive health and reduce chronic disease.

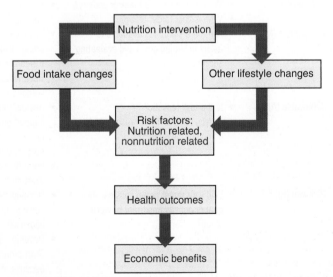

FIG. 10.5 Model for nutrition education. The goal of community nutrition education is to bring about positive changes in food and lifestyle behaviors that lower the risk of chronic disease. (Redrawn from Olendzki MC, Tolpin HG, Buckley EL: Evaluating nutrition intervention in atherosclerosis: some theoretical and practical considerations. *J Am Diet Assoc* 79(7):9, 1981, with permission.)

Implementing a Community Program

Health professionals often encounter nutrition problems in their community that trigger the need for nutrition education and intervention. Developing and implementing a program that will successfully address the problem you have identified requires careful and systematic planning. Program planning involves setting goals and deciding how to meet them. It speaks to the what, where, when, and how the program will be conducted.[37] Successful program planning involves several consecutive steps, as follows:

1. *Assess the needs of the target population and identify existing community resources.* To address individual and family needs you must know the race or ethnicity, educational level, typical household size and composition, language spoken at home, health problems, and income range of your target group. This information can be obtained from county or state census data. Food-related information would include the number of families receiving SNAP benefits or free or reduced-price school lunches and the availability of nearby supermarkets or grocery stores where the target group shops. It is also important to review other local community programs or services addressing similar issues; referrals or expansion to reach the underserved might be appropriate, rather than proposing a new program.

2. *Review all aspects of the problem.* Following your collection of available information, think about the various issues that may influence your approach and ultimate outcome. Teaching children or adults about healthy eating is of no value if they lack the resources to implement what you have recommended. In a school with a large proportion of overweight children, an after-school program focusing on healthy meals and snacks or increasing their physical activity might be a possible intervention. If so, you will need to cooperate with the school food service providers to ensure healthy options at breakfast and lunch. Do the children have access to a safe place to walk or play? If you are working with low-income mothers who receive SNAP benefits, lessons on meal planning can help ensure that food remains available for the entire month. However, do these families have access to a supermarket that offers lower prices and a good selection? Is transportation a hindrance to grocery shopping?

3. *Develop realistic goals and objectives.* A goal is a general statement of what you hope will happen as a result of the program and usually does not include a specific completion date. Objectives are specific statements describing what you plan to do; they must be measurable and include a date for completion. Your action plan will be developed from these objectives. (See Table 10.3 for examples of Specific, Measurable, Achievable, Relevant, and Time Frame (SMART) objectives.)

4. *Develop an action plan.* An action plan is a blueprint for the tasks required to implement your program. It includes who will carry out each task and the resources or assistance required. If the program will be sponsored by your agency or health care facility or school, you will need to identify other participants and gain the approval of the appropriate administrators. If you are working with another professional or community group, their responsibilities and your responsibilities must be carefully defined. If funding is

TABLE 10.3 Developing Smart Objectives

Characteristic	What to Include	Example
Specific (S)	• What is the intended task or activity? • Who is your target group?	• Increase fruit and vegetable intake of Head Start children in your community by increasing servings in meals and snacks at the Head Start Center.
Measurable (M)	• Are there standards available to assist in setting goals and evaluating success?	• Review current menus and snacks; calculate how many servings of fruits and vegetables are being included in meals and snacks and compare with USDA food plan recommendations for the target age group. • Review fruit and vegetable intake goals for this age group at the Healthy People 2020 website and compare with current practices.
Achievable (A)	• Is the task realistic? • Do you have sufficient resources to complete the project?	• Review food budgets within the Head Start program to determine if money is available to support purchase of more fruits and vegetables, or if funds can be reallocated among food groups to make more money available. Will it be necessary to procure additional funds to support proposed menu additions and how or where might they be obtained? • Identify and obtain resources needed to develop and implement in-service training for Head Start staff on greater use of fruits and vegetables in meals and snacks.
Relevant (R)	• Will your target group consider this goal or activity important or worth doing?	• Develop strategies to obtain commitment of Head Start staff to the goal of increased servings of fruits and vegetables (e.g., will they support purchase of more fruit and fewer cookies?). • Develop a presentation describing the health status of the children served by your Head Start program including such parameters as body weight and frequency of days missed because of colds or flu; emphasize the benefits of an improved diet; present to parents, Head Start staff, and potential community sponsors.
Time Frame (T)	• When will project start and end?	• Begin July 1 and end on June 30.

USDA, US Department of Agriculture.
Modified from Centers for Disease Control and Prevention: Develop SMART Ojectives. Public Health Information Network, Communities of Practice Program, Resource Kit, May 2011. https://www.cdc.gov/phcommunities/resourcekit/evaluate/smart_objectives.html.

required, then possible sources and procedures for obtaining resources must be noted. Procurement of teaching materials or food supplies along with any necessary fiscal reporting must be assigned. You and your colleagues need to consider how this program will be marketed so that announcements not only reach the target audience but also encourage their participation. Your chosen location must be safe, comfortable, and easily accessible. Think about how you will evaluate your program and who will collect and protect the confidentiality of the information obtained.

5. *Implement the program.* When your planning is complete, a location secured, necessary funding in place, materials ordered and available, an evaluation plan prepared, and responsibilities assigned, you are ready to proceed. Programs, even well-planned programs, sometimes proceed slowly. Word of mouth about a helpful program, sensitive to individual needs, can build interest and participation.

6. *Evaluate results for future planning.* Program evaluation can include both knowledge and behavior outcomes. Although it is helpful to know if participants have improved their nutrition knowledge, it is more important to know if they made changes in their food choices or food management. For children in the after-school class, rating the number of days they chose water or low-fat milk rather than a sugar-sweetened beverage, or increased their daily steps as measured by a step counter, indicates whether the program led to a potential improvement in health. For SNAP mothers, the number of meals per week that included at least one fruit or vegetable serving or the number of days out of food before receiving their next food stamp allotment impacts their children's well-being. Asking which lessons or activities the participants enjoyed the most or found most helpful is valuable for planning future programs.

Nutrition education is a process, not something that "happens to a person" and immediately changes his or her behavior. It involves small steps that over time improve nutritional status or a disease condition. Community nutrition programs demand close attention to family needs and resources and the knowledge and practical skills required to solve food problems. As noted in Fig. 10.6, persons of all ages can benefit from nutrition education.

Creating a Supportive Learning Environment

Successful community education requires attention to both the social and physical environment. It demands a relationship of trust, respect, and concern. This includes accepting people as they are and where they are in their personal development. It expects a positive environment for participation and discussion. When preparing for your teaching activity, consider the following:

• Use language appropriate to the listener.
• Present information in a way that is easily remembered.
• Provide examples that apply to the listener's personal situation.
• Become familiar with the cultural beliefs, eating patterns, and expectations of your target group

Effective communicators develop skills in analyzing the teaching situation and responding appropriately. Careful listening and observation assist in developing a helping relationship and successful intervention. (To learn more about working with different cultures, see the Focus on Culture box, "Developing Cross-Cultural Competence: A Goal for the Health Professional.")

🌐 FOCUS ON CULTURE

Developing Cross-Cultural Competence: A Goal for the Health Professional

Consider the following situations:

• You are teaching pregnant mothers in a public health clinic and using MyPlate to evaluate their food intake. A Hmong (Vietnamese) mother tells you that she never eats bread, and you are concerned about her servings from the grains group.
• You are working with an older African-American man, and he mentions that his favorite meal is his daughter's homemade Brunswick stew. What foods are included in that dish?

To be effective educators, we need to understand the food patterns of other ethnic, racial, and cultural groups, not just our own. We must acknowledge the health beliefs and values that influence another individual's food choices and nutritional status. The Hmong mother may not eat bread, but she is likely to have rice at every meal and thus more than meet her recommended servings of grains. However, she may be reluctant to take the vitamin and mineral supplements her physician recommended in the belief that they will result in a large infant and difficult delivery. The African-American man obtains important vitamins, minerals, fiber, and protein from his Brunswick stew made with chicken, carrots, tomatoes, white beans, and greens.

Cross-Cultural Situations

Throughout our professional lives, we will experience cross-cultural situations in which we belong to a different race, culture, or ethnic group than that of our supervisors, our colleagues, or the individuals for whom we provide care.

We can begin to develop cross-cultural competence in various ways, as follows:

• *Learn about other cultures by reading, observing, and sharing experiences.* A potluck meal provides an opportunity to share foods and the cultural values surrounding food.
• *Examine your own beliefs and feelings.* Identify and resolve any stereotypes that you may hold about groups other than your own.
• *Consider language training to prepare yourself to work with diverse populations.*

Bibliography

Goody CM, Drago L, editors: *Cultural food practices*, Chicago, 2010, Diabetes Care and Education Dietetic Practice Group, American Dietetic Association.

Kittler PG, Sucher KP, Nahikian-Nelms M: *Food and culture*, ed 6, Belmont, CA, 2012, Wadsworth/Cengage Learning.

McCaffree J: Language: a crucial part of cultural competency, *J Am Diet Assoc* 108:611, 2008.

Tsuji N, Dyck A, Mauldin K, et al: Effect of multicultural cooking classes on cultural competency of university students, *J Acad Nutr Diet* 116(9 Suppl 1):Abstract A-77, 2016.

While, A: Understanding cultural needs, *Br J Community Nurs* 21(4):214, 2016.

FIG. 10.6 People of all ages can benefit from a community nutrition education program. Online nutrition education materials can support continued learning after the formal program is completed. (Copyright 2006 JupiterImages Corporation.)

The physical environment is also important in community education. Look for a location that is familiar to the audience, easily accessible by public transportation, and where your target group will feel comfortable. Choose a setting with adequate space, ventilation, and lighting and free of distractions. You may need to provide child care if your target group includes young families.

A community nutrition education program can consist of a few classes or involve extended individual interaction over weeks or months. For healthy individuals looking to make better food choices in the marketplace, one or two sessions may be adequate. Patients with diabetes, renal disease, or serious heart disease or those at high nutritional risk may require extended classes and follow-up to reach the program goal. Use of technology may be a way to continue learning when formal classes have been completed. (To learn more about use of technology in health education, see the Evidence-Based Practice box, "Text Messaging: Effective Method for Community Education?")

Theories for Behavior Change

Behavioral theories provide a framework for helping us understand why people do what they do and so enable us to target our intervention strategies more effectively.[38,39] Behavior models commonly used in nutrition education have included the health belief model, the concept of self-efficacy, and the stages of change model. We describe each of these next:

- *Health belief model:* Some individuals base their health behavior on how they perceive their vulnerability to a particular disease or condition. Before making a change, this individual would need to (1) consider himself at high risk for developing a condition, (2) regard it as a serious threat to personal well-being, and (3) believe that changing his or her behavior would lessen the risk.[39] A young woman planning a pregnancy might begin using a folate supplement to help prevent a neural tube defect in her infant, or an overweight older adult might begin a walking program to lower his cardiovascular risk.

- *Self-efficacy model:* This theory proposes that behavior change depends on the magnitude of the demands it will make on an individual and his or her perceived ability to cope with the new situation or expected behavior.[40] The greater the person's confidence in his ability to successfully perform the new task or adapt to the new situation, the more likely it is that he will implement the change. Successful interventions work by providing people with the necessary tools or resources to practice the new behavior. A man who formerly ate lunch at a fast food restaurant can learn to prepare a packed lunch that will support his goals of lowering his fat and sodium intake. Helping mothers identify ways to add a vegetable serving to their family's evening meal increases the likelihood the goal of increased vegetable intake will be achieved.

- *Stages of change:* This model was first developed to address smoking cessation[41] but has been used to modify both nutrition and related health behaviors.[42] It proposes that individuals pass through five stages of change or reflection when adopting a new behavior.[41] How people respond to the information presented and the resources needed differ according to stage. Table 10.4 outlines the sequence of stages and role of the health professional as applied to an individual or population.

In practice, theories of behavior change are often used together. Individuals passing through the stages of change are more likely to be successful if given tools that increase their feelings of self-efficacy. As you continue to work in community education, look for clues to indicate your group's current "stage" and let this guide your intervention strategy.

EVIDENCE-BASED PRACTICE

Text Messaging: Effective Method for Community Education?

Identify the Problem: As the cost of face-to-face education continues to rise, health professionals are testing telecommunication methods as cost-effective interventions. The broad availability of cell phones across all socioeconomic and age groups suggests that mobile health (mHealth) may be a strategy to implement evidence-based medicine and support public health. Of American adults, 90% own a cell phone and 81% send text messages. Text messaging is a realistic option because messages can be delivered to any mobile phone.

Review the evidence: A program with the goal of increasing fruit and vegetable consumption among high school youth delivered a daily text message describing the physiological and psychological benefits of five servings a day.[1] Teens receiving the text messages reported an increase in their fruit and vegetable servings as compared with the students who did not receive texts. Regrettably, the intervention lasted for only 2 weeks, so we do not know if the dietary improvement would have continued over time. Regular text messages have also been used in the ongoing treatment of chronic disease.[2-4] More than 350 men and women with diagnosed coronary heart disease received, in addition to their regularly scheduled clinic visits, four text messages per week for 6 months that focused on lifestyle changes relating to diet, physical activity, and smoking cessation. An equal number of patients at the same clinic received the same in-person care but not the text messages. Those receiving the messages reduced their blood low-density lipoprotein (LDL)-cholesterol levels, systolic blood pressure, and body mass index, and increased their physical activity.[2] Daily medication reminders by text message were successful in treating patients with uncontrolled blood pressure.[3,4]

Implement the Findings: Text messaging has been found to be acceptable to target audiences, successful in promoting behavior change, and reasonable in cost. Although we may think of younger individuals as more accommodating of new technology, the mean age of participants in the chronic disease groups described previously was early to late fifties, and less than 5% requested that the text messages be discontinued.[2,3] Among those receiving medication reminders, more than 90% found the messages useful and motivating.[3] Text messages, prepared and delivered in bulk, average 10 to 20 cents each, with the cost of 96 messages over a 6-month period totaling approximately $10.[4] As use of text messaging continues to expand, it will be important to provide messages in multiple languages to accommodate our growing diversity.

References

1. Carfora V, Caso D, Conner M: Randomized controlled trial of a messaging intervention to increase fruit and vegetable intake in adolescents: affective versus instrumental messages, *Br J Health Psychol* 21(4):937, 2016.
2. Chow CK, Redfern J, Hillis GS, et al: Effect of lifestyle-focused text messaging on risk factor modification in patients with coronary heart disease: a randomized clinical trial, *JAMA* 314(12):1255, 2015.
3. Buis L, Hirzel L, Dawood RM: Text messaging to improve hypertension medication adherence in African Americans from primary care and emergency department settings: results from two randomized feasibility studies, *JMIR Mhealth Uhealth* 5(2):e9, 2017.
4. Thakkar J, Kurup R, Laba TL, et al: Mobile telephone text messaging for medication adherence in chronic disease: a meta-analysis, *JAMA Intern Med* 176(3):340, 2016.

TABLE 10.4   Stages of Change Model for Nutrition Behavior as Applied to Three Community Situations[a]

Stage	Behavioral Characteristics	Strategy	Examples of Intervention
Precontemplation	Individuals have no desire or intention to change; may refuse to admit there is a problem	Focus on consciousness-raising; family support may be helpful	A. Public service announcement on need for folate prior to pregnancy B. Poster in school cafeteria about eating fruit for quick energy; discuss healthy snacks in school health class; program for parents on healthy eating for teens C. Patient receives diagnosis of elevated blood pressure at annual physical examination
Contemplation	Individuals recognize there is a problem and have given some thought to what they might do about it—at some time in the future;	Provide information that might be helpful in addressing the problem	A. Provide printed materials describing food or supplement sources of folate in locations frequented by young women. B. Make leaflets available for pick-up in the school cafeteria suggesting a fruit snack that will fit in a backpack; hang posters advertising a website that compares the kcalories in fruit compared to other snacks C. Provide printed materials to patient on how to reduce sodium intake; suggest recipes for herbal mixtures to replace sodium, and reputable websites for more information
Preparation	Individual is getting ready to commit to change; this stage provides the foundation for effective action	Seeks resources or tools to support change	A. Young woman checks availability of supplements when shopping; talks with her pharmacist or physician about options; talks with significant other about options B. Student checks out the price of fruit and availability at the school snack shop or nearby convenience store; talks with parent about putting fruit on the grocery list; looks up the kcalorie content of various fruits on the Internet C. Patient looks for low-sodium recipes on several food websites; talks with physician about safety of salt substitutes; joins a class at the local hospital on healthy eating
Action	Individual has implemented at least one behavior change and is trying to practice it regularly	Encouragement and reinforcement; progress continues despite an occasional relapse	A. Woman takes her folate supplement on most days and tries to have a good folate food source at each meal B. Student participates in the school food service "snack special" of fresh fruit rather than chips C. Patient tries new low-sodium recipes obtained at the hospital healthy eating class; stops adding salt in cooking and adds less salt at the table
Maintenance	Individual has successfully implemented the new behavior for at least 6 months	Continuing encouragement and reinforcement	A. Occasional public service announcement—did you remember your folate today? B. School food service continues to "spotlight" a healthy fruit snack and guarantee availability C. Continued encouragement from health professional with possible improvement in medical condition; reminder posters and new recipe leaflets in doctor's office promoting reducing sodium intake

[a]Example A—Increase folate intake among women of childbearing age to help prevent neural tube defects.
Example B—Increase use of fruit as a snack among high school youth.
Example C—Reduce sodium intake to lower risk of high blood pressure among adults.

Learning and Behavior

Despite our understanding of behavioral theory, the myth still prevails that an increase in knowledge will result in a change in behavior. Learning follows three basic laws:

1. Learning is *personal* and occurs in response to an individual need. People learn only what they believe will be useful to them, and they retain only what they think they will need. Children are accustomed to learning ideas or facts because they are expected to do so; adults pay attention only to those principles for which they believe they have an immediate demand. The sooner a person can put new learning to use, the more likely it will be retained. This highlights the importance of providing an opportunity to practice a behavior before a learning session is completed.
2. Learning is *developmental* and builds on prior knowledge and experience. Find out what the learner already knows and to what past experiences the new knowledge can be related.
3. Learning brings *change*. Nutrition education that focuses on learner needs and goals has the greatest chance for success. Encourage your learners to set personal goals rather than using a prescriptive approach.

The Academy of Nutrition and Dietetics recommends a total diet approach for improving nutrient intake.[43] It is the total diet, not one meal or one food that is important. No one food is a "magic bullet" to health. The three keys are:

- *variety.* Choose many different foods from each food group. Do not eat the same fruits and vegetables or the same protein foods every day.
- *proportionality.* Cover half your plate with fruits and vegetables, with lesser amounts of protein and starch.
- *moderation.* All foods can be included in a healthy diet if used in appropriate amounts and combined with physical activity.

FOOD ASSISTANCE PROGRAMS: OPPORTUNITIES FOR NUTRITION EDUCATION

Families under economic stress often need help in meeting their food needs. Programs funded by local communities or the federal government can supply food directly or increase food-purchasing power to provide added nutrients. Federally funded food assistance programs usually target specific populations, whereas local food banks are likely to serve all age and gender groups.

US Department of Agriculture Programs

The USDA oversees several food assistance programs that reduce food insecurity. They are intended to increase access to food, promote a healthy diet, and implement nutrition education. It is estimated that one in four Americans participates in at least one of the 15 USDA-funded programs at some time during the year.[44] Certain programs are entitlement programs, meaning income guidelines determine eligibility and guarantee participation.

Supplemental Nutrition Assistance Program

The Supplemental Nutrition Assistance Program (SNAP), formerly known as the food stamp program, increases food-purchasing power. SNAP is an entitlement program reaching individuals and families who have incomes within 130% of the federal poverty line. Recent records indicate that nearly 46 million people were receiving SNAP benefits, making this the largest US food assistance program.[44] The average monthly benefit was $127 per person.[44] Although SNAP makes a significant contribution to the food resources of low-income families, many recipients still run out of food before the end of the month and rely on local food pantries for help. (See Appendix D for program details and lists of items that may not be purchased with SNAP benefits.)

Meal Programs for Children

The School Nutrition Program supervised by the USDA is open to all children. Children from families who meet the federal poverty guidelines receive their lunch free or at a reduced cost.[44] When it became apparent that many children were coming to school without breakfast, seriously impeding their ability to learn, the National School Breakfast Program was organized. Children eligible for a free or reduced-cost lunch receive breakfast at the same level of payment. More than 30 million children nationwide participate in the school lunch program daily, and 14 million receive a school breakfast.[44] Local school districts, recreation departments, and nonprofit community groups that sponsor summer education or recreation programs can apply for USDA funds to supply breakfast and lunch meals to their children. These meals are especially important for those who depend on school meals for a significant portion of their nutrient intake. (Current nutrition standards for all USDA meal programs are provided in Appendix D.)

Special Supplemental Nutrition Program for Women, Infants, and Children

The WIC program is administered through state health departments and provides money for food and infant formula through food vouchers or electronic credit. Eligible recipients include (1) low-income mothers who are pregnant, postpartum, or breastfeeding, and (2) their infants and children up to the age of 5. Both income level and nutritional risk determine eligibility. In this respect, WIC differs from entitlement programs such as SNAP and reduced-cost school meals, because income and limited financial resources alone do not guarantee participation. Medical or nutritional risk must be certified by a health care professional for initial and continuing participation, and a federal budgetary ceiling caps national enrollment. Average monthly participation approaches 8 million persons.[44]

Programs for Older Americans

The Nutrition Program for the Elderly (NPE) enacted under the Older Americans Act is open to all adults age 60 and older, but services are targeted to those in greatest social and economic need. Particular attention is directed to low-income, minority, rural, and low-literacy seniors at risk for institutionalization. Federal dollars are supplemented with state and local funds to meet the growing demand. Meals served in congregate settings as well as home-delivered meals are generally provided at noon on weekdays. Individuals receiving home-delivered meals must be certified as homebound by a health or social services professional or be responsible for the care of a homebound family member. Participants are urged to make a donation toward the cost of the meal. Home-delivered meals sponsored by nonprofit community groups have a set charge but usually offer scholarships for those who cannot afford the full price. More than 2.4 million older adults receive meals through these programs.[45]

Nutrition Education Opportunities

Food assistance programs offer unique opportunities for nutrition education. Pregnant and nursing mothers participating in WIC are helped with meal planning and use of allowable WIC foods. School lunch programs present children with examples of well-balanced meals with foods from the protein, fruit, vegetable, grain, and dairy groups; both breakfast and lunch meals include milk or other high-calcium food. Teachers and school health professionals can join together to provide educational experiences that connect the school meal with science and biology, social studies, and health. Appropriate meal planning can help address the growing problem of child obesity and health by limiting fat, sugar, and sodium.[46] For older adults the NPE offers time before or after the meal to address nutrition topics such as limiting sodium intake, low-cost meals for one or two, or good calcium sources.

Expanded Food and Nutrition Education Program/Supplemental Nutrition Assistance Program-Nutrition Education Program

The Expanded Food and Nutrition Education Program (EFNEP)[47] and the Supplemental Nutrition Assistance Program-Nutrition Education Program (SNAP-ED)[48] funded by USDA help limited-resource families learn more about choosing a healthy diet. EFNEP is available to any family falling at or below the federal poverty line, whereas SNAP-ED enrolls families receiving SNAP benefits. These programs serve youth and adults and are delivered by Cooperative Extension agents, paraprofessionals, and volunteers. Experiential lessons offer hands-on opportunities to practice skills in selection of healthy food, food safety, and resource management and encourage physical activity. Individuals are recruited through neighborhood contacts, SNAP offices, and WIC. Group classes, media methods, one-on-one instruction, and educational mailings reach different audiences. More than 2.5 million adults and youth receive direct education through this program each year.[48]

Nutrition and health professionals need to be familiar with local food assistance and education programs and make appropriate referrals.

KEY TERMS

Poverty Line
The minimum amount of income required to provide food, clothing, shelter, and other basic necessities for a family of a given size and composition. This index is used to determine eligibility for government entitlement programs such as SNAP or free or reduced-cost school lunches.

Paraprofessionals
Individuals who do not have a professional degree but work under the supervision of a health professional in providing nutrition education or other health or medical services; paraprofessionals are usually indigenous to the population or community they serve.

TABLE 10.5 Messages for Social Marketing

Audience	Message
Students	"Breakfast at school is cool"
Parents	"Your child needs breakfast"
Teachers	"Your students will do better if they eat breakfast"

Marketing messages should be fitted to the target audience. The messages were used to market a school breakfast program.
Data from Herbold N, Taylor PN: Marketing nutrition programs and services. In Edelstein S, editor: *Nutrition in public health. A handbook for developing programs and services*, Sudbury, MA, 2006, Jones and Bartlett. Modified from messages developed by the Massachusetts Department of Education.

Social Marketing

Social marketing principles can encourage participation in food assistance programs and the adoption of appropriate nutrition behaviors. Social marketing is the practice of applying commercial marketing strategies to the development of educational and public health programs.[49] Just as product advertising creates a need on the part of consumers for a particular food or automobile or article of clothing, so appropriate nutrition and health messages influence individuals to practice healthy behaviors. Table 10.5 describes the messages prepared by a state education department to advertise their school breakfast program, targeting the needs and values of students, parents, and teachers. Social marketing can address barriers associated with a health-related behavior and ways to overcome them. For example, a WIC breastfeeding initiative might emphasize how breastfeeding could be combined with a mother's busy lifestyle. When recommending a food or lifestyle change, consider how it might bring about better health or social well-being.

TO SUM UP

Malnutrition and food scarcity exist worldwide. International agencies support short-term interventions in response to famine and immediate food shortages, and also work with farmers to introduce agricultural practices that will increase the food supply in vulnerable locations. In past years, malnutrition in developing countries usually resulted from an inadequate food supply and nutrient deficiency. However, the worldwide emphasis on dietary sugars and fats has led to a growing obesity and rise in chronic disease prevalence in both developed and developing nations. As a result, developing nations now suffer the double burden of overweight and serious undernutrition within their population. The goal of public health interventions and nutrition education programs worldwide focus on food choices that will lessen the burden of chronic disease. In the US, meal plans developed by USDA offer guidance for meeting nutrient goals on a limited budget, but individuals spending more money on food have higher intakes of micronutrients. Behavioral models help us understand how people change their behavior and assist in developing strategies that lead to positive change. The health belief model, concept of self-efficacy, and stages of change are behavior models often applied to community nutrition programs. Many families under economic stress need help in obtaining the appropriate amounts and types of food. Food assistance programs add to a family's food resources and many also deliver nutrition education. Referral of clients with food needs to appropriate agencies is an important component of nutrition intervention.

■ QUESTIONS FOR REVIEW

1. How would you define "health"? How does it apply to nutrition education?
2. Perform a needs assessment of your county, town, or city. Review race or ethnicity, income, age, household type, employment, language spoken at home, number of families receiving SNAP benefits, and number of children receiving school breakfast and lunch at free or reduced cost. (a) What are food-related issues in your community? (b) What seem to be major causes of these food-related issues? (c) What local food-related programs exist to help meet these needs (include both government-funded agencies and any local food-related charities or services)? (d) Are available programs applicable to diverse population groups? Explain. (To complete this assignment, go to http://www.census.gov and select a state, then county or city to access local census statistics; state departments of education and social services post SNAP and school meal statistics according to locality; local websites are sources of available programs.)
3. Based on your needs assessment, develop a community nutrition program to address one of the issues you identified. Provide an overall goal, specific objectives, an action plan, and criteria you will use to evaluate its success. Name other health professionals, community programs, or facilities that would be potential partners.
4. List the three basic principles of learning. Apply these principles to one of the following situations: (a) a low-income Hispanic mother with limited English skills whose 2-year-old son is underweight for his age or (b) a 71-year-old woman with hypertension who has been told to lower her sodium intake.
5. What is meant by food insecurity? How would you determine if a patient was food insecure?
6. Review the various types of information provided on the food label that describe package contents, freshness, and safe use. Develop a handout to teach these concepts to a low-literacy audience.
7. Using unit pricing, compare the cost per serving of four different ready-to-eat cereals: (a) one sugar-coated cereal, (b) one granola cereal, (c) one whole grain cereal, and (d) one cereal advertised as meeting 100% of the DRIs. Which is the most expensive per serving, and which is the least expensive per serving? Which cereal provides the best nutritional value for the money? Why?
8. Obtain a global positioning satellite (GPS) navigational device or map of your city or county. Using the telephone directory or the Internet, identify supermarkets or discount food stores and input their location. Are there neighborhoods or areas that do not have access to a large grocery store or supermarket? Visit the Food Access Research Atlas maintained by the US Department of Agriculture, and determine if your locality has been designated a food desert (http://www.ers.usda.gov/data-products/food-environment-atlas.aspx#.UUDP1aWhCFI).

REFERENCES

1. Pacific Northwest Foundation: *Definitions of health/wellness*, Pacific Northwest Foundation, 6312 SW Capitol Hwy # 271; Portland, OR 97239. http://www.pnf.org/Definitions_of_Health_C.pdf.

2. Zhang N, Bécares L, Chandola T: Patterns and determinants of double-burden of malnutrition among rural children: evidence from China, *PloS One* 11(7):e0158119, 2016.

3. Nordin SM, Boyle M, Kemmer TM, Academy of Nutrition and Dietetics: Position of the Academy of Nutrition and Dietetics: nutrition security in developing nations: sustainable food, water, and health, *J Acad Nutr Diet* 113:581, 2013.

4. Coleman-Jensen A, Rabbitt M, Gregory C, et al: *Household Food Security in the United States in 2015*, Economic Research Report No. (ERR-215), Washington, DC, September 2016, Economic Research Service, US Department of Agriculture. https://www.ers.usda.gov/publications/pub-details/?pubid=79760.

5. Frongillo EA, Nguyen HT, Smith MD, et al: Food insecurity is associated with subjective well-being among individuals from 138 countries in the 2014 Gallup World Poll, *J Nutr* 147(4):680, 2017.

6. Barquera S, Pedroza-Tobias A, Medina C: Cardiovascular diseases in mega-countries: the challenges of the nutrition, physical activity and epidemiologic transitions, and the double burden of disease, *Curr Opin Lipidol* 27(4):329, 2016.

7. Popkin BM: Nutrition transition and the global diabetes epidemic, *Curr Diab Rep* 15(9):64, 2015.

8. Tzioumis E, Adair LS: Childhood dual burden of under- and overnutrition in low- and middle-income countries: a critical review, *Food Nutr Bull* 35(2):230, 2014.

9. Pan L, Sherry B, Njai R, et al: Food insecurity is associated with obesity among US adults in 12 States, *J Acad Nutr Diet* 112(9):1403, 2012.

10. Bruening M, MacLehose R, Loth K, et al: Feeding a family in a recession: food insecurity among Minnesota parents, *Am J Public Health* 102(3):520, 2012.

11. Pingali PL: Green revolution: impacts, limits, and the path ahead, *Proc Natl Acad Sci U S A* 109(31):12302, 2012.

12. Gorman KS, McCurdy K, Kisler T, et al: Maternal strategies to access food differ by food security status, *J Acad Nutr Diet* 117:48, 2017.

13. Hiza HA, Casavale KO, Guenther PM, et al: Diet quality of Americans differs by age, sex, race/ethnicity, income, and education level, *J Acad Nutr Diet* 113:297, 2013.

14. Aggarwal A, Monsivais P, Drewnowski A: Nutrient intakes linked to better health outcomes are associated with higher diet costs in the US, *PLoS ONE* 7(5):e37533, 2012.

15. Denny S: Is there research to support the statement that healthy diets cost more? *J Acad Nutr Diet* 112:1504, 2012.

16. Rehm CD, Monsivais P, Drewnowski A: Relation between diet cost and Healthy Eating Index 2010 scores among adults in the United States 2007-2010, *Prev Med* 73:70, 2015.

17. US Department of Agriculture: *Cost of food at home. US average at four cost levels*, Washington, DC, January 2017. Center for Nutrition Policy and Promotion. https://www.cnpp.usda.gov/sites/default/files/CostofFoodJan2017.pdf.

18. Personal communication: *Annemarie Kuhns; Economic Research Service, Food Markets Branch*, Washington, DC, US Department of Agriculture. E-mail: amkuhns@ers.usda.gov.

19. US Department of Agriculture, Center for Nutrition Policy and Promotion: *Thrifty food plan: 2006, CNPP-19*, Washington, DC, 2007, US Department of Agriculture. http://www.cnpp.usda.gov/Publications/FoodPlans/MiscPubs/TFP2006Report.pdf.

20. US Department of Agriculture, Center for Nutrition Policy and Promotion: *The low-cost, moderate-cost, and liberal food plans: 2007 Administrative Report, CNPP-20*, Washington, DC, 2007, U.S. Department of Agriculture. http://www.cnpp.usda.gov/Publications/FoodPlans/MiscPubs/FoodPlans2007AdminReport.pdf.

21. US Department of Health and Human Services and US Department of Agriculture: *2015-2020 Dietary Guidelines for Americans*, ed 8, December 2015. https://www.health.gov/dietaryguidelines/2015/.

22. Carlson A, Dong D, Stewart H, et al: *Following dietary guidance need not cost more—but many Americans would need to re-allocate their food budgets*, September 2015, Amber Waves, US Department of Agriculture, Economic Research Service.

23. Stewart H, Jeffrey H, Andrea C, et al: *The cost of satisfying fruit and vegetable recommendations in the dietary guidelines*, EB-27. February 2016, US Department of Agriculture, Economic Research Service.

24. Wolfson JA, Bleich SN: Fruit and vegetable consumption and food values: National patterns in the United States by Supplemental Nutrition Assistance Program eligibility and cooking frequency, *Prev Med* 76:1, 2015.

25. Ng SW, Popkin BM: Monitoring foods and nutrients sold and consumed in the United States: dynamics and challenges, *J Acad Nutr Diet* 112(1):41, 2012.

26. Miller WC, Rogalla D, Spencer D, et al: Community adaptations to an impending food desert in rural Appalachia, USA, *Rural Remote Health* 16(4):3901, 2016.

27. Rimkus L, Isgor Z, Ohri-Vachaspati P, et al: Disparities in the availability and price of low-fat and higher-fat milk in US food stores by community characteristics, *J Acad Nutr Diet* 115(12):1975, 2015.

28. Dutko P, Ver Ploeg M, Farrigan T: *Characteristics and influential factors of food deserts*, Econ Res Rep Num 140, Washington, DC, 2012, Economic Research Service, US Department of Agriculture.

29. US Department of Health and Human Services: *Healthy People 2020: improving the health of Americans, 2020 Topics and Objectives*, Washington, DC, 2014, US Department of Health and Human Services. http://www.healthypeople.gov/2020/topicsobjectives2020/default.aspx.

30. The Food Trust: *The Food Trust, One Penn Center, Suite 900, 1617 John F. Kennedy Blvd*, Philadelphia, PA, 19103, 2012. http://www.thefoodtrust.org.

31. Academy of Nutrition and Dietetics: Practice paper of the Academy of Nutrition and Dietetics: promoting ecological sustainability within the food system, *J Acad Nutr Diet* 113:464, 2013.

32. Feeding America: *Nourishing Healthy Futures: 2016 Annual Report. Feeding America, 35 East Wacker Drive, Suite 2000*, Chicago, Il, 60601, June 30, 2016. http://www.feedingamerica.org/.

33. US Department of Agriculture: *The Emergency Food Assistance Program, Food and Nutrition Service, Nutrition Program Fact Sheet*, June 2016. https://www.fns.usda.gov/sites/default/files/tefap/pfs-tefap.pdf.

34. Micha R, Peñalvo JL, Cudhea F, et al: Association between dietary factors and mortality from heart disease, stroke, and type 2 diabetes in the United States, *JAMA* 317(9):912, 2017.

35. Gerteis J, Izrael D, Deitz D, et al: *Multiple Chronic Conditions Chartbook*, AHRQ Publications No, Q14-0038, Rockville, MD, April 2014, Agency for Healthcare Research and Quality.

36. Goody CM, Drago L, editors: *Cultural food practices*, Chicago, 2010, Diabetes Care and Education Dietetic Practice Group, American Dietetic Association.

37. Moreschi JM: Planning and evaluating nutrition services for the community. In Edelstein S, editor: *Nutrition in public health. A handbook for developing programs and services*, Sudbury, MA, 2006, Jones and Bartlett.

38. Kelley CP, Sbrocco G, Sbrocco T: Behavioral modification for the management of obesity, *Prim Care* 43(1):159, 2016.

39. Martinez DJ, Turner MM, Pratt-Chapman M, et al: The effect of changes in health beliefs among African-American and rural white church congregants enrolled in an obesity intervention: A qualitative evaluation, *J Comm Health* 41:518, 2016.

40. Holli BB, O'Sullivan-Maillet J, Beto JA, et al: *Communication and education skills for dietetics professionals*, ed 5, Philadelphia, 2009, Lippincott Williams & Wilkins.

41. Prochaska JO, Norcross JC, Diclemente CC: *Changing for good: a revolutionary six-stage program for overcoming bad habits and moving your life positively forward*, New York, 1994, Quill.

42. Mastellos N, Gunn LH, Felix LM, et al: Transtheoretical model stages of change for dietary and physical exercise modification in weight loss

management for overweight and obese adults, *Cochrane Database Syst Rev* 5(2):CD008066, 2014.

43. Freeland-Graves JH, Nitzke S, Academy of Nutrition and Dietetics: Position of the Academy of Nutrition and Dietetics: total diet approach to healthy eating, *J Acad Nutr Diet* 113(2):307, 2013.

44. Oliveira, Victor. *The Food Assistance Landscape: FY 2015 Annual Report*, EIB-150, US Department of Agriculture, Economic Research Service, March 2016. https://www.ers.usda.gov/webdocs/publications/44059/56937_eib150.pdf?v=42446.

45. Administration for Community Living: *Aging Integrated Database (AGID), Data-at-a-Glance (SPR)*, 2014, U.S. Department of Health and Human Services. http://www.agid.acl.gov/DataGlance/SPR/.

46. Schober DJ, Carpenter L, Currie V, et al: Evaluation of the LiveWell@ School food initiative shows increases in scratch cooking and improvement in nutritional content, *J Sch Health* 86(8):604, 2016.

47. US Department of Agriculture: *Expanded Food and Nutrition Education Program (EFNEP)*, Washington, DC, 2015, National Institute of Food and Agriculture. https://www.nifa.usda.gov/program/expanded-food-and-nutrition-education-program-efnep.

48. US Department of Agriculture: *SNAP-Ed 2015 FY Supplemental Nutrition Assistance Program Education through the Land-Grant System*, Washington, DC, September 2016, National Institute of Food and Agriculture. https://www.nifa.usda.gov/sites/default/files/resource/SNAP%20Ed%20Report%20-%20Executive%20Summary%20Final%209%2021%2016.pdf.

49. Centers for Disease Control and Prevention: *Gateway to Health Communication and Social Marketing Practice*, Atlanta, GA, January 2016. https://www.cdc.gov/healthcommunication/index.html.

FURTHER READINGS AND RESOURCES

Readings

Robinson E, Harris E, Thomas J, et al: Reducing high calorie snack food in young adults: a role for social norms and health based messages, *Int J Behav Nutr Phys Act* 10:73, 2013.

Utter J, Denny S: Supporting families to cook at home and eat together: findings from a feasibility study, *J Nutr Educ Behav* 48(10):716, 2016.

White AH, Maroto ME: Summer meal programs provide an opportunity for nutrition education and physical activity, *J Acad Nutr Diet* 116(6):905, 2016.

[These articles provide examples of community nutrition interventions.]

Websites of Interest

- Cooperative State Research, Education, and Extension Service, US Department of Agriculture: *SNAP-ED Connection*. This site offers educational materials, recipes, and other resources useful when working with limited-resource audiences. http://www.snap.nal.usda.gov.

- Food and Nutrition Service, US Department of Agriculture. This site offers links to various USDA food assistance programs, including the National School Lunch and Breakfast Programs, the Supplemental Nutrition Assistance Program (SNAP), and the Special Supplemental Nutrition Program for Women, Infants, and Children (WIC). http://www.fns.usda.gov/fns/.

- US Bureau of Census: *FedStats*. This site provides statistical data from all agencies of the federal government including population numbers and demographics, health issues, agriculture, and income parameters; data can be accessed by topic, nation, and state. https://www.fedstats.sites.usa.gov.

- My Plate. This site offers tips for eating on a budget and food shopping. https://www.choosemyplate.gov/budget.

11

Nutrition During Pregnancy and Lactation

Kary Woodruff

ⓔ http://evolve.elsevier.com/Williams/essentials/

In this chapter, we begin a three-chapter sequence on nutrition in health care throughout the life cycle. In each chapter, we will relate principles of nutrition to the remarkable process of human growth and development. As we focus first on the beginning of new life, we examine the prenatal nutritional demands of the pregnant woman and her developing fetus, as well as maternal nutritional needs during lactation. Mother and offspring possess great adaptive abilities to meet nutritional demands during these life cycle stages. Here, we explore the tremendous physiologic changes during pregnancy and lactation and some possible complications. You will see how vital optimal nutrition is for a successful course and outcome.

OUTLINE

Maternal Nutrition and the Outcome of Pregnancy
Health Promotion
  Nutritional Demands of Pregnancy
  Weight Gain During Pregnancy

General Dietary Problems
High-Risk Pregnancies
Complications of Pregnancy
Nutrition During Lactation

MATERNAL NUTRITION AND THE OUTCOME OF PREGNANCY

Early Medical Practice

For centuries in all cultures, a great body of folklore has surrounded pregnancy. Various traditional practices and diets have been followed, many of which have had little factual basis, and much clinical advice has been based only on supposition. For example, early obstetricians even held the notion that semistarvation of the pregnant woman was really a blessing in disguise because it produced a small baby of lightweight who would be easier to deliver. To this end, they used diets restricted in kilocalories (kcalories or kcal), protein, water, and salt. Despite the lack of any scientific evidence to support such ideas, two assumptions, now known to be false, governed practice: (1) the *parasite theory* (i.e., whatever the **fetus** needs it draws from maternal stores despite the maternal diet) and (2) the *maternal instinct theory* (i.e., whatever the fetus needs the pregnant woman instinctively craves and consumes).

Healthy Pregnancy

Until recently, much of the counsel given to pregnant women during the past few decades has been based more on tradition than on scientific fact. Increasing evidence indicates that positive nutritional support of pregnancy, rather than excessive restrictions born of limited knowledge and false assumptions, promotes a successful outcome with increased health and vigor of mothers and their infants. This struggle during the past few decades, particularly to define the "healthy pregnancy," has not been easy. A healthy pregnancy has often been defined

by the birth weight of the newborn, because infant mortality, or death, is lower for infants with birth weights between 2500 and 4000 g.[1]

Two key factors that predict infant birth weight are (1) maternal preconception weight and (2) weight gain during pregnancy.[2] Nutrition and other lifestyle factors affect maternal weight and weight gain; many of these factors, particularly nutrition, are modifiable or may be controlled by the pregnant woman. However, healthy pregnancy may also be viewed in the broader context of social determinants of health, including economic stability, education, social and community context, access to health care, and the physical environment.[3] These other factors contributing to pregnancy outcomes should be considered by the health care community when addressing healthy pregnancies. It is clear that we must assess and support more fully the quality of life of each mother and her family if we are to achieve healthy pregnancy outcomes among women.

Directions for Current Practice

Clinical observations and developing science in nutrition and medicine have provided guidance for healthier pregnancies. Previous false ideas have been refuted, and a sound foundation for current practice has emerged that is evidence based. Guidelines for the nutritional care of pregnant women have been established by the Academy of Nutrition and Dietetics as well as research and recommendations that are published by the American College of Obstetricians and Gynecology.[2,4] Nutritional guidelines for pregnancy and **lactation** for all nutrients are also included in the Dietary Reference Intake (DRI) recommendations published by the Food and Nutrition Board of the Institute of Medicine.[5-9]

The *fetal origins hypothesis*, which later became the *developmental origins of health and disease (DOHaD)*, supports the notion that appropriate nutrition during gestation, or the lack thereof, sets the course for chronic disease in adulthood.[10] Development of cardiovascular disease, hypertension, obesity, type 2 diabetes, metabolic syndrome, and gestational diabetes, among other chronic diseases, has been shown in the offspring of animals experiencing poor nutrition affecting intrauterine growth, as well as in human epidemiologic studies of the relationship between infant anthropometric measurements and adult disease incidence.[1,10] In these epidemiologic studies, infant body size, shape, and weight measurements, as well as measurements of maternal health and pregnancy behaviors, served as indicators of maternal nutrition. Changes in maternal nutrition and other environmental stressors during pregnancy require that the fetus adapt. These adaptations may lead to programming, or the mechanisms through which alterations in gene expression result in permanent changes in organ system structures and functions, resulting in risk of chronic disease. This hypothesis presumes that nutritional insults that occur during critical stages of embryonic and fetal development are most harmful, leading to future disease risk. Evidence supporting the DOHaD paradigm is robust and emphasizes that prevention of chronic diseases later in life begins in early development.[10]

Factors Determining Nutritional Needs

An expanding body of research and the best practices of clinicians reinforce that maternal nutrition is critically important to the mother and the newborn (Fig. 11.1). This lays the necessary foundation for the successful outcome of pregnancy—a healthy mother and infant.[4] Several factors determining nutritional requirements of the mother during pregnancy are well recognized.

Age, Gravida, and Parity

Age plays a major role in pregnancy; the teenage girl adds her own growth and maturation needs to those imposed by pregnancy. Advanced maternal age also presents its own pregnancy risks. In addition, the number of pregnancies (gravida) and the number of viable offspring (parity), as well as the time intervals between them, greatly influence the woman's nutrient reserves, her increased nutritional needs, and the outcome of the pregnancy.

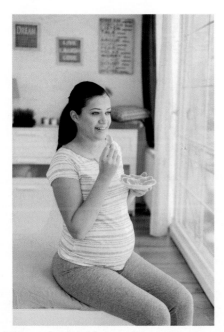

FIG. 11.1 Adequate intake of fruits and vegetables is essential during pregnancy. (Copyright Getty Images.)

Complex Physiologic Interactions of Gestation

Three distinct biologic entities are involved during gestation: the woman, fetus, and placenta, which nourishes fetal growth. Together they form a unique biologic whole. Constant metabolic interactions occur among them. Their functions, although unique, are at the same time interdependent. It is this unique biologic synergism that nourishes and sustains the pregnancy.

Basic Concepts Involved

As a result of our increased knowledge of pregnancy and nutrition, we can provide better nutritional guidance. Three basic concepts form a fundamental framework for assessing maternal nutritional needs and for planning supportive prenatal care.

Perinatal Concept

The prefix *peri-* comes from the Greek root meaning around, about, or surrounding. Thus the word *perinatal* refers more broadly to the scope of factors that surround a birth than merely the 9 months of the physical gestation. Certainly, as nutrition knowledge and understanding have increased, health professionals realize that a woman's life experiences surrounding her pregnancy must be considered. Her nutritional status and food patterns, which have developed over years, and the degree to which she has established and maintained nutritional reserves are all important factors.

Synergism Concept

Synergism describes biologic systems in which two or more factors interact cooperatively to produce a total effect that is better and different from the original parts. Of the many biologic and physiologic examples of synergism, pregnancy is a prime case in point. The mother, fetus, and placenta work synergistically to produce a system that had not existed before; this system now serves to sustain and nurture the pregnancy and its offspring. Through synergism, the physiologic systems of the mother change, and the physiologic norms of the nonpregnant woman no longer apply. For example, a normal physiologic generalized edema of pregnancy is a protective response. It reflects the normal increase in total body water necessary to support the increased metabolic work of pregnancy and is associated with enhanced reproductive performance to better serve the developing offspring.

Life Continuum Concept

In a real sense, throughout her life a woman is providing for the ongoing continuum of life through the food she consumes. Each offspring becomes a part of this continuing process during the pregnancy, when the mother's diet directly sustains growth and development. However, in the broader sense, the mother transfers her nutritional heritage, practices, and beliefs to her growing children, who in the next generation pass on this heritage genetically and culturally. Multigenerational factors carry forward.

HEALTH PROMOTION

Preconception Nutrition

The fact that a woman's health, fitness, nutrition status, and eating habits significantly impact her pregnancy and the health of the fetus underscore the importance of preconception nutrition. The Maternal, Infant and Child objective included in Healthy People 2020 (see Further Readings and Resources at the end of this chapter) addresses the need for improvements in preconception nutrition and health in women in the United States.[11] Preconception counseling is an avenue to such improvements. Related to nutrition, preconception counseling may include screening for medical conditions such as iron deficiency anemia, eating disorders, diabetes, drug-nutrient interactions, and genetic disorders, as well as assessment of current body weight, recent and previous weight changes, body mass index (BMI), fitness and exercise status, folate status, other nutrient intakes, eating patterns, and dietary and botanical supplement use. Evaluation of existing medical conditions such as hypertension, diabetes, thyroid disease, celiac disease, phenylketonuria (PKU), and others is important. Inquiries about the home and family environment, including income, education, safety, lead exposure, and abuse, should also be conducted during preconception counseling so that guidance, recommendations, and referrals may be thoroughly provided. Each of these nutrition, health-related, and environmental factors has documented effects on pregnancy outcome, many of which are adverse. However, preconception counseling and optimal preconception nutrition increase the odds for a healthy pregnancy and desirable infant outcome.

Infertility

Infertility is defined as the failure to conceive after 12 months of engaging in sexual intercourse without using methods of birth control. The prevalence of infertility ranges from 7.0% to 15.5% among the population of women of reproductive ages in the United States.[12] Although many factors, such as nulliparity, older age, lower educational level, and gynecologic conditions, are related to infertility, nutrition-based factors are emerging as additional contributors. For example, obesity or severe underweight in some women delays time to conception,[2,13] and dietary components, including caffeine, alcohol, and specific micronutrients, have been implicated in infertility.[13] An optimal diet may be necessary for fertility.

Excess Body Weight

Approximately 71% of adults in the United States are overweight, and nearly 38% are obese. Hence many women enter their pregnancies with excess body weight. This condition increases the risks of fetal mortality and malformations, excessive weight gain during pregnancy, gestational diabetes, hypertension, and preeclampsia, as well as the likelihood of preterm delivery and infant delivery by cesarean section. Pregnancy is not a time for weight loss because of the energy and nutrient requirements of the woman and fetus. Rather, a woman with excess body weight should moderately and gradually reduce her weight before pregnancy through an individualized energy-restricted diet and exercise plan. Weight gain during pregnancy should then follow recommendations based on BMI as outlined later in this chapter.

Exercise

Women who are physically active before pregnancy should continue exercising, and women who are physically inactive are encouraged to start exercising.[14] In fact, women who engage in prenatal exercise have been shown to have additional health benefits compared with nonexercising women, with benefits extending to the fetus as well. A pregnant woman should strive to achieve approximately 30 minutes of aerobic activity daily to meet a goal of approximately 150 minutes per week.[14] As the woman's body size and shape change throughout the course of pregnancy, exercise type, duration, intensity, and frequency should be adjusted to promote safety for the woman and her fetus (Fig. 11.2). Physical activities not recommended during

FIG. 11.2 Physical activity during pregnancy benefits both the pregnant woman and the fetus. (Copyright 2006 JupiterImages Corporation.)

pregnancy include scuba diving and those with risk of falling or trauma to the abdominal area.

The energy cost of exercise influences the kcalorie needs of the pregnant woman. Adequate kcalories must be consumed to meet the energy cost of exercise and to promote appropriate maternal weight gain and fetal growth and development. Adequate hydration is also vital, and the woman should increase fluid intake during exercise.

NUTRITIONAL DEMANDS OF PREGNANCY

Basic Nutrient Allowances and Individual Variation

Gestation is characterized by exceedingly rapid growth and development. During this 38- to 42-week period, a single fertilized egg cell (ovum) grows into a fully developed infant weighing approximately 3500 g, on average. What nutrients must the woman supply to support this intense period of fetal growth and development? What must her diet provide to meet fetal nutritional demands and her own needs during this critical period?

Pregnancy increases the need for many of the basic nutrients, as indicated by the DRI guidelines from the Food and Nutrition Board of the Institute of Medicine (Table 11.1).[5-9] However, it is important to remember that these are guidelines; individual variances in nutrient needs must be examined for each pregnancy. Individual variations such as basal metabolic rate (BMR), BMI, physical activity, and health status must be considered. In addition, the increased nutrient needs of pregnant adolescents and multifetal pregnancies must be noted. Individual counseling and correct use of nutritional guidelines is imperative.[4] In considering the nutritional needs of the *healthy* pregnant woman, we will review here the macronutrients and selected micronutrients with increased needs, rationale for increased needs, and how such nutrients may be obtained from foods.

Energy Needs

The kcalories must be sufficient to perform the following two functions:
1. Supply the increased energy and nutrient demands created by the increased metabolic workload, including some maternal fat storage and fetal fat storage to ensure an optimal newborn size for survival.
2. Spare protein for tissue building.

The DRI standard recommends an additional 340 kcal/day during the second trimester and 452 kcal/day during the third trimester of pregnancy to supply needs during this time of rapid growth.[6] Total daily kcalorie intake during the second and third trimesters should be based on the woman's nonpregnant estimated energy requirement plus the additional kcalorie need. This primary emphasis on sufficient kcalories is critical to ensure nutrient and energy needs to positively support the pregnancy. Appropriate weight gain during pregnancy indicates whether sufficient kcalories are being consumed. Kcalorie recommendations in the first trimester are not changed.

TABLE 11.1	**Dietary Reference Intakes Per Day of Selected Nutrients for Pregnancy and Lactation**				
	NONPREGNANT GIRL		**NONPREGNANT WOMAN**	**DURING PREGNANCY**	**LACTATION**	
Nutrients	9–13 years 46 kg 101 lb	14–18 years 55 kg 120 lb	19–50 years 63 kg 138 lb	19–50 years	(600 mL/day) first 6 months	(750 mL/day) second 6 months
Kilocalories	2000–2100	2300–2400	2400	No change in first trimester; +340 kcal/day for second trimester and +452 kcal/day for third trimester	+500 kcal/day (170 kcal/day from maternal stores)	+400 kcal/day
Protein (g)	34	46	46	71	71 throughout	
Calcium (mg)	1300	1300	1000	1000 throughout	1000 throughout	
Iron (mg)	8	15	18	27 throughout	9 throughout	
Vitamin A (mcg RAE)[a]	600	700	700	770 throughout	1300 throughout	
Thiamin (mg)	0.9	1.0	1.1	1.4 throughout	1.4 throughout	
Riboflavin (mg)	0.9	1.0	1.1	1.4 throughout	1.6 throughout	
Niacin (mg NE)[b]	12	14	14	18 throughout	17 throughout	
Vitamin C (mg)	45	65	75	85 throughout	120 throughout	
Vitamin D (mcg)	15	15	15	15 throughout	15 throughout	
Folic acid (mcg DFE)[c]	300	400	400	600 throughout	500 throughout	

[a]As retinol activity equivalents (RAEs): One RAE is equal to 1 mcg all-*trans* retinol or 12 mcg β-carotene.

[b]As niacin equivalents (NEs), one NE is equal to 1 mg of niacin or 60 mg of tryptophan.

[c]As dietary folate equivalents (DFEs), one DFE is equal to 1 mcg food folate or 0.6 mcg of folic acid from fortified food (or as a supplement consumed with food) or 0.5 mcg of a supplement taken on an empty stomach.

Data from Food and Nutrition Board, Institute of Medicine: *Dietary reference intakes for calcium, and vitamin D,* Washington, DC, 2011, National Academies Press; Food and Nutrition Board, Institute of Medicine: *Dietary reference intakes for energy, carbohydrate, fiber, fat, fatty acids, cholesterol, protein, and amino acids (macronutrients),* Washington, DC, 2005, National Academies Press; Food and Nutrition Board, Institute of Medicine: *Dietary reference intakes for thiamin, riboflavin, niacin, vitamin B₆, folate, vitamin B₁₂, pantothenic acid, biotin, and choline,* Washington, DC, 1998, National Academies Press; Food and Nutrition Board, Institute of Medicine: *Dietary reference intakes for vitamin C, vitamin E, selenium, and carotenoids,* Washington, DC, 2000, National Academies Press; Food and Nutrition Board, Institute of Medicine: *Dietary reference intakes for vitamin A, vitamin K, arsenic, boron, chromium, copper, iodine, iron, manganese, molybdenum, nickel, silicon, vanadium, and zinc,* Washington, DC, 2000, National Academies Press.

Much of our knowledge regarding the importance of sufficient energy intake during pregnancy arose from records of pregnancy and infant statistics through periods of famine during World War II. Insufficient kcalorie intake during the first trimester of pregnancy was associated with miscarriage and increased incidence of neural tube defects and other metabolic changes, whereas inadequate kcalorie consumption in the second and third trimesters of pregnancy was associated with increased numbers of congenital abnormalities, infants of low birth weight, and infant mortality. Current famine and food insecurity in various locations around the world continue to support these earlier findings regarding the essential need for adequate kcalories during pregnancy to support an optimal infant outcome. Energy needs of pregnancy may be met through a balanced intake of macronutrients.

Protein, Fat, and Carbohydrate Needs

The total amount of protein recommended for a pregnant woman is 71 g/day, an increase of 25 g/day.[6] Protein, with its essential nitrogen, is the nutrient basic to tissue growth. Nitrogen balance studies suggest that a large amount of nitrogen is used by the woman and fetus during pregnancy and emphasize the importance of preconception maternal reserves to meet initial pregnancy needs. More protein is necessary for demands posed by the following:

- Rapid fetal growth
- Enlargement of the uterus, mammary glands, and placenta
- Increase in maternal circulating blood volume and subsequent demand for increased plasma proteins to maintain colloidal osmotic pressure and circulation of tissue fluids to nourish cells
- Formation of amniotic fluid
- Storage reserves for labor, delivery, and lactation

Milk, egg, cheese, soybeans, and meat are complete protein foods of high biologic value. Protein-rich foods also contribute other nutrients, such as calcium, iron, and B vitamins. Additional protein may be obtained from nuts, legumes, and whole grains, with lesser amounts in other plant sources.

An adequate supply of essential fatty acids is also vital throughout pregnancy. Tissue growth, especially the proper development of cell membranes in nerve and brain tissue, and development of organ function, notably cognition and visual acuity, require that essential fatty acids and their converted forms reach the developing fetus in sufficient amounts. Inadequate maternal consumption of essential fatty acids may warrant additional supplementation to maintain adequate levels. However, most pregnant women may consume adequate amounts of linoleic (13 g/day) and α-linolenic (1.4 g/day) acids through consumption of canola, soybean, and walnut oils, in addition to other dietary fat sources.[6] Docosahexaenoic acid (DHA), important for visual and cognitive development, is found in salmon, mackerel, striped bass, and other fish products. Eicosapentaenoic acid (EPA), also found in fish, fish oils, flaxseed, walnuts, and canola oil, is important for blood vessel dilation, blood clotting, and reducing inflammation. Combined DHA and EPA intake of 500 mg/day is recommended.[15] Fish intake during pregnancy is encouraged, with a recommended intake of at least 8 to 12 oz per week, while avoiding fish with a higher methyl mercury content, including albacore tuna, king mackerel, shark, swordfish, and tilefish.[16] (See Chapter 9 for more information on mercury content of fish.)

Carbohydrate intake of at least 175 g/day during pregnancy is important for an adequate supply of glucose and nonprotein energy.[6] Whole grains, legumes, as well as fruits and vegetables, should be consumed to meet maternal and fetal glucose needs and provide fiber for satiety and bowel regulation. Currently, popular low-carbohydrate "diets" are not recommended during pregnancy. These diets do not provide the minimum glucose load required by the maternal and fetal bodies. In general, total daily dietary kcalorie intake should comprise 15% to 20% protein, 25% to 35% fat, and 50% to 60% carbohydrate, keeping in mind the individual needs of the pregnant woman and adequate macronutrient distribution ranges.

Mineral Needs

All of the major and trace minerals play roles in maternal health. Four that have special functions in relation to pregnancy deserve particular attention: (1) calcium, (2) iodine, (3) iron, and (4) zinc.

Calcium

The pregnant woman's DRI recommendation is 1000 mg of calcium per day, the same as the general recommendation for all women ages 19 to 50.[5] Calcium is an essential element for the construction and maintenance of bones and teeth. It is also an important factor in the blood-clotting mechanism and is used in normal muscle action and other essential metabolic activities. Improved absorption of calcium supplies the increased needs arising from the accelerated fetal mineralization of skeletal tissue during the final period of rapid growth. Dairy products are a primary source of calcium. Consumption of milk or equivalent milk foods (cheese, yogurt, and milk powder) or calcium-fortified soy or almond milk is recommended. Additional calcium is obtained from whole or fortified cereal grains and in green leafy vegetables.

Iodine

The recommendation for iodine increases by 70 mcg/day during pregnancy.[8] Iodine is vital for thyroid hormone synthesis and prevention of goiter. The increased need during gestation supports changes in maternal thyroid economy, increased maternal urinary loss, and fetal uptake of iodine. Inadequate iodine consumption may lead to hypothyroidism in the newborn and is often associated with poor and abnormal growth, deficits in cognitive development, and poor motor function. Although infrequently encountered in the United States, infant hypothyroidism may result in cretinism and mental retardation and is one of the most widespread nutrient deficiencies worldwide. Iodine consumption is critical in the first half of pregnancy, and programs designed to provide iodine supplements to women in preconception and prenatal periods in developing countries have been successful in reducing the incidence of infant hypothyroidism. Iodized salt is the primary dietary source for women in developed countries. Seafood is also a noted source of iodine.

Iron

The pregnant woman needs 27 mg of iron per day, a substantial increase beyond her general needs.[8] Some pregnant women may need supplemental iron in addition to increased dietary sources to meet the additional pregnancy requirement. With increased demands for iron, insufficient maternal stores, and inadequate provision through the usual diet, a daily supplement of 30 mg of iron per day may be prescribed. If a woman has iron deficiency anemia at conception, then a larger therapeutic amount of 60 to 120 mg/day of iron may be necessary to reduce the risk of a preterm delivery or low birth weight baby (or both).

During normal pregnancy, maternal circulating blood volume expands by 40%–50% and may increase more with multiple fetuses. This adaptation reduces the strain on the maternal heart, minimizes hemoglobin losses at delivery, and enhances nutrient flow to the fetus. Although red blood cell mass also increases during gestation, this change does not parallel blood volume expansion, resulting in hemodilution of red blood cell mass. Thus specific guidelines are used to determine iron deficiency anemia during pregnancy (see section "Anemia" later in this chapter). Maternal iron is needed to supply iron to the developing placenta and fetal liver. Adequate maternal iron stores also protect the woman against iron losses related to blood loss at delivery.

To assess the amount of iron in dietary supplements, check the percentage of elemental iron in the iron preparation being used. For example, the commonly used compound ferrous sulfate is a hydrated salt ($FeSO_4\ 7H_2O$), which contains 20% iron. It is typically dispensed in tablets containing 195, 300, or 325 mg of the ferrous sulfate compound. Each tablet, then, would contain 39, 60, or 65 mg of iron, respectively. Thus to supply a regular daily supplement of 60 mg of iron, one 300-mg tablet of ferrous sulfate is required (300 mg $FeSO_4$ $7\ H_2O \times 20\% = 60$ mg iron); for a therapeutic dose of 120 mg iron, two 300-mg tablets are required and should be taken separately.

Challenges with routine iron supplementation for pregnant women include unpleasant gastrointestinal side effects (see section "Effects of Iron Supplements" later in this chapter). Of major concern are imbalances with other trace elements, such as zinc and copper, that compete with iron for absorption. Excess iron intake, when not necessary, may actually mask inadequate pregnancy-induced hemodilution. Thus some prenatal clinics follow protocols prescribing regular prenatal vitamins with iron at the first clinic visit and add additional iron supplementation only if hemoglobin falls to 10.5 g/dL or less at any time during the pregnancy.

Although liver is a major food source of iron, liver intake is often avoided during pregnancy. Other food sources include meat and poultry, legumes, dried fruit, green leafy vegetables, eggs, and enriched bread and cereals (see the list of iron-containing foods in Chapter 7).

Zinc

During pregnancy the DRI recommendation for zinc increases from 8 to 11 mg/day.[8] Zinc is vital for enzymatic reactions and is essential to growth and development because of its role in deoxyribonucleic acid (DNA) and ribonucleic acid (RNA) synthesis and protein production. Inadequate zinc consumption during gestation has been associated with low birth weight and congenital malformations. Iron supplementation may inhibit zinc absorption; thus additional dietary sources of zinc are critical when maternal iron supplementation is prescribed. Seafood, eggs, and meat are primary sources of zinc.

Vitamin Needs

Increased amounts of vitamins A, B complex, and C are needed during pregnancy. If these needs are met, then sufficient amounts of vitamins E and K are also provided. The recommended amount of vitamin D does not increase during pregnancy but is important to fetal skeletal development.

Vitamin A

The daily amount of vitamin A recommended for pregnancy is 770 mcg of retinol activity equivalents (RAEs), a slight increase beyond a woman's regular need.[8] For most women in the United States, additional supplementation in not needed. However, malnourished, underweight women and those with multiple pregnancies need more. Vitamin A is an essential factor in cell differentiation, organ formation, maintenance of strong epithelial tissue, tooth formation, and normal bone growth. Liver, egg yolk, butter and fortified margarine, yellow and dark green vegetables, and fruits are good food sources.

Excessive consumption of retinol and retinoic acid, two forms of vitamin A, has been associated with fetal malformations such as heart, facial, and ear defects. Overconsumption is generally related to the use of supplements or medications such as Accutane. Harmful effects are most damaging during the first few months of pregnancy, emphasizing the need for prenatal counseling and appropriate preconception nutrition.

B Vitamins

The need for various B vitamins increases, including thiamin, riboflavin, niacin, pyridoxine, vitamin B_{12}, pantothenic acid, and folate, during pregnancy.[9] The B vitamins are important as coenzyme factors in a number of metabolic activities related to energy production, tissue protein synthesis, and muscle and nerve tissue function; therefore they support the increased metabolic work of pregnancy. B vitamins are typically supplied by a well-balanced diet that supplies adequate kcalories and other nutrients.

There is an increased metabolic need for the B vitamin folate during pregnancy. Folate deficiency usually occurs in conjunction with general malnutrition, making pregnant women in low socioeconomic conditions especially vulnerable. A specific megaloblastic anemia caused by maternal folate deficiency may occur and warrants folic acid supplementation. This added amount is particularly needed in situations in which demands are increased, such as in a multiple pregnancy.

Preconception folic acid supplementation has been shown in randomized clinical trials to greatly reduce a woman's risk of bearing an infant with a neural tube defect, such as spina bifida and anencephaly. These congenital defects result in incomplete formation of the neural tube and develop in the first few weeks of pregnancy when a woman may not know she is pregnant. Each year in the United States approximately 2800 infants are born with spina bifida and anencephaly.[17] The US Public Health Service recommends that all women of childbearing age who are capable of becoming pregnant consume 400 mcg of folic acid per day from food or supplements to prevent such deficiencies. This recommendation is supported in the latest DRI guidelines, which recommend 400 mcg/day for nonpregnant women, rising to 600 mcg/day during pregnancy and 500 mcg/day during lactation.[9] The US Food and Drug Administration (FDA), acting to increase folic acid consumption nationally, mandated in 1998 that enriched cereal grain products be fortified with folic acid. Fortification is estimated to have reduced the prevalence of neural tube defect by 1300 births annually.[17] In addition, orange and pineapple juices, oranges, dark greens, and dried beans are good sources of folic acid. (Review Chapter 6 for more discussion on neural tube defects and their prevention.)

Choline is emerging as a nutrient of greater importance during pregnancy. Adequate choline consumption is necessary for infant neurologic development, and may reduce the risk for neural tube defects.[18] Currently it is recommended pregnant women consume 450 mcg of choline daily, which can be met by consuming eggs and various protein foods.[9] Unfortunately not all prenatal supplements include sufficient choline and so pregnant women are advised to select a prenatal vitamin that contains the recommended amount.

Vitamin C

Ascorbic acid is another vital nutrient for pregnancy. Vitamin C is essential to the formation of intercellular cement material in developing connective tissues and vascular systems. It also enhances the absorption of iron, which is needed for the increased production of hemoglobin. The DRI standard recommends 85 mg/day for the pregnant woman, an increase of 10 mg/day beyond the regular female adult need.[7]

	1st trimester	2nd trimester	3rd trimester
Grains	6 oz per day	7 oz per day	8 oz per day
Whole grains	≥ 3 oz per day	≥ 3½ oz per day	≥ 4 oz per day
Vegetables	2½ cups per day	3 cups per day	3 cups per day
Dark green	1½ cups per week	2 cups per week	2 cups per week
Red and orange	5½ cups per week	6 cups per week	6 cups per week
Beans and peas	1½ cups per week	2 cups per week	2 cups per week
Starchy	5 cups per week	6 cups per week	6 cups per week
Other	4 cups per week	5 cups per week	5 cups per week
Fruits	1½ cups per day	2 cups per day	2 cups per day
Dairy	3 cups per day	3 cups per day	3 cups per day
Protein foods	5 oz per day	6 oz per day	6½ oz per day
Seafood	8 oz per week	9 oz per week	10 oz per week
Oils	5 tsp per day	6 tsp per day	7 tsp per day
Total calories	1800 kcal per day	2200 kcal per day	2400 kcal per day
Discretionary calories	161 kcal per day	266 kcal per day	330 kcal per day

FIG. 11.3 Food intake plan for a pregnant woman based on trimester of pregnancy, age, height, prepregnancy weight, and physical activity using the MyPlate resource (http://www.choosemyplate.gov).

Additional food sources such as citrus fruit and other vegetables and fruits should be included in the woman's diet.

Vitamin D

Women who have adequate exposure to sunlight probably need little additional vitamin D. During pregnancy, because of the demand for calcium and phosphorus presented by the developing fetal skeletal tissue, vitamin D is needed to promote the absorption and use of these minerals. The daily recommended amount for pregnancy is 15 mcg cholecalciferol (600 IU/day), which is the same as for the nonpregnant woman.[5] Food sources include fortified milk, fortified fruit juices, egg yolk, salmon, and fortified margarine.

Dietary Patterns: General and Alternative

General Daily Food Pattern

Two useful and general principles concerning eating habits for all persons also apply during pregnancy, as follows:

1. Eat an appropriate quantity of food.
2. Eat regularly and avoid fasting or skipping meals, especially breakfast.

During pregnancy a variety of familiar foods usually supply the woman's need for added nutrients and make eating pleasurable. The increased quantities of essential nutrients needed during pregnancy may be met through diverse food patterns. The MyPlate resource offers a credible and easily accessible source for a woman to develop an eating plan appropriate for her trimester of pregnancy, age, height, prepregnancy weight, and physical activity level. Fig. 11.3 displays one example of a dietary plan for a pregnant woman.

Lean meats and poultry, fish, dried beans, and nuts provide dietary protein, iron, zinc, and B vitamins for growth of muscles, bones, blood, and nerves; vegetable protein foods also contribute fiber. Milk and dairy products and fortified soy milk provide dietary protein, calcium, and vitamin D to build strong bones, teeth, and healthy nerves and muscles. Grains provide carbohydrates and B vitamins for energy and

healthy nerves, as well as iron for healthy blood. At least one-half of these grains should be whole grain products to provide fiber. Vitamin C–rich fruits and vegetables assist in preventing infection and promoting healing; they also promote iron absorption and act as sources of fiber. Vitamin A–rich fruits and vegetables contribute β-carotene and vitamin A to prevent infection, promote night vision, and prevent constipation. Other fruits and vegetables contribute energy and fiber to the diet. Oils provide vitamin E and essential fatty acids.

Alternative Food Patterns

With the increasing ethnic diversity in the United States, it is especially important to use a woman's personal cultural food patterns in dietary counseling. There is no singular dietary pattern recommended for all pregnant women because intake differs among women from various cultures, belief systems, and lifestyles. Although specific nutrients, not specific foods, are required for a successful pregnancy, these nutrients can be found in a wide variety of food choices. We can counsel our patients to meet their nutrient needs through foods they are already familiar with (see the Case Study box, "A Baby for the Delgados"). A number of resources are available as guides for cultural, religious, and vegetarian food patterns, as well as suggestions for improving transcultural nutrition counseling skills (see Further Readings and Resources at the end of this chapter).

Dietary Supplements

Often, prenatal vitamins are prescribed for pregnant women. These supplements include a variety of vitamins and minerals and are intended to add to nutrient intake from foods rather than replace food and nutrient consumption. Iron and folate are generally the two nutrients that require supplementation during pregnancy. However, some women may need additional nutrients. For example, pregnant women who follow vegan diets and have one or more nutritional deficiencies, smoke cigarettes, use or abuse drugs or alcohol (or both), or have multiple fetuses benefit from prenatal vitamin and mineral supplementation.

Herbal and botanical supplement use during pregnancy is discouraged because of the potentially harmful or unknown effects on the woman and fetus. However, based on cultural and traditional medicine practices and emerging trends, pregnant women may include such products in their daily routines (see the Case Study box, "Nutrition Counseling in Pregnancy"). Reference materials are available regarding the risks associated with use of specific herbals and botanicals during pregnancy (see Further Readings and Resources at the end of this chapter).

KEY TERM

Spina Bifida
A congenital defect in the fetal closing of the neural tube to form a portion of the lower spine, leaving the spine unclosed and the spinal cord open in various degrees of exposure and damage.

CASE STUDY

A Baby for the Delgados

Mrs. Delgado is a 19-year-old married primigravida, who tested positive for urinary human chorionic gonadotropin (hCG) 2 weeks earlier. Mrs. Delgado is 160 cm (5 ft 3 in) tall with an average pregravid weight of 57 kg (125 lb). Her current gestational age is 6 weeks. Her history for chronic disorders and other serious health problems is negative.

During her initial nutrition interview, Mrs. Delgado indicated that the pregnancy was unplanned. She seemed especially worried about the effects of her irregular diet on the baby. As college students, she and her 21-year-old husband had erratic meals, dominated by junk food. Mrs. Delgado's 24-hour diet history revealed an inadequate intake of dark green or red-yellow-orange vegetables and milk products, as well as meat or eggs and citrus fruits. The couple realized that these types of foods were an important part of a nutritious diet but felt inexperienced as cooks and lacked the time and money to prepare healthful meals every day.

At the end of the initial counseling session, the registered dietitian told the couple about a series of prenatal group classes conducted by members of the clinic's perinatal health team, including sessions on pregnancy, labor and delivery, and the care and feeding of the infant. These are attended primarily by a mixture of experienced parents and young, first-time parents to be and are offered as a means of introducing practical aspects of pregnancy and parenting.

The Delgados attended every prenatal group meeting and kept all consequent diet-counseling sessions. Their food choices improved in time, and

Mrs. Delgado's weight gain progressed normally, to a total of 13 kg (28.5 lb) by the time of delivery. The Delgados had a healthy 4 kg (8 lb 13 oz) baby girl.

Questions for Analysis

1. What health professionals ideally should be included on the health care team caring for Mrs. Delgado? Describe the significance of each role to the outcome of her pregnancy. What are the roles of Mr. and Mrs. Delgado?
2. What nutritional deficiencies would you expect in Mrs. Delgado's diet? What practical problems would you expect her to encounter in attempting to improve her diet?
3. Write a 1-day meal plan for Mrs. Delgado, taking into account her lifestyle and schedule, as well as the amounts of nutrients considered adequate for pregnancy.
4. Write a lesson plan for a group session on nutrition during pregnancy. Include a general description, behavioral objectives, content outline, teaching methods and materials, and evaluation tool (or tools) you would use.
5. Would you encourage Mrs. Delgado to breast-feed? If so, then why? What factors would you expect might discourage her from trying? How would you discuss these factors?
6. Write a lesson plan for an infant-feeding session, addressing breast-feeding and bottle-feeding methods. Include the components listed in questions 3 and 4.

CASE STUDY

Nutrition Counseling in Pregnancy

Ms. McLane is a 33-year-old Caucasian woman who is in her 29th week of pregnancy. This is her second pregnancy. During her first pregnancy (at age 29), she gained 24 lb during a normal pregnancy and had a delivery without complications. She is presently 165.1 cm (5 ft 5 in) tall and weighs 81.8 kg (180 lb). Her prepregnancy weight was 72.7 kg (160 lb). Ms. McLane visited her obstetrician before her second pregnancy for prepregnancy planning. She has been consuming a healthy diet and a prenatal vitamin supplement every day. After her first visit to the obstetrician during the current pregnancy (at week 10), Ms. McLane did not return for any further appointments, because of her prior positive experience with pregnancy and belief that she "didn't need anything because the first pregnancy went so well."

Ms. McLane has a positive family history for diabetes, and her mother had gestational diabetes. Ms. McLane should have been screened for gestational diabetes between the 24th and 28th weeks of her current pregnancy; however, this was not done. She experienced frequent urination and fatigue that she reported as "different" from her first pregnancy. This prompted her to return to her obstetrician. The obstetrician completed a full examination and administered an oral glucose tolerance test. One hour after consuming a 100-g solution of glucose, Ms. McLane's blood glucose concentration was 218 mg/dL. She was scheduled for follow-up testing, and gestational diabetes was confirmed. A 2200-kcal/day diabetic diet was prescribed to allow Ms. McLane to control this condition through diet.

Ms. McLane has been referred to you for nutrition counseling. This is now the 31st week of her pregnancy, and she shares with you that a friend suggested that she "use some natural products to help her high blood sugar." In addition to consuming her prenatal supplement on a daily basis, she takes 500 mg of burdock root and 1 tbsp of flaxseed and drinks three cups of

hot fenugreek tea per day. Her prenatal supplement contains 400 mcg of folate, 250 mg of calcium, 40 mg of iron, 100 mg of vitamin C, 5 mcg of vitamin D, 3 mg of thiamin, 3 mg of riboflavin, 4 mg of pyridoxine, 40 mg of niacin, 10 mg of vitamin E, 5 mcg of vitamin B_{12}, 30 mg of zinc, and 10 mg of copper. Completion of a dietary intake analysis shows that Ms. McLane's kcalorie intake is 1750 per day. She reported that she has been nauseated for approximately 2 weeks, so she also added 300 mg of powdered ginger to each cup of the fenugreek tea. She reported some diarrhea and Braxton Hicks contractions during the last week, as well a lack of desire to be physically active.

Questions for Analysis

1. What is Ms. McLane's BMI based on her prepregnancy weight?
2. What is the recommended amount of weight gain for Ms. McLane based on prepregnancy weight and BMI? Has she experienced an appropriate weight gain so far?
3. Is the current level of kcalories appropriate based on her condition of gestational diabetes, BMI, and weight gain?
4. What additional information would you collect from Ms. McLane to complete a nutritional assessment?
5. How would you approach a nutritional intake plan for Ms. McLane?
6. Why would Ms. McLane's friend have recommended burdock root, flaxseed, and fenugreek—why might a pregnant women consider taking botanical supplements? Are botanicals recommended for use during pregnancy?
7. Identify at least five points that you would make during a nutrition counseling session with Ms. McLane. Discuss the priority for the first counseling session with Ms. McLane.

WEIGHT GAIN DURING PREGNANCY

General Amount of Weight Gain

Healthy women produce healthy babies across a wide range of total weight gain. Therefore during pregnancy the nutritional focus should always be on an individualized assessment of need and the quality of weight gain. Recommended weight gain during normal pregnancy is approximately 11 to 16 kg (25–35 lb).[2] Within this average, many individual variations occur. Current recommendations are therefore usually stated in terms of ranges to accommodate variances in needs. An initial base for evaluation is the average weight of the components of pregnancy as shown in Table 11.2. Increasing maternal stores are another important component of growth occurring during this period. Laying down of extra adipose fat tissue is necessary for maternal energy reserves to sustain rapid fetal growth during the latter half of pregnancy, for labor and delivery, and for maintaining lactation after birth. Approximately 1.8 to 3.6 kg (4–8 lb) of adipose tissue is commonly deposited for these needs. The Institute of Medicine (IOM) updated weight gain guidelines for pregnancy in May 2009, using the World Health Organization (WHO) classifications for prepregnancy BMI. The guidelines are as follows[19]:

- Normal-weight women with a BMI of 18.5 to 24.9 should gain from 11.5 to 16 kg (25–35 lb).
- Underweight women with a BMI of less than 18.5 should gain 12.7 to 18.1 kg (28–40 lb).
- Overweight women with a BMI of 25.0 to 29.9 should gain 6.8 to 11.5 kg (15–25 lb).
- Obese women with a BMI of 30.0 or more should gain 5.0 to 9.2 kg (11–20 lb).

The recommendation for adolescent girls is that they should follow the adult BMI guidelines and gain weight within the corresponding range. The recommendation for a woman carrying twins who is of normal BMI is a weight gain range of 16.8 to 24.5 kg (37–54 lb).[19] Overweight women carrying twins should gain 14.2 to 22.8 kg (31–50 lb), whereas obese women carrying twins should gain 11.5 to 19.1 kg (25–42 lb).[19] Compared with less than 10% of single-birth infants, nearly 57% of twin births are premature (gestation of < 37 weeks), 9 times more likely to be very low birth weight (< 1500 g), and almost 9 times more likely to be low birth weight (< 2500 g).[20]

Quality of Weight Gain

An important consideration lies in the nutritional quality of weight gain. The foods consumed should be nutrient dense, not full of empty kcalories, to meet increased nutrient requirements. In addition, in some cases, clinicians have failed to distinguish between weight gained as a result of edema and that resulting from deposition of fat, which provides maternal stores for energy to sustain rapid fetal growth during the latter part of pregnancy and energy for lactation to follow. Analysis of the total tissue gained in an average pregnancy shows that the largest component, 62%, is water. Fat accounts for 31% and protein for 7%. Water is also the most variable component of the tissue gained, accounting for a range of 7 to 8 L (or 7–8 kg), and is distributed among the fetus, placenta, amniotic fluid, uterus, mammary glands, blood, and extracellular fluid.[19] Gravity causes the maternal tissue fluids to pool more in the lower extremities, leading to general swelling of the ankles, which is seen routinely in pregnant women. This fluid retention is a normal adaptive phenomenon designed to support the pregnancy and to exert a positive effect on fetal growth. Maternal connective tissue becomes more hygroscopic as a result of the estrogen-induced changes and thus becomes softer and more easily distended. This facilitates delivery of the infant through the cervix and vaginal canal. In addition, the increased tissue fluid during pregnancy provides a means for handling the increased metabolic workload and circulation of numerous metabolites necessary for fetal growth.

Clearly, severe kcalorie restriction is harmful to the developing fetus and the woman. It is inevitably accompanied by restriction of vitally needed nutrients essential to the growth process. Moreover, weight reduction should never be undertaken during pregnancy. Sufficient weight gain should be encouraged with the use of a nourishing diet.

Rate of Weight Gain

On the whole, approximately 0.5 to 2.0 kg (1.1–4.4 lb) is a target for average weight gain during the first trimester for all pregnant women.[19] Thereafter, the target for average weight gain per week is 0.5 kg (1 lb) for underweight and normal-weight women, 0.3 kg (0.6 lb) for overweight women, and 0.23 kg (0.5 lb) for obese women. Controversy exists as to whether or not obese women, particularly those with grade III obesity, may afford a weight gain that is less than what is recommended by the IOM, and until further evidence is available the current guidelines should be followed.[21] It is only unusual patterns of gain, such as a sudden sharp increase in weight after the 20th week of pregnancy that may signal abnormal water retention, which should be monitored closely, especially if it occurs in conjunction with blood pressure elevation and proteinuria. Conversely, an insufficient or low maternal weight gain during the second or third trimester increases the risk for small for gestational age (SGA) and decreased neonatal fat mass, lean mass, and head circumference.[21]

Weight Gain and Sodium Intake

A moderate amount of dietary sodium is needed for two essential reasons:

1. It is the major mineral required to control the extracellular fluid compartment.
2. This vital body water is increased during pregnancy to support its successful outcome.

Current practice usually follows a regular diet with moderate sodium intake, 1.5 to 2.3 g/day, with light use of salt to taste.[22] Limiting

TABLE 11.2 **Approximate Weight of Components of Normal Pregnancy**	
Components	**Weight**
Fetus	3500 g (7.5 lb)
Placenta	450 g (1 lb)
Amniotic fluid	900 g (2 lb)
Uterus (weight increase)	1100 g (2.5 lb)
Breast tissue (weight increase)	1400 g (3 lb)
Blood volume (weight increase)	1800 g (4 lb) (1500 mL)
Maternal adipose tissue stores	1800–3,600 g (4–8 lb)
TOTAL	10,850–12,650 g (10.9–12.7 kg; 24–28 lb)

KEY TERMS

Hygroscopic
Taking up and retaining moisture readily.

Small for Gestational Age
Infants born at a weight less than the 10th percentile for gestational age.

sodium beyond this general use is contrary to physiologic need in pregnancy and is unfounded. In fact, sodium restriction in pregnancy is associated with low birth weight and low survival rates for the fetus.[23] Maintaining the needed increase in circulating blood volume during pregnancy requires adequate amounts of sodium and protein, as well as adequate fluid intake to prevent dehydration and possible premature contractions.

GENERAL DIETARY PROBLEMS

Functional Gastrointestinal Problems

Nausea and Vomiting

Some general dietary problems temporarily interfere with food and nutrient intake. Most are easily resolved through dietary counseling and with medical attention and have no long-term adverse effects on the quality of maternal weight gain. Symptoms of nausea and vomiting are usually mild and short term, although the term morning sickness is a misnomer in that these symptoms often occur throughout the entire day. At least 50% and up to 80% of all pregnant women, most of them in their first pregnancy, experience this condition, beginning during the 5th or 6th week of the pregnancy and usually ending about the 14th to 16th week.[24] There are a number of contributory factors. Although the exact causes remain unknown, it is thought symptoms are related to hormonal changes that occur early in pregnancy, particularly the increase in the human chorionic gonadotropin hormone (hCG) and estrogens. Other contributors to nausea and vomiting include dietary behaviors, psychological factors, and having a genetic predisposition.[24] Simple treatment generally improves food tolerance. Frequent small, low fat meals and snacks consisting of complex carbohydrates along with some protein are usually more readily tolerated, such as crackers and pretzels with a string cheese. In addition, avoiding strong odors as much as possible may be helpful. Liquids are best taken between meals instead of with meals. Other treatments may include consumption of ginger, vitamin B$_6$, and wearing sea bands.[24]

Hyperemesis

In a small number of pregnant women, approximately 0.3% to 3% of pregnancies, a severe form of persistent nausea and vomiting occurs that does not respond to usual treatment. This condition, *hyperemesis,* begins early in the pregnancy and may last throughout. It may develop into the more serious pernicious form of hyperemesis gravidarum. This persistent condition causes severe alterations in fluids and electrolytes, weight loss, and nutritional deficits, sometimes requiring hospitalization and alternative feeding by enteral or parenteral methods to sustain the pregnancy (see Chapter 19 for more information on nutrition support). First-line treatments including those listed for nausea and vomiting may abate symptoms, but typically medication(s) are needed and require physician supervision.[24]

Constipation

Constipation is experienced by many pregnant women and contributes to discomfort and concern. Placental hormones relax the gastrointestinal muscles, and the pressure of the enlarging uterus on the lower portion of the intestine may make elimination somewhat difficult. Increased fluid intake and the use of naturally laxative foods

---

KEY TERM

Hyperemesis Gravidarum
Severe vomiting during pregnancy, which is potentially fatal.

---

containing dietary fiber, such as whole grains, fruits and vegetables, dried fruits (especially prunes and figs), and other fruits and juices, generally promote regularity. Laxatives should be avoided. Appropriate daily exercise is essential for overall health during pregnancy.

Hemorrhoids

A fairly common complaint during the latter part of pregnancy is that of hemorrhoids. These are enlarged veins in the anus, often protruding through the anal sphincter. This vein enlargement is usually caused by the increased weight of the fetus and its downward pressure. The hemorrhoids may cause considerable discomfort, burning, and itching. Occasionally, they may rupture and bleed under pressure of a bowel movement, causing anxiety. The problem is usually controlled by the dietary recommendations given for constipation. In addition, sufficient rest during the latter part of the day may help relieve some of the downward pressure of the uterus on the lower intestine.

Heartburn or Gastric Pressure

Heartburn is another frequent concern during pregnancy. These discomforts occur particularly after meals and are usually caused by the pressure of the enlarging uterus crowding the stomach, as well as from the relaxing of the gastroesophageal sphincter. Gastric reflux of some of the food mass, now a liquid chyme mixed with stomach acid, may occur in the lower esophagus, causing an irritation and a burning sensation. Although this common complaint has nothing to do with heart action, it receives the name because of the close proximity of the lower esophagus to the heart. The full feeling comes from general gastric pressure, lack of normal space in the area, a large meal, or gas formation. These complaints are usually remedied by dividing the day's food into a series of small meals, avoiding eating large meals at any time, and not lying down after a meal. Comfort is also improved by wearing loose-fitting clothing.

Effects of Iron Supplements

The effects of an iron supplement may include gray or black stools and nausea, constipation, or diarrhea. To mitigate food-related effects, iron supplements should be taken 1 hour before a meal or 2 hours after it, with liquids such as water or orange juice. The absorption of iron is increased with vitamin C and decreased with milk, other dairy foods, eggs, whole grain bread and cereal, and tea. Ferrous fumarate and ferrous gluconate are alternate forms of iron supplements that tend to result in less gastrointestinal distress, although their absorption is less than that of more commonly found forms.

HIGH-RISK PREGNANCIES

Identify Risk Factors Involved

To avoid the consequences of sustained poor nutrition during pregnancy, women at risk need to be identified. In a joint report the American College of Obstetrics and Gynecology and the Academy of Nutrition and Dietetics issued a set of risk factors, shown in Box 11.1, that identify women with special nutritional needs during pregnancy. These nutrition-related factors are based on clinical evidence of inadequate nutrition. However, rather than waiting for clinical symptoms of poor nutrition to appear, a proactive approach would be to identify poor food patterns that will induce nutritional problems and to prevent these problems from developing. On this basis, three types of dietary patterns predict failure to support optimal maternal and fetal nutrition: (1) insufficient food intake, (2) poor food selection, and (3) poor food distribution throughout the day. These patterns, added to the list of risk factors in Box 11.1, can increase one's nutritional risk.

BOX 11.1 Nutritional Risk Factors in Pregnancy

Risk Factors Present at the Onset of Pregnancy

- Age: <15 years old or >35 years old
- Frequent pregnancies: three or more during a 2-year period
- Poor obstetric history or poor fetal performance
- Poverty
- Bizarre or faddist food habits
- Abuse of nicotine, alcohol, or drugs
- Therapeutic diet required for a chronic disorder
- Weight: <85% or >120% of standard weight

Risk Factors Occurring During Pregnancy

- Low hemoglobin (HGB) or hematocrit (HCT): HGB <12 g/dL, HCT <35%
- Inadequate weight gain: any weight loss or weight gain of <1 kg (2 lb)/month after the first trimester
- Excessive weight gain: >1 kg (2 lb)/week after the first trimester

From American College of Obstetrics and Gynecology and American Dietetic Association Task Force on Nutrition: *Assessment of maternal nutrition*, Chicago, 1978, American College of Obstetrics and Gynecology.

Plan Personal Care

After early assessment identifies risk factors, practitioners can then give more careful attention to these women. By working closely with each woman and her personal food pattern and living situation, a food plan can be developed with her to ensure an optimal intake of energy and nutrients to support her pregnancy and its successful outcome.

Recognize Special Counseling Needs

Several special needs require sensitive counseling. These areas of need include the age and parity of the woman; use of harmful agents such as alcohol, cigarettes, drugs, or pica; and socioeconomic problems.

Age and Parity

Pregnancies at either age extreme of the reproductive cycle pose special problems. A recent annual report of the Centers for Disease Control and Prevention (CDC) reported that approximately 249,078 live births occurred to female teenagers.[25] The adolescent pregnancy carries many social and nutrition-related risks associated with increased incidence of low birth weight and perinatal mortality, among other poor outcomes. The obstetric history of a woman is expressed in terms of number and order of pregnancies, or her gravida status. A nulligravida (no prior pregnancy) who is 15 years of age or younger is especially at risk because her own growth is incomplete; therefore sufficient weight gain and the quality of her diet are particularly important.[26] Nutrients of particular concern are those for which the adolescent female requirements are greater than the adult requirements, including calcium, magnesium, phosphorus, and zinc. These nutrients are critical for growth and development of the adolescent, as well as for her fetus. Sensitive counseling provides information and emotional support; it should involve family members or other persons significant to the adolescent. Additionally, the primigravida (an individual with her first pregnancy) who is older than 35 years of age also requires special attention. She may be at greater risk for hypertension, either preexisting or pregnancy induced, and may need more attention to the rate of weight gain and amount of sodium consumed, as well as any drug therapy prescribed. In addition, several pregnancies within a limited

number of years leave a mother drained of nutritional resources and entering each successive pregnancy at increased risk.

Social Habits: Alcohol, Cigarettes, and Drugs

Alcohol, cigarettes, and drugs are three personal habits that may cause fetal damage and are contraindicated during pregnancy. No safe level of alcohol consumption has yet been found for pregnant women. Extensive or habitual alcohol use may lead to one of the fetal alcohol spectrum disorders known as *fetal alcohol syndrome (FAS)*, which is currently a leading cause of mental retardation and is included in the fetal alcohol spectrum disorders.[27] FAS is characterized by growth retardation, malformed facial features, joint and limb abnormalities, cardiac defects, mental retardation, and, in serious cases, death. FAS signs have been seen in animal models as early as the human equivalent of the 3rd week of gestation, when most women are unaware of their pregnancies. Thus moderate-to-heavy drinking among sexually active women of childbearing age may carry potential danger. Even moderate prenatal alcohol exposure has been associated with low birth weight and has effects on a child's psychomotor and cognitive development in the absence of malformations.[27]

Cigarette smoking during pregnancy is also contraindicated. Harmful substances in tobacco and impaired oxygen transport cause fetal damage and special problems of placental abnormalities, leading to increased risk of spontaneous abortion (miscarriage), prematurity, low birth weight, impairment of mental and physical growth, and increased potential mortality. Counseling with women and families who smoke should stress the importance of quitting for pregnancy and beyond.

Drug use, both recreational and medicinal, also poses concerns.[28] Self-medication with over-the-counter drugs carries potential adverse effects. The use of illicit drugs is especially hazardous, exposing the developing fetus to the risks of addiction and possibly human immunodeficiency virus (HIV) from the woman's use of contaminated needles during drug injections. Dangers come not only from the drug itself or contaminated needles but also from impurities contained in illicit drugs. Evaluation of the effects of street drugs (marijuana, cocaine, heroin, methadone) on nutritional status is difficult because of multiple drug use, uncertain purity, unknown dose and timing, and inadequate nutritional status of many drug users. A high incidence of meconium staining (which could relate to fetal damage), poor prenatal weight gain, very short (less than 3 hours) or prolonged labor, operative delivery (cesarean, forceps), and other perinatal problems among marijuana users has been reported. Such outcomes indicate that it is prudent to abstain from drug use during pregnancy.[29]

Abuse from megadosing with basic nutrients such as vitamin A or use of prescription medications such as Accutane during pregnancy may cause fetal damage as previously described.[30] A number of drugs are often prescribed for female patients to treat a variety of psychologic and mental health disorders. However, if taken during pregnancy, many drugs exhibit teratogenic effects. If any of these drugs are taken on a long-term basis for the treatment of serious conditions, such as clinical depression, bipolar disorder, or schizophrenia, then comprehensive medical and psychologic assessment and follow-up is needed throughout the pregnancy. Lithium has been associated with an increased risk for congenital cardiac malformations, goiter, and hypoglycemia, as well as neonatal toxic disturbances such as cyanosis, hypothermia, and bradycardia. A diminished suck reflex will impede attempts to nourish the infant exposed to lithium in utero. Diazepam (Valium) is associated with an abnormal fetal heart rate. The neonate risks delivery by cesarean section, with oral-facial malformations, a depressed Apgar score, and a reluctance to feed. Rats exposed to

KEY TERMS

Nulligravida
A woman who has never been pregnant.

Primigravida
A woman who is pregnant for the first time.

Meconium staining
Resulting from fetal distress, the passing of the first stool by the fetus before birth, resulting in a green-yellow discoloration of the amniotic fluid and often the infant's skin, nailbeds, and umbilical cord at birth; harmful and potentially fatal.

Teratogenic
Causing malformation of an embryo, due to a teratogen (agent or substance that is teratogenic).

diazepam in utero have exhibited abnormal motor skills and arousal processes. Tricyclic antidepressants (e.g., imipramine) have led to morphologic and behavioral abnormalities in rats.

Hydantoin (Dilantin, phenytoin) is used to control seizures caused by epilepsy and other conditions. Even though this drug has been associated with congenital malformations and cognitive impairments, physicians are reluctant to discontinue it for their patients with epilepsy during pregnancy because untreated epilepsy may pose even greater risks to the fetus. Ultimately women with epilepsy need to work with their physician to determine the best course of treatment and should be monitored closely for the duration of their pregnancy.[31]

Thus with the exception of drugs used to treat individuals with seizure disorders or natural replacement therapy (e.g., insulin for persons with type 1 diabetes), most drugs should be avoided during pregnancy to ensure the health of the woman and a safe and healthy pregnancy outcome. The nutrition counselor is well advised to keep up with the most recent findings regarding medications (prescribed, over-the-counter, and street drugs) to evaluate the nutritional status of the woman who uses them and to allow the practitioner and the woman to design a plan of action to safely eliminate the drug, preferably before conception. In addition, evaluation of herbal and botanical supplements, which are not regulated in the same manner as prescription and over-the-counter drugs, is necessary to inform the woman of potential safety issues and to counsel her appropriately.

Caffeine

Caffeine is one of the most commonly consumed drugs worldwide. Caffeine can cross the placenta and enter fetal circulation. Its use at levels of 350 mg/day or greater has been associated with an increased risk of fetal loss and low birth weight infants.[32] Most health agencies recommend that pregnant women limit caffeine consumption from foods, beverages (coffee, tea, cocoa, cola), and medications to less than 300 mg/day to minimize the potential fetal effects of maternal caffeine consumption.[32]

Pica

Pica is the craving and consumption of unusual nonnutritive substances such as laundry starch, clay, dirt, or ice. This practice during pregnancy is more widespread than health care workers have believed, particularly in southern regions of the United States and among specific ethnic and cultural groups. There is a consistent link between pica and iron deficiency, although the direction of causality is unknown.[33] Where these unusual practices exist, they must be appreciated as cultural patterns that require a respectful approach and understanding by health workers who seek to negotiate appropriate behavior changes (see the Focus on Culture box, "Pica During Pregnancy: Cultural Norm of Concern").

FOCUS ON CULTURE

Pica During Pregnancy: Cultural Norm of Concern

Pica is the ingestion of nonfood substances or food components, including but not limited to clay, dirt, chalk, cornstarch, laundry starch, baking powder, baking soda, ice, and freezer frost. These substances are often craved with subsequent consumption. Approximately 23% of pregnant women engage in pica, and the prevalence of this psychobehavioral disorder is greater in rural (compared with urban) areas and in certain cultures.

Normal Cultural Behavior or Pregnancy-Induced Disorder
In some cultures, soil consumption is associated with reproduction and fertility. In a group of women from a variety of ethnic and religious backgrounds living in Kenya, more than 80% reported consumption of approximately 1 cup of soil on a daily basis. In these cultures, pica represents a cultural norm that may increase in prevalence during pregnancy.

Nearly 45% of women born and living in western Mexico engaged in pica during pregnancy, whereas only approximately 30% of Mexican-born women currently residing in California practiced pica during pregnancy. Although pica may be a culturally accepted norm, changes in prevalence may be induced with acculturation into a society where this behavior is less common.

Consequences of Pica and Need for Counseling
A pregnant woman who engages in pica, regardless of cultural background, should be informed about the potential health consequences of pica. It is thought that nutrient deficiencies precipitate pica behaviors, although the exact nature of this relationship is unclear. Regardless, many pica substances are capable of binding nutrients to render them unavailable for absorption. Nutritional anemias may occur, which will have adverse effects on both mother and baby. Exposure to toxins and teratogens from nonfood substances such as battery acid or ashes is also possible. Gastrointestinal perforation, constipation, and microbial infections are additional potential outcomes of pica.

An understanding by the health care practitioner regarding factors leading to pica is vital to affecting changes in behavior. For example, the pregnant woman who believes that a nonfood substance has an essential role in the body's balance or harmony with her environment may be less willing to avoid consumption of that nonfood substance. On the other hand, a pregnant woman who consumes eggshells because of the sensory cravings associated with the texture may be amenable to substituting a crunchy food substance for this nonfood product. Inquiry regarding the history of pica in the pregnant woman is important to identify sources of pica substances and to involve other family members or cultural leaders who may support such behavior; they may need counseling to facilitate appropriate behavior changes. Such nutrition counseling must be delivered in a culturally sensitive and appropriate manner, with emphasis on the importance of behavior changes for an optimal outcome for the infant.

Bibliography
Fawcett EJ, Fawcett JM, Mazmanian D: A meta-analysis of the worldwide prevalence of pica during pregnancy and the postpartum period, *Int J Gynaecol Obstet* 133(3):277, 2016.

Geissler PW, Prince RJ, Levene M, et al: Perceptions of soil-eating and anaemia among pregnant women on the Kenyan coast, *Soc Sci Med* 48(8):1069, 1999.

Njiru H, Elchalal U, Paltiel O: Geophagy during pregnancy in Africa: a literature review, *Obstet Gynecol Surv* 66(7):452, 2011.

Simpson E, Mull JD, Longley E, et al: Pica during pregnancy in low-income women born in Mexico, *West J Med* 173(1):20, 2000.

Socioeconomic Challenges

Special counseling is required for women and young girls facing economic challenges. Numerous studies and clinical observations indicate that lack of prenatal care, often associated with racial prejudices and fears, as well as a lack of adequate financial resources, places the expectant mother in grave difficulty. Special counseling that is sensitive to personal needs is required to help plan resources for care and financial assistance. Resources include programs such as the federally funded Special Supplemental Nutrition Program for Women, Infants, and Children (WIC), described in Appendix D, as well as numerous state and local programs. An example of a community partnership program promoting prenatal care is Stork's Nest, sponsored by the March of Dimes in affiliation with a national women's organization and local community service agencies. Another successful program targeted for low-income women is BabyCare, administered by the Virginia Department of Health (see Further Readings and Resources at the end of this chapter).

COMPLICATIONS OF PREGNANCY

Anemia

Anemia is common during pregnancy. It is often associated with the normal maternal blood volume increase of 40% to 50% and a disproportionate increase in red cell mass of approximately 20%. In the United States, prevalence of iron deficiency is near 18% and iron deficiency anemia is present in 5% of women.[34] Normal values for hemoglobin and hematocrit during pregnancy are 11.5 to 15 g/dL and 32% to 36.5%, respectively. Anemia is far more prevalent among lower–income groups, whom may consume severely insufficient diets. However, anemia is by no means restricted to lower economic groups.

Iron Deficiency Anemia

A deficiency of iron is by far the most common cause of anemia in pregnancy. The total iron cost of a single normal pregnancy is large—approximately 500 to 800 mg. Of this amount, the fetus uses nearly 300 mg. The remainder is used in the expanded maternal blood volume and its increased red blood cells and hemoglobin mass. This iron requirement typically exceeds the available reserves in the average woman. Thus, in addition to including iron-rich foods in the diet, a daily supplement or increased therapeutic dose may be required, as previously described.

Folate Deficiency Anemia

A less common megaloblastic anemia of pregnancy results from folate deficiency. During pregnancy, the fetus is sensitive to folate inhibitors and therefore has increased metabolic requirements for folate. To prevent this anemia the DRI standard recommends 600 mcg of folate per day during pregnancy. Women with poor diets will need supplementation to reach this amount.

Hemorrhagic Anemia

Anemia caused by blood loss may occur during labor and delivery. Blood loss may also occur earlier, as a result of abortion or ruptured tubular pregnancy. Most women undergoing these physiologic problems receive blood via transfusion, and iron therapy may be indicated for adequate replacement for hemoglobin formation.

Hypertensive Disorders of Pregnancy
Relation to Nutrition

Hypertensive disorders of pregnancy (HDP) include chronic hypertension, gestational hypertension, preeclampsia, or preeclampsia superimposed on hypertension. Although the genetic and immune-related causes

of HDP are becoming clearer, diet plays a role in the risk of preeclampsia. For example, diets adequate in calcium and vitamin D and overall rich in fruits, vegetables, and vegetables oils are associated with reduced risk for preeclampsia.[35] Certainly, as many practitioners have observed, HDP are classically associated with poverty, inadequate diet, and little or no prenatal care. HDP, which develop early from the time of implantation of the fertilized ovum into the uterine lining, may be reduced by good prenatal care from the beginning of the pregnancy, which inherently includes attention to sound nutrition. This sound nutritional status which is impacted by nutrition and lifestyle behaviors even before pregnancy provides her with optimal resources for adapting to the physiologic stress of gestation. Her fitness during pregnancy is a direct function of her past state of nutrition and her optimal nutrition throughout pregnancy.

Clinical Symptoms

HDP are defined according to their clinical manifestations, as well as the timing of the onset of symptoms. In addition to hypertension, depending on the condition, there may be abnormal and excessive edema, albuminuria, and, in severe cases, convulsions or coma, a state called eclampsia.

Treatment

Specific treatment varies according to the individual patient's symptoms and needs. Optimal nutrition is a fundamental aspect of therapy in any case. Emphasis is given to a regular diet with adequate dietary protein and calcium, as well as to a diet that is rich in fruits and vegetables, providing magnesium, potassium, and dietary fiber. Correction of plasma protein deficits stimulates the capillary fluid shift mechanism and increases circulation of tissue fluids, with subsequent correction of the hypovolemia. In addition, adequate salt and sources of vitamins and minerals are needed for correction and maintenance of metabolic balance.

Multiple Fetuses

The incidence of multifetal pregnancies has increased in recent decades and presents unique concerns. Infants born from a multifetal pregnancy are more likely to experience intrauterine growth restriction and are at risk for preterm delivery.[36] Thus the nutritional needs of these women must be given special attention. Energy intake must be increased beyond the needs of a single fetus pregnancy so that the recommended weight gain for multiple fetuses is achieved. This increase in energy intake often provides for the additional nutrient demands that exist. Attention to adequate folate intake is critical to reduce risks of low birth weight and preterm delivery. Supplemental iron may be necessary to reduce the incidence of anemia, more commonly found in women with multiple fetuses. Additional calcium and vitamin D are needed with multiple fetuses to promote adequate calcium absorption for optimal bone mineralization in utero. Zinc, magnesium, copper, and pyridoxine supplementation may also be required to support multifetal growth and development.[36]

Maternal Disease Conditions

Preexisting clinical conditions in the woman further complicate pregnancy. In each case, management of these conditions is based on general principles of care related to pregnancy and to the particular disease involved. Examples of such maternal conditions are reviewed here; they are hypertension, diabetes mellitus, PKU, HIV, and eating disorders.

Hypertension

Preexisting hypertension in the pregnant woman can have considerable maternal and fetal consequences. Many of these problems can be prevented by initial screening and continued monitoring by the prenatal nurse, with referral to the clinical nutritionist for a plan of care. The hypertensive disease process begins long before signs and symptoms appear, and later symptoms are inconsistent. Risk factors for hypertension before and during pregnancy are listed in Box 11.2. Nutritional therapy centers on the following three principles:

1. Prevention of weight extremes (i.e., underweight or obesity)
2. Correction of any dietary deficiencies and maintenance of optimal nutritional status during pregnancy
3. Management of any related coexisting disease (e.g., diabetes mellitus, hyperlipidemia)

Sodium intake may be moderate but should not be unduly restricted because of its relation to fluid and electrolyte balances during pregnancy. Initial and continuing client education and a close relationship with the nurse-nutritionist care team contribute to successful management of hypertension and prevent problems that may occur. (For a more detailed discussion of vascular disease, see Chapter 21.)

Diabetes Mellitus and Gestational Diabetes Mellitus

The management of preexisting diabetes in pregnancy presents special problems. However, current improved expectations for the diabetic woman's pregnancy constitute one of the success stories of modern medicine. Contributing factors to this improved outlook include advances in technology for monitoring fetal development, increased knowledge of nutrition and diabetes, and management refinements in tight blood glucose control through self-monitoring.

During pregnancy, glycosuria is not uncommon because of the increased circulating blood volume and its load of metabolites. Routine

screening protocols, typically conducted between the 24th and 28th week of gestation, are used during pregnancy to detect gestational diabetes mellitus (GDM). GDM is an intolerance of carbohydrate such that blood glucose concentration increases during pregnancy. In 95% of cases this carbohydrate or glucose intolerance resolves after delivery. Treatment during pregnancy is important because of the increased risk these women carry for fetal damage during this gestational period.[2] The most common outcome for an infant born to a mother with GDM is macrosomia, a larger than normal body size. Other infant complications include hypoglycemia, jaundice, and trauma at birth. Although GDM occurs in 4% to 9% of the pregnant population, up to 50% of women with pregnancy-induced abnormal glucose tolerance subsequently develop overt diabetes. Team management is required for adequate care of gestational and preexisting types 1 and 2 diabetes mellitus.[37] (See Chapter 22 for a detailed discussion of diabetes care.)

Maternal Phenylketonuria

The successful detection and management of infants with PKU through newborn screening programs in all states have ensured their normal growth and development to adulthood. PKU is a genetic metabolic disease caused by a missing enzyme for the metabolism of the essential amino acid phenylalanine. It is controlled by a special low-phenylalanine diet initiated at birth. It is crucial for a woman with PKU to follow a strict low-phenylalanine diet before conception, to minimize risks of fetal damage in the early cell differentiation weeks of pregnancy.

Human Immunodeficiency Virus

Carefully monitored care throughout pregnancy and after birth is essential for pregnant women infected with HIV. There are two primary goals: (1) to reduce the rate of the disease progression in the woman through nutritional support and (2) to minimize the chance of HIV vertical transmission from mother to infant, either in the womb or after birth via breast-feeding. Poor weight gain and nutrient deficiencies during pregnancy are often found in HIV-positive patients. Although specific nutrient requirements for HIV-infected pregnant women have not been established, these patients may need up to 150% of normal pregnancy intakes of macronutrients and micronutrients. Continued individual monitoring and adjustment are essential. Infants can be infected by HIV during labor and delivery and through breast milk. Where safe alternatives to breast milk are available, such as commercial formula or banked human milk, a decision on breast-feeding depends on the HIV status of the newborn infant. In the United States the CDC and the American Academy of Pediatrics recommend HIV-positive mothers do not breast-feed when the infant is not infected.[38]

Eating Disorders

Eating disorders, specifically anorexia nervosa and bulimia nervosa, have been previously described (see Chapter 8). Diagnosis and treatment of these disorders in the nonpregnant state require multidisciplinary approaches, and even greater consideration with further specialized care is required for a pregnant woman with anorexia or bulimia nervosa. Pregnancy in anorexia nervosa may be less common because amenorrhea is often experienced by these women; however, ovulation and subsequent conception may occur.[39] Compared with anorexia nervosa, pregnancy in a woman with bulimia nervosa may be more likely because of more typical menstrual patterns, weight status, and less restrictive eating. Eating disorders have been linked to spontaneous abortion, poor weight gain, low infant birth weight, premature deliveries, and other adverse fetal outcomes, although conflicting research indicates these effects on pregnancy may be minimal.[39] A team approach that emphasizes nutritional needs of the growing fetus, anticipated maternal body size and shape changes, and postpartum care is critical to a successful course and outcome.[39]

NUTRITION DURING LACTATION

Current Breast-Feeding Trends

Data from the National Immunization Survey show that approximately 80% of mothers initiate breast-feeding.[40] Several factors contribute to this rate of breast-feeding initiation:

- More mothers are informed about the benefits of breast-feeding (Fig. 11.4).
- Practitioners recognize the ability of human milk to meet infant needs (Table 11.3) and promote immune function.[41]
- Maternity wards and alternative birth centers have been modified to facilitate successful lactation.
- Community support is increasingly available, even in workplaces.
- Programs that promote breast-feeding are increasingly responsive to a wider range of maternal socioeconomic conditions and cultural backgrounds.[42]

The WHO recommends breast-feeding be initiated within the first hour of birth, exclusive breast-feeding for the first 6 months, and continued breast-feeding for up to 2 years or beyond.[43] Unfortunately, exclusive breast-feeding declines to 43% and fewer than 22% of mothers by 3 and 6 months, respectively.[40] Solid foods are usually added to the baby's diet at approximately 6 months of age. The Academy of

FIG. 11.4 Breast-feeding can support bonding between the mother and the infant. (Copyright Getty Images.)

Nutrition and Dietetics' position is that breast-feeding should continue for at least the first 12 months of the infant's life.[42]

Cultural factors may influence how women in racial and ethnic groups regard breast-feeding. Although Hispanic and Asian women overall display the highest rates of breast-feeding initiation, Hispanic and Asian subgroups are quite heterogeneous with specific ethnic groups demonstrating much lower breast-feeding rates.[44] Black women, who demonstrate some of the lowest rates of breast-feeding, may be more likely to have negative attitudes toward breast-feeding compared with women in other racial groups, and these women may also face a lack of access to information that supports and promotes breast-feeding.[44] Women of all racial and ethnic groups who search for information about breast-feeding and are more highly educated are more likely to exclusively breast-feed, suggesting that socioeconomic status is correlated to infant feeding choices. Moreover, educational interventions and support systems for breast-feeding can increase the number of women intending to and who actually breast-feed. Women should be educated early and continually about breast-feeding, and health care providers should seek to understand the cultural and socioeconomic influences related to breast-feeding choices among women of racial and ethnic groups.

Nutritional Needs

The physiologic needs of lactation are different from those of pregnancy, and they demand adequate nutritional support (see Table 11.1). The basic nutritional needs for lactation include the following additions to the mother's prepregnancy needs.

Energy

The recommended caloric increase is 330 kcal/day (plus 170 kcal/day from maternal stores) in the first 6 months and 400 kcal/day in the second 6 months of breast-feeding beyond normal energy needs. This makes a daily total of approximately 2700 to 2800 kcal/day for milk production and maternal energy needs, although this value can range according to other anthropometric and lifestyle factors.[6] This additional energy need for lactation is based on the following five factors:

1. *Milk content:* An average daily milk production for lactating women is 780 mL (26 oz). The energy content of human milk averages 0.67 to 0.74 kcal/g. Thus 26 oz of milk has a value of approximately 525 kcal.
2. *Milk production:* The metabolic work involved in producing this amount of milk is approximately 80% efficient and requires from

TABLE 11.3	Selected Nutritional Components of Human Milk (Per 100 mL)			
Milk Component	**Colostrum**	**Transitional**	**Mature**	**Cow's Milk**
Kilocalories	57.0	63.0	65.0	65.0
Vitamins, Fat Soluble				
• A (mcg)	151.0	88.0	75.0	41.0
• D (IU)	—	—	5.0	2.5
• E (mg)	1.5	0.9	0.25	0.07
• K (mcg)	—	—	1.5	6.0
Vitamins, Water Soluble				
• Thiamin (mcg)	1.9	5.9	14.0	43.0
• Riboflavin (mcg)	30.0	37.0	40.0	145.0
• Niacin (mcg)	75.0	175.0	160.0	82.0
• Pantothenic acid (mcg)	183.0	288.0	246.0	340.0
• Biotin (mcg)	0.06	0.35	0.6	2.8
• Vitamin B_{12} (mcg)	0.05	0.04	0.1	1.1
• Vitamin C (mg)	5.9	7.1	5.0	1.1

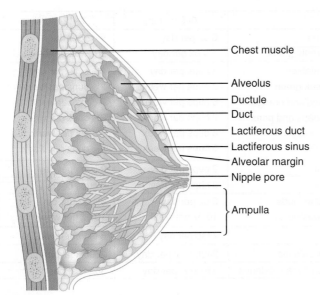

FIG. 11.5 Structural features of the human mammary gland. (From Mahan LK, Escott-Stump S, editors: *Krause's food, nutrition, and diet therapy*, ed 11, Philadelphia, 2004, Saunders.)

Labels: Chest muscle · Alveolus · Ductule · Duct · Lactiferous duct · Lactiferous sinus · Alveolar margin · Nipple pore · Ampulla

400 to 450 kcal. During pregnancy, breast tissues develops for this purpose, stimulated by hormones from the placenta, and forms special milk-producing cells called *lobules* (Fig. 11.5). After birth, maternal production of the hormone prolactin continues this milk-production process, stimulated by the suckling infant. Thus milk production depends on the demand of the infant. The suckling infant stimulates the release of the hormone oxytocin from the pituitary gland, initiating the letdown reflex and the flow of milk from the storage cells to the nipple. This reflex can be inhibited by the mother's fatigue, tension, or lack of confidence, a particular source of anxiety in the new mother. She may be reassured that a comfortable and satisfying feeding routine is usually established in 2 to 3 weeks (see Fig. 11.4).

3. *Maternal adipose tissue storage:* A component of the energy need for lactation (170 kcal/day in the first 6 months) is drawn from maternal adipose tissue stores deposited during pregnancy in normal preparation for lactation. Depending on the adequacy of these stores, additional energy input may be needed in the lactating woman's daily diet.
4. *Exercise:* Moderate to vigorous exercise does not negatively affect milk composition and volume *as long as* adequate energy and fluids are consumed.[14]
5. *Weight loss:* In some women, weight gained during pregnancy may be largely retained and contribute to obesity. Women who breast-feed sometimes have concerns whether a weight-loss program might compromise their breast milk production. Research with overweight women who were exclusively breast-feeding has shown that diet and exercise programs resulting in a weight loss of approximately 0.5 kg/week (approximately 1 lb/week) can support sufficient milk production.[45] However, women who are engaged in weight loss efforts should ensure they are being monitored by their physician.

Protein

The recommendation for protein needs during lactation is 71 g/day during both the first 6 months and the second 6 months.[6] This is approximately a 25-g/day increase from the regular needs of adult women.

Minerals

The DRI standard for calcium during lactation is 1000 mg/day, the same as for the nonpregnant or pregnant adult woman.[5] Calcium that was required during gestation for the mineralization of the fetal skeleton is now diverted into the mother's milk production. Iron, because it is not a major mineral component of milk and because of lactational amenorrhea, does not need to be increased during lactation.

Vitamins

The DRI standard for vitamin C during lactation is 120 mg/day.[7] This is a considerable increase from the regular 75 mg/day for adult women. Increases beyond the mother's prenatal intake are also recommended for vitamin A because it is a constituent of milk[8] and for the B-complex vitamins because they are involved as coenzyme factors in energy metabolism.[9] Therefore the quantities of vitamins needed invariably increase as the kcalorie intake increases.

Fluids

Ample fluid intake is needed and should be based on the mother's urine color. A pale-yellow color of the urine suggests adequate fluid intake. Beverages such as juices and milk contribute fluid and kcalories.[42]

Food Intake

Fig. 11.6 displays an example of a healthy food intake pattern for a breast-feeding woman. In general, 7 oz of grains, at least one-half of which are whole grains; 3 cups of vegetables; 2 cups of fruits; 3 cups of fluid milk or dairy products; 6 to 6.5 oz of lean meats, poultry, fish, dried beans, and nuts per day are recommended to meet nutrient needs during lactation (http://www.choosemyplate.gov).

Dietary Supplements

Many health practitioners recommend that women continue their prenatal vitamin supplements during lactation. Specifically, women with certain health conditions or nutrient needs may require supplements while breast-feeding. For example, mothers who consume vegan diets will need vitamin-B_{12} supplements.[46] Individual recommendations for nutrient supplementation during lactation should be based on a full assessment of the mother's nutritional status and other environmental factors.

Women may desire to use herbal or botanical products as galactogogues (agents that stimulate breast milk production), relaxants, or analgesics. The safety for mother and infant and efficacy of such products during lactation have not been adequately evaluated in randomized, placebo-controlled trials. In general, women should not use herbals and botanicals during lactation; however, some may be appropriate for use within defined quantities. Women considering use of these products should consult with a medical provider or lactation consultant.

Rest and Relaxation

In addition to the increased diet, the nursing mother requires rest, moderate exercise, and relaxation. Postpartum depression (PPD) is increasingly recognized as a specific, and sometimes very serious, condition in mothers. Ranging from "baby blues" to postpartum psychosis, the relationship of this condition with nutritional status is under investigation, although some preliminary research connects poor maternal nutrition quality and symptoms of stress and anxiety.[47] For example, diet quality and other nutrient deficiencies may be linked to PPD (see Evidence-Based Practice box, "Nutrition and Postpartum Depression"). The connections among nutrient needs, PPD, and breast-feeding duration will be of future interest.

	0–6 months	7–12 months
Grains	6 oz per day	9 oz per day
Whole grains	≥ 4 oz per day	≥ 4½ oz per day
Vegetables	3 cups per day	3½ cups per day
Dark green	2 cups per week	2½ cups per week
Red and orange	6 cups per week	7 cups per week
Beans and peas	2 cups per week	2½ cups per week
Starchy	6 cups per week	7 cups per week
Other	5 cups per week	5½ cups per week
Fruits	2 cups per day	2 cups per day
Dairy	3 cups per day	3 cups per day
Protein foods	6 oz per day	6½ oz per day
Seafood	10 oz per week	10 oz per week
Oils	7 tsp per day	8 tsp per day
Total calories	2400 kcal per day	2600 kcal per day
Discretionary calories	330 kcal per day	362 kcal per day

FIG. 11.6 Food intake plan for a breast-feeding woman based on maternal age, height, current weight, and physical activity, infant birth date, and exclusive breast-feeding or combination feeding using the MyPlate resource (http://www.choosemyplate.gov).

Maternal Medical Conditions

Breast-feeding should be encouraged in most mothers (see the Perspectives in Practice box, "Breast-Feeding: The Dynamic Nature of Human Milk"). However, some conditions exist for which it is recommended that women in the United States not breast-feed, including HIV-positive status, active untreated tuberculosis, infant galactosemia, human T-lymphocytic virus, illicit drug use, and with specific chemotherapeutic agents. Other conditions or medications should be discussed with health practitioners.[38,42]

Advantages and Barriers to Breast-Feeding

These factors need to be reviewed with each individual mother in her particular situation so that she can make the informed decision that is best for the infant and herself.

Many nutritional, physiologic, psychological, and practical advantages to breast-feeding exist; six are identified as follows:

1. Human milk composition changes to meet the changing nutrient and energy needs of the infant and provides optimal nutrition for the first months to years of life.
2. Infants experience enhanced immune function and fewer diseases and infections because the mother transfers certain antibodies and immune properties in human milk to her nursing infant.[42]
3. Infants who are breast-fed may experience a reduced risk for the development of allergies. This is related to immunologic properties, the presence of antibodies in human milk, and potentially reduced exposure to allergens.[48]
4. Ease of digestion is greater with breast milk because human milk forms a softer curd in the gastrointestinal tract that is easier for the infant to digest.

EVIDENCE-BASED PRACTICE

Nutrition and Postpartum Depression?

PPD affects approximately 10%–15% of women and can impair a mother's sensitivity, attachment, and parenting style to such an extent that PPD is associated with adverse child outcomes, including cognitive, social, and behavioral development. Although specific causes of PPD are unknown, it is thought to be related to maternal hormone alterations. PPD is a treatable problem. Mild PDD symptoms may be treated with psychosocial strategies including peer support and counseling; psychotherapy can be effective for more moderate depressive symptoms; and pharmacotherapy, including use of Selective Serotonin Reuptake Inhibitors (SSRIs), may be appropriate for more severe symptoms. There is some controversy surrounding use of medications given that small amounts (less than 10% of maternal level) are found in breast milk, but overall the benefits to the mother and her ability to care for her child are believed to outweigh the negative effects.

There has been question as to whether nutritional factors can improve or exacerbate PDD symptoms. Poor iron status was thought to be associated with PPD; however, current research does not support this link. More recently, vitamin D status, omega-3 fatty acid intake, and diet quality are thought to be linked to PDD. Although there is promising research for all three measures, there is inadequate evidence to support vitamin D or omega-3 fatty acid supplementation for treatment of PDD, nor is there sufficient evidence to guide diet quality recommendations to prevent PDD. This is just one example in the field of nutrition that demonstrates the potential for nutrition intervention in treating clinical issues, while research is still clarifying the relationship. However, there are many reasons to encourage women to focus on nutrient-rich diets that include adequate fish intake and to assess for vitamin D sufficiency.

Questions for Analysis

1. Does this evidence suggest that postpartum women should routinely be supplemented with specific vitamins and minerals to prevent PPD?
2. What additional evidence is required to establish practice guidelines regarding nutrition and prevention or treatment of PPD?

Bibliography

Brummelte S, Galea LA: Postpartum depression: etiology, treatment and consequences for maternal care. *Horm Behav* 77:153, 2016.

Gould FJ, Best K, Makrides M: Perinatal nutrition interventions and post-partum depressive symptoms. *J Affect Disord*, 224:2-9, 2016.

Miller BJ, Murray L, Beckmann MM, et al: Dietary supplements for preventing postnatal depression. *Cochrane Database Syst Rev* (10):CD009104, 2013.

Pope CJ, Mazmanian D: Breastfeeding and postpartum depression: an overview and methodological recommendations for future research. *Depress Res Treat* 2016:4765310, 2016.

Stewart DE, Vigod S: Postpartum depression. *N Engl J Med* 375:2177, 2016.

Breast-Feeding: The Dynamic Nature of Human Milk

Human milk is the ideal first food for human infants. Its dynamic nature changes to match growth needs. However, the mother's choice to breast-feed her infant depends on a number of factors, especially for new mothers, who often need information and counseling starting in early pregnancy.

Breast Milk for the Preterm Infant

The levels of nutrients in mother's milk shift according to the gestational age of the infant at birth. Premature infants thrive on breast milk. It is recommended that preterm infants receive human breast milk, including those requiring enteral nutrition, due to the optimal composition of nutrients found in this milk. For example, an analysis of the nutritional quality of preterm milk reveals energy and fat concentrations that are 20% to 30% greater, protein levels 15% to 20% greater, and lactose levels 10% lower than those found in mature milk. Premature milk can meet the preterm infant's nutritional and developmental needs, if the mother is committed to breast-feeding and/or expressing breast milk and feeding by bottle or feeding tube.

Breast Milk During Weaning

Nutrient levels continue to change with time to match changing growth patterns and developing digestive abilities. Mother's milk provides sufficient kcalories and nutrients to keep babies well fed without supplemental formula or food. Even when the infant is being weaned, the nature of human milk ensures adequate nutrients in case the new, solid-food diet cannot meet the child's needs. Human milk collected during gradual weaning has been found to have increased concentrations of protein, sodium, and iron. Lactose levels are lower, possibly so that increased amounts of kcalories can be supplied by fats, a more concentrated source.

Breast Milk and the Cesarean Section Infant

The quality of human milk is not influenced by the delivery method of the infant. Many women fear that a baby born by cesarean section cannot be nursed because they believe that this method of delivery delays or prevents the production of mature milk. Milk production is stimulated by the release of the placenta, which occurs whether the delivery is vaginal or not. Studies confirm that no significant difference exists in the length of time it takes for mature milk to come in after vaginal or cesarean deliveries.

Thus premature or cesarean deliveries should not discourage women from breast-feeding. Mothers should not underestimate the nutritive quality of their milk simply because it does not appear as rich and thick as cow's milk. For the human infant, in nutritional and immunologic terms, breast milk remains the best milk.

Mothers' Facts and Fancies About Breast-Feeding

In early counseling, mothers express a variety of concerns about breast-feeding. Following are a few such statements:

"My Breasts Aren't Big Enough"

When it comes to breast-feeding, small breast size does not indicate insufficient milk production. The only parts of the breast that participate in milk production are the glandular and nervous tissue and the nipple; these are basically the same in all healthy women. The only difference between different breast sizes is the amount of fat tissue the breast contains.

"Breast-Feeding Causes Cancer"

To the contrary, investigators have been looking to breast-feeding as a possible means of preventing certain types of breast and ovarian cancer. Epidemiologic studies suggest a decreased risk for these cancers in women who breast-feed, but additional evidence is needed before a consensus may be reached.

"Breast-Feeding Will Ruin My Figure"

Because the caloric demand of breast-feeding exceeds that of the nonpregnant woman by approximately 400 to 500 kcalories, some women experience a faster return to prepregnancy weight. Oxytocin, the hormone manufactured to stimulate the letdown reflex, also stimulates uterine contractions, helping reduce the uterus to its prepregnancy size more rapidly.

"Breast-Feeding Is Painful"

It may be painful in the first few days or even weeks as mother and baby establish a pattern of feeding and proper latch and release techniques. Milk should not be allowed to collect in the breast to the point of engorgement, the nipples should be kept clean and dry, and a variety of feeding positions may be used while nursing to decrease the chances of having a painful experience. Mastitis is a painful infection of the breast that requires medical attention and often antibiotic treatment.

"Breast Milk Is Not Nutritious"

The thin, bluish appearance of breast milk has some women convinced that it is no more nourishing than water. Refer to Table 11.3; this demonstrates how well breast milk meets the nutritional needs of the infant.

"I Will Have to Change My Diet to Breast-Feed"

Foods that were eaten during pregnancy may be consumed during lactation. Some women report that after they eat onions, cauliflower, cabbage, or other foods their infants do not like the taste of their breast milk. Other women say that eating chocolate or drinking coffee, for example, "makes their babies fussy" when breast-feeding. Scientific evidence does not discourage moderate intake of these foods or drinks and it is the choice of the mother to eliminate these foods to assess if the infant's symptoms improve. A well-balanced diet that includes a variety of colorful foods and fluids is encouraged during breast-feeding.

"I Cannot Go to Work or School if I Breast-Feed"

Breast milk can be stored for up to 5 days in the refrigerator or up to 5 months in the freezer. Many working mothers take advantage of this by expressing their milk and storing it for use by care providers. There are federal and state laws supporting some groups of working mothers that require the workplace to allow for break time for mothers to pump breast milk and a private space for doing so; there are currently efforts to ensure these laws extend to all working mothers. Given that returning to work is often a reason many women discontinue breast-feeding, working mothers need to be educated on how to continue breast-feeding in the workplace.

Other women would like to breast-feed but are worried about special "what if" situations, such as the following:

"What if the Baby Has Down Syndrome?"

Infants with Down syndrome can be nursed; however, it does require time, patience, and the use of slightly different nursing techniques. The mother should be told about the special nursing needs of infants with Down syndrome to avoid disappointment or a feeling of failure should breast-feeding become impractical for her particular living situation.

"What if I Have Twins?"

Although it takes time, patience, and good coordination to breast-feed twins and even triplets, it is possible. The health benefits to these infants may be even greater given that they are more likely to be at risk given the likelihood of prematurity and SGA. Time and fatigue are the most common barriers to breast-feeding multiples and so these mothers will need significant support from those around them.

Continued

PERSPECTIVES IN PRACTICE

Breast-Feeding: The Dynamic Nature of Human Milk—cont'd

"What if I Have Had Breast Surgery?"

Studies on breast augmentation and reduction surgeries have shown mixed results related to successful breast-feeding, and more information is needed in this area. Studies on both breast reduction and breast augmentation surgeries indicate reduced breast-feeding initiation among these women and increased complications with breast-feeding. However, there are postsurgical women who do experience successful breast-feeding. These women should be encouraged to breast-feed and can receive support from a lactation consultant if they experience complications.

"What if I Become Pregnant?"

Some women may purposefully choose to breast-feed to avoid pregnancy, but this is not a dependable contraception method. Women who breast-feed must understand that the lack of a menstrual period during lactation (lactational amenorrhea) does not mean they cannot become pregnant. Contraceptives may be required if another pregnancy is not desired at the current time. If pregnancy occurs, then the woman should discuss appropriate infant-feeding solutions with her health care team, although many women do continue breast-feeding during pregnancy.

Bibliography

American Academy of Pediatrics Section on Breastfeeding: Breastfeeding and the use of human milk, *Pediatrics* 129(3):e827, 2012.

Chung M, Ip S, Yu W, et al: Interventions in primary care to promote breastfeeding: a systematic review, Agency for Healthcare Research and Quality (US) Report No.: 09-05126-EF-1, 2008.

Binns C, Lee M, Low WY: The long-term public health benefits of breastfeeding, *Asia Pac J Public Health* 28(1):7, 2016.

Du Toit G, Foong RM, Lack G: Prevention of food allergy—early dietary interventions, *Allergol Int* 65(4):370, 2016.

Islami F, Liu Y, Jemal A, et al: Breastfeeding and breast cancer risk by receptor status—a systematic review and meta-analysis, *Ann Oncol* 26(12):2398, 2015.

Lessen R, Kavanagh K: Position of the academy of nutrition and dietetics: promoting and supporting breastfeeding, *J Acad Nutr Diet* 115(3):444–449, 2015.

Li DP, Du C, Zhang ZM, et al: Breastfeeding and ovarian cancer risk: A systematic review and meta-analysis of 40 epidemiological studies, *Asian Pac J Cancer Prev* 15(12):4829, 2014.

Position of the American Dietetic Association: Promoting and supporting breastfeeding, *J Am Diet Assoc* 115(3):444, 2015.

Patnode CD, Henninger ML, Senger CA, et al: Primary Care Interventions to Support Breastfeeding: Updated Evidence Report and Systematic Review for the US Preventive Services Task Force, *JAMA* 316(16):1694, 2016.

Roberts CL, Ampt AJ, Algert CS, et al: Reduced breast milk feeding subsequent to cosmetic breast augmentation surgery, *Med J Aust* 202(6):324, 2015.

Thibaudeau S, Sinno H, Williams B: The effects of breast reduction on successful breastfeeding: a systematic review, *J Plast Reconstr Aesthet Surg* 63(10):1688, 2010.

---

5. The convenience and economy of breast milk are greater because the mother is free from the time and expense involved in buying and preparing formula, and her breast milk is always ready and sterile.
6. Breast-feeding provides psychologic bonding because the mother and infant relate to one another during feeding, regular times of rest and enjoyment, and cuddling and fulfillment.[42]

Despite the advantages of breast-feeding, some women face perceived barriers associated with misinformation, cultural influences, family pressures, or outside employment, among other factors. Addressing these barriers, before delivery rather than after, will increase the likelihood that the mother breast-feeds her infant:

- Misinformation, a major barrier, can create negative impressions and ideas. Experienced breast-feeding mothers or lactation consultants can fill this need, especially for young first-time mothers.
- Personal modesty and anxiety, or a fear of appearing immodest in breast exposure, may hinder some mothers from breast-feeding. Sensitive counseling can help allay some of these personal fears. Cultural shifts that create a broader acceptance of breast-feeding will provide increased support for lactating women.
- Family pressures, especially from the husband, not to breast-feed have strong influences on the mother, even though she may want to do so. Initial counseling and education about breast-feeding should include both parents whenever possible. Reasons for negative attitudes can be explored and misinformation clarified with sound education.
- Outside employment, with a limited maternity leave and job loss if the mother does not return to work at that time, can complicate the mother's decision, even though she may want to breast-feed her baby. However, if the mother desires to continue breast-feeding, then it is possible to breast-feed and be employed. After breast-feeding is well established, she can regularly express milk by hand or with a breast pump into sterile disposable nursing bags to use with disposable holder, cap, and nipple ensemble. Rapid chilling and strict sanitation are required, but it can be planned, given the commitment. Some companies provide child care facilities for their employees, recognizing that helping employees with this modern need is good business.

All of these approaches to breast-feeding have real rewards for the infant. In addition, they can strengthen the mother's confidence in her maternal capabilities. The importance of these intangible benefits should not be underestimated.

TO SUM UP

Pregnancy involves synergistic interactions among three distinct biologic entities: (1) the fetus, (2) placenta, and (3) woman. Maternal needs reflect the increasing nutritional demands of the fetus and the placenta, as well as the need to meet maternal needs and to prepare for lactation. Optimal weight gain is recommended during pregnancy to accommodate rapid growth. Diet quality is equally important for healthy pregnancy outcomes.

Common problems occurring during pregnancy include nausea and vomiting, heartburn, and constipation. In most cases they are easily relieved without medication by simple, often temporary, changes in the diet. Serious problems with pregnancy may be associated with preexisting chronic maternal conditions, such as diabetes mellitus, or conditions arising as a result of the physical or metabolic demands of pregnancy, such as iron deficiency anemia and HDP. Unusual or erratic eating habits, age, parity, prepartum weight status, and low income status are among the many related factors that also place the woman at risk for complications.

The Academy of Nutrition and Dietetics strongly encourages public health and clinical efforts that promote breast-feeding to optimize the indisputable nutritional, immunologic, psychologic, and economic benefits. The ultimate goal of prenatal care is a healthy infant and a mother physically capable of breast-feeding her child, should she choose to do so. Human milk provides the essential nutrients in quantities required for optimal infant growth and development. It also supplies immunologic factors that offer protection against infection. Lactation requires an increase in kcalories beyond the needs of pregnancy. Adequate fluid intake is guided by the mother's natural thirst.

QUESTIONS FOR REVIEW

1. List and discuss five factors that influence the nutritional needs of the woman during pregnancy. Which factors would place a woman in a high-risk category? Why?

2. List six nutrients that are required in larger amounts during pregnancy. Describe their special role during this period. Identify four food sources of each.

3. Identify two common problems associated with pregnancy, and describe the dietary management of each.

4. List and describe the screening indicators and risk factors for hypertension and diabetes mellitus during pregnancy.

5. List and discuss five major nutritional factors of lactation.

6. Using the MyPlate resource, determine a food intake plan for a 27-year-old woman who is 5 feet 5 inches tall, weighs 130 pounds, exercises for less than 30 minutes per day, and is exclusively breastfeeding her 2-month-old infant.

REFERENCES

1. Gresham E, Byles JE, Bisquera A, et al: Effects of dietary interventions on neonatal and infant outcomes: a systematic review and meta-analysis, *Am J Clin Nutr* 100(5):1298–1321, 2014.

2. Stang J, Huffman LG: Position of the Academy of Nutrition and Dietetics: Obesity, Reproduction, and Pregnancy Outcomes, *J Acad Nutr Diet* 116(4):677–691, 2016.

3. Maness SB, Buhi ER: Associations between social determinants of health and pregnancy among young people: a systematic review of research published during the past 25 years, *Public Health Rep* 131(1):86–99, 2016.

4. Procter SB, Campbell CG: Position of the Academy of Nutrition and Dietetics: Nutrition and lifestyle for a healthy pregnancy outcome, *J Acad Nutr Diet* 114(7):1099–1103, 2014.

5. Institute of Medicine, Food and Nutrition Board, editors: *Dietary Reference Intakes for calcium and vitamin D*, Washington, DC, 2011, National Academies Press.

6. Institute of Medicine, Food and Nutrition Board, editors: *Dietary Reference Intakes for energy, carbohydrate, fiber, fat, fatty acids, cholesterol, protein, and amino acids (macronutrients)*, Washington, DC, 2005, National Academies Press.

7. Institute of Medicine, Food and Nutrition Board, editors: *Dietary Reference Intakes for vitamin C, vitamin E, selenium, and carotenoids*, Washington, DC, 2000, National Academies Press.

8. Institute of Medicine, Food and Nutrition Board, editors: *Dietary Reference Intakes for vitamin A, vitamin K, arsenic, boron, chromium, copper, iodine, iron, manganese, molybdenum, nickel, silicon, vanadium, and zinc*, Washington, DC, 2000, National Academies Press.

9. Institute of Medicine, Food and Nutrition Board, editors: *Dietary Reference Intakes for thiamin, riboflavin, niacin, vitamin B6, folate, vitamin B12, pantothenic acid, biotin, and choline*, Washington, DC, 1998, National Academies Press.

10. Heindel JJ, Vandenberg LN: Developmental origins of health and disease: a paradigm for understanding disease cause and prevention, *Curr Opin Pediatr* 27(2):248–253, 2015.

11. US Department of Health and Human Services: *Healthy People 2020: framework*, ed 2, Washington, DC, 2010, US Government Printing Office.

12. Thoma ME, McLain, Louis JF, et al: Prevalence of infertility in the United States as estimated by the current duration approach and a traditional constructed approach, *Fertil Steril* 99(5):1324–1331.e1, 2013.

13. Rooney KL, Domar AD: The impact of lifestyle behaviors on infertility treatment outcome, *Curr Opin Obstet Gynecol* 26(3):181–185, 2014.

14. Harrison CL, Brown WJ, Hayman M, et al: The role of physical activity in preconception, pregnancy and postpartum health, *Semin Reprod Med* 34(2):e28–e37, 2016.

15. Jia X, Pakseresht M, Wattar N, et al: Women who take n-3 long-chain polyunsaturated fatty acid supplements during pregnancy and lactation meet the recommended intake, *Appl Physiol Nutr Metab* 40(5):474–481, 2015.

16. US Department of Health and Human Services: *2015–2020 dietary guidelines for Americans*, Washington, DC, 2015, USDA.

17. Williams J, Mai CT, Mulinare J, et al: Updated estimates of neural tube defects prevented by mandatory folic Acid fortification—United States, 1995–2011, *MMWR Morb Mortal Wkly Rep* 64(1):1–5, 2015.

18. Leermakers ET, Moreira EM, Kiefte-de Jong JC, et al: Effects of choline on health across the life course: a systematic review, *Nutr Rev* 73(8):500–522, 2015.

19. Rasmussen KM, Yaktine AL, editors: *Weight gain during pregnancy: reexamining the guidelines*, Washington, DC, National Academics Press, 2009.

20. Martin JA, Hamilton BE, Osterman MJ, et al: Births: final data for 2013, *Natl Vital Stat Rep* 64(1):1–65, 2015.

21. Catalano PM, Mele L, Landon MB, et al: Inadequate weight gain in overweight and obese pregnant women: what is the effect on fetal growth? *Am J Obstet Gynecol* 211(2):137.e1-7, 2014.

22. Institute of Medicine, Food and Nutrition Board, editors: *Dietary Reference Intakes for water, potassium, sodium, chloride, and sulfate*, Washington, DC, 2004, National Academies Press.

23. Sakuyama H, Katoh M, Wakabayashi H, et al: Influence of gestational salt restriction in fetal growth and in development of diseases in adulthood, *J Biomed Sci* 23:12, 2016.

24. Matthews A, Haas DM, O'Mathúna DP, et al: Interventions for nausea and vomiting in early pregnancy, *Cochrane Database Syst Rev* (9):CD007575, 2015.

25. Hamilton BE, Martin JA, Osterman MJ, et al: Births: final data for 2014, *Natl Vital Stat Rep* 64(12):1–64, 2015.

26. Azevedo WF, Diniz MB, Fonseca ES, et al: Complications in adolescent pregnancy: systematic review of the literature, *Einstein (Sao Paulo)* 13(4):618–626, 2015.

27. Cook JL, Green CR, Lilley CM, et al: Fetal alcohol spectrum disorder: a guideline for diagnosis across the lifespan, *CMAJ* 188(3):191–197, 2016.

28. Ayad M, Costantine MM: Epidemiology of medications use in pregnancy, *Semin Perinatol* 39(7):508–511, 2015.

29. Gunn JK, Rosales CB, Center KE, et al: Prenatal exposure to cannabis and maternal and child health outcomes: a systematic review and meta-analysis, *BMJ Open* 6(4):e009986, 2016.

30. McCauley ME, van den Broek N, Dou L, et al: Vitamin A supplementation during pregnancy for maternal and newborn outcomes, *Cochrane Database Syst Rev* (10):CD008666, 2015.

31. Patel SI, Pennell PB: Management of epilepsy during pregnancy: an update, *Ther Adv Neurol Disord* 9(2):118–129, 2016.

32. Chen LW, Wu Y, Neelakantan N, et al: Maternal caffeine intake during pregnancy and risk of pregnancy loss: a categorical and dose-response meta-analysis of prospective studies, *Public Health Nutr* 19(7):1233–1144, 2016.

33. Fawcett EJ, Fawcett JM, Mazmanian D: A meta-analysis of the worldwide prevalence of pica during pregnancy and the postpartum period, *Int J Gynaecol Obstet* 133(3):277–283, 2016.

34. Cantor AG, Bougatsos C, McDonagh M: Routine iron supplementation and screening for iron deficiency anemia in pregnancy, *Ann Intern Med* 163(5):400, 2015.

35. Mol BWJ, Roberts CT, Thangaratinam S, et al: Pre-eclampsia, *Lancet* 387(10022):999–1011, 2016.

36. Luke B: Nutrition for multiples, *Clin Obstet Gynecol* 58(3):585–610, 2015.
37. DeSisto CL, Kim SY, Sharma AJ: Prevalence estimates of gestational diabetes mellitus in the United States, Pregnancy Risk Assessment Monitoring System (PRAMS), 2007-2010, *Prev Chronic Dis* 11:E104, 2014.
38. Lawrence RM: Circumstances when breastfeeding is contraindicated, *Pediatr Clin North Am* 60(1):295–318, 2013.
39. Kimmel MC, Ferguson EH, Zerwas S, et al: Obstetric and gynecologic problems associated with eating disorders, *Int J Eat Disord* 49(3):260–275, 2016.
40. Centers for Disease Control and Prevention: *Breastfeeding among US children born 2002–2012, national immunization surveys.* 2016.
41. U.S.P.S.T. Force, Bibbins-Domingo K, Grossman DC, Curry SJ, et al: Primary Care Interventions to Support Breastfeeding: US Preventive Services Task Force Recommendation Statement, *JAMA* 316(16):1688–1693, 2016.
42. Lessen R, Kavanagh K: Position of the academy of nutrition and dietetics: promoting and supporting breastfeeding, *J Acad Nutr Diet* 115(3):444–449, 2015.
43. WHO: *Infant and young child feeding: Model chapter for textbooks for medical students and allied health professionals*, Geneva, 2009.
44. Jones KM, Power ML, Queenan JT, et al: Racial and ethnic disparities in breastfeeding, *Breastfeed Med* 10(4):186–196, 2015.
45. Amorim Adegboye AR, Linne YM: Diet or exercise, or both, for weight reduction in women after childbirth, *Cochrane Database Syst Rev* (7):CD005627, 2013.
46. Chalouhi C, Faesch S, Anthoine-Milhomme MC, et al: Neurological consequences of vitamin B12 deficiency and its treatment, *Pediatr Emerg Care* 24(8):538–541, 2008.
47. Baskin R, Hill B, Jacka FN, et al: The association between diet quality and mental health during the perinatal period. A systematic review, *Appetite* 91:41–47, 2015.
48. Clarke S: Dietary allergies in breastfed babies, *Community Pract* 88(6):22–23, 2015.

FURTHER READINGS AND RESOURCES

Readings

Dante G, Bellei G, Neri I, Facchinetti F: Herbal therapies in pregnancy: what works? *Curr Opin Obstet Gynecol* 26(2):83, 2014.

Fernandez-Twinn DS, Constancia M, Ozanne SE: Intergenerational epigenetic inheritance in models of developmental programming of adult disease, *Semin Cell Dev Biol* 43:85, 2015.

[Does chronic disease begin in utero? A critical evaluation of evidence to support this hypothesis is provided. Mechanisms underlying metabolic programming of disease origins during in utero development are discussed.]

Harrison CL, Brown WJ, Hayman M, et al: The role of physical activity in preconception, pregnancy and postpartum health, *Semin Reprod Med* 34(2):e28–e37, 2016.

[This publication offers evidence-based and practical guidelines for physical activity recommendations for pregnancy and lactation.]

Kaiser LL, Campbell CG: Practice paper of the academy of nutrition and dietetics: nutrition and lifestyle for a healthy pregnancy outcome, *J Acad Nutr Diet* 114(9):1447, 2014.

[This excellent resource provides helpful guidance for healthy pregnancies, as well as important information for identifying women at nutritional risk.]

Kirkwood NA: *A hospital handbook on multiculturalism and religion: practical guidelines for health care workers*, ed 2, New York, 2005, Morehouse Publishing.

Mangels R: *Everything vegan pregnancy book*, ed 1. Avon, MA, 2011, F+W Media, Inc.

O'Hagan K: *Cultural competence in the caring professions.* London, 2012, Jessica Kingsley Publishers.

[These resources offer facts and insights about culture and religion and implications for eating during pregnancy.]

Stang J, Huffman LG: Position of the Academy of Nutrition and Dietetics: obesity, reproduction, and pregnancy outcomes, *J Acad Nutr Diet* 116(4):677, 2016.

[This position paper published by the Academy of Nutrition and Dietetics examines the effects of obesity on pregnancy outcomes and provides nutrition recommendations to support healthy pregnancy outcomes in this population.]

Websites of Interest

- March of Dimes Birth Defects Foundation. http://www.marchofdimes.org.
- US Department of Health and Human Services, Food and Drug Administration, Center for Food Safety and Applied Nutrition. http://www.fda.gov/AboutFDA/CentersOffices/OfficeofFoods/CFSAN/.
- US Department of Health and Human Services, National Institutes of Health, National Center for Complementary and Integrative Health. https://www.nccih.nih.gov/.
- US Department of Health and Human Services, Office of Disease Prevention and Health Promotion: *Healthy People 2020.* http://www.healthypeople.gov/2020/about/default.aspx.
- Virginia Department of Health, Office of Family Health Services, BabyCare. http//www.alexandriava.gov/health/info/default.aspx?id=81765.

12

Nutrition for Normal Growth and Development

Kary Woodruff

ⓔ http://evolve.elsevier.com/Williams/essentials/

In this second chapter in our life cycle series, we look at growing infants, children, and adolescents. We consider their physical growth and their inseparable psychosocial development at each progressive stage. This unified growth and development nurture the integrated progression of the child into the adult. Within this dual framework of physical and psychosocial development, we consider food and feeding and their vital roles in the development of the whole child. In each age group, we relate nutritional needs and the food that supplies them to the normal physical maturation and psychosocial development achieved in that stage.

OUTLINE

Human Growth and Development
Nutritional Requirements for Growth
Stages of Growth and Development: Age-Group Needs

Health Promotion
　Children and Adolescents: Seeking Fitness

HUMAN GROWTH AND DEVELOPMENT

Individual Needs of Children

Growth may be defined as an increase in body size. Biologic growth of an organism occurs through cell multiplication (hyperplasia) and cell enlargement (hypertrophy). *Development* is the associated process by which growing tissues and organs take on more complex functions. Both processes are part of one whole, forming a unified and inseparable sequence of growth and development. Through these changes a small, dependent newborn is transformed into a fully functioning independent adult. However, each child is a unique entity with individual needs. This is a paramount principle in working with children. Thus we must always seek to discover these individual human needs if we are to help each child reach his or her greatest growth and development potential.[1]

Normal Life Cycle Growth Pattern

The normal human life cycle includes the following four general stages of overall growth and development: (1) infancy, (2) childhood, (3) adolescence, and (4) adulthood.

1. *Infancy:* Growth velocity is rapid during the first year of life, with the rate tapering off in the latter half of the year. By 4 to 6 months of age an infant has typically doubled its birth weight, and at 1 year he or she will likely have tripled it.
2. *Childhood:* During the latent period of childhood, after infancy and before adolescence, the growth rate slows and becomes erratic. During some periods, plateaus are reached. At other times, small spurts of growth occur. This overall growth deceleration affects appetite accordingly. At certain times, children will have little or no appetite; at other times, they will eat voraciously. Parents who know

that this is a normal pattern can relax and avoid making eating a battleground with their children.

3. *Adolescence:* With the beginning of puberty, the second period of growth acceleration occurs. Because of hormonal influences, enormous physiologic changes take place, including growth and maturation of long bones, development of the sex characteristics, and gains in fat and muscle mass.
4. *Adulthood:* In the final stage of a normal life cycle, growth levels off on the adult plateau. Then it gradually declines during old age—the period of senescence.

Measuring Childhood Physical Growth
Growth Charts

Children grow at widely varying individual rates. In clinical practice a child's pattern of growth is compared with percentile growth curves derived from measurements of large numbers of children. Contemporary growth chart grids, developed by the National Center for Health Statistics (NCHS), reflect the growth patterns of breast-fed and formula-fed infants and provide a broad baseline for evaluating growth patterns in children.[2] These charts are based on data from nationally representative samples of children that include various racial and ethnic groups (see Further Readings and Resources at the end of this chapter). Two age intervals are presented: birth to 3 years and 2 to 20 years, with separate curves for boys and girls. A variety of grids monitor growth based on weight and age, length (or stature) and age, weight-for-length (or body mass index [BMI]), and head circumference and age (see the Centers for Disease Control and Prevention website for *CDC Growth Charts: United States* available at the end of the chapter in Further Readings and Resources). Head circumference is a valuable measure in infants, but it is seldom measured routinely after 3 years of age.

Growth charts are essential for tracking the rate of growth over time. A child's measurement within a percentile range on the grid should stay relatively consistent over time. Significant changes, for example weight-for-age decreasing from the 75th percentile down to the 25th percentile, could indicate a medical or health issue such as failure to thrive. Thus frequent measurements of a child's growth allow for an accurate picture of how a child is developing. Directions for use of these growth charts for infants and children with special growth patterns are also available.

The Centers for Disease Control and Prevention recommends that an infant's weight be measured using an infant scale. These may be digital or balance-beam scales. When possible, the infant should be measured in the nude. If a diaper must be worn, weight should be adjusted for its weight. The infant should be gently placed lying supine in the middle of the scale. Infant weight should be recorded to the nearest 0.01 kg. If an infant has difficulty laying still, the weight of the infant may be estimated by weighing an adult holding the infant and subtracting the weight of the adult.

Stature should be measured by recumbent length. An infantometer should be used to measure the length of an infant by laying the infant supine on a horizontal backboard, with the head against the fixed head piece. After the infant's head is gently secured at the head piece in the Frankfort horizontal plane, the infant's legs should be extended by pressing mildly on the knees. The foot piece of the infantometer should then be adjusted to rest securely at the infant's heels. Toes should be pointed upward with feet perpendicular to the foot piece, while the head, shoulders, bottom, and heels lie flat against the backboard. Length is typically measured to the nearest 0.1 cm. Two individuals are generally required to complete measures of recumbent length.

At 2 years of age and beyond, weight should be measured on a standing digital or balance-beam scale to the nearest 0.1 kg. Height should be measured by standing height using a stadiometer. Feet should be flat on the floor or platform with heels together and toes adjusted outward, and body weight should be evenly distributed on both legs. Children should be facing away from the stadiometer, with the head, shoulders, bottom, and heels touching the stadiometer. The head should be aligned in the Frankfort horizontal plane. Hair should be flat. The head piece of the stadiometer should be lowered to rest firmly on the head. The child should then inhale and hold this position during the measurement. Standing height is typically measured to the nearest 0.1 cm. Repeated measurements are typically conducted and averaged at each measurement interval, with the average measurement being recorded. Infants and children should never be left alone during anthropometric measurements.

Nutrition Assessment

Practitioners use the nutrition care process to assess, evaluate, and monitor a child's growth and development, with growth charts and other clinical standards as points of reference. A number of methods and measures, including anthropometry, clinical signs, laboratory tests, and nutritional analysis, may be used as described in Chapter 16.

Motor, Mental, and Psychosocial Development

Motor Growth and Development

Gross motor skills, such as sitting, standing, walking, and running, develop within the first 18 months of life. Fine motor skills gradually develop over a longer period of time. Such control over and coordination of voluntary muscle develops in conjunction with mental, emotional, social, and cultural growth as the child interacts and reacts to sensory stimulants in the environment. Motor skills greatly influence feeding skills and energy needs of the child. For example, the pincer grasp allows toddlers to have better control when handling finger foods. Toddlers and children who are more active and spend more time walking and running generally require more energy.

Mental Growth and Development

Measures of mental growth usually involve abilities in speech and other forms of communication, as well as the ability to handle abstract and symbolic material in thinking. Young children think in very literal terms. As they develop in mental capacity, they can handle more than single ideas, and they can form constructive concepts.

Emotional Growth and Development

Emotional growth is measured in the capacity for love and affection, as well as the ability to handle frustration and anxieties. It also involves the child's ability to control aggressive impulses and to channel hostility from destructive to constructive activities.

Social and Cultural Growth and Development

The social development of a child is measured as the ability to relate to others and to participate in group living and cultural activities. These social and cultural behaviors are first learned through relationships with parents and family, and these relationships greatly influence food habits and feeding patterns. As the child's horizon broadens, relationships are developed with those outside the family, with friends, and with others in the community at school or at religious or other social gatherings. For this reason, a child's play during the early years is a highly purposeful activity.

NUTRITIONAL REQUIREMENTS FOR GROWTH

Energy Needs

During childhood, the demand for kilocalories (kcalories or kcal) is relatively great. However, there is significant variation according to age and

---

Growth Velocity

Rapidity of motion or movement; rate of childhood growth during normal periods of development compared with a population standard.

Growth Deceleration

Period of decreased speed of growth at different points of childhood development.

Growth Acceleration

Period of increased speed of growth at different points of childhood development.

Percentile

One of 100 equal parts of a measured series of values; rate or proportion per hundred.

Growth Chart Grids

Grids comparing stature (length), weight, and age of children by percentile; used for nutritional assessment to determine how their growth is progressing. The most commonly used grids are those of the National Center for Health Statistics (NCHS).

Failure to Thrive

Decelerated or insufficient physical growth associated with abnormal growth and development.

condition. For example, the total daily energy intake of a 5-year-old child is spent in the following way:

- Approximately 50% supplies basal metabolic requirements
- Approximately 5% is used in the thermic effect of food (TEF)
- Approximately 25% goes toward daily physical activity
- Approximately 12% is needed for tissue growth
- Approximately 8% is lost in the feces

Protein Needs

Protein provides amino acids, the essential building materials for tissue growth. As a child grows, the protein requirements per unit of body weight gradually decrease. For example, during the first 6 months of life an infant requires 1.52 g of protein/kg/day.[3] This amount gradually decreases throughout childhood until adulthood, when protein needs are approximately 0.8 g/kg/day.[3] Usually, healthy, active, growing children consume the necessary amounts of kcalories and protein if a variety of food is provided. The Acceptable Macronutrient Distribution Range (AMDR) for dietary protein for children 1 year and older is 10% to 35% of total kcalories.[3]

Essential Fatty Acid Needs

Fat kcalories are important as backup energy sources but are particularly needed to supply linoleic and α-linolenic acids, which are essential fatty acids. Linoleic acid is required for the synthesis of brain and nerve tissue and normal mental development. Infants consuming adequate amounts of breast milk or infant formula in the first 6 months of life and after complementary foods are added in the second 6 months of life are likely to meet their Adequate Intake (AI) for essential fatty acids. Children 1 year and older are recommended to follow the AMDR of 20% to 35% of total kcalories coming from fat.[3]

Carbohydrate Needs

Carbohydrates are the primary energy source and are important in sparing protein for its vital role in tissue formation. Most importantly, carbohydrates provide glucose for essential brain function.[3] The AMDR for dietary carbohydrate is 45% to 65% of total kcalories for children 1 year and older.[3]

Fiber

Many complex-carbohydrate foods also provide dietary fiber. Fiber is important for satiety and bowel regulation and affects blood lipid and glucose concentrations, as well as the vascular system. Fiber may also provide protection against some types of cancer and overweight.[3]

Water Requirements

The infant's relative need for water is greater than that of the adult. The infant's body water content is approximately 70% to 75% of total body weight, whereas in the adult, water contributes only 60% to 65% of total body weight. In addition, a large amount of the infant's total body water is extracellular and more easily lost. Thus prolonged water loss due to diarrhea, as occurs among infants in developing countries given formula prepared from contaminated water, is life threatening and requires immediate oral hydration therapy.[4] Rotavirus is a common cause of diarrhea in infants in many countries. Any infant experiencing diarrhea and fluid imbalance should be immediately examined by a health care professional. The child's water need is related to energy intake and urine concentration. In general, an infant drinks a daily amount of water equivalent to 10% to 15% of body weight, whereas the adult's daily water intake equals 2% to 4% of body weight. A summary of approximate daily fluid needs during the growth years is provided in Table 12.1.[5] In general, infants are able to meet their water needs by consuming breast milk or infant formula. Infant formula

TABLE 12.1 Approximate Daily Fluid Needs During Growth Years

Age	(mL/kg)
0–3 mo	120
3–6 mo	117
6–12 mo	89
1–3 yr	108
4–8 yr	85
9–13 yr	67 (boys)
	57 (girls)
14–18 yr	54 (boys)
	43 (girls)

Data from Food and Nutrition Board, Institute of Medicine: *Dietary References Intakes for water, potassium, sodium, chloride, and sulfate,* Washington, DC, 2004, National Academies Press.

should not be diluted with additional water because this may lead to fluid excess and electrolyte disturbances such as low serum sodium concentration, a potentially life-threatening condition, and long-term may result in failure to thrive in these infants.

Mineral and Vitamin Needs

Minerals and vitamins play essential roles in tissue growth and maintenance, as well as in overall energy metabolism. Positive childhood growth and development depend on an AI of these essential nutrients. For example, rapidly growing young bones require calcium and phosphorus. A radiograph of a newborn's body would reveal a skeleton appearing as a collection of disconnected, separate bones requiring mineralization. Calcium is also needed for tooth development, muscle contraction, nerve excitation, blood coagulation, and heart muscle action. Another mineral of concern is iron, essential for hemoglobin formation and cognitive and psychomotor development. The healthy infant's fetal iron stores are sufficient until 4 to 6 months of age. Thus solid food additions around this time help supply needed iron. Foods such as iron-fortified cereals and meat assist in providing adequate dietary iron. The consumption of iron-fortified formulas and other foods by high-risk children assists in reducing the incidence of iron deficiency anemia among infants and young children.[6] In general, iron supplements are not needed during infancy.

Excess amounts of particular micronutrients are also of concern in feeding children. Excess intake is usually the result of inappropriate use of vitamin or mineral supplements and may occur because of misunderstanding, illiteracy, or carelessness. When supplements are indicated because of a specific and defined medical or nutritional condition, parents must be carefully instructed to use only the amount directed and no more. The following two nutrients pose particular hazards when consumed in excessive amounts:

1. *Vitamin A:* Symptoms of toxicity from excess vitamin A include lack of appetite, slow growth, drying and cracking of the skin, enlargement of the liver and spleen, swelling and pain in the long bones, and bone fragility.
2. *Vitamin D:* Symptoms of toxicity from excess vitamin D include nausea, diarrhea, weight loss, excess urination (especially at night), and eventual calcification of soft tissues, including the renal tubules, blood vessels, bronchi, stomach, and heart.

Summaries of the Dietary Reference Intakes (DRIs) for overall nutritional needs and growth, developed by the Food and Nutrition Board of the Institute of Medicine, are provided in Tables 12.2 to 12.4.

TABLE 12.2 Dietary Reference Intakes for Energy and Protein

	Age (years)	WEIGHT		HEIGHT		Energy (kcal)[a]	Protein (g)
		kg	lb	cm	in		
Infants	0–0.5	6	13	62	24	438–645	9.1
	0.5–1	9	20	71	28	608–844	13.5
Children	1–3	12	27	86	34	768–1683	13
	4–8	20	44	115	45	1133–2225	19
Male subjects	9–13	36	79	144	57	1530–3038	34
	14–18	61	134	174	68	2090–3804	52
Female subjects	9–13	37	81	144	57	1415–2762	34
	14–18	54	119	163	64	1718–2858	46

[a]Varies according to gender, body size, age, and level of physical activity.
Data from Food and Nutrition Board, Institute of Medicine: *Dietary Reference Intakes for energy, carbohydrate, fiber, fat, fatty acids, cholesterol, protein, and amino acids (macronutrients)*, Washington, DC, 2002, National Academies Press.

TABLE 12.3 Dietary Reference Intakes for Vitamins

Age (years)	Vitamin A (mcg RAE)	Vitamin D (mcg)	Vitamin E (mg TE)	Vitamin K (mcg)	Vitamin C (mg)	Thiamin (mg)	Riboflavin (mg)	Niacin (mg NE)	Vitamin B6 (mg)	Folate (mcg)	Vitamin B12 (mcg)
Infants 0–0.5	400	10	4	2	40	0.2	0.3	2	0.1	65	0.4
Infants 0.6–1.0	500	10	5	2.5	50	0.3	0.4	4	0.3	80	0.5
Children 1–3	300	15	6	30	15	0.5	0.5	6	0.5	150	0.9
Children 4–8	400	15	7	55	25	0.6	0.6	8	0.6	200	1.2
Boys 9–13	600	15	11	60	45	0.9	0.9	12	1	300	1.8
Boys 14–18	900	15	15	75	75	1.2	1.3	16	1.3	400	2.4
Girls 9–13	600	15	11	60	45	0.9	0.9	12	1	300	1.8
Girls 14–18	700	15	15	75	65	1.0	1.0	14	1.2	400	2.4

NE, Niacin equivalent; *RAE*, retinal activity equivalent; *TE*, tocopherol equivalent.
From Food and Nutrition Board, Institute of Medicine: *Dietary Reference Intakes for calcium and vitamin D*, Washington, DC, 2011, National Academies Press; Food and Nutrition Board, Institute of Medicine: *Dietary Reference Intakes for thiamin, riboflavin, niacin, vitamin B₆, folate, vitamin B₁₂, pantothenic acid, biotin, and choline*, Washington, DC, 1998, National Academies Press; Food and Nutrition Board, Institute of Medicine: *Dietary Reference Intakes for vitamin C, vitamin E, selenium, and carotenoids*, Washington, DC, 2000, National Academies Press; Food and Nutrition Board, Institute of Medicine: *Dietary Reference Intakes for vitamin A, vitamin K, arsenic, boron, chromium, copper, iodine, iron, manganese, molybdenum, nickel, silicon, vanadium, and zinc*, Washington, DC, 2001, National Academies Press.

TABLE 12.4 Dietary Reference Intakes for Minerals

Age (years)	Calcium (mg)	Phosphorus (mg)	Magnesium (mg)	Iron (mg)	Zinc (mg)	Iodine (mcg)	Selenium (mcg)	Fluoride (mg)
Infants 0–0.5	200	100	30	0.27	2	110	5	0.01
Infants 0.6–1.0	200	275	75	11	3	130	20	0.5
Children 1–3	700	460	80	7	3	90	20	0.7
Children 4–8	1000	500	130	10	5	90	30	1.0
Boys 9–13	1300	1250	240	8	8	120	40	2.0
Boys 14–18	1300	1250	410	11	11	150	55	3.0
Girls 9–13	1300	1250	240	8	8	120	40	2.0
Girls 14–18	1300	1250	360	15	9	150	55	3.0

From Food and Nutrition Board, Institute of Medicine: *Dietary Reference Intakes for calcium and vitamin D*, Washington, DC, 2011, National Academies Press; Food and Nutrition Board, Institute of Medicine: *Dietary Reference Intakes for calcium, phosphorus, magnesium, vitamin D and fluoride*, Washington, DC, 1997, National Academies Press. Food and Nutrition Board, Institute of Medicine: *Dietary Reference Intakes for vitamin C, vitamin E, selenium, and carotenoids*, Washington, DC, 2000, National Academies Press; Food and Nutrition Board, Institute of Medicine: *Dietary Reference Intakes for vitamin A, vitamin K, arsenic, boron, chromium, copper, iodine, iron, manganese, molybdenum, nickel, silicon, vanadium, and zinc*, Washington, DC, 2001, National Academies Press.

STAGES OF GROWTH AND DEVELOPMENT: AGE-GROUP NEEDS

Psychosocial Development

The developmental tasks of choosing and consuming foods flow as an integral part of physical, motor, and psychosocial development. In this section, we discuss food and feeding practices at each stage of childhood and their relationship to normal physical and psychosocial maturation. Developing neuromuscular motor skills enable the child to accomplish related physical activities involved with food. Psychosocial development influences food attitudes, behavior, patterns, and habits.

Throughout the human life cycle, food and feeding not only supply nutrients for physical and motor growth but also play a role in personal and psychosocial development. The nutritional age-group needs of children cannot be understood apart from the child's overall maturation as a unique person. A leading American psychoanalyst, Erik Erikson,[7] has contributed to our understanding of human personality and growth throughout critical periods of development. Erikson identified eight stages in human growth and a basic psychosocial developmental problem with which the individual struggles at each stage.[7] The developmental problem at each stage has a positive ego value and a conflicting negative counterpart, as follows:

1. *Infancy:* trust versus distrust
2. *Toddler:* autonomy versus shame and doubt
3. *Preschooler:* initiative versus guilt
4. *School-age child:* industry versus inferiority
5. *Adolescent:* identity versus role confusion
6. *Young adult:* intimacy versus isolation
7. *Adult:* generativity versus stagnation
8. *Older adult:* ego integrity versus despair

Given favorable circumstances, a growing child develops positive ego strength at each life stage and builds increasing inner resources and strengths to meet the next life crisis. A residue of the negative remains, and in periods of stress, such as an illness, some regression is likely to occur. However, as the child gains mastery at each stage of development, assisted by significant positive and supportive relationships, integration of self-controls takes place. Changes that occur at each stage influence food intake and the interaction of the child with family members, peers, and counselors, as follows[8,9]:

- *Infant:* Infants require appropriate stimulation to thrive; they enjoy seeing different colors, engaging in verbal interactions, and being physically held. Activities such as holding objects, looking at pictures, or hearing nursery rhymes support motor and cognitive development. Their attention span is short, which can create problems at feeding time.
- *Toddler:* Toddlers grow rapidly and begin to demonstrate **autonomy**, with display of temper tantrums or other negative behaviors. They learn behaviors from their parents. They begin to develop language skills and can recall past experiences. Play is an important medium for self-expression and allows the child to express some control over his or her environment.
- *Preschooler:* The preschool years are a time for increasing social experiences, and children begin to interact more with other children. Preschoolers have an increased ability to express themselves and may try to exert control through demands for or refusal of certain foods.
- *School-age child:* The school-age child enters a formal learning environment, and attention span increases. These children are more selective in choosing friends, and peer influence becomes more obvious on food behaviors. As the environment becomes more structured, physical activity may decline, despite the need for play and further coordination of motor skills.
- *Adolescent:* Adolescents become more autonomous in their actions and attempt to exert independence from parental control. Teens perceive themselves to be invulnerable to illness or injury, and risk-taking behaviors involving drugs or alcohol may begin. Obsession with body image may result in inappropriate nutrition practices.

Various related developmental tasks surround each of these stages. These learnings, when accomplished, contribute to successful resolution of the core problem.

Infant (Birth to 1 Year)

Physical Characteristics of a Full-Term Infant

The full-term infant is born after successful growth and development during a normal gestation period of approximately 40 weeks (280 days). During the first year of life the infant generally triples in weight, growing rapidly from an average birth weight of about 3.5 kg (7.5 lb) to a 1-year-old child ready to walk and weighing about 10 kg (22 lb). Thus relative energy requirements during this first year of tremendous growth are high.

Full-term infants have the ability to digest and absorb protein, a moderate amount of fat, and simple carbohydrates. They have some difficulty with starch because amylase, the starch-splitting enzyme, is not produced at birth. However, as starch is introduced, this enzyme begins to function. The renal system functions well in infancy, but more water relative to body size is needed than in the adult to manage the **renal solute load** in urinary excretion. The first baby teeth do not erupt until approximately the fourth month or even much later; therefore food must initially be liquid and later semiliquid.

Nutrition for the Full-Term Infant

The first food for infants, breast milk or infant formula, generally provides all the nutrients required by a healthy infant for the first 6 months of life. Exclusive breast-feeding can, in fact, be adequate for the first 12 months of life (with the exception of iron and vitamin D); however, most mothers choose to supplement their infants' diets with complementary foods around the sixth and as early as the fourth month.[10] Nearly all infants born in a hospital receive an injection of vitamin K shortly after birth to ensure an adequate supply of this nutrient, and infants born at home must also receive supplemental vitamin K. It is recommended to provide vitamin D supplements to breast-fed infants because breast milk may not supply adequate vitamin D to prevent deficiency and the development of rickets.[11,12] This is especially critical in the case of African-American mothers, who demonstrate decreased endogenous synthesis of vitamin D, for mothers who wear special clothing for religious reasons that limits their skin exposure to the sun, or those living at northern latitudes (see the Focus on Culture box, "Nutritional Rickets: Role of Culture"). Overall, breast-feeding mothers should be well nourished to supply optimal levels of nutrients in their milk.[13]

KEY TERMS

Autonomy
The state of functioning independently, without extraneous influence.

Renal Solute Load
Collective number and concentration of solute particles in a solution carried by the blood to the kidney nephrons for excretion in the urine. The particles are usually nitrogenous products from protein metabolism and the electrolyte sodium.

🌐 FOCUS ON CULTURE

Nutritional Rickets: Role of Culture[a]

The eradication of nutritional rickets, or the vitamin D deficiency of childhood, is one of the greatest public health success stories in the United States. Fortification of cow's milk and supplementation of infant formula with vitamin D ensured the virtual disappearance of this nutritional disease by 1970. The understanding of the importance of sunlight exposure in initiating the conversion of inactive vitamin D to active vitamin D, in addition to adequate dietary intake, was monumental. Unfortunately, rickets is on the rise because of a variety of cultural and related behavioral factors.

Factors Linked to Rickets

Several studies describe causes of nutritional rickets. One study found vitamin D deficiency in the umbilical cord blood, which measures the amount of vitamin D passed on to the fetus, in 84% of African-American mothers compared with a deficiency among 22% of Caucasian mothers.[14] Another risk factor of infant vitamin D deficiency includes exclusive and prolonged breast-feeding. Prolonged breast-feeding beyond 6 months *without supplemental vitamin D* provided to the infant may result in low infant vitamin D levels, although recent research indicates that if maternal vitamin D stores of a breast-feeding woman are sufficient, she may pass on adequate amounts of vitamin D in her breast milk. Currently it is unknown how much vitamin D a mother requires to produce milk containing sufficient vitamin D.

Inadequate sunlight exposure, particularly of infants with darkly pigmented skin, is another potential cause of rickets. For example, several case studies and larger epidemiologic investigations have shown a significant prevalence of rickets in African-American infants, even those infants residing in climates with an abundance of sunlight. Other reports have documented rickets in infants required to be fully covered by clothing because of religious or cultural demands.

Rickets has also been documented in infants of lactating mothers who consume vegan diets. Children who are raised on vegan diets or macrobiotic diets may also have vitamin D–deficiency disorders. These diets may be practiced to support cultural, religious, or health beliefs.

Prevention and Treatment of Rickets

Rickets can be easily prevented, but health care practitioners must be able to recognize the clinical signs and symptoms of rickets once developed (see Chapter 6). Dietary intake assessment, along with biochemical and clinical indicators, can be used to evaluate nutritional deficiency diseases. Screening for special diets, infant-feeding method and duration, supplementation, and behaviors related to sunlight exposure of mother and child is necessary. Vitamin D supplementation of the mother, the child, or both is typically decided on a case-by-case basis. Increased sunlight exposure is another avenue to increasing vitamin D concentration in the blood. Culturally sensitive counseling is required for prevention and treatment of nutritional rickets. Targeted public health and community interventions may also help to diminish rickets once again.

Bibliography

Cadario F, Savastio S, Pozzi E, et al: Vitamin D status in cord blood and newborns: ethnic differences, *Ital J Pediatr* 39:35, 2013.

Eldjerou LK, Cogle CR, Rosenau EH, et al: Vitamin D effect on umbilical cord blood characteristics: a comparison between African Americans and Causcasians, *Transfusion* 55(7):1766, 2015.

Halm BM, Lai JF, Pagano I, et al: Vitamin D deficiency in cord plasma from multiethnic subjects living in the tropics, *J Am Coll Nutr* 32(4):215, 2013.

Munns CF, Shaw N, Kiely M, et al: Global consensus recommendations on prevention and management of nutritional rickets, *Horm Res Paediatr* 85:83, 2016.

Sinha A, Cheetham TW, Pearce SH: Prevention and treatment of vitamin D deficiency, *Calcif Tissue Int* 92:207, 2013.

Thiele DK, Senti JL, Anderson CM: Maternal vitamin D supplementation to meet the needs of the breastfed infant: a systematic review, *J Hum Lact* 29(2):163, 2013.

[a]The author thanks Melissa K. Zack for her assistance in creating this box.

Psychosocial and Motor Development

The core psychosocial developmental task during infancy is the establishment of trust in others. Much of the infant's early psychosocial development is tactile in nature from touching and holding, especially with feeding. Feeding is the infant's primary means of establishing human relationships. The close mother-infant or caregiver-infant bonding in the feeding process fills the basic need to build trust. The need for sucking and the development of the oral organs—the lips and mouth—as sensory organs represent adaptations that ensure an adequate early food intake for survival. As a result, food becomes the infant's general means of exploring the environment and is one of the early means of communication. The infant has an additional "nonnutritive" sucking need that is satisfied, especially with the extra effort required in sucking while breast-feeding. As muscular coordination involving the tongue and the swallowing reflex develops, infants gradually learn to eat a variety of semisolid foods, between 4 to 6 months of age. As physical and motor maturation proceed, infants begin to show a desire for self-feeding. When these stages of development occur, the exploration of new motor skills and autonomy should be encouraged. If their needs for food and love are fulfilled in this early relationship with the mother, father, other caregivers, and family members, then trust is developed.

Breast-Feeding

The ideal food for the human infant is human milk.[15] It has specific characteristics that match the infant's nutritional requirements during the first year of life. The process of breast-feeding can be successfully initiated and maintained by most mothers who try. In providing support for mothers who want to breast-feed their babies, experienced nutritionists and nurses, many of whom are certified professional lactation consultants, advise flexibility rather than a rigid approach (see Further Readings and Resources at the end of this chapter). The World Health Organization (WHO) and the United Nations Children's Fund created the Baby-Friendly Hospital Initiative (BFHI)[16,17]; this program has increased the breast-feeding initiation rate of mothers in participating hospitals.[18] Box 12.1 lists the actions that hospitals must carry out to earn BFHI status. Many hospitals use lactation consultants to oversee compliance with the actions and to promote breast-feeding practices that are optimal, yet realistic, for mother and infant.

The mother's breasts, or mammary glands, are highly specialized secretory organs, as indicated in Chapter 11 and illustrated in Fig. 11.5. They are composed of glandular tissue, fat, and connective tissue. The secreting glandular tissue has 15 to 24 lobes, each containing many smaller units called *lobules*. In the lobules, secretory cells called *alveoli* form milk from the nutrient material supplied to them via a rich capillary system. During pregnancy the breasts are prepared for lactation. The alveoli enlarge and multiply, and toward the end of the prenatal period they secrete a thin, yellowish fluid called colostrum, which contains important antibodies and proteins. Hormonal components in breast milk also enhance the maturation of the gastrointestinal (GI) tract. Typically by the end of the first week, mature milk is produced;

BOX 12.1 Prioritizing Breast-Feeding: The Baby-Friendly Hospital Initiative

Actions to Earning Baby-Friendly Hospital Initiative Status
- Write and implement a breast-feeding policy.
- Train health care personnel to support the policy.
- Tell pregnant women how to breast-feed and about its benefits.
- Assist mothers with breast-feeding their newborns in the first 30 minutes after delivery.
- Demonstrate to mothers how to breast-feed and express breast milk.
- Provide only breast milk to infants, unless contraindicated.
- Allow infant to be with mother at all times.
- Educate mothers about on-demand feeding.
- Avoid use of pacifiers or other synthetic nipples.
- Educate mothers about breast-feeding issues and finding support after leaving the hospital.

as the infant grows, the breast milk develops, adapting in composition to meet growth needs.

Breast milk is produced under the stimulating influence of the hormone prolactin from the anterior pituitary gland. After milk is formed, it is carried through converging branches of the lactiferous ducts to reservoir spaces called ampullae or the lactiferous sinus located under the areola, the pigmented area of skin surrounding the nipple. Another pituitary hormone, oxytocin, stimulates the ejection of the milk from the alveoli to the ducts, commonly called the *let-down reflex*. It causes a tingling sensation in the breast and begins the flow of milk. The initial sucking of the baby stimulates this reflex. The newborn rooting reflex, oral need for sucking, and basic hunger drive usually induce and maintain breast-feeding by the healthy mother.

KEY TERMS

Tactile
Pertaining to the touch.

Colostrum
Thin yellow fluid first secreted by the mammary gland a few days before and after childbirth, preceding the mature breast milk. It contains up to 20% protein, including a large amount of lactalbumin, more minerals, and less lactose and fat than in mature milk, and immunoglobulins representing the antibodies found in maternal blood.

Lactiferous Ducts
Branching channels in the mammary gland that carry breast milk to holding spaces near the nipple ready for the infant's feeding.

Ampullae
A general term for a flasklike wider portion of a tubular structure; spaces under the nipple of the breast for storing milk.

Areola
A defined space; a circular area of different color surrounding a central point, such as the darkened pigmented ring surrounding the nipple of the breast.

Rooting Reflex
A reflex in a newborn in which stimulation of the side of the cheek or the upper or lower lip causes the infant to turn its mouth and face to the stimulus.

The mother should follow the baby's lead with an on-demand schedule. The baby's continuing rhythm of need establishes feedings, usually approximately every 2 to 3 hours in the first few weeks after birth.[19,20] The newborn's rooting reflex and somewhat recessed lower jaw are natural adaptations for breastfeeding. The mother should feed from one breast until emptied, and then can switch to the other side. When the baby is satisfied, he or she can be released from the breast. The nipple should air dry to prevent irritation and soreness (see the Focus on Food Safety box, "Ensuring the Safety of Breast Milk and Infant Formula").

The mother's diet and rest are important factors in establishing lactation and breast-feeding. Figure 11.7 suggests a balanced diet to support ample milk production, including food choices from various food groups for meals and snacks (see Chapter 11). Natural thirst guides adequate fluid intake. An adequate energy intake is especially important in the early weeks to establish regular milk production. Rigorous dieting should not be undertaken by breast-feeding mothers.

Breast-feeding may influence feeding behavior and taste preferences into childhood.[21] Acceptance of a wide variety of tastes and preferences for foods may occur if the infant is breast-fed. Odorous compounds, found in foods and beverages, transfer into breast milk; such flavor exposure during breast-feeding often affects acceptance of same-flavored foods in childhood.[21] Studies suggest that breast-fed infants are less likely to become overweight as children compared with infants who are formula-fed.[22,23] Infants who develop a pattern of eating in moderation are less likely to become overweight, and breast-fed infants exhibit better self-regulation of intake than do formula-fed infants. Formula-fed infants may be urged to empty their bottle, even though they may turn away when they are satisfied. Force-feeding is

FOCUS ON FOOD SAFETY

Ensuring the Safety of Breast Milk and Infant Formula

Breast milk or formula can be a source of food-related illness in an infant if these fluids are not properly used and stored. All equipment used in the expression or pumping of breast milk, including pump components and containers, and in the preparation of formula, including scoops and containers, should be sterilized. Most equipment and bottle parts, including synthetic nipples, are dishwasher-safe and may be sterilized in this manner. Alternatively, such components may be sterilized in boiling water for 10 to 12 minutes.

Breast milk may stand at room temperature (77°F or less) for up to 6 hours. Breast milk may be stored for no more than 5 days in a 32°F to 39°F refrigerator or in a self-defrosting freezer for up to 6 months. If not used within these time frames, then breast milk should be discarded. Some lactation consultants use the "5/5/5 rule" for breast milk handling: Use breast milk that has been at room temperature within 5 hours, store breast milk in the refrigerator for no more than 5 days, and maintain breast milk in a freezer for no more than 5 months.

Mixed or reconstituted infant formula may be stored for up to 24 hours in a 32°F to 39°F refrigerator. Formula should not be left to stand at room temperature and cannot be frozen. If mixed formula has been in the refrigerator for more than 24 hours or left at room temperature, then it should be discarded.

Any bottle with unused content should be discarded within 2 hours of when the infant began feeding from the bottle. Additional substances, including honey, sugar, infant cereal, soft drinks, and alcohol, should never be added to a bottle containing breast milk or infant formula.

Data from Centers for Disease Control and Prevention: Proper handling and storage of human milk. https://www.cdc.gov/breastfeeding/recommendations/handling_breastmilk.htm.

less likely to occur in the breast-fed infant but should be avoided in all infants. Feeding should be discontinued at the first sign that the infant has had enough. Children who gain weight more rapidly during the first 4 months of life are more likely to be overweight by middle childhood.

Considerable research suggests that breast-feeding promotes a healthy gut microbiota.[24-26] This genome of microorganisms inhabiting the GI tract known as the gut microbiome plays a role in short- and long-term health promotion and disease prevention. Breast-feeding appears to cultivate health-promoting gut bacteria and may serve to support the maturation of an infant's gut-associated immune system, thereby preventing diarrhea, necrotizing enterocolitis, and even allergies, GI disorders, obesity, and diabetes.[25-27] Breast milk contains oligosaccharides, antimicrobial agents, and immunoglobulins, along with antiinflammatory factors and, of course, nutrients. Breast milk has also been shown to contain certain bacteria that are beneficial to the gut microbiome.[24-27] When possible, infants should be breast-fed.

Bottle-Feeding

Formula feeding may be preferred by some mothers for a variety of reasons. If the mother does not choose to breast-feed or stops breast-feeding before her infant reaches the age of 1 year, then bottle-feeding of an appropriate formula is an acceptable alternative. A variety of commercial formulas that attempt to approximate the composition of human milk are available. Some cow's milk–based formulas are adjusted with whey protein to more nearly approximate the protein ratio in human milk.

A topic of current interest is the nutritional benefit of substantial amounts of the long-chain fatty acids arachidonic acid (ARA) and docosahexaenoic acid (DHA) provided in breast milk. These fatty acids appear to play a special role in cognitive and retinal development and may also be protective against allergic disease risk.[29] Based on the presence of ARA and DHA in human breast milk and the normal metabolic conversion of linoleic acid to ARA and α-linolenic acid to DHA (along with evidence linking ARA and DHA to visual acuity and cognitive development), the US Food and Drug Administration (FDA) approved the addition of these long-chain polyunsaturated fatty acids to infant formula. Because maternal dietary intake of these fatty acids is reflected in breast milk, nursing mothers should be educated on how to consume adequate amounts to support healthy development in their infants. Fatty fish is an excellent source of DHA, and adequate ARA is found in meat, eggs, and dairy foods.

Special formulas have been developed for infants with allergies, lactose intolerance, GI disorders, fat malabsorption, prematurity, or other problems,[30] and several types of constituent proteins and carbohydrates are used. These special formulas include cow's milk protein, soy protein, casein hydrolysate, and elemental formulas (Table 12.5).

TABLE 12.5 Comparison of Types of Formulas Manufactured for Preterm and Full-Term Infants

Class	Brand Names	Calories (kcal/oz)	Carbohydrate Source	Protein Source	Indications
Breast milk		20	Lactose	Human milk	Preferred for all infants
Term formula	Carnation Good Start Enfamil with Iron Similac with Iron	20	Lactose	Cow's milk	Appropriate for most infants
Term formula with DHA & AA	Enfamil Lipil Good Start DHA & ARA Similac Advance	20	Lactose	Cow's milk	Marketed to promote eye and brain development
Preterm formula	Enfamil 24 Premature Preemie SMA 24 Similac 24 Special Care	24	Lactose	Cow's milk	Less than 34 weeks' gestation; weight less than 1800 g
Enriched formula	Enfacare Similac Neosure	22	Lactose	Cow's milk	34–36 weeks' gestation; weight 1800 g or more
Soy formula	Enfamil Prosobee Good Start Soy Similac Isomil	20	Corn based	Soy	Congenital lactase deficiency, galactosemia
Lactose-free formula	Enfamil Lactofree Similac Sensitive	20	Corn based	Cow's milk	Congenital lactase deficiency, primary lactase deficiency, galactosemia, gastroenteritis in at-risk infants
Hypoallergenic formula	Similac Alimentum Enfamil Nutramigen Enfamil Pregestimil	20	Corn or sucrose	Extensively hydrolyzed	Milk protein allergy
Nonallergenic formula	Elecare Neocate Nutramigen AA	20	Corn or sucrose	Amino acids	Milk protein allergy
Antireflux formula	Enfamil AR Similac Sensitive RS	20	Lactose, thickened with rice starch	Cow's milk	Gastroesophageal reflux
Toddler formula	Enfamil Next Step Good Start 2 Similac Go and Grow	20	Lactose	Milk	9–24 months age

AA/AR/ARA, Arachidonic acid; *DHA,* docosahexaenoic acid.

KEY TERMS

Casein Hydrolysate Formulas
Infant formulas composed of hydrolyzed casein, a major milk protein, produced by partially breaking down the casein into smaller peptide fragments, making a product that is more easily digested.

Elemental Formulas
Nutrition support formulas composed of single elemental nutrient components that require no further digestive breakdown and thus are readily absorbed. Infant formula produced with elemental, ready-to-be-absorbed components of free amino acids and carbohydrate as simple sugars.

Hypoallergenic formulas have been developed for infants who are allergic to cow's milk or commercial formulas based on cow's milk and have existing allergy symptoms.[30] Even partially hydrolyzed proteins can provoke an allergic response in infants with hypersensitivity to cow's milk. In the preparation of hypoallergenic formulas, all proteins are completely hydrolyzed to free amino acids. Although some infants allergic to cow's milk tolerate soy formulas, they are not hypoallergenic.

It is estimated that in the United States, approximately 12% of infants are given a soy protein–based formula, typically related to parental preference.[31] Initially, soy protein–based formula was used primarily to feed infants who could not tolerate the protein from cow's milk or the lactose found in standard formulas. However, the use of soy protein–based formulas has been increasing among parents who wish to feed their infants vegetarian diets. In addition, soy protein–based formulas have been used in the management of babies with acute diarrhea. Some controversy surrounds the use of soy protein–based infant formula because of the estrogen-like effects of soy, and the American Academy of Pediatrics recommends the use of soy protein–based infant formula only for infants with galactosemia and lactase deficiency or for infants of caregivers who prefer a vegetarian eating pattern[32] (see the Evidence-Based Practice box, "Food Allergies in Children"). Soy protein–based formula is not recommended as a means of preventing food intolerances or allergies.[33] In the case of a diagnosed cow's milk allergy, a protein hydrolysate formula should be provided to the infant.[34]

Infant formulas are formulated to mimic the nutritional composition of breast milk as closely as possible (although exact replication is simply not possible), and formula ingredients are highly regulated by the FDA.[35]

When feeding formula, the baby should be cradled in the arm as in breast-feeding, keeping the baby's head upright as much as possible to avoid milk running into the ear canals and causing an ear infection. Close human touch and warmth are important. When the infant is obviously satisfied, extra milk should not be forced, regardless of the amount remaining in the bottle. Any remaining formula should be thrown away and not refrigerated for reuse (see the Focus on Food Safety box, "Ensuring the Safety of Breast Milk and Infant Formula"). Infants usually take the amount of formula they need. Most infants are fed on demand versus scheduled, which works out to be approximately every 2 to 3 hours.

Breast-Feeding and Formula-Feeding Combination
Some women desire the flexibility of both breast-feeding and formula-feeding their infants. For example, a mother working outside of the home may choose to breast-feed her infant in the morning before work and in the evening after work and use formula during the day. This combination is possible but is recommended only after an adequate supply of breast milk and infant-feeding pattern have been established. Factors to consider include infant's acceptance of a synthetic nipple and formula's taste, mother's ability or need to express breast milk during the day, and growth of the infant.

EVIDENCE-BASED PRACTICE

Food Allergies in Children

A food allergy is an adverse reaction to a food or food component, brought on by the body's immune system. Foods that most commonly trigger an allergic and immune-based response in children include cow's milk, eggs, wheat, soy, fish, shellfish, peanuts, and tree nuts. Other foods, such as strawberries, may result in an allergic reaction. Signs and symptoms of a food allergy include itching in the mouth, swelling in the oral cavity, tightening of the throat, difficulty breathing, abdominal pain and cramping, vomiting, diarrhea, hives, rashes, and hypotension. In extreme cases, anaphylactic shock may occur. Many children or parents of children may report food intolerances or negative reactions to foods or food components, not triggered by the body's immune system. In these cases, understanding the food-related response is important to determining the severity of the reaction, the origin of the response, and the appropriate course of treatment. All suspected allergic responses as well as intolerances should be addressed with a physician and dietitian. These families should be educated on how to ensure adequate nutrient intake when culprit foods are eliminated from the child's diet.

Given the rise in prevalence of food allergies, many parents want to know what can be done to prevent these diseases. Research supports that exclusive breast-feeding may be protective due to the anti-allergic immune properties and the presence of antibodies found in human milk. In addition, although delayed introduction of common food allergens was previously promoted, recent research indicates there is no additional benefit of the delayed introduction of complementary foods beyond 4 to 6 months of age. In fact, there is mounting evidence that early introduction of common food allergens such as peanuts may actually be protective against allergy development. Further research will provide more specific recommendations.

Questions for Analysis
1. What evidence is needed to distinguish a food allergy from a food intolerance?
2. What is the appropriate course of action for a child who has a suspected food allergy?

Bibliography
Anvari S, Chokshi NY, Kamili QU, et al: Evolution of guidelines on peanut allergy and peanut introduction in infants: a review, *JAMA Pediatr* 171(1):77, 2017.

Du Toit G, Foong RX, Lack G: Prevention of food allergy—early dietary interventions, *Allergol Int* 66(1):159, 2017.

Fleischer DM, Spergel JM, Assa'ad AH, et al: Primary prevention of allergic disease through nutritional interventions, *J Allergy Clin Immunol Pract* 1(1):29, 2013.

Kobernick AK, Burks AW: Active treatment for food allergy, *Allergol Int* 65(4):388, 2016.

Vandenplas Y, De Greef E, Devreker T: Treatment of cow's milk protein allergy, *Pediatr Gastroenterol Hepatol Nutr* 17(1):1, 2014.

Cow's Milk

Regular unmodified cow's milk is not suitable for infants for several reasons, as follows:

- It causes GI bleeding.
- Its renal solute load is too concentrated for the infant's renal system to handle; this leaves too small a margin of safety for maintaining water balance, especially during illness, diarrhea, or hot weather.
- It adversely affects nutrition status.[35] Cow's milk is low in iron, and iron status in the infant is lowered even further by the associated GI bleeding and blood loss caused by the cow's milk. In addition, cow's milk is a poor source of vitamins C and E and essential fatty acids.

To meet the special needs of infants, the American Academy of Pediatrics recommends breast milk or formula as the major food source up to 1 year of age, with a gradual addition of appropriate foods beginning at 4 to 6 months.[20] No need exists for special formulas for older infants; such formulas also present an added expense to the family.

Premature or Small-for-Gestational-Age Infants

Infants born too early or too small have many food-related difficulties to overcome and present a special challenge in feeding. A poor sucking reflex, difficulty in swallowing, small gastric capacity, reduced intestinal motility, tiring easily from eating and being handled, and increased nutrient requirements for catch-up growth all need to be considered. The health team involved in the care of premature or small-for-gestational-age infants is faced with a myriad of decisions to overcome these feeding difficulties. Whenever possible, these infants should be fed breast milk, which may be fortified with additional protein, vitamins, and minerals to the levels found in special formulas developed to meet their particular needs depending upon the degree of prematurity. Delivery of breast milk or formula using tube feeding (enteral feeding) carries less risk of complications than the delivery of nutrients through the veins (parenteral feeding).

A comparison of the nutrient content of breast milk and special formulas for the premature infant is presented in Table 12.5. Formulas developed for the premature infant may have more energy and protein per fluid volume than those developed for the normal infant, as well as increased amounts of calcium, zinc, and the B-complex vitamins. This enriched formula also supports catch-up growth in term infants who are small for their gestational age.[36] Nutrition support of the high-risk infant requires a team approach that includes the pediatrician, nurse, dietitian, and a lactation consultant who can assist the mother and family in developing a routine for expressing and safely storing her breast milk to feed her infant.

Solid Food Additions

Addition of solid food begins the transition from a predominantly liquid diet to a predominantly solid food diet. Nutritional and medical authorities agree that for the first 6 months of life the optimal single food for the infant is human breast milk or an appropriate formula. No nutritional basis exists for introducing solid foods to an infant earlier than 6 months of age; before this age, it may contribute to overfeeding. Until then, the infant does not need any additional food and is not able to adequately handle other foods. In addition to nutritional reasons, developmental reasons exist for delaying the addition of solid foods until the age of 6 months. The following developmental tasks must be mastered before the infant is prepared to receive solid foods:

- The infant can communicate desire and interest in food by opening his or her mouth and leaning forward or, conversely, leaning back or turning away, participating in the feeding process.
- The infant can sit up with support and has good control of the trunk and neck.
- The infant has developed the ability to move food to the back of the mouth for swallowing.

BOX 12.2   Developmental Milestones Associated with Feeding Skills and Practices at Approximate Ages in Infancy[a]

- Suckling, sucking, swallowing—breast milk or infant formula (birth to 6–7 months)
- Controlled head and tongue movements, independent sitting stability, tooth eruption, controlled palmar and pincer grasps, crawling, early verbalization—breast milk or infant formula; infant cereal (iron fortified); pureed fruits, vegetables, and meats (7–9 months)
- Controlled chewing and grasping, additional tooth eruption, use of spoon and "sippy cup"—breast milk or infant formula; infant cereal (iron fortified); well-cooked, smooth, and softly textured vegetables; mashed or sliced fruits; infant crackers (9–10 months)
- Standing and sitting alone, verbalization, controlled gross motor skills, early walking—breast milk or infant formula, infant cereal (iron fortified), bite-sized foods, smooth and textured foods, some "table" foods (10–12 months)

[a]Never introduce honey or cow's milk during infancy; avoid foods and food sizes that present a choking hazard; always have adult supervision of an infant during feeding.

Developmental abilities to use the hands and fingers are required before self-feeding can be initiated. Self-feeding efforts begin first with a whole hand (palmar) grasp and then move to a more refined finger (pincer) grasp by the end of the first year. The first item for self-feeding may be a piece of Melba toast that can be grasped with the whole hand. As solid food is gradually added, the amount of breast milk or formula consumed is reduced accordingly. Box 12.2 lists the developmental milestones that correspond to feeding skills and practices.

Both cultural patterns and the age and educational level of the mother influence infant-feeding practices. Some of these practices, such as adding cereal to the infant's bottle to help the baby sleep through the night, are related more to the convenience of the mother than to the benefit of the infant. Cereal displaces formula when added to the bottle, and the infant might not be able to sleep through the night at an early age. Smaller amounts of food, eaten on

---

KEY TERMS

Small-for-gestational-age
Describes an infant with a weight below the 10th percentile for gestational age.

Palmar Grasp
Early grasp of the young infant, clasping an object in the palm and wrapping the whole hand around it.

Pincer Grasp
Later digital grasp of the older infant; usually picking up smaller objects with a precise grip between thumb and forefinger.

Suckling
Drawing milk from the breast.

Sucking
Drawing liquid into the mouth by suction produced from movements of the oral cavity, tongue, and lips.

a more frequent basis, may contribute to the pattern of eating in moderation.

The traditional transition food is fortified infant cereal—specifically, infant rice cereal mixed with a little milk or formula—because rice cereal has the least potential for allergic reaction. Vegetables, fruits, potato, egg, and meat can be added to the diet in a gradual sequence. No one sequence of food additions must be followed (a general guide is provided in Table 12.6). Single foods are given first, one at a time in small amounts, approximately 5 to 7 days apart, allowing for adverse reactions to be identified. These foods are usually offered before the milk feeding, although it is helpful to ensure the infant is not overly hungry to avoid a fussy baby heading into a new food situation. Individual responses and needs can be a basis for choice. A basic goal during this time is to develop trust between the child and caregiver while having the infant learn to enjoy many different foods. This is the perfect time to introduce a

wide variety of foods because infants appear to be more willing to taste new foods than are toddlers; in fact, the greater the variety of foods presented during this period, the greater the number of foods the infant will accept when they are first presented.[37] This increased acceptance for a wider variety of foods and flavors seems to last for approximately 6 years and supports the benefits of exposures to various flavors early in life.[37]

Many commercial baby foods are now prepared without the addition of sugar, salt, or monosodium glutamate (MSG). Some mothers prefer preparing their own baby food. This can be done by cooking and straining vegetables and fruits and forming a puree using a blender, food processor, or Foley mill. These foods can be frozen in ice cube trays or in 1-tbsp amounts on a cookie sheet. The cubes or individual portions are easily stored in plastic bags in the freezer; then a single portion can be reheated conveniently for use at a feeding. When working with mothers, it is important to stress the need for a clean environment when preparing infant foods to avoid the danger of foodborne illness.

Two foods that require special attention in infant feeding are honey and fruit juices. Honey should never be given to an infant who is younger than 1 year, because it can lead to botulism, a fatal condition in infants. Some fruit juices, including apple, pear, and prune, contain sorbitol, which can lead to diarrhea in infants and toddlers. If given, fruit juice should be limited to no more than 4 oz per day.

Summary Principles

The following two principles should guide the feeding process:
1. Nutrients are needed, not specific foods.
2. Food is a main basis of early learning.

Food not only provides physical sustenance but also fulfills other personal development and cultural needs. Good food habits are formed early in life and continue to develop as a child grows older. By the time infants are approximately 9 or 10 months old, they should be able to eat many family foods that are cooked, chopped, or mashed and simply seasoned, without the need for special infant foods. Throughout the first year of life, the infant's needs for physical growth and psychosocial development will be met by breast milk or formula and a variety of solid food additions, as well as a loving and trusting relationship between parents and child (Fig. 12.1).

TABLE 12.6 **Guideline for Adding Solid Foods to Infant's Diet During the First Year**[a]		
When to Start	**Foods Added**	**Feeding**
Months 6–8	Infant cereal	10 a.m. and 6 p.m.
	Pureed baby foods such as cooked vegetable or fruit; scrambled eggs; potatoes/ sweet potatoes	2 p.m.
	Hard toast that easily dissolves	At any feeding
Suggested Meal Plan for 8 Months to 1 year or Older		
Breakfast	¼–½ cup cereal or mashed egg; ¼–½ cup fruit, diced or pureed; 4–6 oz breast milk/formula	
Snack	4–6 oz breast milk/formula; ¼ cup diced cheese or cooked vegetables	
Lunch	¼–½ cup yogurt or cottage cheese or meat; ¼–½ cup yellow or orange vegetables; 4–6 oz breast milk/formula	
Snack	4–6 oz breast milk/formula; ¼ cup yogurt or diced or pureed fruit	
Dinner	¼ cup diced poultry, meat, or tofu; ¼–½ cup green vegetables; ¼ cup noodles, pasta, rice, or potato; ¼ cup fruit; 4–6 oz breast milk/formula	
Before bed	6–8 oz breast milk/formula or water	

[a]Semisolid foods should be given immediately before milk feeding. One or 2 tsp should be given first. If food is accepted and tolerated well, then the amount should be increased to 1 to 2 tbsp per feeding. Never introduce honey or cow's milk during infancy; avoid foods and food sizes that present a choking hazard; always have adult supervision of an infant during feeding.

Note: Banana or cottage cheese may be used as substitution for any meal.

Healthychildren.org from the American Academy of Pediatrics. https:// www.healthychildren.org/English/ages-stages/baby/feeding-nutrition/ Pages/Sample-One-Day-Menu-for-an-8-to-12-Month-Old.aspx.

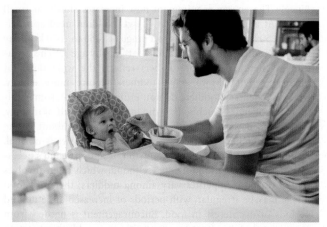

FIG. 12.1 This child is taking a variety of solid food additions and developing wide tastes. Here, feeding serves as a source not only of physical growth but also of psychosocial development. Optimal physical development and security are evident, the result of sound nutrition and loving care. (Copyright Getty Images.)

Toddler (1 to 3 Years)
Physical Characteristics and Growth

After the rapid growth of the first year, the growth rate of children slows. However, although the rate of gain reduces, the pattern of growth produces significant physiological changes. The legs become longer, and the child begins losing "baby fat." Total body water decreases, with a greater amount of intracellular fluids. The young child begins to look and feel less like a baby and more like a child. Relative energy demands are lower because of the decelerated growth rate. However, important muscle development is taking place. In fact, muscle mass development accounts for about one half of the total weight gain during this period. As the child begins to walk and stand erect, more muscle is needed to support these movements. For example, larger muscles are needed in the back, buttocks, and thighs. The overall rate of skeletal growth slows, with increased deposits of mineral in existing bone rather than a lengthening of bones. The increased mineralization strengthens bones to support the increasing body weight. The child may have six to eight teeth at the beginning of the toddler period. By 3 years of age, the remaining deciduous teeth have erupted.

Psychosocial and Motor Development

The psychosocial development of the toddler is pronounced. The core developmental problem is the desire for autonomy. Each child has a profound increasing sense of self, of being a distinct and individual person apart from the parents, not just an extension of them. As physical mobility increases with increased gross and fine motor skill development, the sense of autonomy and independence grows. An expanding curiosity leads to exploration of the environment, and increasingly the mouth is used as a means of exploring. Touch is important, providing the means of learning what objects are like. The constant use of the word "no" reflects the significant struggle between the newly emerging ego needs and the caregiver's control efforts. The child wants to do more and more, but the attention span is fairly short and interest shifts quickly from one thing to another.

Food and Feeding

Physical growth and psychosocial development during the toddler period influence nutrient needs (see Tables 12.2 to 12.4) and food patterns (see the Perspectives in Practice box, "Feeding Toddlers and Preschoolers: Eating Is a Family Affair"), as follows:

- *Energy:* The energy requirement now increases slowly in small spurts. At approximately 1 year of age, children need approximately 850 kcal/day; this rises to a range of 1160 to 1680 kcal/day for boys and 1080 to 1650 kcal/day for girls by age 3.[3] The variation in energy needs for toddlers reflects the wide range of physical activity. More active toddlers require more energy, whereas sedentary toddlers do not. From ages 1 to 2, some children do not eat as much as they did in the second half of infancy. Caregivers may avoid conflict with their toddler about eating if they remember this decrease in need for kcalories is normal, resulting from a slowing in the growth rate and the child's necessary struggle for autonomy and selfhood, which often involves refusal of food. Appetites vary among toddlers; therefore food intake may be irregular, with periods of increased appetite and periods of disinterest in food. Encouragement is needed from caregivers, but constant conflict with the child about eating is futile. A small plate of snacks, including finger-food pieces of raw fruit and cheese kept in the refrigerator or a few crackers on a special colorful plate, can give the child a measure of positive control when hungry. Toddlers will eat when they are hungry.

Positive early experiences help develop appropriate food acceptance patterns.[37]

- *Protein:* In relation to energy needs, protein needs are relatively increased during this stage of life. The toddler requires approximately 13 g of protein per day.[3] Muscle and other body tissues are growing rapidly. Inclusion of animal-based protein foods provides protein with high biologic value. However, toddlers following a balanced and well-planned ovolactovegetarian diet grow just as well and achieve similar growth as their nonvegetarian counterparts.[38] Diets planned for vegan children will need to incorporate soy and legume protein and build on the complementarity of plant proteins (see Chapter 5).

- *Minerals:* Calcium and phosphorus are needed for bone mineralization. The bones are strengthening to keep pace with muscle development and increasing activity. Iron is needed to maintain adequate hemoglobin levels because the increase in body size requires an increasing blood volume. Adequate levels of zinc are necessary to support protein synthesis and cell division. The principle of increasing iron absorption from nonheme sources such as vegetables by including a small amount of heme iron from meat at the same meal, or through inclusion of citric acid–containing foods, (as discussed in Chapter 7) holds true for feeding the toddler.

- *Vitamins:* Fat-soluble and water-soluble vitamins are critical to macronutrient use and growth and development. A variety of foods consumed in proportion to energy needs should provide adequate vitamins to the toddler.

- *Fiber:* As a larger portion of the diet of toddlers comes from solid foods, constipation becomes more prevalent. Adequate fiber of 19 g/day is recommended for children ages 1 to 3 years.[3]

- *Food choices:* Approximately 2 to 3 cups of milk daily is sufficient for the young child's needs. Sometimes, excessive milk intake, a habit carried over from infancy, excludes many solid foods from the diet. As a result, the child may lack iron and develop a so-called milk anemia. Conversely, if a child dislikes milk as a beverage, replacement can be made with cheese, creamed soups, puddings, or milk powder can be used in cooked cereals, mashed potatoes, meat loaf, and casseroles. Calcium-fortified foods can assist in adding calcium to the diet. Offering the child an increasing variety of foods will help develop good food habits; food habits are learned, and little opportunity exists for learning if a child is not exposed to a wide variety of foods. Refined sweets are best avoided, reserving them for special occasions, not for habitual use or to bribe a child to eat.

Summary Principles

The following two important principles should be emphasized when working with caregivers to guide feeding practices during this period:

1. The child needs fewer kcalories but relatively more protein and minerals for physical growth; therefore a variety of foods should be offered in appropriate portion sizes to provide key nutrients. It is important that day care providers and parents work cooperatively to support the development of good food patterns.
2. The child is struggling for selfhood as part of normal psychosocial development. This struggle is expressed in refusing food and the desire to do things for self before being fully able to do them efficiently. If caregivers are patient, offer a variety of foods in small amounts, and encourage some degree of food choice and self-feeding in the child's own ceremonial manner, then eating can be a happy, positive means of development.

If we are to achieve the goal of establishing good food patterns for life, it is especially important to introduce a variety of fruits and vegetables along with grains and meats during this stage of development (Fig. 12.2). One study following nearly 300 children from infancy to

Feeding Toddlers and Preschoolers: Eating Is a Family Affair

Regardless of their ages, children need the same nutrients as adults but in different amounts. The challenge for parents and caregivers is to make available appropriate and appealing foods and to set the time and place for eating. Young children must learn how to make food choices and to decide how much food they consume. We can support parents and caregivers in developing child-feeding strategies based on the developmental needs of their young children. Parents can be reminded that their children are not growing as fast as they did during the first year of life; it follows that they need less food. In addition, a child's energy needs are sporadic; therefore periods of increased food intake will vary with periods of smaller intake. Forcing food during periods of low intake may encourage overeating or food aversion, which can lead to food intake problems later in life.

Amount of Food

Children are not ready for adult-sized portions and may be overwhelmed by large amounts of food on their plate. It is better to serve less food that children are likely to eat and have them ask for more. In planning portion sizes, a good rule of thumb is 1 tbsp of each food for every year of age. When the child begins to play with the food on the plate or seems less interested in eating, remove the plate and provide another activity.

Feeding Frequency

Children do best with a regular feeding schedule; try to keep meals and snacks at regular times. Young children have small stomachs, and it is difficult for them to consume adequate food at one meal to last them until the next meal. They may need to eat 5 or 6 times a day. Try to allow at least 1½ to 2 hours between snacks and meals. When selecting snacks, look for foods that will provide not only additional kcalories but also protein and important vitamins and minerals. Fruit, crackers, raw vegetables (as appropriate), cheese, milk, and cereal are good snacks. It is best if children are not overtired at mealtime; if possible, plan a short rest period immediately before a meal.

What Foods

Over time, it is important for young child to learn to eat a variety of foods. It may be necessary to offer a new food 8 to 10 times, each including at least a taste, before it will be accepted. The child should learn to eat what other family members are eating and not be provided with special foods. However, when planning meals, be sure to have one item that the child likes and will eat. In addition, children are more willing to try a new food if it is accompanied by a favorite food; try to pair such foods at the same meal. Serve dessert, if any, with the main meal rather than later; it should not assume special importance in relation to other foods. Allow your toddler or preschooler to make some choices about foods for meals or snacks, just as older children are able to do. This develops skills in making food choices.

Avoid Forbidding Certain Foods

All foods, including sweets, can be included in a healthy diet for young children if limited in frequency and amount. It is important that children learn how to moderate their intakes of such foods. Excluding certain foods makes them more attractive and may ultimately lead to increased intake when they do become available.

Food Safety

Two major safety considerations in feeding children are avoidance of foodborne illness and the possibility of choking. Young children are very vulnerable to foodborne illness resulting from (1) foods that are not fully cooked, such as hamburger or eggs; (2) foods contaminated by contact with an unwholesome food or other source of bacteria; or (3) improperly stored food with bacterial growth. Eating such foods can lead to serious illness or even death in the young child. Children must be taught at a young age to wash their hands thoroughly after they use the bathroom and before they touch food. Parents should ask about food-handling and other sanitary practices when evaluating the suitability of a caregiver or a care facility.

Children younger than 4 years of age are at greatest risk for choking and death by **asphyxiation**. Foods most likely to cause choking are those that are round and hard and do not dissolve in saliva. Typical items that cause choking are hot dogs, grapes, peanut butter in globs, hard pieces of raw fruits and vegetables, hard candy, or popcorn. Risk of **aspiration** may increase with small grains, such as rice. Young children should always be supervised when eating and should eat sitting down. Running when eating can lead to choking. It is best that children not eat in a moving car unless a second adult, in addition to the driver, is available to assist if needed.

Social Environment at Meal Time

Try to keep mealtime as pleasant as possible. Allow enough time for the young child to eat. Having to hurry adds stress to mealtime and takes away the pleasure of eating, especially for the child who is still learning to self-feed. Be patient about spills or accidents; it takes time to develop feeding skills. Choose appropriate utensils that are unbreakable and easy for the child to grasp. Children are less likely to accept a food that was first introduced in a negative meal situation; therefore make mealtime an enjoyable family time that reinforces positive eating behaviors. Parental modeling is an important influence in encouraging children to try new foods. Toddlers are more likely to taste a new food if they see an adult, especially a familiar adult or parent, eating it. Children model the food choices of parents and caregivers; be sure that others at the table are eating vegetables and drinking milk. Parental modeling is as important in the choice of snacks as it is at mealtime.

Bibliography

Cutler GJ, Flood A, Hannan P, et al: Multiple sociodemographic and socioenvironmental characteristics are correlated with major patterns of dietary intake in adolescents, *J Am Diet Assoc* 111(2):230, 2011.

Kerzner B, Milano K, Maclean WC, et al: A practical approach to classifying and managing feeding difficulties, *Pediatrics* 135(2):344, 2015.

Kleinman RE, Greer FR, editors: *Pediatric nutrition*, ed 7, Elk Grove Village, IL, 2013, American Academy of Pediatrics.

Satter E: *Secrets of feeding a healthy family: how to eat, how to raise food eaters, how to cook*, ed 2, Madison, WI, 2008, Kelcy Press.

Rodenburg G, Kremers SP, Oenema A, et al: Associations of children's appetitive traits with weight and dietary behaviours in the context of general parenting, *PLoS One* 7(12):e50642, 2012.

Scaglioni S, Arrizza C, Vecchi F, et al: Determinants of children's eating behaviors, *Am J Clin Nutr* 94(Suppl 6):S2006, 2011.

age 7 found that at age 2½, children liked eight different vegetables and three fruits; however, by age 7, children ate only half the recommended servings of fruits and vegetables (2½ servings). Importantly, an early liking of fruits and vegetables predicted later intake of these foods.[39] This speaks to the importance of early introduction and exposure to fruits and vegetables to support continued intake later in childhood.

Preschooler (3 to 6 Years)

Physical Characteristics and Growth

As shown in normal childhood growth charts (see the CDC website for *CDC Growth Charts: United* States available at the end of the chapter in Further Readings and Resources), each child tends to settle into a regular genetic **growth channel** as physical growth continues in spurts.

FIG. 12.2 Fruits are an important part of the toddler's diet. (Copyright 2006 JupiterImages Corporation.)

KEY TERM

Asphyxiation
To become unconscious or dead due to an interruption in breathing caused by obstruction, such as food, noxious agent, or allergic reaction.

Aspiration
Taking in of foreign matter, such as food or fluid, into the lungs.

Growth Channel
The progressive regular growth pattern of children, guided along individual genetically controlled channels, influenced by nutritional and health status.

On occasion the child bounds with energy. Play is hard play—running, jumping, and testing new physical resources. At other times, the child will sit for increasing periods of time engrossed in passive types of activities. Mental capacities are developing, and more thinking and exploring of the environment occurs. Energy needs and specific nutrients are shown in Tables 12.2, 12.3, and 12.4. Protein requirements continue to increase as the child grows older. Preschool children need approximately 13 to 19 g/day of good-quality protein,[3] as found in milk, egg, meat, cheese, legumes, and soy. They continue to need calcium and iron to support growth and to build body stores. Because vitamins A and C and folate are often lacking in the diets of preschool children, a variety of fruits and vegetables should be provided. Vitamin D, important for calcium absorption, can be obtained in fortified milk or soy products or by spending time playing outdoors in the sun.

Psychosocial and Motor Development

Each stage of development builds on the previous one. The psychosocial developmental stage for preschool children involves increased socialization and initiative. They are beginning to develop their superego—the conscience. They also have a growing imagination and curiosity. This is a period of increasing imitation. Boys and girls may imitate adults and older siblings who serve as role models. Self-feeding skills increase, and eating takes on increased social aspects. The family mealtime is an important event for socialization, because children imitate their parents and others at the table.[40] Whom a child sees as a role model may have long-term implications in respect to nutrient intake and health. In one study of parental role modeling, parents who served fruits and vegetables as snacks were 5 times more likely to have children meeting the fruit and vegetable intake guidelines.[40]

Food and Feeding

The preschool child is beginning to form definite responses to various types of foods, as follows:

- *Vegetables and fruits:* Fruits are usually well liked. However, of all the food groups, vegetables usually are liked the least by children, yet these foods contain many vitamins and minerals needed for growth. Where space or opportunity exists, involving the young child in the planting and growing of vegetables in a small garden or in containers is an excellent way to draw the child's interest to vegetables to be tasted. Trips to the market or learning activities in the day care setting can help a child see a variety of shapes and colors in vegetables and discover new ones that can be prepared in a variety of ways. It is important to remember that children have a keen sense of taste; therefore flavor and texture are important. Children usually dislike strong vegetables such as cabbage and onions but do like crisp raw vegetables or fruits cut in small pieces to eat as finger foods. Mixed vegetables and fruits are less tolerated than individual ones. Children also react to consistency of vegetables, disliking them when they are overcooked. Tough strings and hard pieces are difficult to chew and swallow and should be removed.

- *Milk, cheese, egg, meat, and legumes:* It is helpful if children can set their own goals of quantities of food. Portions need to be relatively small (see the Perspectives in Practice box, "Feeding Toddlers and Preschoolers: Eating Is a Family Affair"). If children can pour their own milk from a small pitcher into a small glass, then they will drink more. Smaller children like their milk served closer to room temperature, not icy cold. Cheese is a favorite finger food or snack; however, the major source of calcium in this age group is milk. Egg is usually well liked if hard-cooked or scrambled. Meat should be tender and easy to cut and chew; hence ground meat is popular. Ground meat also must be well cooked to ensure safety. (To avoid the risk of foodborne illness that can be fatal in the young child, ground meat should be cooked to a temperature of 160°F, the meat should have a gray-white color, and juices should be clear.)

- *Grains:* A wide variety of grains can be appealing to children who enjoy breads, cereals, and crackers. Whole grains provide important fiber. To avoid unwanted kcalories, presweetened cereals should be used infrequently if at all.

- *Temperature:* Because children prefer their foods lukewarm and not hot, some foods may remain on their plates and become dry and gummy such that the child refuses to eat them. Thus very small portions should be served at a time.

- *Single foods:* Children usually prefer single foods to combination dishes such as casseroles or stews. Preschool is also a period of language learning. Children like to learn names of foods and to be able to recognize and name them on the basis of their shape, color, texture, and taste; these identifiable characteristics need to be retained as much as possible.

- *Finger foods:* Children like to eat food they can pick up with their fingers. Often, a variety of raw fruits and vegetables cut into finger-sized pieces and offered to children for their own selection provide a source of needed nutrition.

- *Food jags and food neophobia:* Because of developing social and emotional needs, preschool children commonly have food jags, refusing to eat all except one particular food. This may last for several days, but it is usually short lived and of no major consequence. Food neophobia, commonly referred to as picky or fussy eating, is the refusal to eat new foods. Strategies for lowering food neophobia include offering new foods with familiar foods, introducing new foods in a playful manner, and continuing to introduce new foods repeatedly.

Summary Principles

The preschool period is one of important growth for the young child. Lifetime food habits are forming. Food continues to play an important part in the developing personality, and group eating becomes significant as a means of socialization. The following two principles should be considered when interacting with preschoolers:

1. The social and emotional environment and companionship at mealtime with family, other caregivers, or other children greatly influence the young child's food intake and diet quality. The child learns food patterns at the family table and follows the examples of food eaten by parents or older siblings.[40] The child may attend a day care or preschool in which group eating occurs. Food habits of preschoolers are greatly affected by peer modeling, and food preferences develop according to what the group is eating. Children in this stage of development may begin to respond to environmental cues encouraging them to consume more food than they need. In a recent review of the literature it was found that 2- and 3-year-olds were adept at self-regulating the amount of food they consumed based on internal cues (i.e., hunger); however, starting at ages 4 and 5, children's energy intake was impacted by the amount of food they were served, with consistent larger portion sizes resulting in increased energy intake, a reflection that these children were overriding their internal cues.[41] In light of the growing numbers of overweight children, we need to encourage parents to be alert to portion size when serving their children's food.

2. Many food preferences and tolerances are established during this period. Exposure to a wide variety of foods in appropriate portion sizes may set the stage for lifetime food habits and associated patterns of health. This stage of growth is also a time for the young child to develop appropriate physical exercise habits, and games that include activities such as skipping or jumping should be encouraged in a safe environment. Physical fitness established at an early age can lower the risk of overweight and obesity in childhood and adulthood, respectively.[42] Encouraging young children to participate in active games rather than sedentary pastimes such as watching videos or television may also support appropriate food patterns (see Further Readings and Resources at the end of this chapter). Exposure to unhealthy food and beverage advertisements increases energy intake and consumption of unhealthy foods.[43] Limiting screen time in the population is encouraged for many health-related reasons.

School-Age Child (6 to 12 Years)
Physical Characteristics and Growth

The school-age period preceding adolescence has been called the *latent time of growth*. During this stage, the rate of growth slows and body changes occur more gradually. By now the body type has been established, and growth rates vary widely. Girls usually outdistance boys in the latter part of this period.

Psychosocial and Motor Development

Psychosocial development during these early school years centers on the formal learning environment and its expectations. Children develop increased cognitive capacity and the ability to problem solve. They learn to cooperate in group activities and begin to experience a sense of adequacy and accomplishment and sometimes the realities of competition. The child begins to move from a dependence on parental standards to those of peers (Fig. 12.3). Pressures are generated for self-control of a growing body, and inappropriate concepts of body image that lead to chronic dieting or eating disorders may take root during this period. Negative attitudes are sometimes expressed; these changes in temperament are evidence of the struggle for growing independence. It is a diffuse period of gangs, cliques, hero worship, pensive daydreaming, emotional stress, and learning cooperation with other

FIG. 12.3 Peers influence the nutrition habits of school-age children. (Copyright 2006 JupiterImages Corporation.)

children. This is also a period during which nutrition and health concepts are being learned.

Food and Feeding

The slowed rate of growth during this period results in a gradual decline in the food requirement relative to body weight. This decline continues until the period just before adolescence. Likes and dislikes are a product of earlier years as well as current peer influences. Family food attitudes are imitated; however, increasing outside activities and influences begin to compete with family mealtimes, and family conflicts may arise.

School and the Learning Environment

Research has established the relationship between sound nutrition and childhood learning.[44] Breakfast is particularly important for the school-age child. It *breaks the fast* of the sleep hours and prepares the child for problem solving and memory in the learning hours at school.[45] The National School Breakfast and Lunch Programs provide nourishing school meals that many children would not otherwise have (see Appendix D). Some studies have documented the positive relationship between breakfast intake and school performance, although methodologic issues among the studies preclude specific statements regarding the effects of breakfast on cognitive performance.[45,46] Programs that increase school breakfast participation have been implemented. School programs guided by the US Department of Agriculture (USDA) help maintain sound nutrition by implementing the 2015 *Dietary Guidelines for Americans* (see Further Readings and Resources at the end of this chapter) into child breakfast and lunch programs. Schools should also take a premier role in promoting lifelong physical activity patterns in children. Health professionals must take leadership roles in their communities to ensure that school meal programs provide positive examples of nutritionally appropriate meal patterns and introduce children to new foods that they may not have tasted previously.[47,48]

The USDA released ChooseMyPlate in 2010 for food guidance in the United States. These program materials continue to assist individuals in identifying energy needs, setting goals for food and nutrient intakes, and developing food intakes based on food groups. The MyPlate Daily Checklist (Fig. 12.4) was developed to build knowledge related to food and nutrient intake along with balance between food intake and physical activity. Classroom-based activities are available on the website of the USDA (https://www.fns.usda.gov/tn/team-nutrition) for implementation in schools.

The school-age child has increasing exposure to positive and negative food habits. Television becomes a powerful source of food information.

Food Group Amounts for 1,600 Calories a Day

Fruits	Vegetables	Grains	Protein	Dairy
1 1/2 cups	**2 cups**	**5 ounces**	**5 ounces**	**2 1/2 cups**
Focus on whole fruits	**Vary your veggies**	**Make half your grains whole grains**	**Vary your protein routine**	**Move to low-fat or fat-free milk or yogurt**
Focus on whole fruits that are fresh, frozen, canned, or dried.	Choose a variety of colorful fresh, frozen, and canned vegetables—make sure to include dark green, red, and orange choices.	Find whole-grain foods by reading the Nutrition Facts label and ingredients list.	Mix up your protein foods to include seafood, beans and peas, unsalted nuts and seeds, soy products, eggs, and lean meats and poultry.	Choose fat-free milk, yogurt, and soy beverages (soy milk) to cut back on your saturated fat.

Limit

Drink and eat less sodium, saturated fat, and added sugars. Limit:

- Sodium to **1,900** milligrams a day.
- Saturated fat to **18 grams** a day.
- Added sugars to **40 grams** a day.

FIG. 12.4 My Daily Food Plan. This daily food plan is intended for a 4- to 8-year-old child of average height and weight who is physically active 30 to 60 minutes each day. (From US Department of Agriculture. https://choosemyplate-prod.azureedge.net/sites/default/files/myplate/checklists/MyPlateDailyChecklist_1600cals_Age4-8.pdf.)

At the same time, positive learning opportunities can occur in the classroom when nutrition education is integrated with other activities and parents provide support and reinforcement at home. An important learning experience can be the preparation of simple meals; interventions that are geared toward increasing a child's involvement in meal preparation show improved dietary quality and eating patterns.[49]

Although declines in physical activity no doubt have contributed to the growing number of overweight children, some researchers have also pointed to changes in eating habits. Research supports that portion sizes as well as the energy density of common foods consumed by children, particularly snacks and sugar-sweetened beverages, have increased drastically over the past several decades.[50] An important message to children should be to eat only when they are hungry; portion size should be moderate, and the best foods are those that are relatively low in kcalories but rich in protein, vitamins, and minerals.

Sound nutrition is especially critical for the child athlete. Children ages 6 to 12 years who are engaged in athletic competition need appropriate nutritional advice from parents, coaches, and trained professionals to meet their energy, protein, and fluid needs for training and competition.[51]

Summary Principles

Growth slows during the school-age years, yet development rapidly continues. Individual- and group-learning experiences greatly influence children. The following two principles should be considered when working with school-age children:

1. Relative energy needs decline, but the quality of the diet is essential to provide the minerals and vitamins essential to school performance and physical demands.
2. The school and home environments must be conducive to assisting 6- to 12-year-olds with making appropriate food and activity choices. These choices should be based on sound evidence related to nutritional needs of the school-age individual.

Adolescent
Physical Characteristics and Growth

During the adolescent period, with the onset of puberty, the final growth spurt of childhood occurs. Maturation during this time varies so widely that chronologic age as a reference point for discussing growth ceases to be useful. **Physiologic age** becomes more important in dealing with individual boys and girls. Adolescent growth accounts for wide fluctuations in physical size, metabolic rate, food needs, and even illness. These capacities can be more realistically viewed only in terms of physiologic growth, often characterized by Tanner stages of pubertal growth.[52]

The profound body changes occurring in the adolescent result from the release of estrogen and testosterone, the sex steroid hormones that regulate the development of the sex characteristics. The rate at which these body changes occur varies widely and is particularly distinct in the growth patterns that emerge between the sexes. In girls, the amount of subcutaneous fat increases, and the hip breadth widens in preparation for childbearing. This fat accumulation and change in body shape are often sources of anxiety to many body-conscious young girls. In adolescent boys, physical growth is manifested by an increased muscle mass and long bone growth. Although the growth spurt in boys occurs later than in girls, boys soon surpass girls in weight and height.

KEY TERM

Physiologic Age
Rate of biologic maturation in individual adolescents that varies widely and accounts more for wide and changing differences in their metabolic rates, nutritional needs, and food requirements than does chronologic age.

Psychosocial and Motor Development

Adolescence is a period marked by turbulence and discovery. On the one hand, teenagers look back to the securities of childhood; on the other hand, they reach for the maturity of adulthood. Emergence of a self-identity is the major psychosocial developmental task of adolescence; the search for self, begun in early childhood, reaches its peak during these years. The profound body changes associated with sexual development and the capability of reproduction also result in changes in body image and resulting tensions in maturing girls and boys. Motor development and skilled coordination is complete.

The identity crisis of the adolescent years, largely revolving around sexual development and preparation for an adult role in a complex society, produces many psychological, emotional, and social pressures. Although the period of most rapid physical growth is relatively short, only 2 or 3 years, the attendant psychosocial development continues during a much longer period. The pressure for peer group acceptance is strong, and fads in fashion and nutrition habits play out this theme. In addition, in a technologically developed society such as the United States, high values are placed on education and achievement. Social tensions and family conflicts are common. These conflicts may have nutritional consequences as teenagers eat away from home more often and develop snacking patterns reflective of personal and peer group choices.

Food and Feeding

With the rapid growth of adolescence comes increased demands for energy, protein, vitamins, and minerals:

- *Energy:* Kcalorie needs increase with the metabolic demands of growth and energy expenditure. Although individual needs vary, males generally require greater kcalories than females, based on their larger body size and increased lean body mass.[3] Sometimes, the large appetite, characteristic of this rapid growth period, leads adolescents to satisfy their hunger with snack foods that are high in sugar and fat and low in essential protein, vitamins, and minerals.
- *Protein:* Adolescent growth needs for protein increase to support the pubertal changes in both sexes and the developing muscle mass particularly prominent in boys. To sustain daily needs and to maintain nitrogen reserves, girls require 46 g/day and boys require 52 g/day.[3]
- *Minerals:* The calcium requirement for all adolescents rises to 1300 mg/day to meet the demands of bone growth. In fact, adolescence is a critical time for the development of bone mass under the influence of the increasing levels of the sex hormones, especially estrogen. Poor bone mineralization in adolescence increases vulnerability to bone fracture at later ages.[53] Menses and consequent iron losses in adolescent females predispose her to iron deficiency anemia. Young female athletes who begin training before menarche and develop primary amenorrhea may in turn have reduced bone mineral density resulting from low estrogen levels. For all young athletes, energy and fluid replacement in any exercise or performance period is essential.[51]
- *Vitamins:* The B vitamins are needed in increased amounts to meet the extra demands of energy metabolism and tissue development. Intakes of vitamins C and A may be low because of erratic food intake and low intake of vegetables and fruits. A higher prevalence of folate deficiency exists among adolescent girls, increasing the risk of neural tube defects (NTDs) in babies born to teenage mothers (see Chapter 6 for a review of NTDs). Vitamin D deficiency has been found to range from 21% in healthy weight children and adolescents to 49% in severely obese children and adolescents, indicating a relationship between vitamin D status and weight status.[54] More prevalent in the winter and spring months

and in African-American and Hispanic adolescent boys and girls,[54] vitamin D deficiency is associated with rickets (overt deficiency) and increased risk of developing osteoporosis, cardiovascular disease, and multiple sclerosis later in life.[54] Use of sunscreens, purposeful avoidance of sunlight exposure, and limited intake of vitamin D–fortified milk contribute to vitamin D deficiency in adolescents. A vitamin D supplement of at least 10 mcg/day is recommended for adolescents who do not consume food sources of vitamin D.[55]

In the development of nutrition intervention programs for teens, it is important to consider their cultural and ethnic backgrounds, recognizing that food habits and problems may differ (see the Case Study box, "Nutrition Program for Adolescents"). Cost is another consideration when making nutritional recommendations to students or parents. Low-income groups demonstrate lower rates of fruit and vegetable intake, and so interventions that target budget-conscious ways to increase intake of these foods are essential.[56] Nutrition counseling must be individualized, taking into consideration both cultural food preferences and other circumstances existing within the family.

Eating Habits

Physical and psychosocial pressures influence adolescent eating behavior (see the Perspectives in Practice box, "Food Habits of Adolescents: Where Do We Begin?"). By and large, males fare better than females.

Their large appetites and the sheer volumes of food they consume usually ensure generally adequate nutrient intakes, but adolescent females may face more challenges. The following two factors combine to increase concerns surrounding nutrition and food intake in adolescent females:

1. *Physiologic sex difference:* Because sexual maturation in females brings about increased fat deposition during the adolescent growth period and because many teenage females are relatively inactive, it is easier for them to gain weight.

2. *Social and personal tensions:* Social pressures dictating thinness sometimes cause adolescent females to follow unwise and self-imposed diets for weight loss. In some cases, actual self-starvation regimens lead to complex and far-reaching eating disorders such as anorexia nervosa and bulimia nervosa (see Chapter 8). These problems, which can assume severe proportions, usually involve a distorted self-image and an irrational pursuit of thinness, even when actual body weight is normal or even less than age norms. In the absence of diagnosed eating disorders, constant dieting can still result in varying degrees of poor nutrition in the adolescent female at the very time in life when her body needs to be building reserves for potential reproduction. The harmful effects that poor eating habits can have on the future course of a pregnancy are clearly indicated in many studies relating preconception nutrition status to the outcome of gestation (see Chapter 11).

CASE STUDY

Nutrition Program for Adolescents

Amanda is a graduate student of clinical nutrition assigned to the "Save Our Senior High" project in a metropolitan community of 300,000 located in the northwestern United States. A representative of the city's educational advisory board approached her institution for assistance in developing a program that addresses three major problems faced by the majority of high school students: (1) popularity of fad diets among athletes, (2) overweight, and (3) iron deficiency anemia.

Amanda and other members of her class met with students of other health professions (medicine, dentistry, nutrition, nursing, social work), as well as several student representatives from the high school, to plan the program. After they developed goals and objectives, they decided that the nutrition topics would be addressed in a series of workshops: Nutrition and Physical Fitness, Food for the Teen Years, and Snack Facts.

The program was introduced to the students through an advance bulletin distributed at the largest high school in the city, where the project was to begin. The bulletin included an article written by Amanda: "Teenage Nutrition: A Seeming Paradox." This article responded to a common concern expressed by adolescents: the apparent preoccupation of school officials with the students' food habits when they, as a group, looked and usually felt very healthy.

Amanda's article stirred a tremendous interest in the student population. Attendance at each session was high, and the discussions were lively. The evaluation results were positive. In reviewing the evaluative data and low cost of the project, the city council asked Amanda and her classmates to repeat the program at two other high schools where these problems were also prevalent. The council approached the school board about the possibility of including the project in the citywide high school curriculum for the coming year.

Questions for Analysis

1. Outline the content of Amanda's article to reflect major points that you would have included.

2. Write a class outline for each workshop, including objectives, major topics, and questions you would expect from the students. What teaching methods and materials would you expect to be most effective in each workshop?

3. What outside influences on eating habits would you expect in this student population? How effective would you expect this educational program to be in influencing a change of behavior in eating habits?

4. Aside from in-school nutrition education programs, describe possible tactics for influencing the eating habits of teenagers.

PERSPECTIVES IN PRACTICE

Food Habits of Adolescents: Where Do We Begin?

Adolescents who have entered their growth spurt seem to eat all the time. The questions for health professionals are "What are they eating?" and "How do we help them improve their choices?" Both the quantity and quality of food are important during this period of rapid growth. Lean body mass increases by approximately 35 kg in boys and 19 kg in girls during these years, and 40% to 60% of adult bone mass is accrued. Generous supplies of iron, zinc, calcium, and essential vitamins, in addition to adequate energy and protein consumption, are needed to support these changes in body size and development.

Food Intake in the Teen Years

Despite the critical nutrient needs in this life stage, national dietary surveys indicate that of all age groups, teens have the poorest diets. Their intakes of calcium, iron, zinc, magnesium, phosphorous, and vitamins A, B_6, C, and E, and folate often fall below recommended levels. Fruit and vegetable consumption is quite low, with only 17% of adolescent males and 14% of adolescent females meeting the recommended intake for vegetables, and 24% of males and 20% of females consuming the recommended amount of vegetables. In addition, almost

Food Habits of Adolescents: Where Do We Begin?—cont'd

20% of adolescents report drinking no milk on a given day, and only 17% of males and 8% of females report consuming the recommended three glasses or more of milk per day. At the same time, most adolescents have excessively high intakes of added sugars, sodium, and fats. Foods such as hamburgers, pizza, tacos, and milkshakes are quite popular among teens, as are foods high in sugar, such as soft drinks and candy, and items high in fat, including pastries, fatty meats, and fried foods, are eaten regularly by many teens. Males and females obtain approximately 33% of their kcalories from added sugars and solid fats. Nearly one-third of adolescents use vitamin-mineral supplements, but the supplement users have better diets and obtain increased intakes of nutrients from food. Teens also indulge in risk-taking behaviors: approximately one-fourth consume tobacco products, one-fourth use marijuana, and approximately one-third report use of alcohol.

Lifestyle, Environment, and Nutritional Behavior

Lifestyle choices in the teen years are influenced by teens' growing need to express their independence and make their own decisions. Adolescents also lead busy lives with school, sports, and jobs. These lifestyle factors need to be considered within a socioecologic perspective of influences on eating behaviors. That is, the social environment, including peers and family, exert strong influences on eating behavior, with peer influence shown to encourage unhealthy eating behaviors. The physical environment is also influential. Thirty-three percent of calories in the teen diet come from "empty calories"—also known as solid fats and added sugars (SoFAS), and stores, schools, and fast foods restaurants contribute 33%, 32%, and 35% of these empty calories, respectively, to the adolescent's diet. Interventions targeting healthy behaviors among this population must address these socioecological factors.

Unfortunately, health is often not an important personal issue at this life stage. A feeling of invulnerability and the idea that they have plenty of time in future years to worry about their health are common in teens. At the same time, body weight and appearance are major concerns for 49% of girls and 43% of boys. The need to be thin causes some adolescent girls to adopt nutritionally inadequate diets or, worse, develop anorexia or bulimia nervosa (see Chapter 8). Adolescent boys trying to increase their muscle mass or "bulk up" may resort to unproven and potentially dangerous supplements or eat high-fat foods in an effort to obtain more kcalories. When working with teens who claim to be dieting, it is necessary to talk with them individually about what kind of diet they are following. For some teens, dieting means drastically reducing their food intake or choosing foods erroneously believed to have special effects on appearance; for others, dieting refers to healthful practices like increasing their intakes of fruits and vegetables or cutting down on fats and sweets.

How Do We Help Teens Improve Their Food Choices?

Improving the food choices of this age group requires the combined efforts of parents, health professionals, food manufacturers, restaurant personnel, and food retailers. An important message to teens is that appropriate food choices, along with regular physical activity, can help to achieve and maintain (1) a healthy weight and positive level of fitness, (2) a high energy level for school and work, and (3) an overall sense of well-being. Physical education and health teachers, nutrition educators, athletic coaches, school nurses, and parents must work together to develop programs that will reach teens at school and on the playing field.

Teens want information that they can use now, not 10 years from now. One topic of immediate use would be educating teens on healthier meal options that are available at fast food restaurants. Snacks such as bananas, oranges, apples, and other fresh fruit; string cheese and nuts; or individual packages of ready-to-eat cereal travel well in a backpack, as do ultrapasteurized milk drinks that do not require refrigeration. Teens should be encouraged to choose simple-to-prepare or carry-along breakfasts, such as ready-to-eat cereal or whole grain bread (or a bagel) with peanut butter. Ready-to-eat cereals, particularly whole grain varieties, may provide a breakfast that is lower in cost, lower in fat, and higher in important nutrients including calcium, iron, vitamins A and D, and folate than fast food breakfast meals, donuts, or toaster pastries.

Because taste is an important factor in food selection for teens, it is important that healthy foods taste good. School cafeteria managers need to produce good-tasting and satisfying food that is attractively served. This means that the school meal must be viewed as an extension of the school's educational mission and supported by teachers and parents. Salad bars have become popular among some teens, and salads "to go" can meet the need of taste and convenience. Recipes that are reduced in fat and sugar but pleasing in taste and texture need to be developed for quantity food programs.

Food manufacturers must be urged to improve the nutrient quality of ready-to-eat main dishes, as well as snack foods. Taste-testing parties with teens that compare lower-fat or reduced-sugar items with less-nutritious products may help to dispel the myth that healthy foods do not taste good. Many popular foods among teens, such as pizza or tacos, can be healthy choices if attention is paid to reducing the levels of ingredients high in fat and saturated fat.

Finally, food retailers who cater to the teen audience must be urged to sell and advertise healthy foods. Some fast food restaurants include orange juice or low fat milk as drink options in combination meals as an alternative to soft drinks. Salads are an option at many fast food outlets, and baked potatoes may be available as an alternative to French fries. A grilled chicken sandwich can be a healthier option than a hamburger. Advertisements for soft drinks or less healthy food items often carry the endorsements of popular sports stars. Such endorsements have been applied to foods such as milk that are important to health and well-being. Community coalitions involving health professionals, educators, and parents concerned about adolescents and their future health will be necessary to bring about needed changes.

Bibliography

Centers for Disease Control and Prevention: Youth Risk Surveillance—United States, *MMWR* 63(4):17, 2013.

Dwyer J, Nahin RL, Rogers GT et al: Prevalence and predictors of children's dietary supplement use: the 2007 National Health Interview Survey, *Am J Clin Nutr* 97(6):1331, 2013.

Gaspar de Matos M, Palmeira AL, Gaspar T, et al: Social support influences on eating awareness in children and adolescents: the mediating effect of self-regulating strategies, *Glob Public Health* 11(4):437, 2016.

Golden NH, Abrams SA, Committee on Nutrition: Optimizing bone health in children and adolescents, *Pediatrics* 134(4):e1229, 2014.

Jackson LW: The most important meal of the day: why children skip breakfast and what can be done about it, *Pediatr Ann* 42(9):184, 2013.

Poti JM, Slining MM, Popkin BM, et al: Where are kids getting their empty calories? Stores, schools, and fast-food restaurants each played an important role in empty calorie intake among US children during 2009-2010, *J Acad Nutr Diet* 114(6):908, 2014.

Slining MM, Popkin BM: Trends in intakes and sources of solid fats and added sugars among US children and adolescents: 1994-2010, *Pediatr Obes* 8(4):307, 2013.

US Department of Agriculture, Agricultural Research Service: Nutrient intakes from food and beverages: mean amounts consumed per individual, by gender and age. What we eat in America, NHANES 2011-2012, 2014.

Watts AW, Lovato CY, Barr SI, et al: A qualitative study exploring how school and community environments shape the food choices of adolescents with overweight/obesity, *Appetite* 95:360, 2015.

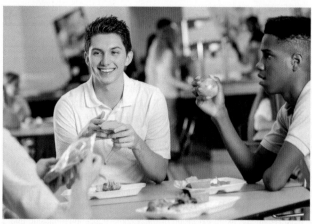

FIG. 12.5 Fruits and vegetables help meet the high nutrient demands during adolescence. (Copyright Getty Images.)

Summary Principles

The following two principles should be considered when intervening with food habits during adolescence:

1. Nutrient demands are high for final growth and development; therefore the quality of the diet is vital (Fig. 12.5).
2. Food choices and eating patterns may be less than optimal because of the many influential factors that affect choices during adolescence.

HEALTH PROMOTION

CHILDREN AND ADOLESCENTS: SEEKING FITNESS

The *Dietary Guidelines for Americans* 2015 provides direction for the development of a healthy diet and lifestyle for all persons age 2 and older.[57] The 2015 edition set goals not only for food patterns in all age groups but also for appropriate physical activity. Many chronic diseases that influence well-being in later life actually begin in childhood. Thus lifestyle practices that promote healthy behaviors related to diet and physical activity must be introduced at an early age, when patterns are being developed that will continue for a lifetime.

Weight Management

Body weight and physical activity are intrinsically related. A regular pattern of exercise beginning in childhood has been shown to promote lifelong heart health and may prevent the accumulation of excess body fat. Nearly one-third of all US children and adolescents are overweight or obese, a number that has been rising steadily over the past few decades.[58] Racial, ethnic, and regional differences are seen in overweight among children. Boys, African Americans, Hispanics, and those living in the Southern states are more likely to be overweight. High-energy diets, coupled with inactivity patterns leading to increased body fat, are associated with the growing incidence of type 2 diabetes in school-age children.

Body fat increases rapidly during the first year of life and then slows until approximately age 6, when a normal increase again occurs in the size and number of body fat cells. For some children, an inappropriate accumulation of body fat begins about this time or even earlier. Fig. 12.6 displays the multifaceted nature of overweight in childhood. Attention must be given to the personal or child characteristics and risk factors, parenting skills and family dynamics, and environmental factors of the community and society that contribute to this complex problem. In general, accumulation of excess body fat can be accelerated by a high energy intake in relation to energy needs or a sedentary life pattern with low energy expenditure.[59] One approach to prevention of inappropriate accumulation of body fat in a child of any age is regular physical activity. The goal is to promote body weight gain within healthy ranges to support normal growth and development.[59] In overweight children and adolescents, the goal is to slow gains in body weight while promoting optimal growth and development.[59]

Physical Activity

Although children and adolescents are typically more active than most adults, many appear to be settling into a sedentary lifestyle more common among adults. The physical activity guideline for children and adolescents is a minimum of 1 hour of aerobic, moderate- to vigorous-intensity physical activity each day. Vigorous-intensity and muscle-strengthening physical activity that is weight bearing and promotes bone health should be completed at least 3 days each week. However, the Youth Risk Behavior Surveillance System (YRBSS) found that only 20% of adolescent females and 41% of adolescent males report meeting the physical activity guideline of engaging in aerobic exercise 60 minutes a day, at least 5 days a week.[60-62] Television,

FIG. 12.6 Ecologic model of predictors of childhood overweight. (Copyright 2001 *Obesity Reviews*. From Davison KK, Birch LL: Childhood overweight: a contextual model and recommendations for future research, *Obes Rev* 2:159, 2001. Reprinted with permission.)

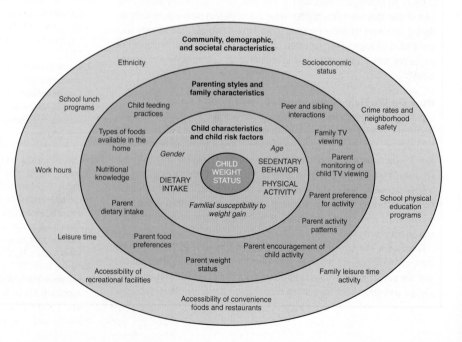

computer games, the Internet, and similar sedentary pastimes are growing in popularity. Watching television for more than 2 hours per day during childhood is related to overweight and the presence of other risk factors for chronic diseases, and the YRBSS found that more than 70% of adolescents exceeded this recommendation.[62,63]

Helping Children Develop an Active Lifestyle

Parents and caregivers, schools, and communities need to work together to increase physical activity among children.[59] Children are more likely to develop an active lifestyle if parents and role models also demonstrate such behavior. Taking your teddy bear for a walk can be a meaningful activity for a preschooler who belongs to a family who walks together regularly. School games and physical education programs should focus on activities such as walking or running that allow all students to participate, rather than on games in which several students are active but the majority sit and watch. Moving away from competitive games that discourage participation by overweight or less-skilled players to such activities as dancing or aerobics that can be done alone to music or in groups after school are worthwhile objectives for physical education. Bike riding and jumping rope are good forms of vigorous exercise. Making school facilities such as a gymnasium or walking track available to families and students after school hours might encourage an increased level of physical activity. Fig. 12.7 illustrates one example of guidelines regarding activity levels for children ages 6 to 11 years.

TO SUM UP

Normal growth and development depend on nutrition to support heightened physiologic and metabolic processes. Nutrition, in turn, depends on a multitude of social, psychological, cultural, and environmental influences that affect individual growth potential throughout the life cycle.

Four types of growth interact during each phase of development: (1) physical, (2) mental, (3) emotional, and (4) sociocultural. Each type of growth must be evaluated when assessing the child's nutrition status and planning an effective counseling approach. Nutritional needs change with each growth period and must be individualized according to the unique growth pattern of every child.

Infants experience rapid growth. They have immature digestive systems and limited ability to absorb and excrete metabolites efficiently. Breast-feeding is preferred during the first year of life. Solid foods are not needed or adequately tolerated until an infant is 4 to 6 months old.

Toddlers (ages 1 to 3 years), preschoolers (ages 3 to 6 years), and school-age children (ages 6 to 12 years) experience the slowed and erratic latent growth of childhood. Their energy requirements per unit of body weight are not as great as those of infants. Their nutritional needs center on protein for growth, with attendant minerals and vitamins. Social and cultural factors influence the

FIG. 12.7 MyActivity Pyramid. (From University of Missouri Extension Publication N386. Reprinted with permission. https://www.extension.missouri.edu/publications/DisplayPub.aspx?P=n386.)

Continued

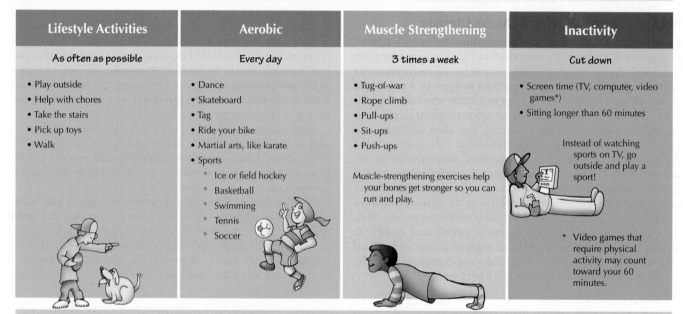

MyActivity Pyramid

Be physically active 60 minutes, up to several hours every day.
Use these suggestions to help meet your goal:

Lifestyle Activities	Aerobic	Muscle Strengthening	Inactivity
As often as possible	**Every day**	**3 times a week**	**Cut down**

Lifestyle Activities
- Play outside
- Help with chores
- Take the stairs
- Pick up toys
- Walk

Aerobic
- Dance
- Skateboard
- Tag
- Ride your bike
- Martial arts, like karate
- Sports
  - Ice or field hockey
  - Basketball
  - Swimming
  - Tennis
  - Soccer

Muscle Strengthening
- Tug-of-war
- Rope climb
- Pull-ups
- Sit-ups
- Push-ups

Muscle-strengthening exercises help your bones get stronger so you can run and play.

Inactivity
- Screen time (TV, computer, video games*)
- Sitting longer than 60 minutes

Instead of watching sports on TV, go outside and play a sport!

* Video games that require physical activity may count toward your 60 minutes.

Find your balance between food and fun:
- Move more. Aim for at least 60 minutes every day.
- Walk, dance, bike, rollerblade – it all counts. How great is that!

This publication is adapted from the USDA's MyPyramid and the 2008 Physical Activity Guidelines for Americans, chapter 3. Funded in part by USDA SNAP.
Running out of money for food? Contact your local food stamp office or go online to *dss.mo.gov/fsd/fstamp*. For more information, call MU Extension's Show Me Nutrition line at 1-888-515-0016.

UNIVERSITY OF MISSOURI
Extension

■ Issued in furtherance of the Cooperative Extension Work Acts of May 8 and June 30, 1914, in cooperation with the United States Department of Agriculture. Director, Cooperative Extension, University of Missouri, Columbia, MO 65211
■ an equal opportunity/ADA institution ■ 573-882-7216 ■ extension.missouri.edu

FIG. 12.7, cont'd

development of food habits in these age groups. Appropriate food behavior by parents and caregivers that can be modeled by children of these ages strongly influences the adoption of good eating habits during these periods of development.

Adolescents (ages 12 to 18 years) experience a second large growth spurt before reaching adulthood. This rapid growth involves sexual maturation and physical growth. During this period, girls increase their body proportion of fat, whereas boys increase their body proportion

of muscle. Reaching peak bone mass is an important milestone for both genders during this period of development. In general, boys (who consume larger amounts of food) more easily achieve the increased kcalorie and nutrient needs of adolescence. In contrast, girls (who may feel social and peer pressure to restrict food intake to avoid weight gain) are less likely to meet their optimal nutrient requirements for growth. This pressure may also inhibit their ability to acquire the nutritional reserves necessary for later reproduction.

QUESTIONS FOR REVIEW

1. How is physical growth measured? What are the NCHS growth charts, and how are they used? What are the limitations of these charts? What are some clinical, biochemical, and dietary measures that are helpful in assessing the nutritional status of infants and children?

2. Describe the physical and psychosocial characteristics of the newborn. What are the capabilities of the newborn's digestive and renal systems, and how do they relate to infant feeding?

3. Why is breast-feeding the preferred method for feeding infants (discuss nutritional and psychosocial factors)? Describe the anatomic and hormonal components that participate in the delivery of breast milk to the nursing infant.

4. You are planning a nutrition education class to prepare pregnant mothers for breast-feeding. Outline the material that you would present, including (a) dietary needs for the new breast-feeding mother and (b) benefits of breast-feeding to the mother.

5. You are counseling a pregnant mother who has decided not to breast-feed. Describe some types of commercial formulas that would provide an appropriate alternative feeding for her infant. Describe the feeding techniques that will be important in meeting the psychosocial needs of her infant.

6. You are working with a mother whose newborn has been found to be allergic to milk proteins. What might be an appropriate food source for this infant?

7. You are working with a low-income mother who has chosen not to breast-feed. She is concerned about the high cost of infant formula and would like to feed her infant cow's milk because it is cheaper. What would you tell her?

8. Outline a general schedule for a new mother to use as a guide for adding solid foods to her infant's diet during the first year of life; indicate both the time of addition and the items to be offered.

9. What changes in physical growth and psychosocial development influence eating habits in the (a) toddler, (b) preschool child, and (c) school-age child? How do these factors influence the nutritional needs of each age group?

10. What factors influence the changing nutritional needs of adolescents? Who is usually at increased nutritional risk during this stage—boys or girls? Why? What nutritional deficiencies may be associated with this vulnerable age?

11. You are the director of a food service program in an elementary school and want to start a nutrition education program. You are working with a science teacher, a social studies teacher, and the school nurse to develop lessons that will connect learning in the classroom with good nutrition in the lunchroom. Visit the USDA's Food and Nutrition Information Center website for Team Nutrition (https://www.fns.usda.gov/tn) to find some ideas and materials that will assist you in this project. Develop a lesson plan for presentation in the science or social studies class that focuses on nutrition or food patterns, and indicate how you will connect this lesson with the lunch program.

REFERENCES

1. Dessi A, Cesare Marincola F, Masili A, et al: Clinical metabolomics and nutrition: the new frontier in neonatology and pediatrics, *Biomed Res Int* 2014:981219, 2014.

2. Ogden CL, Kuczmarski RJ, Flegal KM, et al: Centers for Disease Control and Prevention 2000 growth charts for the United States: improvements to the 1977 National Center for Health Statistics version, *Pediatrics* 109(1): 45–60, 2002.

3. Food and Nutrition Board, Institute of Medicine: *Dietary Reference Intakes for energy, carbohydrate, fiber, fat, fatty acids, cholesterol, protein, and amino acids (macronutrients)*, Washington, DC, 2005, National Academies Press.

4. Dekate P, Jayashree M, Singhi SC: Management of acute diarrhea in emergency room, *Indian J Pediatr* 80(3):235–246, 2013.

5. Food and Nutrition Board, Institute of Medicine: *Dietary Reference Intakes for water, potassium, sodium, chloride, and sulfate*, Washington, DC, 2004, National Academies Press.

6. Kleinman RE: Expert recommendations on iron fortification in infants, *J Pediatr* 167(Suppl 4):S48–S49, 2015.

7. Erikson E: *Childhood and society*, New York, 1963, WW Norton.

8. Cruwys T, Bevelander KE, Hermans RC: Social modeling of eating: a review of when and why social influence affects food intake and choice, *Appetite* 86:3–18, 2015.

9. Mitchell GL, Farrow C, Haycraft E, et al: Parental influences on children's eating behaviour and characteristics of successful parent-focussed interventions, *Appetite* 60(1):85–94, 2013.

10. Smith HA, Becker GE: Early additional food and fluids for healthy breast-fed full-term infants, *Cochrane Database Syst Rev* (8):CD006462, 2016.

11. Bly E, Huntington J, Harper AL: Clinical inquiry. What is the best age to start vitamin D supplementation to prevent rickets in breastfed newborns? Breastfed infants who take vitamin D beginning at 3 to 5 days of life don't develop rickets, *J Fam Pract* 62(12):755–763, 2013.

12. Thiele DK, Senti JL, Anderson CM: Maternal vitamin D supplementation to meet the needs of the breastfed infant: a systematic review, *J Hum Lact* 29(2):163–170, 2013.

13. Valentine CJ, Wagner CL: Nutritional management of the breastfeeding dyad, *Pediatr Clin North Am* 60(1):261–274, 2013.

14. Eldjerou LK, Cogle CR, Rosenau EH, et al: Vitamin D effect on umbilical cord blood characteristics: a comparison between African Americans and Caucasians, *Transfusion* 55(7):1766–1771, 2015.

15. Lessen R, Kavanagh K: Position of the academy of nutrition and dietetics: promoting and supporting breastfeeding, *J Acad Nutr Diet* 115(3): 444–449, 2015.

16. Philipp BL, Merewood A: The baby-friendly way: the best breastfeeding start, *Pediatr Clin North Am* 51(3):761–783, xi, 2004.

17. Tran A: Becoming a baby friendly hospital, *MCN Am J Matern Child Nurs* 42(1):36–42, 2017.

18. Munn AC, Newman SD, Mueller M, et al: The impact in the United States of the baby-friendly hospital initiative on early infant health and breastfeeding outcomes, *Breastfeed Med* 11:222–230, 2016.

19. Prell C, Koletzko B: Breastfeeding and complementary feeding, *Dtsch Arztebl Int* 113(25):435–444, 2016.

20. Lessen R, Kavanagh K: Practice paper of the academy of nutrition and dietetics abstract: Promoting and supporting breastfeeding, *J Acad Nutr Diet* 115(3):450, 2015.

21. Forestell CA: The development of flavor perception and acceptance: the roles of nature and nurture, *Nestle Nutr Inst Workshop Ser* 85:135–143, 2016.

22. Mameli C, Mazzantini S, Zuccotti GV: Nutrition in the first 1000 days: the origin of childhood obesity, *Int J Environ Res Public Health* 13(9): E838, 2016.

23. Singhal A: The role of infant nutrition in the global epidemic of non-communicable disease, *Proc Nutr Soc* 75(2):162–168, 2016.

24. Castanys-Muñoz E, Martin MJ, Vazquez E: Building a beneficial microbiome from birth, *Adv Nutr* 7(2):323–330, 2016.

25. Kashtanova DA, Popenko AS, Tkacheva ON, et al: Association between the gut microbiota and diet: fetal life, early childhood, and further life, *Nutrition* 32(6):620–627, 2016.

26. Andreas NJ, Kampmann B, Mehring Le-Doare K: Human breast milk: a review on its composition and bioactivity, *Early Hum Dev* 91(11):629–635, 2015.

27. Videhult FK, West CE: Nutrition, gut microbiota and child health outcomes, *Curr Opin Clin Nutr Metab Care* 19(3):208–213, 2016.

28. Reference removed in pages.

29. Demmelmair H, Koletzko B: Importance of fatty acids in the perinatal period, *World Rev Nutr Diet* 112:31–47, 2015.

30. Green Corkins K, Shurley T: What's in the bottle? A Review of infant formulas, *Nutr Clin Pract* 31(6), 2016.

31. Rossen LM, Simon AE, Herrick KA: Types of infant formulas consumed in the United States, *Clin Pediatr (Phila)* 55(3):278–285, 2016.

32. Bhatia J, Greer F, American Academy of Pediatrics Committee on Nutrition: Use of soy protein-based formulas in infant feeding, *Pediatrics* 121(5): 1062–1068, 2008.

33. Fleischer DM, Spergel JM, Assa'ad AH, et al: Primary prevention of allergic disease through nutritional interventions, *J Allergy Clin Immunol Pract* 1(1):29–36, 2013.

34. Radlović N, Leković Z, Radlović V, et al: Food allergy in children, *Srp Arh Celok Lek* 144(1-2):99–103, 2016.

35. Martin CR, Ling PR, Blackburn GL: Review of infant feeding: key features of breast milk and infant formula, *Nutrients* 8(5), 2016.

36. Hay WW Jr, Hendrickson KC: Preterm formula use in the preterm very low birth weight infant, *Semin Fetal Neonatal Med* 22(1):15–22, 2017.

37. Fewtrell M, Bronsky J, Campoy C, et al: Complementary Feeding: A Position Paper by the European Society for Paediatric Gastroenterology, Hepatology, and Nutrition (ESPGHAN) Committee on Nutrition, *J Pediatr Gastroenterol Nutr* 64(1):119–132, 2017.

38. Melina V, Craig W, Levin S: Position of the Academy of Nutrition and Dietetics: vegetarian diets, *J Acad Nutr Diet* 116(12):1970–1980, 2016.

39. Fletcher S, Wright C, Jones A, et al: Tracking of toddler fruit and vegetable preferences to intake and adiposity later in childhood, *Matern Child Nutr* 13(2), 2017.

40. Pyper E, Harrington D, Manson H: The impact of different types of parental support behaviours on child physical activity, healthy eating, and screen time: a cross-sectional study, *BMC Public Health* 16(1):568, 2016.

41. Small L, Lane H, Vaughan L, et al: A systematic review of the evidence: the effects of portion size manipulation with children and portion education/training interventions on dietary intake with adults, *Worldviews Evid Based Nurs* 10(2):69–81, 2013.

42. Sisson SB, Krampe M, Anundson K, et al: Obesity prevention and obesogenic behavior interventions in child care: A systematic review, *Prev Med* 87:57–69, 2016.

43. Sadeghirad B, Duhaney T, Motaghipisheh S, et al: Influence of unhealthy food and beverage marketing on children's dietary intake and preference: a systematic review and meta-analysis of randomized trials, *Obes Rev* 17(10):945–959, 2016.

44. Tandon PS, Tovar A, Jayasuriya AT, et al: The relationship between physical activity and diet and young children's cognitive development: a systematic review, *Prev Med Rep* 3:379–390, 2016.

45. Adolphus K, Lawton CL, Champ CL, et al: The effects of breakfast and breakfast composition on cognition in children and adolescents: a systematic review, *Adv Nutr* 7(3):S590–S612, 2016.

46. Adolphus K, Bellissimo N, Lawton CL, et al: Methodological challenges in studies examining the effects of breakfast on cognitive performance and appetite in children and adolescents, *Adv Nutr* 8(1):S184–S196, 2017.

47. Kessler HS: Simple interventions to improve healthy eating behaviors in the school cafeteria, *Nutr Rev* 74(3):198–209, 2016.

48. Merlo C, Brener N, Kann L, et al: school-level practices to increase availability of fruits, vegetables, and whole grains, and reduce sodium in school meals—United States, 2000, 2006, and 2014, *MMWR Morb Mortal Wkly Rep* 64(33):905–908, 2015.

49. Berge JM, MacLehose RF, Larson N, et al: Family food preparation and its effects on adolescent dietary quality and eating patterns, *J Adolesc Health* 59(5):530–536, 2016.

50. Sahoo K, Sahoo B, Choudhury AK, et al: Childhood obesity: causes and consequences, *J Family Med Prim Care* 4(2):187–192, 2015.

51. Purcell LK, Canadian Paediatric Society, Paediatric Sports and Exercise Medicine Section: Sport nutrition for young athletes, *Paediatr Child Health* 18(4):200–205, 2013.

52. Chemaitilly WEO, Witchel SF: Endocrinology. In Zitelli BJ, McIntire S, Nowalk AJ, editor: *Atlas of pediatric physical diagnosis*, Philadelphia PA, 2012, W.B. Saunders.

53. Rizzoli R: Nutritional aspects of bone health, *Best Pract Res Clin Endocrinol Metab* 28(6):795–808, 2014.

54. Turer CB, Lin H, Flores G: Prevalence of vitamin D deficiency among overweight and obese US children, *Pediatrics* 131(1):e152–161, 2013.

55. Smith TJ, Tripkovic L, Damsgaard CT, et al: Estimation of the dietary requirement for vitamin D in adolescents aged 14-18 y: a dose-response, double-blind, randomized placebo-controlled trial, *Am J Clin Nutr* 104(5):1301–1309, 2016.

56. Di Noia J, Cullen KW: Fruit and vegetable attitudes, norms, and intake in low-income youth, *Health Educ Behav* 42(6):775–782, 2015.

57. US Department of Agriculture and US Department of Health and Human Services: *Dietary Guidelines for Americans, 2015 (Policy Document)*, ed 8, Washington, DC, 2015, US Government Printing Office. https://health.gov/dietaryguidelines/2015/guidelines/.

58. Ogden CL, Carroll MD, Kit BK, et al: Prevalence of childhood and adult obesity in the United States, 2011-2012, *JAMA* 311(8):806–814, 2014.

59. Kumar S, Kelly AS: Review of childhood obesity: from epidemiology, etiology, and comorbidities to clinical assessment and treatment, *Mayo Clin Proc* 92(2):251–265, 2017.

60. Iannotti RJ, Wang J: Patterns of physical activity, sedentary behavior, and diet in US adolescents, *J Adolesc Health* 53(2):280–286, 2013.

61. US Department of Health and Human Services: *Physical activity guidelines for Americans*, ed 1, Washington, DC, 2008, US Government Printing Office.

62. Laurson KR, Lee JA, Eisenmann JC: The cumulative impact of physical activity, sleep duration, and television time on adolescent obesity: 2011 Youth Risk Behavior Survey, *J Phys Act Health* 12(3):355–360, 2015.

63. Cameron JD, Maras D, Sigal RJ, et al: The mediating role of energy intake on the relationship between screen time behaviour and body mass index in adolescents with obesity: The HEARTY study, *Appetite* 107:437–444, 2016.

FURTHER READINGS AND RESOURCES

Bruening M, Eisenberg M, MacLehose R, et al: Relationship between adolescents' and their friends' eating behaviors: breakfast, fruit, vegetable, whole-grain, and dairy intake. *J Acad Nutr Diet* 112(10):1608, 2012.

Fewtrell M, Bronsky J, Campoy C, et al: Complementary feeding: a position paper by the European Society for Paediatric Gastroenterology, Hepatology, and Nutrition (ESPGHAN) Committee on Nutrition. *J Pediatr Gastroenterol Nutr* 64(1):119, 2017.

Fletcher A, Bonell C, Sorhaindo A: You are what your friends eat: systematic review of social network analyses of young people's eating behaviours and bodyweight. *J Epidemiol Community Health* 65(6):548, 2011.

Forestell CS: The development of flavor perception and acceptance: the roles of natures and nurture. *Nestle Nutr Inst Workshop Ser* 85:135, 2016.

Howland M, Hunger JM, Mann T: Friends don't let friends eat cookies: effects of restrictive eating norms on consumption among friends. *Appetite* 59(2):505, 2012.

[Adolescents are an important target group for nutrition education. They are highly influenced by their peers and their social networks. Strategies to improve their nutrition and health behaviors may require a multidimensional approach that taps into social structures.]

Kessler HS: Simple interventions to improve health eating behaviors in the school cafeteria. *Nutr Rev* 74(3):198, 2016.

Pedersen S, Gronhoj A, Thogersen J: Following family or friends. Social norms in adolescent healthy eating. *Appetite* 86:54, 2015.

Peralta LR, Dudley DA, Cotton WG: Teaching healthy eating to elementary school students: a scoping review of nutrition education resources. *J Sch Health* 86(5):334, 2016.

Position of the American Dietetic Association: Local support for nutrition integrity in schools. *J Am Diet Assoc* 110(8):1244, 2010.

Position of the Academy of Nutrition and Dietetics: Promoting and supporting breastfeeding. *J Am Diet Assoc* 115(3):444, 2015.

Smith HA, Becker GE: Early additional food and fluids for healthy breastfed full-term infants. *Cochrane Database Syst Rev* 30(8):CD006462, 2016.

Wadhera D, Capaldi Phillips ED, Wilkie LM: Teaching children to like and eat vegetables. *Appetite* 93:75, 2015.

Welker E, Lott M, Story M: The school food environment and obesity prevention: progress over the last decade. *Curr Obes Rep* 5(2):145, 2016.

Witt KE, Dunn C: Increasing fruit and vegetable consumption among preschoolers: evaluation of color me healthy. *J Nutr Educ Behav* 44(2):107, 2012.

[Children attending day care, Head Start, or schools with a breakfast and lunch program receive a major proportion of their meals for the day at that location. This article provides some insight into the role of day care centers and schools in supporting the development of good food habits in children, as well as the role of community health professionals in supporting school food programs in the United States.]

Websites of Interest

- Centers for Disease Control and Prevention: Clinical Growth Charts. https://www.cdc.gov/growthcharts/clinical_charts.htm

- Centers for Disease Control and Prevention, National Center for Chronic Disease Prevention and Health Promotion, Division of Nutrition and Physical Activity. http://www.cdc.gov/nccdphp/dnpa.

- Centers for Disease Control and Prevention, National Center for Health Statistics: *2000 CDC Growth Charts: United States*. http://www.cdc.gov/growthcharts.

- International Lactation Consultant Association. http://www.ilca.org.

- La Leche League International. http://www.llli.org.

- US Department of Agriculture, Food and Nutrition Service, Team Nutrition. http://www.fns.usda.gov/tn/.

- US Department of Agriculture, MyPlate Daily Checklist. http://www.choosemyplate.gov/MyPlate-Daily-Checklist.

- US Department of Agriculture: The MyPlate resource. http://www.choosemyplate.gov.

- US Department of Agriculture, US Department of Health and Human Services, *Dietary Guidelines for Americans*, 2010. http://www.cnpp.usda.gov/dietaryguidelines.htm.

13

Nutrition for Adults: Early, Middle, and Later Years

Eleanor D. Schlenker

ⓔ http://evolve.elsevier.com/Williams/essentials/

This chapter completes our three-chapter sequence on nutrition through the life cycle. After the tumultuous adolescent years come the challenges, opportunities, and concerns of adulthood and maturity. When adolescents come of age, they have three-quarters of their potential years of life still remaining. But the seeds of chronic disease that become apparent in later years are often planted before age 25, a period when risk-taking behaviors and poor attention to diet and positive health habits are commonplace. Yet, public health interventions targeting middle-age and older adults can bring about improvements in health and life expectancy and reduce disease and disability. Although life expectancy continues to rise in the United States, we still fall behind many other countries in projected years of life. As we review the adult life stages—the early, middle, and later years—we will look at individual needs and the role of nutrition in promoting a favorable health advantage.

OUTLINE

ADULTHOOD: CONTINUING GROWTH AND DEVELOPMENT

Adult Development and Aging

The adult years are distinguished by the attainment of optimal function in all body systems and achievement of reproductive capacity. Still, adults continue to grow and develop in various ways. Upon reaching physical maturity, growth marked by increasing numbers of cells and changing body size is halted, and replication, forming new cells to replace old ones, begins. Although the general public holds that aging begins at a certain time in life, such as retirement or when a person begins to "look old," aging encompasses the whole of life as we grow and mature. Two important considerations govern the development and evolution of the physiologic, psychosocial, and nutritional components of life across adulthood:

1. *The individual's genetic makeup:* Gradual aging occurs in all adults, but the *rate* of change is an individual characteristic.
2. *Life history:* Aging is a total life process. Experiences in one stage of life hold importance for well-being in succeeding stages.

Our genes, environment, and lifestyle influence the rate and magnitude of aging changes and progression of chronic disease as we move through the adult years. Even if family history puts us at risk, lifestyle choices and an appropriate food intake enable us to exert some control over our future health and aging. Our cultural and ethnic heritage and accessibility to medical care also influence our long-term health. Each stage of adult life provides the foundation for the one that follows. Harmful health behaviors in the young adult years accelerate physiologic decline, whereas positive lifestyle patterns slow metabolic and physical changes and the progression of any existing disease.

The Nature of Aging

Researchers use the term *aging* to refer to all changes that occur in an individual over time from the moment of conception until death. In the health field, we usually think of aging as those changes that occur later in life and lead to increasing vulnerability, frailty, and risk of death. The term gerontology refers to the study of how and why aging happens, and differs from the term geriatrics, which describes the diseases and medical conditions common to older individuals. Changes in organ systems and the functional decline that occurs with age are controlled by an individual's biologic limits to cell replication, not his age in years. In fact, chronologic age is the least suitable measure of human aging.

KEY TERMS

Replication
To make an exact copy; to repeat, duplicate, or reproduce. In genetics, replication is the process by which double-stranded deoxyribonucleic acid (DNA) makes copies of itself with each separating strand synthesizing a complementary strand. Cell replication is the process by which living cells divide to produce exact copies of themselves.

Gerontology
Study of how and why aging happens.

Geriatrics
Describes the diseases and medical conditions common to older individuals.

Chronologic Age
A person's age in years.

Normal Versus Successful Aging

Experts who study the aging process have defined two types of human aging: normal aging and successful aging. In normal aging, genetic and environmental influences interact to produce degenerative changes in body systems. In successful aging, regressive changes are slowed or prevented by positive lifestyle choices and health interventions. A healthy diet, regular physical activity, a positive mental outlook, appropriate health care, and avoidance of smoking are lifestyle patterns that contribute to successful aging. As we review the food and nutrient intake, lifestyle patterns, and disease risk of young, middle-age, and older adults, consider areas for intervention that will promote successful aging.

ADULT STAGES: YOUNG ADULT (19 TO 40 YEARS)

Physical Characteristics and Lifestyle

After the turbulence of the adolescent years, growth levels off into adult maintenance and stability. The core psychosocial task of the young adult is building relationships outside the core family (Fig. 13.1). Many young adults continue their education or combine classes with full-time or part-time employment. Households are established and individuals may take on the parenting role. With a changing work environment, many find it difficult to meet the expectations of education, work, and family or effectively plan for the future. Young adults ages 18 to 44 are more likely than older adults to feel worried, nervous, or anxious.[1] Some clinicians recommend routine screening in the primary care setting for such risky health behaviors as poor diet, smoking, heavy drinking, and physical inactivity.[2]

Nutritional Needs

The growth patterns of adolescence are strengthened in the adult body. Young men have increased muscle mass and growth in the long bones, and young women develop a greater proportion of subcutaneous fat, genetically intended to support reproduction. Nutritional concerns for the young adult include kilocalories (kcalories or kcal), calcium, iron, and vitamins. Dietary Reference Intakes (DRIs) for adults are found in Tables 13.1 to 13.3):

- *Kcalories:* The Recommended Dietary Allowance (RDA) for sedentary men ages 20 to 40 is estimated to be 2400 kcal, whereas active men in this age range will need 2800 to 3000 kcal.[3] Among women, energy needs range from 1800 to 2000 kcal for those who are sedentary and from 2200 to 2400 kcal for women who are active.[3] Energy needs decrease slightly with each passing decade. Physical activity plays an important role in maintaining energy balance in

FIG. 13.1 The early adult years center on social interaction and building networks outside of family. (Credit: PhotoDisc.)

TABLE 13.1 Dietary Reference Intakes for Energy and Protein for Active Adults[a,b]						
	WEIGHT		**HEIGHT**		**Energy**	**Protein**
Age (years)	kg	lb	cm	in	(kcal)	(g)
Males						
19–30	70	154	177	70	3000	56
31–50	70	154	177	70	2800	56
51–70	70	154	177	70	2600	56
≥71	70	154	177	70	2400	56
Females						
19–30	57	126	163	64	2400	46
31–50	57	126	163	64	2200	46
51–70	57	126	163	64	2000	46
≥71	57	126	163	64	2000	46

[a]Because adults are urged to remain physically active throughout their lives, reference weights remain the same for all adult age categories.
[b]The energy recommendations shown here represent the midpoint of each age range: age 25, age 40, age 60, and age 80. Energy needs in men are expected to decline by 10 kcal per year after the age of 19 and energy needs in women decline by 7 kcal per year.
Data calculated from standards found in Food and Nutrition Board, Institute of Medicine: *Dietary Reference Intakes for energy, carbohydrate, fiber, fat, fatty acids, cholesterol, protein, and amino acids (macronutrients)*, Washington, DC, 2002, National Academies Press, and published in the US Department of Health and Human Services, US Department of Agriculture: *Scientific report of the 2015 Dietary Guidelines Advisory Committee*, Washington, DC, February 2015. https://www.health.gov/dietaryguidelines/2015-scientific-report/.

all adults (Fig. 13.2). Dietary data from the US Department of Agriculture (USDA) indicate the average daily energy intake among US men ages 20 to 30 is approximately 2700 kcal, which over time will lead to weight gain among those with limited physical activity.[4]

- *Protein:* The RDA is 56 g/day for adult men and 46 g/day for adult women,[5] based on an estimated daily need of 0.8 g/kg body weight. Young men are consuming nearly 2 times their RDA, and young women are consuming nearly 1.5 times their RDA.[4]

- *Minerals:* Three minerals—calcium, iron, and potassium—warrant special attention. Young adults need 1000 mg of calcium per day to ensure continued expansion and maintenance of peak bone mass,[6] but only 50% of men and approximately 25% of women in this age group meet the goal,[7] increasing their risk of bone disease and fractures in later life. Iron is a problem for both young men and young women, but for different reasons. Women of childbearing age must offset the iron lost through the menses, making their RDA 18 mg/day,[5] but the mean intake of women ages 20 to 29 is only 13 mg, less than three-fourths the amount needed.[4] In contrast, young men have intakes of nearly 18 mg,[4] more than twice their RDA of 8 mg.[5] Iron intake is closely related to energy intake and the use of fortified cereals, bread, and beef by young men. Fruits and vegetables are major sources of potassium, and low intakes of these foods decrease the supply of this nutrient.[7] Potassium intakes of young men and young women fall well below the DRI.[4,5] Low intakes of potassium coupled with high intakes of sodium likely contribute to the development of hypertension among young adults; 11% of men and 7% of women ages 20 to 34 have high blood pressure.[8]

- *Vitamins:* Vitamin intake is less than optimal in many young adults. Although folate intake from both natural and fortified

TABLE 13.2 Adult Dietary Reference Intakes for Minerals, Electrolytes, and Water

Age (years)	Calcium (mg)	Phosphorus (mg)	Magnesium (mg)	Iron (mg)	Zinc (mg)	Iodine (mcg)	Fluoride (mg)	Potassium (mg)	Sodium (mg)	Water (L/day)
Males										
19–30	1000	700	400	8	11	150	4	4700	1500	3.7
31–50	1000	700	420	8	11	150	4	4700	1500	3.7
51–70	1000	700	420	8	11	150	4	4700	1300	3.7
≥71	1200	700	420	8	11	150	4	4700	1200	3.7
Females										
19–30	1000	700	310	18	8	150	3	4700	1500	2.7
31–50	1000	700	320	18	8	150	3	4700	1500	2.7
51–70	1200	700	320	8	8	150	3	4700	1300	2.7
≥71	1200	700	320	8	8	150	3	4700	1200	2.7

Data from Institute of Medicine, Otten JJ, Hellwig JP, Meyers LD, editors: *Dietary Reference Intakes. The essential guide to nutrient requirements*, Washington, DC, 2006, National Academies Press; Institute of Medicine: *Dietary Reference Intakes for calcium and vitamin D*, Washington, DC, 2011, National Academies Press.

TABLE 13.3 Adult Dietary Reference Intakes for Vitamins

Age (years)	Vitamin A (mcg)	Vitamin D (mcg)	Vitamin E (mg)	Vitamin C (mg)	Thiamin (mg)	Riboflavin (mg)	Niacin (mg NE)	Vitamin B6 (mg)	Folate (mcg)	Vitamin B12 (mcg)
Males										
19–30	900	15	15	90	1.2	1.3	16	1.3	400	2.4
31–50	900	15	15	90	1.2	1.3	16	1.3	400	2.4
51–70	900	15	15	90	1.2	1.3	16	1.7	400	2.4
≥71	900	20	15	90	1.2	1.3	16	1.7	400	2.4
Females										
19–30	700	15	15	75	1.1	1.1	14	1.3	400	2.4
31–50	700	15	15	75	1.1	1.1	14	1.3	400	2.4
51–70	700	15	15	75	1.1	1.1	14	1.5	400	2.4
≥71	700	20	15	75	1.1	1.1	14	1.5	400	2.4

NE, Niacin equivalent.
Data from Institute of Medicine, Otten JJ, Hellwig JP, Meyers LD, editors: *Dietary Reference Intakes. The essential guide to nutrient requirements*, Washington, DC, 2006, National Academies Press; Institute of Medicine: *Dietary Reference Intakes for calcium and vitamin D*, Washington, DC, 2011, National Academies Press.

FIG. 13.2 Energy needs vary according to level of physical activity. (Credit: PhotoDisc.)

sources exceeds the DRI of 400 mcg among certain young women, many do not obtain this amount.[4] Young adults who spend little time in the sun and do not use vitamin D–fortified dairy products or take supplements are low in this vitamin and less able to absorb calcium. Vitamin D status is especially critical in Hispanic and African-American populations because of increased skin pigmentation and lessened ability to synthesize vitamin D.[6]

Food Habits

Restaurant meals at full-service restaurants, fast food and quick-service restaurants, and pizza shops are popular among busy young adults. National surveys indicate that adults ages 20 to 39 consume approximately one-third to one-half of their kcalories in restaurant meals.[9] The work environment also influences the foods consumed and level of physical activity. The availability of sugar-sweetened soft drinks at the workplace and a fast food restaurant within a 5-minute walk or less contributed to a higher rate of obesity.[10] Individuals who found it difficult to obtain healthy food or lacked an opportunity to perform any physical activity in or near the workplace were more likely to be obese (24% in this environment vs. 17% who enjoyed more favorable environments.)[10] In this group of 25-year-olds, 20% ate at a fast food restaurant 3 or more times a week. Sharing meals may be a way to encourage healthier meals in this age group. Young adults who shared meals with others in the same household or with friends had higher intakes of fruits, vegetables, milk, and whole grains.[11] There may be more incentive to prepare a balanced meal if others are eating with you; however, lack of time is a constant barrier to healthful eating for young adults working 40 hours or more per week.

Health and Chronic Disease

Public health leaders are expressing concern about the worsening health profiles of young adults. Risky behaviors such as smoking, low physical activity, and drug and alcohol abuse are not uncommon in this age group.[12] Regrettably, the threat of chronic disease seems remote to an individual with youthful vigor. Unwanted weight gain is also associated with these years. A 10-year follow-up of nearly 2300 young adults, first evaluated as adolescents, found the proportion who were overweight increased from 26% to 52%.[13] The prevalence of overweight was higher among those of lower socioeconomic status who had three or more fast food meals per week, skipped breakfast on most days, and were not meeting recommended levels of physical activity.

Changes in living arrangements and lifestyle associated with new independence make young adults vulnerable to weight gain. However, attitudes and food patterns of a significant other can have positive effects on health behavior. Young women whose significant others practiced positive behaviors were more likely to eat five or more fruits and vegetables daily and complete 3.5 hours of physical activity each week.[14]

The American Heart Association has defined ideal cardiovascular health based on optimal levels of three metabolic factors—blood pressure, blood cholesterol, and blood glucose—along with four behavioral factors—diet, body mass index (BMI), not smoking, and physical activity. Among nearly 6000 men and women with an average age of 36 years, only 1% met all seven criteria.[15] A healthy diet was the criterion most lacking. Fasting glucose met the recommended level among 82% of the group, whereas total blood cholesterol was appropriate in only 62% and blood pressure in only 52%. A healthy dietary intake along with greater physical activity could improve the unfavorable cardiovascular risk profile being recognized in young adults.

ADULT STAGES: MIDDLE ADULT (40 TO 65 YEARS)

Physical Characteristics and Lifestyle

Middle age can bring new challenges and opportunities. Shifts in employment can carry reductions in salary or loss of retirement benefits, wreaking havoc on personal and financial well-being. Some parents experience the "empty nest syndrome" as their children set up their own households, and now have time for their own pursuits, new hobbies, or further education (Fig. 13.3). Others become caregivers to grandchildren or their aging parents. Economic strains are leading to more multigenerational households with parents, their adult children, and grandchildren all living under the same roof.

As individuals move into their 40s, cell replication begins to slow, and men and women start to experience age-related loss of muscle mass, a condition called *sarcopenia*.[16] Although everyone experiences some muscle loss, individuals with low physical activity and inadequate dietary protein lose significant amounts, whereas those practicing strength training lose lesser amounts. The resulting slow but steady decrease in basal metabolic rate (BMR) as active muscle tissue is lost lowers energy needs, adding to the risk of unwanted weight gain.

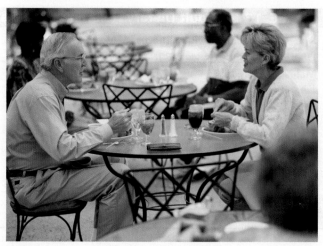

FIG. 13.3 Middle-adult years can be a time for personal growth. (Credit: PhotoDisc.)

Nutritional Needs

Needs for particular nutrients change in the middle adult years (see Tables 13.1 to 13.3), and intake has a critical bearing on chronic disease risk.

- *Kcalories:* Loss of active tissue coupled with a sedentary lifestyle lowers daily energy requirements by an estimated 200 kcal between the ages of 40 and 60,[3] and unless energy intake and activity level are adjusted, body fat will accrue.
- *Minerals:* Calcium intake assumes special importance, particularly for women. Menopause and the loss of estrogen bring about a decrease in calcium absorption and an increase in bone turnover, with a net loss of bone mass and greater risk of fracture. Between ages 51 and 70, the DRI for calcium increases to 1200 mg for women but remains at 1000 mg for men.[6] Optimum intake helps preserve bone mass; however, barely 10% of women ages 51 to 70 are meeting their calcium goal.[7] When the menses cease, iron needs in women drop from 18 to 8 mg, comparable to adult men.[5] Sodium intake declines somewhat in middle age, but 82% of women and 97% of men still exceed the Tolerable Upper Intake Level (UL) of 2300 mg.[7]
- *Vitamins:* The RDA for vitamin D is set at 15 mcg to ensure adequate calcium absorption,[6] but vitamin D continues to be a nutrient of concern. Despite lower milk consumption and more frequent use of sun protection, national surveys indicate increases in vitamin D blood levels among middle age and older individuals.[17] Those authors attribute this improvement in vitamin D status to increased use of vitamin D supplements and possibly more leisure time activities outdoors, but current dietary intake continues to meet barely one-third of the DRI.[4] Vitamin E intake is less than recommended in middle-age adults, despite the need for antioxidant protection as the aging process continues.[4] Vitamin B_6 requirements increase because aging adults use this vitamin less efficiently.[5]

Food Habits

Middle-age adults came to maturity during the early growth of the fast food industry, and, according to a Gallop poll, 44% have at least one meal a week at a fast food restaurant, despite their opinion that "fast food is not good for you."[18] Middle-age adults are also consumers of sugar-sweetened beverages, with men ages 40 to 59 averaging 172 kcal and women 111 kcal per day from this source.[19] Alcohol also adds to the energy intake of both men and

BOX 13.1   Chronic Conditions Reported by Middle-Age Adults

- Hypertension
- Coronary heart disease
- Stroke
- Diabetes
- Cancer
- Arthritis
- Hepatitis
- Kidney dysfunction
- Asthma
- Chronic obstructive pulmonary disease

Modified from Ward BW, Schiller JS, Goodman RA: Multiple chronic conditions among US adults: a 2012 update, *Prev Chronic Dis* 11:E62, 2014.

women. A national survey reported that on drinking days, men had 272 kcal from alcohol and women had 210 kcal; for both genders this equaled approximately 10% of their energy intake for the day.[20]

Intakes of protective foods are less than desirable in this age group. Fewer than one-third of adults ages 45 to 64 consume two or more servings of fruit and three or more servings of vegetables each day. Hispanic and black adults have particularly low intakes of vegetables.[21] Middle-age adults, as compared with young adults, use more dietary supplements, and the supplements being taken reflect new priorities. Multiple vitamin-mineral supplements are used less frequently whereas more adults are using a vitamin D supplement or taking fish oil preparations.[22]

Chronic Disease Risk

The middle adult years hold the key to health in this stage of life and beyond. Those who establish positive health habits as young adults enter their middle years with a minimum of chronic disease. For those who made poor diet and lifestyle choices, cardiovascular disease, diabetes, and cancer are a health risk. Fueled by the obesity epidemic, 31% of persons ages 45 to 64 have one of the chronic conditions noted in Box 13.1, 18% have two, and 14% have three or more. Only 37% have no reportable chronic conditions.[23] Hispanic and Asian persons appear to have a lower incidence of chronic conditions than whites and blacks,[23] although this may reflect a lack of diagnosis rather than the absence of disease. Based on a recent health model, it has been estimated that 45% of deaths from heart disease, stroke, and diabetes are related to dietary characteristics, including high sodium, low nuts/seeds, highly processed meats, low seafood omega-3 fats, low vegetables, low fruits, and high sugar-sweetened beverages.[24] This would reinforce the need for dietary education and intervention among medical patients.

ADULT STAGES: OLDER ADULT (65 TO 85 YEARS)

Aging in America

The first of the baby boomer generation born between 1946 and 1964 have reached and surpassed age 65 and many are facing economic uncertainty and spiraling health care costs. As the older population grows, their influence on our society will continue to mount. The young and middle-age adults that we discussed earlier in this chapter will comprise the older population of 2030 and beyond.

Following are some personal characteristics of the older population and their potential impact on health and nutrition services:

- *Increase in life expectancy*: Life expectancy is a general measure of the overall health of a population.[25] Over the past century, life expectancy at birth rose significantly based on improved sanitation, the discovery of antibiotics, and higher standards of living. Better prevention and treatment of heart disease, cancer, chronic lower respiratory diseases, and stroke, the most common causes of death in persons age 65 and older, has contributed to longer life expectancies. Sixty-five-year-olds can expect to live another 19 years, and 85-year-olds another 6 to 7 years.[25] The 85-and-older group are the fastest-growing age cohort in the United States.

- *Ethnic and racial diversity*: Currently, 78% of the population older than 64 years is white, but this will change. By 2060, 43% of the older US population will be Asian, Hispanic, or black.[25] Nutrition education programs and meal services will need to adjust to different customs, food patterns, and family roles. Growing diversity is also promoting greater interest in complementary and alternative medicine (CAM). (See the Focus on Culture box, "Cultural and Ethnic Differences in Health Practices" for related discussion.)

- *Education*: Eighty-four percent of older adults have completed high school, and 27% have a bachelor's degree or higher[25]; however, older racial and ethnic groups differ widely in levels of education. Only 54% of older Hispanic adults, 75% of older black adults, and 74% of older Asians completed high school, compared with 89% of older whites.[25] Limited ability to read or understand labels on food or medications interferes with appropriate self-care.

- *Income*: Approximately 10% of people ages 65 and older have incomes below the poverty line, and another 23% are low income, falling within 199% of the poverty threshold. However, race and ethnicity are also related to poverty. Black, Hispanic, and Asian older adults are more likely to fall below the poverty line, and older women have lower incomes than older men. Persons over age 74 are more likely to be poor.[25]

- *Living arrangements*: Because women live longer, more older women are widowed and more older men live with a spouse. Thirty-six percent of older women live alone, compared with only 20% of older men.[25] Older single Asian, Hispanic, and black women are more likely to live with other family members, as compared with older, single white women who are more likely to live alone. Only 3.9% of individuals older than 64 years reside in institutional settings, although this rises to 14.7% among those older than 84 years.[25] Older men and women who live alone often have lower incomes and less money to spend on food. They also lack help with meal preparation and may have no support on sick days.

- *Physical disability*: As individuals age, they decline in health, develop physical limitations, and require more health and community services. Chronic diseases such as heart disease, stroke, cancer, and diabetes negatively affect quality of life and contribute to decline in function and the ability to remain independent.[25] Individuals who are unable to stoop, reach over their heads, or lift 10 lb will have difficulty shopping for groceries, preparing meals, or performing housekeeping tasks. Assistance from family members or community service agencies will be required for them to remain in their own homes (Fig. 13.4).

KEY TERM

Life Expectancy
The number of years a person of a given age, gender, race, or ethnic group can expect to live.

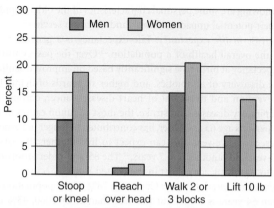

FIG. 13.4 Percent of persons ages 65 and older who require help to perform these tasks. These capabilities are necessary for remaining independent in the community. (Data from Federal Interagency Forum on Aging-Related Statistics: *Older Americans 2012: key indicators of well-being,* Washington, DC, 2012, US Government Printing Office.)

Physiologic Changes in Older Adults

Over time the passage of years brings a gradual waning of physical vigor, work capacity, and strength in the older adult. Physical changes are often minimal immediately following retirement but become more pronounced as individuals move through their 70s and 80s. Lifestyle choices, disease history, and environmental hazards coupled with each person's unique set of genes determine the rate and severity of age-related changes. As a result, older people of the same age are less alike than younger people of the same age, because each has experienced a different set of genetic and environmental influences.

Some individuals are physically old at age 50, whereas others maintain an active pace into their 80s or 90s. All age groups are susceptible to illness and disease, but in younger adults it is more likely an acute problem that runs its course in a few days or weeks. Conditions common to older adults are usually chronic and over time impose limitations on daily activities and lifestyle.

All older adults experience ongoing changes in major organ systems. Physiologic changes that influence nutrient utilization and nutritional status are summarized in the following sections.

Body Composition

Over time, muscle loss affects functional capacity, with the potential loss of independence; reduction in bone mass adds to the risk of fracture. Even if body weight remains unchanged, the older adult has proportionately more fat, making BMI a less reliable estimate in the older adult.[26] Body fat also changes position, moving from the extremities to the trunk, especially the abdomen. This too has implications for health as abdominal fat releases excessive amounts of fatty acids, raising blood lipid and blood insulin levels.

Although some older adults experience weight gain, others experience malnutrition and undergo progressive weight loss, leading to frailty, disability, and increasing mortality risk.[27]

Cardiovascular System

Changes in the heart and vascular system lessen their ability to deliver nutrients and oxygen to working tissues, and remove accumulated waste. The heart weakens as a pump and is less able to respond to increased demands for oxygen during strenuous physical exercise, emotional stress, or acute illness. A drop in the amount of blood pumped with each stroke reduces the blood supply to major organs such as the kidney and lungs. Major arteries, including those that deliver nutrients

---

⊕ FOCUS ON CULTURE

Cultural and Ethnic Differences in Health Practices

Health beliefs and practices often spring from our cultural and ethnic backgrounds. The word *health* was derived from an Anglo-Saxon word meaning *wholeness*, or the interaction of the mind and body in reaching a state of well-being.[1] Many cultures believe that bringing our physical and spiritual beings in harmony with nature is the means to achieving health. In contrast, mainstream medical practices build on biomedicine, applying the sciences of biology, biochemistry, and physiology to the study and treatment of human diseases. Nonconventional approaches used outside of Western medical practice are referred to as alternative health approaches. When used in conjunction with mainstream medical practice, they are referred to as complementary approaches. In general, most individuals who favor alternative procedures use them together with conventional treatment. Many mainstream medical centers are combining alternative and conventional approaches to form what has come to be known as integrative medicine.[2]

The general categories of complementary medicine recognized by the National Center for Complementary and Integrative Health of the National Institutes of Health include *natural products* such as herbs, vitamins, minerals, and probiotics, commonly sold as dietary supplements, and *mind and body practices* such as acupuncture, meditation, massage therapy, yoga, or tai chi.[2] Other complementary approaches include ayurvedic and traditional Chinese medicine which has evolved from ancient times. *Ayur* means longevity and *veda* means knowledge of; this system of medicine uses diet, herbal remedies, and meditation to realign the mind, body, and soul. Ayurvedic botanical remedies used to treat digestive disorders, heart problems, diabetes, and urinary tract disorders were the foundation for many of the drugs currently used in mainstream medicine today.

Many home remedies that make use of herbs and plants have been passed down from generation to generation. Teas made from yellow root or sassafras or ginger are used to relieve stomach distress, and herbal teas prepared from peppermint, chamomile, parsley, and wormwood are used to relieve diarrhea. Tonics made from eggnog or malt are expected to stimulate the appetite or build strength in pale children or pregnant and postpartum women. However, certain alternative practices are hazardous. Preparations containing mercury or lead, brought into the United States from other countries, adversely affect fetal neurodevelopment and can lead to miscarriage or premature birth if consumed during pregnancy.[3]

It is important to know not only what health strategies your patients are observing but also the source of their attitudes and beliefs. Effective approaches combine the strengths of conventional and complementary therapies.

Bibliography

1. Kittler PG, Sucher KP, Nahikian-Nelms M: *Food and culture,* ed 6, Belmont CA, 2012, Wadsworth/Cengage Learning.
2. US Department of Health and Human Services, National Center for Complementary and Integrative Health: *Complementary, alternative, or integrative health: What's in a name?* https://www.nccih.nih.gov/health/integrative-health.
3. Center for Disease Control and Prevention: Lead poisoning in pregnant women who used ayurvedic medications from India—New York City, 2011-2012. *MMWR Morb Mortal Wkly Rep* 61(33):641, 2012.

to the heart muscle itself, stiffen and narrow with atherosclerotic deposition. This stiffening limits arterial stretch when blood is delivered and contributes to the rise in blood pressure common in older age.[28]

Renal System

Aging kidneys are less efficient and require more time to clear waste products from the blood. Urine cannot be concentrated to the same extent; thus increased fluid is required to excrete a given amount of waste. This is why older people receiving high-protein supplements—which produce large amounts of nitrogen-containing waste—require a liberal fluid intake. Fluid balance in aging individuals is poorly regulated at very high or very low intakes of water and sodium.[28]

Respiratory System

The alveoli or air sacs in the aging lung become less elastic, making it more difficult to move air in and out. Other changes in the air sacs reduce the available surface area for exchange of oxygen and carbon dioxide. Widening areas of the lungs no longer participate in gas exchange, and this "dead space" is susceptible to the growth of pathogens, making older persons more vulnerable to upper respiratory conditions and pneumonia. Smoking and air pollution contribute to loss of lung function and a reduced supply of oxygen for normal activity and periods of stress.[28]

Gastrointestinal System

Gastrointestinal changes influence secretions, muscles, and the neural system involved in the digestion of food. Loss of gastric acid interferes with the absorption of vitamin B_{12} and reduces uptake of thiamin, folate, calcium, and iron.[5,6] Changes in neural and muscle function contribute to constipation in frail older adults by increasing the time needed for food to pass through the lower digestive tract. Changes in gastric control systems sometimes result in "early satiety," seriously limiting the amount of food ingested by the older individual, with subsequent malnutrition and weight loss.

Nutritional Requirements

The National Academy of Medicine (formerly the Institute of Medicine) has established two DRI age categories for people older than 50 years[5]: (1) ages 51 to 70; (2) ages 71 and older.

These two categories address the physiologic changes that continue to develop in most people as aging continues. Nutrient absorption and utilization become less efficient, and this is especially apparent in times of illness or stress. Nutrient stores undergo rapid loss and are difficult to replace. Medications can interfere with both food intake and its nutritional benefit. Moreover, at this time we know very little about the interaction between the aging process and chronic disease or how they influence nutritional needs, especially in persons age 85 and older. (See Tables 13.1 to 13.3 to review the DRIs for these age groups.)

Energy and Macronutrients

- *Kcalories:* Energy intake continues to decline from middle to older age, with loss of active tissue and decreased physical activity. The average energy intake of American women drops from 1779 kcal at ages 50 to 59 to 1604 kcal at age 70 and older. In American men, kcalories decrease from approximately 2500 kcal to 2022 kcal in these age groups.[4] Physically active individuals older than 70 will need additional kcalories to support their increased energy expenditure.[3] Measurements of energy expenditure in community-living older adults at age 75 and again at age 82 indicated that both resting metabolic rate (reflective of fat-free mass) and activity level dropped over the intervening years, especially among the men.[29] To develop an understanding of changes in energy needs in very

elderly adults, it will be necessary to undertake repeated measurements in the same individuals.
- *Carbohydrates:* Persons of all ages should obtain 45%–65% of their total energy from carbohydrates, with an emphasis on complex carbohydrates.[5] Diets rich in fiber lessen the need for laxatives in the older adult, and their potential for electrolyte disruption. Complex carbohydrates in vegetables, legumes, and whole grains also help modulate postprandial blood glucose levels.
- *Fats:* Fat intake within the range of 20% to 35% of total kcalories[5] balances the need for essential fatty acids with the disease risk associated with high fat diets. Obtaining more kcalories from healthy fats can help prevent weight loss in frail older adults or restore weight that was lost. Fats are generally well digested and absorbed at older ages, although digestion may be slowed; dividing fat intake among all meals and snacks enhances digestion and utilization.

Protein

- *Protein:* The RDA for protein is set at 0.8 g/kg body weight for younger and older adults[5]; however, this standard remains controversial. The DRI expert committee concluded that healthy older adults use protein as efficiently as healthy younger adults and therefore have no increased need for this nutrient. However, evaluations of protein needs in men and women ranging from ages 65 to 80 and older indicate that intakes of 1.0 to 1.25 g/kg body weight are needed to support nutritional well-being and prevent age-related muscle loss. This is especially true for those with a sedentary lifestyle or increased bed rest.[30-32] Frail or chronically ill elderly or those recovering from surgery or acute illness may require as much as 1.2 to 1.5 g/kg for optimal recovery. For strength training, an intake of 1.2 g/kg body weight or greater is optimum to support muscle building. These protein levels are considered appropriate for all older adults, with the exception of those with severe kidney impairment who require individualized recommendations.[31] It is also best that older adults divide their protein across the day, consuming 25 to 30 g at each meal to ensure maximum utilization of amino acids for muscle building and repair.[16]

Minerals and Electrolytes

- *Calcium:* The calcium DRI for men older than 70 rises from 1000 to 1200 mg as a strategy to reduce bone loss and bone fracture.[6] The recommended intake for women increased from 1000 to 1200 mg at age 51 and continues at this level. Fluid milk, fortified soy milk, fortified juices, and fortified yogurt will supply vitamin D along with calcium.
- *Iron:* Following menopause, the iron requirement of women drops to 8 mg/day, the equivalent of adult men.[5] Iron supplements for both genders are inappropriate unless the individual is being treated for iron deficiency anemia and supplementation is supervised by a physician. In older adults, anemia is more likely related to vitamin B_{12} deficiency or chronic disease than to iron deficiency. (See Chapter 7 for discussion of nutritional anemias.)
- *Potassium:* Various diuretics commonly prescribed for older adults bring about urinary potassium losses that must be replenished by diet. The Adequate Intake (AI) for potassium (4700 mg) can be accomplished with five to nine daily servings of fruits and vegetables.[5] Potassium supplements should be avoided unless recommended and supervised by a physician.
- *Sodium:* Daily intakes should be limited to 2300 mg or less[5] to avoid fluid retention or rise in blood pressure. Meeting this limitation can be difficult for frail older adults who depend on heat-and-serve foods, often high in sodium-containing additives.

Vitamins

- *Folate:* Optimum folate helps prevent a rise in blood homocysteine levels that damage blood vessels and accelerate atherosclerosis.[5]
- *Vitamin B6:* As an active coenzyme in protein synthesis, vitamin B6 is important to the preservation of muscle mass. Vitamin B6 is stored and metabolized mainly in muscle,[5] so the sarcopenia of aging likely changes the body's handling of this nutrient.
- *Vitamin B12:* Age-related decreases in gastric acid hinder the release of vitamin B12 from animal protein foods. Vitamin B12–fortified breads and cereals and juices or vitamin B12 supplements can supply the amount needed to avoid deficiency and prevent megaloblastic anemia and changes in cognitive function.[5]
- *Vitamin D:* To ensure adequate vitamin D levels despite reduced sun exposure and skin synthesis, the RDA increases from 15 mcg (600 IU) for those ages 51 to 70 to 20 mcg (800 IU) for persons beyond age 70.[6] Older individuals who spend most of their time indoors will need vitamin D–fortified foods or supplements. Older adults living in the community were found to obtain on average 350 IU or 40% of their DRI for vitamin D from supplements.[33]

Fluids

Dehydration is a concern for healthy and chronically ill older adults.[34,35] Physiologic changes, effects of disease, medications, and environmental circumstances predispose older people to inadequate fluid intake (Box 13.2). Changes in the hypothalamus alter the thirst mechanism such that older persons do not get thirsty and drink when or as much as they should, and aging kidneys are less able to conserve water to compensate for lower intake. Changes in total body water influence the dilution of medications. Dehydration affects alertness and cognitive function. A geriatric clinician recommends a daily intake of 1.2 to 2 L of fluid for women and 1.2 to 3 L for men[35]; note that these recommendations are slightly higher than the DRI recommendations for the general adult population (see Chapter 7). The general recommendation of 1500 mL/day escalates when outdoor or indoor temperatures rise. Daily fluid needs increase in patients with fever. Individuals suffering from heart disease, renal disease, or respiratory conditions are at elevated risk of dehydration in an overheated environment. At the other extreme, older adults are at risk of overhydration (water intoxication) when fluid intakes are inappropriately high, because excess water is less efficiently excreted.

Older persons and their caregivers should monitor their fluid intake and be alert to signs of dehydration. In long-term care facilities,

---

KEY TERM

Cognitive
Pertaining to mental processes such as memory, judgment, and reasoning.

BOX 13.2 Risk Factors for Dehydration in Older Adults

- Advanced age (85 years and older)
- Loss of thirst sensation
- Problems with mobility
- Confusion or cognitive changes
- Problems in swallowing
- Medications promoting fluid loss (diuretics, laxatives)
- Incontinence leading to self-imposed fluid restriction

Modified from Ferry M: Strategies for ensuring good hydration in the elderly, *Nutr Rev* 63(Suppl 6):S22, 2005. Copyright 2005 International Life Sciences Institute.

---

responsibility for overseeing fluid intake must be assigned and those responsible must be held accountable.

Influences on Food Intake

Many physical, social, and environmental influences relating to the individual and the community converge to support the health and quality of life of older adults. Personal characteristics relating to health, relationships, and economic situation, as well as community resources such as transportation to the grocery store, safe neighborhoods for walking, or available meal programs influence nutritional and physical well-being. Various conditions and situations described next adversely affect food intake in aging adults.

- *Changes in the mouth and esophagus:* Periodontal disease, tooth loss, and poorly fitting dentures (or no dentures) make chewing and eating painful and difficult. Those with few or no teeth consume fewer portions of fruits and vegetables and more soft carbohydrate foods.[34,36] Losses in taste, smell, or sight take away from the enjoyment of eating and influence appetite. As noted in Chapter 2, changes in salivary secretion resulting in xerostomia (dry mouth) make eating and swallowing troublesome. Radiation treatment or stroke damaging the nerves in the head and neck, or complications of diabetes and Parkinson disease interfere with the swallowing reflex and cause fear of choking. Aging changes in the appetite control center of the hypothalamus reduce food intake. (The Case Study box, "An Older Woman Living Alone," provides an example of these problems.)
- *Multiple medications:* Treatment regimens involving multiple drugs (polypharmacy) often lower food intake by producing anorexia, nausea, or unpleasant tastes. Other prescription medications increase appetite, stimulating higher food intake than is desirable. (Nutrient-medication interactions are discussed further in Chapter 18.)
- *Psychosocial distress:* Emotional loss arising from the death of a spouse, physical separation from family and friends, or fear for the future can result in depression and disinterest in food. Older African Americans who expressed a high level of dissatisfaction with their lives had poorer diets, higher in fat and lower in fruits and vegetables; however, social support at mealtime appeared to overcome this disadvantage and improve overall food intake.[37] Older patients with clinically diagnosed depression were found to have poorer diets than those otherwise similar in age, gender, education, chronic disease, and alcohol intake.[38] Older persons living or eating alone, especially men who were unaccustomed to preparing food, may not go to the trouble of planning and cooking a meal and place themselves at nutritional risk. Alcohol sometimes displaces food in the diet. Distorted body image with self-imposed food restriction (anorexia nervosa) occurs in older women and men.
- *Economic problems:* Older adults living in poverty often lack the resources to purchase the quality and quantity of food they should have. Older adults with annual incomes less than $12,000 were more likely to have diets based on fried foods, starchy vegetables, and refined grains.[39] Low-income older adults registering for home-delivered meals were found to have energy intakes only 83% of that recommended.[40] Inadequate housing with nonworking appliances or single room occupancy with no access to food storage or preparation facilities put older individuals at risk.
- *Chronic illness and disability:* Food shopping and meal preparation are difficult or impossible for persons who use a cane or walker, have vision loss, or no longer drive. Those who depend on others for transportation and shop irregularly are often limited in fresh fruits and vegetables and fluid milk. Inappropriately restrictive diets that forbid favorite ethnic or comfort foods lower food intake. Chronic conditions such as diabetes, with growing financial obligations for testing supplies or medications, worsen food insecurity.

An Older Woman Living Alone

Miss E is 81 years old and lives in public housing. Her apartment kitchen has a two-unit cook top and a small refrigerator but very little storage space. She prepares and eats all her meals alone. She has always enjoyed mealtime but now has trouble with food sticking in her throat, so she cooks her food until it is very soft and seldom eats meat. She is very tired much of the time; on days when she is not well enough to fix a meal, she depends on cereal and milk. She likes fruits and vegetables but always buys canned varieties because they are easier to swallow and cost less than fresh or frozen. Miss E shops at a supermarket a half mile from her home. It had been her custom to walk to the market and take the bus home, but it is becoming more difficult to walk, so she rides both ways. She makes the trip twice a week so that she has fewer items to carry at one time. Because she has always liked to walk, Miss E maintained a healthy body weight, but recently she has been losing weight and now worries about her health. She wonders if she should be taking a vitamin or mineral supplement to increase her energy level.

Questions for Analysis

1. What physical changes are influencing Miss E's food intake?
2. What socioeconomic or psychologic changes may be affecting her food intake?
3. Which nutrients are likely to be low in her diet? Why?
4. What might be causing her tiredness?
5. What are your general concerns about Miss E's physical condition? What are the implications of her recent weight loss?
6. Would you recommend that Miss E begin to take a vitamin or mineral supplement? If so, then what might she take? Justify your recommendation.

OLDER ADULTS AT NUTRITIONAL RISK

Frail and chronically ill older adults are vulnerable to declining nutritional status and increasing disability. Caregivers must be alert to developing problems and initiate early intervention to interrupt the progression of a downhill spiral that will be difficult or impossible to reverse.

Inability to Independently Perform Food-Related Activities

Physical disability occurs at all ages as a result of accident, injury, disease condition, or developmental injury, but the majority of individuals with physical limitations are age 65 or older, and problems accelerate with age. Medical conditions associated with functional or cognitive loss include the following:

- *Cardiovascular disease:* Congestive heart failure that results in an inadequate supply of oxygen to muscles, including the heart muscle, limits general movement and self-care.
- *Pulmonary disease:* Chronic obstructive pulmonary disease (COPD) and emphysema cause changes in the alveoli; less air flows in and out of the lungs and breathing becomes difficult.
- *Musculoskeletal disease:* Rheumatoid arthritis is an autoimmune disorder affecting joints in the hands, arms, and feet. Such loss of movement can restrict food shopping, meal preparation, and, in severe cases, self-feeding. Osteoarthritis (degenerative joint disease) limits flexibility in hand motion and makes walking and standing difficult and painful. Osteoporosis and subsequent hip fracture often confine the individual to a wheelchair, with potential loss of independence and institutionalization.
- *Neuromuscular disease:* A cerebrovascular accident (stroke) can result in irreversible paralysis and loss of movement or uncontrolled movement, presenting problems with speech, walking, self-feeding, and self-care. Individuals with cerebral palsy and spina bifida may

have similar problems in self-care, depending on the seriousness of their condition.

- *Progressive neurologic disorders:* Individuals with advancing Parkinson disease who have joint rigidity, body stiffness, and tremors find meal preparation and self-feeding difficult. Multiple sclerosis, myasthenia gravis, and Alzheimer disease are other examples of neurologic disorders that affect food-related activities. (These medical conditions are discussed in greater detail in Part 3, "An Introduction to Clinical Nutrition.")

Chronic conditions with associated disability often require adaptations that may include assistive devices for self-feeding. The ability to self-feed has implications for physical and emotional well-being. Anger, frustration, fear, and a sense of grief can accompany the loss of this fundamental skill. Adequate time to be fed, coupled with the concept of protected meal times, free from interruptions, adds to patient satisfaction and increased food intake.[41] A variety of assistive devices can be purchased or fashioned at little or no cost to help persons with limited range of motion or poor grasp self-feed (Fig. 13.5). (Activity scales used to assess an individual's ability to perform self-care and self-feeding or other tasks related to independent living are described in the Perspectives in Practice box, "Community-Based Long-Term Care: Alternative to Institutionalization")

FIG. 13.5 Various small and inexpensive aids will assist individuals with disabilities in self-feeding. (A) Utensil adaptations help with length, grasp, and range of motion. (B) Plate guards and scoop bowls provide an edge to help place food on the utensil. (From Olson DA, DeRuyter F: *Clinician's guide to assistive technology,* St Louis, 2002, Mosby.)

Community-Based Long-Term Care: Alternative to Institutionalization

At one time, *long-term care* referred to medical, social, or personal services provided to individuals in skilled nursing homes or other resident facilities. Older adults who needed help with daily tasks that could not be provided by family members moved from their homes to a care facility. Currently we emphasize community-based long-term care, initiating support services that will enable older adults to remain in their own homes or with family members. The first step is evaluating the individual's functional and cognitive capabilities that determine a safe and appropriate level of care. Two evaluation scales used to assess an individual's ability to remain independent are the activities of daily living (ADLs) and the instrumental activities of daily living (IADLs).

The ADLs as listed next focus on a person's ability to manage personal care either independently, with some level of help, or not at all:

- Bathing
- Dressing
- Feeding
- Using the toilet
- Transferring between bed and chair

An older adult requiring assistance with personal care may be able to remain in the community if family, paid caregivers, or both are available on a daily basis to provide the help needed.

The IADLs as listed next evaluate an individual's ability to perform meal and housekeeping tasks and other chores required for independent living:

- Preparing meals
- Performing housecleaning chores
- Handling money and balancing a checkbook
- Shopping without help
- Using the telephone
- Leaving home without help

A person able to perform some, if not all, of these tasks may still remain independent if food-related services such as grocery shopping or home-delivered meals can be established.

Evaluations using the ADLs or IADLs are usually performed by a health professional or trained social worker. This may occur at discharge planning after a hospitalization or convalescence. Evaluations can also be requested by family members or health or social service professionals working with the older adult. Ongoing review is provided by a designated case manager who serves as the gatekeeper for professional and support services; he or she monitors any changes in physical or cognitive abilities that require an adjustment in services or level of independence that can be sustained.

Bibliography

Federal Interagency Forum on Aging-Related Statistics: *Older Americans 2016: key indicators of well-being*, Washington, DC, 2016, US Government Printing Office.

Development of Overt Malnutrition

Inadequate intakes of kcalories and protein have been identified in many older adults. For reasonably healthy older adults, energy needs range from 1600 to 2000 kcal for women and 2000 to 2600 kcal for men, depending on lean body mass and level of physical activity.[3] However, many at-risk older adults take in less than these amounts. In a recent national survey,[7] 25% of those older than 70 were found to be taking in fewer than 1250 kcal per day and 10% were taking in less than 1050 kcal.[7] Older adults admitted to a Veterans Affairs facility had energy intakes prior to admission as low as 62% of calculated needs.[42] Inappropriately low kcalorie intake adds to muscle weakness and frailty, compounded when dietary protein must be used for energy. Common chronic conditions such as cancer, cardiac failure, and COPD increase energy needs. In addition, older adults are less able to regulate their energy intake to compensate for day-to-day fluctuations, so temporary reductions in food intake as a result of illness or limited food availability can become the norm, with fewer kcalories consumed and progressive weight loss.[43]

Protein-energy malnutrition occurs in older adults living at home or in long-term care facilities or in the hospital. Among older patients admitted for recuperative care, only 19% were meeting their protein requirement and 41% were taking in less than half their protein DRI, which contributed to their physical deterioration.[42] To ensure an ongoing supply of amino acids for tissue building and maintenance, older adults should be encouraged to spread their protein across all meals.[16] Although the Acceptable Macronutrient Distribution Range (AMDR) for protein is 10% to 35% of total kcalories,[5] intakes at the higher end are best for older adults who consume limited kcalories.

Underweight is a serious condition in older adults; women in their 60s with a BMI less than 18.5 have a mortality risk 2 to 3 times greater than their normal-weight counterparts of similar race and ethnicity,[44] and hospitalized underweight persons have longer stays and greater risk of rehospitalization following discharge.[45] Physicians recommend that older adults maintain a BMI between 22 and 27.[46]

Failure to thrive, a syndrome recognized in young children, has also been identified in older individuals and is characterized by low food intake, unintentional and excessive loss of weight, loss of physical function, and reduced cognitive capacity. Ensuring a sufficient intake of kcalories and protein is key to continued physical and mental well-being.

Chronic Disease and Malnutrition

Medical conditions accentuate the risk of malnutrition. Immune factors called *cytokines*, released in response to chronic disease or tissue injury, not only lower food intake but also interfere with the utilization of available nutrients so that even aggressive efforts at nutrition intervention cannot always reverse the continuing weight loss. Congestive heart failure and cancer cause profound anorexia and wasting, referred to as *cardiac* and *cancer cachexia*. Undernutrition in the aging adult lowers immune function, slows production of red blood cells, and accelerates muscle loss.

Nutrition Screening

Nutrition screening identifies warning signs of malnutrition that initiate a downhill spiral leading to future disability and loss of independence. Nutrition screening takes place in hospitals, long-term care facilities, and the community to seek out older adults at nutritional risk. The Self MNA (Mini Nutritional Assessment for Adults 65 Years of Age and Older) (Fig. 13.6) consists of seven questions that point to inadequate nutrient intake and projected weight loss. It is useful in senior centers, congregate meal sites, physicians' offices, home health

> **KEY TERM**
>
> **Failure to Thrive**
> A syndrome described in older adults that is characterized by loss of body weight and deterioration in physical and cognitive function, and usually caused by inadequate food intake.

Nestlé
Nutrition Institute

Self MNA®
Mini Nutritional Assessment
For Adults 65 years of Age and Older

Last name: _____

First name: _____

Date: _____

Age: _____

Complete the screen by filling in the boxes with the appropriate numbers. Total the numbers for the final screening score.

Screening

A Has your food intake declined over the past 3 months? [ENTER ONE NUMBER]
Please enter the most appropriate number (0, 1, or 2) in the box to the right.

0 = severe decrease in food intake
1 = moderate decrease in food intake
2 = no decrease in food intake

☐

B How much weight have you lost in the past 3 months? [ENTER ONE NUMBER]
Please enter the most appropriate number (0, 1, 2, or 3) in the box to the right.

0 = weight loss greater than 7 pounds
1 = do not know the amount of weight lost
2 = weight loss between 2 and 7 pounds
3 = no weight loss or weight loss less than 2 pounds

☐

C How would you describe your current mobility? [ENTER ONE NUMBER]
Please enter the most appropriate number (0, 1, or 2) in the box to the right.

0 = unable to get out of a bed, a chair, or a wheelchair without the assistance of another person
1 = able to get out of a bed or a chair, but unable to go out of my home
2 = able to leave my home

☐

D Have you been stressed or severely ill in the past 3 months? [ENTER ONE NUMBER]
Please enter the most appropriate number (0 or 2) in the box to the right.

0 = yes
2 = no

☐

E Are you currently experiencing dementia and/or prolonged severe sadness? [ENTER ONE NUMBER]
Please enter the most appropriate number (0, 1, or 2) in the box to the right.

0 = yes, severe dementia and/or prolonged severe sadness
1 = yes, mild dementia, but no prolonged severe sadness
2 = neither dementia nor prolonged severe sadness

☐

Please total all of the numbers you entered in the boxes for questions A-E and write that number here:

☐

FIG. 13.6 Self-MNA Mini Nutritional Assessment *for Adults 65 years of Age and Older.* The *SELF-MNA (Mini Nutritional Assessment)* is a checklist to identify those older individuals in the community who are at nutritional risk. Forms and updates can be accessed at http://www.mna-elderly.com. (Reprinted with the permission of the Société des Produits Nestlé S.A., Vevey, Switzerland, Self-MNA®. All rights reserved. http://www.mna-elderly.com/mna_forms.html)

Continued

Now, please CHOOSE ONE of the following two questions – F1 or F2 – to answer.

Question F1

Height (feet & inches)	Body Weight (pounds)			
4'10"	Less than 91	91-99	100-109	110 or more
4'11"	Less than 94	94-103	104-113	114 or more
5'0"	Less than 97	97-106	107-117	118 or more
5'1"	Less than 100	100-110	111-121	122 or more
5'2"	Less than 104	104-114	115-125	126 or more
5'3"	Less than 107	107-117	118-129	130 or more
5'4"	Less than 110	110-121	122-133	134 or more
5'5"	Less than 114	114-125	126-137	138 or more
5'6"	Less than 118	118-129	130-141	142 or more
5'7"	Less than 121	121-133	134-145	146 or more
5'8"	Less than 125	125-137	138-150	151 or more
5'9"	Less than 128	128-141	142-154	155 or more
5'10"	Less than 132	132-145	146-159	160 or more
5'11"	Less than 136	136-149	150-164	165 or more
6'0"	Less than 140	140-153	154-168	169 or more
6'1"	Less than 144	144-158	159-173	174 or more
6'2"	Less than 148	148-162	163-178	179 or more
6'3"	Less than 152	152-167	168-183	184 or more
6'4"	Less than 156	156-171	172-188	189 or more
Group	**0**	**1**	**2**	**3**

Please refer to the chart on the left and follow these instructions:

1. Find your height on the left-hand column of the chart.

2. Go across that row and circle the range that your weight falls into.

3. Look to the bottom of the chart to find what group number (0, 1, 2, or 3) your circled weight range falls into.

Write the Group Number (0, 1, 2, or 3) here: ☐

Write sum of questions A-E (from page 1) here: ☐

Lastly, calculate the sum of these 2 numbers: ☐

Question F2   DO NOT ANSWER QUESTION F2 IF QUESTION F1 IS ALREADY COMPLETED.

Measure the circumference of your LEFT calf by following the instructions below:

Loop a tape measure all the way around your calf to measure its size.

Record the measurement in inches: _____

If Less than 12 inches, enter "0" in box to the right.

If 12 inches or Greater, enter "3" in box to the right.

☐

© SIGVARIS

Write the sum of questions A-E (from page 1) here: ☐

Lastly, calculate the sum of these 2 numbers: ☐

Screening Score 14 points maximum

12 – 14 points:	Normal nutritional status
8 – 11 points:	At risk of malnutrition
0 – 7 points:	Malnourished

☐

If you score between 0 - 11, please take this form to a healthcare professional for consultation.

FIG. 13.6, cont'd

BOX 13.3 Nutrition Alerts for Older Adults in Long-Term Care

- Involuntary loss of 5% of body weight in 1 month or 10% in 6 months
- Leaving 25% or more of served food uneaten over the past 7 days
- Body mass index ≤21

Modified from Thomas DR, Ashmen W, Morley JE, et al: Nutritional management in long-term care: development of a clinical guideline, *J Gerontol A Biol Sci Med Sci* 55A(12):M725, 2000.

programs, and home-delivered meals programs. Nutrition screening prompts the initiation of intervention strategies to prevent the progression to overt malnutrition. A set of warning signs for use with residents in long-term care facilities is found in Box 13.3.

Community Food Assistance Programs for Older Americans

Several public food assistance programs help older adults meet their food needs. The Supplemental Nutrition Assistance Program (SNAP) extends food-buying power, making food more accessible to adults with limited resources. However, the program having the greatest impact on the nutritional health of older Americans is the national Elderly Nutrition Program, which provides congregate and home-delivered meals to people age 60 and older. (For more information on these programs, see Appendix D.)

Nutrient Supplementation

Healthy older adults who consume a variety of foods, including fortified foods, and meet their DRI for energy and protein are unlikely to require nutrient supplements. However, those with low energy intakes and chronic health problems could benefit from prudent supplementation. Multiple medications, a limited variety of foods, isolation, and little social support put individuals at risk for nutrient deficiency. Nutrient supplements help replenish body stores after critical or debilitating illness.

Decisions relating to nutrient supplementation require an individual assessment and supervision by a health care professional. Individuals who use single-nutrient supplements in addition to multivitamin-multimineral supplements are most at risk for exceeding the UL for one or more nutrients or precipitating dangerous interactions. An evaluation of dietary intake along with biochemical parameters of nutritional status, if available, should provide the basis for any supplement recommendation. Nutritional supplements should add to food, not replace it.

HEALTH PROMOTION

Healthy Food Patterns for Optimum Function

Older Americans are not only living longer but also enjoying robust and active lives. More than 75% of those ages 90 and older still live in the community, and half live alone.[47] Good nutrition and self-care can be key to slowing aging changes and chronic disease. A 16-year follow-up of more than 5000 middle-age individuals reported that those with higher scores on the Healthy Eating Index, a measure of the food servings recommended by MyPlate (http://www.choosemyplate.gov), were more likely to experience *ideal aging*—free of chronic disease with high physical, mental, and cognitive function.[48] Those following a diet high in fats, sweets, refined grains, and red meat had lower odds of ideal aging, regardless of other health behaviors.

Although many persons ages 65 and older meet suggested servings of whole fruits, vegetables, meat, and beans,[21] they can still benefit from appropriate nutrition education. Food guides as described in Chapter 1 can be important as energy needs decline and people eat less food. Food guides promote the selection of foods from all major food groups and help ensure dietary diversity. The Human Nutrition Research Center on Aging at Tufts University has developed a MyPlate for Older Adults that emphasizes eating a wide variety of foods and addresses other issues of particular importance to older adults.[49] A low variety of foods, even nutrient-dense foods, can result in less than the recommended intakes of required nutrients. The image also indicates the need for healthy fats, encourages a liberal fluid intake, and presents ideas for limiting sodium by using low-sodium canned foods and herbs and spices for flavoring (Fig. 13.7). Current public health messages that emphasize lowering fat intake, being sensitive to portion size, and selecting lower-calorie rather than higher-calorie snacks have the goal of preventing inappropriate weight gain among younger and middle-age adults but could be having an unwanted effect on older adults, as many consume fewer kcalories than they should.

Physical Activity for Optimal Function

Physical activity promotes fitness and helps delay age-related changes in functional capacity.

Endurance exercise, the rhythmic use of the large muscles in walking, running, or jogging promotes cardiovascular fitness. For most older individuals, walking is a safe form of endurance exercise that supports cardiovascular health, weight management, and independent living.

Resistance exercise or *strength training* requires the individual to push against or lift a set weight. This brings about an increase in size and strength of muscle fibers, adding to the ability to perform household tasks. Recent evidence suggests that physical changes in functional capacity may actually begin before the age of 50,[50] much earlier than most of us begin to think about it. Accordingly, individuals should take a life span approach to maintaining their basic strength and endurance and not wait until they are no longer able to perform simple tasks. (The Evidence-Based Practice box, "Can Age-Related Loss of Muscle Mass Be Prevented?" examines the benefits of strength training in preventing muscle loss.) (All types of physical activity and related nutritional needs are discussed in Chapter 14.)

EVIDENCE-BASED PRACTICE

Can Age-Related Loss of Muscle Mass Be Prevented?

Define the problem: Muscle fiber atrophy results from a sedentary lifestyle and is worsened by normal aging, reduced secretion of anabolic hormones, and marginal protein intake. By age 70, muscle mass is often half what it was at age 30, with an accompanying decline in muscle strength. At one time, it was assumed that muscle loss in older age was inevitable.

Review the evidence: A classic study carried out by clinicians at the Human Research Center on Aging at Tufts University[1] established that strength training could replace muscle mass in frail nursing home residents as old as 90. All who completed the intervention gained muscle mass but, more importantly, improved their ability to carry out ADLs. Those who, before the program, needed assistance to rise from a chair or walk across the room were able to accomplish those actions without help after completing the program. Although it has been well established that muscle loss can be prevented or regained through strength training, controversy remains as to the protein needed to support the process.

Continued

EVIDENCE-BASED PRACTICE

Can Age-Related Loss of Muscle Mass Be Prevented?—cont'd

A protein intake of approximately 19% of total kcalories has been associated with muscle retention, whereas an intake of only 11% of total kcalories led to significant muscle loss.[2]

Implement the findings: Before beginning strength training, older adults should obtain approval from their health care provider, and seek supervision by a trained health professional. Inactive or frail older adults best begin slowly to avoid injury. To ensure sufficient protein for muscle-building, a dietary goal of 1.2 g/kg body weight or 18% to 20% of total kcalories is appropriate.[3] Protein synthesis is enhanced if the training session is followed with a meal containing 25 to 30 g of protein.[4] (A sample meal providing 25 g of protein would include 1 cup of reduced-fat or skim milk, a sandwich including 2 ounces of turkey, 2 ounces of tuna fish or two eggs, and 1 cup of baby carrots.) Community centers often offer supervised strength training programs for older adults. Guides for beginning an exercise program at home are available free from the National Institute on Aging at https://go4life.nia.nih.gov/free.

Bibliography

1. Fiatarone MA, Marks EC, Ryan ND, et al: High intensity strength training in nonagenarians: effects on skeletal muscle, *JAMA* 263:3029, 1990.
2. Wolfe RR, Cifelli AM, Kostas G, et al: Optimizing protein intake in adults: interpretation and application of the recommended dietary allowance compared with the acceptable macronutrient distribution range, *Adv Nutr* 8:266, 2017.
3. Cermak NM, Res PT, de Groot LCPGM, et al: Protein supplementation augments the adaptive response of skeletal muscle to resistance-type exercise training: a meta-analysis, *Am J Clin Nutr* 96:1454, 2012.
4. Evans WJ, Boccardi V, Paolisso G: Perspective: dietary protein needs of elderly people: protein supplementation as an effective strategy to counteract sarcopenia, *J Am Med Dir Assoc* 14(1):67, 2013.

MyPlate for Older Adults

Fruits & Vegetables

Whole fruits and vegetables are rich in important nutrients and fiber. Choose fruits and vegetables with deeply colored flesh. Choose canned varieties that are packed in their own juices or low-sodium.

Healthy Oils

Liquid vegetable oils and soft margarines provide important fatty acids and some fat-soluble vitamins.

Herbs & Spices

Use a variety of herbs and spices to enhance flavor of foods and reduce the need to add salt.

Fluids

Drink plenty of fluids. Fluids can come from water, tea, coffee, soups, and fruits and vegetables.

Grains

Whole grain and fortified foods are good sources of fiber and B vitamins.

Dairy

Fat-free and low-fat milk, cheeses and yogurts provide protein, calcium and other important nutrients.

Protein

Protein rich foods provide many important nutrients. Choose a variety including nuts, beans, fish, lean meat and poultry.

Remember to Stay Active!

Tufts UNIVERSITY   JEAN MAYER USDA HUMAN NUTRITION RESEARCH CENTER ON AGING   HNRCA   **AARP** Foundation

FIG. 13.7 MyPlate for Older Adults. The MyPlate for Older Adults was adapted from the MyPlate developed for the general public to draw attention to the specific needs of the older adult. http://hnrca.tufts.edu/myplate/# (Reprinted with the permission of the Human Nutrition Research Center on Aging, Tufts University, and the American Association for Retired Persons Foundation.)

TO SUM UP

Nutrient needs throughout adult life respond to the ebb and flow of continuing maturation and gradual decline. In young adults, nutrients support the physical body that has reached its full potential and build reserves for active living. Lifestyle patterns formed by young adults often continue throughout life, and sedentary living and unwanted weight gain are concerns. Middle age begins the period of physical decline, although changes occur slowly at the onset. Losses of muscle and bone mass influence functional capacity and threaten independent living in later years. Attention to protein, calcium, and vitamin D, along with participation in endurance and resistance exercise, slows these processes. Patterns of healthy eating, regular physical activity, and avoidance of smoking or other addictive behaviors, established early in life, support successful aging and the delay of degenerative changes. Nutrient needs in advanced age are influenced by changes in body composition, organ function, and chronic disease and are often complicated by associated malnutrition and weight loss. Physical disability, poverty, chewing or swallowing problems, isolation and depression, and multiple medications lower food intake and add to nutritional risk in later life. The Self MNA offers a tool to identify at-risk older adults and educate individuals and communities in preventive care.

QUESTIONS FOR REVIEW

1. Select one of the adult age groups, and describe its physical characteristics, psychosocial development, general socioeconomic status, and nutritional needs. What do you see as the most urgent topic for health promotion in this age group? Why?

2. You are working with a 32-year-old man who lives alone. He has a demanding job with no time to exercise and eats fast food most of the time. He has gained 15 lb over the past 2 years and is concerned about his overall health. What questions should you ask before making any diet or lifestyle recommendations? What diet and lifestyle recommendations might be compatible with his current lifestyle?

3. You are working with a middle-age adult who is overweight, sedentary, and eats mostly meat, bread, potatoes, and desserts. Does this person represent normal aging or successful aging? How would you approach this individual about his health and what suggestions would you have for improvement?

4. What is meant by the aging process? Describe how physiologic changes occurring in advanced age might influence food intake or nutritional status.

5. Discuss the economic status, ethnic and racial composition, and living arrangements of the aging population. How might these factors influence the older adult's diet or health status? What are the implications for health and support services? Describe the individual in this age group that you would consider to be at greatest risk. Why did you choose him or her?

6. Interview a family member, neighbor, or friend who is older than 65. What are some changes in health, living arrangements, or employment/retirement that have influenced his or her lifestyle over the past 10 years? How have these changes affected his or her eating habits?

7. You are helping a 75-year-old retired couple on a limited income with their diet. Both appear to be underweight, and you suspect that their food supplies are limited. Using the Healthy US-Style Eating Pattern or the Healthy Mediterranean Style Eating Pattern develop a 2-day menu of meals and snacks that will supply each food group in the appropriate amounts for their age, gender, and activity level. How might you increase their energy intake and still remain within the AMDR for the three macronutrients? (USDA Food Patterns and Calorie Recommendations can be accessed at http://www.cnpp.usda.gov/USDAFoodPatterns.htm.)

8. Identify a food-related program for older adults in your community and interview the director to determine (a) the target audience, (b) the types and amounts of food provided, (c) any major problems associated with implementation of the program, and (d) the major successes of the program.

REFERENCES

1. Centers for Disease Control and Prevention: QuickStats: percentage of adults aged ≥18 years who often felt worried, nervous, or anxious, by sex and age group—National Health Interview Survey, United States, 2010-2011, *MMWR Morb Mortal Wkly Rep* 62(10):197, 2013.

2. Webb MJ, Kauer SD, Ozer EM, et al: Does screening for and intervening with multiple health compromising behaviours and mental health disorders amongst young people attending primary care improve health outcomes? A systematic review, *BMC Fam Pract* 17:104, 2016.

3. US Department of Health and Human Services and US Department of Agriculture: *2015-2020 Dietary Guidelines for Americans*, ed 8, December 2015.

4. US Department of Agriculture, Agricultural Research Service: *Table 1. Nutrient Intakes from Food and Beverages: Mean Amounts Consumed per Individual, by Gender and Age, in the United States, 2013-2014. What We Eat in America, NHANES 2013-2014*, 2016. https://www.ars.usda.gov/ARSUserFiles/80400530/pdf/1314/Table_1_NIN_GEN_13.pdf.

5. Institute of Medicine, Otten JJ, Hellwig JP, Meyers LD, editors: *Dietary Reference Intakes. The essential guide to nutrient requirements*, Washington, DC, 2006, National Academies Press.

6. Institute of Medicine: *Dietary Reference Intakes for calcium and vitamin D*, Washington, DC, 2011, National Academies Press.

7. US Department of Health and Human Services, US Department of Agriculture: *Scientific Report of the 2015 Dietary Guidelines Advisory Committee*, Washington, DC, February 2015. https://www.health.gov/dietaryguidelines/2015-scientific-report/.

8. Center for Disease Control and Prevention: *High blood pressure facts*, Atlanta, GA, 2016. https://www.cdc.gov/bloodpressure/facts.htm.

9. US Department of Agriculture, Agricultural Research Service: *Table 53. All Restaurants: Percent Reporting, Mean Amounts and Percent of Selected Nutrients from Foods Obtained from all Restaurants by Gender and Age, in the United States, 2013-2014. What We Eat in America, NHANES 2013-2014*, 2016. https://www.ars.usda.gov/ARSUserFiles/80400530/pdf/1314/Table_53_RST_GEN_13.pdf.

10. Watts AW, Laska MN, Larson NI, et al: Millennials at work: Workplace environments of young adults and associations with weight-related health, *J Epidemiol Community Health* 70(1):65, 2016.

11. Larson N, Fulkerson J, Story M, et al: Shared meals among young adults are associated with better diet quality and predicted by family meal patterns during adolescence, *Public Health Nutr* 16(5):883, 2013.

12. Olson JS, Hummer RA, Harris KM: Gender and health behavior clustering among US young adults, *Biodemography Soc Biol* 63(1):3, 2017.

13. Watts AW, Mason SM, Loth K, et al: Socioeconomic differences in overweight and weight-related behaviors across adolescence and young adulthood: 10-year longitudinal findings from Project EAT, *Prev Med* 87:194, 2016.

14. Berge JM, MacLehose R, Eisenberg ME, et al: How significant is the 'significant other'? Associations between significant others' health behaviors and attitudes and young adults' health outcomes, *Int J Behav Nutr Phys Act* 9:35, 2012.

15. Oikonen M, Laitinen TT, Magnussen CG, et al: Ideal cardiovascular health in young adult populations from the United States, Finland, and Australia and its association With cIMT: The International Childhood Cardiovascular Cohort Consortium, *J Am Heart Assoc* 2(3):e000244, 2013.

16. Paddon-Jones D, Campbell WW, Jacques PF, et al: Protein and healthy aging, *Am J Clin Nutr* 101(6):S1339, 2015.

17. Schleicher RL, Sternberg MR, Lacher DA, et al: The vitamin D status of the US population from 1988 to 2010 using standardized serum concentrations of 25-hydroxyvitamin D shows recent modest increases, *Am J Clin Nutr* 104(2):454, 2016.

18. Dugan A: *Fast food still major part of US diet. Gallup World Headquarters, 901 F Street*, Washington, DC, August 6, 2013. http://www.gallup.com/poll/163868/fast-food-major-part-diet.aspx?version=print.

19. Rosinger A, Herrick K, Gahche J, et al: *Sugar-sweetened beverage consumption among US Adults, 2011-2014*, NCHS Data Brief 270, Hyattsville, MD, January 2017, National Center for Health Statistics, US Department of Health and Human Services. https://www.cdc.gov/nchs/data/databriefs/db270.pdf.

20. Breslow RA, Chen CM, Graubard BI, et al: Diets of drinkers on drinking and nondrinking days: NHANES 2003-2008, *Am J Clin Nutr* 97:1068, 2013.

21. Hiza HA, Casavale KO, Guenther PM, et al: Diet quality of Americans differs by age, sex, race/ethnicity, income, and education level, *J Acad Nutr Diet* 113(2):297, 2013.

22. Kantor ED, Rehm CD, Du M, et al: Trends in dietary supplement use among US adults From 1999-2012, *JAMA* 316(14):1464, 2016.

23. Ward BW, Schiller JS, Goodman RA: Multiple chronic conditions among US adults: A 2012 update, *Prev Chronic Dis* 11:e62, April 17, 2014.

24. Micha R, Peñalvo JL, Cudhea F, et al: Association between dietary factors and mortality from heart disease, stroke, and type 2 diabetes in the United States, *JAMA* 317(9):912, 2017.

25. Federal Interagency Forum on Aging-Related Statistics: *Older Americans 2016: key indicators of well-being*, Washington, DC, 2016, US Government Printing Office.

26. Camina Martín MA, de Mateo Silleras B, Redondo del Río MP: Body composition analysis in older adults with dementia. Anthropometry and bioelectrical impedance analysis: a critical review, *Eur J Clin Nutr* 68(11):1228, 2014.

27. Verlaan S, Ligthart-Melis GC, Wijers SLJ, et al: High prevalence of physical frailty among community-dwelling malnourished older adults. A systematic review and meta-analysis, *J Am Med Dir Assoc* 18(5):374–382, 2017.

28. Kane R, Ouslander JG, Abrass I, et al: *Essentials of Clinical Geriatrics*, ed 7, New York, 2013, McGraw Hill.

29. Cooper JA, Manini TM, Paton CM, et al: Longitudinal change in energy expenditure and effects on energy requirements of the elderly. Health ABC study, *Nutr J* 12:73, 2013.

30. Volpi E, Campbell WW, Dwyer JT, et al: Is the optimal level of protein intake for older adults greater than the recommended dietary allowance? *J Gerontol A Biol Sci Med Sci* 68(6):677, 2013.

31. Bauer J, Biolo G, Cederholm T, et al: Evidence-based recommendations for optimal dietary protein intake in older people: A position paper from the PROT-AGE Study Group, *J Am Med Dir Assoc* 14(8):542, 2013.

32. Galvan E, Arentson-Lantz E, Lamon S, et al: Protecting skeletal muscle with protein and amino acid during periods of disuse, *Nutrients* 8(7): e404, 2016.

33. Murphy SP, Wilkens LR, Monroe KR, et al: Dietary supplement use within a multiethnic population as measured by a unique inventory method, *J Am Diet Assoc* 111:1065, 2011.

34. Bernstein M1, Munoz N, Academy of Nutrition and Dietetics: Position of the Academy of Nutrition and Dietetics: food and nutrition for older adults: promoting health and wellness, *J Acad Nutr Diet* 112:1255, 2012.

35. Morley JE: Dehydration, hypernatremia, and hyponatremia, *Clin Geriatr Med* 31(3):389, 2015.

36. Zhu Y, Hollis JH: Tooth loss and its association with dietary intake and diet quality in American adults, *J Dent* 42(11):1428, 2014.

37. Wickrama KAS, Ralston PA, O'Neal CW, et al: Life dissatisfaction and eating behaviors among older African Americans: the protective role of social support, *J Nutr Health Aging* 16(9):749, 2012.

38. Payne ME, Steck SE, George RR, et al: Fruit, vegetable, and antioxidant intakes are lower in older adults with depression, *J Acad Nutr Diet* 112:2022, 2012.

39. Hsiao PY, Mitchell DC, Coffman DL, et al: Dietary patterns and diet quality among diverse older adults: the University of Alabama at Birmingham study of aging, *J Nutr Health Aging* 17(1):19, 2013.

40. Racine EF, Lyerly J, Troyer JL, et al: The influence of home-delivered Dietary Approaches to Stop Hypertension meals on body mass index, energy intake, and percent of energy needs consumed among older adults with hypertension and/or hyperlipidemia, *J Acad Nutr Diet* 112:1755, 2012.

41. Beck M, Birkelund R, Poulsen I, et al: Supporting existential care with protected mealtimes: patients' experiences of a mealtime intervention in a neurological ward, *J Adv Nurs* 73(8):1947, 2017.

42. Dennis RA, Johnson LE, Roberson PK, et al: Changes in activities of daily living, nutrient intake, and systemic inflammation in elderly adults receiving recuperative care, *J Am Geriatr Soc* 60:2246, 2012.

43. Roberts SB, Rosenberg I: Nutrition and aging: changes in the regulation of energy metabolism with aging, *Physiol Rev* 86:651, 2006.

44. Chen Z, Klimentidis YC, Bea JW, et al: Body mass index, waist circumference, and mortality in a large multiethnic postmenopausal cohort-results from the Women's Health Initiative, *J Am Geriatr Soc* 65(9):1907, 2017.

45. Marshall S, Young A, Bauer J, et al: Malnutrition in geriatric rehabilitation: prevalence, patient outcomes, and criterion validity of the scored patient-generated Subjective Global Assessment and the Mini Nutritional Assessment, *J Acad Nutr Diet* 116(5):785, 2016.

46. Thomas DR, Ashmen W, Morley JE, et al: Nutritional management in long-term care: development of a clinical guideline, *J Gerontol A Biol Sci Med Sci* 55(12):M725, 2000.

47. US Bureau of Census: *Census Bureau releases comprehensive analysis of fast-growing 90-and-older population, Newsroom release*, November 17, 2011. https://www.census.gov/newsroom/releases/archives/aging_population/cb11-194.html.

48. Akbaraly T, Sabia S, Haggar-Johnson G, et al: Does overall diet in midlife predict future aging phenotypes? A cohort study, *Am J Med* 126(5):411, 2013.

49. Human Nutrition Research Center on Aging, Tufts University and American Association for Retired Persons Foundation: *My Plate For Older Adults*, Boston MA, 2015. http://hnrca.tufts.edu/myplate/.

50. Hall KS, Cohen HJ, Pieper CF, et al: Physical performance across the adult life span: Correlates with age and physical activity, *J Gerontol A Biol Sci Med Sci* 72(4):572, 2017.

FURTHER READINGS AND RESOURCES

Readings

Bailey RL, Gahche JJ, Miller PE, et al: Why US adults use dietary supplements. *JAMA Intern Med* 173(5):355, 2013.

Jahns L, Conrad Z, Johnson LK, et al: Diet quality is lower and energy intake is higher on weekends compared with weekdays in midlife women: a 1-year cohort study, *J Acad Nutr Diet* 117(7):1080, 2017.

Laska MN, Hearst MO, Lust K, et al: How we eat what we eat: identifying meal routines and practices most strongly associated with healthy and unhealthy dietary factors among young adults, *Public Health Nutr* 18(12):2135, 2015.

[These authors address lifestyle and demographic factors that influence food intake in adults.]

Bruening M, Argo K, Payne-Sturges D, et al: The struggle is real: a systematic review of food insecurity on postsecondary education campuses, *J Acad Nutr Diet* 117(11):1767, 2017.

Hernandez DC, Reesor L, Murillo R: Gender disparities in the food insecurity-overweight and food insecurity-obesity paradox among low-income older adults, *J Acad Nutr Diet* 117(7):1087, 2017.

[These authors focus on food insecurity issues in both younger and older adults.]

Websites of Interest

- Administration on Aging (AoA); Administration for Community Living (ACL). This site describes many programs and health-related materials to assist older adults. https://www.acl.gov/programs.

- National Institutes of Health (NIH). The NIH Health Information site contains materials on healthy lifestyles; individual locations focus on teens, men, and women's health. https://www.nih.gov/health-information/science-based-health-wellness-resources-your-community.

- National Institute on Aging (NIA). This site includes updates on aging research along with numerous publications available to older adults and their families. https://www.nia.nih.gov/health.

- Eldercare Locator: *Federal Websites*. This site includes many topics of interest to older adults and their caregivers such as health, retirement, and housing options. https://eldercare.acl.gov/Public/Resources/Federal_Websites.aspx.

Nutrition and Physical Fitness

Kary Woodruff

http://evolve.elsevier.com/Williams/essentials/

Nutrition and physical fitness are integral to overall health, weight management, and disease prevention. In an increasingly fast-paced and technology-dependent society, making regular physical activity part of a busy life requires commitment. Physical fitness is a vital cornerstone in the preventive approach to controlling chronic disease in modern society. We examine first how nutrition provides energy for muscle action; then we apply principles to enhancing fitness and athletic performance by providing evidence-based recommendations for nutrition practices that support physical activity and exercise. "Good food choices will not make a mediocre athlete into a champion, but poor food choices may prevent the potential champion from realizing his/her potential."[1]

OUTLINE

PHYSICAL ACTIVITY, MODERN CIVILIZATION, AND CHRONIC DISEASE

Physical Fitness and Health

The Centers for Disease Control and Prevention (CDC) defines *physical activity* as any bodily movement produced by the contraction of skeletal muscles that increases energy expenditure above a basal level.[2] Examples of physical activity include walking or riding a bike as a form of transportation, using the stairs instead of the escalator, or manual labor such as carpentry work, gardening, or farming. Physical activity differs from *exercise* based on the structure and purpose. *Exercise* is a subcategory of physical activity that is planned, structured, repetitive, and purposive in that improving or maintaining one or more components of physical fitness is the objective.[2] People engage in exercise for the purpose of training, competing, and keeping organs and bodily functions healthy. Examples of exercise include aerobic classes, jogging, running, swimming, cycling, weight training, tennis, and other such bouts of planned activities with the intention of improving overall physical fitness.

Physical fitness is defined by the CDC as the ability to carry out daily tasks with vigor and alertness, without undue fatigue, and with ample energy to enjoy leisure-time pursuits and respond to emergencies. Physical fitness includes a number of components consisting of cardiorespiratory endurance (aerobic power), skeletal muscle endurance, skeletal muscle strength, skeletal muscle power, flexibility, balance, speed of movement, reaction time, and body composition.[2]

Physical inactivity is a global health problem and is 1 of the 10 leading risk factors for global mortality as estimated by the World Health Organization (WHO).[3] In fact, physical inactivity is considered to be comparable to obesity and smoking as a leading risk factor for

mortality.[4] Increased participation in regular physical activity as a part of everyday life remains a national health goal. The US Department of Health and Human Services (USDHHS) in its report *Healthy People 2020* has set health-related goals for Americans in nutrition and physical fitness. The 2020 target is to reduce the percentage of adults who do not engage in any leisure-time physical activity to 32.6% or less. Current progress reports indicate that only 20.6% of adults meet the minimum recommendation of aerobic physical activity and muscle-strengthening activity on a regular basis.[5] All *Healthy People 2020* objectives are available at http://www.healthypeople.gov/2020/.

Health promotion, disease prevention, and disease management require attention to the related roles of nutrition and physical fitness. The US Department of Agriculture (USDA) has published national dietary guidelines every 5 years since 1980. Starting with the *Dietary Guidelines for Americans 2010,*[6] the Physical Activity Guidelines (2008) have been included. These guidelines encourage all people to focus on healthy eating patterns, to be physically active each day, and to aim for a healthy weight. The 2015 *Dietary Guidelines* encourage Americans to prevent and/or reduce overweight and obesity through improved eating and physical activity and to increase physical activity and reduce time spent in sedentary behaviors.[7]

Modern Developed Nations and Chronic Disease

Over time and many generations, daily life in developed nations has evolved from agriculture-based societies requiring constant physical exertion to a more sedentary standard of living. Poor nutrition and inactivity contribute to a host of illnesses, the so-called diseases of modern civilization, including cardiovascular disease, type 2 diabetes, metabolic syndrome, and some forms of cancer. Substantial research

261

supports both the preventive and therapeutic roles of a healthy diet and physical activity on such chronic diseases.[8,9]

BODY IN MOTION

Nature of Energy

The term *energy* refers to the body's ability, or power, to do work. The energy required to do work takes several different forms: mechanical, chemical, electrical, radiant, nuclear, and heat. Energy, like matter, can neither be created nor destroyed. It can only be changed into another form; therefore energy is constantly cycled in the body and environment. We also speak of energy as being potential or kinetic. Potential energy is stored energy, ready to be used. Kinetic energy is active energy, being used to do work. Physical activity requires appropriate nutrition to supply the substrate fuels, which along with oxygen and water, meet widely varying levels of energy demands for body action.

Muscle Physiology

Muscle Structure. The synchronized action of millions of specialized cells that comprise our skeletal muscle mass makes possible all forms of physical activity. A finely coordinated series of small bundles within the muscle fibers (Fig. 14.1) produce a smooth symphony of action through simultaneous and alternating contraction and relaxation. These successively smaller muscle structures include the following:

- *Fasciculi:* A small bundle of nerve or muscle fibers.
- *Muscle fiber:* Muscle cells composed of bundles of still smaller strands called *myofibrils.*

- *Myofibril:* The basic unit of a muscle cell, the myofibril strand, is made up of the smallest of all the fiber bundles, called *myofilaments.* Muscular contraction occurs here.
- *Myosin* and *actin:* Within each myofilament are the contractile proteins, myosin, actin, and titin which are the smallest moving parts of the muscle.

Muscle Action. Inside the muscle fiber, *myofibrils* run the length of the cell. Myofibrils contain the contractile proteins, myosin, actin, and titin, which interact in the presence of calcium to shorten the cell (and the muscle). The muscle shortening causes movement in different directions at the joint. When the calcium is pumped out of the surrounding fluid, the cell then relaxes to return the muscle elastically to its resting length. This alternating process of muscle contraction and relaxation can continue until muscle glycogen is depleted and muscle fatigue occurs.

Fuel Sources. At rest, fuel sources include a mix of carbohydrate and fat. During exercise, carbohydrate is the primary fuel, with fat providing energy at lower intensities and for exercise of longer duration. Protein is a fuel of last resort and is used only when the other fuels are exhausted. The high-energy compound driving body cells is adenosine triphosphate (ATP), the energy currency of the cell. Various forms of energy are required for successive energy needs:

- *Immediate energy:* High-power or immediate energy demands over a short time depend on ATP being readily available within the muscle tissue. This amount is used rapidly, and a

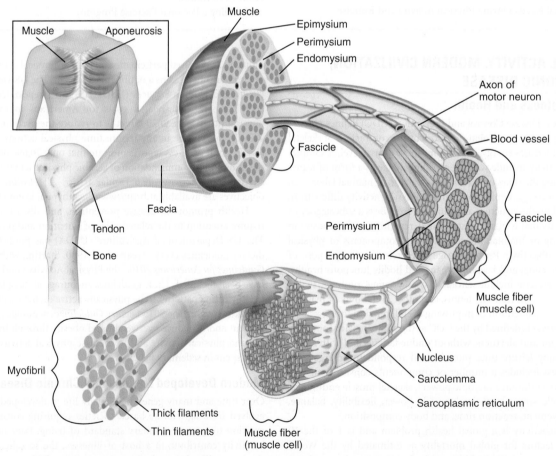

FIG. 14.1 Skeletal muscle, showing the progressively smaller bundles within bundles. (From Thibodeau GA, Patton KT: *Anatomy & physiology,* ed 5, St Louis, 2003, Mosby.)

backup compound, creatine phosphate (CP), replenishes ATP. These high-energy compounds will sustain exercise for up to 10 seconds.

- *Short-term energy:* For anaerobic bursts like sprints and weight lifting (between 10 and 180 seconds), muscle glycogen and blood glucose provide the only available fuel source through the glycolytic pathway. Although the amount of available glucose is small, it is an important rapid source of energy for brief muscular effort.

- *Long-term energy:* Exercise continuing more than 2 to 3 minutes requires an oxygen-dependent, or aerobic, energy system, and thus a constant supply of oxygen in the blood is necessary. The mitochondria, organelles within the cell, produce large amounts of ATP. The ATP is produced mainly from glucose and fatty acids and supplies the continued energy needs of the body (Fig. 14.2).

Exercise intensity also affects the preferred fuel source for active muscles. Sustained, low-intensity exercises rely primarily on triglycerides for energy through the aerobic pathway. As intensity increases, the source of energy gradually shifts to carbohydrates and makes more use of the glycolytic and CP systems (Table 14.1).

Nutrients become depleted during continued exercise as the body draws on its stored energy. As demands for ATP increase, the body metabolizes blood glucose and muscle glycogen to provide energy via anaerobic glycolysis. However, with prolonged exercise of increased intensity, the levels of these nutrients fall too low to sustain the body's demands. Without a resupply of nutrients, fatigue follows, and exercise cannot continue.

Oxygen Use and Physical Capacity

The most profound limit to exercise is the person's ability to deliver oxygen to the tissues and use it for energy production. This vital ability depends on the fitness of the pulmonary and cardiovascular systems. Because the heart is a muscle, aerobic exercise strengthens it, enabling it to pump more blood per beat, a capacity called *stroke volume.* The cardiac output—how much the heart pumps out in a given period of time—depends on the amount of blood per contraction and on the cardiac rate, which is the number of contractions in a given time. The following factors are influential in fitness level:

- *Cardiovascular fitness:* Cardiovascular fitness is defined in terms of aerobic capacity, which depends on the body's ability to deliver and use oxygen in sufficient quantities to meet the demands of increasing levels of exercise. Oxygen uptake increases with exercise intensity until either the demand is met or the ability to supply it is exceeded. The maximum rate the body can take in oxygen, or aerobic capacity, is called the *VO₂max*—the maximum uptake volume of oxygen. This capacity determines the intensity and duration of exercise that a person can perform. Starting from at rest, a steep rise in oxygen consumption occurs at the onset of exercise. After several minutes the body reaches equilibrium between the energy required by the exercising muscles and the aerobic energy-producing system. The aerobic capacity of an individual, or their VO_2, is measured in terms of milliliters of oxygen consumed per kilogram of body weight per minute. This relative measurement allows people of differing sizes to be compared equally.

- *Genetic influence:* A person's aerobic capacity is somewhat determined by their genetic propensity for exercise response.[10] In other words, physiologic gains and cardiovascular adaptation from the same exercise program will vary among individuals based on their specific genetics.

- *Age:* In general, maximal aerobic capacity declines gradually with age and is largely the result of age-related losses in lean body mass due to decreased physical activity levels.

- *Body composition and gender:* Gender differences in aerobic capacity reflect differences in body composition. In general, men have a higher aerobic capacity due to their larger lean body mass, the metabolically active body tissue. These highly metabolic tissues of the body use more oxygen than other tissues such as fat. However, when oxygen consumption is expressed relative to lean body mass instead of body weight, men and women have a similar aerobic capacity. In general, women carry more body fat, a gender difference in body composition that serves critical biologic functions (see Chapter 8). Essential structural and functional body fat in women is 8% to 12% of their body weight (compared with 3%–5% in men).[11] In addition, because women must, of course, carry their entire body weight as part of their total workload, their performance will be affected accordingly.

FIG. 14.2 Contribution of the different energy systems during exercise of increasing duration. The anaerobic energy system provides adenosine triphosphate *(ATP)* to the working myofilaments from ATP–creatine phosphate *(CP)* stores and the lactate or glycolytic path. The aerobic system supplies ATP from mitochondria, which require oxygen to burn carbohydrates and fats. (Redrawn from Nieman DC: *Exercise testing and prescription,* ed 5, Boston, 2003, McGraw-Hill.)

TABLE 14.1	**Effect of Intensity on Fuel Type**
Exercise Intensity	**Fuel used by Muscle**
<30% VO₂max (easy walking)	Carbohydrates at first, then largely muscle fat stores with durations over 30 min
40%–65% VO₂max (jogging, brisk walking)	Fat and carbohydrate used evenly
75% VO₂max (running)	Mainly carbohydrate
≥80% VO₂max (sprinting)	Nearly 100% carbohydrate

KEY TERM

Aerobic Capacity (VO₂)
Milliliters of oxygen consumed per kilogram of body weight per minute; influenced by body composition and fitness level.

NUTRITIONAL NEEDS DURING PHYSICAL ACTIVITY AND EXERCISE

All six classifications of nutrients in human nutrition (carbohydrates, protein, fat, vitamins, minerals, and water) are essential components in meeting the body's energy and hydration needs for physical activity and exercise.

Carbohydrates

Carbohydrates as Fuel Substrate. The chief macronutrient providing energy throughout exercise is carbohydrate. Carbohydrates are the necessary energy source for anaerobic activity. Carbohydrate fuels come from two sources: (1) circulating blood glucose and (2) glycogen stored in muscle and liver tissue. Liver glycogen primarily contributes to blood glucose homeostasis, whereas muscle glycogen is used for the specific muscle in which it is stored.

Carbohydrates in the Diet. Carbohydrates are the preferred energy source. Carbohydrate energy should contribute 45% to 65% of the kilocalories (kcalories or kcal) in the daily diet. Athletes' carbohydrate needs are expressed relative to body weight and range from 5 to 12 g of carbohydrate per kg of body weight (g/kg body weight), depending upon sport type, training volume, and other sport-related factors.[11] In general, complex carbohydrates (starches) are preferable to simple carbohydrates (monosaccharides and disaccharides). Starches break down gradually and help maintain blood glucose levels more evenly (avoiding low blood glucose drops), as well as maintain glycogen storage as a constant primary fuel. Simple sugars, however, can supply important immediate energy particularly before and during endurance events or high-intensity exercise.

In prolonged bouts of intense or endurance exercise, studies have found that diets low in carbohydrate have proven to be less effective at maintaining energy homeostasis and pace.[12,13] A low-carbohydrate diet decreases the body's capacity for work, which intensifies over time. Athletes on a low-carbohydrate diet are susceptible to fatigue, ketoacidosis, and dehydration. Conversely, a high-carbohydrate diet enhances muscle glycogen concentrations and exercise performance.[13,14] In addition, carbohydrate supplementation during exercise bouts of at least 60 to 90 minutes improves whole body carbohydrate oxidation and metabolic efficiency.[14,15] Therefore athletes consuming carbohydrate foods before and during exercise maintain glucose concentrations and rates of glucose oxidation necessary to exercise strenuously and delay fatigue.

Carbohydrate loading is a common practice among endurance athletes that is intended to encourage muscles to deposit maximum glycogen stores prior to an endurance event lasting longer than 90 minutes for extra stored energy. The initial protocol for glycogen loading was a two-step procedure. First, athletes consumed a diet low in carbohydrates, while simultaneously exercising at high intensity; thus muscle glycogen stores were rapidly depleted. In the second step, athletes did just the opposite; they gradually decreased exercise intensity and volume while consuming a diet high in carbohydrates (approximately 70%–75% of total caloric intake). However, recent research has demonstrated that high glycogen stores can be achieved in the absence of the initial depletion step. The current carbohydrate loading protocol includes a carbohydrate consumption of 10 to 12 g/kg over a 36- to 48-hour period.[14] Table 14.2 illustrates one sample day of carbohydrate loading providing 11 g/kg/day. Because every gram of glycogen stored requires 2.7 mL of water, potential side effects may occur. Extra water weight in muscles may result in

bloating, or tight or sore muscles that could ultimately hinder performance. Athletes are encouraged to experiment with carbohydrate loading before their competitive events to ensure comfort and personal benefits.

Although there was previously question as to whether the glycemic index or glycemic load (see Chapter 3) of a carbohydrate food had an effect on performance, it is now accepted that neither glycemic index nor load impacts exercise performance or metabolic response when carbohydrate and energy intake are appropriate.[11]

Fat

Fat as Fuel Substrate. Fatty acids serve as a fuel source from dietary intake and adipose tissue. In the presence of oxygen, fatty acids are oxidized to provide energy. The rate at which this can occur is determined in part by the rate of mobilization of fatty acids from storage, but not all stored fat is alike. The body stores fat in two ways: (1) depot fat in adipose tissue, which is destined for transport back and forth to other tissues as needed for energy, and (2) essential fat in metabolically active tissue, such as bone marrow, heart, lungs, liver, spleen, kidneys, intestines, muscles, and nervous system, which is reserved in these places for necessary structural and functional use only. Although storage depot fat in men and women is approximately comparable, essential fat reserves are significantly different; they are about 3 times greater in women.

Fat in the Diet. Fat, as a fuel substrate, is drawn from the body's adipose tissue in response to increasing activity of the enzyme

TABLE 14.2 One Day of Carbohydrate Loading for 155-lb Males (Providing 11 g/kg per body weight)		
Meal	**Food**	**Carbohydrate (g)**
Breakfast	Whole wheat raisin bagel	55
	2 tbsp raspberry jam	18
	1 large banana	31
	2 cups orange juice	57
	1 cup low fat strawberry yogurt	43
A.M. snack	1 Clif bar	49
	16 ounces Gatorade	31
Lunch	Turkey sandwich: 2 slices whole wheat bread, 4 slices turkey, 2 slices tomatoes, 1 tbsp mustard	28
	1 box raisin	34
	1 cup pretzels	32
	2 cups grape juice	75
P.M. snack	Low fat blueberry muffin	57
	1.5 cups apple juice	42
Dinner	1 large roasted yam	56
	4 ounces grilled chicken	0
	1 cup corn	34
	1 cup grapes	16
	2 cups low fat chocolate milk	55
Evening snack	1.5 cups Raisin Bran	71
	1.5 cup skim milk	18
	1 large apple	29
	Total	847

hormone-sensitive lipase (HSL). HSL activity rises as blood insulin levels decrease, allowing for the mobilization of fatty acids throughout the body. It is not necessary to specifically consume extra fat to maintain the body's adipose tissue, because excess kcalories from all macronutrients will be converted to fat and stored. On the other hand, a moderate level of fat is necessary in the diet for the absorption of fat-soluble vitamins and to ensure adequate intake of the essential fatty acids (linoleic and α-linolenic acids). An extremely low fat intake can be medically dangerous by creating a deficiency of the essential fatty acids. The standard recommendation that 20% to 35% of kcalories come from fat, per the Acceptable Macronutrient Distribution Range (AMDR), is ample for most healthy individuals including athletes. Athletes should be discouraged from a fat intake of less than 20% of kcalories in the diet.[11]

Protein

Protein as Fuel Substrate. Although some amino acids can feed into the basic energy cycle, protein makes a relatively insignificant and inefficient contribution to energy during exercise under normal circumstances. However, in glycogen-depleted muscles, more protein will be used as a fuel substrate.[16]

Protein in the Diet. A daily intake of 0.8 to 1 g of protein/kg of body weight is sufficient to meet the general needs of sedentary individuals. This amounts to the recommended daily dietary intake for adults, with 10% to 35% of the kcalories in the diet coming from protein. However, the optimal dietary protein intake for active individuals ranges from 1.0 to 1.6 g/kg, and for athletes an intake of 1.2 to 2.0 g/kg is desired to stimulate muscle protein synthesis and maintain lean body mass.[11,16] As athletes increase their total kcalorie intake to meet elevated energy needs, a balanced varied diet will provide proportionally more protein and is typically adequate to cover the additional needs.[17]

There is no indication that protein or amino acids from dietary supplements are necessary to meet needs or are superior to whole food forms of protein. A well-balanced diet can easily meet dietary protein needs for the active person and the athlete (see Chapter 5). Excess protein in the diet cannot be stored in the body as amino acids; thus protein is converted to fat, and the amine portion (nitrogen) must be excreted.

Micronutrients

Vitamins and Minerals as Catalytic Cofactors. Vitamins and minerals cannot be used as fuel substrates. They are not oxidized or expended in the process of energy production. However, vitamins and minerals are essential as catalytic cofactors in enzyme reactions.

Vitamins and Minerals in the Diet. Increased physical exertion during exercise or athletic training does not require a greater intake of vitamins and minerals beyond current recommendations. A well-balanced diet will supply adequate amounts of vitamins and minerals, and exercise may improve the body's efficient use of them. For example, because athletes have an increased dietary need for energy, their larger kcalorie intake from high-quality food sources will boost their general intake of vitamins and minerals. However, if an athlete is restricting calories, vitamin and mineral deficiencies are possible. Energy-restricting behaviors often result in avoidance of animal products such as meat and dairy, which are particularly rich sources of calcium, iron, and zinc. In addition, some athletes may be at risk for vitamin D

deficiency, particularly those training indoors or living at higher latitudes.

Conversely, multivitamin and mineral supplementation does not improve physical performance in healthy athletes who eat a well-balanced diet. Furthermore, the potential side effects of toxicity are well known (see Chapters 6 and 7).

Hydration: Water and Electrolytes

Water and Dehydration. Controlled studies in experimental settings have shown that dehydration limits exercise capacity in endurance and resistance activities.[18,19] The effects of dehydration depend on many factors, such as exercise environment, psychologic stressors, gender, body composition, intensity and duration of exercise, body temperature, level of fitness, and preexercise state of hydration (see the Case Study box, "Fluid and Energy Needs for Endurance Athletes"). In cases of severe dehydration, athletes may experience problems such as cramps, delirium, vomiting, hypothermia, and hyperthermia. By establishing euhydration before athletic events and consuming fluid replacement beverages during events warranting fluid replacement, these problems can be prevented. Adequate fluid intake and access to rehydration fluids should be planned for all types of athletes, not just individuals who participate in endurance events. Some strategies to increase fluid intake by athletes are provided in Box 14.1.

Cause of dehydration. ATP production results in significant heat release within the working muscle. During moderate-intensity physical activity, most individuals maintain a body temperature within a desirable range. However, during intense exercise or exercise in hot environments, heat production may exceed the body's acceptable temperature range for performance and the body's heat tolerance capacity.[18] Sweating is our primary mechanism for dissipating body heat. The major source of fluid loss in sweat is plasma fluid. High-intensity or long-endurance events (especially in hot climates) can cause the loss of several liters of water as sweat to regulate body temperature. Unless this fluid is replaced, consequences from dehydration and heat illness may result.

Prevention of dehydration. To prevent dehydration, athletes are advised to (1) establish euhydration at least several hours before activity; (2) drink during exercise to avoid excessive water loss, defined as 2% to 3% body weight loss from water; and (3) replace fluid loss after completion of exercise.[18,19] The American College of Sports Medicine, Academy of Nutrition and Dietetics, and Dietitians of Canada recommend that athletes develop a customized fluid replacement protocol that meets their needs and preferences

---

BOX 14.1 Strategies for Sports Team Members to Increase Fluid Intake

- Establish a regular schedule; drink during warm-up exercises and between periods of play.
- Give each player a sports squeeze bottle.
- Supply players with a sports drink that tastes good during exercise.
- Make available a choice of fluids to drink.
- Offer cool fluids.
- Avoid carbonated beverages because athletes tend to drink less when the beverage is carbonated.

From Palumbo CM: Nutrition concerns related to the performance of a baseball team, *J Am Diet Assoc* 100(6):704, 2000. Copyright with permission from the American Dietetic Association.

(e.g., fluid temperature, taste preferences).[11] Measuring weight before and after activity is an easy and appropriate method to estimate fluid loss in sweat. Water volume and body weight are equivalent (i.e., 16 oz of water = 1 lb of weight); thus one can assume that weight lost during activity is equivalent to the volume of water lost. Hydration with fluids containing glucose and sodium reduces urinary fluid loss. Therefore, during longer events (particularly those lasting more than 2 hours), fluids with mild solutions of sodium are recommended to help reduce fluid loss and prevent dehydration.[18]

Sodium. In the 1960s researchers believed that sodium losses exceeded water loss during vigorous activity with substantial sweat production. However, sweat is more dilute than internal fluids, and thus we lose proportionately more water than sodium. In most instances, sodium losses are replaced with the athlete's next meal. However, for ultra endurance events lasting more than 2 hours, fluid replacements including sodium are fundamental in preventing sodium losses and reducing the risk of hyponatremia.[18] Therefore the current recommendations state that during longer and more demanding endurance events, especially in warm or humid environments, a mild sodium and glucose (5%–10% glucose solution) sports drink that has rapid gastric emptying and intestinal absorption times may be beneficial.[11,19] A number of specialty sports drinks are now available with replacement electrolytes (see the Evidence-Based Practice box, "Sorting Out the Sports Drinks Saga").

CASE STUDY

Fluid and Energy Needs for Endurance Athletes

Lucy is a 34-year-old female training for a marathon race of 26.2 miles. She is 5 ft 5 in tall and currently weighs 120 lb. On her long runs of more than 3 hours, she has been drinking water, approximately 30 oz, and consuming one GU (an energy supplement containing 100 kcal from simple sugar) at the 2-hour mark. Lucy is coming to you for advice because she is becoming increasingly weak and nauseous toward the end of her runs. She reports feeling light-headed and irritable on her long training days. Lucy states that she is eating a tuna fish sandwich with 4 oz of tuna mixed with 3 tbsp of mayonnaise on whole wheat bread approximately 20 minutes before her run.

Questions for Analysis
1. What sources of fuel is Lucy predominately using in this type of exercise?
2. How can Lucy assess how much fluids she losses during her run so that she can come up with an appropriate fluid replacement strategy?
3. On what time schedule would you recommend that she consume her fluid and carbohydrate?
4. What would you recommend regarding Lucy's preexercise meal?
5. Should Lucy consider electrolyte replacement, or will plain water be sufficient as a beverage of choice?

EVIDENCE-BASED PRACTICE

Sorting Out the Sports Drinks Saga

Problem: Sorting through the many available sports drinks and the plethora of claims that accompany each one is no easy task. Ultimately we need to answer these questions: How much and what kind of a sports drink is needed during physical activity and exercise?

The first well-known commercially available sports drink was a solution called *Gatorade,* a beverage its developers named for their university's football team. They reasoned that if they analyzed the sweat of their players, they could then replace the lost minerals and water in a drink containing some flavoring, coloring, and sugars to make it acceptable, and it would taste better and have more benefits than plain water. Although Gatorade is beneficial for some athletes, most do not need it during general exercise.

However, what endurance athletes do need, especially in hot weather, is water and fuel in the form of carbohydrates. For athletes losing substantial amounts of water and sodium through sweat, electrolyte replacement is also an important consideration. Hyponatremia, although rare, can be fatal. The most common cause of hyponatremia in endurance athletes results from excess sodium loss through sweat combined with fluid replacement of plain water. Water dilutes the plasma sodium even more, exacerbating the condition. Thus sports drinks with simple carbohydrates and electrolytes are beneficial for endurance athletes.

Another category of sports drinks on the market adds large amounts of vitamins and minerals to their solutions. All of these extra vitamins do not help an athlete's performance, and on a hot day a perspiring athlete could easily consume a megadose in four or five bottles. Athletes who eat well-balanced diets with enough kcalories to maintain energy balance do not need additional vitamin or mineral supplementation.

A third category of beverages promoted to enhance athletic performance includes energy drinks. These products should not be confused with sports drinks; although sports drinks have a proven performance benefit in specific athletic contexts, energy drinks do not demonstrate this benefit and carry with them the potential to impair performance. Not only is the glucose concentration higher than the recommended amount, which could result in serious gastrointestinal symptoms, but these products also contain added stimulants and chemicals that are poorly regulated. Consumption of these products should be discouraged, particularly in relation to physical activity.

As a general guide, it is worth the time to sort out the costs and claims made by sports drink manufacturers. These products are not for everyone. Although special sports drinks may meet the needs of athletes competing in physically demanding endurance events, they are not required by those participating in less demanding sports activities. Water is the best solution for regular needs, and it costs far less.

Bibliography

Position of the Academy of Nutrition and Dietetics, Dietitians of Canada, and the American College of Sports Medicine: Nutrition and athletic performance, *J Acad Nutr Diet* 116(3):501, 2016.

NUTRITION AND ATHLETIC PERFORMANCE

Exercise and Energy

Exercise raises the body's kcalorie expenditure and has the additional benefit of helping to regulate appetite to meet these needs. Table 14.3 gives some examples of the amount of kcalories spent in various activities. The replenishment of glycogen reserves is important for athletes such as long-distance runners who compete in endurance events and need a steady supply of energy within the muscle. When exercise

TABLE 14.3 Approximate Energy Expenditure Per Hour During Various Activities

Activity	Kcalories per hour[a]
Sleeping	63
Lying/sitting, awake	70
Standing, relaxed	84
Rapid typing, sitting	105
Dressing and undressing	140
Walking slowly (24 min/mile)	210
Water aerobics	280
High-impact aerobics	490
Football, flag/touch	560
Walking very fast (12 min/mile)	560
Stair, treadmill	630
Swimming, vigorous effort	700
Running (8 min/mile)	875

[a]For an adult weighing 70 kg (154 lb).
From Nix S: *Williams' basic nutrition & diet therapy,* ed 14, St Louis, 2013, Elsevier.

levels rise from mild or moderate amounts up to strenuous levels, kcaloric needs also rise to supply needed fuel.

Active people, even athletes, require no more dietary fat than their inactive counterparts. Carbohydrate is the preferred fuel and is also needed in the recovery period. Complex carbohydrate forms (i.e., starches) sustain energy needs and supply added fiber, vitamins, and minerals. Protein is also required in greater amounts. The recommended composition of energy nutrients to support physical activity in highly active people is as follows[11]:

- *Carbohydrate:* 5 to 12 g/kg body weight per day based on sport type and intensity and duration of training volume
- *Protein:* 1.2 to 2.0 g/kg of body weight, depending upon the athlete's volume of training, inclusion of resistance training, and state of energy balance
- *Fat:* 20% to 35% of total kcalories

Pregame and Training Meals. Protein and fat delay the emptying of the stomach, and neither contributes to the glycogen stores needed during exercise. Therefore the ideal pregame meal is approximately 1 to 4 g of carbohydrate per kg of body weight consumed within 1 to 4 hours before the event, allowing adequate time for digestion and absorption.[12] A sample meal is illustrated in Box 14.2. This meal should be high in complex carbohydrates, moderate in protein, and with little fat or fiber. Good food choices include pasta, bread, bagels, fruit, and cereal with nonfat milk or milk substitute. Throughout the period of vigorous training, a high-carbohydrate diet with 6 to 12 g/kg

BOX 14.2 Sample Pregame Meal

This sample pregame meal includes approximately 234 g of carbohydrates, is high in complex carbohydrates, and is low in protein, fat, and fiber:

- 1½ cups white rice (302 kcal, 66 g carbohydrate)
- 2 tbsp teriyaki sauce (28 kcal, 5 g carbohydrate)
- ½ cup steamed green peas (62 kcal, 11 g carbohydrate)
- 1 slice French bread, large (281 kcal, 55 g carbohydrate)
- 1 baked sweet potato, large (260 kcal, 60 g carbohydrate)
- 1 cup grape juice (152 kcal, 37 g carbohydrate)

of body weight a day is recommended. All athletes should experiment with their own level of tolerance during training sessions.

Energy During Exercise. For activities lasting less than 1 hour, most athletes do not need exogenous sources of energy during the exercise period. However, performance is enhanced during longer endurance events with the interval consumption of carbohydrates. The American College of Sports Medicine, the Academy of Nutrition and Dietetics, and the Dietitians of Canada recommend eating or drinking approximately 30 to 60 g of carbohydrate per hour during long events.[11] It is most effective to consume equal amounts of the preferred food every 15 to 20 minutes throughout the event rather than consuming the entire 30 to 60 g at once. Athletes should experiment with various forms of carbohydrate before competition to determine what is best tolerated. A large variety of sports drinks, gels, and other forms of carbohydrates are available from which the athlete may choose. The food of choice should provide carbohydrates primarily from glucose, with little or no fat, protein, or fiber.

Energy After Exercise: Recovery. Proper nutrition continues to play an integral role in the recovery process. Fluid carbohydrates, and protein consumed within 30 to 60 minutes after a glycogen-depleting endurance event will result in improved glycogen and muscle protein synthesis and muscle recovery than if those same replacement nutrients were consumed 2 hours or more after the event.[20] Rehydration beverages should contain sodium to support fluid retention and comprise 125% to 150% of the fluids that were lost during exercise. Postexercise foods should include approximately 1 to 1.2 g/kg of carbohydrate per body weight each hour for 4 to 6 hours to support muscle glycogen resynthesis, and 20 to 30 g of high quality protein to promote muscle protein synthesis.[21]

Myths and Misinformation. Athletes and their coaches are particularly susceptible to myths and claims about foods and dietary supplements, relentlessly searching for the competitive edge (see the Focus on Culture box, "The Winning Edge—or Over the Edge?"). Knowing this, marketers unremittingly exploit this hunt. Manufacturers sometimes make distorted and false claims about products. For example, pangamic acid was marketed as "vitamin B$_{15}$," although it is not a vitamin at all and carried claims about its ability to enhance oxygen transport during exercise, to lessen muscle fatigue, and to increase endurance. Naturally, if such a compound existed, then it would be of interest to athletes and their trainers. However, scientific research has exposed these claims as unfounded.[22,23] Nevertheless, products and advertisements still appear for "vitamin B$_{15}$," although it is currently illegal to distribute pangamic acid in the United States.

Training and Precompetition Abuses Among Athletes

Weight-Control Measures. The sport of wrestling has a long history of widely fluctuating weight patterns among its athletes. Wrestlers often restrict food and fluid intake to qualify for a weight classification that is less than their off-season weight, seeking to gain advantages in strength, speed, and leverage over a smaller opponent. This practice of "making weight" still seems to be an ingrained tradition that produces large, frequent, and rapid weight-loss and regain cycles, with methods such as dehydration, food restriction, and loss of food and fluid through induced vomiting and use of laxatives and diuretics. Such disordered eating affects normal growth, and progressive dehydration impairs regulation of body temperature and cardiovascular function. Other sports such as bodybuilding, gymnastics, and lightweight

⊕ FOCUS ON CULTURE

The Winning Edge—or Over the Edge?

Athletes and their coaches have become increasingly aware that the percentage of body fat versus the percentage of lean body mass is an influential factor on athletic performance. There is the belief that each extra pound of body fat an athlete carries into competition is nonproductive weight because the muscles, the lean body mass, provide the strength, agility, and endurance required to win.

Because of this pressure, many athletes strive to achieve as low a percentage of body fat as possible. However, in reaching for such a goal, many young athletes develop an abhorrence of body fat, resulting in food aversion and the undertaking of excessive weight-loss regimens. These beliefs are commonly reinforced by those surrounding young athletes: coaches, teammates, and parents. Such an all-consuming focus may result in compulsive behaviors, driving the athlete to set unrealistic goals, and leading to abusive weight loss behaviors.

Such excessive voluntary weight loss practices in young athletes are not usually the result of chronic emotional problems, as with other psychologic eating disorders. The reasons typically are more performance driven, resulting from an accumulation of immediate and short-term goals and concerns. These athletes usually respond well to counseling and can reverse these unhealthy behaviors with the support of concerned friends and teammates.

Yet for a few individuals, the reversal of these risky behaviors is not so simple. There is research to indicate that athletes who engage in dieting behaviors are more likely to develop a psychological eating disorder. Although it is not exactly understood why some athletes progress to pathologic eating behaviors and others do not, it is believed that there is a conflux of cultural, individual, biochemical, and psychological risk factors predisposing certain individuals. The culture of an athlete's sport can enhance this pressure, whether it is real or perceived, to maintain a low body weight or low percentage of body fat. Furthermore, some athletes have personal characteristics such as perfectionism and high-achievement orientation which allow them to excel in their sport but may also contribute to their increased eating disorder risk. These individuals typically require therapeutic counseling as well as working with a physician and sports dietitian to address these deep-rooted beliefs and behaviors.[24]

Compulsive dieting, as in anorexia nervosa, is a serious psychologic disorder; on the other hand, compulsive training is seen by society as a positive personality trait demonstrating commitment. In reality, both may be symptomatic of unstable self-concepts and attempts to establish a firm sense of identity. They are perceptual disorders: individuals with anorexia nervosa believe that they are not thin enough; compulsive exercisers believe that they are not exercising adequately. For these individuals, no goal, once attained, is sufficiently satisfying. Such striving, often despite physical contraindications, has resulted in permanent disabilities and even death.

The danger of athletic pressure leading to eating disorders was highlighted by the 1994 death from anorexia nervosa of 22-year-old Christy Henrich, a world-class American gymnast. At 4 ft 10 in (147 cm) and 95 lb (43 kg), Christy won a silver medal at the 1989 US National Championships. She was known as a perfectionist who pushed herself hard, a characteristic that, when extreme, is often associated with eating disorders in athletes. She felt compelled to lose more weight and at times limited herself to only an apple a day even while continuing to train. Because of her eating disorder, she eventually lost the strength to perform and was forced to retire from competition. She weighed only 60 lb (27 kg) when she died. Although her death marked the first time an American gymnast had died from an eating disorder, such problems are widely known in competitive women's gymnastics, especially at the national and international levels.

It should be noted that such risk factors are not true for all competitive athletes, nor are such risk factors confined to competitive athletes. Although athletes seem to have a higher prevalence than their nonathletic peers, not all sports carry the same risks. Aesthetic sports such as figure skating and gymnastics, weight class sports like martial arts or wrestling, and endurance sports such as distance running and cycling carry a higher risk of disordered eating and eating disorders due to the pressures to maintain a low body weight. Female athletes are at higher risk than their male counterparts. Any athlete suspected of having an eating disorder should receive multidisciplinary treatment.[26]

Bibliography

Obituary: Christy Henrich 1972–1994, *Int Gymnast* 36(10):48–49, 1994.

---

rowing may follow similar routines, especially before competition. In sports that favor lean bodies, it is not uncommon for young preadolescent girls, who wish to maintain a small body size in the face of advancing age, to reduce food intake and body fat which may ultimately develop into an eating disorder.[24] As a result, a cascade of events may follow: impaired growth, delayed puberty, primary or secondary amenorrhea from low estrogen levels, disruption or delay in bone density development, and even osteoporosis.[25] A similar pattern has been observed among young long-distance runners, cheerleaders, and dancers.[26]

Drug Abuse. From ancient Greek runners and discus throwers in the first Olympian contests to top competitors from around the world in current Olympic events, athletes have experimented with various ergogenic aids in their eternal search for the competitive edge or the perfect body. Modern athletes—from professional football players to their aspiring high school counterparts—are still trying to find the magic potion in everything from bee pollen and seaweed to freeze-dried liver flakes, gelatin, amino acid supplements, and ginseng. Such efforts have been worthless in most cases but fortunately not

particularly harmful. However, in the case of anabolic-androgenic steroids, human growth hormone, and insulin-like growth factor, which are now epidemic in the sporting world, great danger and even death may lie ahead for the user.[27] These dangers include cardiovascular health risk, impaired liver function, disturbances in normal steroid production, increased aggression and hostility, mood disturbances, and additional disturbances in psychologic and dermatologic conditions.[27]

The use of legal pharmacologic agents in an illegal manner has created a black market network, which adds criminal jeopardy and street preparation impurities to the drug's inherent dangers. Abuse of anabolic steroids in the United States has moved from its early use among bodybuilders and invaded almost all areas of athletics, beginning as early as adolescence.[28] In addition, other abuses amplify the dangers of steroids. For example, diuretics are often abused by athletes to rapidly lose water weight and to dilute the urine in attempt to mask the use of other banned substances during drug screenings.[29]

Risks for Female Athletes

Some female athletes who enter highly competitive and demanding sports face health risks related to anemia and low bone mineral density (BMD) if their diets do not adequately meet their nutrient and energy needs. These risks are especially prevalent for female athletes in sports with intensive training and endurance events, such as gymnastics, running, cycling, and other endurance events. Highly skilled dancers and those performing in aesthetic sports face similar risks.

Sports Anemia and Iron Deficiency Anemia. Normal hemoglobin values are approximately 12 to 15.5 g/dL for women and 13.5 to 17.5 g/dL for men. Iron deficiency anemia is defined as hemoglobin levels less than these ranges. As baseline plasma volume increases with aerobic training, the concentration of hemoglobin (found within red blood cells) is reduced as a percentage of total blood. Such a situation is more appropriately referred to as *sports anemia* rather than iron deficiency anemia, because the total volume of red blood cells is normal. Additional iron intake, whether through food or supplementation, is not needed in sports anemia. However, care must be taken to appropriately distinguish sports anemia from other forms of true anemias.

True iron deficiency anemia is typically a result of inadequate iron in the diet, decreased iron absorption, or increased iron losses. Absolute and functional levels of iron deficiency are particularly of concern for elite athletes.[30] Reduced hemoglobin in an athlete's blood means reduced oxygen-carrying capacity with negative implications for aerobic capacity and the ability to sustain an exercise workload.[30] Accordingly, one of the first implications for iron deficiency anemia is exertional fatigue. Unless a woman is experiencing amenorrhea, she will have cyclic menstrual loss of iron. Some iron is lost in profuse sweating and occasionally because of intravascular hemolysis, which is the rupture of red blood cells caused by the stresses of heavy exercise, although neither is believed to be a major contributor to iron loss. Regular evaluation of dietary iron intake and iron status among athletes is warranted.

Low Bone Mineral Density. An inadequate diet, intentionally or not, combined with an interrupted menstrual cycle can lead to low

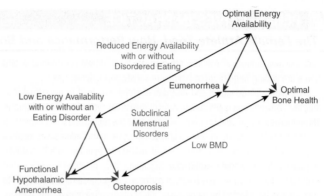

FIG. 14.3 Spectra of the female athlete triad. The three interrelated components of the female athlete triad are energy availability, menstrual status and bone health. Energy availability directly affects menstrual status, and in turn, energy availability and menstrual status directly influence bone health. Optimal health is indicated by optimal energy availability, eumenorrhea and optimal bone health, whereas, at the other end of the spectrum, the most severe presentation of the female athlete triad is characterized by low energy availability with or without an eating disorder, functional hypothalamic amenorrhoea and osteoporosis. An athlete's condition moves along each spectrum at different rates depending on her diet and exercise behaviors. *BMD,* bone mineral density. (Adapted with permission from Lippincott Williams and Wilkins/Wolters Kluwer Health: Medicine and Science in Sport and Exercise.)

BMD (**osteopenia**). In some cases the bone loss may progress to a state of osteoporosis at an abnormally young age. Low BMD is a component of the *female athlete triad* (Fig. 14.3) and results from three contributing factors: (1) low energy availability, (2) menstrual dysfunction, and (3) bone loss. The Perspectives in Practice box, "The Female Athlete Triad: How Performance and Social Pressure Can Lead to Low Bone Mass," illustrates the contributing factors that ultimately lead to injury and impaired health.

PERSPECTIVES IN PRACTICE

The Female Athlete Triad: How Performance and Social Pressure Can Lead to Low Bone Mass

The female athlete triad is a medical condition that includes any one of the three components: (1) low energy availability with or without disordered eating, (2) menstrual dysfunction, and (3) low BMD. Low energy availability is likely the underlying cause, and if left untreated, low BMD may progress to osteoporosis and menstrual dysfunction may lead to functional hypothalamic amenorrhea. Health consequences of the triad are numerous and include musculoskeletal and cardiovascular damage, as well as impaired endocrine, gastrointestinal, renal, and neuropsychiatric functioning.[25] Women in top physical form may be more susceptible to social and performance pressures leading to disordered eating habits and consequently, low energy availability. The dilemma facing female athletes currently is how to maintain optimal physical performance while not provoking health risks.

Women who participate in competitive endurance sports, such as long-distance running or cycling; who are judged partially on physical appearance, such as in ice skating, diving, and gymnastics; or who participate in weight class sports such as lightweight rowing are more likely to be preoccupied with

their weight and to have self-image issues. Social and competitive pressures for a woman to be thin can contribute to her sense of imperfection (for both athletes and nonathletic females). These demands and pressures can lead to disordered eating patterns, which in combination with strenuous exercise may result in low energy availability. This drop in energy will negatively affect the performance of the athlete through adverse effects on physical and muscular fitness.[31] Although low energy availability may be inadvertent (the athlete is unaware of their low energy intake), it may be the result of disordered eating behaviors that may eventually progress to a psychological eating disorders. Examples include bulimia nervosa, characterized by binge eating followed by compensatory mechanisms; or anorexia nervosa, characterized by the inability to consume sufficient calories for daily requirements. These disorders may, in turn, progress to additional health problems, including depression, seizures, cardiac arrhythmia, myocardial infarction, or other health complications. Contributing factors to eating disorders include weight cycling and dieting pressure, personality factors, early start of sport-specific training, traumatic events,

Continued

and coaching behavior.[26] Athletes often equate leanness with performance, and some are willing to go to great lengths to satisfy perfectionist needs.

Inadequate caloric intake and disordered eating may lead to menstrual dysfunction. Amenorrhea is the suppression of menstrual cycles to a level of zero to three menses a year, and primary amenorrhea is the repression of all menstrual cycles until after age 16. In some highly competitive sports, adolescent females may actually strive to delay the onset of puberty to maintain small, childlike physiques. Some women experience oligomenorrhea, or sporadic cycles that occur 3 to 9 times a year. The levels of estrogen and progesterone that regulate menses can be affected by metabolism, intensive exercise, stress, and particularly low energy availability.

Menstrual dysfunction plays a causative role in low BMD. Low BMD is the leading cause of stress fractures and injuries throughout the body, some of which may be irreversible. If left untreated, low BMD may eventually progress to osteoporosis. Before the age of 30, bone density reaches its peak, and it is vital for young women to strive for dense bones in early adulthood to maintain healthy bone density later in life. If the density of bones is compromised, then osteopenia occurs; if severe enough, it can be a signal of future osteoporosis. Porous bones increase the likelihood of stress fractures and injuries, and women are more likely to incur such injuries than men.

However, some studies indicate that weight-bearing activities, such as gymnastics, seem to actually improve bone density, even perhaps in vertebrae, and they may help to prevent density decreases later in life. Nonetheless, the problem facing female athletes who are eating improperly is that the decline in BMD is amplified as menstrual cycles continue to be erratic. Weight-bearing sports will not overcome the tendency for participants to have low BMD if diet and exercise levels are not balanced.

The primary goal of treatment is to achieve optimal energy availability by increasing caloric intake, decreasing exercise, or both. Weight restoration

may also be required. Nutrient supplementation may be indicated to maximize bone growth and avert endothelial dysfunction involving calcium and vitamin D, although supplementation alone will not improve BMD or address the underlying metabolic problems. In general, oral contraceptive therapy is not recommended because it may mask menstrual dysfunction and does not appear to improve BMD.[25]

Only improved energy intake can improve BMD and menstrual function. Athletes should receive treatment from a sports dietitian, a therapist in the presence of an eating disorder, and a sports physician. Gradually caloric intake should be increased until sufficient. Ideal body weight is individual, depending on height and skeletal structure, and one specific weight goal should not exist for all female athletes. An appropriate body weight can be determined by a sports dietitian and medical provider.

The societal and competitive pressures that may cause low energy availability must be addressed. Asking female athletes to sacrifice their health for an unrealistic body image projected on them by others (as well as their coaches' and trainers' desire for vicarious victory) must not alter what constitutes acceptable eating habits. In our current weight-conscious society, the emphasis must not be on a perfect image, size, or body but rather on the perfect balance of health and training. The female athlete's skeletal integrity, and potentially her cardiovascular function, suffers as she resorts to drastic measures in her aspiration for an overly lean physical image.

The need to educate trainers, athletes, and health professionals about the consequences of neglected nutrition is imperative. Young female athletes must understand that deprivation of life's essential nutrients results in significant bodily harm.

An estimated 40% to 60% of a woman's normal BMD for her lifetime develops during adolescence when her sex hormone estrogen becomes active. Diet and hormones must work in concert. Calcium intake must be adequate, as well as normal functioning of the female estrogen cycle to stimulate osteoblastic activity (bone growth). Unfortunately, many young females restrict their diets in an effort to control their weight, growth, and body fat, with resulting inadequate dietary energy and calcium. Some females may have more profound eating disorders, such as anorexia nervosa. At the same time, intense athletic training in women can lead to primary amenorrhea or secondary amenorrhea as a result of low energy availability. Amenorrhea is more common in athletes than in nonathletes; it is especially prevalent among aesthetic, endurance, and weight-class sports.[26] When athletic training begins before normal menarche, the onset of puberty and its associated growth and developmental patterns may be delayed. Such delays include the secondary sex characteristics shaping the female figure. Consequently, normal estrogen levels may be depressed. As a result, these young women athletes are at a high risk for low BMD and stress fractures.[26] Injuries and fractures can interrupt or permanently end an athletic career, and bone mineral loss may be irreversible and become a lifelong risk.

KEY TERMS

Amenorrhea
The absence of menses (menstrual cycle) entirely or no more than three periods in a year; associated with lower-than-normal estrogen levels in women.

Osteoporosis
Abnormal thinning of bone, producing a porous, fragile, latticelike bone tissue of enlarged spaces that is prone to fracture or deformity.

Ergogenic
Tendency to increase work output; various substances that increase work or exercise capacity and output.

Osteopenia
Below-normal level of BMD, which increases the risk of stress fractures; the bone thinning is not as severe as that found in osteoporosis.

Primary Amenorrhea
Amenorrhea delay of menarche past the age of 16.

Secondary Amenorrhea
Cessation of the normal menstrual cycle after menarche.

HEALTH PROMOTION

BUILDING A PERSONAL EXERCISE PROGRAM

Exercise is a critical component in health promotion and disease prevention. The current *Physical Activity Guidelines for Americans* state the following[32]:

Children and Adolescents: Participate in 60 minutes (1 hour) or more of physical activity daily.

- Most of the 60 or more minutes a day should be either moderate- or vigorous-intensity aerobic physical activity and should include vigorous-intensity physical activity at least 3 days a week. Table 14.4 describes the classifications of exercise intensity.
- As part of their 60 or more minutes of daily physical activity, children and adolescents should include muscle-strengthening physical activity on at least 3 days of the week.
- As part of their 60 or more minutes of daily physical activity, children and adolescents should include bone-strengthening physical activity on at least 3 days of the week. (See Chapter 12 for more information about children and physical activity.)

Adults: Avoid inactivity. Some physical activity is better than none, and adults who participate in any amount of physical activity gain some health benefits.

- For substantial health benefits, adults should do at least 150 minutes (2 hours and 30 minutes) a week of moderate-intensity, or 75 minutes (1 hour and 15 minutes) a week of vigorous-intensity aerobic physical activity, or an equivalent combination of moderate- and vigorous-intensity aerobic activity. Aerobic activity should be performed in episodes of at least 10 minutes, and preferably it should be spread throughout the week.
- For additional and more extensive health benefits, adults should increase their aerobic physical activity to 300 minutes (5 hours) a week of moderate intensity, or 150 minutes a week of vigorous intensity aerobic physical activity, or an equivalent combination of moderate- and vigorous-intensity activity. Additional health benefits are gained by engaging in physical activity beyond this amount.
- Adults should also do muscle-strengthening activities that are moderate or high intensity and involve all major muscle groups on 2 or more days a week because these activities provide additional health benefits.

Older Adults: The guidelines for adults also apply to older adults. In addition, the following guidelines are just for older adults:

- When older adults cannot do 150 minutes of moderate-intensity aerobic activity a week because of chronic conditions, they should be as physically active as their abilities and conditions allow.
- Older adults should do exercises that maintain or improve balance if they are at risk of falling.
- Older adults should determine their level of effort for physical activity relative to their level of fitness.
- Older adults with chronic conditions should understand whether and how their conditions affect their ability to do regular physical activity safely.

Exercise and Disease Prevention

Coronary Heart Disease. Exercise reduces risks for heart disease in several ways related to heart function, blood cholesterol levels, and oxygen transport:

- *Heart muscle function:* Exercise, especially aerobic conditioning, strengthens the heart, thereby enabling the heart to pump more blood per beat (stroke volume). A heart strengthened by exercise has an increased aerobic capacity (i.e., the heart can pump more blood per minute without an undue increase in the heart rate). Therefore exercises that rely primarily on the aerobic oxygen system for energy, such as walking, jogging, and workouts on light cardiopulmonary exercise machines, improve heart function.
- *Blood lipid levels:* Aerobic exercise programs improve blood lipid profiles by lowering total cholesterol (TC), low-density lipoproteins (LDLs), the TC/high-density lipoprotein (HDL) ratio, and triglycerides. When aerobic training is combined with a prudent diet, the improvements in lipid profile are even more significant.[32a,33]
- *Oxygen-carrying capacity:* Exercise also enhances the circulatory system by increasing the oxygen-carrying capacity of the blood. As training continues, a person's VO2max will improve, thus increasing the efficiency of oxygen use and uptake.

Hypertension. The risk for cardiovascular complications increases continuously with increasing levels of blood pressure. Hypertension is indicated when the systolic blood pressure is greater than 130 mm Hg, the diastolic blood pressure is greater than 80 mm Hg, or both. Exercise is one of the most effective nondrug treatments for treating and reducing the risk of hypertension.[34,35] Even for persons with moderate to severe hypertension, exercise has proven to be an important adjunct to drug therapy, offsetting adverse drug effects and lowering medication requirements. Normal rises in blood pressure occur during dynamic (e.g., walking, cycling) and resistance (i.e., strength training) exercise. Both forms of exercise are beneficial for individuals with hypertension. However, exercisers should avoid holding their breath during the exertion phase of heavy weight lifting to prevent severe stress on the cardiovascular system, especially those with diagnosed hypertension.

Diabetes. Resistance and endurance-type exercise programs help to maintain glucose homeostasis in patients with impaired glucose tolerance and type 2 diabetes.[36] Physically active lifestyles are especially beneficial for individuals with type 2 diabetes to reduce the risk of chronic complications associated with the disease.[36] Exercise improves the action of a person's naturally produced insulin by increasing the sensitivity of insulin receptor sites on cells. In managing type 1 diabetes mellitus, the type of exercise and when it is done must

TABLE 14.4 Classification of Exercise Intensity			
Intensity	% Maximum Heart Rate	%VO2max	Perceived Exertion
Light	57–63	37–45	Very light to fairly light
Moderate	64–76	46–63	Fairly light to somewhat hard
Vigorous	77–95	64–90	Somewhat hard to very hard

Modified from Garber CE, Blissman B, Deschenes MR: American College of Sports Medicine position stand. Quantity and quality of exercise for developing and maintaining cardiorespiratory, musculoskeletal, and neuromotor fitness in apparently healthy adults: guidance for prescribing exercise, *Med Sci Sports Exerc* 43(7):1334–1359, 2011.

be balanced with food and insulin to prevent reactions caused by drops in blood glucose. (See Chapter 22 for a more detailed discussion of diabetes.)

Weight Management. Although exercise alone is not generally sufficient to obtain or maintain weight loss, it is an important aspect of a healthy lifestyle that supports fitness and a healthy weight. Furthermore, when moderate to vigorous physical activity is combined with nutrition intervention (decreased caloric intake), weight loss is greatest compared with weight loss resulting from the two behaviors individually. Exercise is particularly important in supporting weight maintenance (see Chapter 15).[37]

Stress Management. Exercise helps to reduce stress-related eating. Exercise training has also shown improvements in heart rate, heart rate variability, and cortisol levels that are produced in the body by stress, thus helping to reduce a major risk factor in the development of chronic disease.[38]

Bone Disease. Weight-bearing exercises improve bone mineralization, thus reducing the risk of bone weakness and of potential osteoporosis.

Mental Health. Extended aerobic exercise stimulates the production of brain opiates, which are substances called *endorphins*. These natural substances decrease pain (this is how aspirin works, by stimulating production of endorphins) and improve the mood, including an exhilarating kind of "high."

Assessment of Personal Health and Exercise Needs

There are many options for exercise and activity. Choosing the best form depends on individual health, personal needs, the aerobic benefits involved, and personal enjoyment.

Assessing Health and Personal Needs. In planning an exercise program, it is important to assess individual health status, personal needs, present level of fitness, and resources available. Discussing an exercise program with a medical practitioner is always recommended, and getting a medical clearance before beginning an exercise program is especially important for older individuals and those with chronic disease. It is wise to start slowly and build gradually rather than risk injury and discouragement. Moderation and consistency are key.

Beginning a Program. Many options exist regarding where, what, when, and how one exercises. It is important to evaluate these options before committing to any one routine. A golden rule for success is that if a person enjoys the activity they are doing, then they are much more likely to make it part of their everyday schedule. Some individuals benefit from joining a fitness facility where they feel encouraged by others. However, others may shy away from fitness facilities for fear of discomfort. Keeping the following questions in mind while designing an exercise program can be helpful:

1. Which is better, a fitness facility or a home program?
   - Is external encouragement helpful in maintaining a regular exercise schedule? Is company and interaction with others desirable during exercise, or is exercising alone preferable?
   - Is sticking to a schedule ideal and easy, or is it more realistic to work around other obligations and exercise when and where possible?
   - Is a fitness facility located near home or work? Is it affordable?

- Is the office or home in an area that can provide uninterrupted bouts of exercise?
2. What type of exercise best fits the needs of you or your client?
   - It is important for everyone to determine independently what he or she *likes* to do. If the exercise chosen is not fun, then the patient or client will soon stop doing it, making it of no benefit. Encourage someone who has little exposure to various forms of physical activity to experiment with a variety of activities before committing to one.
   - While exercising at a fitness facility, would your client or patient enjoy aerobic exercise on a bike, on a treadmill, or in a group class?
   - If your client or patient is considering exercising at home, you can ask other questions: Do you live in an area where you can run, walk, or bike? If not, then do you have access to a stationary bike, treadmill, or other aerobic machine? Videos and DVDs can also provide great at-home exercise opportunities. Try to choose an activity that he or she can stick with throughout the year, or choose a variety of activities that can be alternated during various seasons. For instance, perhaps swimming or biking work well in the summer, whereas running or participating in aerobic classes would work in the winter.
   - For strength training, fitness facilities usually provide an assortment of free weights and resistance machines. Always encourage your client or patient to ask for help if he or she is not sure how to correctly perform any exercise. Resistance training can be done effectively at home as well, with a combination of resistance bands, small hand weights, or even cans of beans!

Frequency, Intensity, and Duration. To achieve aerobic benefits from exercise, it is recommended that individualized exercise prescriptions meet the following levels of intensity and duration[39]:

- *Frequency:* 5 or more days per week of moderate exercise, or 3 or more days per week of vigorous exercise, or a combination of moderate and vigorous exercise on 3 to 5 days per week.
- *Intensity:* Moderate and/or vigorous intensity is recommended for most adults (see Table 14.4).
- *Duration:* 30 to 60 minutes per day (150 minutes per week) of purposeful moderate exercise, or 20 to 60 minutes per day (75 minutes per week) of vigorous exercise, or a combination of moderate and vigorous exercise per day is recommended for most adults. Less than 20 minutes per day of exercise can be beneficial, especially in previously sedentary persons. If exercise is broken into short periods, the accumulated duration should be 30 minutes or more daily in bouts of 10 minutes or more each period.

Types of Exercise

Many types of exercise exist from which a participant may choose. Many of them are enjoyable and healthful but do not reach aerobic levels. For example, golf is a passion for many and gets them outdoors, but it is far too slow and sporadic to be aerobic. It is best to have a variety of exercises in any exercise plan (Fig. 14.4). Even though many sports do not reach aerobic levels, if they are enjoyable they should be included.

Aerobic Exercise. Forms of exercise that can be sustained at a necessary level of intensity to provide aerobic benefits include such activities as swimming, running, jogging, bicycling, and aerobic dancing routines and workouts (Table 14.5). The exercise performed should be

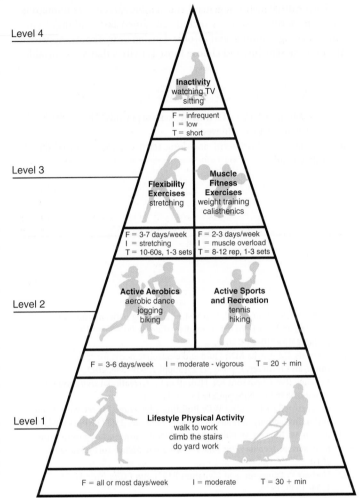

FIG. 14.4 Physical activity pyramid. (Modified with permission from Corbin CB, Lindsey R: *Fitness for life,* ed 5, Champaign, IL, 2005, Human Kinetics, pp. 64.)

Level 4

Inactivity
watching TV
sitting

F = infrequent
I = low
T = short

Level 3

Flexibility
Exercises
stretching

Muscle
Fitness
Exercises
weight training
calisthenics

F = 3-7 days/week
I = stretching
T = 10-60s, 1-3 sets

F = 2-3 days/week
I = muscle overload
T = 8-12 rep, 1-3 sets

Level 2

Active Aerobics
aerobic dance
jogging
biking

Active Sports
and Recreation
tennis
hiking

F = 3-6 days/week   I = moderate - vigorous   T = 20 + min

Level 1

Lifestyle Physical Activity
walk to work
climb the stairs
do yard work

F = all or most days/week   I = moderate   T = 30 + min

TABLE 14.5 Examples of Aerobic Exercises for Physical Fitness[a]	
Type of Exercise	**Aerobic Forms**
Ball playing	Handball
	Racquetball
	Squash
Bicycling	Stationary
	Touring
Dancing	Aerobic routines
	Ballet
	Disco
Jumping rope	Brisk pace
Running or jogging	Brisk pace
Skating	Ice skating
	Roller skating
Skiing	Cross-country
Swimming	Steady pace
Walking	Brisk pace

[a]Maintained at aerobic level for at least 30 minutes total.

regular, purposeful, continuous and rhythmic in nature, and involve the major muscle groups.[39] Perhaps the simplest and most popular form of stimulating exercise is walking. If the pace is fast enough to elevate the pulse and maintain it, then walking can be an excellent form of aerobic exercise. Walking is convenient, available, and appropriate for most people; in addition, it requires no equipment other than good walking shoes.

Resistance Exercise. Resistance types of exercises are designed to increase muscle strength and endurance. An ideal program would consist of several exercises with 8 to 12 repetitions of each, focusing on the major muscles of the body, performed 2 to 3 days per week. For an individual whose primary goal is to gain strength and power, the repetitions should be of high intensity (60%–80% of 1 repetition max). For improved endurance, a lower weight should be used that will allow at least 15 to 20 repetitions before muscle fatigue.[39]

Weight-bearing exercises, such as walking, jogging, aerobic dancing, or jumping rope, are important for bone structure and strength. In each of these exercises, muscles are working against gravity. Bones will adapt to the environment and load put on them during weight-bearing exercises to build more bone cells and increase bone density.

Flexibility Exercises and Stretching. Flexibility exercises and stretching are recommended for all age groups. Selecting a variety of stretches that target each of the major muscle-tendon units is ideal to help maintain joint mobility, stability, and balance. Stretching and holding the stretch for 10 to 60 seconds at a point of tightness is recommended at least 2 to 3 days a week.[39]

TO SUM UP

The energy molecule of the body is ATP, and the powerhouse of the cell is the mitochondrion. The cell replenishes ATP through CP. These two high-energy phosphate compounds are in limited supply. They can produce energy for a brief initial period only and need to be replenished for exercise to continue. Initially, additional energy is produced by anaerobic glycolysis, with energy made available for continued exercise by the body's aerobic system. The process of glycolysis metabolizes only carbohydrate substrate, furnished by either blood glucose or stored glycogen. Dietary carbohydrate is necessary to replenish these fuel sources. Protein contributes little to energy for exercise, whereas the body's ability to burn fat as fuel depends on the level of fitness and intensity of exercise. The higher the body's efficiency in using oxygen, the more fatty acids will contribute to the energy supply. Even in the best-trained athletes, fatty acid oxidation must be accompanied by glucose metabolism.

Contrary to popular belief, exercise does not require an increased intake of vitamins or minerals. The body's increased needs are well supplied by a normal healthy diet. Exercise increases the body's need for kcalories, carbohydrates, protein, and water. Cold water taken in small, frequent amounts is the best way to prevent dehydration in most athletic events and exercise. In most cases, electrolytes lost in sweat are replaced by a diet of adequate quality and quantity. A mild sodium and glucose solution (4%–8%) may supply fluid and fuel to sustain energy during longer endurance events. Some athletes use harmful practices such as food and fluid deprivation for controlling weight, as well as such ergogenic aids as illegal steroid drugs for bulking muscles.

The optimal diet for the athlete is moderate in protein and fat, with 5 to 12 g/kg of body weight per day coming from carbohydrates. The pregame meal should be small, having little or no protein or fat and relying mainly on complex carbohydrates.

The health benefits of general and aerobic exercise are numerous. Excellent aerobic exercises include sustained fast walking, swimming, jogging, running, and aerobic dancing or workouts. Approach any exercise sensibly, and choose those activities that are enjoyable.

QUESTIONS FOR REVIEW

1. What are the component muscle structures, and how do they produce muscular action?
2. What type of substrate fuel does the body use for immediate energy needs? For short-term needs? For long-term needs?
3. How does oxygen relate to physical activity capacity and aerobic effect?
4. Outline the nutrition and physical fitness principles to discuss with an athlete. Plan a diet for this client that would meet nutrient and energy needs.
5. Why is fluid balance vital during exercise periods? How is water and electrolyte balance achieved?
6. Describe the short-term and long-term consequences of female athlete triad.

REFERENCES

1. Maughan RJ, Shirreffs SM: Nutrition for sports performance: issues and opportunities, *Proc Nutr Soc* 71(1):112–119, 2012.
2. Centers for Disease Control and Prevention: *Physical activity, glossary of terms*, 2015.
3. World Health Organization: *Physical Activity Fact Sheet.* 2016. http://www.who.int/mediacentre/factsheets/fs385/en/.
4. Lee IM, Shiroma EJ, Lobelo F, et al: Effect of physical inactivity on major non-communicable diseases worldwide: an analysis of burden of disease and life expectancy, *Lancet* 380(9838):219–229, 2012.
5. McGuire S: Centers for Disease Control and Prevention. State indicator report on Physical Activity, 2014. Atlanta, GA: US Department of Health and Human Services; 2014, *Adv Nutr* 5(6):762–763, 2014.
6. US Department of Health and Human Services, US Department of Agriculture, US Dietary Guidelines Advisory Committee: *Dietary guidelines for Americans, 2010*, ed 7, Washington, DC, 2010, HHS publication, pp xi, 95.
7. US Department of Health and Human Services, US Department of Agriculture: *Dietary Guidelines for Americans 2015–2020*, 2016.
8. Chiuve SE, Cook NR, Shay CM, et al: Lifestyle-based prediction model for the prevention of CVD: the Healthy Heart Score, *J Am Heart Assoc* 3(6):e000954, 2014.
9. Ford ES, Bergmann MM, Boeing H, et al: Healthy lifestyle behaviors and all-cause mortality among adults in the United States, *Prev Med* 55(1):23–27, 2012.
10. Rice TK, Sarzynski MA, Sung YJ, et al: Fine mapping of a QTL on chromosome 13 for submaximal exercise capacity training response: the HERITAGE Family Study, *Eur J Appl Physiol* 112(8):2969–2978, 2012.
11. Thomas DT, Erdman KA, Burke LM, Position of the Academy of Nutrition and Dietetics, Dietitians of Canada, and the American College of Sports Medicine: Nutrition and Athletic Performance, *J Acad Nutr Diet* 116(3):501–528, 2016.
12. Hawley JA, Leckey JJ: Carbohydrate dependence during prolonged, intense endurance exercise, *Sports Med* 45(Suppl 1):S5–S12, 2015.
13. Williams C, Rollo I: Carbohydrate nutrition and team sport performance, *Sports Med* 45(Suppl 1):S13–S22, 2015.
14. Burke LM, Hawley JA, Wong SH, et al: Carbohydrates for training and competition, *J Sports Sci* 29(Suppl 1):S17–S27, 2011.
15. Cole M, Coleman D, Hopker J, et al: Improved gross efficiency during long duration submaximal cycling following a short-term high carbohydrate diet, *Int J Sports Med* 35(3):265–269, 2014.
16. Phillips SM: Dietary protein requirements and adaptive advantages in athletes, *Br J Nutr* 108(Suppl 2):S158–S167, 2012.
17. Erdman KA, Tunnicliffe J, Lun VM, et al: Eating patterns and composition of meals and snacks in elite Canadian athletes, *Int J Sport Nutr Exerc Metab* 23(3):210–219, 2013.
18. Shirreffs SM, Sawka MN: Fluid and electrolyte needs for training, competition, and recovery, *J Sports Sci* 29(Suppl 1):S39–S46, 2011.
19. Kenefick RW, Cheuvront SN: Hydration for recreational sport and physical activity, *Nutr Rev* 70(Suppl 2):S137–S142, 2012.
20. Spaccarotella KJ, Andzel WD: Building a beverage for recovery from endurance activity: a review, *J Strength Cond Res* 25(11):3198–3204, 2011.
21. Beelen M, Burke LM, Gibala MJ, et al: Nutritional strategies to promote postexercise recovery, *Int J Sport Nutr Exerc Metab* 20(6):515–532, 2010.
22. Herbert V: Pangamic acid ("vitamin B15"), *Am J Clin Nutr* 32(7):1534–1540, 1979.
23. Currell K, Moore DR, Peeling P, et al: A-Z of nutritional supplements: dietary supplements, sports nutrition foods and ergogenic aids for health and performance - part 28, *Br J Sports Med* 46(1):75–76, 2012.
24. Sundgot-Borgen J, Meyer NL, Lohman TG, et al: How to minimise the health risks to athletes who compete in weight-sensitive sports review and position statement on behalf of the Ad Hoc Research Working Group on Body Composition, Health and Performance, under the auspices of the IOC Medical Commission, *Br J Sports Med* 47(16):1012–1022, 2013.
25. Joy E, De Souza MJ, Nattiv A, et al: 2014 female athlete triad coalition consensus statement on treatment and return to play of the female athlete triad, *Curr Sports Med Rep* 13(4):219–232, 2014.
26. Bratland-Sanda S, Sundgot-Borgen J: Eating disorders in athletes: overview of prevalence, risk factors and recommendations for prevention and treatment, *Eur J Sport Sci* 13(5):499–508, 2013.
27. Momaya A, Fawal M, Estes R: Performance-enhancing substances in sports: a review of the literature, *Sports Med* 45(4):517–531, 2015.
28. Woolf J, Swain P: Androgenic anabolic steroid policy and high school sports: results from a policy Delphi study, *Int J Sport Policy* 6(1):89–106, 2014.
29. Cadwallader AB, Murray B: Performance-enhancing drugs I: Understanding the basics of testing for banned substances, *Int J Sport Nutr Exerc Metab* 25(4):396–404, 2015.
30. Clénin GE, Cordes M, Huber A, et al: Iron deficiency in sports—definition, influence on performance and therapy, *Schweiz Z Sportmed* 64(1):6–18, 2016.
31. El Ghoch M, Soave F, Calugi S, et al: Eating disorders, physical fitness and sport performance: a systematic review, *Nutrients* 5(12):5140–5160, 2013.
32. Centers for Disease Control and Prevention: *Physical activity guidelines for Americans*, Washington, DC, 2008, US Department of Health and Human Services.

32a. Gordon B, Chen S, Durstine JL: The effects of exercise training on the traditional lipid profile and beyond, *Curr Sports Med Rep* 13(4):253–259, 2014.

33. Pattyn N, Cornelissen VA, Eshghi SR, et al: The effect of exercise on the cardiovascular risk factors constituting the metabolic syndrome: a meta-analysis of controlled trials, *Sports Med* 43(2):121–133, 2013.

34. Börjesson M, Onerup A, Lundqvist S, et al: Physical activity and exercise lower blood pressure in individuals with hypertension: narrative review of 27 RCTs, *Br J Sports Med* 50(6):356–361, 2016.

35. Pescatello LS, MacDonald HV, Lamberti L, et al: Exercise for hypertension: a prescription update integrating existing recommendations with emerging research, *Curr Hypertens Rep* 17(11):87, 2015.

36. Röhling M, Herder C, Stemper T, et al: Influence of acute and chronic exercise on glucose uptake, *J Diabetes Res* 2016:2868652, 2016.

37. Raynor HA, Champagne CM: Position of the academy of nutrition and dietetics: Interventions for the treatment of overweight and obesity in adults, *J Acad Nutr Diet* 116(1):129–147, 2016.

38. Klaperski S, von Dawans B, Heinrichs M, et al: Effects of a 12-week endurance training program on the physiological response to psychosocial stress in men: a randomized controlled trial, *J Behav Med* 37(6):1118–1133, 2014.

39. Garber CE, Blissmer B, Deschenes MR, et al: American College of Sports Medicine position stand. Quantity and quality of exercise for developing and maintaining cardiorespiratory, musculoskeletal, and neuromotor fitness in apparently healthy adults: guidance for prescribing exercise, *Med Sci Sports Exerc* 43(7):1334–1359, 2011.

FURTHER READINGS AND RESOURCES

Readings

Garber CE, Blissmer B, Deschenes MR, et al: American College of Sports Medicine position stand. Quantity and quality of exercise for developing and maintaining cardiorespiratory, musculoskeletal, and neuromotor fitness in apparently healthy adults: guidance for prescribing exercise. *Med Sci Sports Exerc* 43(7):1334–1359, 2011.

[This position stand paper provides guidelines for individualized exercise prescription for healthy adults.]

Thomas DT, Erdman KA, and Burke LM: Position of the Academy of Nutrition and Dietetics, Dietitians of Canada, and the American College of Sports Medicine: Nutrition and Athletic Performance. *J Acad Nutr Diet* 116(3):501–528, 2016.

[This joint position statement emphasizes the importance of nutrition in physical activity, athletic performance, and recovery from exercise. The experts specifically address nutrient and fluid needs, body composition, supplements and ergogenic aids, and the roles and responsibilities of health care professionals.]

Websites of Interest

- American College of Sports Medicine. http://www.acsm.org.
- National Coalition for Promoting Physical Activity. http://www.ncppa.org.
- Sports, Cardiovascular, and Wellness Nutrition, dietetic practice group of the Academy of Nutrition and Dietetics. http://www.scandpg.org.
- US Department of Health and Human Services, *Physical Activity and Health: A Report of the Surgeon General.* http://www.cdc.gov/nccdphp/sgr/sgr.htm.

15

The Complexity of Obesity: Beyond Energy Balance

Joyce Gilbert

ⓔ http://evolve.elsevier.com/Williams/essentials/

In this chapter, we look at the complex issue of obesity. In recent years the prevalence of obesity has grown to epidemic proportions. Linked as a risk factor for many chronic disorders in the United States, the magnitude of this health care problem and its effect on the health care system are immense.

OUTLINE

Realities of Obesity
Energy Intake, Energy Expenditure, and Development
  of Obesity
Obesity as a Disease

Beyond Energy Balance
Epidemiologic Model
Overview of Treating the Disease of Obesity
Health Promotion

We are living in a time when the number of **overweight** individuals is increasing more rapidly than ever before. This chapter is intended to help you understand this problem. Using an epidemiologic model of the interactions between environmental agents and the human host to explain **obesity**, we explore food, medications, physical inactivity, toxins, and viruses as environmental agents that act on the genetically programmed host to disturb energy balance and cause obesity. Large portion size, high-fat intake, sugar-sweetened beverages, and labor-saving innovations all play a role in the toxic environment that leads to obesity. The genetic, physiologic, and psychological responses of the host determine whether or not this "toxic environment" will produce obesity. Reversing the current trends of obesity requires a new look at the limits of the energy balance concept and a better understanding of how environmental factors acutely and chronically change responses of the susceptible host so that obesity is manifested.

KEY TERMS

Overweight
A body mass index (BMI) of 25 or greater (weight [kg]/height^2 [m^2])

Obesity
An excess amount of body fat. A body mass index (BMI) of 30 or greater (weight [kg]/height^2 [m^2]). Three subclasses of obesity are defined as follows:
- Class 1 = BMI 30–34.9 kg/m^2
- Class 2 = BMI 35–39.9 kg/m^2
- Class 3 = BMI >40 kg/m^2

REALITIES OF OBESITY

During the early part of the 20th century, the **prevalence** of obesity increased slowly; however, around 1980 it began to increase more rapidly.[1-4] As illustrated in Fig. 15.1, the rise in the rate of obesity has continued to the present time. In the period between 2009 and 2010 the prevalence of obesity was 35.7%.[1]

Although historically a greater percentage of women have been obese, the latest data indicate no significant difference in prevalence between men and women at any age. Overall, adults aged 60 and older are more likely to be obese than younger adults. Among men, there was no significant difference in obesity prevalence by age. However, among women, 42.3% of those ages 60 and older are obese compared with 31.9% of women ages 20 to 39.[1] Moreover, African-American (59%) and Hispanic women (41%) have a higher prevalence of obesity than Caucasian women (33%). This racial disparity is larger in women than in men.[2] Overweight is also higher among people who make less money and have less education than it is among those who have a higher education and income.[3] Children are also affected by obesity. The prevalence was approximately 5% in 1960 but has increased to 17% in 2010.[1,5]

Obesity increases the risk of developing many chronic diseases including type 2 diabetes mellitus, coronary heart disease, hypertension, gallbladder disease, certain forms of cancer, and sleep-breathing disorders.[4] Prominent among these is type 2 **diabetes mellitus**. This disease most often occurs in overweight or obese adolescents and adults and presages a bleak future, particularly for children as the complications of blindness, heart disease, renal failure, and amputation disable them in the next 20 or so years. Through the development of chronic diseases, being overweight reduces life expectancy and shortens life span by 3 to 7 years for a 40-year-old individual with a **body mass index (BMI)** of 30 or more.

Obesity increases the cost of health care, which has now been estimated to be as high as $147 billion per year. Moreover, in the United States approximately one-half of the costs are paid by Medicare and Medicaid, suggesting that taxpayers foot the bill for much of the costs of obesity.[5,6] The frequency of hospital and medical office visits

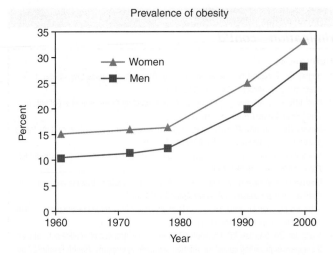

Prevalence of obesity

NHES I	NHANES	NHANES II	NHANES III	NHANES III
1960–1962	1970–1974	1976–1980	1988–1994	1999–2000

FIG. 15.1 Graph illustrating the prevalence of obesity. The *red line* shows the prevalence of obesity for women and the *green line* for men, using data from several surveys of obesity done by the US government beginning in the years 1960 to 1962. Obesity rose slowly from 1960 until approximately 1980, when the rate for men and women began to increase. (Data from National Center for Health Statistics: *National Health and Nutrition Examination Survey I, 1960–1962 and National Health and Nutrition Examination Surveys 1970–1974, 1976–1980, 1988–1994, and 1999–2000*, Hyattsville, MD, 1960–2000, Centers for Disease Control and Prevention.)

increases with increasing body weight. The use of drugs and surgery to treat the complications associated with obesity also increases.

Fortunately, risks associated with obesity are generally ameliorated by modest weight loss. A weight loss of 5% to 10% of initial body weight is sufficient to reduce the development of diabetes in people with **prediabetes** by up to 58%.[7] Weight loss that is maintained is an effective treatment for hypertension. Risks from abnormal blood lipids (dyslipidemia) are also reduced with weight loss.[8]

For children and adults, a social **stigma** is associated with a weight problem.[9] Overweight children are less liked as playmates and tend to view themselves less favorably than normal-weight children. Children

are often teased at school by being labeled "fatty" and other derogatory terms. Such disparaging remarks often jeopardize feelings of self-confidence. Many overweight children and adults are traumatized by the stigma of obesity. Adults experience prejudice in social and economic situations. Measures of quality of life show that the obese score lower on many scales and that weight loss improves their quality of life (see the Focus on Culture box, "Antifat Bias: The Last Acceptable Form of Cultural Discrimination").

KEY TERMS

Prevalence
This term relates the number of individuals with a particular condition at a particular time to the total number of people. If 10 people were overweight in a population of 1000, then this would indicate a prevalence of 1%.

Diabetes Mellitus
A disease defined by a high level of glucose in the blood, which often appears in the urine if it is high enough. Two general types of diabetes mellitus exist: type 1, which refers to the disease normally diagnosed in younger individuals (younger than 30 years of age) in which the pancreas cannot produce enough insulin and thus not enough circulating insulin exists; and type 2, which refers to the disease normally diagnosed in older individuals who are often overweight or obese and in which more than enough circulating insulin exists but relatively poor response to this insulin occurs.

Body Mass Index (BMI)
Body weight in kilograms divided by the height in square meters (kg/m^2). It can be calculated from pounds and inches as $703 \times$ body weight in pounds $\div$ by the height in inches squared. This measurement is the common method used to define overweight and obesity.

Prediabetes
A condition also known as *impaired glucose tolerance* and defined as a fasting glucose between 100 and 126 mg/dL and a blood glucose between 140 and 199 mg/dL 2 hours after ingestion of 75 g of glucose.

Stigma
A mark or identification marking. In this context it is an increased body fat that is obvious to the viewer and that elicits emotional feelings, which are usually negative.

🌐 FOCUS ON CULTURE

Antifat Bias: The Last Acceptable Form of Cultural Discrimination

Our culture idealizes slimness and denigrates obesity. Discrimination based on weight bias has been recognized in many different areas of our society, including representation of obese persons in our culture. Common stereotypes of obese persons include the following:
- Warm
- Dependable
- Gluttonous
- Lazy
- Stupid
- Worthless

Popular messages in the media promote fat jokes and idealization of thin women and muscular men. Unfortunately, it appears that it is socially acceptable in the United States to assume that obese people are fully responsible for their condition. However, do health care professionals, who are trained to understand

that obesity is caused by hereditary and environmental factors and is not merely a function of personal behavior (e.g., overeating, lack of exercise), express this same bias? Regrettably, research shows that health professionals are not immune to overt or inherent antifat bias. The very people who are responsible for caring for individuals who are obese demonstrated the following attitudes toward obese patients[1-8]:
- Family practice physicians described obese patients with negative terms such as *lacking self-control*.
- Physicians reported that they would feel more negatively toward overweight patients and spend less time with them but would order more tests.
- Nurses reported the following:
- Feeling uncomfortable caring for obese patients
- Being "repulsed" by obese persons
- Having a preference not to care for obese patients

Continued

🌐 FOCUS ON CULTURE

Antifat Bias: The Last Acceptable Form of Cultural Discrimination—cont'd

- Medical students described obese patients as follows:
- Less attractive
- More depressed
- Less compliant
- Registered dietitians and dietetic students reported negative attitudes toward obese individuals.
- Overweight and obese women are less likely to be screened for cervical and breast cancer.

Thus it appears the physical and psychological consequences of obesity may stem from not only Western culture's weight-related bias and stigma but also from the biases of health professionals. Obviously, Schwartz and colleagues[6] were right when they said, "Much more work is needed to understand and ameliorate this bias."

How about you? Are you part of the solution or part of the problem?

To tackle the hazards of obesity for children, adolescents, and adults, we need to adopt effective strategies for prevention and, where prevention fails, for treatment of obesity.

References

1. Bagley CR, Conklin DN, Isherwood RT, et al: Attitudes of nurses toward obesity and obese patients, *Percept Mot Skills* 68:954, 1989.
2. Hebl MR, Xu J: Weighing the care: physicians' reaction to the size of a patient, *Int J Obes Relat Metab Disord* 25:1246, 2001.
3. Loomis GA, Connolly KP, Clinch CR, et al: Attitudes and practices of military family physicians regarding obesity, *Mil Med* 166:121, 2001.
4. Maroney D, Golub S: Nurses' attitudes toward obese persons and certain ethnic groups, *Percept Mot Skills* 75:387, 1992.
5. Oberrieder H, Walker R, Monroe D, et al: Attitude of dietetics students and registered dietitians toward obesity, *J Am Diet Assoc* 95:914, 1995.
6. Schwartz M, Chambliss HO, Brownell KD, et al: Weight bias among health professionals specializing in obesity, *Obes Res* 11:1033, 2003.
7. Teachman BA, Gapinski KD, Brownell KD, et al: Demonstrations of implicit anti-fat bias: the impact of providing causal information and evoking empathy, *Health Psychol* 22:68, 2003.
8. Wigton RS, McGaghie WC: The effects of obesity on medical students' approach to patients with abdominal pain, *J Gen Intern Med* 16:262, 2001.

ENERGY INTAKE, ENERGY EXPENDITURE, AND DEVELOPMENT OF OBESITY

One easy way to view the problem of obesity is with the aid of a teeter-totter, a childhood toy. On one side is the amount of food we eat expressed in calories (joules). On the other side is the energy we expend during the day for our various activities, which includes the energy needed to heat our bodies and keep them at 37°C (98.6°F), the energy needed to keep our hearts beating, our brains working, our kidneys filtering blood, our intestines digesting food, and all other essential body processes whether we are awake or not. Energy is also used for physical activity when we sit, stand, walk, run, or do other activities. When the two sides of the teeter-totter are in balance (i.e., when the energy on one side is equal to the energy on the other side), we are in "energy balance." As long as we are in energy balance, we will not gain or lose weight. Overweight develops when the energy on the intake side is more than on the expenditure side, which can occur because energy intake rises, because energy expenditure falls, or both. The conservation of energy implied by the energy balance equation is often referred to as the *first law of thermodynamics* applied to human energy consumption and expenditure. This law was first demonstrated for human beings more than 100 years ago, and no reason exists to doubt that it provides the overall framework for understanding the way in which obesity develops. However, as we will show, the problem of obesity lies in the details of the relation of energy intake and energy expenditure.

OBESITY AS A DISEASE

Obesity is a disease. What do we mean by this? A disease has several components. First, it has a cause. As noted previously, this is the result of an imbalance between energy intake and energy expenditure. It has clinical signs and symptoms such as increased amount of fatness that is usually visible to the eye. No one would have difficulty distinguishing between an overweight and normal-weight individual walking down the street. Obesity also has a "pathology," by which we mean the presence of some unique features that allow one to diagnose it under a microscope, at an autopsy examination, or by defined blood tests. For obesity this is the enlarged fat cell.

All forms of obesity have as one characteristic an enlargement of the individual fat cells all over the body. The adult human has close to 60 billion fat cells. As people gain weight, the first change in these cells is to enlarge to accommodate the extra fat. As the cells reach their maximal size, additional cells may be recruited to store the extra fat. Fat cells are very remarkable. They not only store vast amounts of energy for later use, but they are also part of the larger endocrine cellular system that secretes products into the bloodstream that have effects elsewhere. In the case of fat cells, many secreted products can affect blood clotting (plasminogen activator inhibitor-1 [PAI-1]), the removal of fats from the blood (lipoprotein lipase), inflammation (interleukin-1 [IL-1], IL-6, tumor necrosis factor-α [TNF-α]), blood pressure (angiotensinogen), and energy balance (leptin). The release of this latter hormone—leptin—is an important signal from the fat cells to the brain about the amount of body fat. Circulating levels of leptin are directly related to amount of body fat. Until the amount of body fat reaches a "critical" level in women, menstruation does not occur. In many women who are ballet dancers or gymnasts, with small amounts of body fat, menstrual periods cease because leptin levels are too low. The many hormones produced and secreted from the fat cells in the body produce the pathophysiologic responses that lead to the associated diseases we described previously. Thus obesity can be described as an endocrine disease.

KEY TERMS

Calories

The amount of heat energy needed to raise the temperature of water from 14°C to 15°C. Because this is a small unit, we usually use *kilocalories*, which are 1000 of these small calories (see also *joule*).

Joules

Units of energy. The International System of Units uses joules in place of calories to refer to food energy, and most nutrition journals require its use instead of calories (1 kcal = 4.184 kilojoules [kJ], often rounded to 4.2 kJ for ease in calculation). A 1000-kcal diet would be equivalent to a 4200-kJ or 4.2-MJ (megajoule) diet.

BEYOND ENERGY BALANCE

There is no doubt that obesity results from energy imbalance and that we can predict the magnitude of the weight change over time if we know the net energy balance. However, it is what the energy balance concept does not tell us that is most important in dealing with obesity. The first law of thermodynamics does not tell us anything about the regulation of food intake or the way in which genes are involved in this process. It does not help us understand why men and women distribute fat in different places on their bodies or how fat distribution changes with age. The first law of thermodynamics also does not help us understand why some drugs produce weight gain whereas others produce weight loss, or why weight loss stops after a period of treatment with diet or medication. Understanding these mechanisms will allow us to tackle the epidemic of obesity.

One problem with the concept of energy balance is that we are never in complete energy balance for any length of time. To study energy balance, healthy men were housed in small, sealed rooms so that their respiratory gasses could be measured to determine energy expenditure (respiration calorimetry). Food intake and exercise were manipulated to get as close as possible to zero energy balance (i.e., when energy intake equals energy expenditure).[10,11] In fact, the difference was rarely closer than 50 kcal/day, or approximately 2.5% out of an intake of 2000 kcal/day. The values of energy imbalance for these healthy men ranged from 50 to 150 kcal/day. Had these differences been maintained for 1 year, these men would be expected to gain approximately 2.5 kg (5.5 lb) at the smaller error and 7.5 kg (16.5 lb) at the larger error.

To keep from gaining weight, we must make "corrective" responses in energy intake or energy expenditure to counterbalance the error that occurred on previous days. These corrective responses around a weight of relative stability make it look as though "weight regulation" exists. For some people the oscillations around this balance point can keep weight stable for many years. For others a slow upward drift occurs in this regulatory point, and weight is gradually gained. If you are fortunate enough to have robust corrective responses, then you can maintain a stable weight over many years. If it is not stable, then the following two strategies are available:

1. *Conscious control:* This method is exhibited in some people who have a pattern of eating called *restrained eating.*
2. *Regular weighing:* This second and perhaps best way to maintain weight over a long period is to weigh oneself regularly at the same time of day on an accurate scale and address weight increases in a timely fashion by adjusting energy intake.

Because we are never in energy balance, we need to view energy balance as an ideal, not a realistic goal to be obtained by counting calories.

From the perspective of energy balance, the solution to obesity should be simple: eat less and exercise more. The truth of this advice was shown by Kinsell and colleagues[12] for overweight individuals housed in a metabolic ward and provided with all their food. During the course of several months, these patients ate diets with 1200 kcal/day. After the initial rapid weight loss because of rebalancing body fluids, subsequent weight loss was linear and was not affected by wide variations in fat, carbohydrate, and protein content of the diet. More recent studies using foods tagged with a nonradioactive isotopic carbon-13 showed that weight loss increased in relation to how well subjects adhered to a diet.[13] Thus it is adherence to diets, not diets themselves, that makes the difference.

Another limitation to the concept of energy balance as the cause of obesity is the implication that if you are getting fatter, then it is your fault. You need only to control your calorie intake (food) and calorie expenditure to control the problem, which implies that we should blame our children for their obesity. This notion seems grossly inappropriate. If obesity were easily controlled by moderating calorie intake, then the US military would not discharge up to 5000 men and women yearly for failing to meet its weight standards. If loss of livelihood is not sufficient motivation to lose weight, then the problem must be more complex.

In the very rare instance of leptin deficiency in humans, the cure of obesity involves treatment with leptin. This concept demonstrates a genetic basis for some obesity, more than simply lack of willpower.[14] Although simple in theory, applying the ideas of energy balance and calorie counting to body weight control has proven unsuccessful. More than 95% of people using dietary, behavior, and lifestyle approaches to lose weight regained it within less than 5 years.[15]

EPIDEMIOLOGIC MODEL

The current epidemic can be viewed from the perspective of an epidemiologic model shown in Fig. 15.2. Food, low physical activity, drugs, viruses, and toxins are the environmental agents that facilitate the development of obesity. One or more of these factors acting on a susceptible host can produce obesity. Using this model, we can approach the problem by manipulating either the environment or the host.

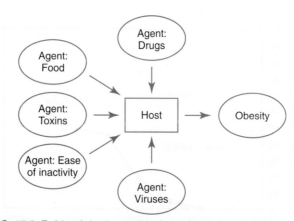

FIG. 15.2 Epidemiologic model of obesity. In this model the agent that produces obesity is "food" or food-related products. If food is in limited supply, then obesity does not develop. The food that is ingested interacts with the host. In a susceptible host the toxic effects of food produce obesity, the disease.

Environmental Agents

Food and Its Costs as a Major Environmental Agent. Several components of our food supply may be important in determining whether or not obesity develops. The first of these is the size of food packages and restaurant portions. Convincing evidence indicates that when larger portion sizes are provided, more food is eaten. Portion sizes have dramatically increased in the past 40 years[16] and now need reduction. Sugar-sweetened beverages that contain 10% high-fructose corn syrup (HFCS) are available in 12-, 20-, 32-, and 44-oz containers and provide 150, 250, 400, or 550 kcal, respectively, if the entire drink is consumed. Prepackaged foods list the calories per serving, but the package often contains more than one serving, encouraging consumption of more than the recommended serving size.

Patterns of food consumption have changed during the past 30 years. The most striking change from 1970 to 2010 has been the rising consumption of HFCS.[17] HFCS is now used as the caloric sweetener in almost all soft drinks, as well as in reconstituted juice drinks and many solid foods. The rise in HFCS consumption occurred over the same time interval as the rapid rise in the prevalence of obesity.[18] On the one hand, this relationship may be strictly coincidental. However, on the other hand, it may not be (Fig. 15.3). Fructose is sweeter than either glucose or sucrose, a molecule that is a combination of fructose and glucose. In addition, HFCS is a solution of fructose and glucose as separate molecules, and thus it differs in osmotic properties from a solution with the same concentration of sucrose.[19]

The intake of sugar-sweetened beverages has been related to the epidemic of obesity.[17-19] Ludwig and colleagues[20] reported that the intake of soft drinks was a predictor of initial BMI in children in the Planet Health Study. They also showed that higher soft drink consumption predicted an increase in BMI; during nearly 2 years of follow-up, those with the highest soft drink consumption at baseline had the highest increase in BMI. A Danish study[21] showed that individuals who consumed calorically sweetened beverages during 10 weeks gained weight, whereas subjects drinking the same amount of artificially sweetened beverages lost weight. In one study, children who were focusing on reducing intake of "fizzy" drinks and replacing them with water showed slower weight gain than those not advised to reduce the intake of fizzy drinks.[22] These studies strongly suggest that calorie-containing soft drinks could play a role in the epidemic of obesity. If so, then their consumption should be curtailed, particularly for very young children, and for schoolchildren, for whom beverages are a ready source of energy with few other nutrients.

Dietary fat is another component that may be related to the epidemic of obesity.[23,24] Fats contain more than twice the energy of carbohydrates (9 kcal/g). Foods combining fat and sugar may be a particular problem because they are often very palatable and usually inexpensive.[25] The Leeds Fat Study shows that people who were high-fat consumers have an increased incidence of obesity.[26] Providing palatable low-fat foods is important.

Several studies now show that when infants were given breast milk as the sole source of nutrition for more than 3 months, their risk of obesity was significantly reduced at the time of entry into school and in adolescence compared with infants who were not breast-fed or who were breast-fed for less than 3 months.[27,28] The composition of the breast milk may be important. Over the past 50 years the proportion of n-6 fatty acids in human milk has increased, reflecting changes in dietary fat composition. The amount of n-3 fatty acids in breast milk has remained constant. A higher amount of n-6 fatty acids provides prostaglandin derivatives that stimulate fat cell proliferation in infants.[27,29,30] This is a concept that needs further evaluation. The rate of weight gain between ages of 2 and 12 years also predicts future obesity; those children who gain the most weight have the highest risk of becoming obese. Monitoring weight change early can be predictive of future obesity.

Calcium intake is another dietary factor that may be related to the development of obesity in children and adults. The level of calcium intake in population studies is inversely correlated with the risk of being overweight. In other epidemiologic studies and in feeding trials, higher dietary calcium is associated with reduced BMI or reduced incidence of insulin resistance.[31,32] Calcium supplementation does not appear to be as effective as calcium from dairy products and other foods.

The cost of food is another factor in the cause of obesity. The price of items we buy influences our choices and the amount we buy. During the period from 1960 to 1980 the price of food rose more slowly than the other components in the consumer price index. Real wages also rose, providing additional money for consumption, some of which could buy a wider variety of healthy foods such as fresh fruits and vegetables, fish, and dairy products. This period was a time when the rise in the prevalence of obesity was slow. However, between 1983 and 2009 the relative cost increase in these food items was much faster than the foods with higher energy density, which contain more fat and sugar. In this period the price of fresh fruits and vegetables rose 190%, fish by 100%, and dairy products by 82%. Contrast this with sugar and sweets, which increased 66%; fats and oils, 70%; and carbonated beverages, 32%.[5] This means that your food dollar will buy relatively more food energy if the foods contain more sugar and fat or are carbonated beverages.

Low Levels of Physical Activity. Epidemiologic data show that low levels of physical activity and watching more television predict higher body weight.[33] Studies suggest that individuals in American cities where they had to walk more tended to weigh less than those living in other cities. Low levels of physical activity also increase the risk of early mortality. The Aerobic Center Longitudinal Study was carried out with more than 80,000 individuals over a period of 35 years. Several studies based on this cohort addressed both the independent and combined effects of adiposity and fitness on death rate. These studies demonstrated that low fitness resulted in a greater risk of mortality than fatness, whereas fitness diminished the impact of fatness on mortality.[34] It is thus better to be thin than fat and to be physically active rather than inactive.

FIG. 15.3 The consumption of high-fructose corn syrup (HFCS) and sugar (cane, sucrose) over the years when the obesity epidemic developed. (Copyright 2005, George A. Bray, Baton Rouge, LA.)

Drugs and Chemicals That Produce Weight Gain. Several drugs can cause weight gain, including a variety of hormones and psychoactive agents.[35] The degree of weight gain is generally not sufficient to cause substantial obesity, except occasionally in patients treated with high-dose corticosteroids, as well as some psychoactive drugs such as valproate. These drugs can also cause insulin resistance and increase the risk of developing type 2 diabetes mellitus.

Cessation of smoking is another environmental agent that will affect body fat stores. Partially mediated by nicotine withdrawal, a weight gain of 1 to 2 kg (2.2 to 4.4 lb) is seen in the first few weeks and is often followed by an additional 2- to 3-kg weight gain over the next 4 to 6 months, resulting in an average weight gain of 4 to 5 kg or more.[36]

Viruses as Environmental Causes of Obesity. The injection of several viruses into the central nervous system (CNS) produces obesity in mice. Findings of antibodies to one of the adenoviruses (Ad-36) in larger amounts in obese humans raises the possibility that viruses are involved in some cases.[37] The adenoviral syndrome can be replicated in nonhuman primates and is characterized by modest obesity and a low circulating cholesterol concentration. Further studies are needed to establish that a syndrome of obesity associated with low concentrations of cholesterol clearly exists in human beings. If so, then this would enhance the value of the epidemiologic model.

Toxins. In experimental animals, exposure in the neonatal period to monosodium glutamate (MSG), a common flavoring ingredient in food, produces obesity. A similar effect of reduction in glucose can also produce obesity, suggesting that the brain of the growing animal, and possibly that of human beings, may respond with damage to the "metabolic sensors" that regulate food needs. In human beings, we know that body fat stores many "toxic" chemicals that are mobilized with weight loss. The metabolic rate can be reduced by organochlorine molecules,[38] and conceivably prolonged exposure to many chlorinated chemicals in our environment has affected metabolic pathways and energy metabolism.

Host

Genetic Factors. Several kinds of research indicate that genetic factors are important in regulating body weight and in whether we develop obesity. The first is family studies. For more than 75 years we have known that individuals from families with overweight parents are likely to be overweight. In contrast, individuals from families in which the parents are lean are likely to be lean. Adoption studies in which children are traced to their birth families show that the children are more like their biologic parents than like the parents who adopted them. Finally, studies in identical and nonidentical twins provide the icing on the cake, so to speak. When identical twins who have been reared in separate families from birth are identified, they are found to be more like each other than are nonidentical twins similarly reared apart. From these data we can place the role of genetic factors between 35% and 70% of the inheritance of obesity, meaning that if one individual in a given environment becomes overweight, it is highly likely that his or her identical twin would also become overweight. If one twin resists obesity, then the other identical twin would be very likely to also resist obesity.

Further insight into the genetic causes of obesity has come from the cloning of several genes that produce obesity in human beings. Leptin, identified in 1994, was the first of these important gene products to be identified. As noted previously, it is produced in adipose tissue and secreted into the blood in relation to the amount of body fat.[39] Leptin-deficient individuals are massively obese from childhood. When they are treated with leptin, food intake falls and body fat is mobilized until body weight is nearly normalized, indicating that this is an important metabolic pathway for which the gene has been identified. This genetic defect is extremely rare, and most obese people have an appropriate level of circulating leptin for their size, indicating that there is an error in leptin signaling either with the leptin receptor or a downstream pathway.

The most common single gene defect in obese children and adults is in the melanocortin-4 receptor, a key regulator of food intake.[39,40] When this receptor is inactive, food intake is nearly as high as when leptin is deficient. When this receptor is only partially inactivated, the food intake is only modestly beyond control levels.

Several other rare genetic defects have been identified in the regulatory process for controlling food intake that, when abnormal, lead to obesity. These basic biologic insights tell us that body fat has important regulation that is largely, if not completely, independent of willpower.

Intrauterine Imprinting. Several intrauterine events may lead to obesity later in life, probably because of fetal imprinting as a result of early exposure that affects brain plasticity. The Dutch winter famine of 1945 showed that starvation of infants in utero could affect long-term postnatal weight status. Another example is the infants of mothers who smoked during pregnancy; these infants have an increased risk of becoming overweight during their first three decades of life when compared with infants of mothers who did not smoke during pregnancy.[41] Similarly, infants of mothers who have diabetes are at higher risk of developing obesity than infants born to mothers who did not have diabetes during pregnancy.[42] Infants who are small for their birth date are at higher risk of developing central adiposity and diabetes than normal-weight infants. Finally, experimental studies teach us that exposure to high levels of insulin during the period of brain plasticity can lead to obesity later in life.

Physiologic Control. To maintain a stable body weight over time, the body must correct daily errors in energy balance. A number of physiologic factors are known to disturb this correction. Overall, low metabolic rate may also predict future weight gain,[43] but conversely, a high rate of carbohydrate oxidation, as measured by a high respiratory quotient (RQ) predicts future weight gain.[44] One explanation is that when carbohydrate oxidation is higher than carbohydrate intake, carbohydrate stores are depleted, and we must eat to replace them. Obese individuals who have lost weight are less effective

---

KEY TERMS

Incidence

The number of new cases of a particular condition that develop over time. If among 1000 people, 10 people who were not overweight initially become overweight in 1 year, then the incidence rate would be 10 cases per 1000 person-years.

Energy density

The amount of energy or calories in a food compared with the weight of the food.

Insulin

Hormone produced by the pancreas that lowers blood glucose by enhancing its entry into cells.

in increasing fat oxidation in the presence of a high-fat meal than normal-weight individuals are, and this may be one reason why they are so susceptible to weight regain.

Fat cells in our body serve two major functions: (1) They store and release fatty acids ingested from food or from liver or fat cells, and (2) they secrete many important hormones and chemicals. The discovery of leptin catapulted the fat cell into the arena of endocrine cells.[45] In addition to leptin, the fat cell secretes a variety of other peptides (lipoprotein lipase, adipsin [complement D], complement C, adiponectin, TNF-α, IL-6, PAI-1, angiotensinogen, bradykinin, and resistin). The fat cell also releases other metabolites such as lactate, fatty acids, glycerol, and prostacyclin. Our understanding of fat cells as important endocrine cells continues to expand.

Production of cortisol from inactive cortisone in fat cells by the enzyme 11β-hydroxysteroid dehydrogenase type 1 may be important in determining the quantity of visceral adipose tissue.[46] Changes in this enzyme may contribute to the risk menopausal women face in developing more visceral fat. High levels of this enzyme keep the quantity of cortisol in visceral fat high, providing a fertile environment for the development of new fat cells.

Increased visceral fat seems to result in a high level of proinflammatory cytokines. The ratio of visceral fat is proportional to the risk for development of metabolic and cardiovascular problems associated with obesity. Interestingly, if a substantial amount of visceral fat is surgically removed, then insulin resistance is immediately improved.[47]

Information about hunger and satiety comes from the gastrointestinal (GI) tract, where several peptides signal the body to stop or start eating. Ghrelin has received attention because, in contrast to other GI hormones, it stimulates food intake.[48] Levels of ghrelin are low in obesity, except for Prader-Willi syndrome, suggesting that it may play a role.

The brain is a receiver, transducer, and transmitter of information about hunger and satiety. Several neurotransmitter systems are involved in regulation of food intake.[49] Serotonin receptors modulate the quantity of food eaten and macronutrient selection, and their loss through genetic targeting produces obesity. Peptide neurotransmitters also play a very important role in the regulation of feeding. Sleep deprivation is one way to enhance the release of peptides that produce hunger.[50,51] In young men allowed to sleep only 4 hours per night for 2 days, leptin decreased and ghrelin increased relative to the pattern seen with 10 hours of sleep on each of 2 nights.

OVERVIEW OF TREATING THE DISEASE OF OBESITY

Prevention of the Current Epidemic

The epidemic of obesity occurs on a genetic background that has not changed significantly in the past 100 years and certainly not since the epidemic began 30 years ago. Nonetheless, it is clear that genetic factors play a critical role in the susceptibility of becoming obese in a "toxic environment."[52] One analogy is that "genes load the gun and a permissive or toxic environment pulls the trigger." Modification of environmental factors that act on our ancient genes must be the strategy to prevent the disease. The belief that this can be done by the individual alone is to miss the argument of how environmental factors have acted on these genes to produce the current epidemic, with major emphasis on the imprinting of the plastic brain of the growing child and adolescent.

We argue that the first law of thermodynamics has lulled us into the uncomfortable position of believing that individuals, through willpower, increased food choices, or more places to exercise can overcome the current epidemic of obesity. Cognitive approaches relying on individual commitment and resolve have been unsuccessful in stemming the epidemic, and nothing suggests that they will be more successful in the future.

We also argue that it is what the first law of thermodynamics does not tell us that is important. In this context it is the unconscious host systems on which environmental factors operate that produces the disease. If the vending machines now in schools contained beverages with no added sugar or HFCS, then available calories would be reduced. We have argued that the exposure of young children to HFCS may produce detrimental imprinting of the brain, making obesity more likely and more difficult to control.

At least three preventive strategies are available to deal with the epidemic: (1) education, (2) regulation, and (3) modification of the food supply. Education in the school curriculum about good nutrition and healthy weight would be beneficial in helping all children learn how to select appropriate foods. School breakfast and lunch programs should match the educational messages.

It is unwise to rely on educational strategies alone, because they have not prevented the obesity epidemic. Regulation is a second strategy. Regulating an improved food label would be one good idea. Regulations on appropriate serving sizes in packages and nutrition information provided by restaurants might be part of the solution. Headway is being made in these areas due to public pressure.

Modification in some components of the food system is a third and most important strategy. Because the energy we eat comes from food, we need to modify this system to provide less energy density if we are to succeed in combating the epidemic of obesity.

Treatment of Overweight People When Prevention Fails

A detailed discussion of treatment for obesity is beyond the scope of this chapter, but a few general comments about the major approaches are essential because they involve food intake and exercise. Although prevention is unlikely to be successful by relying solely on individual initiative, treatment requires individual initiative. For any change to occur, the individual must be ready for change. This idea of "stages of change" is a key component of any individual approach. The overweight person must be aware that he or she has a problem and must have moved beyond the stage of precontemplation (i.e., the stage of denial before a person is willing to do something about a problem) and into a stage of contemplation and then to action. When overweight individuals are in this state, they are ready to move forward. Their options are diet, exercise, behavioral therapy, medication, and surgery. These are the principal approaches available to those who have a weight problem that they want to address. The use of diet, exercise, and behavioral therapy are appropriate for all levels of overweight.

Dietetic professionals can play an important role in all of these approaches. First, the educated dietetic professional needs to be keenly aware of the complexity of the obesity problem. The dietitian obviously cannot alter the genetic makeup of an individual but is able to address the environmental aspects that serve to exacerbate the situation. Simply handing out diet sheets will not work. Helping obese patients requires attention to their overall diet history, current eating and activity patterns, and behavioral obstacles that either cause problems or prevent change. Although quick weight loss may be a patient's immediate desire, permanent lifestyle changes should be the primary objective. Tips for addressing this have been outlined by Bray and Champagne (Box 15.1).[53] Finally, the dietitian can be an instrument of change by appealing to policymakers to modify environmental conditions, such as the school vending machine situation cited previously.

BOX 15.1   Practice Points for the Clinical Dietitian

- *Focus on personal history:* More than ever, the personal history of the patient is a critical focus area for the dietitian in clinical practice who deals with patients diagnosed with the metabolic syndrome. In particular, assessment of past dietary habits using a valid food frequency questionnaire is warranted. The current dietary practices of the patient can help highlight target areas; collecting a food record for as many days as the patient is willing to keep it will be instrumental in future counseling efforts.
- *Obtain thorough information:* Encouraging the patient to provide as much dietary information as possible will make a measurable difference in the accuracy of the dietary data for evaluation purposes. Remember to focus on the fact that no judgments will be formed; you are simply identifying areas of diet for which you will be targeting change.
- *Assess exercise habits:* Physical activity patterns are useful for designing the total lifestyle program. The dietitian may choose to collect a physical activity

questionnaire from the patient and, in addition, provide the patient with an activity monitor to assess actual physical activity steps for a more accurate appraisal of daily activity levels.
- *Customize:* For increased success, dietary treatment needs to be highly individualized. It may be helpful to include a variety of weight loss strategies, such as meal replacements (for quicker initial weight loss), slightly higher protein diets, low fat diets, and perhaps even a Mediterranean diet approach. An important point to remember: What works for one patient may not necessarily be ideal for another.
- *Consult the physician:* Working with the patient's physician to provide the ideal combination of diet, physical activity suggestions, behavior changes, and medication (if prescribed by the physician) is key to the patient's success.
- *Follow-up:* Regular evaluations to monitor patient progress are key to weight management by the physician and the dietitian in clinical practice.

Data from Bray GA, Champagne CM: Obesity and the metabolic syndrome: implications for dietetics practitioners. *J Am Diet Assoc* 104:86, 2004.

Diet. Popular diets have been published for more than 150 years; obviously, if any diet were significantly better than the others, it would have "won the battle" and the others would have disappeared. Popular diets can be grouped into several categories: low-energy (calorie) diets, low-fat diets, low-carbohydrate diets, and high-protein diets. A summary of data abstracted by the US Department of Agriculture (USDA) is shown in Table 15.1.

Several popular diets, including the Atkins Diet (low carbohydrate), the Ornish (low fat), Weight Watchers, and the Zone diet (high protein), were recently compared and found to produce comparable weight loss, suggesting that none of these diets is better than the other.[54] A randomized clinical trial that compared reduced-calorie diets with different macronutrient targets (low or high fat, average or high protein, low or high carbohydrate) determined that any type of reduced-calorie diet can be effective in achieving weight loss.[55]

Exercise. Increased movement, both modest and vigorous, is a way to increase energy expenditure that will burn fat deposits. Human beings expend approximately two-thirds of their energy with basal activities, including maintaining body temperature, and only approximately one-third in various activities. Thus to expend a significant number of calories through exercise takes time. As a rule of thumb, approximately 100 kcal are expended for each mile walked. If it takes 15 minutes to walk a mile, then you could expend up to 400 kcal in an hour of brisk walking. From a practical point of view, it is often easier to eat 400 kcal less than to exercise for the extra 400 kcal. Despite the relatively large effort to burn a considerable amount of energy with physical activity, people who exercise more have been shown to have greater weight loss maintenance than did those who exercised less.[56] This observation may be due to an increase in lean mass with the physically active, which would increase basal energy expenditure.

Behavioral Therapy. Since their introduction in 1967, behavioral approaches to helping overweight individuals focus on the issues that revolve around eating have been a cornerstone in the treatment of obesity. These techniques are adapted from psychologic learning theory, in which rewarding appropriate behavior tends to reinforce that behavior. The process involves familiarity with the activities associated with learning and providing consequences of eating, as well as rewards that reinforce appropriate behaviors. Among the successful techniques in this area are self-monitoring, increased physical activity, and eating a lower-fat diet. People who are successful at maintaining a lowered body weight over time use these and other techniques.

Medication. Currently only six medications are approved by the US Food and Drug Administration (FDA) for the treatment of obesity. These include five drugs that have been approved only for short-term use (**benzphetamine** [Didrex], **diethylpropion** [Tenuate], **phendimetrazine** [Adipost, Anorex-SR, Appecon, Bontril PDM, Bontril Slow Release, Melfiat, Obezine, Phendiet, Plegine, Prelu-2, Statobex], **phentermine** [Adipex-P, Fastin, Ionamin, Obenix, Obephen, Oby-Cap, Oby-Trim, Panshape M, Phentercot, Phentride, Pro-Fast HS, Pro-Fast SA, Pro-Fast SR, Teramine, Zantryl], and a combination of phentermine and **topiramate** [Qsymia]) and two drugs that have been approved for longer-term use—**orlistat** (Alli, Xenical) and **lorcaserin** (Belviq).

Researchers believe that all of the drugs except for orlistat work by modifying the neurotransmitters in the CNS. Some of these drugs work in part by binding to molecules on the surface of brain cells (neurons) that transport neurotransmitters back into these neurons after they have been secreted. Because the short-term drugs are related to the addictive drug amphetamine, albeit quite indirectly, the US government regulates their use through the Drug Enforcement Administration (DEA). Topiramate was originally sold as an anticonvulsant medication

---

TABLE 15.1   Features of the Major Diets Used by Americans

Type of Diet	Calories	Fat, g (%)	Carbohydrate, g (%)	Protein, g (%)
Typical American diet	2200	85 (35)	274 (50)	82 (15)
High-fat, low-carbohydrate diet	1400	94 (60)	35 (10)	105 (30)
Moderate-fat diet	1450	40 (25)	218 (60)	54 (15)
Low-fat and very-low-fat diet	1450	16–24 (10–15)	235–271 (65–75)	54–72 (15–20)

Modified from Freedman MR, King J, Kennedy E: Popular diets: a scientific review, *Obes Res* 9(Suppl):1S, 2001, with permission from NAASO, The Obesity Society.

that was found to have the side effect of weight loss by increasing feelings of fullness, making foods taste less appealing, and increasing energy expenditure. In clinical studies with these drugs, the weight loss is approximately 4 to 5 kg (8.8 to 11 lb) more than with placebo controls after 6 to 12 months of treatment. To be eligible for use of medications, an individual needs to have a BMI greater than 30 kg/m^2, unless associated problems exist, such as diabetes, heart disease, high blood pressure, or other problems that would benefit from weight loss. In that case the lower limit for use of medications may be 27 kg/m^2 (see the Diet-Medications Interactions table, "Drugs Used to Treat Obesity").

Orlistat contrasts with these centrally acting drugs. It works in the intestine to block an enzyme called *lipase,* which is produced and secreted from the pancreas. At clinically used doses, it blocks digestion of approximately one-third of the dietary fat. This dietary fat then passes through the intestinal tract and exits the body in the feces. When used improperly, this drug can produce significant GI tract symptoms. In clinical studies this drug produces 2 to 4 kg (4.4 to 8.8 lb) more weight loss than placebo-treated groups and appears to be slightly less effective than the other types of drugs.[57]

Surgery. Use of bariatric surgery for treatment of obesity has expanded greatly with the rising obesity rate.[58] Several different types of operations are currently in use for treatment of obesity. Usually the stomach is restricted, part of the small intestine is bypassed, or both. To be eligible for surgical intervention, an overweight individual needs to have a BMI greater than 40 kg/m^2, unless the person has associated diseases such as diabetes, heart disease, sleep apnea, or osteoarthritis, in which case the BMI for considering therapy can be lowered to 35 kg/m^2. Gastric bypass is associated with the near-elimination of type 2 diabetes and improvements in cardiovascular risk factors, sleep apnea, and quality of life. Side effects include dumping syndrome, which produces nausea, flushing, bloating, and extreme diarrhea. Weight loss after surgery is greatest over the first 12 months and continues until approximately 18 months. Patients lose an average of 60% of excess weight after gastric bypass and 40% after gastric restriction. At 2 years after surgery, 30% of patients have regained some weight.[59] Weight regain is associated with reduced remission of type 2 diabetes. Bariatric surgery patients should participate in nutrition education and support group programs to ameliorate weight regain. More data are needed on the long-term effects of bariatric surgery.

DIET-MEDICATIONS INTERACTIONS

Drugs Used to Treat Obesity

Generic Name	Trade Name	Mechanism of Action	Food-Drug Interactions
Benzphetamine	Didrex	Appetite suppressant, stimulates central nervous system, and decreases appetite (similar to amphetamine); short-term use only	Alcohol may increase the dizziness effects of this medicine
Diethylpropion	Tenuate, Tenuate Dospan		
Phendimetrazine	Adipost, Anorex-SR, Appecon, Bontril PDM, Bontril Slow-Release, Melfiat, Obezine, Phendiet, Plegine, Prelu-2, Statobex		A reduced-calorie diet must be followed while using an appetite suppressant to lose weight. In addition, to keep the lost weight from returning, changes in diet and exercise must be continued after the weight has been lost
Phentermine	Adipex-P, Fastin, Ionamin, Obenix, Obephen, Oby-Cap, Oby-Trim, Panshape M, Phentercot, Phentride, Pro-Fast HS, Pro-Fast SA, Pro-Fast SR, Teramine, Zantryl		
Phentermine/ Topiramate	Qsymia	Appetite suppressant, makes foods taste less appealing, and increases energy expenditure	Alcohol produces several interactions with this medication
Orlistat	Alli, Xenical	Blocks fat from being absorbed in intestine	This drug prevents the absorption of some dietary fat. It should be taken during the meal or within 1 hour of eating and may decrease absorption of fat-soluble vitamins from food. A multivitamin supplement should be taken once a day at least 2 hours before or after taking orlistat
			The diet should contain no more than 30% of calories as fat; more fat in the diet will increase side effects
			Patients who have diabetes mellitus may need to have their insulin or oral hypoglycemic agents adjusted
			Patients may experience gas with leaky bowel movements, inability to hold bowel movements, increased bowel movements, oily bowel movements, and oily spotting of underclothes
Lorcaserin	Belviq	Works on serotonergic system	A reduced-calorie diet must be observed in conjunction with the medication to lose weight and keep it off
			Extreme caution is warranted with other serotonergic drugs such as antidepressants or antipsychotics

KEY TERMS

Benzphetamine
One of the appetite-suppressant drugs that has been approved for more than 30 years for short-term use but that is regulated by the US DEA because of potential for addictive abuse (trade name, Didrex).

Diethylpropion
One of the appetite-suppressant drugs that has been approved for more than 30 years for short-term use but that is regulated by the DEA because of potential for addictive abuse (trade name, Tenuate).

Phendimetrazine
One of the appetite-suppressant drugs that has been approved for more than 30 years for short-term use but that is regulated by the DEA because of potential for addictive abuse; trade names, Adipost, Anorex-SR, Appecon, Bontril PDM, Bontril Slow Release, Melfiat, Obezine, Phendiet, Plegine, Prelu-2, and Statobex.

Phentermine
One of the appetite-suppressant drugs that has been approved for more than 30 years for short-term use but that is regulated by the DEA because of potential for addictive abuse; trade names, Adipex-P, Fastin, Ionamin, Obenix, Obephen, Oby-Cap, Oby-Trim, Panshape M, Phentercot, Phentride, Pro-Fast HS, Pro-Fast SA, Pro-Fast SR, Teramine, and Zantryl.

Topiramate
Originally used as an anticonvulsant, drug was approved in 2012 to be used in combination with phentermine for weight loss under the trade name Qsymia.

Orlistat
Drug (trade name, Xenical) that partially blocks pancreatic lipase, thus decreasing digestion of dietary fat. It is available by prescription and over the counter; trade names, Alli and Zenical.

Lorcaserin
Drug (trade name, Belviq) approved as an appetite suppressant in 2012 that works through a serotonergic pathway.

Pancreas
Gland located near the duodenum and small intestine that has two sets of cells: (1) acinar cells, which secrete digestive enzymes into the intestine, and (2) beta cells, which produce and secrete insulin into the blood.

HEALTH PROMOTION

Our lives are constrained by the laws of nature—gravity, momentum, and thermodynamics—with which we have been dealing in this chapter. The strategies we take to deal with the influence of these laws on our lives include education, regulation, and product design. Deaths from the effects of the laws of momentum produced by automobile accidents provide a glimpse into the strategies we could use to minimize this effect. They also provide insights into the strategies that may be needed to deal with the epidemic of obesity. Although the laws of momentum or the laws of thermodynamics cannot be changed, their effect on producing automobile accidents and obesity can be mitigated. This goal can be achieved through better education about driving and about nutritional needs to prevent obesity. Just as educating drivers about the dangers of speeding and not wearing seatbelts may not always cause a change in behavior, educating people about the dangers of being overweight and energy balance may not affect the diet of many people. Education can be complemented in the case of cars by regulations that require seat belts, air bags, and other safety devices. In the case of obesity, it can be complemented by limiting access to large portion sizes and to high-energy–density foods, as well as creating an environment in which physical activity is more prevalent. Finally, product design to make cars safer partly addresses the driving problem, just as modifying the types of foods that are available and food prices may help to combat the obesity epidemic by redesigning the food environment.

TO SUM UP

Obesity is a chronic, relapsing disease characterized by an accumulation of excess body fat caused by habitual consumption of more energy than is used. Normally, physiologic systems hold the body in energy balance, but environmental factors such as food, medications, physical inactivity, toxins, and viruses can interact with the host's genetic predisposition to gain weight. Obesity is a major health issue because it increases the risk for many other chronic diseases (especially type 2 diabetes), raises health care costs, and may produce psychologic stress. The increased prevalence of obesity in the past few decades has been attributed to a "toxic environment" of abundant high-energy foods with little need for physical activity. Reversing this trend requires a better understanding of how environmental factors affect the development of obesity and a redesigning of these factors.

Acknowledgments

The author thanks George A. Bray and Catherine M. Champagne for their contributions to this chapter in previous editions.

QUESTIONS FOR REVIEW

1. Why is obesity considered to be a disease?
2. What are the psychological, pathologic, and financial effects of obesity?
3. Why are adipose cells considered to be endocrine cells?
4. Explain how portion sizes may contribute to obesity.
5. How does high-fructose corn syrup contribute to obesity?
6. What is the function of leptin?
7. What have twin studies shown about obesity?
8. What are three prevention strategies for dealing with the obesity epidemic?
9. What is the most effective popular diet?
10. What criteria must a person meet to qualify for weight loss surgery?

REFERENCES

1. Ogden CL, Carroll MD, Kit BK, et al: Prevalence of obesity in the United States, 2009-2010, *NCHS Data Brief* (82):1–8, 2012.
2. Flegal KM, Carroll MD, Kit BK, et al: Prevalence of obesity and trends in the distribution of body mass index among US adults, 1999-2010. *JAMA* 307:491, 2012.
3. Wang Y, Beydoun MA: The obesity epidemic in the United States—gender, age, socioeconomic, racial/ethnic, and geographic characteristics: a systematic review and meta-regression analysis, *Epidemiol Rev* 29:6, 2007.
4. Kopelman PG: Obesity as a medical problem, *Nature* 404:635, 2000.
5. Finkelstein EA, Strombotne KL: The economics of obesity, *Am J Clin Nutr* 91:1520S, 2010.

6. Trogdon JG, Finkelstein EA, Hylands T, et al: Indirect costs of obesity: a review of the current literature, *Obes Rev* 9:489, 2008.

7. Knowler WC, Barrett-Connor E, Fowler SE, et al: Reduction in the incidence of type 2 diabetes with lifestyle intervention or metformin, *N Engl J Med* 346:393, 2002.

8. Unick JL, Beavers D, Bond DS, et al: The long-term effectiveness of a lifestyle intervention in severely obese individuals, *Am J Med* 126(236):242, 2013.

9. Puhl RM, King KM: Weight discrimination and bullying, *Best Pract Res Clin Endocrinol Metab* 27:117, 2013.

10. de Jonge L, Nguyen T, Smith SR, et al: Prediction of energy expenditure in a whole body indirect calorimeter at both low and high levels of physical activity, *Int J Obes Relat Metab Disord* 25:929, 2001.

11. Smith SR, de Jonge L, Zachwieja JJ, et al: Concurrent physical activity increases fat oxidation during the shift to a high-fat diet, *Am J Clin Nutr* 72:131, 2000.

12. Kinsell LW, Gunning B, Michaels GD, et al: Calories do count, *Metabolism* 13:195, 1964.

13. Lyon XH, Di VV, Milon H, et al: Compliance to dietary advice directed towards increasing the carbohydrate to fat ratio of the everyday diet, *Int J Obes Relat Metab Disord* 19:260, 1995.

14. Licinio J, Caglayan S, Ozata M, et al: Phenotypic effects of leptin replacement on morbid obesity, diabetes mellitus, hypogonadism, and behavior in leptin-deficient adults, *Proc Natl Acad Sci U S A* 101:4531, 2004.

15. Stern JS, Hirsch J, Blair SN, et al: Weighing the options: criteria for evaluating weight-management programs, The Committee to Develop Criteria for Evaluating the Outcomes of Approaches to Prevent and Treat Obesity, *Obes Res* 3:591, 1995.

16. Young LR, Nestle M: Reducing portion sizes to prevent obesity: a call to action. *Am J Prev Med* 43:565, 2012.

17. Bray GA, Popkin BM: Calorie-sweetened beverages and fructose: what have we learned 10 years later, *Pediatr Obes* 8:242, 2013.

18. Morgan RE: Does consumption of high-fructose corn syrup beverages cause obesity in children? *Pediatr Obes* 8:249, 2013.

19. Stanhope KL, Schwarz JM, Havel PJ: Adverse metabolic effects of dietary fructose: results from the recent epidemiological, clinical, and mechanistic studies, *Curr Opin Lipidol* 24:198, 2013.

20. Ludwig DS, Peterson KE, Gortmaker SL: Relation between consumption of sugar-sweetened drinks and childhood obesity: a prospective, observational analysis, *Lancet* 357:505, 2001.

21. Raben A, Agerholm-Larsen L, Flint A, et al: Meals with similar energy densities but rich in protein, fat, carbohydrate, or alcohol have different effects on energy expenditure and substrate metabolism but not on appetite and energy intake, *Am J Clin Nutr* 77:91, 2003.

22. James J, Thomas P, Cavan D, et al: Preventing childhood obesity by reducing consumption of carbonated drinks: cluster randomised controlled trial, *BMJ* 328:1237, 2004.

23. Astrup A, Ryan L, Grunwald GK, et al: The role of dietary fat in body fatness: evidence from a preliminary meta-analysis of ad libitum low-fat dietary intervention studies, *Br J Nutr* 83(Suppl 1):S25–S32, 2000.

24. Bray GA, Popkin BM: Dietary fat intake does affect obesity! *Am J Clin Nutr* 68:1157, 1998.

25. Drewnowski A, Rehm CD: Energy intakes of US children and adults by food purchase location and by specific food source, *Nutr J* 12:59, 2013.

26. Blundell JE, Macdiarmid JI: Fat as a risk factor for overconsumption: satiation, satiety, and patterns of eating, *J Am Diet Assoc* 97:S63–S69, 1997.

27. Beyerlein A, Toschke AM, von Kries R: Breastfeeding and childhood obesity: shift of the entire BMI distribution or only the upper parts? *Obesity* 16:2730, 2008.

28. von Kries R, Koletzko B, Sauerwald T, et al: Breast feeding and obesity: cross sectional study, *BMJ* 319:147, 1999.

29. Young BE, Johnson SL, Krebs NF: Biological determinants linking infant weight gain and child obesity: current knowledge and future directions, *Adv Nutr* 3:675, 2012.

30. Muhlhausler BS, Ailhaud GP: Omega-6 polyunsaturated fatty acids and the early origins of obesity, *Curr Opin Endocrinol Diabetes Obes* 20:56, 2013.

31. de Oliveira Freitas DM, Stampini Duarte Martino H, Machado Rocha Ribeiro S, et al: Calcium ingestion and obesity control, *Nutr Hosp* 27:1758, 2012.

32. Huang L, Xue J, He Y, et al: Dietary calcium but not elemental calcium from supplements is associated with body composition and obesity in Chinese women, *PLoS One* 6:e27703, 2011.

33. Erik LC, Poulton R, Welch D, et al: Programming obesity and poor fitness: the long-term impact of childhood television, *Obesity (Silver Spring)* 16:1457, 2008.

34. Hainer V, Toplak H, Stich V: Fat or fit: what is more important? *Diabetes Care* 32(Suppl 2):S392–S397, 2009.

35. Heal DJ, Gosden J, Jackson HC, et al: Metabolic consequences of antipsychotic therapy: preclinical and clinical perspectives on diabetes, diabetic ketoacidosis, and obesity, *Handb Exp Pharmacol* (212):135, 2012.

36. O'Hara P, Connett JE, Lee WW, et al: Early and late weight gain following smoking cessation in the Lung Health Study, *Am J Epidemiol* 148:821, 1998.

37. Esposito S, Preti V, Consolo S, et al: Adenovirus 36 infection and obesity, *J Clin Virol* 55:95, 2012.

38. Tremblay A, Chaput JP: About unsuspected potential determinants of obesity, *Appl Physiol Nutr Metab* 33:791, 2008.

39. Zhang Y, Scarpace PJ: The role of leptin in leptin resistance and obesity, *Physiol Behav* 88:249, 2006.

40. O'Rahilly S, Farooqi IS, Yeo GS, et al: Minireview: human obesity—lessons from monogenic disorders, *Endocrinology* 144:3757, 2003.

41. Toschke AM, Ehlin AG, von Kries R, et al: Maternal smoking during pregnancy and appetite control in offspring, *J Perinat Med* 31:251, 2003.

42. Dabelea D, Pettitt DJ, Hanson RL, et al: Birth weight, type 2 diabetes, and insulin resistance in Pima Indian children and young adults, *Diabetes Care* 22:944, 1999.

43. Astrup A, Gotzsche PC, van de Werken K, et al: Meta-analysis of resting metabolic rate in formerly obese subjects, *Am J Clin Nutr* 69:1117, 1999.

44. Zurlo F, Lillioja S, Esposito-Del Puente A, et al: Low ratio of fat to carbohydrate oxidation as predictor of weight gain: study of 24-h RQ, *Am J Physiol* 259:E650–E657, 1990.

45. Spiegelman BM, Flier JS: Obesity and the regulation of energy balance, *Cell* 104:531, 2001.

46. Hochberg Z, Friedberg M, Yaniv L, et al: Hypothalamic regulation of adiposity: the role of 11beta-hydroxysteroid dehydrogenase type 1, *Horm Metab Res* 36:365, 2004.

47. Esposito K, Giugliano G, Scuderi N, et al: Role of adipokines in the obesity-inflammation relationship: the effect of fat removal, *Plast Reconstr Surg* 118:1048, 2006.

48. Altman J: Weight in the balance, *Neuroendocrinology* 76:131, 2002.

49. Blundell JE, Goodson S, Halford JC: Regulation of appetite: role of leptin in signalling systems for drive and satiety, *Int J Obes Relat Metab Disord* 25(Suppl 1):S29–S34, 2001.

50. Van Cauter E, Holmback U, Knutson K, et al: Impact of sleep and sleep loss on neuroendocrine and metabolic function, *Horm Res* 67(Suppl 1):2, 2007.

51. Spiegel K, Tasali E, Penev P, et al: Brief communication: sleep curtailment in healthy young men is associated with decreased leptin levels, elevated ghrelin levels, and increased hunger and appetite, *Ann Intern Med* 141:846, 2004.

52. Rankinen T, Zuberi A, Chagnon YC, et al: The human obesity gene map: the 2005 update, *Obesity (Silver Spring)* 14:529, 2006.

53. Bray GA, Champagne CM: Obesity and the metabolic syndrome: implications for dietetics practitioners, *J Am Diet Assoc* 104:86, 2004.

54. Dansinger ML, Gleason JA, Griffith JL, et al: Comparison of the Atkins, Ornish, Weight Watchers, and Zone diets for weight loss and heart disease risk reduction: a randomized trial, *JAMA* 293:43, 2005.

55. Sacks FM, Bray GA, Carey VJ, et al: Comparison of weight-loss diets with different compositions of fat, protein, and carbohydrates, *N Engl J Med* 360:859, 2009.

56. Anderson JW, Konz EC, Frederich RC, et al: Long-term weight-loss maintenance: a meta-analysis of US studies, *Am J Clin Nutr* 74:579, 2001.

57. Rodgers RJ, Tschop MH, Wilding JP: Anti-obesity drugs: past, present and future, *Dis Model Mech* 5:621, 2012.

58. Noria SF, Grantcharov T: Biological effects of bariatric surgery on obesity-related comorbidities, *Can J Surg* 56:47, 2013.

59. Hsu LK, Benotti PN, Dwyer J, et al: Nonsurgical factors that influence the outcome of bariatric surgery: a review, *Psychosom Med* 60:338, 1998.

PART 3

Introduction to Clinical Nutrition

16

Nutrition Assessment and Nutrition Therapy in Patient Care

Joyce Gilbert

ⓔ http://evolve.elsevier.com/Williams/essentials/

In this chapter, we focus on the Nutrition Care Process (NCP), which is the foundation of nutrition therapy. Information gathered during nutrition assessment is used to establish goals for nutrition intervention. Once interventions are initiated, monitoring and evaluation function as the point of reference from which to determine efficacy of treatment. Nutrition assessment is defined as a "process used to evaluate nutritional status, identify disorders of nutrition, and determine which individuals need nutrition instruction and/or nutrition support."[1] Because no single test measures nutritional status, nutrition assessment draws from numerous indexes to provide a complete picture of nutritional health.[2]

OUTLINE

Role of Nutrition in Clinical Care
Nutrition Screening and Assessment
Nutrition Diagnosis

Nutrition Intervention: Food Plan and Management
Evaluation: Quality Patient Care

ROLE OF NUTRITION IN CLINICAL CARE

Nutrition therapy plays an essential role in disease management, health care, and preventive health care and should be provided by a qualified nutrition professional.[2,3] Comprehensive nutrition assessment provides the necessary foundation for appropriate nutrition therapy based on identified needs. Nutrition assessment and nutrition therapy promote multiple goals: assisting patients in recovery from illness or injury, helping persons maintain follow-up care to promote health, and helping control health care costs.[4] Registered dietitians (RDs) use their expertise and skills to make sound clinical judgments and to work effectively with the clinical care team. These professionals provide an essential component for successful management of the patient's plan of care.

Nutritional Status

Nutritional status can be established by measuring indicators of nutrient stores. Variations of nutrient stores result in changes in nutritional status when nutrient needs and nutrient use are increased or alterations in nutrient intake occur. Inadequacy or excess of a particular nutrient produces physiologic alteration in the body.[2]

Malnutrition

Many patients are malnourished when admitted to the hospital, whereas others may develop malnutrition during their hospital stay.[5] Hospitalized patients with hypermetabolic and physiologic stress of illness or injury can be at risk for malnutrition from increased nutritional needs. Hospital operating guidelines that provide for nutrition screening on admission, combined with follow-up monitoring, will identify patients at malnutrition

risk and provide essential medical nutrition therapy.[2] However, potential problems arising from hospital routines may contribute to a lack of adequate nourishment in some cases, including the following:

- Highly restricted diets remaining on order and unsupplemented too long
- Unserved meals because of interference of medical procedures and clinical tests
- Unmonitored patient appetite

Each injured or ill patient is a unique person and requires special treatment and care. A formidable array of staff persons seeks to determine needs and implement what each patient requires as appropriate care. When individual human needs are met with personal care, within the context of carefully developed care protocols, patients will not feel intimidated and powerless.

Undernutrition: Undernutrition subsequent to insufficient intake; altered digestion; or absorption of protein, energy, or both (calories); is called *protein-energy malnutrition (PEM)* or *protein-calorie malnutrition (PCM)*. Characteristics include weight loss, fat loss, muscle wasting and weakness, impaired immune function, poor wound healing, and reduction of protein synthesis.[1]

Overnutrition: More than two-thirds of American adults are overweight or obese,[6] making these conditions the two most common forms of overnutrition.[1] Overweight is defined as body mass index (BMI) greater than 25 and obesity as BMI greater than 30 (Box 16.1). Both are associated with a number of health risks, including coronary heart disease, type 2 diabetes mellitus, certain cancers (breast, endometrial, colon), hypertension, dyslipidemia, stroke, gallbladder disease, liver disease, sleep apnea, osteoarthritis, and infertility.[7]

BOX 16.1   Body Mass Index

Calculating Body Mass Index (BMI)

$$BMI = \frac{Weight\ (kg)}{Height^2\ (m)}\ \ or\ \ BMI = \frac{Weight\ (lb)}{Height^2\ (in)} \times 704.5$$

Example: An individual weighs 65 kg (143 lb) and is 1.7 m (5 ft 7 in) tall. BMI = $65/(1.7)^2$ = 22.5 kg/m^2

Classification of BMI

Underweight: <18.5
Normal: 18.5–24.9
Overweight: 25.0–29.9
Obese: ≥30.0
Extreme obesity: ≥40.0

From Moore MC: *Pocket guide to nutrition assessment and care,* ed 6, St Louis, 2009, Mosby.

NUTRITION SCREENING AND ASSESSMENT

Patients at nutritional risk need to be identified to allow provision of high-quality nutrition care.[8] Poor nutritional status may create complications that may lead to increased morbidity and mortality, length of stay, and cost of care.[9] Identification of nutrition risk is accomplished through the process of nutritional assessment. However, before patients can be assessed, they must first be identified. Identification takes place through the process of nutrition screening, the entry into the NCP (Box 16.2).[10,11]

Nutrition Screening

Nutrition screening is defined as "the process of identifying characteristics known to be associated with nutrition problems with the purpose of identifying individuals who are malnourished or at nutritional risk."[8,11] In long-term care, assessments must be completed on all residents within 14 days of admission, but it is not

BOX 16.2   The Academy of Nutrition and Dietetics' Nutrition Care Process: Definition of the Nutrition Care Process

Providing nutrition care using the Nutrition Care Process (NCP) from the Academy of Nutrition and Dietetics (AND) (formerly the American Dietetic Association [ADA]) begins when a patient is recognized as being at nutritional risk and requires additional support to attain or maintain positive nutritional status. The NCP is defined as "a systematic problem-solving method that dietetics professionals use to critically think and make decisions to address nutrition-related problems and provide safe and effective quality nutrition care." It is composed of the following four separate but interrelated and associated steps:

1. Nutrition assessment
2. Nutrition diagnosis
3. Nutrition intervention
4. Nutrition monitoring and evaluation

Each step builds on the preceding one, but the process is not necessarily linear. The International Dietetics and Nutrition Terminology is a standardized language used to describe the results of each step of the model. Standardized language allows for appropriate, accurate, ongoing, relevant, and timely documentation of nutrition care. Fig. 16.1 provides a visual illustration of the NCP model.

Step 1: Nutrition Assessment

Techniques such as those outlined in the chapter are used to systematically obtain information necessary to determine or reassess whether or not a nutrition problem (or diagnosis) exists. If so, then the problem is diagnosed using a PES (problem, etiology, signs and symptoms) statement in step 2 of the NCP (see Fig. 16.1).

Step 2: Nutrition Diagnosis

Before nutrition intervention can take place, the nutrition problem (or problems) must be identified. This is accomplished with the nutrition diagnosis. Standardized language is used to make the nutrition diagnosis clear to other nutrition and health care professionals. When the nutrition problem has been identified, it is labeled with a specific, standardized diagnostic term. The nutrition diagnosis statement or PES statement is organized in three distinct parts: (1) the problem (P); (2) the etiology, or cause, of the problem (E); and (3) the signs and symptoms associated with the problem (S). Typically, nutrition diagnoses fall into three categories or domains:

1. Intake
2. Clinical
3. Behavioral-environmental

The following is an example of how a nutrition diagnosis is written:

A disordered eating pattern is *related to* harmful beliefs about food and nutrition *as evidenced by* the reported use of laxatives after meals and statements that calories are not absorbed when laxatives are used.

Step 3: Nutrition Intervention

Intervention begins once the nutritional diagnosis is identified. It is generally aimed at the etiology (E) of the nutrition diagnosis and is directed at reducing or eradicating effects of the signs and symptoms (S). Nutrition interventions are intended to modify a nutrition-related problem and comprise two interconnected components: (1) planning and (2) implementation. Nutrition diagnoses are prioritized in the planning component, whereby implementation is the "action phase." The plan is communicated and carried out, data continue to be collected, and nutrition interventions are revised as necessary. Four categories or domains of nutrition intervention have been identified:

1. Food and/or nutrient delivery
2. Nutrition education
3. Nutrition counseling
4. Coordination of care

Step 4: Nutrition Monitoring and Evaluation

The point of this step in the NCP is to measure improvement made by the patient in meeting nutrition care goals. Patients' progress is examined by determining if the nutrition intervention is being executed and by providing evidence that the intervention *is* or *is not* altering the patients' nutritional status. Nutrition monitoring and evaluation terms are organized into four categories or domains:

1. Food- and nutrition-related history
2. Biochemical data, medical tests, and procedures
3. Anthropometric measurements
4. Nutrition-focused physical findings

In summary, the NCP allows for continuous treatment alteration. As patients' conditions change, so do diagnoses, plans, and interventions. If patients do not respond to interventions, then new interventions can be developed for them. However, it is important to remember that any and all nutrition interventions should be planned in consultation with patients, as well as with their caregivers or significant others. For more detailed information regarding the NCP, refer to the following Bibliography.

Bibliography

American Dietetic Association: *International Dietetics and Nutrition Terminology (IDNT) Reference Manual. Standardized language for the nutrition care process,* ed 4, Chicago, 2013, American Dietetic Association.

American Dietetic Association: Nutrition Care Process and Model Part 1: the 2008 update, *J Am Diet Assoc* 108:1113, 2008.

American Dietetic Association: Nutrition Care Process Part II: using the International Dietetics and Nutrition Terminology to document the Nutrition Care Process, *J Am Diet Assoc* 108:1287, 2008.

Lacey K, Pritchett E: Nutrition Care Process and model: ADA adopts road map to quality care and outcomes management, *J Am Diet Assoc* 103(8):1061, 2003.

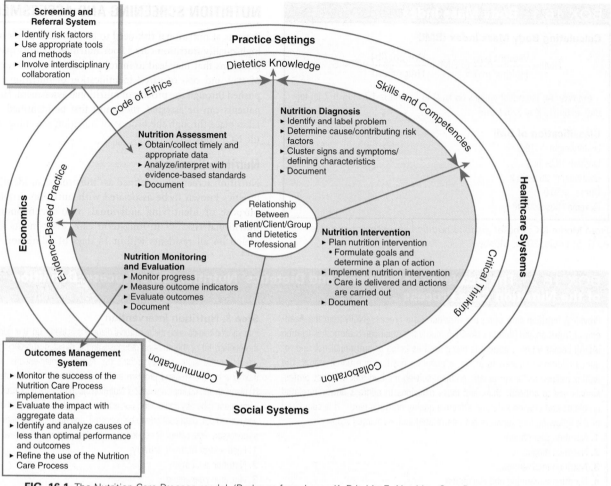

Screening and Referral System
▸ Identify risk factors
▸ Use appropriate tools and methods
▸ Involve interdisciplinary collaboration

Practice Settings

Dietetics Knowledge

Code of Ethics

Skills and Competencies

Nutrition Assessment
▸ Obtain/collect timely and appropriate data
▸ Analyze/interpret with evidence-based standards
▸ Document

Nutrition Diagnosis
▸ Identify and label problem
▸ Determine cause/contributing risk factors
▸ Cluster signs and symptoms/ defining characteristics
▸ Document

Economics

Evidence-Based Practice

Relationship Between Patient/Client/Group and Dietetics Professional

Nutrition Intervention
▸ Plan nutrition intervention
  • Formulate goals and determine a plan of action
▸ Implement nutrition intervention
  • Care is delivered and actions are carried out
▸ Document

Healthcare Systems

Critical Thinking

Nutrition Monitoring and Evaluation
▸ Monitor progress
▸ Measure outcome indicators
▸ Evaluate outcomes
▸ Document

Outcomes Management System
▸ Monitor the success of the Nutrition Care Process implementation
▸ Evaluate the impact with aggregate data
▸ Identify and analyze causes of less than optimal performance and outcomes
▸ Refine the use of the Nutrition Care Process

Communication

Collaboration

Social Systems

FIG. 16.1 The Nutrition Care Process model. (Redrawn from Lacey K, Pritchitt E: Nutrition Care Process and model: ADA adopts road map to quality care and outcomes management, *J Am Diet Assoc* 103[8]:1061, 2003, with permission from the American Dietetic Association [ADA].)

possible or necessary to complete a full nutrition assessment on every patient hospitalized in acute care. However, it is necessary to have a system in place to quickly identify patients at risk for nutrition problems, such as malnutrition or nutritional risk.[2] The Joint Commission requires that nutrition screening be performed within 24 hours of inpatient admission when applicable for the patient's condition.[12]

Nutrition screening can be executed by RDs, dietetic technicians, dietary managers, nurses, physicians, or other trained personnel.[2,8,9] Whether or not RDs are engaged in performing nutrition screening, they are responsible for providing input regarding the development of suitable screening parameters to make certain the screening process addresses the correct parameters.[8] The nutrition screening process has the following characteristics[13]:

- May be completed in any setting
- Facilitates completion of early intervention goals
- Includes collection of relevant data on risk factors and interpretation of data for intervention and treatment
- Determines need for a nutrition assessment
- Is cost-effective

Each facility or setting is responsible for determining the most appropriate mechanism for screening patients. It is important to identify patients at nutritional risk.[14] After individuals are identified, a nutrition assessment can be performed, and personalized intervention can

then be planned and implemented.[1] Certain criteria are used for nutrition screening[1,14]:

- Weight (i.e., BMI greater than 25 or less than 18.5)
- Unintentional weight loss of 10% or more of usual body weight within 6 months or 5% of usual body weight in 1 month
- Nausea and vomiting
- Chewing and swallowing ability
- Diagnosis or presence of chronic disease
- Increased metabolic requirements (e.g., trauma, burns, systemic infection)
- Food allergies
- Diet
- Altered intake (e.g., recent surgery, serious illness, parenteral or enteral nutrition)
- Inadequate intake expected to continue 7 days or longer
- Laboratory data (i.e., albumin, hematocrit)

If patients have been hospitalized for an extended length of time, they should be rescreened.[14] It is vital that a patient at nutritional risk is referred to an RD who will conduct the nutrition assessment, make nutrition diagnoses, and provide nutrition care.

Nutrition Assessment

Nutrition assessment is "a systematic approach to collect, record, and interpret relevant data from patients, clients, family members, caregivers and other individuals and groups. [It] is an ongoing, dynamic process that involves initial data collection as well as continual reassessment and analysis of the patient's/client's status compared to specified criteria."[10] The fundamental purpose of nutrition assessment in general clinical practice is to determine the following three factors:

1. Overall nutritional status of the patient
2. Current health care needs—physical, psychosocial, and personal (see Diet-Medications Interactions box, "Assess Your Knowledge of Food-Drug Interactions")
3. Related factors influencing these needs in the person's current life situation

The first step in nutrition assessment, as with assessing any situation to determine needs and actions, is to collect pertinent information, which will act as a database, for use in identifying needs. The clinical dietitian, assisted by other health care team members as needed, uses several basic types of activities for nutrition assessment of patients' needs, as follows:

- Anthropometric data
- Biochemical tests
- Clinical observations
- Diet evaluation and personal histories (i.e., medical, social, medications) (See the Focus on Culture box, "Cultural Stereotyping: Melting Pot or Salad Bowl?")

DIET-MEDICATIONS INTERACTIONS

Assess Your Knowledge of Food-Drug Interactions

Medications can treat and cure many health problems, but they must be taken properly to be effective. Many medications interact with foods, beverages, alcohol, and caffeine to make them less effective or cause dangerous side effects. Assess your knowledge of food-drug interactions by answering the following questions:

1. do risk of food-drug interactions exists when taking over-the-counter medications.
   a. True.
   b. False.
2. Your neighbor, Greta, has serious allergies. Her physician prescribed an antihistamine to control her symptoms. Which of the following labels might appear on her prescription bottle?
   a. Take on an empty stomach.
   b. Take with food.
   c. Take only at bedtime.
   d. Take with coffee.
3. The previously mentioned label is on Greta's prescription antihistamine because:
   a. Effectiveness is increased when taken on an empty stomach.
   b. Effectiveness is increased when taken with food.
   c. The drug is metabolized more efficiently when taken at bedtime.
   d. Caffeine enhances absorption of the medication.
4. Your other neighbor, Abdul, has a horrible headache from studying too hard last night. He asks you if he should take his over-the-counter nonsteroidal antiinflammatory drug (NSAID) on an empty stomach or with a meal. He should take the NSAID with food because:
   a. These medications can irritate the stomach.
   b. Food will increase effectiveness.
   c. It is easier to remember to take them with a meal.
5. Combining NSAIDs or acetaminophen with alcohol will:
   a. Decrease stomach irritation.
   b. Increase risk of liver damage.
   c. Protect the liver from the effects of alcohol.
   d. Have no effect whatsoever.
6. Your cousin Vinny is dining on a super-sized meal at the local fast food restaurant. Which of the following prescription medications should he avoid taking with the meal because high fat meals may increase levels in the body?
   a. Hydrochlorothiazide (diuretic)
   b. Tetracyclines (antibiotic)
   c. NSAIDs
   d. Some forms of theophylline (bronchodilator)
7. Grandma Minnie takes a diuretic to control hypertension. Her physician told her this drug could cause hypokalemia. Which of the following foods should she eat on a regular basis to avoid hypokalemia?
   a. Hamburgers and hot dogs
   b. Twinkies and Ding Dongs
   c. Low fat dairy products
   d. Bananas, oranges, and potatoes
8. Uncle Joe is taking captopril (an angiotensin-converting enzyme [ACE] inhibitor) for his high blood pressure. He cannot remember if his physician told him to take the captopril with a meal or on an empty stomach. What can you tell him?
   a. Take it with meals to increase absorption.
   b. Take it 1 hour before or 2 hours after meals so as to not affect absorption.
   c. Take it with breakfast but not with dinner.
9. Your roommate's cousin's uncle is taking a "statin" medication to lower serum cholesterol. Which of the following statements is true about statin medications?
   a. Avoid drinking large amounts of alcohol because it may increase risk of liver damage.
   b. Take with breakfast to enhance absorption.
   c. Take with the evening meal to decrease absorption.
10. High doses of vitamin E may prolong clotting time and increase risk of bleeding. Large doses of vitamin E should be avoided when taking which of the following drugs?
    a. Warfarin (anticoagulant)
    b. Lovastatin (3-hydroxy-3-methylglutaryl coenzyme A [HMG-CoA] reductase inhibitor)
    c. Furosemide (diuretic)
    d. NSAIDs
11. Your cousin Bunny is taking oral contraceptives. Which of the following drugs may decrease effectiveness of "the pill," thereby increasing her chance of pregnancy?
    a. Anticoagulants
    b. NSAIDs
    c. Antibiotics
    d. Antidepressants
12. Bunny's pet turtle, Speedy, died. She wants to take St. John's wort because her roommate told her it would help with her depression. Are there any problems with her taking St. John's wort while she is taking oral contraceptives?
    a. No. St. John's wort is an herb and sold at the Universal Nutrition Center at the mall. Herbal and dietary supplements cannot be sold if they are not safe.
    b. Yes. St. John's wort will decrease effectiveness of the oral contraceptives.
13. Mr. Wilson is very excitable and nervous. Which of the following might be an explanation for this?
    a. He took Cipro (quinolone) with his morning coffee.
    b. He took penicillin at breakfast, which included yogurt.
    c. He took aspirin on an empty stomach.
    d. He just received a call from the Internal Revenue Service (IRS) to schedule an audit of last year's tax return.

Continued

DIET-MEDICATIONS INTERACTIONS

Assess Your Knowledge of Food-Drug Interactions—cont'd

14. Curt is taking tetracycline to control acne. Which of the following should he avoid?
    a. Dairy products
    b. Antacids
    c. Vitamins containing iron
    d. All of the above
15. Your favorite aunt, Constance, takes a monoamine oxidase inhibitor (MAOI). Her pharmacist cautioned her about eating foods high in tyramine (an amino acid). Why?
    a. MAOIs combined with tyramine cause hiccups.
    b. A rapid, potentially fatal decrease in blood pressure can occur.
    c. A rapid, potentially fatal increase in blood pressure can occur.
    d. None of the above will happen. Her pharmacist is mistaken.
16. Your nervous neighbor, Biff, takes alprazolam (Xanax), an antianxiety drug. He was told he should not take the Xanax with Mountain Dew. Why?
    a. Carbonation in the soft drink will enhance effects of the Xanax.
    b. Carbonation in the soft drink will decrease effects of the Xanax.
    c. Caffeine in Mountain Dew may lessen the antianxiety effect of Xanax.
    d. Caffeine in the Mountain Dew may enhance the antianxiety effect of Xanax.
17. Kevin just found out his stomach pain is being caused by excess acid production that caused an ulcer. His physician prescribed a histamine blocker and told him to avoid alcohol. Why?
    a. Alcohol is a gastric irritant, which will make it more difficult for the stomach to heal.
    b. Alcohol decreases the effectiveness of the histamine blocker.

c. Alcohol increases the effectiveness of the histamine blocker.
d. Kevin's physician does not want any of her patients to drink alcohol.
18. Grandpa Moe takes digoxin for his heart condition. Your cousin Sunshine brought him ginseng on her last visit. Should he take ginseng with the digoxin?
    a. Yes. Herbal products are natural and safe.
    b. No. Ginseng falsely elevates plasma digoxin levels.
    c. It does not matter.
19. Trixie has a bad case of poison ivy. The physician gave her a prescription for Medrol, a corticosteroid to stop the itching. She cannot remember if the physician told her to take the Medrol on an empty stomach or with food. Can you help her?
    a. It does not matter if Trixie takes it on an empty stomach or not.
    b. Trixie should take the medicine on an empty stomach to decrease stomach irritation.
    c. Trixie should take the Medrol with food or milk to decrease stomach upset.
20. Great Uncle John takes nitroglycerin (nitrate) for chest pain. Which of the following can add to the blood vessel–relaxing effect of nitrates and cause dangerously low blood pressure?
    a. Milk and dairy products
    b. Fruits and vegetables
    c. Alcohol
    d. Meats and cheeses

Answers: 1. b; 2. a; 3. a; 4. a; 5. b; 6. d; 7. d; 8. b; 9. a; 10. a; 11. c; 12. b; 13. a; 14. d; 15. c; 16. c; 17. a; 18. b; 19. c; 20. c.

FOCUS ON CULTURE

Cultural Stereotyping: Melting Pot or Salad Bowl?

Do all Southerners eat grits? Do all those who practice the Jewish religion follow orthodox food laws? Do all people of Hispanic origin eat tortillas and beans? Should you address your patient informally (by his or her first name) or more formally (e.g., Mrs. Garcia or Mr. Sato)? If your patient does not look you in the eye while talking, is he or she being deceitful or showing respect? Why do you need to know the answer to these questions and others?

The population of the United States is growing increasingly culturally diverse. Between 2000 and 2010, the Hispanic population grew by 43% and the Asian population grew by 45.6%. Almost 25% of the total population is non-Anglo American. By 2043, although non-Hispanic Caucasians will be the largest single ethnic group, no group will make up a majority of the population. By 2060, minority groups, which currently make up 37% of the total population, will grow to 57% of the total US population. So what does this mean to you?

In terms of nutrition assessment and nutrition counseling, cultural diversity is a fact. Cultural competency is a necessity. Cultural competency is more than recognizing and accepting cultural diversity. It is a skill critical to all dietitians and health care professionals. What good does it do to conduct a nutrition assessment or provide nutrition education if the patient's cultural background is not considered? Culture includes language, lifestyle, values, beliefs, and attitudes. These and other elements of culture influence how patients might experience illness, how they might access health care, and how they get well.

To deliver culturally competent care, dietitians and health care providers must understand beliefs, values, traditions, and cultural practices. There are differences in the dominant American cultural **paradigm**, the Anglo-American culture, and more traditional cultural populations.

There was a time when minorities in the United States tended to imitate the dominant middle-class culture, but this is no longer the case. Individual and

cultural expression are becoming desirable. It is an expression of respect to learn about different cultures, to develop flexibility in how to approach clients and patients, and to develop cultural competency.

How Culturally Competent Are You?[a]

1. When the patient and dietitian come from different cultural backgrounds, the nutrition history obtained may not be accurate.
   a. True.
   b. False.
2. Which of the following are the correct ways to communicate with a patient through an interpreter?
   a. Making eye contact with the interpreter when you are speaking, then looking at the patient while the interpreter is telling the patient what you said.
   b. Speaking slowly, pausing between words.
   c. Asking the interpreter to further explain the patient's statement to get a more complete picture of the patient's condition.
   d. None of the above.
3. Which of the following statements is not true?
   a. Friendly (nonsexual) physical contact is an important part of communication for many Latin-American people.
   b. Many Asian people think it is disrespectful to ask questions of a health care professional.
   c. Most people of African heritage are either Christian or follow a traditional religion.
   d. Eastern Europeans are highly diverse in terms of customs, language, and religion.

Cultural Stereotyping: Melting Pot or Salad Bowl?—cont'd

4. Which of the following is good advice for a health care professional attempting to use and interpret nonverbal communication?
   a. The provider should recognize that a smile may express unhappiness or dissatisfaction in some cultures.
   b. To express sympathy, a health care professional can lightly touch a patient's arm or pat the patient on the back.
   c. If a patient will not make eye contact with a health care professional, then it is likely the patient is hiding the truth.
   d. When a language barrier exists, the provider can use hand gestures to bridge the gap.

5. Some symbols—a positive nod of the head, a pointing finger, a "thumbs-up" sign—are universal and can help bridge the language gap.
   a. True.
   b. False.

6. A female Muslim patient may avoid eye contact, physical contact, or both because:
   a. She does not want to spread germs.
   b. Muslim women are taught to be submissive.
   c. Modesty is very important in Islamic tradition.
   d. She does not like the health care professional.

7. When a patient is not compliant with prescribed nutrition therapy after several visits, which of the following approaches is *not* likely to lead to compliance?
   a. Involving family members.
   b. Repeating the instructions very loudly and several times to emphasize the importance of the nutrition therapy.
   c. Agreeing to a compromise in the recommended nutrition therapy.
   d. Spending time listening to discussions of folk and alternative remedies.

8. If a family member speaks English and the patient's native language and is willing to act as interpreter, then this is the best possible solution to the problem of interpreting.
   a. True.
   b. False.

9. Which of the following is *true?*
   a. People who speak the same language have the same culture.
   b. The people living in the African continent share the main features of African culture.
   c. Cultural background, diet, religious, and health practices, as well as language, can differ widely within a given country or part of the country.
   d. An alert health care professional can usually predict a patient's health behaviors by knowing what country he or she comes from.

10. Out of respect for a patient's privacy, the health care professional should always begin a relationship by seeing an adult patient alone and drawing the family in as needed.
    a. True
    b. False

Answers: 1. a; 2. d; 3. c; 4. a; 5. b; 6. c; 7. b; 8. b; 9. c; 10. b.

Bibliography

Betterley C: Increasing cultural competency of nutrition educators through travel study programs, Unpublished paper, 2001.

Brannon C: Cultural competency—values, traditions, and effective practice, *Today's Dietitian* 6(11):14, 2004. http://www.todaysdietitian.com/newarchives/td_1104p14.shtml.

Curry KR: Multicultural competence in dietetics and nutrition, *J Am Diet Assoc* 100:1142, 2000.

Stein K: Moving cultural competency from abstract to act, *J Am Diet Assoc* 110:S21, 2010.

US Census Bureau: *Census 2010 data for the United States*, Washington, DC, 2010, US Government Printing Office. http://www.census.gov.

aQuiz modified from Management Sciences for Health and the US Department of Health and Human Services, Health Resources and Administration, Bureau of Primary Healthcare: *The provider's guide to quality & culture*, Boston, 2008, Management Sciences for Health. Retrieved from: www.erc.msh.org/mainpage.cfm?file=1.0.htm&module=provider&language=English.

KEY TERM

Paradigm
A pattern or model serving as an example; a standard or ideal for practice or behavior based on a fundamental value or theme.

Each part of this approach is important because no single parameter directly measures individual nutritional status or determines problems or needs. Furthermore, the overall resulting impression must be interpreted within the context of the patient's own social and health factors, because these factors have the potential to alter his or her nutritional requirements. The procedures outlined here provide a good base in general practice.

Anthropometric Measurements. Anthropometric measurements are measurements of body size, weight, and proportions. These measurements can be used to assess nutritional status, as well as growth and development of infants and children; they are useful tools for monitoring the effects of nutritional intervention.[9]

Weight. One of the most important measurements in nutritional assessment is body weight. It is used to predict energy expenditure in prediction equations[9] (see the Evidence-Based Practice box, "What is the Best Prediction Equation to Determine Energy Needs?"). Hospitalized patients should be weighed at consistent times—for example, before breakfast after the bladder has been emptied. Clinic patients should be weighed without shoes in light, indoor clothing or an examining gown. For accuracy, use regular clinic beam scales with nondetachable weights (Fig. 16.2). Additional weight attachment is available for use with very obese persons. Metric scales with readings to the nearest 20 g provide specific data; however, the standard clinic scale is satisfactory. Scales should be checked frequently and calibrated every 3 or 4 months for continued accuracy. The weight of nonambulatory (unable to stand or walk) individuals can be measured using a bed or chair scale (Fig. 16.3).

After careful reading and recording of the patient's weight, ask about usual body weight. Interpret the patient's present weight in terms of the percentage of usual body weight. Check for any recent weight loss: 1% to 2% in the past week, 5% during the past month, 7.5% during the previous 3 months, or 10% in the past 6 months are significant. Unintentional weight loss greater than these rates can be severe. Unexplained weight loss is a problem with persons of any age. It is particularly important in older adults because it may be a clue to depression or a wasting disease such as cancer and needs to be on record and followed up. Values charted in the patient's record should indicate the percentage of weight change.

EVIDENCE-BASED PRACTICE

What is the Best Prediction Equation to Determine Energy Needs?

Assessment of energy needs is a necessary component in the NCP. Indirect calorimetry is the "gold standard" for determining resting metabolic rate (RMR) and is accurate within 5% in most cases. However, because indirect calorimetry is not always available, prediction equations are commonly used to determine RMR.

The four prediction equations most commonly used in clinical practice are as follows:

Mifflin-St. Jeor

Men	RMR = (9.99 × wt in kg) + (6.25 × ht in cm) − (4.92 × age in yr) + 5
Women	RMR = (9.99 × wt in kg) + (6.25 × ht in cm) − (4.92 × age in yr) − 161

Harris-Benedict

Men	RMR = 66.47 + (13.75 × wt in kg) + (5.0 × ht in cm) − (6.75 × age in yr)
Women	RMR = 665.09 + (9.56 × wt in kg) + (1.84 × ht in cm) − (4.67 × age in yr)

Owen

Men	RMR = 879 + (10.2 × wt in kg)
Women	RMR = 795 + (7.18 × wt in kg)

World Health Organization/Food and Agriculture Organization/United Nations University (WHO/FAO/UNU)

Age (yr)	Weight Only
Men	
18–30	15.3 × wt in kg + 679
31–60	11.6 × wt in kg + 879
>60	13.5 × wt in kg + 487
Women	
18–30	14.7 × wt in kg + 496
31–60	8.7 × wt in kg + 829
>60	10.5 × wt in kg + 596

Age (yr)	Weight and Height (m)
Men	
18–30	(15.4 × wt in kg) − (27 × ht in m) + 717
31–60	(11.3 × wt in kg) + (16 × ht in m) + 901
>60	(8.8 × wt in kg) + (1128 × ht in m) − 1071
Women	
18–30	(13.3 × wt in kg) + (34 × ht in m) + 35
31–60	(8.7 × wt in kg) − (25 × ht in m) + 865
>60	(9.2 × wt in kg) + (637 × ht in m) − 302

Of the four equations listed, the Mifflin-St. Jeor equation was found to be the most accurate in estimating basal metabolic rate (BMR). The oldest prediction equation in clinical use, Harris-Benedict, was found to systematically overestimate basal energy expenditure (BEE) by at least 5%. The Owen equation underestimates RMR approximately 21% of the time and overestimates RMR 6% of the time. Accuracy of the WHO/FAO/UNU equations could not be evaluated because of how the equations have been validated. For more details about the research of these prediction equations, refer to the Frankenfield manuscripts cited in the bibliography.

Bibliography

Food and Agricultural Organization/World Health Organization/United Nations University: *Energy and protein requirements, Report of a Joint FAO/WHO/UNU expert consultation,* World Health Organization Technical Report Series 724, Geneva, Switzerland, 1985, WHO.

Frankenfield DC, Muth ER, Rowe WA: The Harris-Benedict studies of human basal metabolism: history and limitations, *J Am Diet Assoc* 98(4):439, 1998.

Frankenfield D, Roth-Yousey L, Compher C: Comparison of predictive equations for resting metabolic rate in healthy nonobese and obese adults: a systematic review, *J Am Diet Assoc* 105(5):775, 2005.

Harris JA, Benedict FG: *A biometric study of basal metabolism in man,* Washington, DC, 1919, Carnegie Institute of Washington, Pub No 279.

Mifflin MD, St Jeor ST, Hill LA, et al: A new predictive equation for resting energy expenditure in healthy individuals, *Am J Clin Nutr* 51:241, 1990.

Owen OE, Holup JL, D'Alessio DA, et al: A reappraisal of the caloric requirements of men, *Am J Clin Nutr* 46:875, 1987.

Owen OE, Kavle E, Owen RS, et al: A reappraisal of caloric requirements in healthy women, *Am J Clin Nutr* 44:1, 1986.

Length and stature. Measurements of length and stature (height) are easily obtained anthropometric measures. They are the most sensitive indicators of growth and development in infants and children.[9]

If possible, use a fixed measuring stick or tape on a true vertical flat surface. Have the patient stand as straight as possible, without shoes or hat, heels together, and looking straight ahead. Heels, buttocks, shoulders, and head should be touching the wall or vertical surface of the measuring rod. Read the measure carefully, and compare it with previous recordings. Children younger than 2 years should be measured using a stationary headboard and movable footboard (Fig. 16.4).

FIG. 16.2 Balance beam scale. (From Jarvis C: *Physical examination and health assessment*, ed 6, St Louis, 2012, Elsevier Saunders.)

FIG.16.3 Bed scale. (From Grodner M, Long S, Walkingshaw BC: *Foundations and clinical applications of nutrition: a nursing approach*, ed 5, St Louis, 2012, Elsevier.)

FIG. 16.4 Measuring a baby's stature. (From Mahan LK, Escott-Stump S: *Krause's food, and the nutrition care process*, ed 13, Philadelphia, 2012, Elsevier Saunders.)

Note growth of children or the diminishing height of adults. Metric measures of height in centimeters provide a smaller unit of measure than inches.

Although it is always preferable to obtain standing measurements,[9] this is not always possible. Several alternative measures can provide values for estimating height and weight of persons confined to bed:

- *Knee height* (Fig. 16.5) has been shown to correlate well with stature.[17-19] Measurement is taken with the person lying in the supine position. The left leg is measured with knee and ankle at a 90-degree angle using a specialized sliding caliper. Measurements are then entered into one of the following validated equations[15,17]

Men:

$$\text{Stature (cm)} = [2.02 \times \text{knee height (cm)}] - (0.04 \times \text{age}) + 64.19$$

Women:

$$\text{Stature (cm)} = [1.83 \times \text{knee height (cm)}] - (0.24 \times \text{age}) + 84.88$$

- To estimate height of a nonambulatory person who has no skeletal abnormalities or contractures, *recumbent bed measurement* can be taken by marking the base of the heels and top of the crown on the bed sheet (Fig. 16.6) on which the patient is resting in a straight line. The distance between these two lines can be measured with a tape measure.
- *Arm span* measurement taken from sternal notch to the longest finger on the dominant hand is reliable in individuals with no contractures, spinal deformities, and who can fully extend their arms. To estimate stature, multiply the number obtained by 2.[15,16]

Body mass index. BMI is a ratio of weight to height and has been correlated with overall mortality and nutritional risk.[2,15] It does not estimate body composition (lean body mass or adiposity); however, it is a reliable indicator of total body fat (see Box 16.1), which is related to the risk of disease.[20] Although BMI measurements are valid for men and women, they do have some limits[15,20]:

- BMI has not been validated in acutely ill patients.
- BMI may overestimate body fat in individuals who have a muscular build.
- BMI may underestimate body fat in older adults and others who have lost muscle mass.

Standardized growth charts for children can be found on the Centers for Disease Control and Prevention (CDC) website (http://www.cdc.gov/nchs/about/major/nhanes/growthcharts/clinical_charts.htm). These growth charts show percentile rankings of height and weight for age and weight for height, as well as BMI for age.[1]

Waist circumference. Waist circumference is inexpensive, easy to perform, and assesses abdominal fat content. BMI and waist circumference highly correlate with obesity and risk for disease, and both should be used to classify overweight and obesity, as well as to estimate disease risk.[1,15,21] Circumference greater than 40 inches in men and greater than 35 inches in women indicates risk for disease. It should be noted that visceral adiposity may vary among racial and ethnic groups.[1]

Biochemical (Laboratory) Measurements. Biochemical (or laboratory) tests are a useful adjunct in measuring and managing nutritional status, but their use can be problematic.[9] Precise interpretation

FIG. 16.6 Recumbent bed length. (From Lee RD, Nieman DC: *Nutritional assessment,* ed 4, Boston, 2007, McGraw-Hill.)

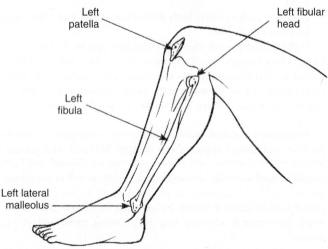

Left patella

Left fibular head

Left fibula

Left lateral malleolus

FIG. 16.5 Knee height measurement. (From Lee RD, Nieman DC: *Nutritional assessment,* ed 4, Boston, 2007, McGraw-Hill.)

necessitates awareness of the appropriate test, as well as nutritional and nonnutritional factors that have the potential to alter blood chemistries. Significant nonnutritional factors to be considered include disease processes, treatments, procedures, medications, and hydration status.[22] The most commonly used methods for assessing and monitoring nutritional status and planning nutrition care in clinical practice are listed here. General ranges for normal values are given in standard texts.

Protein assessment. Usually, biochemical assessment of protein status has been undertaken from the standpoint of two protein compartments: (1) somatic and (2) visceral proteins.[9] Somatic protein is found within skeletal muscle, and visceral proteins are found in body organs, red blood cells, white blood cells, and serum proteins. Both protein pools are metabolically active, meaning the body can tap into these stores if necessary.[9] Obviously use of any proteins stored in the body means the protein is no longer available for bodily functions like synthesis of antibodies, hormones, and other vital components. In addition, no single laboratory test or group of tests is sensitive, specific, or both for protein malnutrition. Evaluation of serum proteins necessitates simultaneous assessment of nutrient intake, physical findings, and clinical condition.[22]

Serum proteins. Serum protein concentrations can be helpful in determining protein status, risk of medical complications, and response to nutritional intervention with limitations.[9,22] A number of factors other than inadequate protein intake affect serum protein concentrations (Table 16.1).

Somatic proteins. Somatic proteins can be measured using anthropometric measures such as midarm muscle area, midarm circumference, and overall body weight.[2] A laboratory test that can be used for estimating body muscle mass is 24-hour urinary creatinine excretion.[10]

When assessing biochemical measurements, it is important to consider that a review of serial laboratory data is recommended. Direction and speed of change are more important than static value. Improvement in nutrition parameters does not always confer clinical benefit. Treat the person, not the laboratory value.[22]

Clinical Observations and Nutrition Physical Assessment. Certain information used to assess nutritional status is taken from physical examinations performed by physicians and nurses. Furthermore, RDs perform nutritional physical examinations to assess patients for signs and symptoms consistent with malnutrition or specific nutrient deficiency.[2] Techniques used in nutritional physical examinations are summarized in Table 16.2.

Clinical signs of malnutrition. Careful attention to physical signs of possible malnutrition provides an added dimension to the overall assessment of general nutritional status. A guide for a general examination of such signs is given in Table 16.3. A careful description of any such observations is documented in the patient's medical record.

TABLE 16.1 Laboratory Measures of Serum Proteins

Serum protein	Function	Comments
Albumin		
Normal: 3.5–5.0 g/dL	Maintains plasma oncotic	Not sensitive or specific for acute protein malnutrition or response to nutrition
Depletion:	pressure, carrier for	therapy; affected by hydration status, disease state, clinical condition
Mild: 3.0–3.4 g/dL	small molecules	Can be used as prognostic indicator of morbidity, mortality, and severity
Moderate: 2.4–2.9 g/dL		of illness
Severe: <2.4 g/dL		
Half-life ~14–20 days		
Transferrin		
Normal: 200–400 g/dL	Binds iron in plasma	Inversely correlated with body's iron stores; elevated concentration often indi-
Depletion:	and transports to bone	cates early iron deficiency
Mild: 150–200 mg/dL	marrow	Will decrease during acute illness
Moderate: 100–149 mg/dL		Verify with laboratory whether lab is direct measurement or calculated
Severe: <100 mg/dL		
Half-life ~8–10 days		
Prealbumin (transthyretin, thyroxin-binding prealbumin)		
Normal: 16–40 mg/dL	Carrier protein for thyroxin	Influenced less by intravascular fluid volume
Depletion:	Combined with retinol-	Not affected as early or as significantly with liver disease (compared with
Mild: 10–15 mg/dL	binding protein,	albumin)
Moderate: 5–9 mg/dL	transports vitamin A	More likely to be reflection of recent dietary intake than accurate indicator of
Severe: <5 mg/dL		nutritional status
Half-life ~2–3 days		

Modified from (compiled from components in tables and text) Moore MC: *Pocket guide to nutrition assessment and care,* ed 6, St Louis, 2009, Mosby; Lee RD, Nieman DC: *Nutritional assessment,* ed 4, Boston, 2007, McGraw-Hill; Thompson CW: Laboratory assessment. In Charney P, Malone AM, editors: *ADA pocket guide to nutrition assessment,* ed 2, Chicago, 2009, American Dietetic Association.

TABLE 16.2 Nutritional Physical Examination

Technique	Skill	Purpose
Inspection	Systematic visual inspection	Monitor changes to normal features
Auscultation	Using a stethoscope and naked ear to identify deviations from standard sounds	Evaluate sounds produced by heart, lungs, and gastrointestinal (GI) tract such as bowel sounds
Palpation	Examination of the body using touch	Reveal conditions that have nutritional implications such as abdominal tenderness, ascites, distention, peripheral edema, nail integrity, and skin turgor
Percussion	Use of sound to distinguish deviations from standard sounds created by presence of body organs and cavities	Identify gastric air bubble, intestinal air, or fluid present in lungs

Data from Nelms MN, Sucher K, Long S: *Understanding nutrition therapy and pathophysiology,* Belmont, CA, 2007, Wadsworth.

TABLE 16.3 Clinical Signs of Nutritional Status

Area of Concern	Possible Deficiency	Possible Excess
Hair		
Dull, dry, brittle	Pro	
Easily plucked (with no pain)	Pro	
Hair loss	Pro, Zn, biotin	Vit A
Flag sign (loss of hair pigment in strips around head)	Pro, Cu	
Head and Neck		
Bulging fontanel (infants)		Vit A
Headache		Vit A, D
Epistaxis (nosebleed)	Vit K	
Thyroid enlargement	Iodine	

Continued

TABLE 16.3   Clinical Signs of Nutritional Status—cont'd

Area of Concern	Possible Deficiency	Possible Excess
Eyes		
Conjunctival and corneal xerosis (dryness)	Vit A	
Pale conjunctiva	Fe	
Blue sclerae	Fe	
Corneal vascularization	Vit B$_2$	
Mouth		
Cheilosis or angular stomatitis (lesions at corners of mouth, Fig. 16.7A)	Vit B$_2$	
Glossitis (red, sore tongue)	Niacin, folate, vit B$_{12}$, and other B vit	
Gingivitis (inflamed gums)	Vit C	
Hypogeusia, dysgeusia (poor sense of taste, distorted taste)	Zn	
Dental caries	Fluoride	
Mottling of teeth		Fluoride
Atrophy of papillae on tongue	Fe, B vit	
Skin		
Dry, scaly	Vit A, Zn, EFAs	Vit A
Follicular hyperkeratosis (resembles gooseflesh)	Vit A, EFAs, B vit	
Eczematous lesions	Zn	
Petechiae, ecchymoses	Vit C, K	
Nasolabial seborrhea (greasy, scaly areas between nose and lip)	Niacin, vit B$_{12}$, B$_6$	
Darkening and peeling of skin in areas exposed to sun	Niacin	
Poor wound healing	Pro, Zn, vit C	
Nails		
Spoon-shaped nails (see Fig. 16.7B)	Fe	
Brittle, fragile	Pro	
Heart		
Enlargement, tachycardia, failure	Vit B$_1$	
Small heart	Energy	
Sudden failure, death	Se	
Arrhythmia	Mg, K, Se	
Hypertension	Ca, K	
Abdomen		
Hepatomegaly	Pro	Vit A
Ascites	Pro	
Musculoskeletal Extremities		
Muscle wasting (especially temporal area)	Energy	
Edema	Pro, vit B$_1$	
Calf tenderness	Vit B$_1$ or C, biotin, Se	
Beading of ribs, or "rachitic rosary" (child)	Vit C, D	
Bone and joint tenderness	Vit C, D, Ca, P	
Knock-knee, bowed legs, fragile bones	Vit D, Ca, P, Cu	
Neurologic		
Paresthesias (pain and tingling or altered sensation in the extremities)	Vit B$_1$, B$_6$, B$_{12}$, biotin	
Weakness	Vit C, B$_1$, B$_6$, B$_{12}$, energy	
Ataxia, decreased position and vibratory senses	Vit B$_1$, B$_{12}$	
Tremor	Mg	
Decreased tendon reflexes	Vit B$_1$	
Confabulation, disorientation	Vit B$_1$, B$_{12}$	
Drowsiness, lethargy	Vit B$_1$	Vit A, D
Depression	Vit B$_1$, biotin, B$_{12}$	

Ca, Calcium; *Cu,* copper; *EFAs,* essential fatty acids; *Fe,* iron; *K,* potassium, *Mg,* magnesium; *Na,* sodium; *P,* phosphorus; *Pro,* protein; *Se,* selenium; *Vit,* vitamin(s); *Zn,* zinc.
Data from Moore MC: *Pocket guide to nutrition assessment and care,* ed 6, St Louis, 2009, Mosby, pp 60–63.

FIG. 16.7 Examples of Findings in Malnourished States. (A) Cheilosis or angular stomatitis; (B) spoon-shaped nails. (From Moore MC: *Pocket guide to nutrition assessment and care*, ed 6, St Louis, 2009, Mosby.)

Dietary Assessment

Collecting information. A careful nutrition history, including nutrition information related to living situation and other personal, psychosocial, and economic problems, is a fundamental part of nutrition assessment. Obtaining accurate information about basic food patterns and actual dietary intake is not simple because some individuals misreport or underreport what they eat. Each method of diet evaluation has particular strengths and limitations.[9] However, a sensitive practitioner may obtain useful information by using one or more of the basic tools described in Table 16.4.

TABLE 16.4	Strengths and Limitations of Techniques Used to Measure Dietary Intake		
Technique	**Brief Description**	**Strengths**	**Limitations**
24-hour food record	Trained interviewer asks respondent to recall, in detail, all food and drink consumed during a period of time in the recent past.	Requires <20 min to administer Inexpensive Easy to administer Can provide detailed information on types of foods consumed Low respondent burden More objective than dietary history Does not alter usual diet Useful in clinical settings	One recall rarely illustrative of typical intake Underreporting and overreporting problems Dependent on memory Omissions of sauces, dressings, and beverages can lead to low estimates of energy intake Data entry sometimes labor intensive
Food record or diary	Respondents record, at the time of consumption, the identity and amounts of all foods and beverages consumed for a period of time, usually ranging from 1 to 7 days.	Does not rely on memory Can provide detailed intake data Can provide information about eating habits Multiple-day data more representative of usual intake Reasonably valid up to 5 days	Requires high degree of cooperation Subject must be literate Takes more time to obtain data Act of recording may alter usual intake
Food frequency questionnaires	Respondents indicate how many times a day, week, month, or year they usually consume foods using a questionnaire consisting of a list of approximately >150 foods or food groups that are important contributors to the population's intake of energy and nutrients.	Can be self-administered Machine readable Modest demand on respondents Relatively inexpensive May be more representative of usual intake than a few days of diet records	May not represent usual food or portion sizes chosen by respondent Intake data can be compromised when multiple foods are grouped within single listings Depends on ability of respondent to describe diet
Diet history	Respondents are interviewed by a trained interviewer about number of meals eaten per day, their appetites, their food dislikes, the presence or absence of nausea and/or vomiting, the use of nutritional supplements and/or herbal products, cigarette smoking, as well as habits related to sleep, rest, work, and exercise.	Assesses usual nutrient intake Can detect seasonal changes Data on all nutrients can be obtained Can correlate well with biochemical measures	Lengthy interview process Requires highly trained interviewers May overestimate nutrient intake Requires cooperation of respondent with ability to recall usual diet

Modified from Lee RD, Neiman DC: *Nutrition assessment*, ed 4, Boston, 2007, McGraw-Hill.

Evaluation of dietary intake. Valid patient care planning requires analysis of all nutrition data collected. On this basis, problems requiring solutions can be identified. A detailed analysis of all available nutrition information helps determine nutrition diagnosis, any primary or secondary nutritional disease, and any underlying nutrition-related conditions.

Medical tests used for nutrition assessment are generally reliable in persons of any age, but conditions in older adult patients may interfere and need to be considered in evaluating test results. For example, laboratory values are affected by hydration status, presence of chronic diseases, changes in organ function, and drugs. Nutrition assessment is an important part of the general health care of everyone, especially older adults. Health outreach programs for older persons, such as those in rural areas, can use brief, easily administered tools for screening and assessing nutritional status and risk of malnutrition as part of geriatric care.

NUTRITION DIAGNOSIS

Nutrition diagnosis is not to be confused with medical diagnosis. Medical diagnosis is a disease or pathologic condition that can be treated or prevented, and the diagnosis does not change as long as the condition exists.[8] Nutrition diagnosis is "a food and nutrition professional's identification and labeling of an existing nutrition problem that the food and nutrition professional is responsible for treating independently."[10] Nutrition diagnoses provide a mechanism for dietetics practitioners to document the link between nutrition assessment and nutrition intervention and to set realistic and measurable expected outcomes for patients. Identifying diagnoses also assists dietetics practitioners in establishing priorities when planning nutrition care.[23] More than one nutrition diagnosis is possible, and nutrition diagnoses change as patients' nutritional needs change.[8,10] Each nutrition diagnosis should be accompanied by an intervention and monitoring strategy.[10] Nutrition diagnoses are dependent on evidence-based practice and standardized language.[2,8] More information on evidence-based practice is available for Academy of Nutrition and Dietetics (AND) members (formerly the American Dietetic Association [ADA]) at http://www.adaevidencelibrary.com/default.cfm.

More than 60 nutrition diagnoses have been developed through use of standardized language and are grouped into three categories: (1) intake, (2) clinical, and (3) behavioral-environmental. Standardized language provides a means for dietetics professionals to communicate with each other, as well as with other health care professionals. It is a fundamental part of the NCP and assists dietetics professionals in better documenting nutrition care.[23] See Box 16.2 for more in-depth information and to determine how a nutrition diagnosis is written.

NUTRITION INTERVENTION: FOOD PLAN AND MANAGEMENT

Basic Concepts of Nutrition Therapy

Nutrition therapy is always based on normal nutritional requirements and personal needs for each particular patient. It is modified only as the specific disease in the specific individual necessitates. When planning and counseling for nutrition care, this is an important initial fact to grasp and impart to patients and clients. For example, it is a great source of encouragement to the parents of a child newly diagnosed with diabetes to know the food plan will be based on individual growth and development needs and will make use of regular foods.

Disease Application. Principles of a nutrition therapy will be based on modifications of nutritional components of the normal diet as a particular disease condition may require. These changes may include the following types of modifications:

- *Nutrients:* modification of one or more of the basic nutrients—protein, carbohydrate, fat, minerals, and vitamins
- *Energy:* modification in energy value as expressed in kilocalories (kcalories or kcal)
- *Texture:* modification in texture or seasoning, such as liquid or low residue

Individual Adaptation. Nutrition therapy may be theoretically correct and have well-balanced food plans, but if these plans are unacceptable to the patient, they will not be followed. A workable plan for a specific person must be based on individual food habits within the specific personal life situation. This can be achieved only through careful planning with the patient, or with the parents of a child who requires a special diet, based on an initial interview to obtain a diet history, knowledge of personal food habits, living conditions, and food security. In this way, diet principles can be understood and motivation secured. Regardless of the problems, nutrition therapy is valid only to the extent that it involves this kind of knowledge, as well as these particular skills and insights. Individual adaptations of the diet to meet individual needs are imperative for successful therapy.

Routine House Diets

A schedule of routine "house" diets, based on some type of cycle menu plan, is usually used in hospitals for patients who do not require a special diet modification. According to general patient need and tolerance, the diet order may be liquid (clear liquid), soft (in texture), and regular (a full, normal-for-age diet) (Table 16.5).

Managing the Mode of Feeding

Depending on the patient's condition, the clinical dietitian may manage nutrition therapy by using any one of the following four feeding modes.

1. *Oral diet.* As long as possible, of course, regular oral feeding is preferred. Supplements are added if needed. According to the patient's condition, he or she may need assistance in eating.
2. *Enteral nutrition and tube feeding.* If a patient is unable to eat but the gastrointestinal (GI) tract can be used, enteral delivery, or tube feeding, may provide needed nutrition support. A number of commercial formulas are available.
3. *Peripheral nutrition.* If the patient cannot take in food or formula via the GI tract, intravenous feeding is used. Solutions of dextrose, amino acids, vitamins, and minerals, with lipids as appropriate, can be fed through peripheral veins when the need is not extensive or long term.
4. *Total parenteral nutrition (TPN).* If the patient's nutritional need is great and support therapy may be required for a longer time, parenteral feeding through a large central vein is needed. Placement of this catheter is a special procedure. More concentrated special solutions can be used and monitored by a nutrition support team. Formulas are determined by the dietitian and physician, and they are prepared by trained pharmacists. This specialized nutrition support method was originally used only in hospitals, but advances in TPN administration now allow its use in many health care settings and even at home with some patients.

TABLE 16.5 Routine Hospital Diets

Food	Clear Liquid	Soft	Regular
Soup	Clear fat-free broth, bouillon	Same, plus all cream soups	All
Cereal		Cooked cereal, cornflakes, rice, noodles, macaroni, spaghetti	All
Bread		White bread, crackers, Melba toast, zwieback	All
Protein foods		Eggs (not fried), mild cheese, cottage and cream cheese, fowl, fish, sweetbreads, tender beef, veal, lamb, liver, bacon, gravy	All
Vegetables		Potatoes (baked, mashed, creamed, steamed, scalloped), tender cooked whole bland vegetables, fresh lettuce, tomatoes	All
Fruit and fruit juices	Fruit juices (as tolerated), flavored fruit drinks	Same, plus cooked fruit (peaches, pears, applesauce, peeled apricots, white cherries), ripe peaches, pears, bananas, orange and grapefruit sections without membrane	All
Desserts and gelatin	Fruit-flavored gelatin, fruit ices, and Popsicles	Same, plus plain sponge cakes, plain cookies, plain cake, puddings, pie made with allowed foods	All
Miscella-neous	Soft drinks (as tolerated), coffee and tea, decaffeinated coffee and tea, cereal beverages (e.g., Postum), sugar, honey, salt, hard candy, Polycose (Ross Laboratories), residue-free supplements	Same, plus mild salad dressings	All

KEY TERMS

Enteral
A mode of feeding that uses the GI tract; oral or tube feeding.

Parenteral
A mode of feeding that does not use the GI tract; instead it provides nutrition by intravenous delivery of nutrient solutions.

EVALUATION: QUALITY PATIENT CARE

General Considerations

When the NCP is carried out, patient care activities need to be considered in terms of nutrition diagnosis and treatment objectives, as well as the extent to which each of the care activities helps meet the particular goals of the patient and family. This evaluation is continuous and thorough, and it requires careful, objective documentation (see the Case Study box, "Nutrition Assessment and Therapy for a Patient with Cancer"). It seeks

CASE STUDY

Nutrition Assessment and Therapy for a Patient With Cancer

Esther is a 160-cm (5 ft 4 in) tall, medium-frame, 43-year-old patient recovering from a gastrectomy performed 8 days ago to treat gastric cancer. Her weight has dropped gradually for the past 4 months, from an average of 59 kg (130 lb) before her illness began. She continues to observe a full-liquid diet, consuming 60 to 120 mL (2 to 4 oz) of milk every few hours, plus one or two soft-boiled eggs each day. Today Esther informed the nutritionist that she consumed a total of 721 mL (24 oz) of milk and two eggs.

In reviewing Esther's records, the clinical dietitian found the following nutrition assessment data: weight, 46.8 kg (103 lb); triceps skinfold, 10 mm; and midarm circumference, 17 cm. Laboratory values include serum albumin, 3 g/dL; total iron-binding capacity (TIBC), 230 mcg/dL; lymphocytes, 1200 cells/mm³ (23%); hematocrit, 35%; and hemoglobin, 10.5 g/dL. Urinalysis (24 hours) included blood urea nitrogen, 16 g; and creatinine, 1.75 g.

After reviewing the data, the clinical dietitian calculated nitrogen balance, transferrin, and creatinine-height index, which were recorded on the patient chart. Basal energy expenditure (BEE) needs, as well as the kcalories and protein needed to overcome catabolism, were also calculated, along with estimates for additional vitamin and mineral requirements.

The clinical dietitian noted the physician had ordered chemotherapy for the patient, continuing after discharge, and recommended use of TPN, also to be continued after discharge, as a means of meeting Esther's nutritional needs. In addition, the clinical dietitian planned ways of meeting any feeding problems that often accompany chemotherapy, such as sore

mouth, nausea, and food intolerances. Observing a carefully prepared protocol developed by the hospital nutrition support team, Esther and her husband were instructed in procuring and using the home TPN treatment. The clinical dietitian also provided follow-up counseling for Esther and her husband at the office and in the group sessions for cancer patients and their families.

Questions for Analysis

1. Use a nutrition assessment data summary sheet from your hospital (or design your own) to record pertinent data given in this case study. What additional data would you collect? How would it be obtained?
2. For each test listed on your data sheet, explain what it measures and how that information contributes to an understanding of Esther's status.
3. What specific nutritional needs (nutrition diagnoses) can you identify in this case? List them in order of priority.
4. Calculate Esther's nitrogen balance and transferrin for day 8. Why are these indexes important to assessing her nutritional status?
5. What is Esther's creatinine-height index? How does it reflect her nutritional status?
6. What nutrition problems do you expect Esther to experience after discharge? How could they be resolved? What community agencies might contribute to her sense of well-being after discharge?

to validate care while it is being given, as well as determine the effectiveness of a particular course of care. Various areas need to be investigated, as follows:

- *Estimate the achievement of nutrition therapy goals:* What is the effect of diet or mode of feeding on the illness or patient's situation? Does a need exist for any change in nutrient ratios of diet or formula as originally calculated, in meal distribution pattern, or in feeding mode?
- *Judge the accuracy of intervention actions:* Does a need exist to change any of the NCP components? For example, is it necessary to change the type of food or feeding equipment, environment for meals, procedures for counseling, or types of learning activities for nutrition education and self-care procedures?
- *Determine the patient's ability to follow the prescribed nutrition therapy:* Do any hindrances or disabilities exist that prevent the patient from observing the treatment plan? What is the effect of nutrition therapy on the patient, family, or staff? Were the necessary nutrition assessment procedures for collecting nutrition data carried out correctly? Do patient and family understand the information given for self-care? Have community resources required by the patient and family been available and convenient for use? Has any needed food assistance program been sufficient to meet needs for the patient's ongoing care?

TO SUM UP

The basis for an accurate assessment of the patient's nutritional needs begins with the individual patient and family. Physical, psychologic, social, economic, and cultural factors in and out of the clinical setting all play a role in evaluating the patient's health status and any possible problems with the nutrition care plan.

Nutrition assessment is based on a broad foundation of pertinent data, including food and drug uses and values. Effectiveness of an assessment based on analysis of these data depends on effective communication with the patient, family members, and significant others in the development of an appropriate care plan, as well as with other members of the health care team. The patient's medical record is a basic means of communication among health care team members.

Nutrition therapy, based on a combination of personal and physiologic needs of the patient, requires a close working relationship among nutrition, medical, and nursing staff in the health care facility. The nurse's schedule offers many opportunities to reinforce nutrition principles of the diet. Nutrition therapy does not end with the patient's discharge. Outpatient nutrition services, appropriate social services, and food resources in the community help meet the continuing needs of patients and their families.

▌QUESTIONS FOR REVIEW

1. Identify and discuss possible effects of various psychological factors on the outcome of nutrition therapy.
2. Outline a general procedure for assessing the nutritional needs of a 65-year-old widower hospitalized with coronary heart disease. Include the appropriate community agencies that you would refer the patient to for follow-up care, services, and information.
3. Describe commonly used anthropometric procedures, as well as laboratory and urine tests for nutritional status information, in

terms of the significance of the measure or test (i.e., what is being measured, what the results tell you).
4. Select several clinical signs used to assess nutritional status, and describe what each sign shows in a malnourished person and why.
5. Describe the nature and purpose of quality assurance plans for standards of nutrition care.

REFERENCES

1. Moore MC: *Pocket guide to nutrition assessment and care,* ed 6, St Louis, 2009, Mosby.
2. Nelms M: Assessment of nutrition status and risk. In Nelms MN, Sucher K, Long S, editors: *Understanding nutrition therapy and pathophysiology,* Belmont, CA, 2007, Wadsworth.
3. American Dietetic Association: Position of the American Dietetic Association: integration of medical nutrition therapy and pharmacotherapy, *J Am Diet Assoc* 110:950, 2010.
4. Wolf AM, Siadaty M, Yaeger B, et al: Effects of lifestyle intervention on health care costs: Improving Control with Activity and Nutrition (ICAN), *J Am Diet Assoc* 107:1365, 2007.
5. Fessler TA: Malnutrition: a serious concern for hospitalized patients, *Today's Dietitian* 10(7):44, 2008.
6. Weight-Control Information Network: *Overweight and obesity statistics,* Bethesda, MD, 2012, National Institute of Diabetes and Digestive and Kidney Diseases. http://www.win.niddk.nih.gov/statistics/index.htm.
7. Centers for Disease Control and Prevention: *Overweight and obesity: causes and consequences,* Atlanta, GA, 2012, Centers for Disease Control and Prevention. http://www.cdc.gov/obesity/adult/causes/index.html.
8. Lacey K, Pritchitt E: Nutrition Care Process and model: ADA adopts road map to quality care and outcomes management, *J Am Diet Assoc* 103(8):1061, 2003.
9. Lee RD, Nieman DC: *Nutritional assessment,* ed 6, Boston, 2012, McGraw-Hill.
10. American Dietetic Association: Nutrition Care Process and Model Part 1: The 2008 Update, *J Am Diet Assoc* 108:1113, 2008.
11. Identifying patients at risk: ADA's definitions for nutrition screening and nutrition assessment, *J Am Diet Assoc* 94:838, 1994.
12. The Joint Commission: Standards FAQ Details: *Nutritional, Functional and Pain Assessments and Screens,* Oakbrook Terrace, Ill., 2008, The Joint Commission. http://www.jointcommission.org/standards_information/jcfaq.aspx?ProgramId=39.
13. Identifying patients at risk: ADA's definitions for nutrition screening and nutrition assessment, *J Am Diet Assoc* 94(8):838, 1994.
14. Charney P, Marian M: Nutrition screening and nutrition assessment. In Charney P, Malone AM, editors: *ADA pocket guide to nutrition assessment,* ed 2, Chicago, 2009, American Dietetic Association.
15. Lefton J, Malone AM: Anthropometric assessment. In Charney P, Malone AM, editors: *ADA pocket guide to nutrition assessment,* ed 2, Chicago, 2009, American Dietetic Association.
16. National Heart, Lung, and Blood Institute: *Obesity education initiative,* Bethesda, MD, 2012, National Heart, Lung, and Blood Institute, National Institutes of Health. http://www.nhlbi.nih.gov/health/public/heart/obesity/lose_wt/risk.htm.
17. Chumlea WC, Guo SS, Steinbaugh ML: Prediction of stature from knee height for black and white adults and children with application to mobility-impaired or handicapped persons, *J Am Diet Assoc* 94:1385, 1994.

18. Cockram DB, Baumgartner RN: Evaluation of accuracy and reliability of calipers for measuring recumbent knee height in elderly people, *Am J Clin Nutr* 52:397, 1990.

19. Muncie HI, Sobal J, Hoopes JM, et al: A practical method of estimating stature of bedridden female nursing home patients, *J Am Geriatr Soc* 35:285, 1987.

20. Mitchell CO, Lipschitz DA: Arm length measurement as an alternative to height in the nutrition assessment of the elderly, *JPEN J Parenter Enteral Nutr* 6:226, 1982.

21. American Dietetic Association Evidence Analysis Library: *Adult weight management guidelines*, Chicago, 2014, American Dietetic Association. http://www.adaevidencelibrary.com.

22. Thompson CW: Laboratory assessment. In Charney P, Malone AM, editors: *ADA pocket guide to nutrition assessment*, ed 2, Chicago, 2009, American Dietetic Association.

23. American Dietetic Association: *International Dietetics and Nutrition Terminology (IDNT) reference manual. Standardized language for the nutrition care process*, ed 4, Chicago, 2013, American Dietetic Association.

FURTHER READINGS AND RESOURCES

Readings

American Dietetic Association: Position of the American Dietetic Association: integration of medical nutrition therapy and pharmacology, *J Am Diet Assoc* 103(10):1363, 2003.

American Dietetic Association: Position of the American Dietetic Association: ethical and legal issues in nutrition, hydration, and feeding, *J Am Diet Assoc* 108(5):873, 2008.

Websites of Interest

- Nestle Nutrition, Clinical Resources and Tools. This site provides tools and resources to help identify, assess, and select appropriate products to address the nutrition challenges of patients. http://www.nestle-nutrition.com/Clinical_Resources/Default.aspx.

- US Department of Agriculture, Food and Nutrition Information Center, Dietary Analysis and Intake Calculators. This site, hosted by the Food and Nutrition Information Center (FNIC) at the National Agricultural Library (NAL), provides links to numerous diet-analysis tools. http://www.fnic.nal.usda.gov/dietary-guidance/interactive-tools

Metabolic Stress

Joyce Gilbert

ⓔ http://evolve.elsevier.com/Williams/essentials/

In this chapter, various surgical procedures are discussed, with a focus on surgical procedures and situations that could have a large nutritional consequence, particularly thermal injuries (or burns). An understanding of the surgical procedure performed, with knowledge of nutritional and absorptive function and capacity of the alimentary tract, is imperative to providing optimal nutrition care of surgery patients (see the Focus on Culture box, "Physiologic Changes Related to the Aging Process That Can Affect Surgery"). An understanding of the body's response to metabolic stress is also important when determining optimal timing and type of nutrition intervention for the patient.

OUTLINE

Nutritional Needs of General Surgery Patients
Nutritional Concerns for Patients Undergoing Alimentary Canal
  Surgery

Nutritional Needs in Thermal Injuries
Health Promotion
Immunonutrition

NUTRITIONAL NEEDS OF GENERAL SURGERY PATIENTS

Preoperative Nutrition

The nutritional needs of surgery patients vary based on several factors, including the patient's disease process, other comorbidities, and baseline nutritional status. Many general surgery patients are adequately nourished preoperatively and therefore do not have any special nutrient requirements (see the Perspectives in Practice box, "Energy and Protein Requirements in General Surgery Patients"). The disease itself often lends to poor nutrient intake and a hypermetabolic state that places the patient at nutritional risk. Malnutrition is associated with altered immune function, poor wound healing, and increased morbidity and mortality rates.[1] Researchers estimate that more than 50% of hospitalized patients are malnourished on hospital admission and hospital discharge.[2-5] For optimal outcome a malnourished patient should be nutritionally repleted for 7 to 10 days before surgery, if time permits.[6] Unless the gastrointestinal (GI) tract is nonfunctional, nutrient provision should be provided enterally rather than parenterally.[7] The following are some guidelines:

- *Energy:* Adequate calories should be consumed to prevent loss of endogenous stores of carbohydrate, fat, and protein. Carbohydrates should constitute the majority of calories (50%-60%). A minimum of approximately 150 g of carbohydrates per day is needed for central nervous system (CNS) function.
- *Protein:* Most patients do not have excessive preoperative protein requirements, but body stores should be assessed. Adequate protein status is imperative to facilitate optimal wound healing.
- *Vitamins and minerals:* Any deficiency state such as anemia should be corrected. Electrolytes and fluids should be normalized and in balance with correction of dehydration, acidosis, or alkalosis.

One often-overlooked factor is the use of medicinal herbs. Many patients do not think to disclose the ingestion of herbal supplements when they are asked about medications during the preoperative interview, but some of these substances can complicate surgery. (Some common herbal supplements that can cause complications during surgery are listed in the Diet-Medications Interactions box, "Medicine or Poison?")

Immediate Preoperative Period

Typical dietary preparation for surgery involves giving nothing by mouth 8 to 12 hours before surgery. The rationale is to ensure the stomach is empty of food and liquids to prevent vomiting or aspiration during surgery or anesthesia recovery. In an emergency situation, gastric suction is used to remove stomach contents. With surgery involving the GI tract, food and fecal matter may interfere with the procedure itself and cause contamination. Therefore before lower GI surgery, a low-residue diet may be prescribed to reduce fecal residue. Although restricting dietary intake may decrease the risks associated with anesthesia, it can also impair the patient's ability to respond to the metabolic stress of surgery. To reduce surgical stress and postoperative complications the use of an enhanced recovery after surgery (ERAS) protocol is important.[8] An ERAS protocol attenuates the surgical stress response and accelerates postoperative recovery.[9]

Postoperative Nutrition

Nutrient provision in the postoperative period depends on several factors, including the surgical procedure performed and anticipated time to resumption of oral intake, complications of surgery and postoperative clinical status, and preoperative nutritional status. The well-nourished patient undergoing elective surgery will typically resume

🌐 FOCUS ON CULTURE

Physiologic Changes Related to the Aging Process That Can Affect Surgery

Physiologic Change	Effects	Potential Postoperative Complications
Cardiovascular ↓ Elasticity of blood vessels ↓ Cardiac output ↓ Peripheral circulation	↓ Circulation to vital organs Slower blood flow	Shock (hypotension), thrombosis with pulmonary emboli, delayed wound healing, postoperative confusion, hypervolemia, decreased response to stress
Respiratory ↓ Elasticity of lungs and chest wall ↓ Residual lung volume ↓ Forced expiratory volume ↓ Ciliary action Fewer alveolar capillaries	↓ Vital capacity ↓ Alveolar volume ↓ Gas exchange ↓ Cough reflex	Atelectasis, pneumonia, postoperative confusion
Urinary ↓ Glomerular filtration rate ↓ Bladder muscle tone Weakened perineal muscles	↓ Kidney function Stasis of urine in bladder Loss of urinary control	Prolonged response to anesthesia and drugs, over hydration with intravenous fluids, hyperkalemia, urinary tract infection, urinary retention
Musculoskeletal ↓ Muscle strength Limitation of motion	↓ Activity	Atelectasis, pneumonia, thrombophlebitis, constipation or fecal impaction
Gastrointestinal ↓ Intestinal motility	Retention of feces	Constipation or fecal impaction
Metabolic ↓ γ-Globulin level ↓ Plasma proteins	↓ Inflammatory response	Delayed wound healing, wound dehiscence or evisceration
Immune System Fewer killer T cells ↓ Response to foreign antigens	↓ Ability to protect against invasion by pathogenic microorganisms	Wound infection, wound dehiscence, pneumonia, urinary tract infection

From Keeling AW, Muro A, Long BC: Preoperative nursing. In Phipps WJ, Cassmever VL, Sands JK, editors: *Medical-surgical nursing: concepts and clinical practice*, ed 5, St Louis, 1995, Mosby.

🌐 PERSPECTIVES IN PRACTICE

Energy and Protein Requirements in General Surgery Patients

The nutritional needs of general surgery patients vary based on several factors, including the patient's disease process, other comorbidities, surgery to be performed, and baseline nutritional status. For example, compare the following patient situations.

Adequately Nourished Preoperative Patient

For the patient with normal energy and nitrogen balance, approximately 25 kcal/kg/day and 0.8 to 1.0 g/kg/day of protein should maintain these balances.

Adequately Nourished Postoperative Patient

If no complications have occurred after surgery, then energy requirements remain about the same—25 kcal/kg/day. Protein requirements increase slightly because of increased metabolism and need for wound healing in the postoperative period to 1.0 to 1.1 g/kg/day.

Adequately Nourished Stressed Patient

This patient is assumed to have adequate nutrient stores; therefore replenishment is not the goal. Metabolic stress increases metabolic and catabolic rates, making energy and protein needs elevated. Energy needs are estimated at 25 to 30 kcal/kg/day and protein needs, 1.2 to 1.5 g/kg/day. Postoperatively the patient should be reassessed, and protein needs may increase up to 2 g/kg/day.

Nutritionally Depleted Nonstressed Patient
Upcoming Surgery: Gastrointestinal Tract Resection Resulting from Obstruction

Because of reduced dietary intake, this patient's nutrient stores (mostly glycogen and fat) may be depleted. In the nonstressed state, protein stores are spared for the most part. Energy needs are similar to those of the nourished preoperative patient at 25 kcal/kg/day. However, protein needs are slightly elevated to 1.0 to 1.2 g/kg/day. Postoperatively this patient's energy needs will remain near the same at 25 kcal/kg/day, but protein needs are increased to 1.2 to 1.5 g/kg/day.

Nutritionally Depleted Stressed Patient

This patient has elevated requirements for energy and protein because of cytokine and hormonal shifts causing a hypermetabolic and hypercatabolic state.

Continued

PERSPECTIVES IN PRACTICE

Energy and Protein Requirements in General Surgery Patients—cont'd

Energy needs are 25 to 30 kcal/kg/day, with caution to avoid overfeeding. Overfeeding in a hypermetabolic state can result in hyperglycemia, hypercarbia, hepatic steatosis, and overall immune suppression. Protein needs are elevated to 1.5 to 2.0 g/kg/day. Postoperatively the nutrient needs remain about the same. At this point the goal is to minimize loss of lean body mass, not to replenish it. Once the patient is stable and anabolic, calories can be increased to 35 kcal/kg/day as needed for rehabilitation.

Bibliography

ASPEN Board of Directors and the Clinical Guidelines Task Force: Guidelines for the use of parenteral and enteral nutrition in adult and pediatric patients, *JPEN J Parenter Enteral Nutr* 26(Suppl 1):1SA–138SA, 2002.

Frankenfield D: Energy and macrosubstrate requirements. *American Society for Enteral and Parenteral Nutrition: The science and practice of nutrition support: a case-based core*, ed 3, Dubuque, IA, 2001, Kendall/Hunt.

DIET-MEDICATIONS INTERACTIONS

Medicine or Poison?

"Poisons and medicines are oftentimes the same substances given with different intents."

Peter Mere Latham (1789-1875)

Medicinal herbs and pharmaceutical drugs: Both can be therapeutic at one dose and toxic at another. Patients may not think to include herbal supplements when reporting medications used during the preoperative interview. Possible surgical complications vary depending on the herbal supplement used. Following are some common herbal supplements that may cause surgical complications.

Herb	Common Uses	Possible Surgical Complication
Danshen *(Salvia miltiorrhiza)*	Antibacterial, antihepatotoxin, mild sedative, antiinflammatory	May cause bleeding
Dong quai *(Angelica sinensis)*	Menstrual disorders, menopause	May cause bleeding (interferes with warfarin)
Echinacea *(Echinacea purpurea)*	Prevent and treat common cold, treat infections, enhance wound healing	May interfere with effectiveness of immunosuppressant drugs given to prevent transplant rejection; may interfere with body's immune functioning after surgery; could impair wound healing
Ephedra[a] *(Ma huang, herbal ecstasy, Chinese ephedra)*	Sinus congestion, weight loss (ephedrine/caffeine)	May cause cardiovascular problems (increased heart rate, arrhythmias, heart attack or stroke); interaction with anesthesia can lead to abnormal heartbeat. For patients taking maintenance doses of MAOIs, interaction with anesthesia and MAOIs may result in life-threatening hypertension and coma
Feverfew *(Tanacetum parthenium)*	Migraine headaches (prophylaxis), RA	May cause bleeding
Garlic *(Allium* spp.)	Atherosclerosis, hyperlipidemia, hypertension, antithrombotic effects, chemoprevention, insect repellant, antimicrobial	May cause bleeding or interfere with normal clotting
Ginkgo *(Ginkgo biloba)*	Alzheimer disease and non-Alzheimer dementia, ordinary age-related memory loss, improving memory and mental function in the young, intermittent claudication, premenstrual syndrome, altitude sickness, tinnitus	May cause bleeding
Ginseng *(Panax ginseng)*	Enhancing immunity, improving mental activity, diabetes, athletic performance	May cause bleeding (interferes with warfarin)
Goldenseal *(Hydrastis canadensis)*	Antimicrobial, expectorant	May cause or worsen hypertension
Kava *(Piper methysticum)*	Anxiety	May enhance sedative effects of anesthesia
Licorice[b] *(Glycyrrhiza glabra)*	Peptic ulcer disease, expectorant/antitussive	May increase blood pressure
St. John's wort *(Hypericum perforatum)*	Major depression of mild to moderate severity, polyneuropathy	Can increase or decrease effect of some drugs used during and after surgery
Valerian *(Valeriana officinalis)*	Insomnia, anxiety	May interfere with effects of anesthesia

Bibliography

Bratman S, Girman AM: *Mosbys handbook of herbs and supplements and their therapeutic uses*, St Louis, 2003, Mosby.

Escott-Stump S: *Nutrition and diagnosis-related care*, ed 6, Philadelphia, 2007, Lippincott Williams & Wilkins.

Fugh-Berman A: Herb-drug interactions, *Lancet* 355:134, 2000.

Kuhn MA, Winston D: *Winston and Kuhn's: Herbal therapy and supplements: a scientific and traditional approach*, ed 2, Philadelphia, 2007, Lippincott Williams & Wilkins.

Mayo Clinic Staff: *Herbal supplements and surgery: what you need to know*, Rochester, MN, 2003, Mayo Foundation for Medical Education and Research. http://www.mayoclinic.com.

[a]Ephedra was banned by the US Food and Drug Administration (FDA) in December 2003.
[b]Most licorice candy contains little or no herbal licorice. Consumers should consult the product ingredients. "Licorice flavoring" is safer than "licorice extract" or "natural licorice" for these purposes.
Note: Different herbs stay in the body for different lengths of time. An individual taking herbs may need to stop taking them 1 or 2 weeks before surgery.
MAOIs, Monoamine oxidase inhibitors; *RA*, rheumatoid arthritis.

oral feeding by postoperative day 3 to 7, depending on return of bowel function. In this situation, supplemental nutrition in the form of enteral and parenteral nutrition is not indicated. The malnourished patient who is undergoing elective or emergency surgery and not anticipated to be able to meet his or her nutritional needs orally for a period of 7 to 10 days should receive specialized nutrition support.[6] This nutrition support should be provided enterally rather than parenterally to minimize incidence of complications.[6] Duration of this therapy will then depend on the patient's clinical status and transition to an adequate oral dietary consumption.

Energy Requirements

In the immediate postoperative period, especially in the critically ill, the goal of nutrition support is maintenance of current lean body mass, not repletion, and should serve as an adjunct to other critical therapies. Numerous factors are present that limit the effectiveness of exogenously administered nutritional substrates in preventing catabolism regardless of the level of support. It should not be expected to convert a catabolic, septic patient into an anabolic state at this time. Many undesirable metabolic complications can occur in attempting to do so, such as hypercapnia, hyperglycemia, hypertriglyceridemia, hepatic steatosis, and azotemia.[7,10-13] Once the hypermetabolic process is corrected, anabolism is favored and repletion can occur.

Multiple methods are available for determining energy requirements. Indirect calorimetry involves actual measurement of energy expenditure and remains the "gold standard."[14] However, many disadvantages to this method exist, including increased cost, the potential for improperly trained personnel, inaccurate readings in patients with an FiO_2 (fraction of inspired oxygen) of 50% or more, the possibility of malfunctioning chest tubes and endotracheal tubes, and the occurrence of bronchopleural fistulas. Because of these flaws, many institutions do not have the technology available and rely on predictive equations. Predicting energy needs can be difficult because of uncertainties regarding multiple factors of energy expenditure (Table 17.1).[15] Predictive equations (Box 17.1) may overestimate energy needs for those mechanically ventilated and sedated, and neuromuscular paralysis can decrease energy requirements by as much as 30%.[16-18] Calculated results are only as accurate as the variables used in the equation. Obesity and resuscitative water weight complicate use of these equations and lead to a tendency for overfeeding.[19] It is unclear

Extent of Body Reserves of Nutrients

Nutrient	Time Required to Deplete Reserves in Well-Nourished Individuals
Amino acids	Several hours
Carbohydrate	13 hours
Sodium	2–3 days
Water	4 days
Zinc	5 days
Fat	20–40 days
Thiamin	30–60 days
Vitamin C	60–120 days
Niacin	60–180 days
Riboflavin	60–180 days
Vitamin A	90–365 days
Iron	125 days (women), 750 days (men)
Iodine	1000 days
Calcium	2500 days

From Guthrie HA: *Introductory nutrition*, ed 7, St Louis, 1989, Mosby.

TABLE 17.1 Influences on Resting Energy Expenditure

Clinical Condition	REE (%)[a]
Elective Uncomplicated Surgery	Normal
Major Abdominal, Thoracic, and Vascular Surgery	
• ICU + mechanical ventilation	105-109 ± 20-28
Cardiac Surgery	
• ICU + mechanical ventilation	119 ± 21
Multiple Injury	
• ICU + mechanical ventilation	138 ± 23
• Spontaneous ventilation	119 ± 7
Head and Multiple Injury	
• ICU + mechanical ventilation	150 ± 23
Head Injury	
• ICU + spontaneous ventilation	126 ± 14
• ICU + mechanical ventilation	104 ± 5
Infection	
• Sepsis + spontaneous ventilation	121 ± 27
• ICU + septic shock + mechanical ventilation	135 ± 28
• Sepsis + mechanical ventilation	155 ± 14
• Septic shock + mechanical ventilation	102 ± 14
• Multiple injury + sepsis + mechanical ventilation + TPN	191 ± 38

[a]Values are percentage of reference value (±SD [standard deviation]). *ICU*, Intensive care unit; *REE*, resting energy expenditure; *TPN*, total parenteral nutrition.
Modified from Chiolero R, Revelly JP, Tappy L: Energy metabolism in sepsis and injury. *Nutrition* 13(Suppl):45S, 1997, with permission from Elsevier.

BOX 17.1 Selected Methods for Estimating Energy Requirements

Harris-Benedict Basal Energy Expenditure (BEE) Equation

Male: $66.5 + 13.8(W) + 5.0(H) - 6.8(A)$

Female: $655.1 + 9.6(W) + 1.9(H) - 4.7(A)$,

where W is weight (in kilograms); H, height (in centimeters); and A, age (in years).

Note: To predict total energy expenditure (TEE), add an injury/activity factor of 1.2–1.8 depending on the severity and nature of illness.

Ireton-Jones Energy Expenditure Equations (EEEs)
Spontaneously Breathing Patients

$EEE(s) = 629 - 11(A) + 25(W) - 609(O)$

Ventilator-Dependent Patients

$EEE(v) = 1784 - 11(A) + 5(W) + 244(G) + 239(T) + 804(B)$,

where EEE is given in kcal/day; v, ventilator dependent; s, spontaneously breathing; A, age (in years); W, body weight (in kilograms); G, gender (female = 0, male = 1); V, ventilator support (present = 1, absent = 0), T, diagnosis of trauma (present = 1, absent = 0); B, diagnosis of burn (present = 1, absent = 0); and O, obesity >30% more than ideal body weight (from 1959 Metropolitan Life Insurance tables; present = 1, absent = 0).

as to whether ideal body weight (IBW) or actual body weight should be used in predictive energy equations. It has been reported that obese patients should receive 20 to 30 kilocalories (kcalories or kcal)/kg IBW per day,[20] as well as use of adjusted body weight, particularly in those weighing more than 130% IBW.[21] Predictive equations have been developed to account for obesity, using actual body weight, as well as trauma, burns, and ventilatory status.[21] Patiño, and colleagues[22] reported a hypocaloric-hyperproteinic nutrition regimen provided during the first days of the flow phase of the adaptive response to injury, sepsis, and critical illness. The regimen consists of a daily supply of 100 to 200 g of glucose and 1.5 to 2.0 g of protein per kilogram IBW. Overall, energy requirements for surgery patients range from 20 to 35 kcal/kg usual body weight per day.[23]

Protein Requirements

Dietary protein is required to build new and maintain existing body tissue and has many functions in the body. Protein can also be oxidized directly for adenosine triphosphate (ATP) and is critical to the body's ability to perform gluconeogenesis. Therefore protein is an important energy substrate in addition to its role in tissue building and repair.

Protein requirements in the surgical patient are typically elevated, particularly in the critically ill. Increased requirements are the result of the need for tissue synthesis and wound healing, maintenance of oncotic pressure, adequate blood volume, maintenance of immune function, and energy substrate. Stressed critically ill patients require protein in the range of 1.5 to 2.0 g/kg/day.[22] Achieving positive nitrogen balance is nearly impossible immediately after metabolic insult, but after the primary insult is controlled or resolved, positive nitrogen balance is feasible. Protein requirements do not decrease with increasing age. Short-term inadequate protein intake in older adults has been shown to change skeletal muscle transcript levels that may lead to muscle wasting.[24] Reduction in lean body mass and obligatory loss of protein during physiologic stress increase protein requirements for critically ill older patients to requirements similar to those for younger patients.[25,26] Protein tolerance, as opposed to protein requirement, often determines amount of protein delivered. Onset of azotemia (i.e., impaired renal or hepatic function) signals the need to reduce protein delivery. Most studies that examined graded protein intakes in septic, injured, or burned patients have found no protein-sparing benefit to giving protein in excess of the previous recommendations.[27]

Fluid Requirements

Water is the medium within which all systems and subsystems function. It is necessary in digestion, absorption, transport, and use of nutrients, as well as in elimination of toxins and waste products. Total body fluid can be compartmentalized into two reservoirs: intracellular and extracellular. The intracellular compartment includes all water within the cell membrane and provides the environment for the metabolic reactions that take place in cells. The extracellular compartmental water includes all water external to cell membranes and allows nutrients to flow into cells and cellular waste products to return to the bloodstream. Water also provides structure to cells and is a vital component of thermoregulation. Water is the most abundant substance in the human body, accounting for approximately 60% of body weight of men and 50% of body weight of women. The majority of water

KEY TERM

Sepsis
Presence in the blood or other tissues of pathogenic microorganisms or their toxins; conditions associated with such pathogens.

TABLE 17.2 Normal Daily Fluid Gains and Losses in Adults

Fluid Gains		Fluid Losses	
Sensible		**Sensible**	
Food	1000 mL	Urine	1500 mL
Fluid	1200 mL	Feces	100 mL
		Sweat	50 mL
Insensible		**Insensible**	
Oxidative metabolism	350 mL	Skin	500 mL
		Lungs	400 mL
Total	2550 mL	Total	2550 mL

Reprinted from Gottschlich MM, Fuhrman M, Hammond K, et al: *The science and practice of nutrition support: a case-based core curriculum.* Dubuque, IA, 2001, Kendall/Hunt, p. 55.

intake comes from ingested fluid and food; a small amount is produced as a by-product of metabolic processes, primarily carbohydrate metabolism. The main source of water loss is in the form of urine. However, sizable amounts are also lost insensibly through skin and respiratory tract. Smaller amounts of water are lost in sweat and feces (Table 17.2).

Normal body water requirements can be estimated using a variety of methods. The National Research Council (NRC) recommends 1 mL/kcal energy expenditure for adults with average energy expenditure living under average environmental conditions. Fluid requirements increase with several conditions, including fever, high altitude, low humidity, profuse sweating, watery diarrhea, vomiting, hemorrhage, diuresis, surgical drains, and loss of skin integrity (e.g., burns, open wounds).

Therefore fluid balance is of vital concern after surgery. Patients often receive large volumes of fluid intraoperatively. These volumes are normally eliminated postoperatively, but occasionally the patient may require diuretics to facilitate this. Typically, surgical patients are provided with intravenous fluids until oral intake is resumed and tolerated to maintain fluid balance. Daily weight measurement of the patient provides a guideline for fluid balance.

Vitamin and Mineral Requirements

Adequate levels of vitamins and minerals are very important for optimal postoperative recovery. Vitamin C serves many functions in the body. In addition to being an antioxidant, it is required for synthesis of collagen (the structural protein found in skin, bone, tendon, and cartilage), carnitine, and neurotransmitters, as well as for immune-mediated and antibacterial functions of white blood cells. Vitamin C is also required for the scar tissue, which aids in wound healing. Iron is an essential component of the following: (1) hemoglobin, which is necessary for oxygen transport; (2) myoglobin, which is necessary for muscle iron storage; (3) and in cytochromes, which transport electrons through the respiratory chain resulting in the oxidative production of cellular energy. Vitamin K is essential in the blood-clotting cascade by activating inactive clotting factors resulting in the formation of fibrin. Surgical patients with elevated enteric losses (e.g., ostomy, stool, fistula) are at risk for several trace element deficiencies (e.g., zinc, copper). If losses exceed 800 mL/day, then extra supplementation of micronutrients should be considered. Various GI operations may also place a surgical patient at risk for several micronutrient deficiencies, depending on the amount of remaining small intestine, the location of bowel resection, and the functional status of remaining GI tract.[1]

Diets
Oral Diet
The preferred route of nutrient delivery is for the patient to be able to consume adequate nutrients through an oral diet. Fortunately the majority of surgical patients can accomplish this by postoperative day 7 at the latest. Routine intravenous fluids are intended to provide hydration and electrolytes, not energy and protein requirements. For example, 1 L of routine intravenous fluids of a 5% dextrose solution provides 50 g of dextrose, with an energy value of only 170 kcal; no protein is provided. If adequate calories and protein are not consumed, then the patient's diet may be supplemented. Often the addition of between-meal feedings that consist of soft, high-protein foods is adequate. However, sometimes commercially available oral supplements may be provided because they are a concentrated source of energy, protein, and vitamins and minerals.[28] Not all patients tolerate these supplements, because they tend to be very sweet, and patients develop taste fatigue. Every effort should be made to maximize the patient's diet for his or her diet preferences to improve inadequate dietary consumption.

Routine Postoperative Diets
A diet order is typically prescribed postoperatively after the patient exhibits adequate bowel function (e.g., flatus, bowel sounds present). Historically the first diet order is a clear liquid diet (Box 17.2). This

---

BOX 17.2 Typical Foods in Postoperative Diets

Clear Liquid
- Broth
- Clear juice (apple, grape, cranberry)
- Gelatin
- Sodas (Sprite, ginger ale)
- Tea
- Coffee

Full Liquid
- Juice (any)
- Milk
- Milkshakes
- Ice cream
- Cream soups
- Thinned oatmeal, corn grits
- Scrambled eggs (in some institutions)
- Oral liquid nutritional supplements (e.g., Ensure, Boost)

Soft/Regular
- Juice
- Canned fruits
- Cooked vegetables
- Soft meats (baked chicken, stews, roasts)
- Scrambled eggs
- Pancakes, biscuits, muffins
- Soups
- Soft sandwiches (egg, tuna, chicken salad, turkey, ham, and cheese)
- Soft starches (mashed potatoes, pasta, rice)
- Milk, tea, coffee
- Ice cream
- Puddings, yogurt
- Soft desserts (cake, pies, soft cookies)

---

diet contains hyperosmolar fluids, calories from primarily simple sugars, very little protein, and a fair amount of sodium and chloride. Because this diet is incomplete and very unpalatable, patients should be advanced to either a full liquid or soft/regular diet as soon as the clear liquid diet is tolerated. These diets are complete diets in that calorie, protein, and vitamin and mineral requirements can be met if adequate amounts are consumed. Recently this historical diet progression after GI surgery was challenged.[29] Patients randomized to a regular diet as their first postoperative diet after abdominal surgery had equal tolerance and improved nutrient intake compared with those receiving a clear liquid diet.

Specialized Nutrition Support
If an oral diet is not tolerated or feasible, then enteral or parenteral nutrition may be provided. Enteral nutrition is indicated for patients with an adequately functional GI tract and oral nutrient intake that is insufficient to meet estimated needs.[6] Enteral nutrition maintains nutritional, metabolic, immunologic, and barrier functions of the intestines; it is less expensive and safer than parenteral nutrition.[30] A series of studies of patients with GI cancer suggests parenteral nutrition increased the overall risk of postoperative complications by 10%. However, parenteral nutrition administered 7 to 10 days before surgery decreases postoperative complications by approximately 10%. Wound healing and surgical recovery may be impaired if parenteral nutrition is not begun within 5 to 10 days after surgery in patients unable to eat or tolerate enteral feeding. Although enteral nutrition is the preferred route of nutrient delivery, it is not innocuous. Some situations exist in which enteral feeding is not feasible (Box 17.3), and therefore parenteral nutrition should be used. Expected length of therapy, clinical condition, risk of aspiration, and medical expertise usually determine route of administration and type of access for tube feedings. Multiple methods for obtaining enteral access exist (Box 17.4), all of which carry various levels of required expertise, risk, and expense. Nasoenteric or oroenteric tubes are generally used when therapy is anticipated to be of short duration (e.g., less than 4 weeks) or for interim access before placement of a long-term device. Long-term access requires a percutaneous or surgically placed feeding tube. It is not always clear when enteral nutrition will be tolerated. If the needs of the individual are not met enterally, then parenteral nutrition may be implemented for either full nutrient provision or concurrently with enteral delivery to provide the balance of nutrients not tolerated.

The majority of postoperative surgical patients can tolerate a standard enteral formulation that provides their energy and protein

---

BOX 17.3 Indications for Parenteral Nutrition

Indications
- Bowel obstruction
- Persistent intolerance of enteral feeding (e.g., emesis, diarrhea)
- Hemodynamic instability
  Major upper gastrointestinal (GI) bleed
- Ileus
- Unable to safely access intestinal tract

Relative Indications
- Significant bowel wall edema
- Nutrient infusion proximal to recent GI anastomosis
- High-output fistula (>800 mL/day)

BOX 17.4 Methods of Enteral Access

Short Term (<4 weeks)
Nasoenteric Feeding Tube
- Spontaneous passage
- Bedside prokinetic agent

Active Passage
- Bedside assisted
- Endoscopic
- Fluoroscopic
- Operative

Long Term (>4 weeks)
Percutaneous Feeding Tube
- Percutaneous endoscopic (PEG)
- Gastric (PEG)
- Gastric/jejunal (PEG/jejunostomy)
- Direct jejunal (DPEJ)

Laparoscopic
- Gastrostomy
- Jejunostomy

Surgical
- Gastrostomy
- Jejunostomy

TABLE 17.3 Common Gastrointestinal Operations and Nutritional Consequences

Location	Potential Consequences
Esophagus	
Resection/replacement	Weight loss because of inadequate intake
Gastric pull-up	↑ Protein loss because of catabolism
Colonic interposition	May require enteral/parenteral nutrition until oral intake appropriate
	Antidumping diet; may malabsorb fat/fat-soluble vitamins, simple sugars, and various vitamins/minerals
	Early satiety because of reduced storage capacity (gastric pull-up)
Stomach	
Partial gastrectomy/ vagotomy	Early satiety because of reduced storage capacity
	Delayed gastric emptying of solids because of stasis
	Rapid emptying of hypertonic fluids
Total gastrectomy	Weight loss because of dumping/malabsorption, early satiety, anorexia, inadequate intake, unavailability of bile acids and pancreatic enzymes because of anastomotic changes
	Malabsorption may lead to anemia, metabolic bone disease, protein-calorie malnutrition
	Bezoar formation
	Vitamin B_{12} deficiency because of lack of intrinsic factor
Intestine[a]	
Proximal	Malabsorption of vitamins/minerals (Ca^{2+}, Mg^{2+}, iron, vitamins A and D)
Gastric bypass	Protein-calorie malnutrition from malabsorption because of dumping, unavailability of bile acids and pancreatic enzymes because of anastomotic changes
	Bezoar formation
Distal	Malabsorption of vitamins or minerals (water soluble—folate, vitamins B_{12}, C, B_1, B_2, pyridoxine)
	Protein-calorie malnutrition because of dumping
	Fat malabsorption
	Bacterial overgrowth if ileocecal valve resected
Colon	Fluid and electrolyte (K^+, Na^+, Cl^-) malabsorption

[a]Note that consequences may occur only with extensive disease process and resection.

---

requirements. Recent research studies have evaluated use of "immune-enhancing" enteral formulas in postoperative GI cancer patients, trauma patients, and patients with critical illness. These formulas are supplemented with various immune-enhancing nutrients, including L-arginine, L-glutamine, omega-3 fatty acids, nucleic acids, and various vitamins and minerals. When these diets were used in these surgical populations, decreases in infectious complications and hospital length of stay were noted.[6,31]

NUTRITIONAL CONCERNS FOR PATIENTS UNDERGOING ALIMENTARY CANAL SURGERY

The digestive tract is a metabolically active organ involved in digestion, absorption, and metabolism of many nutrients; therefore various surgical interventions involving the GI tract can result in malabsorption and maldigestion and nutritional deficiencies (Table 17.3).

Head and Neck Surgery

These patients often present for surgery malnourished because of their disease state. Many times, surgical intervention is required because of a tumor that may be inhibiting the patient's ability to chew and swallow normally. Typically, loss of this ability is what makes the patient seek medical attention. Patients with head and neck cancer usually have a long history of alcohol and tobacco use, which may also affect optimal nutritional status.

Depending on the patient's treatment, optimization of nutrition preoperatively is ideal. This also depends on the individual's disease progression and ability to swallow. Many times, preoperative treatment involves radiation, chemotherapy, or both to reduce the tumor size. In these situations, the ability to swallow may worsen because of negative side effects of these therapies. Ideally, placement of a percutaneous endoscopic gastrostomy (PEG) feeding tube can

be performed to allow for nutrition, hydration, and medication administration to maintain or improve (or both) nutritional status preoperatively. The patient may also still be able to swallow soft foods or liquids, which should be maximized for caloric and protein density. If a PEG tube is not placed preoperatively, then it can be placed intraoperatively or a nasoenteric tube may be placed. These feeding tubes are then used postoperatively until the patient is able to resume an oral diet.

Esophageal Surgery

Several medical conditions affecting the esophagus can prevent swallowing and thus nutrient intake. Common conditions include corrosive injuries and perforation, achalasia, **gastroesophageal reflux disease (GERD)**, and partial or full obstruction caused by cancer, congenital abnormalities, or strictures. These conditions usually require surgical intervention involving removal of a segment or the entire esophagus (see the Case Study box, "The Patient with Esophageal Cancer"). The esophageal tract is then replaced with either the stomach (gastric pull-up) or the intestine (colonic and jejunal interposition). A gastric pull-up procedure involves drawing the stomach up to the esophageal

stump, causing displacement of the stomach into the thoracic cavity. This procedure results in a reduction of stomach volume capacity, with potential delayed gastric emptying and **dumping syndrome** (Fig. 17.1). The colonic and jejunal interposition procedure involves forming a new conduit by anastomosing the selected portion of bowel between the esophagus and stomach. Complications after this procedure include swallowing difficulties, strictures, and leakage at the anastomotic site.

CASE STUDY

The Patient with Esophageal Cancer

Kevin is a 54-year-old accountant seen by his family physician for pain with swallowing and difficulty swallowing solid foods for the past 6 weeks. This has resulted in continued weight loss and fatigue. Kevin was referred to the GI medicine service for further evaluation. After a series of tests that included endoscopy and biopsy, Kevin was found to have esophageal cancer with the tumor lying in the midesophagus. He was then referred to the GI surgery service for surgical evaluation.

A medical history revealed that Kevin smoked two packs of cigarettes per day, drank three martinis per day, and was cachectic. A referral was sent to the dietitian for nutritional evaluation and recommendations for optimizing his nutritional status for surgery. A nutrition history revealed that during the past 6 weeks, Kevin's diet had progressively decreased in consistency to the point where he could tolerate only liquids and some soft solid foods such as mashed potatoes, oatmeal, and applesauce. At a height of 178 cm (5 ft 10 in), Kevin's weight had dropped from 80 kg (176 lb) to 63 kg (139 lb), leaving him at 79% of his usual body weight. His blood work revealed a serum albumin level of 3.0 g/dL and prealbumin of 13.2 mg/dL. He no longer could stand long enough to make himself a meal and had to take a bath rather than shower because he became too tired. Kevin was not currently taking any medications because he could not swallow them. His current diet order was a full liquid diet.

Assessment of calorie and protein requirements estimated that Kevin required approximately 1800 kcal (basal energy expenditure + 25%) and 75 to 95 g of protein (1.2 to 1.5 g/kg) daily. Because he could eat some solid foods, the

dietitian changed him to a soft diet. The dietitian modified Kevin's diet so that it contained soft, high protein–containing solids and liquids that Kevin stated he could eat and ordered a 48-hour calorie count. A liquid multivitamin was also provided. Kevin was now able to eat enough calories and protein for 14 days preoperatively that he gained 3 kg (7 lb); his albumin increased to 3.1 g/dL, and prealbumin increased to 17 mg/dL.

Kevin underwent an esophagectomy with a gastric pull-up. A feeding jejunostomy tube was placed intraoperatively. Kevin was started on low-rate enteral feedings on postoperative day 2, which were gradually advanced to his goal requirements during the next 2 days. He was not allowed to eat until postoperative day 7 after a swallowing study for anastomotic evaluation. Once Kevin's diet was initiated and tolerated, his tube feedings were provided nocturnally because he was not able to consume 100% of his nutritional needs orally. He was discharged home with an oral postgastrectomy diet and nocturnal tube feedings to provide approximately 50% of his nutritional needs for 10 days, at which time his nutrition would be reevaluated.

Questions for Analysis

1. Evaluate the preoperative nutrition assessment data. Why were the particular energy and protein assessment factors chosen?
2. What dietary modifications accompany a postgastrectomy diet?
3. Why was Kevin placed on a postgastrectomy diet when his stomach was not resected?
4. At what point should his enteral tube feedings be discontinued?

KEY TERMS

Malabsorption
Malabsorption is a syndrome in which normal products of digestion do not traverse the intestinal mucosa and enter the lymphatic or portal venous branches.

Maldigestion
Maldigestion, which may be clinically similar to malabsorption, describes defects in the intraluminal phase of the digestive process caused by inadequate exposure of chyme to bile salts and pancreatic enzymes. Clinical symptoms of malabsorption include diarrhea, steatorrhea, and weight loss. Laboratory signs include depressed serum fat-soluble vitamin levels, accelerated prothrombin time, hypomagnesemia, and hypocholesterolemia. Patients with symptoms of malabsorption should have a laboratory workup to determine the presence and level of nutrient loss.

Gastroesophageal Reflux Disease
Describes symptoms that result from reflux of gastric juices, and sometimes duodenal juices, into the esophagus. Symptoms include substernal burning (heartburn), epigastric pressure sensation, and severe epigastric pain. Prolonged and severe gastroesophageal reflux disease (GERD) can lead to esophageal bleeding, perforation, strictures, Barrett epithelium, adenocarcinoma, and

pulmonary fibrosis (from aspiration). Conservative dietary therapy involves weight reduction; restriction of carbonated beverages, caffeine, fatty foods, peppermint, chocolate, and ethanol; small frequent meals; and wearing of loose clothing to promote symptomatic relief.

Dumping Syndrome
Constellation of postprandial symptoms that result from rapid emptying of hyperosmolar gastric contents into the duodenum. The hypertonic load in the small intestine promotes reflux of vascular fluid into the bowel lumen, causing a rapid decrease in the circulating blood volume. Rapid symptoms of abdominal cramping, nausea, vomiting, palpitations, sweating, weakness, reduced blood pressure, tremors, and osmotic diarrhea occur. Symptoms of early dumping begin 10 to 30 minutes after eating; late dumping syndrome occurs 1 to 4 hours after a meal. Late dumping is a result of insulin hypersecretion in response to the carbohydrate load dumped into the small intestine. Once the carbohydrate is absorbed, the hyperinsulinemia causes hypoglycemia, which results in vasomotor symptoms such as diaphoresis, weakness, flushing, and palpitations. Individuals who have undergone GI surgery resulting in a reduced or absent gastric pouch are more prone to dumping syndrome.

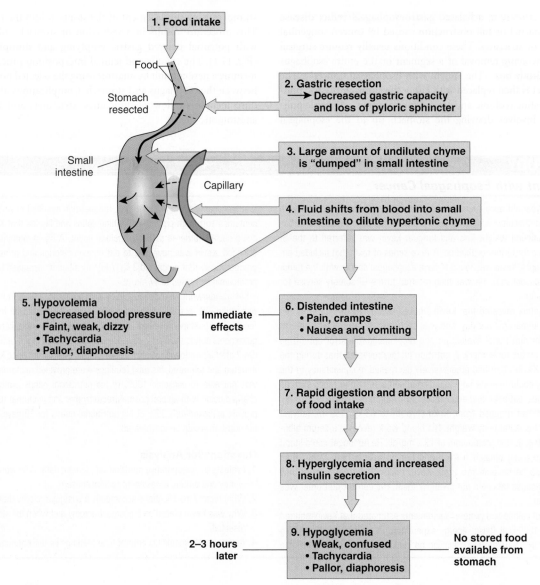

1. Food intake

Food

Stomach
resected

2. Gastric resection
→ **Decreased gastric capacity and loss of pyloric sphincter**

Small
intestine

Capillary

3. Large amount of undiluted chyme is "dumped" in small intestine

4. Fluid shifts from blood into small intestine to dilute hypertonic chyme

5. Hypovolemia
• **Decreased blood pressure**
• **Faint, weak, dizzy**
• **Tachycardia**
• **Pallor, diaphoresis**

Immediate
effects

6. Distended intestine
• **Pain, cramps**
• **Nausea and vomiting**

7. Rapid digestion and absorption of food intake

8. Hyperglycemia and increased insulin secretion

2–3 hours
later

9. Hypoglycemia
• **Weak, confused**
• **Tachycardia**
• **Pallor, diaphoresis**

No stored food available from stomach

FIG. 17.1 Dumping syndrome (postgastrectomy). (From Gould BE: *Pathophysiology for health professions,* ed 2, Philadelphia, 2002, Saunders.)

Preoperative nutrition for these patients may be a tolerated oral diet (often liquids because of dysphasia and obstruction). If a patient is unable to consume his or her full nutrient needs orally, then a feeding tube may be placed if the esophagus is not obstructed. A PEG tube is not indicated if a gastric pull-up procedure is to be performed, because the stomach is used to make the esophageal conduit and a hole resulting from a gastrostomy tube would be contraindicated. These patients may require preoperative parenteral nutrition if the esophagus is obstructed. Intraoperatively, a jejunal feeding tube may be placed to allow for postoperative enteral nutrition until the anastomosis heals and oral intake is resumed. If enteral access is not obtained intraoperatively, then parenteral nutrition is indicated because these patients may not resume oral intake for 7 to 10 days.

For patients with chronic GERD, a Nissen fundoplication procedure may be performed. This is the most commonly performed antireflux procedure operation for patients with gastroesophageal reflux refractory to medical management. This procedure involves wrapping the stomach around the base of the esophagus, near the lower esophageal sphincter; this places pressure and narrows the lower esophageal opening to prevent reflux (Fig. 17.2). Patients are typically placed on a

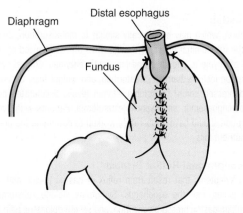

Diaphragm

Distal esophagus

Fundus

FIG. 17.2 Nissen fundoplication. (From Lewis SM, Heitkemper MM, Dirksen SR: *Medical-surgical nursing: assessment and management of clinical problems,* ed 5, St Louis, 2000, Mosby.)

CHAPTER 17 Metabolic Stress **313**

pureed diet for 2 weeks after this procedure, with small frequent meals, no gulping of liquids, and crushed or liquid medications. After this time, solid foods are gradually added to the diet with future avoidance of bread products, nuts, and seeds because these can become lodged in the lower esophagus and cause an obstruction.

Gastric Surgery

A number of nutrition problems may develop after gastric surgery, depending on the type of surgical procedure and the patient's response. Several indications exist for gastric surgery, including tumor removal, ulcer disease, perforation, hemorrhage, **Zollinger-Ellison syndrome, gastric polyposis,** and **Ménétrier disease (giant hypertrophic gastritis).** A **vagotomy** is often performed to eliminate gastric acid secretion. Vagotomy at certain levels can alter the normal physiologic function of the stomach, small intestine, pancreas, and biliary system. Total gastric and truncal vagotomy procedures impair proximal and distal motor function of the stomach. Digestion and emptying of solids are retarded, whereas emptying of liquids is accelerated.[32] These vagotomy procedures are commonly accompanied by a drainage procedure (antrectomy or pyloroplasty) that helps the stomach empty. Nutrition complications associated with vagotomy and pyloroplasty include dumping syndrome, steatorrhea, and bacterial overgrowth.

A total gastrectomy involves removal of the entire stomach. A storage reservoir may be created using a section of jejunum. A subtotal or partial gastrectomy involves removal of a portion of the stomach accompanied by a reconstructive procedure. A Billroth I (gastroduodenostomy) involves an anastomosis of the proximal end of the intestine (duodenum) to the distal end of the stomach (Fig. 17.3). A Billroth II (gastrojejunostomy) involves an anastomosis of the stomach to the side of the jejunum, which creates a blind loop (Fig. 17.4). Any gastric surgery carries some potential for development of malnutrition. Common consequences include weight loss, dumping syndrome,

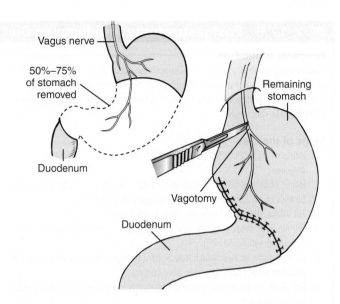

FIG. 17.3 Billroth I (gastroduodenostomy). (From Lewis SM, Heitkemper MM, Dirksen SR: *Medical-surgical nursing: assessment and management of clinical problems,* ed 5, St Louis, 2000, Mosby.)

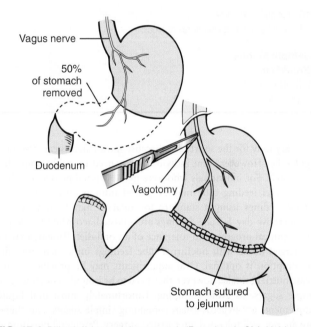

FIG. 17.4 Billroth II (gastrojejunostomy). (From Lewis SM, Heitkemper MM, Dirksen SR: *Medical-surgical nursing: assessment and management of clinical problems,* ed 5, St Louis, 2000, Mosby.)

malabsorption, anemia, and metabolic bone disease. Dumping syndrome, epigastric fullness, nausea, and vomiting often occur in the early postoperative period. These symptoms are managed with dietary modifications and antiemetic medications.[32]

In general, after gastric surgery, small, frequent oral feedings are resumed according to the patient's tolerance (Box 17.5). For the first 2 weeks after surgery, soft, bland foods with a low fiber content should be consumed in small portions. Simple sugars, lactose, and fried foods should be avoided; beverages should be consumed at least 30 minutes before and after meals; and foods high in complex carbohydrates and protein should be emphasized. In general, these diet modifications are

---

KEY TERMS

Anastomosis
A surgical joining of two ducts to allow flow from one to the other.

Sphincter
A circular band of muscle fibers that constricts a passage or closes a natural opening in the body (e.g., lower esophageal sphincter, pyloric sphincter).

Zollinger-Ellison Syndrome
A condition characterized by severe peptic ulceration, gastric hypersecretion, elevated serum gastrin, and gastrinoma of the pancreas or the duodenum. Total gastrectomy may be necessary.

Gastric Polyposis
An abnormal condition characterized by the presence of numerous polyps in the stomach.

Ménétrier Disease (Giant Hypertrophic Gastritis)
Rare disease characterized by large folds of nodular gastric rugae that may cover the wall of the stomach, causing anorexia, nausea, vomiting, and abdominal distress.

Vagotomy
Cutting of certain branches of the vagus nerve, performed with gastric surgery, to reduce the amount of gastric acid secreted and lessen the chance of recurrence of a gastric ulcer.

BOX 17.5   Postgastrectomy Antidumping Diet

Principles of the Diet

After surgery some discomfort or diarrhea may occur. Therefore to reduce the likelihood of those symptoms, a healthy, nutritionally complete diet should be observed. Each person may react to food differently. Foods should be reintroduced into the diet slowly.

Steps of the Diet

1. Intake of complex carbohydrates is unlimited (e.g., bread, vegetables, rice, potatoes).
2. Intake of simple sugars (e.g., sugar, candy, cake, pies, jelly, honey) should be kept to a minimum. Artificial sweeteners may be used.
3. Fat intake should be moderate (30% of total calories).
4. Protein (e.g., meats, legumes) consumption should be unlimited because it helps with wound healing.
5. Milk contains lactose, which may be hard to digest. Introduce milk and milk products slowly several weeks after surgery.
6. Eat small, frequent meals, approximately six meals per day, to avoid loading the stomach.
7. Limit fluids to 4 oz (½ cup) during mealtimes. This prevents the rapid movement of food through the upper gastrointestinal (GI) tract.
8. Drink fluids 30 to 45 minutes before and after eating to prevent diarrhea.
9. Relatively low-roughage foods and raw foods are allowed as tolerated after postoperative day 14.
10. Eat and chew slowly.
11. Avoid extreme temperatures of foods.

Sample Menus

Breakfast
Scrambled egg, 1
Toast, 1 slice
Margarine, 1 tsp
Low-sugar jelly, 1 tsp
Banana, 1 small

Midmorning Snack
Canned fruit, water packed, ½ cup
Graham crackers, 2 squares

Lunch
Bread, 2 slices
Ham, 2 oz
Cheese, 1 oz
Mustard, 2 tsp
Canned fruit, water packed, ½ cup
Yogurt, sugar free, 4 oz

Midafternoon Snack
Saltine crackers, 3 squares
Peanut butter, 1 tbsp

Dinner
Chicken breast, 3 oz
Mashed potatoes, ½ cup
Green beans, ½ cup
Margarine, 2 tsp
Yogurt, sugar free, 4 oz

Evening Snack
Pudding, sugar free, ½ cup
Vanilla wafers, 3 pieces

necessary only for the short term because most patients can resume a regular diet. However, some individuals may need an antidumping diet indefinitely. For individuals who were malnourished preoperatively, a small bowel feeding tube may be placed intraoperatively. Low-rate enteral feedings using a standard formulation may be initiated on postoperative day 1. Tube feedings are adjusted according to the patient's clinical progress and tolerance of an oral diet. Patients may be discharged home with nocturnal tube feedings until their oral diet consumption is optimal. Oral supplements may be provided to increase nutrient intake; however, they need to be isotonic, containing no simple sugars, to avoid dumping. Unfortunately, most oral liquid supplements are hyperosmolar, containing simple sugars, and therefore are not well tolerated after gastric surgery. Parenteral nutrition is indicated only if enteral access is not available and the patient is malnourished and not able to tolerate adequate nutrients orally.

Anemia is a common consequence of gastric surgery. Anemia can be attributed to a deficiency or malabsorption of one or more nutrients, including iron, vitamin B_{12}, and folate. Assimilation of vitamin B_{12} requires liberation of the vitamin from protein and binding of the vitamin to intrinsic factor, both of which occur in the stomach. Failure of either of these reactions to occur results in vitamin B_{12} malabsorption, which, with time, produces anemia.[32] Total gastrectomy patients require periodic intramuscular vitamin B_{12} injections. Metabolic bone disease can be a late complication of gastric surgery. The cause of metabolic bone disease varies with the surgical procedure. The Billroth II procedure is associated with more complications than the Billroth I because it bypasses the duodenum and upper jejunum (the site of calcium absorption). Procedures that destroy the pylorus can result in

rapid gastric emptying, which may contribute to development of metabolic bone disease. Rapid gastric emptying not only reduces absorption time but also, when fats are malabsorbed, can lead to formation of insoluble calcium soaps.[32] Fat malabsorption can also lead to vitamin D malabsorption, which leads to impaired metabolism of calcium and phosphorus.

Intestinal Surgery

Surgical resections of the small and large intestine are usually well tolerated. If excessive amounts of bowel are removed, then nutritional consequences can arise, depending on the location resected. If more than 50% of the small intestine is removed, then short bowel syndrome may occur. This syndrome is characterized by severe diarrhea or steatorrhea, malabsorption, and malnutrition, depending on the amount of remaining small intestine, the site of the resection, and the functional status of the remaining GI tract. Often the patient may require long-term parenteral nutrition to maintain his or her nutritional status and fluid and electrolyte balance (see Chapter 19).

Pancreaticoduodenectomy (Whipple Procedure)

In cases of ampullary, duodenal, and pancreatic malignancies, a pancreaticoduodenectomy may be performed. This procedure, one of the most difficult and technically demanding in GI surgery, involves resecting the distal stomach, distal common duct, pancreatic head, and duodenum. Three anastomoses must be performed: (1) pancreaticojejunostomy, (2) choledochojejunostomy, and (3) gastrojejunostomy (Billroth II). In the past few years a pyloric-sparing Whipple procedure has become more prominent, resulting in a Billroth I anastomosis.

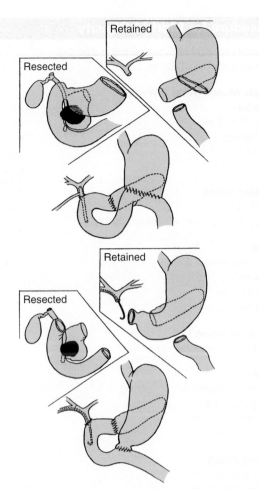

FIG. 17.5 Whipple procedure. (From Hardy JD, editor: *Hardy's textbook of surgery,* ed 2, Philadelphia, 1988, Lippincott Williams & Wilkins.)

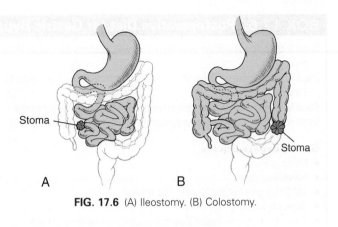

FIG. 17.6 (A) Ileostomy. (B) Colostomy.

FIG. 17.7 (A) Vertical banded gastroplasty *(VBG).* (B) Roux-en-Y gastric bypass.

This procedure carries fewer postoperative nutritional concerns than the other, which results in a Billroth II anastomosis (Fig. 17.5).

Ileostomy and Colostomy

In cases of intestinal lesions, obstruction, or inflammatory bowel disease of the entire colon or when diversion of fecal matter is required, an ileostomy or a colostomy may be the treatment of choice. These procedures involve creation of an artificial anus on the abdominal wall by incision into the colon or ileum and bringing it out to the surface, forming a stoma (Fig. 17.6). A pouch is placed externally over the stoma to collect fecal matter. In general, patients with ostomies should eat regular diets. Foods that are gas forming or difficult to digest may be avoided to reduce undesired side effects. In the case of high-output ostomies (more than 800 mL/day), patients may need to avoid hypertonic, simple sugar–containing liquids and foods; fatty foods; and foods with a high amount of insoluble fiber to reduce outputs.

Bariatric Surgery

In the past several years, surgery for treatment of obesity has become more prevalent. Probably the most common procedure for weight loss in the world is the vertical banded gastroplasty (VBG), or gastric stapling (Fig. 17.7A). This technique is performed under general anesthesia and requires approximately 4 to 5 days in the hospital postoperatively. The VBG procedure limits food intake by creating a small pouch (½ oz) in the upper stomach, with a narrow outlet (½ in) reinforced by a mesh band to prevent stretching. The pouch fills quickly and empties slowly with solid food, producing a feeling of fullness. Overeating results in pain or vomiting, thus restricting food intake. This procedure is preferred for those people who engage in "bulk" or "binge" eating. The disadvantage of this procedure is that weight loss is not as great as that with other procedures. It does not restrict the intake of high-caloric liquids, and the pouch can stretch with overeating. As a result, 20% of people do not lose weight, and only half of people lose at least 50% of their excess weight with a VBG.

The Roux-en-Y gastric bypass (see Fig. 17.7B) is a combination of gastric stapling and intestinal bypass. It promotes weight loss by (1) restricting the amount of food a person can ingest by reducing the holding capacity of the stomach and (2) interfering with complete absorption of nutrients by shortening the length of small intestine through which the food travels. Unlike the VBG, this procedure discourages intake of high-calorie sweets by producing nausea, diarrhea, and other unpleasant symptoms. With this procedure a small gastric pouch (15 mL) is made near where stomach and esophagus meet. The small pouch and remainder of the stomach are divided from each other with staples. An opening is made in the pouch where a portion of the small intestine is connected. This new connection between the pouch and the small intestine is called a *Roux-en-Y limb.* Food then travels down the esophagus and bypasses nearly all of the stomach and first 2 feet of small intestine. Complications related to gallstones, which tend to form during rapid weight loss, can be prevented by

BOX 17.6 Postoperative Diet for Gastric Bypass Procedure for Morbid Obesity

Stage I: clear liquids—Begin once liquids allowed; continue for two to three meals

Stage II: gastric bypass—Begin after clear liquids tolerated; liquids continue for 3-4 weeks

Stage III: pureed—Begin after postoperative week 4; continue for 1-2 weeks

Stage IV: soft, solids—Begin after postoperative week 6; continue indefinitely

Gastric Bypass Liquids
- Nonfat milk
- Blenderized soups
- 100% fruit juice (diluted ½ water and ½ juice)
- Vegetable juice (e.g., V8, tomato)
- Sugar-Free Carnation Instant Breakfast powder mixed with nonfat milk
- Grits, oatmeal, cream of wheat, mashed potatoes (thinned down enough that it could go through a straw)
- Nonfat, sugar-free milkshakes
- Thinned baby food
- Sugar-free drinks (e.g., sodas, tea)

Eating Guidelines
- Small meals: each feeding should be 4 oz total (½ cup)
- Six to eight feedings per day to consume adequate nutrients
- An hour between meals and drinking fluids
- Eat slowly/chew food well; each feeding should last at least 30 minutes
- Avoid sugars (i.e., sucrose, honey, corn syrup, fructose) and sugar-containing beverages, foods, and candy
- Low-fat foods only (avoid fried foods, gravies, excessive margarine, butter, high-fat meats, and breads)
- Eat high-protein foods (e.g., milk, yogurt, soft meats, eggs)
- Avoid soft, calorie-dense foods (e.g., ice cream, chocolate, cheese, cookies)
- Avoid obstructive foods (e.g., tough, fibrous red meat; bread made from refined flour; celery; popcorn; nuts; seeds; membranes of citrus fruits)

- Take daily complete multivitamin (liquid or chewable)
- Calcium supplements (1500 mg/day)

Sample Menus (After 8 Weeks)
Breakfast
Banana, ¼ medium
Scrambled egg, 1 egg
Toast, white, ½ slice
Margarine, ½ tsp

Morning Snack
Graham crackers, 2
Pudding, sugar free made with nonfat milk, ½ cup

Lunch
Broiled chicken breast, 2 oz
Carrots, boiled, ¼ cup
Margarine, 1 tsp
Pasta salad, ¼ cup

Afternoon Snack
Canned fruit, water packed, ½ cup

Dinner
Baked or broiled fish, 2 oz
Green beans, ¼ cup
Potato, baked, ½ small
Margarine, ½ tsp

Evening Snack
Cheese, American, 1 oz
Saltine crackers, 2 squares

Note: Consume nonfat milk or yogurt between meals, throughout the day. Eat and drink no more than 2 to 3 oz at a time for a daily total of 2 cups.

removal of the gallbladder. This procedure is intended for people who "graze" during the day on high-calorie and sugar-containing foods, and eat large amounts. Box 17.6 lists a sample meal plan after gastric bypass surgery.

Like any major abdominal operation, these bariatric surgical procedures carry risks such as bleeding, infection, bowel blockage because of scar tissue formation, hernia through the incision, and anesthesia risks. The most serious risk is leakage of fluid from the stomach or intestines, which can result in abdominal infection and reoperation. Additional risks are directly related to being obese; these include blood clots in legs or lungs, pneumonia, and cardiac complications. Less immediate risks are ulcers in the stomach or intestine, dumping syndrome, bezoar formation, obstruction of stoma, and malnutrition from too-rapid weight loss and loss of vitamins and minerals. Some people (10%-15%) experience some complications from the gastric bypass; death may occur from complications in 1% to 2% of patients. Because this procedure is not risk free, strict criteria for eligibility should be made. In general, candidates are those who have at least 100-lb excess body weight (or a body mass index [BMI] of 40 kg/m^2 or greater) and have significant obesity-related medical problems and for whom all other serious attempts at weight reduction have failed. A thorough medical and nutritional-behavioral evaluation is necessary to determine eligibility.

Other Related Problems
Enteric Fistulas

Enteric fistulas are abnormal communications between a portion of the intestinal tract and another organ (internal) or between the intestinal tract and the surface of the body (external or enterocutaneous).[32] The most common sites of origin are the pancreas and the large and small intestines. The majority of enteric fistulas result from surgical wound dehiscence or necrosis from bowel ischemia. Inflammatory bowel disease, cancer, trauma, and radiation to the abdomen can also lead to fistula development.

KEY TERMS

Bariatric
A term used to describe the field of medicine that focuses on the treatment and control of obesity and diseases associated with obesity.

Bezoar
A hard ball of hair or vegetable fiber that may develop within the stomach and intestines; can cause an obstruction, requiring removal. Formed because of reduced gastric motility, decreased gastric mixing and churning, and reduced gastric secretions.

Several metabolic complications can arise as a result of an enteric fistula, including fluid and electrolyte losses, malnutrition, and sepsis. A retrospective analysis of patients with small bowel fistulas found a lower mortality rate, increased spontaneous fistula closures, and increased rate of surgical closures in those receiving parenteral nutrition.[33] The route of nutrition intervention depends on the location of the fistula. Proximal fistulas may require that a patient be placed on parenteral nutrition if enteral access distal to the fistula cannot be achieved. This is because eating, and thus nutrients in the proximal bowel, stimulates GI secretions, thereby complicating fistula management and the likelihood of spontaneous fistula closure. Fistulas located in the distal bowel, particularly the colon, may have low output (less than 500 mL/day) and thus allow for oral intake of low-residue or even elemental feedings. High-output fistulas (more than 500 mL/day) most likely will not close spontaneously and require surgical correction.

Chylous Ascites and Chylothorax

Chylous leaks into the peritoneal and thoracic cavities can follow surgical injury or trauma to the lymphatic ducts and obstruction because of cancer or congenital anomalies. Leakage of chyle into the abdominal or thoracic cavity can cause ascites, pleural effusions, abdominal pain, anorexia, hypoalbuminemia, hyponatremia, hypocalcemia, hypocholesterolemia, and elevated alkaline phosphatase.[32] Chylous leaks may resolve with conservative management, although surgical repair can be required to ligate the duct. Conservative management involves reducing the chyle flow, which is normally 1500 to 5500 mL/day. Dietary intake (fat and fluid), blood pressure, and portal blood flow contribute to the production of chyle. Dietary manipulation is the main means of reducing chyle flow. Because dietary long-chain triglycerides (LCTs) are incorporated into chylomicrons, restriction of these fats in the diet is imperative. Depending on severity of the chyle leak and patient's response, the patient may be allowed oral dietary intake with no LCTs, enteral feeding with no LCTs, or parenteral nutrition. Medium-chain triglycerides (MCTs) are allowed enterally because these are absorbed directly via the portal vein, not the lymphatic system. A diet without or limited to less than 4% of calories as LCTs is not advised for more than 10 to 14 days because it lacks essential fatty acids (linoleic and linolenic acid), causing the patient to develop a deficiency. Resolution of lymphatic leaks conservatively can take up to 6 weeks; therefore adequate nutrition during this period is important to maintain nutritional status.

KEY TERM

Chyle
The fat-containing, creamy white fluid that is formed in the lacteals of the intestine during digestion; it is transported through the lymphatics and enters the venous circulation via the thoracic duct.

NUTRITIONAL NEEDS IN THERMAL INJURIES

Patients with trauma and burns exhibit similar metabolic alterations as previously described, but metabolic alterations often occur to a much greater extent. Few traumatic injuries result in a hypermetabolic state comparable with that of a major burn. An understanding of the cause of metabolic response and implications for nutritional requirements is necessary with traumatic and burn injuries for a nutrition care plan to be designed to minimize the effects of hypermetabolism and hypercatabolism, as well as for support immunocompetence to be developed.

TABLE 17.4   Ebb and Flow Phases

	Ebb Phase	Flow Phase
Hormonal and nonhormonal	↑ Glucagon ↑ Adrenocorticotropic hormone (ACTH)	↑ Counterregulatory hormones (epinephrine, norepinephrine, glucagon, cortisol) ↑ Insulin ↑ Catecholamines ↑ Cytokines (TNF-α, IL-1, IL-2, and IL-6)
Metabolic	Circulatory insufficiency, ↑ heart rate (vascular constriction) ↓ Digestive enzyme production ↓ Urine production	Hyperglycemia ↓ Protein synthesis/amino acid efflux ↑ Gluconeogenesis ↑ Glycogenolysis ↑↑ Urea nitrogen excretion/net (−) nitrogen balance
Clinical outcomes	Hemodynamic instability	Fluid and electrolyte imbalances Mild metabolic acidosis ↑ Resting energy expenditure

IN, Interleukin; *TNF,* tumor necrosis factor.
Modified from Cresci G, Martindale R: Nutrition in critical illness. In Berdanier C, editor: *Handbook of nutrition and food,* Boca Raton, FL, 2002, CRC Press; Cresci G: Metabolic stress. In Matarese L, Gottschlich M, editors: *Contemporary nutrition support practice,* ed 2, Philadelphia, 2003, Saunders.

Metabolic Response to Injury

Stressed patients undergo several metabolic phases as a series of ebb and flow states reflecting a patient's response to the severity of the stress. The initial ebb phase occurs immediately after injury and is associated with shock. If the injured patient survives, then the ebb phase evolves into the flow phase. Table 17.4 lists hormonal, metabolic, and clinical outcome comparisons between the two phases.

Clinical efforts in the ebb phase are focused on maintaining heart action and blood circulation. The flow state is a hyperdynamic phase in which substrates are mobilized for energy production while increased cellular activity and hormonal stimulation are noted. An energy expenditure distinction exists for each phase, making the goals of nutrition therapy variable depending on the stage in question. During the ebb phase a decrease in metabolic needs occurs. Typically, because of hemodynamic instability and need for resuscitation, nutrition intervention is not pursued during this phase. The flow phase brings hypermetabolism, yielding increased proteolysis and nitrogen loss, accelerated gluconeogenesis, hyperglycemia and increased glucose use, and retention of salt and water. Mobilization of protein, fat, and glycogen is believed to be mediated through release of cytokines such as tumor necrosis factor-a (TNF-a); interleukin-1 (IL-1), IL-2, and IL-6; and counterregulatory hormones such as epinephrine, norepinephrine, glucagon, and cortisol. Circulating levels of insulin are also elevated in most metabolically stressed patients, but responsiveness of tissues to insulin, especially skeletal muscle, is severely blunted. Researchers believe this relative insulin resistance to be caused by the effects of the counterregulatory hormones. The hormonal milieu normalizes only after the injury or metabolic stress has resolved. As long as the patient is in a hyperdynamic catabolic state, optimal nutrition support is needed but can only at best approach zero nitrogen balance in attempts to minimize further protein wasting.

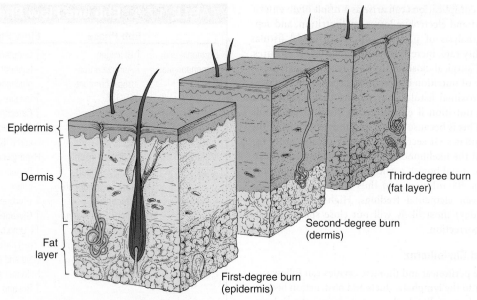

FIG. 17.8 Depth of skin area involved in burns.

Burn Wounds

Size and depth of the burn wound affect its healing process and overall prognosis (Fig. 17.8). Burns are usually classified by degree using the **rule of nines**, as follows:

1. *First-degree burns:* **erythema** involving cell necrosis above the basal layer of the epidermis
2. *Second-degree burns:* erythema and blistering, and necrosis within the dermis
3. *Third-degree burns:* full-thickness skin loss, including fat layer
4. *Fourth-degree burns:* exposed bone and tendon

Burns of first- and second-degree depths generally reepithelialize without surgical intervention. Third-degree burns will not heal independent of excision and grafting. Fourth-degree burns typically involve the use of muscle flaps, because skin grafting onto bone is not a viable therapy option.

Extent of the burn directly affects fluid resuscitation, surgical needs, immunocompetence, metabolic sequelae, and nutrition intervention. Second- and third-degree burns covering 15%-20% or more of the total body surface area (TBSA), or 10% in children and older adults, usually cause extensive fluid loss and require intravenous fluid and electrolyte replacement therapy. Burns of severe depth covering more than 50% of the TBSA are often fatal, especially in infants and older adults. Thermal injury permits the loss of heat, water, nitrogen, whole proteins, and micronutrients through the open wound. Loss of the protective skin barrier allows microorganisms to access subcutaneous tissue and potentiates systemic infectious processes, contributing to the postburn hypermetabolic state. Loss of plasma volume and electrolytes through the open wound predispose the burned patient to acid-base imbalance and cardiovascular, pulmonary, and renal instability. Adequate fluid and electrolyte resuscitation during the first 24 to 48 hours of postburn hypovolemia is essential for hemodynamic stability. Extensive fluid shifts, unique to burn injury, drive the characteristic edema process of resuscitation by increasing intracellular and interstitial fluid volumes. Fluids given during the resuscitative period should be titrated in accordance with urine output to prevent overresuscitation and underresuscitation. The replacement of extracellular sodium chloride, most commonly in the form of **lactated Ringer solution**, is obligatory for successful resuscitation.[34]

In addition, certain herbs and botanicals have been suggested for use in patients with thermal injuries. (For an outline of these herbs and additional information on their efficacy, safety, and possible interaction with other drugs, see the Complementary and Alternative Medicine [CAM] box, "Feel the Burn?")

Nutrition Therapy After Burn Injury

Thermal injury induces hypermetabolism of varying intensity and duration depending on extent and depth of the body surface affected, presence of infection, and efficacy of early treatment. Energy requirements peak at approximately postburn day 12 and typically slowly normalize as the percentage of open wound decreases with reepithelialization or skin grafting.

Energy

Burn patients require individualized nutrition plans to provide optimal energy and protein to accelerate muscle and protein synthesis and minimize proteolysis. Numerous predictive equations are used to estimate energy needs. Several studies have reviewed the accuracy of predictive equations in determining energy requirements in burn

---

KEY TERMS

Rule of Nines
Describes the percentage of the body surface represented by various anatomic areas. For example, each upper limb, 9%; each lower limb, 18%; anterior and posterior trunk, each 18%; head and neck, 9%; and perineum and genitalia, 1%.

Erythema
Redness of the skin produced by coagulation of the capillaries.

Lactated Ringer Solution
Sterile solution of calcium chloride, potassium chloride, sodium chloride, and sodium lactate in water administered to replenish fluid and electrolytes.

🌿 COMPLEMENTARY AND ALTERNATIVE MEDICINE (CAM)

Feel the Burn?

The following herbs and botanical supplements have been suggested for use with thermal injury.

Herb/Botanical and Use in Burns	Efficacy	Safety Issues	Drug Interactions
Aloe (*Aloe vera*) Aloe is a topical gel used to heal burns and reduce burn pain.	It may help heal abrasions and burns; research indicates aloe significantly delays healing of deep surgical wounds.	It produces an occasional allergic reaction and may lower blood glucose levels. Aloe is considered safe, but comprehensive safety studies are lacking.	None are known. Aloe gel may be a useful adjuvant therapy when combined with hydrocortisone acetate cream. If gel is taken internally, then it can reduce absorption of many medications.
Echinacea (*E. purpurea, E. pallida, E. angustifolia*) Echinacea is used topically to enhance wound healing.	Several research studies have provided evidence that various *Echinacea* species can significantly reduce the duration and severity of illness, but little demonstration of efficacy in wound healing is reported.	Oral Echinacea causes few side effects; most common reports include bad taste and minor GI symptoms.	*E. angustifolia* (the most popular species in North America) root might inhibit cytochrome P_{450} 3A4 (CYP3A4).
Garlic (*Allium* spp.) Garlic is used orally and topically to fight infections.	Little research, if any, is available to substantiate this claim.	Garlic is on the FDA's GRAS list. Raw garlic taken in excessive doses can cause numerous symptoms such as stomach upset, heartburn, nausea, vomiting, diarrhea, flatulence, facial flushing, rapid pulse, and insomnia. Topical garlic can cause skin irritation, blistering, even third-degree burns.	When taken with anticoagulants, NSAIDs, antiplatelet agents, or other herbs that exert anticoagulation effects (feverfew, ginkgo), garlic may increase bleeding time. Blood glucose level may be decreased with hypoglycemic agents.
Gotu kola (*Centella asiatica*) Gotu kola is used in Europe as treatment for scarring.	No substantial evidence exists to support this claim.	Rare allergic reactions occur to topical gotu kola.	None are known.
Plantain (*Plantago ovata, P. psyllium, P. lanceolata, P. major*) Plantain is used topically for skin inflammation.	Efficacy has not been validated scientifically.	Plantain is safe; long-term use shows no toxicity.	None are known.
St. John's wort (*Hypericum perforatum*) Hypericum tincture or oil is used topically for inflammation and burns.	It speeds healing of burns.	Noted side effects are related to ingestion of the herb.	Interactions are related to ingestion of the herb.

Bibliography

Bascom A, Breiner MA, Brigs M, et al: *Professional guide to complementary and alternative therapies*, Springhouse, PA, 2001, Springhouse.

Bratman S, Girman AM: *Mosby's handbook of herbs and supplements and their therapeutic uses*, St Louis, 2003, Mosby.

Escott-Stump S: *Nutrition and diagnosis-related care*, ed 6, Philadelphia, 2007, Lippincott Williams & Wilkins.

Kuhn MA, Winston D: *Winston and Kuhn's: Herbal therapy and supplements: a scientific and traditional approach*, ed 2, Philadelphia, 2007, Lippincott Williams & Wilkins.

FDA, Food and Drug Administration; *GI,* gastrointestinal; *GRAS,* generally recognized as safe; *NSAIDs,* nonsteroidal antiinflammatory drugs.

patients. Consensus indicates that predictive equations tend to overestimate energy expenditure; therefore the preferred method of determining energy requirements is by using indirect calorimetry. If indirect calorimetry is not available in the clinical situation, then resting energy expenditure (REE) can be estimated at 50% to 60% more than the Harris-Benedict equation for burns of more than 20% of TBSA.[32]

Carbohydrate

During the flow phase of metabolic stress, hyperglycemia is present because of the increased glucagon-to-insulin ratio that activates gluconeogenesis. Tissue insulin resistance further exacerbates glucose intolerance. Despite these metabolic aberrations, carbohydrate should be the primary energy source provided for the burned patient. For burns exceeding 25% TBSA, carbohydrate should comprise 60% to 65% of the calories.[34] Patients should be monitored closely for hyperglycemia and glucosuria, with exogenous insulin provided to maintain blood glucose levels at less than 180 mg/dL.[6] Complications of hyperglycemia include osmotic diuresis with resulting dehydration and hypovolemia, lipogenesis, fatty liver, and carbon dioxide (CO_2) retention inhibiting ventilatory weaning.

Protein

Trauma, burns, and sepsis initiate a cascade of events that leads to accelerated protein degradation, decreased rates of synthesis of selected proteins, and increased amino acid catabolism and nitrogen loss. Clinical consequences of these metabolic alterations can increase morbidity and mortality rates of patients, causing serious organ dysfunction and impaired host defenses. Therefore trauma and burn patients require increased amounts of protein in attempts to minimize endogenous proteolysis, as well as to support the large losses from wound exudate. Providing 20% to 25% of calories as protein to those with burns of greater than 25% TBSA promotes improved nutrition laboratory values, immunity, nitrogen balance, and survival.[35] Overall recommendations are to provide protein in the amount of 1.5 to 2.0 g/kg body weight, but rarely up to 3.0 g/kg body weight per day in an attempt to minimize protein losses. Providing these increased levels of protein requires continuous monitoring of fluid status, blood urea nitrogen, and serum creatinine because of high renal solute load. In addition to the quantity of protein provided, protein quality is also significant. The use of protein of high biologic value is preferred for burn patients. Consumption of whey protein has been recommended more than the use of casein because of its beneficial effects on burned children, improvement in tube-feeding tolerance, enhanced solubility at low gastric pH, increased digestibility, and improved nitrogen retention. Pharmacologic doses of the single amino acids arginine and glutamine have also been explored regarding their benefit in critical illness and burns.

Fat

Lipid is an important component of a trauma or burn patient's diet for many reasons; at 9 kcal/g, it is an isosmotic concentrated energy source for these patients. Dietary lipid is also a carrier for fat-soluble vitamins, as well as a provider of the essential fatty acids linoleic and linolenic acid. Even though lipids are required in critical illness, excess lipid can be detrimental. Excessive lipid administration has been associated with hyperlipidemia, fatty liver immunosuppression, and impaired clotting ability. For burn and multiple trauma patients, the recommended amount of total fat delivery is 12% to 15% of total calories. A minimum of 4% of calories in the diet should consist of essential fatty acids to prevent deficiencies, which often equates to approximately 10% of total calories as fat, because most sources do not solely contain essential fatty acid. Formulations supplemented with fish oil, a rich source of omega-3 fatty acids (eicosapentaenoic acid [EPA] and docosahexaenoic acid [DHA]), and canola oil (α-linolenic acid) are of particular interest for their potential antiinflammatory and immune-enhancing benefits.[36]

Vitamins and Minerals

Micronutrients function as coenzymes and cofactors in metabolic pathways at the cellular level. With increased energy and protein demands associated with traumatic and burn injury, one would also expect an increased need for vitamins and minerals. In addition, increased nutrient losses from open wounds and altered metabolism, absorption, and excretion would also be suspect for requirements beyond that of the Recommended Dietary Allowance (RDA). Various vitamins and minerals have also been found to aid with wound healing, immune function, and other biologic functions. Unfortunately, little concrete data are available to support exact requirements during these hypermetabolic states. However, in addition to a daily multivitamin, burn patients may benefit from additional vitamin A (5000 IU/1000 kcal of enteral nutrition),

vitamin C (500 mg twice daily), and zinc (45 mg elemental zinc per day).

Nutrient Delivery

Oral intake is generally adequate in children and adults with burns of less than 25% TBSA and in young children and infants with less than 15% TBSA. Adequate oral intake can be achieved by providing patient food preferences; high-calorie, high-protein supplements; and modular calorie and protein enhancement of foods.[34] However, patients with burns of greater than 25% TBSA often require enteral tube feeding. Gastric feedings are frequently interrupted in burn patients for multiple reasons such as the presence of gastric ileus, dressing changes, physical therapy, prone positioning, respiratory treatments, and surgery. Enteral feeding is well tolerated in burn patients when delivered in the small intestine because the small bowel maintains its absorptive capacity. Therefore a nasoenteric feeding tube is preferred. Small bowel feeding may also reduce incidence of aspiration. Enteral nutrient delivery should be initiated as soon as possible after injury (during the resuscitative period). Early enteral feedings, within the first 6 hours after the burn, have been shown to decrease the level of catabolic hormones, improve nitrogen balance, maintain gut mucosal integrity, lower the incidence of diarrhea, and decrease hospital stay.[37] A full-strength, intact protein formula at low rate (20 to 30 mL/h) advanced by 5 to 20 mL/h to the desired volume is typically tolerated.[34] Parenteral nutrition is indicated only if enteral nutrition is not tolerated or grossly inadequate, because it has been associated with metabolic and immunologic complications.[37] Whenever possible, low-rate enteral feedings should accompany parenteral nutrition to prevent villous atrophy.

HEALTH PROMOTION

IMMUNONUTRITION

It is known that malnutrition leads to suppressed immune responses. Providing nutrition support using standard enteral formulations has shown improvements in various clinical indexes of nutritional status when adequate calories and protein are given; however, a lack of demonstrated effect is seen on morbidity and mortality. During the past 20 years the field of immunology has exploded and expanded into nearly every area of medicine, including nutrition. Certain dietary components have been classified as *immune-enhancing nutrients*. Compared with standard nutrients, an immune-enhancing nutrient is a substance that provides positive effects on the immune system when provided in certain quantities. A distinct attribute of immune-enhancing agents is a modulation of the humoral and cellular immune function resulting in a reduction of systemic inflammatory response syndrome (SIRS) and postoperative infection rates.[38] Of the many immune-enhancing nutrients identified in human clinical trials, the ones that appear to be most beneficial are L-arginine, L-glutamine, nucleotides, omega-3 fatty acids (EPA and DHA), and various vitamins and minerals (zinc and vitamins A, E, and C). Several special enteral nutrient formulations have been categorized as immune-enhancing formulations (IEFs). Each of these formulas contains various combinations or levels (or both) of these immune-enhancing nutrients.[39]

Immune-Enhancing Formulations

Glutamine is known to be a major fuel source for rapidly dividing cells such as enterocytes, reticulocytes, and lymphocytes. In normal metabolic states, glutamine is a nonessential amino acid. However, during times of metabolic stress, glutamine is implicated as being conditionally essential because it is needed for the maintenance of gut metabolism, structure, and function. Despite the accelerated skeletal muscle release of amino acids, blood glutamine levels are not increased after burns. In fact, decreased plasma glutamine levels have been reported after severe burn, multiple trauma, or multiple organ failure.[40]

A number of studies have shown beneficial effects with supplemental glutamine, its precursors (ornithine α-ketoglutarate, α-ketoglutarate), or glutamine dipeptides (alanine-glutamine, glycine-glutamine). These studies deliver glutamine in pharmacologic doses of 25% to 35% of the dietary protein. Supplemental glutamine has been shown to have multiple benefits that include increased nitrogen retention and muscle mass, maintenance of the GI mucosa and its permeability, preserved immune function and reduced infections, and preserved organ glutathione levels. These protective effects of glutamine supplementation could have significant effects on morbidity and mortality rates in trauma and burn patients. Research continues on the safety and cost-effectiveness of glutamine supplementation in trauma and burns.

Arginine, like glutamine, is considered a conditionally essential amino acid. Arginine is the specific precursor for nitric oxide production, as well as a potent secretagogue for anabolic hormones such as insulin, prolactin, and growth hormone. Under normal circumstances, arginine is considered a nonessential amino acid because it is adequately synthesized endogenously via the urea cycle. However, research suggests that during times of metabolic stress, optimal amounts of arginine are not synthesized to promote tissue regeneration or positive nitrogen balance.

Studies in animals and humans have investigated the effects of supplemental arginine in various injury models. Positive outcomes from supplementation include improved nitrogen balance, wound healing, and immune function, as well as increased anabolic hormones (insulin and growth hormone). The outcomes are of special interest in the posttrauma and postburn patient during the flow phase, when enhancement of these processes would yield the greatest advantage. However, despite these positive effects, caution with excessive arginine supplementation is warranted in burn patients because of its potential adverse effects on nitric oxide production.

Even though lipids are required, excess lipid can be detrimental. Excessive lipid administration has been associated with hyperlipidemia, fatty liver immunosuppression, and impaired clotting ability. All long-chain fatty acids share the same enzyme systems because they are elongated and desaturated, with each pathway competitive in nature based on substrate availability. Dietary fatty acids modulate the phospholipid cell membrane composition and the type and quantities of eicosanoids produced. Prostaglandins of the 3 series (PGE_3) and series 5 leukotrienes have proved to be antiinflammatory and immune-enhancing agents. In addition, PGE_3 is a potent vasodilator. These concepts have received considerable attention for the potential of n-3 fatty acids to enhance immune function and reduce acute and chronic inflammation.

In most standard enteral formulations, the fat source is predominantly n-6 fatty acids, with a portion coming from MCTs. Formulations supplemented with fish oil, a rich source of n-3 fatty acids (EPA and DHA), and canola oil (α-linolenic acid) are available. Clinical trials using these formulations have shown positive benefits in patients with psoriasis, rheumatoid arthritis (RA), burns, sepsis, and trauma. Researchers believe these results are caused by alterations in eicosanoid and leukotriene production, with decreased arachidonic acid metabolites (e.g., PGE_2), as well as increased production of the less biologically active trienoic prostaglandins and pentaenoic leukotrienes.

Clinical Outcomes with Immune-Enhancing Formulas

Trauma Outcomes

IEFs have been used in trauma patients and are associated with decreased incidence of intraabdominal abscess, multiple organ failure, infections, and SIRS, as well as decreased hospital length of stay and days of therapeutic antibiotic use.

Intensive Care Unit and Sepsis Outcomes

The intensive care unit population involves a very heterogeneous group, making data interpretation difficult. This population involves differing severity and pathologic processes of various disease states. Studies conducted with this population contain differences in study design and methods of reporting data, adding to the complexity of comparing results between investigations. A few studies have been conducted with various diagnoses, such as cardiac failure, pulmonary failure, transplantation, trauma, and GI surgery. Positive outcomes in the form of decreased incidence of infections, requirement for mechanical ventilation, incidence of bacteremia, and length of stay were reported when using IEFs.

Surgery Outcomes

Research in surgical populations using IEFs has been performed with preoperative, postoperative, or combined nutrition therapies. The majority of procedures performed in these studies involved upper GI cancer or head and neck cancer surgery. Significantly improved outcomes in the IEF groups include fewer infections and wound complications, decreased severity of complications, and shorter postoperative and hospital length of stay.[41]

Other Populations (Burns, Head Injury, HIV, and AIDS)

In patient populations comprising those with burns, head injury, or HIV and AIDS, the study of the use of IEFs is limited. Currently only two studies investigating the effect of IEFs on immune function and nutritional status of patients with AIDS have been published. Improved weight gain was found in one of the studies when IEF was provided (but not in the other study).[42] Burn patients appear to benefit when provided with IEFs, exhibiting decreased infections and length of hospital stay. Head injury patients theoretically should benefit from IEFs because of severe hypermetabolism and the likelihood of infectious complications. However, no clinical data are available to support this theory. More research using IEFs in these populations is needed.

TO SUM UP

The nutritional status of the patient should be addressed before the patient is even considered for surgery. If the patient has any nutrient deficiencies, these should be corrected before surgery if time allows. Postoperatively the patient should be provided with nutrition as soon as feasible to improve surgical outcomes.

Postoperative nutrition may be supplied in a number of ways. The oral route is preferred; however, often it is not feasible or adequate to support metabolic needs. Enteral or parenteral nutrition may be provided for those unable to achieve adequate nutrient intake and absorption orally. Enteral feeding is preferred to parenteral feeding. Because alimentary tract surgery often alters the flow of nutrients, resulting in several potential metabolic and nutrition complications, postoperative diets are described to help minimize these effects.

QUESTIONS FOR REVIEW

1. Discuss the requirements for energy, protein, vitamins and minerals, and the means of providing them during the various stages of surgery (preoperative, immediately preoperative, postoperative).
2. Describe potential nutritional consequences that may result after surgery of the head and neck, esophagus, stomach, and intestine.
3. Develop a menu plan for a patient undergoing gastric bypass surgery for morbid obesity; include all phases of the diet progression.
4. Describe metabolic alterations that occur during metabolic stress.
5. Develop a nutrition care plan for a patient who has sustained third-degree burns covering 40% TBSA.

REFERENCES

1. Klein S, Kinney J, Jeejeebhoy K, et al: Nutrition support in clinical practice: review of published data and recommendations for future research directions. National Institutes of Health, American Society for Parenteral and Enteral Nutrition, and American Society for Clinical Nutrition, *JPEN J Parenter Enteral Nutr* 21:133, 1997.
2. Vitello J: Prevalence of malnutrition in hospitalized patients remains high, *J Am Coll Nutr* 12:589, 1993.
3. Naber TH, Schermer T, de Bree A, et al: Prevalence of malnutrition in non-surgical hospitalized patients and its association with disease complication, *Am J Clin Nutr* 66:1232, 1997.
4. Coats K, Morgan SL, Bartolucci AA, et al: Hospital-associated malnutrition: a reevaluation 12 years later, *J Am Diet Assoc* 93:27, 1993.
5. Kelly IE, Tessier S, Cahill A, et al: Still hungry in hospital: identifying malnutrition in acute hospital admissions, *Q J Med* 93:93, 2000.
6. ASPEN Board of Directors and the clinical Guidelines Task Force: Guidelines for the use of parenteral and enteral nutrition in adult and pediatric patients, *JPEN J Parenter Enteral Nutr* 26(Suppl 1):1SA, 2002.
7. VATPN Cooperative Study: Perioperative total parenteral nutrition in surgical patients, *N Engl J Med* 325:525, 1991.
8. Gustafsson O, Ljungqvist O: Perioperative nutritional management in digestive tract surgery. In Toulson M, Correia D, Gassull M, editors: *Nutrition and the gastrointestinal tract*, ed 5, Baltimore, 2011, Lippincott Williams & Wilkins.
9. Ren L, Zhu D, Wei Y, et al: Enhanced recovery after surgery (ERAS) program attenuates stress and accelerates recovery in patients after radical resection for colorectal cancer: a prospective randomized controlled trail, *World J Surg* 36(2):407–414, 2012.
10. Cerra FB, Benitez MR, Blackburn GL, et al: Applied nutrition in ICU patients: a consensus statement of the American College of Chest Physicians, *Chest* 111:769, 1997.
11. Klein CJ, Stanek GS, Willes CE: Overfeeding macronutrients to critically ill adults: metabolic complications, *J Am Diet Assoc* 98:795, 1998.
12. Pomposelli JJ, Baxter JK, Babineau TJ, et al: Early postoperative glucose control predicts nosocomial infection rate in diabetic patients, *JPEN J Parenter Enteral Nutr* 22:77, 1998.
13. Pomposelli JJ, Bistrian BR: Is total parenteral nutrition immunosuppressive? *New Horiz* 2:224, 1994.
14. Flancbaum L, Choban PS, Sambucco S, et al: Comparison of indirect calorimetry, the Fick method, and prediction equations in estimating the energy requirements of critically ill patients, *Am J Clin Nutr* 69:461, 1999.
15. Chioléro R, Revelly JP, Tappy L: Energy metabolism in sepsis and injury, *Nutrition* 13(Suppl 9):45S, 1997.
16. Frankenfield DC, Rowe WA, Smith JS, et al: Validation of several established equations for resting metabolic rate in obese and nonobese people, *J Am Diet Assoc* 103:1152, 2003.
17. Frankenfield DC, Roth-Yousey L, Compher C: Comparison of predictive equations for resting metabolic rate in healthy nonobese and obese adults: a systematic review, *J Am Diet Assoc* 105:775, 2005.
18. Barton RG: Nutrition support in critical illness, *Nutr Clin Pract* 9:127, 1994.
19. Cutts ME, Dowdy RP, Ellersieck MR, et al: Predicting energy needs in ventilator-dependent critically ill patients: effect of adjusting weight for edema or adiposity, *Am J Clin Nutr* 66:1250, 1997.
20. Marik P, Varon J: The obese patient in the ICU, *Chest* 113:492, 1998.
21. Ireton-Jones CS, Turner WW Jr, Liepa GU, et al: Equations for estimation of energy expenditures in patients with burns with special reference to ventilatory status, *J Burn Care Rehabil* 13:330, 1992.
22. Patiño JF, de Pimiento SE, Vergara A, et al: Hypocaloric support in the critically ill, *World J Surg* 23:553, 1999.
23. Cresci GA, Martindale RG: Nutrition support in trauma. In Koretz, RL, editor: *American Society for Enteral and Parenteral Nutrition: The science and practice of nutrition support: a case-based core curriculum*, ed 3, Dubuque, IA, 2001, Kendall/Hunt.
24. Thalacker-Mercer AE, Fleet JC, Craig BA, et al: Inadequate protein intake affects skeletal muscle transcript profiles in older humans, *Am J Clin Nutr* 85:1344, 2007.
25. Campbell WW, Crim MC, Dallal GE, et al: Increased protein requirements in elderly people: new data and retrospective reassessments, *Am J Clin Nutr* 60:501, 1994.
26. Campbell WW, Johnson CA, McCabe GP, et al: Dietary protein requirements of younger and older adults, *Am J Clin Nutr* 88:1322, 2008.
27. Dabrowski G, Rombeau JL: Practical nutritional management in the trauma intensive care unit, *Surg Clin North Am* 80:921, 2000.
28. Keele AM, Bray MJ, Emery PW, et al: Two-phase randomized controlled clinical trial of postoperative oral dietary supplements in surgical patients, *Gut* 40:393, 1997.
29. Jeffery KM, Harkins B, Cresci GA, et al: The clear liquid diet is no longer a necessity in the routine postoperative management of surgical patients, *Am Surg* 62:167, 1996.
30. Lipman TO: Grains or veins: is enteral nutrition really better than parenteral nutrition? A look at the evidence, *JPEN J Parenter Enteral Nutr* 22:167, 1998.
31. Heyland DK, Novak F, Drover JW, et al: Should immunonutrition become routine in critically ill patients? A systematic review of the evidence, *JAMA* 286:944, 2001.
32. Sullivan M, Alonso E: Gastrointestinal and pancreatic disease. In Matarese L, Gottschlich M, editors: *Contemporary nutrition support practice*, Philadelphia, 1998, Saunders.
33. Himal HS, Allard JR, Nadeau JE, et al: The importance of adequate nutrition in closure of small intestinal fistulas, *Br J Surg* 61:724, 1974.
34. Mayes T, Gottschlich M: Burns and wound healing. In Koretz, RL, editor: *American Society for Enteral and Parenteral Nutrition: The science and practice of nutrition support: a case-based core curriculum*, ed 3, Dubuque, IA, 2001, Kendall/Hunt.
35. Alexander JW, MacMillan BG, Stinnett JD, et al: Beneficial effects of aggressive protein feeding in severely burned children, *Ann Surg* 192:505, 1980.
36. Khorram-Sefat R, Behrendt W, Heiden A, et al: Long-term measurements of energy expenditure in severe burn injury, *West J Med Surg* 23:115, 1999.
37. Rose J, Shires T, Langer B, et al: Advances in burn care. In Cameron J, editor: *Advances in surgery*, vol 30, Chicago, 1996, Mosby-Year Book.
38. Cerantola Y, Hübner M, Grass F, et al: Immunonutrition in gastrointestinal surgery, *Br J Surg* 98:37, 2011.
39. Hillhouse J: Immune-enhancing enteral formulas: effect on patient outcome, *Support Line* 23:16, 2001.
40. Martindale RG, Cresci GA: The use of immune enhancing diets in burns, *JPEN J Parenter Enteral Nutr* 25(Suppl 2):S24, 2001.
41. Sax HC: Effect of immune enhancing formulas (IEF) in general surgery patients, *JPEN J Parenter Enteral Nutr* 25(Suppl 2):S19, 2001.
42. Schloerb PR: Immune-enhancing diets: products, components, and their rationales, *JPEN J Parenter Enteral Nutr* 25(Suppl 2):S3, 2001.

FURTHER READINGS AND RESOURCES

Readings

Cerra FB: How nutrition intervention changes what getting sick means, *JPEN J Parenter Enteral Nutr* 14(Suppl 5):164, 1990.
[*This article provides a good review of three basic factors that influence what is observed at an ill patient's bedside when considering the effects of nutrition intervention: (1) the disease process inherent in the metabolic response to injury, (2) the presence of starvation, and (3) the presence of the nutrition intervention.*]

Hustler DA: Nutritional monitoring of a pediatric burn patient, *Nutr Clin Pract* 6:11, 1991.
[*This experienced dietitian-specialist on a burn center team provides a case report of a young boy who sustained mostly full-thickness burns on 56% of his total body surface area (TBSA). She describes in detail the challenge of initial evaluation and therapy, constant close monitoring, and appropriate responses to changing needs.*]

Tynes JJ, Austhof SI, Chima CS, et al: Diet tolerance and stool frequency in patients with ileoanal reservoirs, *J Am Diet Assoc* 92(7):861, 1992.

[*This brief report of a survey of patients with ileoanal reservoirs provides helpful background information about this recently developed alternative surgical procedure to the ileostomy, with practical guidance for nutritional management and patient counseling.*]

Websites of Interest

- American Academy of Physical Medicine and Rehabilitation. This is the website of the only organization exclusively serving physicians who specialize in physical medicine and rehabilitation. http://www.aapmr.org.
- American Botanical Council. The American Botanical Council is an independent, not-for-profit research and education organization dedicated to providing accurate and reliable information for consumers, healthcare practitioners, researchers, educators, industry, and the media. http://www.herbalgram.org.
- National Center for Complementary and Alternative Medicine. Lead agency of the US government for scientific research on diverse medical and health care systems, practices, and products not generally considered part of conventional medicine. http://www.nccam.nih.gov/.

18

Drug-Nutrient Interactions

Joyce Gilbert

ⓔ http://evolve.elsevier.com/Williams/essentials/

In this chapter, which continues our clinical nutrition sequence, we look briefly at some main effects of combining food and nutrients with drugs. We will see how these interactions affect nutrition therapy. Currently consumers are generally better informed about drug misuse. However, many are dangerously uninformed or misinformed about the specific drugs they may be taking, especially in relation to the food they eat. All members of the health care team must have knowledge of drug actions and nutrition to make the wisest and most effective use of drugs and nutrition therapy. Here we examine some of these drug-nutrient effects and how these interactions affect nutrition therapy and education.

OUTLINE

Drug-Nutrient Problems in Modern Medicine
Drug Effects on Food and Nutrients
Food and Nutrient Effects on Drugs

Nutrition-Pharmacy Team
Health Promotion
  "The Pain Reliever Doctors Recommend Most"

DRUG-NUTRIENT PROBLEMS IN MODERN MEDICINE

Problem Significance: Causes, Extent, and Effects

Medications and food interact in various ways. Various nutrients interfere with the medication's absorption and efficacy. In addition, medications can disturb ingestion, digestion, and absorption of nutrients. During this century, unprecedented medical progress has resulted in decreased childhood mortality rates and increased life expectancy. As we live longer, the incidence of chronic diseases such as cardiovascular disease, type 2 diabetes mellitus, hypertension, and arthritis will continue to increase, often in a comorbid manner. Furthermore, treatment of these and other chronic diseases often involves long-term use of medications, often resulting in polypharmacy, in addition to alternative and herbal therapies (see the Focus on Culture box, "Are We Speaking the Same Language?").[1] To this we can then add the large volume of nonprescription drugs that Americans purchase without a physician's guidance (Fig. 18.1).

Drug Use and Nutritional Status
Drug Administration

Drugs are administered several different ways. The administration route depends on the chemical properties of the drug, desired effect, and patient characteristics that affect administration of the drug. Drug administration routes are described in Table 18.1.

Older Adults at Risk

All of us, at any age, risk harmful drug-drug or drug-nutrient interactions. However, older adults are particularly vulnerable, and this will only become more prevalent. Currently, adults older than age 65

represent approximately 14% of the US population. It is projected this number will increase to 20% to 22% by 2050.[2] Older adults take a much larger percentage of prescription and nonprescription medications than their younger counterparts (Fig. 18.2). Several factors contribute to an increased risk among older adults, including the following[3]:

- They are likely to be taking more drugs for longer periods to control chronic diseases.
- Their drugs are likely to be more toxic.
- They respond to drugs with increased variability.
- They have less capability of handling drugs efficiently.
- Their nutritional status is more likely to be deficient.
- They are more likely to make increased errors in self-care because of illness, mental confusion, or lack of drug information.

As a result of these problems, concerned physicians, nutritionists, pharmacists, and nurses are increasingly working together as a team to provide drug and nutrition education and therapy on a more sound basis. A number of drug-nutrient interactions demand this type of teamwork in patient care.[1]

Nutritional Status

Poor nutritional status can have a major effect on risk for complications of drug-nutrient reactions. Nutrient-drug mechanisms that influence nutritional status include those affecting the following:

- Stimulated or suppressed appetite
- Decreased intestinal absorption
- Increased renal excretion
- Competition or displacement of nutrients for carrier protein sites
- Interference with synthesis of a necessary enzyme, coenzyme, or carrier

🌐 FOCUS ON CULTURE

Are We Speaking the Same Language?

Consider the following prescription label directions written half in English and half in Spanish:

Aplicarse once cada dia til rash is clear.

What does it mean to you? If you do not read Spanish, then it probably does not mean much (although you can pick out the words *once* and *til rash is clear*). In addition, if you study this phrase hard enough, then you might figure out it says something about using the medication once a day until the rash is gone.

If you read Spanish, then the meaning may be entirely different. *Once* means 11 in Spanish. If this is a mild topical medication, then perhaps no permanent harm would result if you used it 11 times a day. However, if this is an oral medication, then the results could be fatal.

Many people using prescription or over-the-counter (OTC) medications, herbal products, or vitamin and mineral supplements use a language other than English as their primary language. Foreign-born individuals make up 11% of the US population. The majority of immigrants are of Hispanic origin. Although many members of these groups have good reading and writing skills in their native languages, they may not possess the same skills in English. How then are they supposed to read and understand directions regarding how to take medications or supplements? How can they adhere to a prescribed medical regimen if they are unable to read the label? This language barrier may make the individuals more susceptible to food-drug interactions.

Another barrier to health is literacy. More than 40% of patients with chronic illnesses are functionally illiterate. Almost 25% of all adult Americans read at or below a fifth-grade level, whereas medical information is typically written at a tenth-grade level or greater. The National Adult Literacy Survey (NALS) found almost 25% of patients with inadequate functional health literacy did not know how to take medications.

Limited health literacy and language barriers have many consequences. Patients who do not understand prescription directions and instructions for preventive care and self-care may make the following mistakes:

- Incorrect doses (e.g., improper infant formula preparation and feeding)
- Incorrect schedules of administration (e.g., 4 times a day vs four pills at 1 time)
- Incorrect routes of administration (e.g., teens who have misunderstood directions for contraceptive jelly and have eaten it on toast every morning to prevent pregnancy)

Low health literacy risk groups include pediatric patients, older adult patients, and patients with language barriers. Pediatric patients are at increased risk of incorrect doses. Older adult patients take multiple medications, which increases risk for errors. In addition, patients older than age 60 may have hearing loss, memory loss, short attention span, and low energy levels, thus exacerbating the problems. Patients who speak English as their second language are vulnerable to misinterpretation of information.

Following are some solutions to this problem:

- Provide written materials in several languages and at a fifth-grade reading level or lower.
- Offer small amounts of information at a time.
- Avoid using "medical speak" (medical terms that are used every day in the clinical setting but are unfamiliar to patients).
- Employ a multilingual staff.
- Have patients repeat instruction to ensure the message was received and understood.
- Use identifiers such as time-of-day references (e.g., "Take one tablet in the morning when you wake up and the second tablet at bedtime.").
- Use visual images when possible.

Bibliography

Hardin LR: Frontline pharmacist: counseling patients with low health literacy, *Am J Health Syst Pharm* 62:364, 2005.

Institute for Safe Medication Practices: *Hospitals need to take action now to reduce threat of medication errors with magnesium sulfate, ISMP Medication Safety Alert!* http://www.ismp.org/recommendations/high-alert-medications-acute-list.

Institute for Safe Medication Practices: *To promote understanding, assume every patient has a health literacy problem, ISMP Medication Safety Alert!* http://www.ismp.org/recommendations/confused-drug-names-list.

Literacy Partners of Manitoba: *Literacy and health resources,* Manitoba, Canada, 2005, Literacy Partners of Manitoba. https://www.health.mb.literacy.ca/health.htm.

National Institute for Literacy: *Literacy fact sheets: scope of the literacy need,* Washington, DC, 2001, National Institute for Literacy. http://www.factfinder.census.gov/servlet/DatasetMainPageServlet?_program=ACS&_submenuid=&_lang=en&_ts=%29.

US Census Bureau: *Profile of selected social characteristics: 2000, Census 2000 supplementary survey summary tables,* Washington, DC, 2001, US Government Printing Office.

Wallendorf M: Literally literacy, *J Consum Res* 27:505, 2001.

FIG. 18.1 Prescription and nonprescription drugs have become part of American life. (Copyright 2006 JupiterImages Corporation.)

- Hormonal effects on genetic systems
- Drug delivery system
- Components in drug formulation

In general, drugs are grouped according to primary action. In the following sections, we review the various effects of drugs on food and nutrients and the effects of food and nutrients on drugs. In each case, we give some examples for your reference in patient care.

DRUG EFFECTS ON FOOD AND NUTRIENTS

Drug Effects on Food Intake

Appetite Changes. The following drugs may stimulate appetite, weight gain, or both[4]:

- *Antihistamines:* These drugs can lead to marked increase in appetite and subsequent weight gain. Cyproheptadine hydrochloride (Periactin) is an antihistamine also used as an appetite stimulant.

TABLE 18.1   Drug Administration Routes

Administration Route	Characteristics
Oral	Requires ability to swallow and absorb the medication
Sublingual	Medication placed under tongue to dissolve; absorbed quickly across mucous membrane
Buccal	Medication placed in cheek to dissolve; absorbed quickly across mucous membrane
Parenteral	Injection in circulatory system
Subcutaneous (SC)	Injection under the skin
Intradermal (ID)	Injection under outermost layer of skin
Intramuscular (IM)	Injection into muscle
Intraperitoneal (IP)	Injection into peritoneal cavity
Intravenous (IV)	Injection into a vein
Topical	Applied to skin
Inhalation	Medication breathed into respiratory system
Ophthalmic	Placement of medication into eye
Otic	Placement of medication into ear
Epidural	Placement of medication into spinal fluid
Intrathecal	Placement of medication into membrane surrounding central nervous system (CNS)

Data from Nelms M: Pharmacology. In Nelms MN, Sucher K, Long S, editors: *Understanding nutrition therapy and pathophysiology,* Belmont, CA, 2007, Wadsworth.

FIG. 18.2 Older adults make up a large percentage of those taking prescription and nonprescription medications in the United States.

- *Antianxiety drugs:* Some drugs in this classification may lead to hyperphagia, or excessive eating. Some of these drugs include chlordiazepoxide hydrochloride (Librium), diazepam (Valium), and alprazolam (Xanax).
- *Tricyclic antidepressants:* Tricyclic antidepressants and most antipsychotic drugs such as amitriptyline hydrochloride (Elavil), olanzapine (Zyprexa), chlorpromazine hydrochloride (Thorazine), and clozapine (Clozaril) may promote appetite and lead to significant weight gain.
- *Insulin:* Hypoglycemia can occur in persons with type 1 diabetes if food is not taken immediately after their insulin injection

(see Chapter 22). If some food is not readily available to counteract the rapid progression of the unrelieved severe hypoglycemia, then coma and death occur. If excess food is consumed to avoid or treat hypoglycemia, then weight gain may occur.
- *Steroids:* Anabolic steroids, including testosterone, promote nitrogen retention, increased lean body mass, and subsequent weight gain.

The following drugs may depress appetite[4]:
- *Selective serotonin reuptake inhibitors (SSRIs):* This class of antidepressants may cause anorexia and weight loss; an example is fluoxetine (Prozac). (See the Case Study box, "Drug-Herb Interaction," for an application of the use of SSRIs.)
- *Amphetamines:* These drugs act as stimulants to the central nervous system (CNS) and have the effect of depressing the desire for food, thus leading to marked loss of weight. For this reason, they have been used in the past as appetite-depressant drugs in the treatment of obesity. However, long-term use of these drugs for such treatment has caused problems, such as addiction. For this reason, amphetamines are rarely used now for this purpose. Children taking amphetamines show dose-dependent growth retardation.

CASE STUDY

Drug-Herb Interaction

Ivanna is a 20-year-old exchange student from Germany. She lives with three roommates and is in her junior year at the local university. Ivanna is seeking medical attention at the urging of her roommates, who report her mood has become increasingly depressed during the past two semesters. She has become withdrawn and moody but is otherwise a healthy young woman. She is 5 ft 11 in tall and weighs 160 lb on admission.

Ivanna reports a 5-lb weight loss in the past 3 months. She takes oral contraceptives, smokes a half of a pack of cigarettes per day, and drinks four to five beers on the weekends. Her mother has been treated for depression with St. John's wort by the family physician in Germany for the past 10 years. Her admitting diagnosis is depression. Physician's orders are as follows: Zoloft, 50 mg every day, referral to house psychologist for counseling, and nutrition consult for her poor eating habits.

Questions for Analysis
1. Ivanna's physician ordered Zoloft to treat her depression. Zoloft is a selective SSRI. Are there any pertinent nutritional considerations when using this medicine?

2. How do SSRIs work?
3. During the diet history, you ask Ivanna if she uses any OTC vitamins, minerals, or herbal supplements. She tells you her mother suggested she try *Hypericum perforatum* (St. John's wort) because in Germany it is prescribed to treat depression. Ivanna did as her mother suggested because it is available without prescription in the United States. What is St. John's wort?
4. How is St. John's wort used in the United States?
5. How does St. John's wort work as an antidepressant?
6. Does St. John's wort have any side effects?
7. How is St. John's wort regulated in the United States? How is it used in Europe?
8. What is your immediate concern regarding Ivanna's use of St. John's wort?

Data from Nelms MN, Long S, Lacey K: *Medical nutrition therapy: a case study approach,* ed 3, Belmont, CA, 2008, Wadsworth.

• *Alcohol:* Abuse of alcohol can lead to loss of appetite, reduced food intake, and malnutrition. The anorexia, or loss of appetite, can stem from various effects of alcoholism such as gastritis, hepatitis, cirrhosis, ketosis, pancreatitis, alcoholic brain syndrome, drunkenness, and withdrawal symptoms. The resulting reduced food intake can then lead to malnutrition, which further complicates the anorexia.

Taste and Smell Changes

Drugs such as the tricyclic antidepressant amitriptyline (Elavil) may impair salivary flow, causing dry mouth along with a sour or metallic taste.[4] The antibiotic clarithromycin (Biaxin) is secreted into saliva, causing a bitter taste.[4] Antibiotics such as tetracycline may suppress natural oral bacteria, resulting in oral yeast overgrowth or candidiasis. Metronidazole (Flagyl), an antibiotic, may cause dysgeusia (abnormal or impaired sense of taste) by causing a metallic taste in the mouth.[4] Antineoplastic medications (cisplatin or methotrexate) may damage rapidly growing cells, causing stomatitis, glossitis, or esophagitis (or a combination of these problems)[4] (see the Perspectives in Practice box, "Counseling Patients About Potential Food-Medication Interactions").

Gastrointestinal Effects

Many drugs can affect the stomach and cause nausea, vomiting, bleeding, or ulceration; intestinal peristalsis; or changes in intestinal flora. Nonsteroidal antiinflammatory drugs (NSAIDs) such as aspirin (acetylsalicylic acid [ASA]), ibuprofen (Advil, Motrin), and naproxen (Aleve, Anaprox) cause stomach irritation.[4] Sometimes the irritation is so severe as to cause sudden and serious gastric bleeding.[4] Anticholinergic medications (antipsychotics, antidepressants, antihistamines) slow peristalsis, resulting in constipation. Ciprofloxacin (Cipro) is an antibiotic that can allow for the overgrowth of *Clostridium difficile,* resulting in pseudomembranous colitis.[4]

PERSPECTIVES IN PRACTICE

Counseling Patients About Potential Food-Medication Interactions

- Provision of relevant medication information: drug name, drug indications, duration of therapy
- Information detailing how to take the medication
- Probable side effects and dietary suggestions to lessen symptoms
- Nutritional difficulties that may develop, particularly if dietary intake is poor
- Dietary alteration that may change drug action
- Food and beverages to avoid or consume in moderation while taking the medication
- Implications of alcohol ingestion
- Potential for interactions involving medications and vitamin and mineral supplements (or other food supplements)
- Significance of staying on a special diet prescription for treatment of medical condition
- Individualization of dietary prescription to that person only
- Consultation with prescribing physician before modifying drug or diet prescription
- Consultation with a registered dietitian (RD) for in-depth nutrition information
- Consultation with a registered pharmacist (RPh) for questions regarding drug action or possible side effects

Data from Pronsky ZM: *Food medication interactions,* ed 15, Birchrunville, PA, 2008, Food-Medication Interactions.

Drug Effects on Nutrient Absorption and Metabolism
Nutrient Absorption

A number of drugs can increase nutrient absorption and thus benefit nutritional status. For example, cimetidine (Tagamet), a gastric antisecretory agent, helps patients with bowel resection in several ways.[4] The drug reduces gastric acid and volume output; it also lowers duodenal acid load and volume and reduces jejunal flow.[4] It maintains the pH of secretions and decreases fecal fat, nitrogen, and volume, thus improving absorption of macronutrients.[4] This drug is therefore helpful in the treatment of various gastrointestinal (GI) disorders, including peptic ulcer disease (see Chapter 20).[4] On the other hand, prolonged use of cimetidine may cause decreased absorption of vitamin B_{12}, thiamin, and iron.[4]

A number of drugs can contribute to primary malabsorption. Questran (antihyperlipidemic, bile acid sequestrant [cholestyramine]) binds vitamins A, D, E, and K in the GI tract, preventing absorption of these nutrients.[4] Colchicine, a drug used in the treatment of gout, leads to vitamin B_{12} deficiency, causing megaloblastic anemia.[4] Alcohol abuse can provoke malabsorption of thiamin and folic acid, causing peripheral neuritis and anemia.[4] Laxatives can produce severe malabsorption, leading to conditions such as osteomalacia.[4]

Secondary malabsorption may also be drug induced. For example, the antibiotic neomycin causes tissue changes in the intestinal villi, precipitates bile salts, prevents fat breakdown by inhibiting pancreatic lipase, and decreases bile acid absorption.[4] These effects can lead to steatorrhea and failure to absorb the fat-soluble vitamins A, D, E, and K.[4] Malabsorption of vitamin D in turn leads to a calcium deficiency. Other drugs cause malabsorption of folic acid or impair its use. For example, methotrexate, used in cancer chemotherapy, is a folic acid antagonist that impairs the intestinal absorption of calcium.[4] Summaries of medications that affect food and nutrients can be found in Table 18.2.

Mineral Depletion

Certain drugs can lead to mineral depletion through induced GI losses or renal excretion[5]:

- *Diuretics:* Diuretic drugs are intentionally used to reduce levels of excess tissue water and sodium, but they may also result in loss of other minerals, such as potassium, magnesium, and zinc. Potassium deficiency brings weakness, anorexia, nausea, vomiting, listlessness, apprehension, and sometimes diffuse pain, drowsiness, stupor, and irrational behavior. However, potassium-retaining diuretics such as spironolactone, as well as overuse of potassium supplementation, may cause the opposite effect of hyperkalemia.
- *Chelating agents:* Penicillamine attaches to metals and can lead to the deficiency of such key trace elements as zinc and copper.
- *Alcohol:* Abuse of alcohol can lead to diminished levels of potassium, magnesium, and zinc.
- *Antacids:* These commonly used OTC medications are of concern because they can produce phosphate deficiency, with symptoms of anorexia, malaise, paresthesia, profound muscle weakness, and convulsions, as well as calcification of soft tissues from the prolonged hypercalcemia.
- *Aspirin:* Salicylates such as ASA (aspirin) can induce iron deficiency by causing low-level blood loss from erosions in the stomach or intestinal tissue when taken incorrectly (see section "Health Promotion" for discussion).

KEY TERMS

Paresthesia
Abnormal sensations such as prickling, burning, and crawling of skin.

TABLE 18.2	**Medications Affecting Food and Nutrients**			
Drug Class	**Examples**	**Action**	**Nutrients Affected**	**How to Avoid**
Alcohol, particularly excessive use	Beer, wine, spirits	Increases turnover of some vitamins; substitution of alcohol for food	Vitamin B_{12}, folate, and magnesium	Limit alcohol consumption to <2 drinks per day for men, <1 drink per day for women
Analgesic, NSAID, and antiinflammatory agents	Salicylates (aspirin), ibuprofen (Motrin, Advil), naproxen (Anaprox, Aleve, Naprosyn), acetaminophen (Tylenol)	Increases loss of vitamin C and competes with folate and vitamin K	Vitamin C, folate, vitamin K	Increase intake of foods high in vitamin C, folate, and vitamin K; take with 8 oz water
Antacid agents	Aluminum antacids, H_2 blockers	Inactivates thiamin; decreases absorption of some nutrients	Thiamin (B_1)	Foods containing thiamin (B_1) should be consumed at a different time; depends on antacid; possibly magnesium, phosphorus, iron, vitamin A, and folate Take antacid after meals; take iron, magnesium, or folate supplements separately by 2 hours; take separately from citrus fruit or juices or calcium citrate by 3 hours
Antiulcer agents (histamine blockers)	Ranitidine (Zantac), cimetidine (Tagamet), famotidine (Pepcid)	Decreases vitamin absorption	Vitamin B_{12}	Consult physician or RD regarding vitamin B_{12} supplementation
Antibiotic agents	Tetracycline, ciprofloxacin (Cipro)	Chelation of minerals; ingestion with caffeine may increase excitability and nervousness	Calcium, magnesium, iron, and zinc; caffeine	Take tetracycline at least 1 h before or 2 h after a meal; do not take with caffeine-containing products
Antineoplastic agents	Methotrexate	Causes mucosal damage, which may cause decreased nutrient absorption	Folate and vitamin B_{12}, (also see Antibiotic Agents)	Consult physician or RD regarding supplementation
Anticholinergic agents	Amitriptyline (Elavil), chlorpromazine (Thorazine)	Saliva thickens and loses ability to prevent tooth decay	Fluids	Increase intake of fluids
Anticonvulsant agents	Phenobarbital, phenytoin (Dilantin)	Increases metabolism of folate (possibly leading to megaloblastic anemia), vitamin D (especially in children), and vitamin K	Folate, vitamin D, and vitamin K	Increase folate, vitamins D and K intake
Antidepressant agents	Lithium carbonate, Lithane, Lithobid, Lithonate, Lithotabs, Eskalith	May cause metallic taste, nausea, vomiting, dry mouth, anorexia, weight gain, and increased thirst	Fluids	Drink 2–3 L of water per day and take with food, consistent sodium intake
Antihyperlipidemic agents	Cholestyramine (Questran), colestipol (Colestid)	Binds bile salts and nutrients	Fat-soluble vitamins (A, D, E, K), folate, vitamin B_{12}, and iron	Include rich sources of these vitamins and minerals in diet
Antituberculosis agents	Isoniazid (INH)	Inhibits conversion of vitamin B_6 to active form	Vitamin B_6	Vitamin B_6 supplementation is necessary to prevent deficiency and peripheral neuropathy
Corticosteroid agents	Prednisone, Solu-Medrol, hydrocortisone	Increases excretion	Protein, potassium, calcium, magnesium, zinc, vitamin C, and vitamin B_6	Increase intake of foods high in protein, potassium, calcium, magnesium, zinc, vitamin C, and vitamin B_6
Loop diuretic agents	Furosemide (Lasix)	Increases mineral excretion in urine	Potassium, calcium, magnesium, zinc, sodium, and chloride	Include fresh fruits and vegetables in diet
Thiazide diuretic agents	Hydrochlorothiazide (HCTZ)	Increases excretion of most electrolytes, but enhances reabsorption of calcium	Potassium, calcium, magnesium, zinc, sodium, chloride, and calcium	Increase intake of foods high in potassium, calcium, magnesium, zinc, sodium, and chloride
Potassium-sparing diuretic agents	Triamterene (Dyrenium)	Hyperkalemia	Potassium	Avoid potassium-based salt substitutes

TABLE 18.2	Medications Affecting Food and Nutrients—cont'd			
Drug Class	**Examples**	**Action**	**Nutrients Affected**	**How to Avoid**
Laxative agents	Fibercon, Mitrolan	Decreases nutrient absorption	Vitamins and minerals	Consult physician or RD regarding supplementation
Sedative agents	Barbiturates	Increases metabolism of vitamins	Folate, vitamin D, vitamin B_{12}, thiamin, and vitamin C	Increase intake of foods high in folate, vitamin D, vitamin B_{12}, thiamin, and vitamin C
Mineral oil	Agoral Plain	Decreases absorption	Fat-soluble vitamins (A, D, E, K), betacarotene, calcium, phosphorus, and potassium	Take 2 h apart from food and fat-soluble vitamins
Oral contraceptive agents	Estrogen/progestin	May cause selective malabsorption or increased metabolism and turnover	Vitamin B_6 and folate	Increase foods high in B_6 and folate

NSAID, Nonsteroidal antiinflammatory drug; *RD,* registered dietitian.
Data from Anderson J, Bland SE: Drug-food interactions, *J Pharm Soc Wisc* 28, 1998; Bobroff LB, Lentz A, Turner RE: *Food/drug and drug/nutrient interactions: what you should know about your medications,* Gainesville, 1994, University of Florida Cooperative Extension Service, Institute of Food and Agricultural Science. https://www.edis.ifas.ufl.edu; Food and Drug Administration/National Consumers League: *Food & drug interactions,* Washington, DC, US Government Printing Office. https://www.nclnet.org/Food%20&%20Drug.pdf.

Vitamin Depletion

Certain drugs act as metabolic antagonists and can cause deficiencies of the vitamins involved.

- *Vitamin antagonists:* Various drugs have been used successfully to treat disease because they are antagonists of certain vitamins and thus can control key metabolic reactions in which that vitamin is involved. For example, warfarin (Coumadin) anticoagulants inhibit regeneration of vitamin K, which is necessary for blood clotting. In addition, some cancer chemotherapy drugs such as methotrexate have multiple antagonist effects on folate metabolism, thus inhibiting the synthesis of cell reproduction substances—deoxyribonucleic acid (DNA) and ribonucleic acid (RNA)—and protein. In a similar manner, the antimalaria drug pyrimethamine inhibits the action of folate in protein synthesis.

Special Adverse Reactions

Several reactions are related to specific drug interactions with particular nutrients, as follows:

- *Monoamine oxidase inhibitors (MAOIs):* These antidepressant drugs can increase the vascular effect of simple vasoactive amines, such as tyramine and dopamine, from food.[5] The resulting tyramine syndrome is marked by headache, pallor, nausea, and restlessness. With increased absorption, symptoms may escalate to apprehension, sweating, palpitations, chest pain, fever, and increased blood pressure, at times, although rarely, to the extent of hypertensive crisis and stroke.
- *Flushing reaction:* A number of drugs react with alcohol to produce a flushing reaction along with dyspnea and headache. CNS depressants, including hypnotic sedatives, antihistamines, phenothiazines, and narcotic analgesics, may cause a loss of consciousness if taken in combination with alcohol. Extreme caution must be exercised with these medications, and patients should be alerted to the dangers of mixing them with alcohol.
- *Hypoglycemia:* Drugs such as chlorpropamide (Diabinese) and similar oral medications used to control type 2 diabetes mellitus are hypoglycemic agents. They precipitate a rapid release of insulin, which may provoke a hypoglycemic reaction. This response of a rapidly reduced blood glucose level is especially strong when the drugs are used with alcohol. Symptoms of hypoglycemia include weakness, mental confusion, and irrational behavior. If not treated, then loss of consciousness can follow.

- *Disulfiram reaction:* The drug disulfiram, commonly called Antabuse, is used in the treatment of alcoholism. It combats alcohol consumption by producing extremely unpleasant side effects when taken with alcohol. Within 15 minutes, flushing ensues, followed by headache, nausea, vomiting, and chest or abdominal pain. Other drugs, including aldehyde dehydrogenase inhibitors, may have a similar effect.

FOOD AND NUTRIENT EFFECTS ON DRUGS

Physiologic Factors in Drug Absorption

Absorption of drugs is a complex matter. Physiologic events are important in a number of ways.

Solution

Before an orally administered tablet or capsule can dissolve, it must first disintegrate. The absorption of the drug, either from solution in acid gastric secretions or in the more alkaline medium of the intestine, may be more or less complete, depending on its degree of solubility (see the Evidence-Based Practice box, "Grapefruit 'Juices' Certain Medications"). Food may affect eventual drug absorption at any of these points. Table 18.3 provides some examples of drugs that are

---

KEY TERMS

Vasoactive
Having an effect on the diameter of blood vessels.

Flushing Reaction
Short-term reaction resulting in redness of neck and face.

Dyspnea
Labored, difficult breathing.

Disulfiram
White to off-white crystalline antioxidant; inhibits oxidation of the acetaldehyde metabolized from alcohol. It is used in the treatment of alcoholism, producing extremely uncomfortable symptoms when alcohol is ingested after oral administration of the drug.

EVIDENCE-BASED PRACTICE

Grapefruit "Juices" Certain Medications

Almost all oral drugs are subject to first-pass metabolism. That is, any substance the body views as a toxin (e.g., drugs, alcohol) goes through the liver via hepatic portal circulation, thus removing some of the active substance from blood before it enters general circulation. This means a fraction of the original dose of the drug will not be "available" to systemic circulation because it has undergone biotransformation. In other words, the bioavailability of the drug has been altered, or lowered. One mechanism responsible for this is an enzyme system found in the intestinal wall and liver. The cytochrome P_{450} 3A4 (CYP3A4) system, specifically CYP3A4-mediated drug metabolism, is responsible for first-pass metabolism of many medications. Most medications are lipid soluble and readily absorbed. However, to eliminate toxins (i.e., drugs) from the body, the CYP3A4 system either breaks them down in the gut or changes the drug into a more water-soluble version in the liver, allowing it to be eliminated via urine.

Where does grapefruit juice come into play? Grapefruit juice blocks the CYP3A4 enzyme in the wall of the small intestine, thus increasing the bioavailability of the drug. This means an increased serum drug level, which may cause unpleasant consequences, including side effects, toxicity, or both.

What is it in grapefruit juice that does this? The precise chemical nature of the substance responsible for inhibiting the gut wall CYP3A4 enzyme is unknown, but it is believed that more than one component present in grapefruit juice may contribute to the inhibitory effect on CYP3A4.

A single glass (8 oz) of grapefruit juice has the potential to increase bioavailability and enhance beneficial or adverse effects of a broad range of medications. These effects can persist up to 72 hours after grapefruit consumption, until more CYP3A4 has been metabolized. Interactions have been found between grapefruit juice and drugs, as outlined in the following table.

Interactions Between Grapefruit Juice and Medications

Category	Generic Name	Brand Name	Effect
Antihypertensive (calcium channel blockers) agents	Felodipine	Plendil	Flushing, headache, tachycardia, decreased blood pressure
	Nifedipine	Procardia, Adalat	
	Nimodipine	Nimotop	
	Nisoldipine	Sular	
	Nicardipine	Cardene	
	Isradipine	Dyna Circ	
	Verapamil	Calan, Isoptin	Same as previously stated plus bradycardia and AV block
Nonsedating antihistamine agents	Astemizole	Hismanal	No studies available; recommendation is to avoid taking grapefruit juice with astemizole
Immunosuppressant agents	Cyclosporine	Neoral, Sandimmune, SangCya	Kidney toxicity, increased susceptibility to infections
	Tacrolimus	Prograf	
Statin (HMG-CoA reductase inhibitors) agents	Atorvastatin	Lipitor	Headache, GI complaints, muscle pain, increased risk of myopathy
	Lovastatin	Mevacor	
	Simvastatin	Zocor	
Caffeine			Nervousness, overstimulation
Antianxiety, insomnia, or antidepressant agents	Buspirone	BuSpar	Increased sedation
	Diazepam	Valium	
	Alprazolam	Xanax	
	Midazolam	Versed	
	Triazolam	Halcion	
	Zaleplon	Sonata	
	Carbamazepine	Tegretol	
	Clomipramine	Anafranil	
	Trazodone	Desyrel	
Protease inhibitor agents	Saquinavir	Fortovase, Invirase	Doubles bioavailability, resulting in increased efficacy or toxicity depending on dose and patient variability
Sexual dysfunction agents	Sildenafil	Viagra	Delayed absorption (takes longer to become effective)
Medications Considered Safe for Use with Grapefruit			
	Cetirizine	Zyrtec, Reactine	
	Fexofenadine	Allegra	
	Fluvastatin	Lescol	
	Loratadine	Claritin	
	Pravastatin	Pravachol	

AV, Atrioventricular; *GI*, gastrointestinal; *HMG-CoA*, 3-hydroxy-3-methylglutaryl coenzyme A.

EVIDENCE-BASED PRACTICE

Grapefruit "Juices" Certain Medications—cont'd

Bibliography

Bailey DG, Malcolm J, Arnold O, et al: Grapefruit juice-drug interactions, *Br J Clin Pharmacol* 46(2):101, 1998.

Guo L, Fukuda K, Ohta T, et al: Role of furanocoumarin derivatives on grapefruit juice–mediated inhibition of human CYP3A activity, *Drug Metab Dispos* 28:766, 2000.

Ho PC, Saville DJ, Wanwimolruk S: Inhibition of human CYP3A4 activity by grapefruit flavonoids, furanocoumarins and related compounds, *J Pharm Pharm Sci* 4(3):217, 2001.

Hyland R, Roe EG, Jones BC, et al: Identification of the cytochrome P450 enzymes involved in the N-demethylation of sildenafil, *Br J Clin Pharmacol* 51:239, 2000.

Jetter A, Kinzig-Schippers M, Walchner-Bonjean M, et al: Effects of grapefruit juice on the pharmacokinetics of sildenafil, *Clin Pharmacol Ther* 71(1):21, 2002.

Kane GC, Lipsky JJ: Drug-grapefruit juice interactions, *Mayo Clin Proc* 75:933, 2000.

Pronsky ZM: *Food medication interactions*, ed 15, Birchrunville, PA, 2008, Food-Medication Interactions.

Schmiedlin-Ren P, Edwards DJ, Fitzsimmons ME, et al: Mechanisms of enhanced oral availability of CYP3A4 substrates by grapefruit constituents. Decreased enterocyte CYP3A4 concentration and mechanism-based inactivation by furanocoumarins, *Drug Metab Dispos* 25(11):1228, 1997.

University of Illinois Chicago College of Pharmacy Drug Information Center: *Grapefruit juice interactions*, Chicago, 2005, University of Illinois. https://www.uic.edu/pharmacy/services/di/grapefru.htm.

TABLE 18.3 Foods and Nutrients Affecting Medications

Drug Class	Examples	Use	Action	Food/Nutrients	How to Avoid
Alcohol, particularly excessive use	Beer, wine, spirits	Lower inhibitions, CNS depressant	Slows absorption	Food	Consume alcohol with food or meals
Analgesic and NSAID agents	Salicylates (aspirin), ibuprofen (Motrin, Advil), naproxen (Anaprox, Aleve, Naprosyn), acetaminophen (Tylenol)	Pain and fever	Alcohol ingestion increases hepatotoxicity, liver damage, or stomach bleeding	Alcohol	Limit alcohol intake to <2 drinks per day for men, <1 drink per day for women
Antiulcer agents (histamine blockers)	Cimetidine (Tagamet)	Ulcers	Increased blood alcohol levels, reduced caffeine clearance	Alcohol, caffeine-containing foods and beverages	Limit caffeine intake; limit alcohol intake to <2 drinks per day for men, <1 drink per day for women
Antibiotic agents	Ciprofloxacin (Cipro)	Infection	Decreases absorption	Dairy products	Avoid dairy products
Anticoagulant agents	Warfarin (Coumadin)	Blood clots	Reduced efficacy, increased anticoagulation	Vitamins K and E (supplements) may reduce efficacy, alcohol and garlic may increase anticoagulation	Consistent intake of foods high in vitamin K: broccoli, spinach, kale, turnip greens, cauliflower, Brussels sprouts; avoid high dose of vitamin E (400 IU or more)
Antineoplastic agents	Methotrexate	Cancer	Increased hepatotoxicity with chronic alcohol use	Alcohol	Avoid alcohol
Antiemetic agents	Amitriptyline HCl (Elavil), chlorpromazine HCl (Thorazine)	Antidepressant; antipsychotic/antiemetic	Increased sedation	Alcohol	Avoid alcohol
Anticonvulsant agents	Phenobarbital	Seizures, epilepsy	Increased sedation	Alcohol	Avoid alcohol
Antidepressant agents: MAOIs	Phenelzine (Nardil), tranylcypromine (Parnate)	Depression, anxiety	Rapid, potentially fatal increase in blood pressure	Foods or alcoholic beverages containing tyramine	Avoid beer; red wine; American processed, cheddar, bleu, Brie, mozzarella, and Parmesan cheeses; yogurt; sour cream; beef or chicken liver; cured meats such as sausage and salami; game meats; caviar; dried fish; avocados; bananas; yeast extracts; raisins; sauerkraut; soy sauce; miso soup; broad (fava) beans; ginseng; caffeine-containing products (colas, chocolate, coffee, tea)
Antihistamine agents	Fexofenadine (Allegra), loratadine (Claritin), cetirizine (Zyrtec), astemizole (Hismanal)	Allergies	Increases drowsiness and slows mental and motor performance	Alcohol	Use caution when operating machinery/driving

Continued

TABLE 18.3   Foods and Nutrients Affecting Medications—cont'd

Drug Class	Examples	Use	Action	Food/Nutrients	How to Avoid
Antihypertensive agents	ACE-inhibitors, angiotensin II receptor antagonists, β-blockers, verapamil HCl	Hypertension	Reduced effectiveness	Natural licorice (Glycyrrhiza glabra) and tyramine-rich foods	Avoid these foods
Antihyperlipidemic agents (HMG-CoA reductase inhibitors) or statin agents	Atorvastatin (Lipitor), lovastatin (Mevacor), pravastatin (Pravachol), simvastatin (Zocor)	High serum LDL-cholesterol	Enhances absorption, increases risk of liver damage	Food/meals, alcohol	Lovastatin should be taken with evening meal to enhance absorption; avoid large amounts of alcohol
Antiparkinsonian agents	Levodopa (Dopar, Larodopa)	Parkinson disease	Decreased absorption	High-protein foods (eggs, meat, protein supplements), vitamin B_6	Spread protein intake equally in 3–6 meals per day to minimize reaction; avoid vitamin B_6 supplements or multivitamin supplement in doses <10 mg
Antituberculosis agents	Isoniazid (INH)	Tuberculosis	Reduced absorption with foods, increased hepatotoxicity and reduced INH levels with alcohol	Alcohol	Take on empty stomach, avoid alcohol
Bronchodilator agents	Theophylline (Slo-Bid, Theo-Dur)	Asthma, chronic bronchitis, emphysema	Increased stimulation of CNS; alcohol can increase nausea, vomiting, headache, and irritability	Caffeine, alcohol	Avoid caffeine-containing foods/beverages (chocolate, colas, teas, coffee); avoid alcohol if taking theophylline medications
Corticosteroid agents	Prednisolone (Pediapred, Prelone), methylprednisolone (Solu-Medrol), hydrocortisone	Inflammation/itching	Stomach irritation	Food	Take with food or milk to decrease stomach upset
Hypoglycemic agents	Chlorpropamide (Diabinese), metformin (Glucophage)	Diabetes	Severe nausea and vomiting	Alcohol	Avoid alcohol

ACE, Angiotensin-converting enzyme; *CNS*, central nervous system; *HMG-CoA*, 3-hydroxy-3-methylglutaryl coenzyme A; *LDL*, low-density lipoprotein; *MAOIs*, monoamine oxidase inhibitors; *NSAID*, nonsteroidal antiinflammatory drug.
Data from Bland SE: Drug-food interactions, *J Pharm Soc Wisc* 28, 1998; Bobroff LB, Lentz A, Turner RE: *Food/drug and drug/nutrient interactions: what you should know about your medications,* Gainesville, 1994, University of Florida Cooperative Extension Service, Institute of Food and Agricultural Science. https://www.edis.ifas.ufl.edu; Brown CH: Overview of drug interactions. *US Pharm* 25(5), 2000. https://www.uspharmacist.com; Food and Drug Administration/National Consumers League: *Food & drug interactions,* Washington, DC, US Government Printing Office. https://www.nclnet.org/Food%20&%20Drug.pdf.

better used when taken without food and those that should be taken with food. The drug then passes through the intestinal mucosa and liver circulation before entering systemic circulation. In the systemic blood circulation system, it may be subject to metabolism, deactivation, and elimination through the so-called first-pass mechanism.

Stomach-Emptying Rate. Composition of the diet affects the rate at which food enters the small intestine from the stomach. Slow emptying of food from the stomach has the effect of doling out small portions of a drug, creating more optimal saturation rates on the absorptive sites in the small intestine. Fats, high temperatures, and solid meals prolong the time the food stays in the stomach. Food usually increases secretion of bile, acid, and gut enzymes. It also enhances intestinal motility and splanchnic blood flow. Certain food particles may adsorb drugs.

Clinical Significance. Whether these physiologic events have clinical significance depends on the extent of the effect and nature of the drug. A small change in absorption is critical for a drug with a steep dose response curve but perhaps unnoticeable for a drug with a wide range of effective concentrations. In general, the amount of absorption is clinically more important than the rate of absorption because it has increased effect on the steady-state plasma concentration of the drug after multiple doses.

Effects of Food on Drug Absorption

Increased Drug Absorption. In summary, the following five basic circumstances contribute to increased absorption of a drug:
1. *Dissolving characteristics:* When a drug does not dissolve rapidly after it has been taken, the time it remains in the stomach with food is prolonged. This increased time in the stomach may increase its effective dissolution and consequent absorption. In some instances

the drug may not dissolve properly because of either the drug or gastric pH, and it is excreted, thus decreasing absorption of the drug.

2. *Gastric-emptying time:* Delayed emptying of food from the stomach can have the effect of doling out small portions of a drug, creating more optimal saturation rates on the absorption sites in the small intestine.

3. *Nutrients:* Some nutrients can promote absorption of certain drugs. For example, high-fat diets increase absorption of the antifungal drug griseofulvin. This drug is fat soluble, and high-fat diets stimulate the secretion of bile acids, which aid in absorption of the drug. Vitamin C, as well as gastric acid, enhances iron absorption. Studies indicate that citrus fruit reduced lipoprotein oxidation in persons who consumed a high-saturated fat diet.[6] Anticoagulant drugs interact with dietary factors, and a consistent dietary intake of vitamin K is important.[7,8] Folic acid supplementation is needed when phenytoin is used for seizure control in patients with epilepsy.[9]

4. *Blood flow:* Food intake increases splanchnic blood flow carrying any ingested drugs. This direct circulation to abdominal visceral organs stimulates absorption and results in an increased availability of the accompanying drugs.

5. *Nutritional status:* In addition to the presence of specific nutrients, nutritional status may also affect the bioavailability of certain drugs in different ways. For example, the antibiotic chloramphenicol is absorbed more slowly in children with protein-energy malnutrition, but elimination of the drug is slower in well-nourished children. In both cases the effect is a net increased bioavailability of the drug.

Decreased Drug Absorption

Absorption of some drugs is delayed or reduced by the presence of food:

- *Aspirin:* Absorption of aspirin is reduced or delayed by food. It should be taken on an empty stomach with ample water, preferably cold (see section "Health Promotion" for discussion).
- *Tetracycline:* Nutritional status may also have an effect on drug absorption. For example, tetracycline absorption is impaired in malnourished individuals. Absorption of this commonly used antibiotic is also hindered when it is taken with milk, as well as with antacids or iron supplements. The drug combines with these materials to form new insoluble compounds that the body cannot absorb, causing loss of the minerals involved (i.e., calcium or iron).[6]
- *Phenytoin:* The presence of protein inhibits absorption of phenytoin. Carbohydrate increases its absorption, but fat has no effect.

Effects of Food on Drug Distribution and Metabolism
Carbohydrates and Fat

Dietary carbohydrates and fat, especially their relative quantities, influence liver enzymes that metabolize drugs. For example, the presence of fat increases the activity of diazepam (Valium). Fat increases the concentration of the unbound active drug by displacing it from binding sites in plasma and tissue protein.

Licorice

Licorice, a sweet-tasting plant extract used in making chewing tobacco, candy, and certain drugs, causes sodium retention and increased hypertension.[10] A person being treated for hypertension needs to avoid any natural licorice-containing product. The active ingredient in licorice is glycyrrhizic acid, which is named for its natural plant source, *Glycyrrhiza glabra,* meaning sweet root, a member of the legume family. An analog of this active part of licorice is marketed under the trade

FIG. 18.3 Examples of cruciferous vegetables. (Copyright 2006 Jupiter-Images Corporation.)

names Biogastrone and Duogastrone, which are widely used, especially in Europe, for healing gastric ulcers, but hypertension is a side effect.

Indoles

Indoles in cruciferous vegetables (e.g., cabbage, Brussels sprouts, broccoli, cauliflower) (Fig. 18.3) can speed up the rate of drug metabolism. They apparently induce mixed-function oxidase enzyme systems in the liver.

Cooking Methods

The method of cooking foods may alter rate of drug metabolism. For example, charcoal broiling increases hepatic drug metabolism through enzyme induction.

Vitamin Effects on Drug Action
Vitamin Effects on Drug Effectiveness. Pharmacologic doses or large megadoses beyond nutritional need of vitamins decrease blood levels of drugs when vitamins interact with the drugs. For example, large doses of folate or pyridoxine can reduce the blood level and

---

KEY TERMS

Indoles
Compounds produced in the intestines by the decomposition of tryptophan; also found in the oil of jasmine and clove.

Cruciferous
Bearing a cross; botanical term for plants belonging to the botanical family Cruciferae or Brassicaceae, the mustard family, so called because of crosslike four petaled flowers; name given to certain vegetables of this family, such as broccoli, cabbage, Brussels sprouts, and cauliflower.

effectiveness of anticonvulsive drugs such as phenytoin (Dilantin) or phenobarbital that are used for seizure control. Unwise self-medication with large drug-level doses of vitamins can cause severe toxic complications (see the Complementary and Alternative Medicine [CAM] box, "At Least It's Natural!"). On the other hand, vitamins themselves may become important medications when used as part of the medical treatment for a secondary deficiency induced by a childhood genetic or metabolic disease. Such is the case with biotin in treating certain organic acidemias or with riboflavin in treating certain defects in fatty acid metabolism.

✿ COMPLEMENTARY AND ALTERNATIVE MEDICINE (CAM)

At Least It's Natural!

The US Food and Drug Administration (FDA) does not regulate herbal remedies and dietary supplements, so the purity, potency, and safety of these products can and do vary. Manufacturers' claims of efficacy and safety are not subject to the same rigorous testing mandatory for medications. It is likely for herbs and dietary supplements to be contaminated with other herbs, pesticides, herbicides, and other products during growth, harvesting, preparation, and storage. Moreover, active chemical components in the herb may not be standardized. This leads to dissimilar potencies from lot to lot or even from capsule to capsule within the same lot. Safety, toxicity, and the likelihood of adverse interactions with other medications or treatments frequently have not been tested, particularly in children. Patients who are contemplating use of herbs and dietary supplements should proceed with caution and seek out products only from reliable manufacturers.

The reason many people give for using herbal remedies and food supplements is based in tradition (e.g., the Chinese have been using it for thousands of years!), as well as in their belief in the extensive and aggressive marketing claims that tout certain herbal remedies as "miracle cures," regardless of the lack of scientific data available to support such statements. Many turn to herbal remedies because they are considered natural and therefore seen as harmless. However, it is important to remember that hemlock, nightshade, mistletoe berries, belladonna, and poison ivy are all "natural" plants. What many do not realize is that the term *natural* is not synonymous with *safe*—especially when they combine herbs with medications.

Herb	Traditional Use[a]	Drug(s) that Interact With the Herb	Adverse Effects/Drug Interactions
Chamomile (English) (*Chamaemelum nobile, Matricaria recutita*)	Indigestion, reduce tension, and induce sleep; eczema, irritation of mucous membranes after chemotherapy or radiation (for cancer)	Anticoagulants: heparin, warfarin (Coumadin)	May increase bleeding time
		Benzodiazepines: alprazolam (Xanax), chlordiazepoxide (Librium), diazepam (Valium), flurazepam (Dalmane), lorazepam (Ativan), temazepam (Restoril), triazolam (Halcion)	Binds to benzodiazepine receptors, which may alter effect of drug
		Central nervous system (CNS) depressants: alcohol, anticonvulsants, antiemetics, antihistamines, antipsychotics, antivertigo drugs, barbiturates, hypnotics, opioids, tricyclic antidepressants, paraldehyde (Paral)	May add to sedative effect
Chasteberry (*Vitex agnus-castus*)	Premenstrual syndrome (PMS), menopausal symptoms, amenorrhea, and other menstrual irregularities; fibrocystic breasts	Hormone replacement therapy, oral contraceptives	Herb binds to estrogen receptor, may counteract oral contraceptives
Dong quai (*Angelica sinensis*)	Menstrual irregularities, menopausal complaints	Anticoagulants	May increase bleeding time; if using concurrently, then obtain prothrombin time and International Normalized Ratio (INR) to rule out interactions
Echinacea (*Echinacea angustifolia, E. pallida, E. purpurea*)	Decrease duration of colds	Immunosuppressants: azathioprine, basiliximab, cyclosporine, daclizumab, interferon, muromonab CD3, mycophenolate, sirolimus, tacrolimus, corticosteroids	May decrease immunosuppressant effect
Ma huang, ephedra (*Ephedra sinica, E. equisetina, E. intermedia*)	Bronchodilator, decongestant, CNS stimulant, diuretic	Amitriptyline (Elavil)	Drug may decrease hypertensive effect of ephedrine
		Anticonvulsants	Sympathomimetic effects, which may interfere with drug
		General anesthetics	
		Caffeine and other xanthine alkaloids	Concurrent use may result in arrhythmias
		Monoamine oxidase inhibitors (MAOIs)	Increased effects and potential toxicity
		Antihypertensives: angiotensin-converting enzyme (ACE) inhibitors, α-blockers, angiotensin II receptor blockers, β-blockers, calcium channel blockers, diuretics	Increased sympathomimetic effects
			May decrease effectiveness of drug caused by stimulant effect
		Insulin/oral hypoglycemic agents	Possible hyperglycemia with concurrent use
		Methylphenidate (Ritalin)	May displace drug from adrenergic neurons, which may decrease effectiveness of drug
		Morphine	Increases analgesic effect
		Oxytocin (Pitocin)	Possible hypertension

🌿 COMPLEMENTARY AND ALTERNATIVE MEDICINE (CAM)

At Least It's Natural!—cont'd

Herb	Traditional Use[a]	Drug(s) that Interact With the Herb	Adverse Effects/Drug Interactions
Evening primrose oil (*Oenothera biennis L*)	PMS, eczema, diabetic neuropathy, fibrocystic breasts, rheumatoid arthritis (RA)	Phenothiazines: chlorpromazine (Thorazine), fluphenazine (Prolixin), prochlorperazine (Compazine), promethazine hydrochloride (Phenergan)	May increase risk of seizures
		Anticoagulants	May increase risk of bleeding
Ginkgo (Ginkgo biloba)	Improved blood flow, protection against free-radical damage, attention-deficit hyperactivity disorder (ADHD), dementia, macular degeneration, mental performance	Aspirin or Coumadin	May increase risk of bleeding
Ginseng American (*Panax quinquefolius*) Panax or Asian (*Panax ginseng*)	ADHD, stress reduction, chronic fatigue syndrome, fibromyalgia, age-related memory loss, menopausal cloudy thinking	Insulin/oral hypoglycemic agents Oral contraceptives/hormone replacement therapy General anesthetics Caffeine and other stimulants Immunosuppressants MAOIs	May enhance hypoglycemic effect May alter effectiveness of exogenous hormones Should be discontinued 7 days before surgery; herb increases risk of hypoglycemia and bleeding Red ginseng (steamed) may be additive to stimulant effect Ginseng has immunostimulant activity and should not be used concurrently Potentiates phenelzine, causing manic symptoms
Kava (or kava-kava) (*Piper methysticum*)	Sleep disorders, antianxiety, tension headaches, menopausal anxiety, fibromyalgia	Alprazolam (Xanax) Alcohol, tranquilizers (barbiturates), and antidepressants Antiparkinsonian drugs	Synergistic CNS activity of alprazolam May potentiate action May increase tremors and make medications less effective May reduce intestinal absorption
Senna (*Cassia senna*)	Laxative, weight loss	Any drug Antiarrhythmics Corticosteroids Digoxin/cardiac glycosides Diuretics	May reduce intestinal absorption May potentiate drug May cause hypokalemia May increase effects May interfere with potassium-sparing effect
St. John's wort	Depression, seasonal affective disorder	Theophylline and β₂-agonists Selective serotonin reuptake inhibitors (SSRIs)	Possibility of increased anxiety Serotonin syndrome (sweating, agitation, tremor)
Valerian (*Valeriana officinalis*)	Sleep disorders, ADHD, menstrual cramps	Sedatives, barbiturates, CNS depressants, general anesthetics, thiopental	May intensify effects

[a]Not an exhaustive listing.
Data from Kemper K, Gardiner P, Chan E: "At least it's natural." Herbs and dietary supplements in ADHD, *Contemp Pediatr* 9:116, 2000. https://www.contemporarypediatrics.com; Kemper K, Gardiner P, Conboy LA: Herbs and adolescent girls: avoiding the hazards of self-treatment, *Contemp Pediatr* 3:133, 2000. https://www.contemporarypediatrics.com; Kuhn MA, Winston D: *Herbal therapy and supplements. A scientific and traditional approach*, ed 2, Philadelphia, 2007, Lippincott Williams & Wilkins.

Control of Drug Intoxication

Riboflavin is useful in treating boric acid poisoning. Boric acid combines with the ribitol side chain of riboflavin and is excreted in the urine. In addition, vitamin E combats pulmonary oxygen toxicity. Premature human infants at risk for development of bronchopulmonary dysplasia by oxygen treatment have been protected by vitamin E administration during the acute phase of respiratory distress requiring oxygen treatment.

NUTRITION-PHARMACY TEAM

A decade or so ago, hospitalized patients as a whole were less severely ill than they are nowadays. Now, however, as a reflection of our more complex medical system and economic reform efforts, patients who are hospitalized are more acutely ill. They are more at risk for nutritional deficits and more likely to develop malnutrition, which leads to increased lengths of stay and increased costs. The task of monitoring

TABLE 18.4	Adverse Drug Reactions Caused by Alcohol and Specific Foods		
Type of Reaction	**Drugs**	**Alcohol/Foods**	**Effects**
Flushing	Chlorpropamide (diabetes), griseofulvin, tetrachloroethylene	Alcohol	Dyspnea, headache, flushing
Disulfiram reaction	Aldehyde dehydrogenase inhibitors: disulfiram (Antabuse), calcium carbamide, metronidazole, nitrofurantoin, sulfonylureas	Alcohol, foods containing alcohol	Abdominal and chest pain, flushing, headache, nausea and vomiting
Hypoglycemia	Insulin-releasing agents: oral hypoglycemic drugs	Alcohol, sugar, sweets	Mental confusion, weakness, irrational behavior, unconsciousness
Tyramine reaction	Monoamine oxidase inhibitors (MAOIs): antidepressants such as phenelzine, procarbazine, isoniazid (isonicotinic acid hydrazide)	Foods containing large amounts of tyramine: cheese, red wines, chicken liver, broad beans, yeast	Cerebrovascular accident, flushing, hypertension

Modified from Roe DA: Interactions between drugs and nutrients. *Med Clin North Am* 63:985, 1979; Roe DA: *Diet and drug interactions*, ed 2, New York, 1979, AVI Books.

food and drug interactions is complex and requires team responsibilities. Coordinating the pharmacy, food service, and clinical nutrition minimizes adverse drug-nutrient interactions (Table 18.4).

Hospitals and other health care facilities concentrate on key processes and functions, such as drug-nutrient interactions in this case, rather than traditional strictly compartmentalized tasks of departments. Current standards continue to focus on departmental or service roles, but this is changing because of economic necessity, as well as philosophy of care. This changing focus is being shaped, for example, in the work of The Joint Commission.[11]

The Joint Commission's accreditation manual reflects the philosophy that key functions often involve different disciplines coming together as partners with clearly defined responsibilities. The team of clinical dietitians and clinical pharmacologist is clearly one of these partnerships. Current guidelines mandate monitoring of drug therapy and counseling with patients about adverse drug-nutrient interactions.[11]

HEALTH PROMOTION

THE PAIN RELIEVER DOCTORS RECOMMEND MOST

Aspirin (Fig. 18.4) has a venerable history. Being a buffered form of salicylic acid, it is a modified version of an ancient folk remedy of willow bark that had been used for many hundreds of years for fever, aches, and pain. However, the acetyl group in ASA makes aspirin easier on the stomach than willow bark.

Aspirin is an analgesic agent, an effect enhanced in combination with caffeine,[12] that is used for the relief of minor aches and pains. Its

mechanism of action is through inhibition of certain prostaglandins (see Chapter 4). The prostaglandins have a profound influence on a spectrum of physiologic functions, including blood clotting, blood pressure, inflammatory process, contraction of voluntary muscles, and transmission of nerve impulses (Table 18.5).

Studies implicate aspirin in alleviating many disorders, dangers, and discomforts, including the following:

- Risk of repeated transient ischemic attacks (TIAs), or little strokes, is reduced by 50% in men (but not in women) who have already had one.
- Many studies indicate aspirin is effective in reducing risk for myocardial infarction.
- Aspirin is one of the most effective antiinflammatory drugs and is effective in long-term treatment of arthritis.
- Aspirin may play a role in inhibiting spread of some cancers through its action of inhibiting production of prostaglandin E_2.
- Aspirin's effect as an anticoagulant is important in treatment of phlebitis and other clot-related disorders.
- Aspirin may be effective in promoting sleep. Many scientists now believe aspirin is as effective as most prescription sedatives, and it has far fewer and less serious side effects.

It is important to remember aspirin is a drug. Many of the benefits of aspirin stem from its systemic, wide-reaching effects on metabolism, which may have unforeseen, short- and long-term detrimental results. We do know that aspirin is to be strictly avoided by persons with hemophilia. In addition, allergic reactions to aspirin can be severe. Aspirin seems to be implicated in asthma. Children are especially vulnerable to side effects and should not be given aspirin without a physician's instructions.

Aspirin is an irritant to the stomach and intestine. Its continuous use is associated with low-level chronic loss of iron caused by mucosal erosion. This can lead to iron deficiency anemia. Aspirin has been linked to birth defects, especially when it is taken later in the course of pregnancy. It increases risk of infant and neonatal mortality, low birth weight, and intracranial hemorrhage.

The best way to take aspirin is on an empty stomach with a full glass of water. This is important: absorption of aspirin is facilitated by a large volume of liquid and inhibited by the presence of food. In addition, taking aspirin—especially on an empty stomach—without a large fluid intake invites erosion of the stomach lining.[13] However, aspirin should never be taken when using alcohol because it increases the bioavailability of alcohol, raising the blood concentration and thus the effect of alcohol on brain centers.[14]

FIG. 18.4 Aspirin remains one of the most popular pain relievers in the United States. (Copyright 2006 JupiterImages Corporation.)

TABLE 18.5 Is There a Difference in Pain Relievers?

Analgesic	EFFECTS		Other Effects	Trade Names
	Pain Relief	Fever Reduction		
Aspirin (acetylsalicylic acid [ASA])	✓	✓	Antiinflammatory Reduces blood clotting Gastric irritation May cause Reye syndrome in children with viral infection Allergic reaction	Ascriptin, Bayer, Bufferin, Ecotrin
Acetaminophen	✓	✓	Large doses can injure the liver or kidneys Use by persons who have three or more alcoholic drinks per day may cause liver damage	Tylenol
Ibuprofen	✓	✓	Antiinflammatory Gastric irritation Reduces blood clotting Worsens existing kidney problems	Advil, Motrin IB
Naproxen sodium	✓	✓	Antiinflammatory Reduces blood clotting Worsens existing kidney problems	Aleve
Ketoprofen	✓	✓	Antiinflammatory Gastric irritation Use by persons who have three or more alcoholic drinks per day may cause gastric bleeding	Orudis, Orudis KT

Data from Mayo Clinic Staff: *Over-the-counter pain reliever guide: compare before choosing,* Rochester, MN, 2005, Mayo Foundation for Medical Education and Research. https://www.mayoclinic.com.

TO SUM UP

Drugs can have multiple effects on the body's absorption, metabolism, retention, and nutrient status. They can provoke adverse reactions in combination with certain foods and can influence appetite, either repressing it or artificially stimulating it. Drugs can either increase an individual's absorption of nutrients or, more commonly, decrease absorption, sometimes leading to clinical deficiencies. Drugs can also induce mineral and vitamin deficiencies by their mode of action.

Just as drugs affect our use of food, food affects our use of drugs. Food can affect the absorption of drugs in a variety of ways. Foods also have an effect on subsequent distribution and metabolism of drugs. Vitamins may interfere with drug effectiveness, especially if they are taken in large doses. On the other hand, large doses of specific vitamins can be effective in countering certain toxicity conditions or a specific secondary deficiency induced by a genetic disease.

QUESTIONS FOR REVIEW

1. Name four ways food may affect drug use, and give examples of each.
2. If your patient were using a prescribed MAOI such as tranylcypromine sulfate (Parnate), what foods would you instruct the patient to avoid?
3. What is the most effective way to take aspirin? With what type of liquid should it be taken? Should it be taken with or without food? Why?
4. What foods would you suggest to a hypertensive patient on the diuretic drug hydrochlorothiazide (HCTZ) as good sources of potassium replacement?
5. Outline suggestions you would discuss with a patient experiencing a drug-induced taste loss. How would you explain the cause of the taste loss?

REFERENCES

1. Cresci G: Patient history. In Charney P, Malone AM, editors: *ADA pocket guide to nutrition assessment,* ed 2, Chicago, 2009, American Dietetic Association.
2. US Census Bureau: *Profiles of general demographic characteristics,* Washington, DC, 2006, US Government Printing Office. Retrieved April 11, 2009 from www.census.gov/.
3. Nelms M: Pharmacology. In Nelms MN, Sucher K, Long S, editors: *Understanding nutrition therapy and pathophysiology,* Belmont, CA, 2007, Wadsworth.
4. Pronsky ZM: *Food medication interactions,* ed 15, Birchrunville, PA, 2008, Food-Medication Interactions.
5. Merriman SH: Monoamine oxidase drugs and diet. *J Hum Nutr Diet* 12:21, 1999.
6. Harats D, Chevion S, Nahir M, et al: Citrus fruit supplementation reduces lipoprotein oxidation in young men ingesting a diet high in saturated fat: vitamin E presumptive evidence for an interaction between vitamins C and E in vivo, *Am J Clin Nutr* 67(2):240, 1998.
7. Harris JE: Interaction of dietary factors with oral anticoagulants: review and applications, *J Am Diet Assoc* 95(5):580, 1995.
8. Booth SL, Charnley JM, Sadowski JA, et al: Dietary vitamin K and stability of oral anticoagulation: proposal of a diet with constant vitamin K content, *Thromb Haemost* 77(3):408, 1997.
9. Lewis DP, Van Dyke DC, Willhite LA, et al: Phenytoin-folic acid interaction, *Ann Pharmacother* 29(7-8):726, 1995.

10. Morris DJ, Davis E, Latif SA, et al: Licorice, chewing tobacco, and hypertension, *N Engl J Med* 322:849, 1990.

11. The Joint Commission: *2012 Comprehensive accreditation manual for hospitals: the official handbook (CAMH)*, Oakbrook Terrace, IL, 2012, The Joint Commission.

12. Schachtel BP, Fillingim MD, Lane AC, et al: Caffeine as an analgesic adjuvant, *Arch Intern Med* 151:733, 1991.

13. Koch PA, Schultz CA, Wills RJ, et al: Influence of food and fluid ingestion on aspirin bioavailability, *J Pharm Sci* 67(11):1533, 1978.

14. Roine R, Genry RT, Munõz RH, et al: Aspirin increases blood alcohol concentration in humans after ingestion of ethanol, *JAMA* 264(18):2406, 1990.

FURTHER READINGS AND RESOURCES

Websites of Interest

- American Academy of Family Physicians. This consumer-focused site provides links to the Family Doctor website. http://www.familydoctor.org/121.xml.
- Center for Food-Drug Interaction Research and Education. This site, cosponsored by the University of Florida and Tufts University, provides education about risk and potential significance of food-drug interactions based on scientifically founded evidence. http://www.druginteractioncenter.org/.
- Grapefruit-Drug Interactions. Created for pharmacists and other allied health professionals, this page is designed to provide up-to-date information in the large body of research on grapefruit-drug interactions. http://www.powernetdesign.com/grapefruit/.
- Medline Plus. This site has gathered facts from the National Library of Medicine, National Institutes of Health, and other government agencies and health-related organizations to provide information on thousands of prescription and over-the-counter medicines. http://www.nlm.nih.gov/medlineplus/druginformation.html.
- Rx List. *The Internet Drug List, sponsored by WebMD.* This site provides food-drug interaction information for consumers and health professionals. http://www.rxlist.com/.
- US Pharmacist. *U S Pharmacist* is a monthly journal dedicated to providing up-to-date, authoritative, peer-reviewed clinical articles relevant to contemporary pharmacy practice in a variety of settings. http://www.uspharmacist.com/.

19

Nutrition Support: Enteral and Parenteral Nutrition

Pamela Charney

(e) http://evolve.elsevier.com/Williams/essentials/

In this chapter, we look at alternate modes of feeding to provide nutrition support for patients with special needs. We examine ways of feeding when the gastrointestinal (GI) tract can be used—enteral nutrition (EN) given orally or through a feeding tube. Then we review nutrient feeding directly into a vein when the GI tract cannot be used—parenteral nutrition (PN). Malnutrition, preexisting and hospital-induced, is a serious concern in hospitalized patients, especially those with critical illness or injury. Nutrition care provided by a skilled nutrition support team or clinician can have a positive effect on patient survival and recovery. This chapter will examine EN and PN support formulas, solutions, and delivery systems for use in hospital and home.

OUTLINE

NUTRITION ASSESSMENT

Nutrition Support and Degree of Malnutrition

It is an easier task to maintain nutrition than to replenish body stores lost due to malnutrition. The effect of uncomplicated starvation on the body, even during relatively brief periods, is well documented.[1] The small amount of glycogen stored in the liver is a crucial immediate energy source. Glycogen breakdown for fuel begins 2 to 3 hours after a meal, and glycogen stores are depleted after 30 hours of fasting in the absence of metabolic stress. Release of amino acids from body tissue proteins begins after 4 to 6 hours of fasting to provide a source of blood glucose. In addition, fatty acids are mobilized from the body's adipose tissues to provide keto acids as a principal fuel for heart, brain, and other vital organs. As adaptation to starvation occurs, the body relies less on amino acids from protein for fuel and uses more ketones from fat to meet metabolic needs. This reduces nitrogen losses and preserves lean body mass. During critical illness, this adaptation to insufficient energy to meet needs does not occur. Severely ill patients rely heavily on large amounts of glucose and protein for fuel. They often have elevated insulin levels, which inhibit mobilization of fat for energy production and thus increase reliance on the carbon skeleton of amino acids from protein, leading to urinary nitrogen loss of 10 to 15 g/day or more that continues unchecked. Critical illness can lead to severe depletion of lean body mass. Nutrition provided during critical illness reduces but does not reverse the process.

For example, two healthy people are hiking in the mountains and get lost. They have a limited supply of food but adequate water available from mountain streams. Hiker #1 is severely injured in a fall while the two are searching for the way back to civilization. Both have an inadequate food supply to meet their energy needs. Hiker #2 will initially use glycogen stores followed by breakdown of lean body mass and fat for energy needs. However, after several days the body will decrease its use of protein for energy and start relying on fat so that lean body mass is preserved as long as possible. This is the adaptation to starvation. Hiker #1 will not adapt to starvation. He will continue to use protein for energy and rely much less on fat for fuel and thus will lose more lean body mass during the period of inadequate energy supply than Hiker #2.

Any medical treatment has less chance of success if the patient is malnourished. The patient who becomes malnourished during hospitalization (iatrogenic malnutrition) has been referred to as *the skeleton in the hospital closet*, with several reports of general malnutrition among hospitalized patients.[2-6] Lack of adequate nutrition to meet metabolic demands is increasingly recognized as a serious concern in medical and surgical patients. Malnutrition is the end result when nutrient intake does not meet nutrient needs over some period. Braunschweig and colleagues[6] reported that as many as 54% of patients admitted to the hospital were malnourished and 31% of these patients declined nutritionally during hospitalization.

In addition, many medical and surgical diagnoses are associated with nutritional risk through impact on nutrient requirements, ability to consume nutrients, or by changing nutrient metabolism. Deterioration of a patient's nutritional status during hospitalization may contribute to increased length of hospital stay, development of comorbidities, and increased cost.[6] Persons with underlying chronic disease or traumatic injury and older adults are particularly at risk. Thus assessment, appropriate intervention, monitoring, and reassessment of nutritional status become important parts of overall care, especially for hospitalized patients (see Chapter 16). For the severely malnourished patient, especially those facing problems such as organ failure or extensive surgery, adequate and consistent provision of nutrition support is indicated. The guiding principle for provision of nutrition support is "if the gut works, then use it." Studies have shown when patients are fed appropriately enterally rather than parenterally, they experience fewer infectious complications and shorter lengths of stay and recover more rapidly.[7-9]

It is strongly recommended that nutrition risk screening be completed within 24 hours of hospital admission. The purpose of the initial nutrition screen is to quickly identify potential nutrition diagnoses, including malnutrition, so that interventions can be initiated as soon as possible. When risk for nutrition problems is identified through the admission nutrition screen, the registered dietitian (RD) should be consulted.

The RD conducts the initial nutrition assessment and performs ongoing monitoring of nutritional status. Initial assessment data supply the necessary basis for (1) identifying patients who require nutrition intervention, (2) determining an appropriate nutrition support route (i.e., enteral or parenteral), (3) calculating the patient's nutrient requirements, (4) determining specific formulations to meet those requirements, and (5) identifying measurable nutrition-related outcomes for determining if the nutrition care plan is appropriate and effective. Once therapy begins, careful monitoring maintains optimal therapy and discourages metabolic, septic, and GI complications.

Guidelines for Nutrition Assessment

Nutrition assessment is done through a standard approach and includes five key parameters: (1) evaluation of nutrient intake and adequacy, (2) nutrition-focused physical assessment, (3) biochemical laboratory data, (4) anthropometrics, and (5) comprehensive review of medical and surgical histories. Information obtained from the nutrition assessment is used to diagnose nutrition problems.[10,11] Nutrition assessment techniques and parameters are described in detail in Chapter 16. However, standard nutrition assessment parameters are adversely affected by critical illness and inflammatory response. Weight is often affected by fluid status and may no longer reflect usual or current body weight. However, experienced nutrition support RDs are able to evaluate the patient's "dry weight" by an accounting of the fluid volume infused (1 L of water weighs 1 kg). There are no laboratory values that accurately reflect nutrition status. Clinicians must rely primarily on subjective global assessment (Box 19.1) and astute clinical judgment to perform and interpret assessment of nutritional status.[5,12] Subjective global assessment focuses on history and physical examination.[5] This technique eliminates the ambiguity and nonspecific, nonsensitive nature of laboratory values during critical illness and inflammation.

KEY TERMS

Enteral
A feeding modality that provides nutrients, either orally or by tube feeding through the gastrointestinal (GI) tract.

Parenteral
A feeding modality that provides nutrient solutions intravenously rather than through the GI tract.

BOX 19.1 Subjective Global Assessment Components

History
- Change in weight
- Change in dietary intake
- Gastrointestinal (GI) symptoms
- Functional capacity
- Nutritional requirements of disease

Physical Assessment
- Loss of subcutaneous fat
- Muscle loss
- Fluid retention
- Ankle and sacral edema
- Ascites

Data from Detsky AS, McLaughlin JR, Baker JP, et al: What is subjective global assessment of nutritional status? *JPEN J Parenter Enteral Nutr* 11(1):8, 1987. Reprinted with permission of SAGE Publications.

History

History includes all aspects of the patient's health: weight change, nutrient intake, GI function and symptoms, functional capacity, and diagnosis and its nutritional effect. The clinician should identify whether the patient has experienced an intentional or nonintentional weight change from normal or usual weight and the time frame during which the weight change occurred. Quantifying weight loss is not always easy, particularly if the patient has lost lean body mass, but weight is unchanged because the patient is retaining fluid as occurs with end-stage liver, heart, and kidney diseases. Current or actual body weight (ABW) and height are interpreted according to changes from usual body weight (UBW) and the percentage of recent weight change:

$$\text{Percent UBW} = \text{ABW} \div \text{UBW} \times 100$$

$$\text{Percent weight change} = [(\text{UBW} - \text{ABW}) \div \text{UBW}] \times 100$$

The amount of recent weight change is compared with values associated with malnutrition (Table 19.1).

Changes in appetite and dietary intake must be assessed to identify overall nutrient adequacy of the diet and potential contributing factors for reported weight loss. It is important to identify diet modifications observed and nutritional supplements consumed by the patient. The clinician must verify whether nutritional supplements are being taken in addition to meals or used as a meal replacement. It should be remembered that it is not enough to simply order these supplements: They

TABLE 19.1 Categorization of Severity of Weight Loss by Percentage of Weight Lost Over Time

Time Period	Significant Weight Loss (%)	Severe Weight Loss (%)
1 Week	1–2	>2
1 Month	5	>5
3 Months	7.5	>7.5
6 Months	10	>10

Modified from the American Society for Parenteral and Enteral Nutrition (ASPEN): Nutritional and metabolic assessment of the hospitalized patient. *JPEN J Parenter Enteral Nutr* 1(1):11, 1977. Reprinted with permission of SAGE Publications.

must be consumed, and when consumed they must not take the place of food. GI function determines the ability to assimilate nutrients. The presence of nausea, vomiting, diarrhea, and anorexia inhibits nutrient intake and availability. Assessment of functional capacity of the patient determines whether the patient can perform activities of daily living (ADLs), completely or in part, or if the patient is bedridden and totally dependent on others for care. Medical and surgical history entails examination of the past and current medical problems and enables the clinician to identify potential risks for nutrient inadequacies, deficiencies, excesses, and toxicities.

Physical Examination

During the physical assessment, the clinician looks for signs of muscle and fat wasting. Inspection of the upper body can identify temporal, clavicular, and torso wasting of skeletal muscle mass and subcutaneous fat. Signs of edema and ascites indicate inability to keep fluid in the vascular space with subsequent interstitial fluid accumulation. Physical signs and symptoms are then correlated to the patient's disease process and current medical condition.

Basal Energy Expenditure

More than 200 different formulas have been proposed for use in estimating energy requirements. At this time, if indirect calorimetry is not available, the Mifflin-St. Jeor regression equation is recommended for use in most care settings. Daily energy requirements are estimated by combining basal energy expenditures (BEEs), disease and injury energy needs, and physical activity (see Chapter 8).

The Mifflin-St. Jeor equation uses measures of weight in kilograms, height in centimeters, and age in years to calculate resting energy expenditure (REE)[13]:

$$\text{Women: REE} = (10 \times \text{wt}) + (6.25 \times \text{ht}) - (5 \times \text{age}) - 161$$

$$\text{Men: REE} = (10 \times \text{wt}) + (6.25 \times \text{ht}) - (5 \times \text{age}) + 5$$

For example, the REE for a 35-year-old woman, weighing 60 kg (132 lb), standing 165 cm (5 ft 5 in) is calculated as follows:

$$(10 \times 60) + (6.25 \times 165) - (5 \times 35) - 161$$
$$= 600 + 1031 - 175 - 161 = 1295 \text{ kcal/day}$$

The term *REE* is often used interchangeably with BEE in discussing basal energy needs. In general, energy provision to critically ill patients should not exceed 20% beyond the BEE/REE. However, metabolic conditions such as severe burns or head injury create energy needs up to 50% to 100% beyond BEE.

Energy requirements for hospitalized patients on nutrition support vary with amount of metabolic stress but generally range from 20 to 35 kcal/kg.[14] Regardless of the calculation used to estimate energy expenditure, it is important to monitor the effect of nutrients provided to determine changes needed to maintain or replete the patient. Energy and nutrients are adjusted based on patient tolerance and desire versus actual response to nutrient provision. Remember that estimations of energy requirements are simply that—an estimation. Frequent follow-up and feeding adjustments ensure that desired therapeutic goals are met more so than which formula is used to estimate requirements.

The more malnourished a patient is, the more carefully resumption of nutrition should be done. Refeeding syndrome is a life-threatening response to overaggressive provision of energy to a patient who has been chronically starved. Hallmark symptoms of refeeding are a shift of electrolytes from blood into the cell, resulting in decreased blood levels of potassium, phosphorus, and magnesium, along with increased blood glucose levels and fluid retention.[15] The end result can be cardiac collapse and death. Refeeding syndrome is entirely preventable through early identification of risk combined with appropriate monitoring of serum electrolyte levels, with replacement as needed.

Critically ill patients with major trauma, sepsis, and inflammation demonstrate catabolism (i.e., breakdown of body tissue) resulting in a net loss of body mass. When protein is broken down, the nitrogen component of amino acids is released and excreted in urine. Nitrogen lost in urine can be as high as 15 to 30 g over 24 hours. This can result in a negative nitrogen balance if the patient is losing more nitrogen in urine than is provided from protein in the diet. Catabolic periods with losses of lean body mass are inevitable after trauma and extensive surgery. The catabolic process increases nutrient demand and requirements. Initiating nutrition support in these patients reduces, but does not eliminate, negative nitrogen balance that occurs after traumatic injury or critical illness.

Nitrogen Balance

Nitrogen balance studies are calculations that estimate the amount of catabolism. The patient's intake of protein (nitrogen) is subtracted from nitrogen output through urinary and insensible losses:

$$\text{Nitrogen balance} = \text{Nitrogen intake} - \text{Nitrogen loss}$$

$$\text{Nitrogen intake} = \text{Protein intake} \div 6.25$$
(6.25 g of protein yields 1 g nitrogen.)

$$\text{Nitrogen loss} = \text{Urinary urea nitrogen} + 4$$
(Estimated insensible losses of nitrogen.)

For example, a patient receiving 50 g of protein per day in an enteral tube feeding is getting 8 g of nitrogen per day (50 g ÷ 6.25 = 8 g). If that individual's nitrogen losses are 10 g per 24 hours (6 g in urine per nitrogen balance study + 4 g of insensible losses), then the patient's nitrogen balance is −2 g/24 hours. Increasing protein in the enteral tube feeding to more than 62.5 g protein per day will result in a positive nitrogen balance.

However, nitrogen balance calculation is not accurate with renal failure or retained nitrogen such as elevated blood urea nitrogen (BUN). Other sources of nitrogen such as blood products, as well as the loss of nitrogen from wounds, stool, nasogastric suction, and bleeding, must also be taken into account when calculating nitrogen balance. The 4 g of insensible nitrogen loss may not be an accurate estimate and could affect the accuracy of the results. Measurement of urinary urea nitrogen (UUN) requires an accurate 24-hour urine collection. Accurate 24-hour urine collections are very difficult to obtain in clinical settings, even in patients who have urinary catheters in place. Because of this and the expense associated with measurement of UUN, routine use of nitrogen balance cannot be recommended in clinical practice.

Hepatic Proteins as Nutrition Indicators

In the past, serum levels of the hepatic transport proteins, albumin, transferrin, and prealbumin, were used to determine the patient's nutritional status. During critical illness, hepatic production of albumin, transferrin, and prealbumin is decreased in favor of increased production of acute-phase reactants required for survival.[12,16] A decreased serum value of albumin, prealbumin, or transferrin therefore signifies an inflammatory process (or how sick the patient is) and does not provide information about the patient's nutritional status or response to nutrition therapy. These proteins are better used as prognostic indicators of the patient's risk of complications (morbidity) and death (mortality). It is no longer recommended that serum hepatic transport protein levels be used to assess nutritional status or to monitor response to nutrition support.

Management of Nutrition Support Patients

Management of nutrition support is ideally performed by an official interdisciplinary nutrition support committee or team composed of designated members from the departments of medicine, surgery, nutrition, nursing, and pharmacy.[17] Each team member should be certified in nutrition support by an accrediting body such as the National Board of Nutrition Support Certification and the Board of Pharmaceutical Specialties. The American Society for Parenteral and Enteral Nutrition (ASPEN) has developed standards of practice for nutrition support professionals and interdisciplinary nutrition support competencies.[18-22] However, in many facilities, nutrition support management is overseen by an informal collection of interested clinicians, a sole nutrition support practitioner, or no one person in particular. Standards of The Joint Commission and the Accreditation Manual for

Hospitals (AMH) have focused on key multidisciplinary processes that ensure performance of nutrition screening and assessment to promote quality patient outcomes.[23] (For additional considerations surrounding nutrition support, see the Focus on Culture box, "What's Religion Got to Do With It?")

Baseline nutrition data obtained before starting nutrition support provide a means of measuring effectiveness of treatment. At designated periods during therapy, certain tests are repeated to monitor the patient's course and reduce metabolic complications. Specific protocols vary in different medical centers. However, a general guide for standard monitoring data is summarized in Box 19.2.[24]

In general, clinicians give primary importance to the following three major monitoring parameters: (1) serial weights to determine the adequacy of total energy provision and to monitor fluid status, (2) physical examination for micronutrient adequacy and changes in body fat and muscle mass, and ultimately (3) improvement in clinical and functional status.

🌐 FOCUS ON CULTURE

What's Religion Got To Do With It?

"That was not a natural death. It was an imposed death," said Cardinal Renato Martino, a top Vatican official. "When you deprive somebody of food and water, what else is it? Nothing else but murder." In this impassioned statement, the cardinal was referring to the landmark battle over the life of Terri Schiavo after her death after nearly 2 weeks without any nutrition support. More than 15 years had passed since Terri Schiavo had suffered severe brain damage stemming from heart failure and had relied on enteral nutrition (EN) for survival ever since. The legal decision to stop her tube feeding created a national uproar and sparked many debates over end-of-life issues, including nutrition support. The Catholic Church fervently opposed the legal action taken and was especially vocal in the events surrounding Terri Schiavo's death because she was Catholic.

What role does religion have in issues such as nutrition support? In this section, we will encapsulate beliefs of three religions, focusing on end-of-life issues, particularly nutrition support.

Catholicism

Because Catholics believe they are stewards of their bodies and life is to be respected, the act of withholding nutrition support is not something to be taken lightly. However, bodily life is not to be maintained at all costs. The late Pope John Paul II wrote: "Certainly there is a moral obligation to care for oneself and allow oneself to be cared for, but this duty must take account for concrete circumstances. It needs to be determined whether the means of treatment available are objectively proportionate to the prospects for improvement."

In short, withdrawal of nutrition support is not condemned, but rather only recommended when quality of life is so low that nutrition is of absolutely no benefit. Although it is hard to know where the point of "no benefit" is, it is the duty of a Catholic to promote a social order in which a certain level of responsibility exists for those who are marginalized or in a vegetative state. Each case merits special consideration, and in most cases, nutrition is considered a basic form of care likened to warmth and cleanliness.

Judaism

According to Judaism, life possesses an intrinsic value as a divine gift of creation. As in Catholicism, humans are thought to be only a temporary steward of the body and therefore must treat the body with utmost respect and sensitivity. Jewish law mandates humans must do everything in their power to heal themselves when ill and must also strive to save the lives of others. However, this obligation applies only to those therapies that have a

reasonable chance of success, and, although some believe tube feeding is equivalent to medical treatments, Jewish tradition disagrees with this opinion. According to Jewish authorities, nutrition in any form is a basic human need and should be provided to all patients unless feeding itself causes suffering. Consequently, Jewish law further accentuates feeding must be done in a kind and compassionate manner, emphasizing the importance this religion places on nourishment.

Islam

Not unlike the other religions mentioned in this section, in Islam humans are thought of as stewards of their bodies, which are viewed as a gift from God. Sanctity of life is a monumental principle, and every moment of life is deemed precious and must be preserved. Even so, death is believed to be a natural part of life, and treatment does not have to be provided if it merely prolongs the final stages of a terminal illness. Nutrition support—especially EN—is considered part of basic care rather than a treatment; therefore it is a religious obligation to provide nourishment unless such an act shortens life.

Religion and end-of-life issues like nutrition support are complicated and sensitive matters that must be approached with understanding and tolerance. People from different religious backgrounds can have varying views on this subject that can drastically affect the choice of care provided. The Terri Schiavo case brought to life a plethora of issues that will not likely be resolved any time soon; however, when dealing with nutrition support cases, it is important to consider the implications that the patient's religion can have for your decisions and actions.

Bibliography

Associated Press: Vatican: Schiavo's death "cruel." *Fox News* March 31, 2005 (News broadcast).

Clarfield AM, Gordon M, Markwell H, et al: Ethical issues in end-of-life geriatric care: the approach of three monotheistic religions—Judaism, Catholicism, and Islam. *J Am Geriatr Soc* 51:1149, 2003.

Cooley M: Faith, ethics help many in agonizing dilemma. *The Spokesman-Review* A1, 2005.

Huggins C: *Survey finds physicians willing to allow patients' religion to trump medical advice*, New York, 2005, Reuters Health (News release).

Jotkowitz A, Clarfield A, Slick S: The care of patients with dementia: a modern Jewish ethical perspective, *J Am Geriatr Soc* 53:881, 2005.

Sunshine E: Sunshine, Truncating Catholic tradition: Florida bishops avoid full consideration of ethical issues in Schiavo case. *Natl Cathol Report* 41:23, 2005. From http://www.natcath.com/NCR_Online/archives2/2005b/040805/040805k.php.

BOX 19.2 Clinical Parameters to Monitor During Nutrition Support

Daily I/O
Daily weights
Physical examination
Temperature, pulse, respirations
Laboratory parameters:

- Acid-base status
- Blood urea nitrogen (BUN)
- Complete blood cell count (CBC)
- Creatinine
- Electrolytes
- Glucose
- International normalized ratio (INR)
- Liver function tests
- **Osmolarity**, serum and urine
- Platelet count
- Prothrombin time (PT)
- Triglyceride level
- Urinary urea nitrogen
- Urine specific gravity
- Vitamins and minerals

KEY TERM

Osmolarity
The number of millimoles of liquid or solid in a liter of solution; parenteral nutrition solutions given by central vein have an osmolarity around 1800 mOsm/L; peripheral parenteral solutions are limited to 600 to 900 mOsm/L (dextrose and amino acids have the greatest effect on a solution's osmolarity).

All baseline and monitoring data are recorded in the patient's medical record, along with all enteral and parenteral solution orders.

No evidence-based "rules" exist for the time to start nutrition support with either EN or PN. Determination of when to initiate nutrition support depends on the patient's nutritional status and the anticipated time period before oral diet can be resumed and tolerated. The ASPEN guidelines[7] recommend that nutrition support should be considered when the patient has had an inadequate oral intake for 7 to 14 days or the patient's oral intake is anticipated to remain inadequate for 7 to 14 days. A 5- to 10-day timeline is recommended for critically ill patients. Other guidelines available to identify when to feed are the "rule of five" and amount of weight loss. The rule of five states that if a patient has

had no food for 5 days and is unable to tolerate an oral diet for an additional 5 days, nutrition support should be considered to reduce the risk of developing malnutrition. The weight loss rule stratifies patients according to the percentage of weight loss of their usual total body weight over a designated period (see Table 19.1). Patients who have undergone severe weight loss and are unable to tolerate oral nutrition for 5 to 7 days or longer are candidates for nutrition support.

ENTERAL NUTRITION VERSUS PARENTERAL NUTRITION

Debate continues concerning evidence-based effectiveness of PN and EN support. Questions focus on what constitutes early EN, how to select the most appropriate enteral tube feeding formula according to each patient's specific disease state, what is the preferred method of formula delivery, and which factors contribute to enteral tube feeding–related complications, such as diarrhea or respiratory problems.[25,26] In all cases when the GI tract is functioning, EN support should be used to restore or maintain an optimal state of nutrition. PN should be reserved for patients with a nonfunctional GI tract or an inadequately functional GI tract that prevents the patient from meeting nutrient needs enterally. In some cases, the patient can take some enteral feeding, but impairment in either digestive or absorptive capacity requires supplementation with parenteral therapy. The Veterans Affairs Cooperative Study showed perioperative nutrition support was beneficial for severely malnourished patients but contributed to increased complications in mild to moderately malnourished patients.[27] However, patients enrolled in the Veterans Affairs Cooperative Study were fed significantly more than estimated requirements, which may have contributed to complications. The GI tract should always be the first choice for nutrition support. Fig. 19.1 provides an algorithm for determining the route of nutrition support.[7]

PN is associated with risk for serious complications, as shown in Box 19.3. Reliance on PN when the GI tract is functional can contribute to disuse of the GI tract, with subsequent bacterial overgrowth, hepatic abnormalities, deterioration of GI integrity with subsequent migration of intestinal bacteria into the systemic circulation, and sepsis. Patients reliant solely on PN are at risk for septic and hepatic complications that can contribute to morbidity and mortality. The GI tract is the body's largest immune organ. (To learn more about probiotics and how they contribute to EN and PN, see the Evidence-Based Practice box, "Probiotics.") GI disease that prevents or reduces use of the GI tract may itself contribute to adverse effects often associated with PN. Therefore it may not be the route of feeding, but rather the inability to use the gut that increases infectious and metabolic complications.[28]

EVIDENCE-BASED PRACTICE

Probiotics

The popularity of probiotics has increased greatly in recent years, but the truth is that probiotics have been the subject of research for some time now. In fact, probiotics have been researched so often that a joint effort by the Food and Agriculture Organization of the United Nations (FAO) and World Health Organization (WHO) established guidelines for the evaluation of probiotics in food in October 2001.[1]

Probiotics have been defined as "live microorganisms that, when administered in adequate amounts, confer a health benefit on the host."[1] Some of the confirmed positive consequences of ingested probiotics include enhanced lactose digestion for individuals with lactose intolerance, reduced incidence of sepsis, and enhanced

hepatic function for patients with alcohol-related or hepatitis C–related cirrhosis, to name just a few.[1,2] The negative side effects of probiotic ingestion are, at best, rare and limited to individuals with underlying medical conditions.[1]

Intestinal microflora survive by consuming very small amounts of indigestible food that people eat. The waste products of the microflora can be beneficial, including the production of vitamin K and medium-chain fatty acids, which the host can use.[3] During periods of fasting, or when the diet does not supply sufficient nutrition for the microflora, they decrease in number.

Periods of fasting and decreased gastric motility are often found hand in hand with patients on parenteral nutrition (PN) or enteral nutrition (EN). Decreased

Continued

EVIDENCE-BASED PRACTICE

Probiotics—cont'd

gastric motility is also a common and serious problem in critically ill patients. The decreased motility can affect EN efforts, resulting in atrophy of intestinal mucosa, sepsis, and multiple organ failure. Although probiotics have not been found to effectively reverse the effects of inhibited gastric motility, they have been proven effective in managing all forms of diarrhea. To understand the importance of effectively managing diarrhea, see the *Case Study* box at the end of this chapter.

Because of the nature of numerous procedures performed in hospitals, many patients are, at least in the short term, left in a fasting state for the purpose of surgical preparation, as well as for other reasons. Probiotics have been shown to have beneficial effects on patients during fasting periods, and administration of probiotics can help maintain nutritional status, including enhanced recovery from malnutrition and reduced mucosal atrophy, at least in animal models.[4]

However, probiotics may have little clinical significance in critically ill patients. In one study the probiotic *Lactobacillus plantarum* 299v was enterally fed to critically ill patients.[3] A significantly delayed attenuation of systemic inflammatory response syndrome (SIRS) was found in the treatment group versus the probiotic group, although the design of the study could not confirm this delayed attenuation was caused by the probiotics.

The end result of the study concluded that probiotics may play a hand in delaying SIRS but could not reduce morbidity or mortality in critically ill patients.

In the end, consumer acceptance and researcher curiosity are spurring the demand for more research into the beneficial effects of probiotics. Probiotics are being studied at an increasing rate, and research is showing promising results; however, not enough consistent information is available to make a professional recommendation to use probiotics in the treatment of patients on EN or PN. Perhaps with more time, probiotics may find a place in assisting those on EN or PN, but for now we will simply have to accept that probiotics have a place only in the intestines of the healthy.

References

1. *FAO/WHO guidelines for the evaluation of probiotics in food. Joint FAO/WHO Working Group report on drafting guidelines for the evaluation of probiotics in food*, London, Ontario, 2002, pp 1–11.
2. O'Brien A, Williams R: Nutrition in end-stage liver disease: principles and practice, *Gastroenterology* 134:1729, 2008.
3. McNaught CE, Woodcock NP, Anderson AD, et al: A prospective randomized trial of probiotics in critically ill patients, *Clin Nutr* 24:211, 2005.
4. Dock DB, Latorraca MQ, Aguilar-Nascimento JE, et al: Probiotics enhance recovery from malnutrition and lessen colonic mucosal atrophy after short-term fasting in rats, *Nutrition* 20:473, 2004.

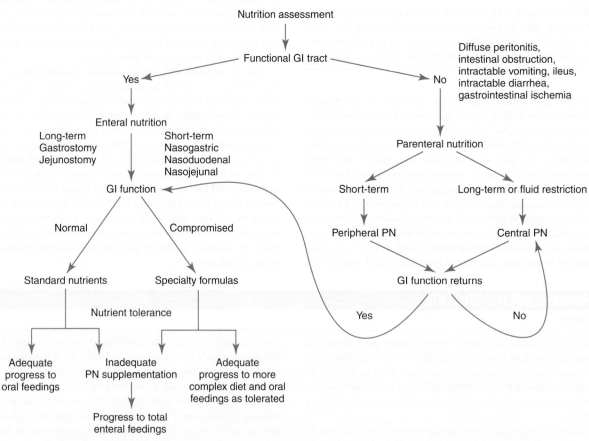

FIG. 19.1 Route of administration of specialized nutrition support. *GI,* Gastrointestinal; *PN,* parenteral nutrition. (Reprinted from ASPEN Board of Directors: *Clinical pathways and algorithms for delivery of parenteral and enteral nutrition support in adults,* Silver Spring, MD, ASPEN, 1998, p 5.)

BOX 19.3   Complications Associated With Parenteral Nutrition

Catheter-Related Complications
- Air embolism
- Catheter embolization
- Catheter occlusion
- Improper tip location
- Phlebitis
- Pneumothorax
- Sepsis
- Venous thrombosis

Gastrointestinal Complications
- Fatty liver
- Gastric hyperacidity
- GI atrophy
- Hepatic cholestasis

Metabolic Complications
- Acid-base imbalance
- Electrolyte abnormalities
- Essential fatty acid deficiency
- Fluid imbalance
- Glucose intolerance
- Metabolic bone disease
- Mineral abnormalities
- Overfeeding
- Refeeding syndrome
- Triglyceride elevation

ENTERAL TUBE FEEDING IN CLINICAL NUTRITION

Modes of Enteral Nutrition Support

Many patients with a functioning GI tract do not or cannot eat a sufficient amount of nutrients by mouth to restore, repair, or maintain physiologic systems or body tissues. The first option for providing adequate nutrition should be to deliver nutrients orally. The patient can be given small, frequent, nutrient-dense meals. If oral intake remains suboptimal despite attempts to increase nutrient intake via diet changes, then enteral tube feeding can be initiated to meet nutrient and energy requirements. If it is not feasible to use the GI tract for feeding or if the GI tract cannot effectively provide consistent and adequate nutrition, then PN may be an appropriate feeding modality. Therefore the following questions must be answered:
- Does the patient require nutrition support?
- What is the optimal route of feeding: oral, tube feeding, or parenteral?
- Will the enteral route alone be sufficient to meet nutrient and energy requirements?
- What type of formula is needed, and how should it be provided?
- Does the patient require long-term nutrition support?

Oral Diet

When a patient does not consume a nutritionally complete diet, the energy value of foods in the oral diet can be increased according to patient tolerance and preference with added sauces, seasonings, and dressings. Frequent, less bulky, concentrated small meals may be helpful so that the patient is not overwhelmed or discouraged by a tray full of food. If a patient is on a modified diet (e.g., a low-fat, low-sodium, or diabetic diet), then liberalization of the diet as much as is medically feasible can help improve oral intake. For example, changing from a regimented 1800-kcal diabetic diet to a carbohydrate-counting diet allows the patient more flexibility in food selection. In some cases it may be necessary to liberalize to an unrestricted or regular diet to increase oral intake. Depending on the patient's condition and food preferences, snacks, milkshakes, or oral liquid nutritional supplements can be provided between meals. It is important to ensure frequent patient visits when ordering liquid nutritional supplements, because taste fatigue can happen fairly rapidly when patients are receiving two to six cans of an oral nutritional supplement per day. In addition, patients may use their nutritional supplements as meal replacements, therefore not increasing overall energy and nutrient intake. It is important to offer a variety of snacks and nutritional supplements in different flavors to maintain adequate consumption. Some facilities, particularly those specializing in long-term care, have found that dispensing oral nutritional supplements in small amounts of 30 to 60 mL during times when medications are administered improved oral nutritional supplement intake and nutrient delivery.[29,30]

Enteral Tube Feeding

If a sufficient oral intake of nutrients and energy is not possible, then the next option is EN by tube feeding, either as a supplement to oral dietary intake or as the sole source of nutrition.

Indications for Enteral Tube Feeding

ASPEN has published guidelines for indications for nutrition support.[7] Enteral tube feeding is indicated for patients who are (or who are likely to become) malnourished and unable or unwilling to consume adequate nutrition by mouth. Factors that affect the decision to provide enteral tube feeding include the patient's preadmission nutritional status, risk for malnutrition based on current disease or condition, ability to consume a nutritionally complete oral diet, and functional status of the GI tract. Research found no benefit to aggressive early enteral tube feeding for patients who were not malnourished versus those who waited 6 days to begin an oral diet.[31]

ENTERAL TUBE FEEDING FORMULAS

Complete Enteral Tube Feeding Formulas

Blenderized Formulas

Prior to the availability of commercial enteral formulas, enteral formulas were prepared by blenderizing regular diets and using broth or gravy to thin the mixture enough to flow through feeding tubes. Currently the majority of enteral tube feedings in health care facilities are given with a defined, commercially prepared enteral tube feeding formula. However, financial or personal reasons may motivate a patient or family to use blenderized formulas for home enteral tube feeding. Many feel that emotional comfort may be achieved by using home-prepared enteral formulas. With proper attention given to nutrient content and sanitary precautions, use of home-prepared enteral formulas can be safely done. Care should be taken to ensure that homemade formulas are prepared properly to avoid tube clogging, bacterial contamination, and inconsistent nutrient adequacy. The blenderized formula must be given into the stomach and requires a normal GI tract to digest and absorb the nutrients contained in the formula.

Commercial Enteral Tube Feeding Formulas

In contrast to homemade enteral formulas, commercial enteral tube feeding formulas provide sterile, nutritionally complete, homogenized solutions suitable for small-bore enteral feeding tubes. Enteral tube feeding formulas are available as polymeric, semielemental or oligomeric, and elemental or monomeric formulas (Table 19.2).[32] It is important to

TABLE 19.2   Categories and Macronutrient Sources for Various Types of Enteral Formulas

Type of Formula	Protein Sources	Carbohydrate Sources	Fat Sources	kcal/ mL	Protein Content	Nonprotein Calorie-to-Nitrogen Ratio	Examples
Intact (Polymeric)							
	Calcium and magnesium caseinates	Maltodextrin	Medium-chain triglycerides	1–2	30–84 g/L	75–177:1	Boost (No)
		Corn syrup solids					Compleat (No)
	Sodium and calcium caseinates	Sucrose	Canola oil				Fibersource (No)
		Cornstarch	Corn oil				Isocal (No)
	Soy protein isolate	Glucose polymers	Lecithin				Isosource (No)
	Calcium potassium caseinate	Sugar	Soybean oil				Jevity (R)
		Vegetables	Partially hydrogenated				Nutren (Ne)
	Delactosed lactalbumin	Fruits	soybean oil				Osmolite (R)
	Egg white solids	Nonfat milk	High-oleic safflower				Resource (No)
	Beef		oil				TwoCal HN (R)
	Nonfat milk		Beef fat				Ultracal (No)
Hydrolyzed (Oligomeric or Monomeric)							
	Enzymatically hydrolyzed whey or casein	Hydrolyzed cornstarch	Medium-chain triglycerides	1–1.33	21–52.5 g/L	67–282:1	Advera (R)
							AlitraQ (R)
	Soybean or lactalbumin hydrolysate	Sucrose	Sunflower oil				Criticare HN (No)
		Fructose	Lecithin				Crucial (Ne)
	Whey protein	Maltodextrin	Soybean oil				Peptamen (Ne)
	Soy protein hydrolysate	Tapioca starch	Safflower oil				Perative (R)
		Glucose oligo-saccharides	Corn oil				Tolerex (No)
			Coconut oil				Vital HN (R)
			Canola oil				Vivonex Plus (No)
			Sardine oil				
Modular							
Protein	Low-lactose whey and casein	—	—	Per 100 g 370–424	Per 100 g 75–88.5	—	Casec (No)
							ProMod (R)
	Calcium caseinate						Resource Protein
	Free amino acids						Powder (No)
Carbohydrate	—	Maltodextrin	—	Per 100 g 380–386	—	—	Moducal (No)
		Hydrolyzed cornstarch					
Fat	—	—	Safflower oil	Per 1 tbsp 67.5–115	—	—	MCT Oil (No)
			Polyglycerol esters of fatty acids				Microlipid (No)
			Soybean oil				
			Lecithin				
			Medium-chain triglycerides				
			Fish oil				

Ne, Nestle; *No,* Novartis; *R,* Ross.
Modified from Gottschlich MM, Shronts EP, Hutchins AM: Defined formula diets. In Rombeau JL, Rolandelli RH, editors: *Clinical nutrition: enteral and tube feeding*, ed 3, Philadelphia, 1997, Saunders.

keep abreast of products currently available because new formulations and enteral tube feeding products are constantly being developed. Polymeric enteral tube feeding formulas require digestion and are available with and without fiber. Macronutrients and micronutrients of a polymeric tube feeding formula can be modified for specific needs of patients with various disease states. Semielemental or oligomeric tube feeding formulas are partially digested or hydrolyzed. Smaller molecules increase the osmolality of the formula. Elemental or monomeric tube feeding formulas are completely predigested and require only absorption

for assimilation into the body. These formulas have the highest osmolality, lowest viscosity, and worst taste of all enteral tube feeding formulas. Enteral tube feeding formulas will also vary according to nutrient density from 1 to 2 kcal/mL. More concentrated formulas are designed for patients with fluid intolerance, such as those with renal, hepatic, or cardiac failure, as well as for patients who desire less volume or fewer feedings per day. However, if patients who receive a concentrated enteral tube feeding formula do not have fluid restrictions, it is imperative to provide adequate water so that they do not become dehydrated.

Nutrient Components

Carbohydrates

Approximately 50% to 60% of the energy in the American diet comes from carbohydrates, the vast majority of this from starches and sugars. Carbohydrates are the body's primary energy source (see Chapter 3). Although large starch molecules are well tolerated and easily digested by most patients, their relative insolubility creates problems in enteral tube feeding formulas. Thus smaller sugars formed by partial or complete breakdown of cornstarch and other glucose polymers are common tube feeding formula components (see Table 19.2).[32] Very few enteral tube feeding formulas contain lactose, because lactose intolerance is common among hospitalized patients. Tube feeding formulas can also contain soluble and insoluble fiber. Considerable controversy exists as to the benefit of providing fiber in enteral tube feeding formulations.[25,32] Insoluble fiber increases stool volume and thus is used to treat problems with gastric motility such as constipation or diarrhea. Soluble fiber has been promoted to improve blood sugar control, reduce serum cholesterol levels, and maintain colon health. The focus on maintaining normal intestinal bacteria has resulted in increased research and availability of prebiotics and probiotics given with or in enteral tube feeding formulas. Prebiotics, nondigestible food components, provide fuel to enhance repletion of normal bacteria found in the GI tract, whereas probiotics, live nonpathogenic microbes, are designed to repopulate by providing "good" bacteria directly to the GI tract.[33] The strain of probiotic and combination of strains most effective depends on the therapeutic intent (see Evidence-Based Practice box, "Probiotics" for more information).

Protein

Protein content of standard enteral tube feeding formulas is designed to maintain body cell mass and promote tissue synthesis and repair (see Chapter 5). Biologic quality of dietary protein depends on its amino acid profile, especially its relative proportions of essential amino acids. To supply these needs, the following three major forms of protein are used in nutrition support enteral tube feeding formulas: (1) intact proteins, (2) hydrolyzed proteins, and (3) crystalline amino acids (see Table 19.2).[32]

1. *Intact proteins:* Intact proteins are the complete and original forms as found in foods, although protein isolates such as lactalbumin and casein from milk are intact proteins that have been separated from their original food source. These larger polypeptides and proteins must be broken down further (digested) before they can be absorbed.
2. *Hydrolyzed proteins:* Hydrolyzed proteins are protein sources that have been broken down by enzymes into smaller protein fragments and amino acids. These smaller products—tripeptides, dipeptides, and free amino acids—are absorbed more readily into the blood circulation.
3. *Crystalline amino acids:* Pure crystalline amino acids are readily absorbed, particularly when combined in a mix of dipeptides and tripeptides. The small size of the amino acid results in an increase in osmolality of the formula. Amino acids result in a bitter-tasting formula. If an elemental tube feeding formula is used as an oral supplement, then it requires flavoring aids or special preparation methods to improve taste (e.g., pudding, frozen slush, Popsicle). However,

despite flavorings, the taste can still be unacceptable to a sick patient or can quickly lead to taste fatigue and refusal by the patient.

Fat

The major roles of fat in an enteral tube feeding formula are to supply a concentrated energy source, essential fatty acids, and a transport mechanism for fat-soluble vitamins. Major forms of fat used in standard formulas are butterfat in milk-based mixtures; vegetable oils from corn, soy, safflowers, or sunflowers; medium-chain triglycerides (MCTs); and lecithin (see Table 19.2).[32] Vegetable oils supply a rich source of the essential fatty acids—linoleic and linolenic acids. Researchers continue to examine outcomes related to enteral tube feeding formulas containing various combinations of short-chain fatty acids, medium-chain fatty acids, and omega-3 fatty acids (see Chapter 4).[34,35]

Vitamins and Minerals

Standard whole-diet commercial tube feeding formulas provide 100% of the Recommended Dietary Allowance (RDA) and Dietary Reference Intake (DRI) for vitamins and minerals when the formula is provided at a specific volume per day. The volume required to provide the RDA-DRI varies with each tube feeding formula and the nutrient requirements of the patient. Delivery of a reduced volume and use of diluted formulas may require supplementation with vitamin and mineral preparations. Patients with nutrient deficiencies may require supplementation of specific vitamins and minerals in addition to the standard vitamin and mineral composition of the enteral tube feeding formula. Several enteral tube feeding formulas are designed for specific patient populations and contain micronutrients designed to meet the requirements of the particular disease state or condition.

Physical Properties

After selecting a tube feeding formula according to the patient's nutritional requirements and GI function, the clinician must consider physical properties of the formula that can affect tolerance. Individual intolerance is reflected in delayed gastric emptying, abdominal distention, cramping and pain, diarrhea, or constipation. A factor often evaluated when a patient demonstrates intolerance is osmolality of the enteral tube feeding formula. Osmolality is based on concentration of the formula and defined as number of osmotic particles per kilogram of solvent (water), energy-nutrient density, and residue content. However, no evidence indicates that enteral tube feeding formula osmolality is the primary contributor to formula intolerance. Enteral tube feeding formulas can approximate 600 mOsm, whereas some medications are 4000 mOsm or more. Signs and symptoms of enteral tube feeding intolerance, of which diarrhea is the most common, are more often related to inappropriate tube feeding techniques or drug interactions.

Medical Foods for Special Needs

Certain tube feeding formulas designed for special nutrition therapy are called medical foods. The US Food and Drug Administration (FDA) first recognized the concept of medical foods as distinct from drugs in 1972, when the first special formula was developed for treatment of the genetic disease phenylketonuria (PKU) in newborns (see Chapter 12). The definition of medical foods remained rather murky as medical research developed an increasing number of special formulas. The Orphan Drug Act has defined *medical food* as a food that is formulated to be consumed or administered enterally under the supervision of a physician and that is intended for the specific dietary management of a disease or condition for which distinctive nutritional requirements, based on recognized scientific principles, are established by medical evaluation. The Orphan Drug Act was subsequently incorporated into the reformed Nutrition Labeling and Education Act of 1990.

An explosion of specialty enteral tube feeding formulas has occurred over the past 10 years. Several products are available in each category of disease- or condition-specific formulation: (1) end-stage renal disease, (2) hepatic disease, (3) pulmonary disease, (4) diabetes mellitus, (5) malabsorption syndromes, (6) immunoincompetence, (7) oncology, and (8) metabolic stress. Every patient with one of the previous diagnoses does not need a specialty tube feeding formula. Indications for specialty tube feeding formulas are limited to a small subset of patients within each disease state classification for which a specialty formula is designed. Considerable debate exists regarding the treatment value and cost-effectiveness of specialty tube feeding formulas; therefore scientific evidence to support their use is needed before use can be recommended.[25]

Modular Enteral Tube Feeding Formulas

Commercially available, nutritionally complete enteral formula products for tube feeding are designed with a fixed ratio of nutrients to meet general standards for nutritional needs. However, some patients' particular needs are not met by these standard fixed-ratio tube feeding formulas, and they require an individualized modular formula. An individual formula, composed completely of modular components, is planned, calculated, prepared, and administered with the expertise of the RD. Modular enteral components are listed in Table 19.2. However, the more common use of modular components is the addition of carbohydrate, fat, or protein to a commercial formula to individualize the calorie and protein content of the formula for the patient. For example, additional protein powder can be added to increase the amount of protein per liter, or more carbohydrate or fat can be added to increase energy concentration. Other modular nutrients such as fiber and probiotics or prebiotics can also be added to the feeding regimen but should be given separately through the feeding tube and not added directly to the commercial tube feeding formulation. Every component added to an enteral tube feeding formula can increase the osmolality and viscosity of the formula and contribute to feeding intolerance, bacterial contamination, or clogging of the feeding tube.

In the past it was common practice to add blue food dye to tube feeding formulas to detect aspiration of formula into the trachea and lungs. Concern exists as to safety, specificity, and sensitivity of blue dye in identifying aspiration in tube-fed patients.[36-38] The addition of blue food dye increases risk of bacterial contamination, false-positive occult stool test, discoloration of the skin and body fluids, and death. In addition, no standardization exists for how much food dye to add per liter of tube feeding formula, with formula hues ranging from pale to cobalt blue. Methylene blue should not be added to tube feeding formulas because it can adversely affect cellular function.[39] Colored dyes are not diagnostic for aspiration, are potentially harmful, and should not be added to tube feedings.[38] Nonrecumbent positioning (elevating the head of the bed 30–40 degrees) is an evidence-based method for aspiration prevention and should be emphasized in all tube-fed patients.[38]

ENTERAL TUBE FEEDING DELIVERY SYSTEMS

Tube Feeding Equipment

Nasoenteric Feeding Tubes

Small-bore nasoenteric feeding tubes, generally from 8 to 10 French, made of softer, more flexible polyurethane and silicone materials, have replaced former large-bore stiff tubing. Small-bore feeding tubes are more comfortable for patients and permit the infusion of commercially available enteral tube feeding formulas. Nasoenteric tubes can be inserted into either the stomach or beyond the pyloric valve into the small intestine (Fig. 19.2).[40] Distal placement of a feeding tube beyond the ligament of Treitz into the jejunum is often preferred for patients with a history or risk of aspiration, impaired gastric emptying, depressed gag reflex, neurologic impairment, and critical illness.[26] Feeding tube insertion can be done blindly at the bedside or using radiographic visualization. Placement of a feeding tube should be performed by experienced, trained personnel. Feeding tube placement is an invasive procedure and carries the risk of misplacement into the lungs, as well as perforation of the GI tract. During placement, aspirates of GI contents can be checked for pH and enzyme concentration, as well as visually inspected to reduce the number of radiographs required to determine when the desired location has been reached.[41] However, no tube feeding should be infused until feeding tube placement is confirmed by radiography.

Tube Feeding Enterostomies

Nasoenteric tube placement is usually indicated for short-term therapy. However, for enteral feeding anticipated to last more than 3 to 4 weeks, surgically or endoscopically placed enterostomies are preferred (see Fig. 19.2),[40] as follows:

- *Esophagostomy:* A cervical esophagostomy can be placed at the level of the cervical spine to the side of the neck after head and neck surgeries for cancer or traumatic injury. This removes the discomfort of

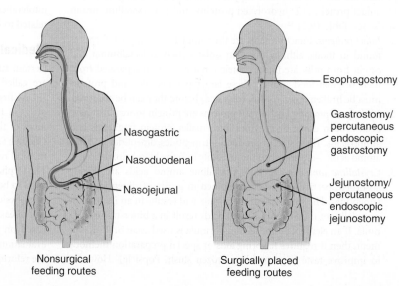

FIG. 19.2 Types of enteral feeding routes. (From Rolin Graphics in Grodner M, Anderson SL, DeYoung S: *Foundations and clinical applications of nutrition: a nursing approach,* ed 2, St Louis, 2000, Mosby.)

Nasogastric

Nasoduodenal

Nasojejunal

Nonsurgical feeding routes

Esophagostomy

Gastrostomy/ percutaneous endoscopic gastrostomy

Jejunostomy/ percutaneous endoscopic jejunostomy

Surgically placed feeding routes

a nasoenteric tube, and the entry point can be concealed under clothing. Esophagostomies are only rarely used.

- *Gastrostomy:* A gastrostomy tube is surgically or endoscopically placed in the stomach if the patient is not at risk for aspiration and has normal gastric motility.
- *Jejunostomy:* A jejunostomy tube is surgically or endoscopically placed past the ligament of Treitz in the jejunum, the middle section of the small intestine. This procedure is indicated for patients with neurologic impairment, a risk or history of aspiration, an incompetent gag reflex, or gastric dysfunction. Gastric dysfunction can be related to gastric atony, gastroparesis, gastric cancer, gastric outlet obstruction, or gastric ulcerative disease.

Care and Maintenance of Enteral Feeding Tubes

Enteral feeding tubes should be flushed routinely with water to maintain patency and prevent clogging. Tap water is generally sufficient. If concern exists regarding safety of the water source or if the patient is immunosuppressed, then sterile water may be used to flush the feeding tube. Standard flushing volumes are 30 mL of water every 4 hours during continuous feedings. Water flushes for intermittent and bolus enteral feedings are a minimum of 30 mL immediately after each feeding. The amount of water flushed through the tube is adjusted according to the patient's fluid requirements and tolerance. Larger fluid volumes will be needed for patients who cannot drink water for hydration; smaller fluid volumes are needed for patients on fluid restrictions.

General Comfort Tips for Patients With Nasoenteric Tube Feedings

- *Thirst, oral dryness:* Lubricate lips, chew sugarless gum, brush teeth, rinse mouth frequently with water, and suck lemon drops occasionally. If a small amount of water by mouth is permitted, then let ice cubes melt in the mouth to soothe mouth and esophagus.

- *Tube discomfort:* Gargle with a mixture of warm water and mouthwash, gently blow the nose, and clean the tube regularly with water-soluble lubricant.
- *Tension, fullness:* Relax and breathe deeply after each tube feeding infusion.
- *Loud stomach noises:* Take feedings in private.
- *Limited mobility:* Change positions in bed or chair, and walk around the house or hospital corridor. Perform range-of-motion exercises while confined to bed.
- *General gustatory distress with feeding:* Warm or chill the tube feeding formula.
- *Persistent hunger:* Chew a favorite food, then spit it out; chew gum; or suck lemon drops.
- *Inability to drink:* Rinse the mouth frequently with water or other liquids.

Ideally no medications should be put down small-bore feeding tubes, because medications are a primary contributor to feeding tube clogs. However, the reality of life often requires administration of medications via feeding tubes. Flush with 30 mL of water before and after medication administration. Each medication should be administered separately with 5 mL of water flushed through the tube between each medication. Check with a pharmacist when determining which medications are compatible with administration through a feeding tube (see the Diet-Medications Interactions box, "Drug-Nutrient Interactions"). Medications should never be added directly to the tube feeding formula because of the risk of drug-nutrient interactions. Warm water, a 30- to 60-mL syringe, and a pumping action can be used to dislodge a clog within the feeding tube. No evidence supports the use of other liquids such as soft drinks or juices to declog feeding tubes.[42] A pancreatic enzyme and bicarbonate mixture may be effective against formula clogs but will not dissolve medication clogs.[43]

💊 DIET-MEDICATIONS INTERACTIONS

Drug-Nutrient Interactions

Relatively few clinical studies are available that document drug-nutrient interactions associated with enteral feeding solutions. In spite of this, potential consequences of interactions should not be taken lightly. Medication administration in patients receiving EN support have increased risk for complications that can interfere with administration of nutrition, alter the bioavailability of a given drug, or cause long-term vitamin and mineral deficiencies due to drug-nutrient interactions.

Physical interferences with nutrition support are problems related to manipulation of the delivery system of nutrition support or the drug before it enters the body. Physical interferences are the most commonly reported problems and include but are not limited to occlusion of the feeding tube related to medication administration, manipulation of solid-dose forms of drugs, and exposure of photosensitive drugs to light for extended periods of time. No medication is formulated to be administered in combination with EN support; therefore the composition can sometimes alter viscosity of enteral feeding solutions and cause occlusion of the feeding tube. Furthermore, when crushing a solid-dose pill for administration through a feeding tube, there is a risk of occlusion, and the bioavailability of the medication and its time release properties will be altered considerably. Any type of drug added to a feeding solution will have longer exposure to ultraviolet light than if taken orally, which in some cases can compromise therapeutic effects.

The composition of enteral formulas differs considerably from orally fed diets. Enteral feeds contain increased concentrations of proteins, vitamins, and minerals, which can bind drugs or alter the mechanism by which they are metabolized. Closely related, but resulting in a more long-term effect, are vitamin and mineral binding. Chronic problems such as osteoporosis can develop over time as a result

of an interaction that goes unnoticed. The following is a brief list of some classically noted drug-nutrient interactions related to EN support.

Drug	Interaction	Possible Remedy
Phenytoin	Probable cause of interaction is the binding of phenytoin to caseinate proteins found in enteral feeds, preventing its absorption from the gastrointestinal (GI) tract.	Withhold feedings for 2 h after administration of phenytoin. Increased dose might be in order.
Quinolones	Concurrent administration of a quinolone and enteral feed could compromise antimicrobial efficiency. This is related to the divalent cations found in enteral nutrition (EN) formulas.	Withhold feedings 1 h before and 1 h after administration of quinolones. Increase dose when converting from intravenous to oral form.
Warfarin	Decreased bioavailability of this drug results from high binding of warfarin to proteins found in EN. In addition, vitamin K was formerly found to reverse anticoagulant effects of warfarin, but most current enteral feeds contain little or no vitamin K.	Avoid concurrent administration of warfarin and EN solutions. Choose EN supplements that contain limited vitamin K content.

Continued

◆ DIET-MEDICATIONS INTERACTIONS

Drug-Nutrient Interactions—cont'd

Working as a team with physicians, nurses, speech pathologists, and pharmacists can substantially reduce interactions stemming from EN support. By educating those who administer and prescribe medications, risks involved can be controlled and monitored correctly.

Bibliography

ASPEN Board of Directors: Section IX: drug nutrient interactions. *J Parenter Enter Nutr* 26:1, 2002.

British Association for Parenteral and Enteral Nutrition, The British Pharmaceutical Nutrition Group: *Drug administration via enteral feeding tubes: a guide for general practitioners and community pharmacists*, Redditch, UK, 2001, BAPEN.

Finch C, Self T: Medication and enteral tube feedings: clinically significant interactions. *J Crit Illn* 16:20–21, 2001.

Fitzgerald M: What do I need to know about drug interactions with enteral feeding? *Medscape Nurses* 7:1, 2005. From http://www.medscape.com/viewarticle/498270.

Tube Feeding Containers and Pumps

The enteric tube feeding system includes the formula container, connection tubing, and often an infusion pump. A variety of tube feeding containers and feeding sets is available. Tube feeding formulas can be administered by syringe, gravity drip, or a volumetric pump. A pump may be needed for more accurate control, which is essential for tube feedings given directly into the small intestine, tube feedings infused at slow rates, and tube feedings using more viscous formulas. Critically ill patients should also be tube fed by volumetric pump to increase tolerance to EN support.

Tube feeding delivery systems are categorized as either *open* or *closed*. An open delivery system involves pouring a volume of formula from a can or mixing bowl (or container) into an empty tube feeding bag, syringe, or infusion container. The infusion bag or container is reopened and refilled periodically with more formula. Clean technique is required when decanting the tube feeding formula into the bag and when handling the tubing connections. Formula hang time is limited to 8 hours or less.[23,44] Hang time is further reduced if additives such as protein powder are placed into the formula. The tube feeding infusion bag should be rinsed with sterile water before initial filling and subsequent refilling with formula.[23] The tube feeding administration set, tubing and infusion bag, should be changed every 24 hours. The primary benefit of the open system is the ability to modulate the tube feeding formula.

The closed system is composed of a sterile vessel that is purchased prefilled with tube feeding formula. The container is spiked and connected to an infusion pump. Hang time is expanded to 24 to 48 hours (refer to manufacturer's guidelines for hang time of product being used). Benefits of the closed system are a reduction of time, labor, and contamination risk.[45,46] Caveats of the closed system are its increased cost and the inability to modulate the formula. Regardless of the system used, good hand washing is essential to reduce bacterial contamination. Clinicians working with patients on tube feedings need to be familiar with different delivery systems, types of enteral feeding tubes, and features of enteral feeding pumps to determine which products are preferable for their facility and patient population.

Infusion of Enteral Tube Feeding

Tube feedings can be provided via bolus, intermittent, or continuous infusion through a feeding tube. Selection of the feeding schedule should be based on the patient's clinical condition. All enteral tube feedings should be initiated at full strength. Tolerance to tube feeding has not been shown to be improved with dilution of the formula.[47] Enteral tube feedings should be introduced gradually and progressed per patient tolerance. Gastric tube feedings can be given as bolus, intermittent, or continuous feedings. Small bowel tube feedings are usually given as continuous feedings, although patients on home nutrition support may use intermittent small bowel feedings.

Bolus tube feeding is generally initiated with 120 to 240 mL of formula every 3 to 4 hours and increased by 120 to 240 mL every 8 to 12 hours, depending on the level of illness and tolerance. The infusion period is relatively short, 10 to 20 minutes, and is infused through a syringe or from a bag by the flow of gravity.[48] The infusion should not exceed 40 to 60 mL/min. Gravity infusion is controlled by a roller clamp, raising or lowering the formula container, or advancing the plunger into the syringe.

Intermittent tube feedings are similar to bolus feedings but are given over a longer time period of 30 to 60 minutes every 3 to 6 hours. The enteral tube feeding formula is placed in a bag with rate controlled by a roller clamp. This method is used to provide periodic gastric feedings to patients who do not tolerate the more rapid infusion of a bolus feeding. The maximum amount of formula given by bolus or intermittent feedings varies from 240 to 500 mL per feeding and is based on patient tolerance and requirements.

Continuous tube feedings are provided over a defined period, with the formula infused by gravity or pump. Continuous feedings can be given over 24 hours or cycled over a shorter period, such as 8 to 20 hours per day. Enteral tube feeding tolerance is generally better in critically ill patients who are fed continuously regardless of whether fed into the stomach or small bowel.

All patients fed through a feeding tube should have the head of the bed elevated 30 to 45 degrees to reduce the risk of aspiration.[49] Patients fed with a tube into the small bowel can still aspirate gastric contents and may require concomitant gastric decompression during small bowel feeding.[50] Patients who must lie flat or in Trendelenburg position should have enteral feedings stopped.

MONITORING THE TUBE-FED PATIENT

Monitoring of the tube-fed patient should focus on transitioning to an oral diet and reducing or eliminating dependency on tube feeding. All patients being nourished by tube feeding should be carefully monitored for signs and symptoms of enteral tube feeding intolerance. Tolerance to enteral tube feeding is determined by GI signs of vomiting, abdominal distention or bloating, and frequency and consistency of bowel movements. If problems occur, then the tube feeding formula may need to be replaced, the infusion rate adjusted,

KEY TERM

Viscous

Physical property of a substance dependent on the friction of its component molecules as they slide by one another; viscosity.

or the method of administration changed until tolerance improves and symptoms subside. In most instances the tube feeding formula itself is not the causative agent for the intolerance. Residual volume and diarrhea are two parameters that are often used to determine tolerance to tube feeding. Both are terms that have no standardized definition within each institution, much less nationwide standard definitions.

Diarrhea is generally defined by the person cleaning it up and can be based on volume, frequency, or consistency of the stools (or a combination of these factors). Fourteen definitions of diarrhea are found in the literature.[51] Commonly used definitions are more than three stools per day or more than 500 mL of stool per day for 2 consecutive days.[52] Each health care facility should define diarrhea and then create an algorithm or protocol for treatment to reduce unnecessary interruptions of enteral feeding.[52] The most common cause of diarrhea in the tube-fed patient is medications, primarily antibiotics and medications containing sorbitol (see the Health Promotion section later in this chapter for a discussion).

The interpretation of *residual volume* is also often determined by caregiver experience and not evidence-based guidelines. Enteral feeds are interrupted for gastric residual volumes ranging from 50 to 200 mL.[53] Although some still advocate for close monitoring of gastric residual volumes, a recent research study found that problems with accuracy of measurement make it possible to safely feed patients without frequent monitoring of residual volume.[54] If residual volumes are measured, high residual volumes should be correlated with the presence of physical signs of intolerance before stopping enteral feeding. Another study found that if patients were given a prophylactic prokinetic agent, then a residual volume of 250 mL was tolerated.[55] The ASPEN Guidelines[7] and the Canadian Clinical Practice Guidelines[56] state a high residual volume is more than 500 mL for two consecutive checks. In contrast, according to a survey of intensive care unit (ICU) nurses, the nurses believed a residual volume greater than 100 mL was excessive.[57] A patient with a history of aspiration or reflux is at risk of aspiration regardless of the volume of gastric residuals; therefore residual volumes do not always correlate with risk of aspiration.

GI aspirates that contain gastric enzymes and hydrochloric acid (HCl) required for digestion, electrolytes, enteral formula, and fluid should be returned to the patient after determining the volume. However, if doing so would make the patient uncomfortable or if the volume removed exceeds 300 mL, then the residuals should be discarded and rechecked in 1 to 2 hours. The feeding tube should be flushed with 30 mL water after checking and returning residuals to be sure gastric contents with digestive enzymes are no longer within the lumen of the feeding tube. Patient tolerance of tube feeding formula, state of hydration, and nutritional response to tube feeding should be monitored using data collected from a variety of sources, including laboratory, anthropometric, physical and clinical assessment, and nursing records. Protocols for enteral tube feeding can provide guidelines for troubleshooting problems and improve nutrient delivery.[58,59]

Clinical and Laboratory Parameters to Monitor

Blood glucose levels should be monitored daily or more frequently in patients who have diabetes or are at risk for diabetes. It is important not to overfeed patients on nutrition support. Historically, insulin has been provided as needed to maintain serum glucose level at less than 200 mg/dL. Some research indicates that glycemic control between 110 mg/dL[60] and 140 mg/dL[61] can significantly reduce mortality and morbidity in ICU patients. However, tight blood glucose control increases risk for hypoglycemia. Because many patients are not aware of

the signs/symptoms of hypoglycemia, blood glucose should be checked every 3 to 4 hours when target blood glucose levels are less than 140 mg/dL.

Daily weights, compared with a baseline weight before start of the tube feeding, along with daily input and output measures, are essential for an accurate assessment of patient tolerance and nutrient adequacy. Routine monitoring also includes serum tests for potassium, sodium, chloride, carbon dioxide (CO_2), and creatinine, as well as BUN and complete blood count (CBC), along with periodic tests for urine specific gravity. Sudden weight changes can indicate fluid imbalance and need to be investigated. (See Box 19.2 for a list of nutrition support monitoring parameters.)

Hydration Status

Signs of volume deficit or dehydration include weight loss, poor skin turgor, dry mucous membranes, and low blood pressure from decreased blood volume. Patients also demonstrate increased serum levels of sodium, albumin, hematocrit, and BUN, as well as elevated urine specific gravity levels. Severe dehydration is critical and life threatening. Fluid requirements can be estimated by several available formulas, such as 1 mL of water per kcalorie or 30 to 35 mL/kg. Water content of the enteral tube feeding formula and the amount of water given with medications and routine flushing of the feeding tube, as well as the patient's medical condition, are taken into consideration when determining the patient's fluid requirements. Fluids must be monitored for adequacy and adjusted as necessary to attain and maintain adequate hydration. Patients with large fluid losses from fistulas, ostomies, and drains may require intravenous hydration in conjunction with enteral tube feeding nutrition.

Signs of volume excess or overhydration include weight gain, edema, jugular vein distention, elevated blood pressure, and decreased serum levels of sodium, albumin, BUN, and hematocrit. Patients with renal, cardiac, and hepatic impairment may require less fluid than other patients.

Documentation of the Enteral Nutrition Tube Feeding

The patient's medical record is an essential means of communication among members of the health care team. The health care team is involved in actions and documentation related to (1) all ongoing nutritional analyses of actual tube feeding formula intake; (2) tolerance of the formula and any complications; (3) desired versus actual intake; (4) urine and stool output; (5) recommendations for adjustments in tube feeding formula, routine tube flushing, and method and rate of delivery; and (6) education of patient and family.

PARENTERAL FEEDING IN CLINICAL NUTRITION

PN should be reserved for patients who are unable to receive adequate nutrition via the oral or enteral route. ASPEN has published general guidelines to determine when PN support is appropriate.[7] Indications and contraindications for PN are listed in Box 19.4.

Basic Technique

Guidelines for ordering PN are given in Box 19.5, and an example of a basic PN solution is given in Box 19.6. PN refers to any intravenous feeding method. Nutrients are infused directly into the blood when the GI tract cannot or should not be used. The following two parenteral routes are available (Fig. 19.3)[62]:

1. *Central parenteral nutrition (CPN):* A large central vein is used to deliver concentrated solutions for nutrition support. Osmolarity of central vein parenteral formulas can be as high as 1700 to 1900 mOsm/L.

BOX 19.4   Indications and Contraindications for Parenteral Nutrition

Indications

1. Nonfunctional gastrointestinal (GI) tract
   a. Obstruction
   b. Intractable vomiting or diarrhea
   c. Short bowel syndrome
   d. Paralytic ileus
2. Inability to adequately use GI tract
   a. Slow progression of enteral nutrition (EN)
   b. Limited tolerance of EN
3. Perioperative condition
   a. Severely malnourished
   b. Nothing by mouth (NPO) for at least 1 week before surgery

Contraindications

1. No central venous access
2. Grim prognosis when parenteral nutrition (PN) will be of no benefit
3. EN is an alternative means of support

Conditions Previously Treated With PN That Benefit From Enteral Feeding

1. Inflammatory bowel disease
2. Pancreatitis

Modified from Fuhrman MP: Parenteral nutrition. *Diet Edge* 2(1):53, 2001.

BOX 19.5   Guidelines for Ordering Parenteral Nutrition

1. Determine that the patient has central intravenous access.
2. Identify amount of energy, protein, and fluid desired.
3. Determine desired distribution of dextrose and lipids.
4. Indicate additives desired.
   a. Vitamins
   b. Minerals
   c. Electrolytes
   d. Medications
   e. Sterile water
5. Determine infusion rate based on compounded volume and time of infusion.

BOX 19.6   Example of a Basic Parenteral Nutrition Formula for a 65-kg Patient Providing Approximately 25 kcal/kg and 1.2 g Protein/kg

Base Solution

70% Dextrose	350 mL	245 g	833 kcal
10% Amino acids	800 mL	80 g	320 kcal
20% Lipid	250 mL	50 g	500 kcal
TOTAL	**1400 mL**		**1653 kcal**

Additives

Standard Electrolytes	Amount per day
Sodium chloride	20 mEq
Sodium acetate	50 mEq
Potassium chloride	30 mEq
Potassium phosphate	30 mEq (20 mmol phosphorus)
Calcium gluconate	10 mEq
Magnesium sulfate	10 mEq
Multivitamin preparation	10 mL
Trace element preparation	1 mL
Medications	
Regular insulin	Only with hyperglycemia
H$_2$ antagonists	Dose depends on H$_2$ antagonist and renal functions
Famotidine 40 mg	

High formula osmolarity requires infusion of the formula into a large vessel with rapid blood flow. A central line generally originates from the subclavian, internal jugular, or femoral vein, with the tip in the superior vena cava, right atrium of the heart, or inferior vena cava. Central line access can also be achieved with a peripherally inserted central catheter (PICC) that is inserted in the basilic vein, with the tip in the superior vena cava or right atrium.

2. *Peripheral parenteral nutrition (PPN):* A smaller peripheral vein, usually in the distal arm or hand, is used to deliver less-concentrated solutions for periods less than 14 days. Osmolarity of PPN is limited to 900 mOsm/L or less to reduce risk of thrombophlebitis in smaller vessels of the upper distal extremities.[63]

Parenteral Nutrition Development

The pioneering work of American surgeons such as Jonathan Rhodes and Stanley Dudrick in the late 1960s propelled PN from theory into reality.[64] Further developments of the surgical technique, equipment,

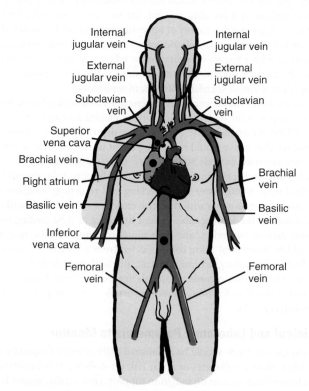

FIG. 19.3 Sites of central venous access for parenteral nutrition. (From Fuhrman MP: Management of complications of parenteral nutrition. In Matarese LE, Gottschlich MM, editors: *Contemporary nutrition support practice: a clinical guide*, Philadelphia, 1998, Saunders.)

and solutions to meet nutritional requirements of catabolic illness and injury, as well as development of certain antibiotics and diuretics, led to widespread use and continuing development of PN.[25,65] PN was preferentially used to treat critically ill patients until a resurgence in EN in the 1990s, when more was learned about the importance of maintaining GI integrity. PN is associated with potentially serious mechanical, metabolic, and GI complications (see Box 19.3). PN should be used judiciously to minimize the risks involved. PPN can be used in many cases as a viable alternative for brief periods for patients without central vein access.[66]

Basic factors govern decisions about use of PN: availability and functional capacity of the GI tract, prognosis, and availability of central intravenous access.[7] The cost of PN is generally more than that of enteral feeding, and institutions have demonstrated cost savings when inappropriate use of PN is decreased.[67,68] Patients must have central intravenous access to receive PN, with one port designated exclusively for PN. Thus careful assessment of each situation should weigh benefits and burdens of providing PN for nutrition support.

Indications for PN include inability to access or the malfunction of the GI tract. Patients may have inadequate absorption of nutrients in the GI tract because of reduced bowel length or inflammation. Examples of indications for PN are obstruction, fistula, severe inflammation, intractable vomiting or diarrhea, or GI bleeding (see Box 19.4). If the GI tract is functional but the patient cannot or will not consume sufficient nutrients orally, then enteral tube feeding should be considered. Many conditions that had been previously thought to be an indication for PN are treated with enteral tube feeding, such as pancreatitis, severe malnutrition, ileus, and coma.

Candidates for Parenteral Nutrition

PN should be reserved for patients unable to receive or tolerate adequate nutrients via the enteral route. On the basis of these general considerations, a number of clinical situations suggest a need for aggressive PN support:

- *Preoperative nutrition intervention:* This measure may benefit moderately to severely malnourished patients who can receive nutrition support for a minimum of 7 to 14 days preoperatively who cannot be fed orally or enterally.[7] Surgery should never be delayed simply for nutrition support. The Veterans Affairs Cooperative Study[27] demonstrated the greatest benefit of perioperative PN was experienced by severely malnourished patients. Third-party payers do not routinely pay for preoperative nutrition support.
- *Postoperative surgical complications:* Complications that often result in initiation of PN are prolonged paralytic ileus and obstruction; stomal dysfunction; short-bowel syndrome; enterocutaneous, biliary, or pancreatic fistula; chylothorax; chylous ascites; and peritonitis. However, reports exist of successful enteral feeding with short bowel syndrome, fistula, and chylous leaks when patients are given an elemental or semielemental, low-fat enteral formula.[69-71] PN is not indicated in patients who can resume EN within 7 to 10 days postoperatively.[7]
- *Bowel inflammation:* Intractable gastroenteritis, regional enteritis, ulcerative colitis, extensive diverticulitis, and radiation enteritis may require PN if the GI inflammation is severe and prolonged.[7] Studies have shown that in some cases enteral feeding can be feasible and beneficial in diseases with bowel inflammation.[72]
- *Malabsorption:* Nutrient losses and interference with nutrient absorption occur with chemotherapy and radiation therapy. The malabsorption that is associated with severe GI inflammation, acute severe pancreatitis, and massive burns can exceed the ability to meet nutrient requirements enterally.

> **KEY TERM**
>
> **Fistula**
> Abnormal connection between two internal organs, an internal organ and the skin, or an internal organ and a body cavity.

Peripheral Parenteral Nutrition

In general, decisions to use PPN instead of CPN are based on energy demands, anticipated time of use, and availability of intravenous access. Characteristics of PPN include caloric value generally less than 2000 kcal/day, of which 50% to 60% is provided by lipids; infusion volume of 2 to 3 L (dilution of the formula is required for peripheral vein tolerance); and use of infusion for less than 14 days.[66] PPN cannot be used when the patient has problems with fluid retention or hyperlipidemia.

PARENTERAL SOLUTIONS

Parenteral Nutrition Prescription

The PN prescription and plan of care are based on the calculation of basic nutritional requirements plus additional needs resulting from the patient's level of illness or injury, malnutrition, and physical activity. An example of a basic PN formula is shown in Box 19.6. The same principles of nutrition therapy are applied whether the patient is fed enterally or parenterally. Nutritional needs are fundamental—energy, protein, electrolytes, minerals, and vitamins. Guidelines are available that address PN labeling, compounding, formulations, stability, and filtering.[73] The guidelines are designed to reduce errors and complications in prescribing, preparing, labeling, and infusing parenteral solutions.

Preparation of the Parenteral Nutrition Solution

A variety of PN component solutions exist, with varying concentrations and nutrient compositions. Standard components of PN can include dextrose, lipids, amino acids, electrolytes, vitamins, minerals, and medications. In an attempt to contain costs, many facilities are using "premixed" PN solutions that do not allow customization. When PN is compounded with modular components, there is an ability to adjust dextrose, lipid, and protein independent of each other, the energy provided to meet estimated or measured energy needs should include total energy (kcalories) from carbohydrate, fat, and protein (Table 19.3). Estimated and measured energy equations are based on total energy (kcalories) requirements.

Protein-Nitrogen Source

Nitrogen is supplied by essential and nonessential crystalline amino acids in the PN solution. Standard commercial amino acid solutions range in concentration from 3% to 20%. Standard amino acid solutions are appropriate for almost all adult patients receiving PN. Protein has an energy value of 4 kcal/g (see Table 19.3) and usually provides 10% to 20% of the total energy provided in PN.

In addition to standard amino acid solutions, two specialized amino acid solutions have been formulated for specific disease states. The two disease-specific formulas are more expensive than standard solutions, and their effectiveness has not been demonstrated. One type is enriched with the branched-chain amino acids (BCAAs) isoleucine, leucine, and valine, and is designed for patients with liver failure. A renal failure formula contains only essential amino acids to prevent the development of hyperuremia. Neither disease-specific formula has been found to improve outcomes in these patient populations.[7] However, infusion of BCAA may be beneficial in a very small population of patients with chronic hepatic encephalopathy that is unresponsive to drug therapy.[7] It is important to note that this specialized, expensive

TABLE 19.3 Caloric Value Per Milliliter of Parenteral Components

Nutrient	Concentration (%)	kcal/mL
Dextrose	70.0	2.38
	50.0	1.85
Lipids	30.0	3.0
	20.0	2.0
	10.0	1.1
Amino acids	15.0	0.6
	10.0	0.4
	8.5	0.34

TABLE 19.4 Micronutrients and Parenteral Nutrition for Adults

Micronutrients	Standard Daily Amounts
Electrolytes	
Potassium (K)	1–2 mEq/kg
Sodium (Na)	1–2 mEq/kg
Phosphate (HPO$_4$)	20–40 mmol
Magnesium (Mg)	8–20 mEq
Calcium (Ca)	10–15 mEq
Acetate	Balance with chloride to maintain acid-base balance
Chloride	Balance with acetate to maintain acid-base balance
Vitamins	
Vitamin A	3300 IU
Vitamin D	200 IU
Vitamin E	10 IU
Vitamin K	150 mcg
Thiamin (B$_1$)	6 mg
Riboflavin (B$_2$)	3.6 mg
Niacin (B$_3$)	40 mg
Folic acid	600 mcg
Pantothenic acid	15 mg
Pyridoxine (B$_6$)	6 mg
Cyanocobalamin (B$_{12}$)	5 mcg
Biotin	60 mcg
Ascorbic acid (vitamin C)	200 mcg
Trace Elements	
Chromium	10–15 mcg
Copper	0.3–0.5 mcg
Iodine	Not routinely provided
	50 mcg for pregnant women
Iron	Not routinely provided
	25–50 mg per month without blood loss
Manganese	60–100 mcg
Selenium	20–60 mcg
Zinc	2.5–5.0 mg
Molybdenum	Not routinely provided

Data from Fuhrman MP: Complication management in parenteral nutrition. In Matarese LE, Gottschlich MM, editors: *Contemporary nutrition support practice: a clinical guide*, ed 2, Philadelphia, 2003, Saunders; Task force for the revision of safe practices for parenteral nutrition: Safe practices for parenteral nutrition. *JPEN J Parenter Enteral Nutr* 28(Suppl):S39, 2004; American Medical Association, AMA Department of Foods and Nutrition: Multivitamin preparations for parenteral use: a statement by the Nutrition Advisory Group. *JPEN J Parenter Enteral Nutr* 3:258, 1979; Parenteral multivitamin products; drugs for human use; drug efficacy study implementation; amendment (21 CFR 5.70). *Fed Register* 65:21200, 2000; Expert Panel for Nutrition Advisory Group, AMA Department of Foods and Nutrition: Guidelines for essential trace element preparations for parenteral use. *JAMA* 241:2051, 1979.

amino acid formulation should never be used as the first line of treatment and never in place of medical treatment of encephalopathy.

A third type of specialized amino acid formula is designed specifically for the needs of pediatric patients and is selected based on the age and nutrient requirements of the child.

Carbohydrate-Dextrose

Dextrose is the most common and least expensive source of energy used for PN support. Dextrose is available in concentrations ranging from 2.5% to 70%. Hypertonic solutions of 50% to 70% dextrose are often used in PN formulations and provide 50 or 70 g of dextrose per 100 mL, respectively. Glucose used in PN support is commercially available as dextrose monohydrate ($C_6H_{12}O_6H_2O$), which has an energy value of 3.4 kcal/g versus the energy value of 4 kcal/g of dietary glucose ($C_6H_{12}O_6$). The caloric values of dextrose solutions are given in Table 19.3. The initial dextrose content of PN should not exceed 200 g. Gradual introduction of dextrose enables the clinician to evaluate blood sugar response and, if necessary, institute insulin therapy. The amount of dextrose provided is increased to goal according to patient tolerance and should not exceed 5 mg/kg/min.

Fat Lipids

Lipid emulsions provide a concentrated energy source, 9 kcal/g, as well as the essential fatty acids linoleic and linolenic acid. A minimum of 4% to 10% of the daily energy intake should consist of fat to prevent essential fatty acid deficiency. Lipids are available in 10% (1.1 kcal/mL), 20% (2 kcal/mL), and 30% (3 kcal/mL) products (see Table 19.3). A 500-mL bottle of 10%, 20%, or 30% fat emulsion provides 550, 1000, and 1500 kcal, respectively. Commercial lipid emulsion products consist of soybean and safflower oils combined or soybean oil alone. The content of lipid in a parenteral solution is usually limited to 20% to 30% of total energy because lipids have been reported to adversely affect the immune system.[74] However, infusion of lipids over 24 hours may limit this adverse effect. Research on alternative lipid sources includes forms such as short-chain fatty acids, medium-chain fatty acids, omega-3 fatty acids, and blended or structured lipids. However, these alternatives are not available for commercial use in the United States. Lipid emulsions can be infused separately through the Y-port of the intravenous catheter (piggybacked) or combined with the dextrose and amino acid base in what is called a *total nutrient admixture* (TNA) or *3-in-1*.[73]

Electrolytes

The body maintains a balance of fluid and electrolytes in intracellular and extracellular spaces of all tissues to maintain homeostasis (see Chapter 7). Electrolyte status is affected by disease state and metabolic condition of the patient. Electrolytes in PN formulas are based on normal electrolyte balance with adjustments according to individual patient requirements. Electrolytes should be routinely monitored to determine electrolyte requirements in PN.

In general, basic electrolyte recommendations are shown in Table 19.4, with chloride and acetate balanced among the salts. Commercial amino acid formulations are available with or without added electrolytes. Amounts of electrolytes present in the amino acid solution must be taken into account when calculating additions of electrolytes for a specific patient. Guidelines for electrolyte management include the following:

1. Identify and correct any preexisting deficits before initiating PN.
2. Determine the cause of electrolyte abnormalities.
3. Replace excessive fluid and electrolyte losses.
4. Monitor and assess electrolyte status daily.

Depending on requirements for electrolyte replacement, it may be necessary to give additional electrolytes outside the PN, because limitations exist regarding what can be added to a parenteral solution based on solution stability and compatibility.[70] Selected electrolytes can be omitted from the parenteral solution when serum levels exceed normal values, such as potassium and phosphorus with renal failure. Electrolyte levels should be checked in all patients before starting PN and routinely throughout PN therapy.

Vitamins

Vitamin requirements are based on normal standards (see Chapter 6), with adjustments made according to metabolic states that require either more or less of a specific vitamin. All patients on PN should receive vitamins daily. Serum levels of vitamins should be monitored in patients requiring long-term PN or when deficiencies or excesses are suspected.

The Nutrition Advisory Group of the American Medical Association has established guidelines for parenteral administration of 12 vitamins: A, D, E, thiamin, riboflavin, niacin, pantothenic acid, pyridoxine, folic acid, biotin, cyanocobalamin, and ascorbic acid (see Table 19.4).[75] Multivitamin infusion preparations based on these guidelines are commercially available. Vitamin K has not historically been a component of any injectable vitamin formulation for adults. The FDA mandated changes in parenteral vitamin formulations that included addition of 150 mcg of vitamin K to injectable multivitamin preparations.[76] It will be important to monitor International Normalized Ratio (INR) levels, particularly for patients on anticoagulation therapy started or stopped on PN containing vitamin K. An injectable multivitamin preparation without vitamin K is also available.

Trace Elements

The American Medical Association has set guidelines for the addition of four trace elements in PN solutions: zinc, copper, manganese, and chromium (see Table 19.4).[77] Trace element preparations are available with combinations of the aforementioned four trace elements only, the standard four plus selenium, or the standard four plus selenium, molybdenum, and iodine. Each trace element is also available as a single injectable mineral product. A growing amount of literature demonstrates the importance of providing selenium to PN patients who are critically ill[78,79] and those who require long-term PN.[80] Iron is not routinely added to PN because of incompatibility with intravenous lipids, as well as the potential adverse effects of iron dextran. Other forms of intravenous iron have fewer adverse effects but are not approved for addition to the PN solution. Intravenous iron should only be given to patients with iron deficiency anemia and administered apart from the PN admixture or added to a 2-in-1 PN solution.[73] A dose of 25 to 50 mg of iron dextran once a month should be sufficient to meet iron needs in a patient without blood loss.[73]

Patients on long-term PN without trace element supplementation are at risk for micronutrient deficiencies.[80,81] In addition, reports exist of excess trace element levels with infusion of standard trace element preparations.[82] Patients who require long-term PN should be routinely monitored for potential trace element deficiencies and toxicities.

Medications

Medications often added to PN include insulin, H_2 antagonists, heparin, metoclopramide, and octreotide. Inclusion of these medications and others will depend on each institution's guidelines and protocols for addition of medications to PN solutions. Many issues exist concerning compatibility, bioavailability, efficacy, interactions, and safety when including medications in PN solutions. Consult a pharmacist whenever considering the addition of a medication to PN solutions.

PARENTERAL NUTRITION DELIVERY SYSTEM

Equipment

Strict aseptic technique throughout PN administration by all health care personnel is absolutely essential. This includes (1) solution preparation by the pharmacist, (2) surgical placement of the venous catheter by the physician, (3) care of the catheter site and all external equipment, and (4) administration of the solution by the nurse. At every step of the PN process, strict infection control is a primary responsibility of all health care professionals.

Venous Access

Surgical placement of the venous catheter is done by the physician at the bedside or in a surgical suite, using local or general anesthesia. Intravenous catheters are available with single, double, triple, or quadruple lumens. Inconsistent data exist as to whether the number of lumens contributes to the risk of catheter-related infection.[83-85] Catheters are also categorized as either *temporary* or *permanent.* Temporary catheters involve a direct percutaneous puncture into a major vessel and are used short-term during hospitalization. Permanent catheters are designed for long-term use and are available as implanted ports, tunneled catheters, and PICCs. The tip of a central venous catheter is located in the inferior or superior vena cava, which leads directly into the heart (see Fig. 19.3).[62] Placement of the catheter tip in the vena cava allows infusion of concentrated solutions, 5 times the concentration of blood plasma, to be infused at a rate of 2 to 3 mL/min. Hypertonic solutions are immediately diluted by the large blood flow of 2 to 5 L/min in the vena cava.

Catheter-related sepsis is a serious complication, particularly with the increase in colonization of resistant strains of microorganisms that limit available treatment options. Antibiotic-impregnated catheters and dressings are available and are associated with reduced catheter-related septic complications.[86-88] Filters (0.22 μm) on intravenous catheter tubing prevent infusion of not only particulate matter but also certain microorganisms.[73] However, a larger filter (2.1 μm) that is less effective against microorganisms must be used with PN containing lipids. Clinicians must use aseptic technique when inserting and caring for intravenous catheters.

Solution Infusion and Administration

Volumetric infusion pumps should be used to deliver the parenteral solution at a constant rate to prevent metabolic complications. Protocols for external delivery system tubing changes are provided by infection control guidelines. Routine flushing of intravenous catheters is recommended to maintain catheter patency. Needleless intravenous access devices reduce risk of needlestick injuries but can increase risk of catheter-related infections. According to the Intravenous Nurses Society standards of practice, needleless devices should be changed every 24 hours, the injection port should be disinfected with alcohol before accessing, and all junctions should be secured with Luer-Lok, clasps, or threaded devices.[89]

Infusion of PN is generally over 24 hours, particularly in the critically ill. PN is usually cycled for patients at home or who need "time off" during hospitalization for physical therapy or other routine

PERSPECTIVES IN PRACTICE

Parenteral Nutrition Administration

Of all the various ways of nourishing the human body—normal eating, liquid diets, enteral nutrition (EN), and parenteral nutrition (PN)—PN requires the highest level of skilled and precise administration. A risk of potentially life-threatening complication and infection exists. Trained nutrition support clinicians are central to the success of PN. The nutrition support nurse administers the PN solution according to the nutrition support team protocol, monitoring the entire PN system frequently to see that it is operating accurately.

Specific clinical protocols will vary somewhat, but they usually include the following points:

- *Schedule carefully:* PN volume can vary from 1 to 3 L and should be infused with an infusion pump. The infusion rate is based on the total volume of the compounded solution.
- *Monitor closely:* Note metabolic effects of glucose and electrolytes. Blood glucose levels should not exceed 200 mg/dL during initiation of PN and should not exceed 110 to 150 mg/dL when the patient is stable on the formula. First-day formulas generally contain no more than 200 g dextrose. Monitor glycemic tolerance closely, particularly the first couple of days, as the feeding is advanced. Electrolyte status and glucose levels should be determined before and throughout PN administration. Increase energy provision only as patient tolerates macronutrient content.
- *Make changes cautiously:* Monitor and report the effect of all changes, and proceed slowly.
- *Maintain a constant rate:* Keep to the correct hourly infusion rate, with no "catch-up" or "slow-down" effort to meet the original volume order.
- *Discontinue PN:* Reduce the rate by one-half for 1 hour before discontinuing. If patient has had insulin added to PN and is not receiving enteral tube feeding, then monitor for rebound hypoglycemia (check serum glucose 2 h after stopping PN infusion).

activities. PN can be cycled over 10 to 12 hours if desired and if the patient can tolerate the larger volume over a shorter period. The rate of infusion is based on the final compounded volume and length of time the infusion is to be given. Administration of PN should be adjusted based on the patient's response and tolerance to the regimen (see the Perspectives in Practice box, "Parenteral Nutrition Administration"). When PN is being discontinued, the infusion rate should be cut by one-half for 1 hour and then stopped. Abrupt interruption of PN infusion may require hanging 10% dextrose to prevent possible rebound hypoglycemia.[73]

Monitoring

Complications of PN include catheter, GI, and metabolic problems (see Box 19.3). In the hands of well-trained PN clinicians, risks can be minimized and complications controlled.[90] Specific evidence-based protocols, updated periodically, guide continuing assessment and monitoring.[91] Every patient on PN should undergo a routine nutrition reassessment with adjustments made in the feeding regimen according to the patient's metabolic and nutritional needs. Every effort should be made to transition the patient from PN to enteral tube feeding or oral diet whenever feasible or appropriate. Providing at least a portion of energy via the GI tract may help reduce the adverse effects associated with PN.[62]

HOME NUTRITION SUPPORT

Patients who are discharged with home nutrition support and those who started on nutrition support while in the home require special consideration. Several factors must be evaluated to ensure that the home environment is safe and the patient and family are able and willing to accept the responsibility of home infusion therapy. The home should have refrigeration, running water, electricity, and adequate storage for supplies. The patient and family must be capable of and willing to learn techniques required to administer and manage the feeding access. It is also important that the patient and family accept responsibility to comply with the infusion regimen so that the patient receives nutrients as prescribed. Ongoing communication occurs among the patient, physician, and home infusion provider, but ultimately the patient must self-manage the therapy and work closely with the home nutrition support team. The Oley Foundation (http://www.oley.org) provides a network of support for patients on chronic, long-term home enteral and parenteral therapies. Reimbursement for services must be confirmed before sending a patient home on nutrition support. The process can require additional diagnostic testing and documentation for the patient to qualify, particularly when Medicare is the source of reimbursement.

Home Enteral Tube Feeding
Patient Selection

Developments in enteral tube feeding formulas and portable, lightweight infusion equipment have simplified home tube feeding and made it easier to manage. As a result, the number of patients who receive home tube feeding continues to grow as a means of cutting hospital costs and allowing earlier family support at home. The success of home infusion of enteral tube feeding relies on the education and training of patient and family.[92]

Teaching Plan

Educating the patient and family for home infusion of enteral tube feeding is a team responsibility. This team may be hospital based or affiliated with the home infusion company that will manage the patient's care after discharge. The RD, nurse, and pharmacist develop and carry out a teaching plan, which includes topics and related tasks in preparing patients and families for discharge on home enteral feeding (Box 19.7).[87] The goal is to promote self-care and monitoring.

The hospital or home infusion company should provide a teaching manual with illustrations to guide the teaching-learning process and that can be used as a reference at home. The teaching plan should start as soon as the decision for home tube feeding is made. A social worker identifies and, if possible, resolves any personal, psychosocial, safety, or economic issues with home infusion.

Finally, the teaching plan should allow sufficient time before discharge for the patient and family to demonstrate competency in administering the tube feeding formula and recording all necessary

---

BOX 19.7 Home Enteral Tube Feeding Education Topics and Tasks

- Which enteral formulation is used and why
- How to prepare the tube feeding formula for infusion
- How to infuse the formula through the feeding tube
- How to correctly use and troubleshoot problems with the equipment
- How much water and how often to flush the feeding tube
- How to care for the tube site
- How to recognize tube feeding formula intolerance
- How to avoid and treat complications
- How to give medications and other separate nutrients through the feeding tube
- When to call the physician or home infusion provider

information about formula and fluid intake, formula tolerance, and complications. Directions for recording information are included in the home infusion manual. Records are reviewed regularly by the home nutrition support team and the patient's physician.

Follow-up Monitoring

The plan for follow-up monitoring should be guided by specific protocols developed by the home infusion provider for laboratory, clinical, and home nutrition assessments. The home nutrition support team checks the patient's progress and works with the patient and family to troubleshoot any problems that arise and make required adjustments in the formula or tube feeding plan. Whenever feasible and appropriate, the RD works closely with the patient and family to transition from tube feeding to oral intake. A study by Silver and colleagues[93] reported older adults who received home enteral tube feeding with no consistent clinical follow-up experienced complications associated with unscheduled health care visits and readmissions to the hospital. This study demonstrated the potential for improving outcomes with more frequent monitoring, reassessment, and intervention by a home nutrition support team that includes an RD.

Home Parenteral Nutrition

The patient sent home with PN requires education and training on the provision of PN in the outpatient setting. In the hands of knowledgeable and capable patients and their families, home PN allows mobility and independence. Equipment used in the home is small and portable, fitting in a backpack and allowing patients to resume normal activities. The patient and family must be trained to use aseptic technique for adding micronutrients and medications to the solution and for accessing the intravenous catheter or port. Special equipment, solutions, and guidelines for training and supervising patients and families have been developed and are successfully used by hundreds of patients. Ongoing assessment of GI function must be performed to determine if the patient is ready to transition to enteral feedings (either oral or via feeding tube). Patients are also monitored closely for the development of complications associated with long-term PN infusion.

A study in complex inflammatory bowel disease patients demonstrated home PN could be successfully used to delay or avoid surgery.[94] The study also found anxiety about managing PN at home decreased for most of the patients after 1 week at home.

▌HEALTH PROMOTION

TROUBLESHOOTING DIARRHEA IN TUBE-FED PATIENTS

Diarrhea is one of the most common complications associated with tube feeding, yet the reported incidence ranges widely, from as little as 2% to as much as 70% in general patient populations to as high as 80% in ICU patients. Questions that relate to this wide variance and that plague investigators apparently center on definition and cause. However, the ultimate bottom line for patients, their families, and health insurers is the cost of the clinical search for the cause of diarrhea in these patients and the appropriate method of treatment. Although clinicians search for an effective treatment, diarrhea results in reduced energy intake, dehydration, electrolyte abnormalities, and skin breakdown. Diarrhea also causes the patient discomfort, embarrassment, and frustration.

Problem of Definition

Several definitions of enteral feeding–related diarrhea have been used in the literature. However, little agreement exists concerning which definition most accurately reflects diarrhea that requires intervention. Common definitions include output of more than 500 mL on 2 consecutive days or more than three stools per day. From a nursing standpoint, collection and measurement of stool outputs are much less desirable than tracking the number of occurrences. However, the true definition of diarrhea may need to reflect consistency and volume and not just the number of stools per 24 hours. Most institutions do not have a standard definition for diarrhea; therefore in most cases, diarrhea is defined by the person cleaning it up. Diagnosis of the cause of diarrhea and subsequent treatment consume time and health care resources. Meanwhile the patient is losing fluid, electrolytes, and nutrients through uncontrolled stool output. This can further exacerbate impaired nutritional status. Diarrhea not only takes a physical and nutritional toll on the patient but also has a psychologic effect of embarrassment and humiliation from an inability to control bodily functions and the loss of privacy.

A recently reported case of unexplained diarrhea in a tube-fed patient illustrates the difficult—and often expensive—search for the cause (see the Case Study box, "Case of the Costly Chase").

Factors Contributing to Diarrhea

Reported causes of diarrhea in tube-fed patients also vary. The finger of blame for diarrhea usually is pointed at the tube feeding formula. This results in manipulation of the formula—selection and concentration and infusion methods—usually to no avail, because feeding intolerance is generally a manifestation, not the cause, of diarrhea. A variety of causes for diarrhea have been reported. The most common contributors to diarrhea in tube-fed patients are medications or some aspect of the patient's condition. However, many times a combination of events or therapies (not a single contributor) results in diarrhea.[51,52,85-98]

Formula

Tube feeding formula osmolality or concentration and rate of delivery are often blamed for instigating diarrhea. However, reports have shown no increase in the incidence of diarrhea when the formula concentration varied widely from 145 to 430 mOsm/L, and no significant association has been made between malabsorption and formula osmolality or rate of delivery. Formulas that provide more than 30% of total kcalories as fat have been associated with an increased incidence of diarrhea, whereas those providing 20% fat rarely were involved. Further study of fat composition is needed, specifically comparing MCTs versus long-chain triglycerides (LCTs) and omega-3 versus omega-6 fatty acids. Studies of the role of fiber in tube feedings have had conflicting results. No consistency is seen in the types and amount of fiber in enteral tube feeding formulas. Soluble fiber can increase colonic absorption of water. However, when the fiber given to a patient is increased rapidly, the patient will experience flatulence, abdominal distention, and constipation. Reviewers have found that studies thus far have been few, the models used have been variable, limitations were substantial, and the conclusions of investigators were mixed. In general, the amount and type of fiber in enteral formulas are not significant enough to prevent or contribute to diarrhea.[51,52,95-98]

Bacterial Contamination

Studies have shown the more manipulation and additives, such as modular components, that are added to an enteral formula, the more likely the formula will become contaminated. Tube feeding formula hang time, open versus closed delivery systems, and preparation technique can affect the risk of bacterial contamination of the enteral tube feeding formula. Formula added to open delivery systems should hang no longer than 8 hours (and for even shorter periods of time if additives are combined with the formula). Closed systems that use

Case of the Costly Chase

A reported case of unexplained diarrhea in a tube-fed patient illustrates the difficult, and often costly, search for the cause. Max was a 55-year-old man who had had an aortic aneurysm and undergone emergency surgery to repair it. In the intensive care unit (ICU), the postoperative course was complicated by respiratory problems requiring ventilator assistance. He was administered a bronchodilator drug, theophylline, in tablet form, crushed and administered by nasogastric tube with water. When Max was started on an enteral tube feeding with an isotonic formula, crushed theophylline tablets were changed to a sugar-free theophylline solution. Within a day Max began to have progressive abdominal distention and continuous liquid diarrhea. To rule out an abdominal catastrophe related to the aneurysm or surgery, a computed abdominal tomography scan, an aortogram, and colonoscopy were performed, but all of these studies produced normal results.

Despite stopping the enteral tube feeding, the distention and diarrhea continued. Stool specimens were tested for fecal leukocytes, parasites, and *Clostridium difficile* toxin, and an enteric pathogen culture was prepared. All were nondiagnostic. Extensive additional serum and urine tests, as well as a sigmoidoscopy with rectal biopsy, gave no clue. Then stool electrolytes and osmolality measures suggested an osmotic diarrhea. Because Max was not receiving enteral tube feedings, his physicians thought a secretory bacterial toxin was probably causing continuing diarrhea, so the previous studies were repeated to confirm the osmotic nature of the diarrhea. In addition, all medications were reviewed, but none appeared to be the cause.

Because the continued diarrhea prohibited enteral tube feeding and Max needed to be fed, parenteral nutrition (PN) was ordered. This move immediately brought an automatic nutrition support service consultation, which included assessment of medications. This evaluation revealed that the sugar-free theophylline solution was 65% sorbitol.

Sorbitol is a polyhydric alcohol used as a sweetener in many sugar-free products such as dietetic foods and chewing gum. Because sorbitol is considered an "inactive" ingredient, the package label and insert contained no information about it. Sorbitol content was obtained by contacting the manufacturer.

However, fortunately for Max, the nutrition support team did know the components of the medication and found the hidden culprit. The registered dietitian (RD) knew sorbitol in larger doses acted as a laxative. Calculations of the regular daily amount of theophylline Max was taking showed he was receiving nearly 300 g of sorbitol daily when the usual laxative dose was only 20 to 50 g. The nutrition support team immediately recommended that this sorbitol-sweetened solution of theophylline be discontinued and a sorbitol-free form of the medication be used instead. Almost immediately the diarrhea began to decrease, and in 3 days it was gone.

The extent of this costly chase was revealed in Max's hospital bill. He had continued to receive the faulty drug for almost half of his 3-month hospital stay, during which time the diarrhea prevented enteral tube feeding and he had to have the more expensive PN. The PN cost $5000 more than enteral feedings would have cost for the same period. In addition, all the extensive investigations to find the cause of the diarrhea cost $5300, which together with the indirect costs for extra days of care and supplies made a total hospital bill of approximately $200,000.

Causes of diarrhea in tube-fed patients are many, but in the hands of a skilled nutrition support team, the formula is seldom one of them. It is often found in the medications. Just remember what this medication's hidden ingredient—sorbitol—cost Max.

Data from Wong K: The role of fiber in diarrhea management. *Support Line* 20:16, 1998.

containers prefilled with formula can hang 24 to 48 hours. The fewer times any system is handled and opened, the less chance exists for contamination. Commercial formula manufacturers are making formulas now that contain microbial inhibitors to reduce the risk of bacterial contamination of the enteral formula itself.[51,52,95-98]

Infusion Method

Intragastric feedings are associated with an increased incidence of diarrhea. Infusion of a large amount of energy into the stomach stimulates the colon to secrete water, sodium, and chloride, with resulting inability of the colon to absorb nutrients.[51,52,95-98]

Patient's Condition

Malnourished or critically ill patients are more susceptible to mucosal tissue breakdown and malabsorption leading to diarrhea. Hypoalbuminemia has also been reported to be a potential cause of diarrhea because of its effect on reducing colloidal osmotic pressure within blood vessels, which could lead to edema of the intestinal mucosa, malabsorption, and diarrhea. However, no correlation has been found between patients with hypoalbuminemia and incidence of diarrhea. Patients with pancreatic insufficiency, celiac disease, short bowel syndrome, fecal impaction, diabetes mellitus, or GI inflammation are at increased risk for diarrhea.[51,52,95-98]

Medications

Multiple medications routinely given to hospitalized patients have been related to diarrhea. Antibiotics are most often associated with GI side effects. However, patients more susceptible to developing diarrhea are those who are critically ill and on multiple medications.

Extensive treatment with antibiotics and disuse of the GI tract contribute to a change in the bacterial milieu of the intestine, with proliferation of the enteric pathogen *Clostridium difficile*. Other medications associated with development of diarrhea are H$_2$ blockers, lactulose or laxatives, magnesium-containing antacids, potassium and phosphorus supplements, antineoplastic agents, and quinidine. Medications are often hyperosmolar and require dilution before infusion through a feeding tube. In general, drug reactions may relate to the metabolically active agent or to another ingredient added for its physical properties in the form of the drug, such as tablet or liquid (as the case in the *Case Study* box illustrates). Probiotics, nonpathogenic lactic acid bacteria, are receiving more attention as a potential treatment of diarrhea and as a means of preventing bacterial overgrowth and *C. difficile* infections.[51,52,95-98]

TO SUM UP

For patients with functioning GI tracts, EN support has proven to be a potent tool against present or potential malnutrition. EN support is achieved by an oral diet with nutrient-dense supplementation or alternately by tube feeding when the patient cannot, will not, or should not eat. Commercial tube feeding formulas with or without modular enhancement provide complete nutrition when provided in adequate amounts. Enteral tube feeding can be provided through nasoenteric or enterostomy feeding tubes with an open or closed delivery system. Tubing and container adaptations and development of small, mobile infusion pumps, together with a comprehensive teaching plan for patient and family and follow-up monitoring by a clinical team, allow many patients the option of home tube feeding.

For patients with a dysfunctional GI tract, PN is a life-sustaining therapy. This feeding method depends heavily on biomedical technology for the development of tubes, bags, pumps, and other equipment for feeding nutrients directly into the vein. The route of entry may be a large central vein for intravenous feeding over a long period or a smaller peripheral vein for feeding less-concentrated solutions for a shorter period. Home PN is successfully used by many patients with the support of family, friends, and a home nutrition support team.

QUESTIONS FOR REVIEW

1. Describe several types of patient situations in which enteral tube feeding may be indicated. What nutrition assessment procedures may help identify these individuals?
2. Describe nutrient components of a typical complete polymeric enteral formula. How does it differ from a modular formula? How does it differ from a semielemental and an elemental formula?
3. Define PN, and identify examples of conditions in which it would be used.

The following questions apply to the case of a man referred to nutrition support services. Imagine you are caring for this patient.

While on a long transport haul as a truck driver, a previously healthy 45-year-old man was in an accident in which he sustained a severe abdominal injury that required extensive surgical repair and left the GI tract unavailable for use for an undetermined period. He is referred to the nutrition support team for PN. Early in this care he asks you how this feeding works.

4. How would you describe and explain the PN feeding process?
5. What nutrition assessment parameters would be beneficial in identifying his risk of developing malnutrition and his tolerance of parenteral therapy?
6. List typical components of a basic PN formula he may require, and describe the purpose of each to help reassure him of its adequacy and importance.
7. Sufficient energy (kcalorie) intake is essential to immediately meet his metabolic needs after surgery. Assume a normal preinjury weight (175 lb) and height (70 in) and an added stress factor of 1.2 times his BEE. Calculate his total energy requirement, using the Harris-Benedict equation and the Mifflin-St. Jeor equation. Compare the results.
8. Define hepatic proteins, and describe why they are not appropriate indicators of nutritional status. How can you monitor the effectiveness of the PN formula in meeting his nutrition support needs for recovery?

REFERENCES

1. Borum PR: Nutrient metabolism. In Gottschlich MM, Fuhrman T, Hammond K, editors: *The science and practice of nutrition support: a case-based core curriculum,* Dubuque, IA, 2001, Kendall/Hunt Publishing.
2. Butterworth CE: The skeleton in the hospital closet, *Nutr Today* 9:4, 1974.
3. Bistrian BR, Blackburn GL, Hallowell E, et al: Protein status of general surgical patients, *JAMA* 230:858, 1974.
4. Naber TH, Schermer T, de Bree A, et al: Prevalence of malnutrition in nonsurgical hospitalized patients and its association with disease complications, *Am J Clin Nutr* 66:1232, 1997.
5. Kang MC, Kim JH, Ryu SW, et al. Prevalence of malnutrition in hospitalized patients: A multi-center cross-sectional study, *J Korean Med Sci* 33(2): e10, 2018.
6. Braunschweig C, Gomez S, Sheean PM, et al: Impact of declines in nutritional status on outcomes in adult patients hospitalized for more than seven days, *J Am Diet Assoc* 100:1316, 2000.
7. A.S.P.E.N. Board of Directors: Clinical guidelines for the use of parenteral and enteral nutrition in adult and pediatric patients, *J Parenter Enteral Nutr* 33:255–259, 2009.
8. Berkelmans GH, vanWorkum F, Weijs TJ, et al: The feeding route after esophagectomy: a review of the literature, *J Thorac Dis* 9(Suppl 8): S785–S791, 2017.
9. Luo Z, Wang J, Zhang Z, Li H, Huang L, Qiao Y, et al: Efficacy of early enteral immunonutrition on immune function and clinical outcome for postoperative patients with gastrointestinal cancer, *J Parenter Enteral Nutr* 2017. doi:10.1177/0148607117715439.
10. Charney P: Nutrition screening vs nutrition assessment: how do they differ? *Nutr Clin Pract* 23(4):366–372, 2008.
11. Lacey K, Pritchett E: Nutrition care process and model: ADA adopts road map to quality care and outcomes management, *J Am Diet Assoc* 103:1061, 2003.
12. Fuhrman MP, Charney P, Mueller CM: Hepatic proteins and nutrition assessment, *J Am Diet Assoc* 104:1258, 2004.
13. Mifflin MD, St. Jeor ST, Hill LA, et al: A new predictive equation for resting energy expenditure in healthy individuals, *Am J Clin Nutr* 51(2):241, 1990.
14. Frankenfield DC, Rowe WA, Smith JS, et al: Validation of several established equations for resting metabolic rate in obese and nonobese people, *J Am Diet Assoc* 103:1152, 2003.
15. Owers EL, Reeves AI, Ko SY, et al: Rates of adult acute inpatients documented as at risk of refeeding syndrome by registered dietitians, *Clin Nutr* 34(1):134–139, 2015.
16. Friedman AN, Fadem SZ: Reassessment of albumin as a nutritional marker in kidney disease, *J Am Soc Nephrol* 21:223–230, 2010.
17. Meyer J, Lund D, Smith J, et al: Benefits of a nutrition support service in an HMO setting, *Nutr Clin Pract* 16:25, 2001.
18. DiMaria-Ghalili RA, Gilbert K, Lord L, et al: Standards of nutrition care and professional performance for nutrition support and generalist nurses, *Nutr Clin Pract* 31(4):527–547, 2016.
19. Tucker A, Ybarra J, Bingham A, et al: American Society for Parenteral and Enteral Nutrition standards of practice for nutrition support pharmacists, *Nutr Clin Pract* 30(1):139–146, 2015.
20. Mascarenhas M, August DA, Delegge M, et al: Standards of practice for nutrition support physicians, *Nutr Clin Pract* 27(2):295–299, 2012.
21. Brantley SL, Russell MK, Mogensen KM, et al: American Society for Parenteral and Enteral Nutrition and Academy of Nutrition and Dietetics revised 2014 standards of practice and standards of professional performance for registered dietitians in nutrition support, *Nutr Clin Pract* 29(6):792–828, 2014.
22. Ukleja A, Freeman KL, Gilbert K, et al: Standards for nutrition support: adult hospitalized patients, *Nutr Clin Pract* 25(4):403–414, 2010.
23. The Joint Commission Board of Directors: *Comprehensive accreditation manual for hospitals,* Oakbrook Terrace, IL, 2014, The Joint Commision.
24. Fuhrman MP: Parenteral nutrition: a clinician's perspective, *Diet Edge* 2(1):53, 2001.
25. Bankhead R, Boullata J, Brantley S, et al: Enteral nutrition practice recommendations, *J Parenter Enteral Nutr* 33(2):122–167, 2009.
26. Roth JL, Clohessy S: Administration of enteral nutrition: initiation, progression, and transition. In Rolandelli RH, editor: *Clinical nutrition: enteral and tube feeding,* ed 4, Philadelphia, PA, 2005, Saunders.
27. Veterans Affairs Total Parenteral Nutrition Cooperative Study Group: Perioperative total parenteral nutrition in surgical patients, *N Engl J Med* 325:525, 1992.
28. Jeejeebhoy KN: Total parenteral nutrition: potion or poison? *Am J Clin Nutr* 74:160, 2001.
29. Lewis DA, Boyle K: Nutritional supplement use during medication administration: selected case studies, *J Nutr Elder* 17(4):53, 1998.
30. Elia M, Parsons EL, Cawood AL, Smith TR, Stratton RJ: Cost effectiveness of oral nutritional supplements in older malnourished care home residents, *Clin Nutr* 2017. doi:10.1016/j.clnu.2017.02.008.

31. Watters JM, Kirkpatrick SM, Norris SB, et al: Immediate postoperative enteral feeding results in impaired respiratory mechanics and decreased mobility, *Ann Surg* 266:369, 1997.

32. Charney P, Russell M: Enteral formulations: standard. In Rolandelli RH, editor: *Clinical nutrition: enteral and tube feeding*, ed 4, Philadelphia, PA, 2005, Saunders.

33. Matarese LE, Seidner DL, Steiger E, et al: The role of probiotics in gastrointestinal disease, *Nutr Clin Pract* 18:507, 2003.

34. Gadek JE, DeMichele SJ, Karlstad MD, et al: Effect of enteral feeding with eicosapentaenoic acid, α-linolenic acid, and antioxidants in patients with acute respiratory distress syndrome, *Crit Care Med* 27:1409, 1999.

35. Consensus recommendations from the US: Summit on Immune-Enhancing Enteral Therapy, *J Parenter Enteral Nutr* 25:S61, 2001.

36. Metheny NA: Preventing respiratory complications of tube feedings: Evidence-based practice, *Am J Crit Care* 15(4):360–369, 2006.

37. Lucarelli MR, Shirk MB, Jultan MW, et al: Toxicity of Food, Drug, and Cosmetic Blue #1 dye in critically ill patients, *Chest* 125(2):793–795, 2004.

38. Maloney JP, Ryan TA: Detection of aspiration in enterally fed patients: a requiem for bedside monitors of aspiration, *J Parenter Enteral Nutr* 26:S34, 2002.

39. Klein L: Is blue dye safe as a method of detection for pulmonary aspiration? *J Am Diet Assoc* 104(11):1651–1652, 2004.

40. Moore MC, editor: *Enteral nutrition. Mosby's pocket guide series: nutritional care*, ed 4, St Louis, 2001, Mosby.

41. Metheny NA, Stewart BJ, Smith L, et al: pH and concentration of bilirubin in feeding tube aspirates as predictors of tube placement, *Nurs Res* 48(4):189, 1999.

42. Dandeles LM, Lodolce AE: Efficacy of agents to prevent and treat enteral feeding tube clogs, *Ann Pharmacother* 45(5):676–680, 2011.

43. Bourgault AM, Heyland DK, Drover JW, et al: Prophylactic pancreatic enzymes to reduce feeding tube occlusions, *Nutr Clin Pract* 18(5):398–401, 2003.

44. Marian M, Carlson SJ: Enteral formulations. In Merritt R, DeLegge MH, Holcombe B, editors: *A.S.P.E.N. nutrition support practice manual*, Silver Spring, MD., 2005, American Society for Parenteral and Enteral Nutrition.

45. Phillips W, Roman B, Glassman K: Economic impact of switching from an open to a closed enteral nutrition feeding system in an acute care setting, *Nutr Clin Pract* 28(4):510–514, 2013.

46. Herlick SJ, Vogt C, Pangman V, et al: Comparison of open versus closed systems of intermittent enteral feeding in two long-term care facilities, *Nutr Clin Pract* 15:287, 2000.

47. Keohane PP, Attrill H, Love M, et al: Relation between osmolality of the diet and gastrointestinal side effects in enteral nutrition, *Br Med J (Clin Res Ed)* 288:678, 1984.

48. Lysen LK: Enteral equipment. In Matarese LE, Gottschlich MM, editors: *Contemporary nutrition support practice: a clinical guide*, ed 2, Philadelphia, PA., 2003, Saunders.

49. Ibáñaez J, Peñafiel A, Raurich JM, et al: Gastroesophageal reflux in intubated patients receiving enteral nutrition: effect of supine and semirecumbent positions, *J Parenter Enteral Nutr* 16:419, 1992.

50. Cogen R, Weinryb J, Pomerantz C, et al: Complications of jejunostomy tube feeding in nursing facility patients, *Am J Gastroenterol* 86:1610, 1991.

51. Mobarhan S, Demeo M: Diarrhea induced by enteral feeding, *Nutr Rev* 53:67, 1995.

52. Kim SH, Park CM, Seo JM, et al: The impact of implementation of an enteral feeding protocol on the improvement of enteral nutrition in critically ill adults, *Asia Pac J Clin Nutr* 26(1):27–35, 2017.

53. Emami Zeydi A, Sharafkhani M, Armat MR: Gastric residual volume: Rethinking the threshold, *Crit Care Nurse Q* 39(4):387–388, 2016.

54. Ozen N, Tosun N Yamanel L, Altintas ND, et al: Evaluation of the effect on patient parameters of not monitoring gastric residual volumes in intensive care unit patients on a mechanical ventilator receiving enteral feeding: a randomized clinical trial, *J Crit Care* 33:137–144, 2016.

55. Pinilla JC, Samphire J, Arnold C, et al: Comparison of gastrointestinal tolerance to two enteral feeding protocols in critically ill patients: a prospective, randomized trial, *J Parenter Enteral Nutr* 25:81, 2001.

56. Heyland DK, Dhaliwal R, Drover JW, et al: Canadian clinical practice guidelines for nutrition support in mechanically ventilated, critically ill adult patients, *J Parenter Enteral Nutr* 27:355, 2003.

57. Mateo MA: Nursing management of enteral tube feeding, *Heart Lung* 25:318, 1996.

58. Wikjord K, Dahl V, Søvik S: Effects on nutrition practice after implementation of a flow chart based nutrition support protocol in an intensive care unit, *Nurs Open* 4(4):282–291, 2017.

59. Heyland DK, Dhaliwal R, Day A, et al: Validation of the Canadian clinical practice guidelines for nutrition support in mechanically ventilated, critically ill adult patients: results of a prospective observational study, *Crit Care Med* 32:2260, 2004.

60. van den Berghe G, Wouters P, Weekers F, et al: Intensive insulin therapy in critically ill patients, *N Engl J Med* 345:1359, 2001.

61. Krinsley JS: Effect of an intensive glucose management protocol on the mortality of critically ill adult patients, *Mayo Clin Proc* 79:992, 2004.

62. Fuhrman MP: Complication management in parenteral nutrition. In Matarese LE, Gottschlich MM, editors: *Contemporary nutrition support practice: a clinical guide*, ed 2, Philadelphia, PA, 2003, Saunders.

63. Derenski K, Catlin J, Allen L: Parenteral nutrition basics for the clinician caring for the adult patient, *Nutr Clin Pract* 31(5):578–595, 2016.

65. Dudrick SJ, Wilmore DW, Vars HM, et al: Can intravenous feeding as the sole means of nutrition support growth in the child and restore weight loss in an adult? *Ann Surg* 169:974, 1969.

65. Klein S, Kinney J, Jeejeebhoy K, et al: Nutrition support in clinical practice: review of published data on recommendations for future directions, *J Parenter Enter Nutr* 21(3):133, 1997.

66. Gura KM: Is there still a role for peripheral parenteral nutrition? *Nutr Clin Pract* 24(6):709–717, 2009.

67. Trujillo EB, Young LS, Chertow GM, et al: Metabolic and monetary costs of avoidable parenteral nutrition use, *J Parenter Enteral Nutr* 23:109, 1999.

68. Speerhas RA: Five year follow-up of a program to minimize inappropriate use of parenteral nutrition, *J Parenter Enteral Nutr* 25:S4, 2001.

69. Yin J, Wang J, Yao D, et al: Is it feasible to implement enteral nutrition in patients with enteroatmospheric fistulae? A single-center experience, *Nutr Clin Pract* 29(5):656–661, 2014.

70. Joly F, Dray X, Corcos O, et al: Tube feeding improves intestinal absorption in short bowel syndrome patients, *Gastroenterology* 136(3):824–831, 2009.

71. Spain DA, McClave SA: Chylothorax and chylous ascites. In Gottschlich MM, Fuhrman T, Hammond K, editors: *The science and practice of nutrition support: a case-based core curriculum*, Dubuque, IA, 2001, Kendall/Hunt Publishing.

72. Kelly DG, Nehra V: Gastrointestinal disease. In Gottschlich MM, Fuhrman T, Hammond K, editors: *The science and practice of nutrition support: a case-based core curriculum*, Dubuque, IA, 2001, Kendall/Hunt Publishing.

73. Task force for the revision of safe practices for parenteral nutrition, et al: Safe practices for parenteral nutrition, *J Parenter Enteral Nutr* 28(Suppl 6):S39, 2004.

74. Seidner DL, Mascioli EA, Istfan NW, et al: Effect of long-chain triglyceride emulsions on reticuloendothelial system function in humans, *J Parenter Enteral Nutr* 13:614, 1989.

75. American Medical Association, AMA Department of Foods and Nutrition: Multivitamin preparations for parenteral use: a statement by the Nutrition Advisory Group, *J Parenter Enteral Nutr* 3:258, 1979.

76. Parenteral multivitamin products; drugs for human use; drug efficacy study implementation; amendment (21 CFR 5.70), *Fed Regist* 65:21200, 2000.

77. Expert Panel for Nutrition Advisory Group, AMA Department of Foods and Nutrition: Guidelines for essential trace element preparations for parenteral use, *JAMA* 241:2051, 1979.

78. Forceville X, Vitoux D, Gauzit R, et al: Selenium, systemic immune response syndrome, sepsis, and outcome in critically ill patients, *Crit Care Med* 26:1536, 1998.

79. Angstwurm MAW, Schottdorf J, Schopohl J, et al: Selenium replacement in patients with severe systemic inflammatory response syndrome improves clinical outcome, *Crit Care Med* 71:1807, 1999.

80. Cohen HJ, Brown MR, Hamilton D, et al: Glutathione peroxidase and selenium deficiency in patients receiving home parenteral nutrition: time course for development of deficiency and repletion of the enzyme activity in plasma and blood cells, *Am J Clin Nutr* 49:132, 1989.

81. Fuhrman MP, Herrmann V, Masidonski P, et al: Pancytopenia following removal of copper from TPN, *J Parenter Enteral Nutr* 24:361, 2000.

82. Masumoto K, Suita S, Taguchi T, et al: Manganese intoxication during intermittent parenteral nutrition: report of two cases, *J Parenter Enteral Nutr* 25:95, 2001.

83. Pemberton LB, Lyman B, Lander V, et al: Sepsis from triple- vs single-lumen catheters during total parenteral nutrition in surgical or critically ill patients, *Arch Surg* 121:591, 1986.

84. Farkas JC, Liu N, Bleriot JP, et al: Single- versus triple-lumen central–catheter-related sepsis: a prospective randomized study in a critically ill population, *Am J Med* 93:277, 1992.

85. Savage AP, Picard M, Hopkins CC, et al: Complications and survival of multilumen central venous catheters used for total parenteral nutrition, *Br J Surg* 80:1287, 1993.

86. Maki DG, Stolz SM, Wheeler S, et al: Prevention of central venous catheter-related bloodstream infection by use of an antiseptic-impregnated catheter: a randomized, controlled trial, *Ann Intern Med* 127:257, 1997.

87. Veenstra DL, Saint S, Sullivan SD, et al: Cost-effectiveness of antiseptic-impregnated central venous catheters for the prevention of catheter-related bloodstream infection, *JAMA* 282:554, 1999.

88. Centers for Disease Control and Prevention: Guidelines for the prevention of intravascular catheter-related infections, *MMWR Morb Mortal Wkly Rep* 51(RR–10):1, 2002.

89. Intravenous Nurses Society: Infusion nursing standards of practice, *J Intraven Nurs* 23(Suppl 6):S1, 2000.

90. Dodds ES, Murray JD, Texler KM, et al: Metabolic occurrences in total parenteral nutrition patients managed by a nutrition support team, *Nutr Clin Pract* 16:78, 2001.

91. Klein CJ, Stanek GS, Wiles CE, et al: Nutrition support care map targets monitoring and reassessment to improve outcomes in trauma patients, *Nutr Clin Pract* 16:85, 2001.

92. American Society for Parenteral and Enteral Nutrition Board of Directors: Standards for home nutrition support, *Nutr Clin Pract* 14:151, 1998.

93. Silver HJ, Wellman NS, Arnold DJ, et al: Older adults receiving home enteral nutrition: enteral regimen, provider involvement, and health care outcomes, *J Parenter Enteral Nutr* 28:92, 2004.

94. Evans JP, Steinhart AH, Cohen Z, et al: Home total parenteral nutrition: an alternative to early surgery for complicated inflammatory bowel disease, *J Gastrointest Surg* 7:562, 2003.

95. Bowling TE: Enteral-feeding-related diarrhea: proposed causes and possible solutions, *Proc Nutr Soc* 54:579, 1995.

96. Ringel AF, Jameson GL, Foster ES: Diarrhea in the intensive care patient, *Crit Care Clin* 11:465, 1995.

97. Wong K: The role of fiber in diarrhea management, *Support Line* 20:16, 1998.

98. Williams MS, Harpter R, Magnuson B, et al: Diarrhea management in enterally fed patient, *Nutr Clin Pract* 13:225, 1998.

FURTHER READINGS AND RESOURCES

American Society for Parenteral and Enteral Nutrition Board of Directors and Task Force on Standards for Specialized Nutrition Support of Hospitalized Adult Patients: Standards for Specialized Nutrition Support: Adult hospitalized patients. *Nutr Clin Pract* 17:384, 2002.

ASPEN Board of Directors and the Clinical Guidelines Task Force: Guidelines for the use of parenteral and enteral nutrition in adult and pediatric patients. *JPEN J Parenter Enteral Nutr* 26(Suppl):1SA, 2002.

Heyland DK, Dhaliwal R, Drover JW, et al: Canadian clinical practice guidelines for nutrition support in mechanically ventilated, critically ill adult patients. *JPEN J Parenter Enteral Nutr* 27:355, 2003.

Task Force for the Revision of Safe Practices for Parenteral Nutrition and the A.S.P.E.N. Board of Directors: Safe practices for parenteral nutrition. *JPEN J Parenter Enteral Nutr* 28(Suppl):S30, 2004.

Websites of Interest

- Academy of Nutrition and Dietetics. The world's largest organization of food and nutrition professionals committed to improving the nation's health and advancing the profession of dietetics through research, education, and advocacy: http://www.eatright.org.
- American Society for Parenteral and Enteral Nutrition (ASPEN). An interdisciplinary organization involved in provision of clinical nutrition therapies including parenteral and enteral nutrition: http://www.nutritioncare.org.
- CIGNA Medicare. This site offers free Medicare training for clinicians regarding Medicare qualifications for home enteral and parenteral nutrition: http://www.cignamedicare.com/webtraining.
- Dietitians in Nutrition Support. Dietetic practitioners integrating the science of enteral and parenteral nutrition to provide appropriate nutrition support to individuals in inpatient and outpatient settings: http://www.dnsdpg.org.
- The Oley Foundation. This nonprofit organization provides information and psychosocial support of consumers of home parenteral and enteral nutrition: http://www.oley.org.

20

Gastrointestinal Diseases

Dorothy Chen-Maynard

http://evolve.elsevier.com/Williams/essentials/

In this chapter, we consider diseases of the gastrointestinal (GI) tract and surrounding accessory organs—the liver, gallbladder, and pancreas. Digestion and absorption of food are accomplished through a series of intimately interrelated actions among and within these organ systems. Therefore disease or malfunction at any point interferes with this finely interwoven process, adequate nutrition needs to be provided either through quantitative or qualitative modifications of food provided to the patient. The GI tract is a sensitive mirror of the individual human condition. Its physiologic function often reflects physical and psychological conditions. In this chapter, these basic functions, healing process, nutrition therapy indicated, and individual's needs or dietary modifications will be discussed. The Complementary and Alternative Medicine box, "Alternative Treatments for Diseases of the Gastrointestinal Tract," outlines the effectiveness of alternative treatments for diseases of the GI tract.

OUTLINE

Digestive Process
Problems of the Mouth and Esophagus
Problems of the Stomach and Duodenum
Disorders of the Small Intestine

Disorders of the Large Intestine
Diseases of the Gastrointestinal Accessory Organs
Health Promotion

DIGESTIVE PROCESS

When food is taken into the mouth, the act of eating stimulates the GI tract into accelerated action. Throughout the digestive process, the systems and the functions are highly coordinated and interactive (Fig. 20.1). Secretory functions provide the necessary environment and agents for chemical digestion. Peristalsis and gravity move the food mass along. Nutrients are absorbed into circulation and carried to cells that take up what is needed to nourish the body. Emotional factors influence overall individual response patterns. This highly individual and interrelated functional network forms the basis for nutrition therapy in disease.

After food is taken into the mouth and masticated (forming a bolus), swallowing occurs, allowing the bolus to pass from the laryngopharynx into the esophagus entrance at the upper esophageal sphincter (UES) (Fig. 20.2). Food is pushed through the esophagus by gravity and involuntary muscular movements, called *peristalsis*, controlled by the medulla oblongata. Circular

muscle fibers contract, constricting the esophageal wall, thereby squeezing the bolus toward the stomach. The lower esophageal sphincter (LES) muscle at the entry to the stomach forms a controlling valve, relaxing to receive the bolus and then closing to hold each bolus for some initial digestive action of enzymes. Stomach cells produce enzymes to partially break down food particles and other secretions to protect themselves from being broken down. Passage of food from mouth to stomach takes approximately 4 to 8 seconds.

Chyme (semiliquid mass) is released by the stomach through the pyloric sphincter into the duodenum, the first section of the small intestine, where most digestion occurs. A number of small intestine and accessory organ conditions may interfere with normal food passage and digestive processes and create malabsorption problems. These overall conditions vary widely, from brief periods of functional discomfort to serious disease and complete obstruction. In making nutrition therapy recommendations for food choices and feeding mode, the dietetics practitioner will take into account the degree of dysfunction.

🌸 COMPLEMENTARY AND ALTERNATIVE MEDICINE (CAM):

Alternative Treatments for Diseases of the Gastrointestinal Tract

What Is Known From the Scientific Evidence About CAM Modalities for Gastrointestinal Disorders?

No well-documented herbal treatments exist for gastrointestinal (GI) disorders, although use of probiotics to treat Crohn disease shows some promise.

What CAM Therapies Might Be Used to Treat GI Disorders?

The table contains some of the common herbs used for GI ailments and their effectiveness based on scientific finding as reported on National Center for Complementary and Integrative Health of the National Institute of Health website https://www.nccih.nih.gov/health/herbsataglance.htm.

GI Disorder	Herb	Scientific Name	Active Ingredient	Efficacy	Side Effects and/or Risks
Cirrhosis	Milk thistle (plant)	*Silybum marianum*	Silymarin (found in the fruit)	Results are inconsistent. Does not appear to be effective against hepatitis virus	It is generally well tolerated but can cause laxative effects and allergic reactions in people allergic to ragweed, chrysanthemum, marigold, and daisy. People with diabetes should use caution due to possible hypoglycemia
Crohn's disease	Fish oil	Docosahexaenoic acid (DHA), eicosapentaenoic acid (EPA), omega-3 fatty acids, omega-3 oils		Results are mixed as to whether or not fish oil helped keep the disease controlled in patients who were in remission. Existing data do not support routine maintenance treatment of celiac disease	Safe but possible risk of bleeding complications
Dyspepsia, colitis	Curcumin/Turmeric	*Curcuma longa*	Polyphenol	It stimulates contraction of the gallbladder; it provides full or partial relief of symptoms	It could present risks in individuals with gallbladder disease. Maximum safe doses in individuals with severe hepatic or renal disease are not known
Hepatitis C virus (HCV)	Milk thistle (plant)	*Silybum marianum*	Silymarin (found in the fruit)	Although some benefits might be seen, none are definitively beneficial in treating HCV	Maximum safe doses in individuals with severe hepatic or renal disease are not known
	Licorice root (plant)	*Glycyrrhiza glabra*	Glycyrrhizin	Injectable form might have antiviral properties in vitro and has the potential for reducing some of short-term effects, such as fatigue and GI functions, and long-term complications of chronic HCV in patients who do not respond to interferon. It does not reduce the amount of HCV in patients' blood.[a]	Licorice intake over a long period of time can lead to hypertension, salt and water retention, swelling, depletion of potassium, headache, and/or sluggishness. In addition, it can worsen ascites and can interact with certain drugs (diuretics, digitalis, antiarrhythmic agents, and corticosteroids) (see Chapter 18)
	Thymus extract (gland)	(Should not be confused with the prescription drug thymosin α_1)	Peptides from thymus glands of cows or calves, sold as dietary supplements	Very little research exists, but no studies found the product beneficial for patients with HCV	Thrombocytopenia (a drop in number of platelet cells in blood) is possible. Concern exists regarding possible contamination from diseased animal parts (people on immunosuppressive drugs should use caution)
	Schisandra (plant)	*Schisandra chinensis, S. sphenanthera*	Extracts from its fruits	Some antioxidant effects are possible. No reports exist regarding the safety and effectiveness of using schisandra alone to treat HCV in humans	It is found as an ingredient in herbal formulas and considered generally safe. In some patients it may cause heartburn, acid indigestion, decreased appetite, stomach pain, or allergic skin rashes

Continued

🌸 COMPLEMENTARY AND ALTERNATIVE MEDICINE (CAM):

Alternative Treatments for Diseases of the Gastrointestinal Tract—cont'd

GI Disorder	Herb	Scientific Name	Active Ingredient	Efficacy	Side Effects and/or Risks
	Colloidal silver	Silver	Metallic element	Silver has no known function in the human body and is not an essential mineral supplement. Claims of silver "deficiency" in the body are unfounded	Silver builds up in body tissues: argyria—a bluish gray discoloration of the body, especially skin, other organs, deep tissues, nails, and gums. Argyria is not treatable or reversible. Other possible complications include neurologic problems (e.g., seizures), kidney damage, stomach distress, headaches, fatigue, and skin irritation. It might interfere with absorption of the following drugs: penicillamine, quinolones, tetracyclines, and thyroxine. Not safe to use
Irritable bowel syndrome (IBS)	Peppermint oil	*Mentha piperita*	Menthol	It provides antispasmodic properties and might provide some relief from cramp and abdominal pain	Enteric-coated peppermint is believed to be reasonably safe in healthy adults; nonenteric-coated peppermint oil can cause heartburn. Maximum doses in individuals with severe hepatic or renal disease are not known
	Probiotics	*Lactobacillus plantarum*	Acidophilus	Evidence of efficacy is mixed; it might reduce intestinal gas and pain	No known safety issues exist
	Flaxseed	*Linum usitatissimum*	Lignans, α-linolenic acid	It helps relieve constipation, abdominal pain, and bloating	It is not associated with any significant adverse effects
Nausea	Ginger	*Zingiber officinale*		It is as effective for motion sickness as standard pharmaceutical agents. In addition, it is effective in reducing nausea in pregnancy	No drug interactions are known. Ginger should be used with care in patients using anticoagulant or antiplatelet agents
Peptic ulcer disease (PUD)	Licorice, deglycyrrhizinated (DGL)	*Glycyrrhiza glabra*	DGL is a specially processed form of licorice that does not produce pseudohyperaldosteronemia	No evidence indicates that DGL eradicates *Helicobacter pylori*; it may protect gastric lining from NSAID-induced gastritis. It is no more effective than antacids in providing relief	It may reduce testosterone levels in men. The maximum safe doses in those with severe hepatic or renal disease are not known. Licorice appears to potentiate topical and oral corticosteroids. It should be used with caution in patients taking thiazide or loop diuretics and/or digitalis
	Probiotics	*Lactobacillus plantarum*	Acidophilus	It exerts inhibitory action on *H. pylori* but not enough to eradicate the bacterium. It may be a useful adjunct to standard antibiotic therapy	No known safety issues exist
Ulcerative colitis (UC)	Probiotics	*Escherichia coli* spp.	Nonpathogenic strain of *E. coli*	It can prevent acute attacks of UC as effectively as Mesalazine	No known safety issues exist
	Essential fatty acids	DHA, EPA, omega-3 fatty acids, omega-3 oils	Fish oils	It might be helpful for reducing symptoms of UC; regular use does not appear to help prevent disease flare-ups	Safe but possible risk of bleeding complications.
	Essential fatty acids	Omega-6 fatty acid GLA	Evening primrose oil	Somewhat beneficial in preventing flare-ups	Safe but possible risk of bleeding complications.

ᵃSee http://www.nccam.nih.gov/health/licoriceroot.

GLA, γ-linolenic acid; *NSAID,* nonsteroidal antiinflammatory drug

Data from National Center for Complementary and Alternative Medicine: *CAM and hepatitis C: a focus on herbal supplements,* NCCAM Pub No D422, Bethesda, MD, 2008, NCCAM. From: http://www.nccam.nih.gov/health/hepatitisc/hepatitiscfacts.htm; Bratman S, Girman AM: *Mosby's handbook of herbs and supplements and their therapeutic use,* St Louis, 2003, Mosby.

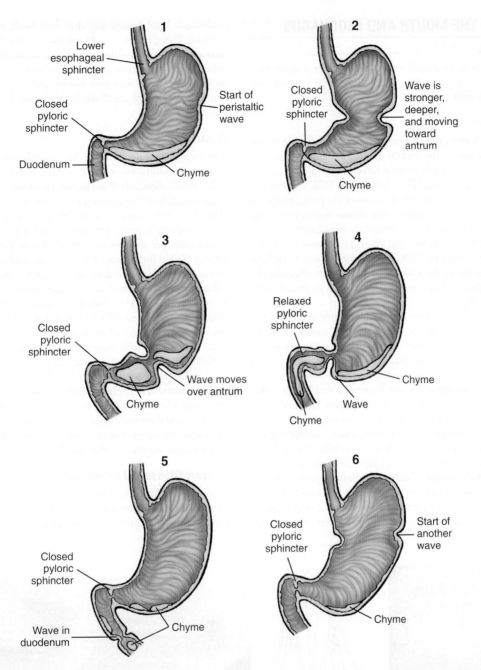

FIG. 20.1 Peristaltic waves force chyme toward the pyloric sphincter. Meanwhile, a small amount of chyme is squirted into the duodenum, and the remainder is forced back into the stomach, where further mixing occurs. (From Monahan FD, Neighbors M: *Medical-surgical nursing: foundations for clinical practice*, ed 2, Philadelphia, 1998, Saunders.)

FIG. 20.2 Parts of the mouth, pharynx, and esophagus involved in the swallowing process. (From Wardlaw GM, Insel PM: *Perspectives in nutrition*, ed 2, New York, 1993, McGraw-Hill.)

PROBLEMS OF THE MOUTH AND ESOPHAGUS

Mouth Problems

Teeth and jaw muscles in the mouth work together to break down food into a form that can be easily swallowed. Conditions that interfere with this process interfere with nutritional intake.

Tissue Inflammation

Tissues of the mouth often reflect a person's basic nutritional status. In malnutrition, tissues of the mouth deteriorate and become inflamed and are more vulnerable to local infection or injury, causing pain and difficulty with eating. These conditions (Fig. 20.3) in the oral cavity include (1) gingivitis, inflammation of the gums, involving the mucous membrane with its supporting fibrous tissue circling the base of the teeth (see Fig. 20.3A); (2) stomatitis, inflammation of the oral mucosa lining the mouth (see Fig. 20.3B); (3) glossitis, inflammation of the tongue (see Fig. 20.3C); and (4) cheilosis, a cracking and dry scaling process at the corners of the mouth affecting the lips and corner angles, making opening the mouth to receive food difficult (see Fig. 20.3D).

These oral tissue problems may also be nonspecific and unrelated to nutritional factors. In some cases, gingivitis and stomatitis occur in mild form in relation to another disease or stress. Occasionally a severe form of acute necrotizing ulcerative gingivitis occurs. It is caused by a specific infectious bacterium, *Fusobacterium nucleatum*, often in conjunction with the spirochete *Treponema vincentii*; it is also known as *Vincent disease,* from the Paris physician Henri Vincent (1862–1950), who first identified the disease process. Gums around the bases of teeth become puffy, shiny, and tender, overlapping the teeth margins. Affected gums often bleed, especially during tooth brushing. This serious condition destroys gum tissue and supporting tissues of the teeth and requires a course of antibiotic treatment.

Mouth pain in these conditions often causes decreased food intake. Maintaining adequate nutritional intake then becomes a major problem. In general, patients are given high-protein, high-energy (calorie or kcal) liquids and then soft foods, usually nonacidic and without strong spices so as to avoid irritation. Temperature extremes may also be avoided if they cause pain. Gradually foods are increased according to toleration, and foods are often supplemented with vitamins and minerals. In severe disease, use of a mouthwash containing a mild topical local anesthetic before meals helps relieve the pain of eating.

Dental Problems

The incidence of dental caries has recently been reduced in children and young adults. However, it is still present in many children and older adults, especially those unable to afford regular dental care, and causes tooth loss and chewing problems. In older adults, periodontal disease is a major cause of tooth loss. If dental caries is untreated or if dental hygiene is poor, then gum tissue at the base of the teeth becomes damaged and pockets form between the gums and the teeth. Dental plaque forms from a sticky deposit of mucus, food particles, and bacteria. Plaque hardens into calculus, a mineralized coating developed from plaque and saliva. These hardened particles then collect in pocket openings at the base of the teeth where bacteria attack periodontal tissue. The result is bacterial erosion of bone tissue surrounding affected teeth and subsequent tooth loss. Preventive care through daily dental care with fluoridated toothpaste, careful flossing, and periodic plaque removal by a dental professional forms the best approach. Extensive tooth loss leads to the need for tooth replacement with dentures. In many older adults, these dentures become ill fitting, especially when weight loss occurs, and hinder adequate chewing. All of these dental problems need to be reviewed as part of the physical assessment in any patient's nutrition history so that food textures and forms can be adjusted to individual needs.

Salivary Glands and Salivation

Disorders of the salivary glands affect eating because saliva carries an amylase that begins starch breakdown and is vital in moistening food to facilitate chewing. Problems may arise from infection, such

FIG. 20.3 Tissue inflammation of the mouth. (A) Gingivitis. (B) Stomatitis. (C) Glossitis. (D) Cheilosis. ([A] From Murray PR, Rosenthal KS, Pfaller MD: *Medical microbiology,* ed 2, St Louis, 1994, Mosby; [B] from Doughty DB, Broadwell-Jackson D: *Gastrointestinal disorders,* St Louis, 1993, Mosby; [C] courtesy Hoffbrand AV, Pettit JE, Vyas P: *Color atlas of clinical hematology,* ed 4, Philadelphia, 2010, Saunders; [D] from Lemmi FO, Lemmi CAE: *Physical assessment findings,* Philadelphia, 2000, Saunders.)

as infection with the mumps virus that attacks the parotid gland. Other problems come from excessive salivation, which occurs in numerous disorders affecting the nervous system, such as Parkinson disease, and from local disorders such as mouth infections or injury. Problems may arise from any disease or drug that causes overactivity of the parasympathetic division of the autonomic nervous system, which controls the salivary glands.

Conversely, lack of salivation, which causes xerostomia (dry mouth), may be a temporary condition caused by fear, salivary gland infection, or action of anticholinergic drugs that hinder the normal action of neurotransmitters. Clients with dry mouth best tolerate moist, soft foods with added gravies and sauces. Permanent xerostomia is rare but does occur in Sjögren syndrome, a symptom complex of unknown cause thought to be an abnormal immune response. It occurs in middle-aged or older women and is marked by dry mouth and enlargement of the parotid glands; it is often associated with rheumatoid arthritis (RA) or radiation therapy. Difficulty occurs in swallowing and speaking; problems also include tooth decay and interference with taste. Salty foods dry the mouth and should be avoided. Chewing gum or sucking on sugarless candy can increase salivary secretions. Extreme mouth dryness may be partially relieved by spraying the inside of the mouth with an artificial saliva solution.

Swallowing Disorders

Most people take swallowing for granted. Each day we eat, chew, and swallow without giving it a second thought. However, the process of swallowing involves highly integrated actions of mouth, pharynx, and esophagus (see Fig. 20.2). Swallowing difficulty, known medically as *dysphagia*, is a fairly common problem arising from many causes, including stroke, aging, developmental disabilities, and nervous system diseases. It may be only temporary, such as a piece of food lodged in the back of the throat, for which the abdominal thrust is appropriate first aid, or it may be involved with insufficient production of saliva and xerostomia. Such dysfunctional swallowing often causes individuals to aspirate food particles, in turn causing coughing and choking episodes. Dysphagia is of concern for many reasons. Foods may enter the trachea and aspirate into the lungs, allowing bacteria to multiply, leading to pneumonia. Clients with dysphagia are usually referred to a special interdisciplinary team that includes a physician, speech pathologist, nurse, clinical dietitian, physical therapist, and an occupational therapist, with special training in swallowing problems. Thin liquids are the most difficult food form to swallow. Depending on the level of dysphagia, liquids may need to be thickened. Thickening agents include baby rice, commercially prepared thickeners, potato flakes, or mashed potatoes. Levels of thickness include thick (yogurt or pudding consistency) and medium thick (nectar consistency).

Esophageal Problems
Central Problems

The esophagus is a long, muscular tube lined with mucous membranes that extends from the pharynx, or throat, to the stomach (see Fig. 20.2). It is bounded on both ends by circular muscles, or sphincters, that act as valves to control food passage. The upper sphincter remains closed except during swallowing, thus preventing airflow into the esophagus and stomach. Disorders along the tube that may disrupt normal swallowing and food passage include esophageal spasm (uncoordinated contractions of the esophagus), esophageal stricture (a narrowing caused by a scar from previous inflammation, ingestion of caustic chemicals, or a tumor), and esophagitis (an inflammation). These problems hinder eating and require medical attention through dilation, stretching procedures, or surgery to widen the tube, or drug therapy.

Lower Esophageal Sphincter Problems

Defects in the operation of the LES muscles may come from changes in smooth muscle itself or from nerve-muscle hormonal control. In general, these LES problems arise from spasm, stricture, or incompetence.

Achalasia

If the LES does not relax normally when presented with food during swallowing, the uncommon condition of achalasia (*a* meaning without and *chalasia* meaning relaxation) occurs. A primary esophageal motility ailment, achalasia is characterized by absence of esophageal peristalsis and failure of the LES to relax on swallowing. These aberrations bring about a functional obstruction at the gastroesophageal junction. Signs and symptoms characterizing achalasia are dysphagia (most common), regurgitation, chest pain, heartburn, and weight loss.[1]

The exact cause of achalasia is unknown, but it is thought to be an autoimmune disorder, infectious agent, or both.[1] Medical intervention and treatments are outlined in Table 20.1. Nutritional requirements of patients with achalasia vary with severity of the disease and approach to treatment. In general, nutrient-dense liquids and semisolid foods, taken at moderate temperatures, in small quantities, and at frequent intervals, are usually tolerated by patients with achalasia.[2]

Gastroesophageal Reflux Disease

Gastroesophageal reflux disease (GERD), backflow or regurgitation of gastric contents from the stomach into the esophagus, is a very

---

TABLE 20.1 Medical Interventions and Treatment of Achalasia

Type	Description and Efficacy
Pharmacologic: calcium channel blockers, nitrates, phosphodiesterase inhibitors	This intervention is used to reduce LES pressure and is of limited value
Mechanical: dilation by pneumatic balloons	This intervention involves esophageal dilation to decrease LES pressure. It is successful in decreasing LES pressure in 42%–85% of patients
Botulism toxin: Botox	This intervention decreases LES pressure by blocking the release of neurotransmitters at presynaptic cholinergic nerve endings. The best results have been seen in patients with vigorous achalasia. Effective duration of treatment varies but takes 6–12 months in most patients
Surgical: esophageal myotomy	This intervention—surgery—is considered to be the primary treatment. The procedure involves controlled division of muscle fibers of the lower esophagus and proximal stomach, followed by a partial fundoplication to prevent reflux. It relieves symptoms in 80%–100% of patients

LES, Lower esophageal sphincter.
Data from Pohl D, Tutuian R: Achalasia: an overview of diagnosis and treatment, *J Gastrointest Liver Dis* 16(3):297, 2007.

🔹 DIET-MEDICATIONS INTERACTIONS

Potential Food Interactions With Drugs Used to Treat Heartburn

Drugs and nutrients share related characteristics in the body. They are most often absorbed from the same sites in the intestine. Both can alter physiologic processes, and both can be toxic in high doses. Drugs used to treat heartburn, GERD, and peptic ulcer disease (PUD) are commonly used. Many are available without prescription. Following is a discussion of common drug-nutrient and herb-drug interactions.

Antacids and Alginates

Antacids may have an effect on absorption of vitamins and iron. Antacids should be taken at least 2 hours before or after iron preparations. The effect of aluminum-containing antacids may be decreased by high-protein meals. Prolonged antacid use, along with excessive consumption of calcium, may cause high calcium levels and result in serious metabolic disease. Antacids may impair folate absorption, which may increase the risk of neural tube defects and congenital anomalies of the heart, palate, and urinary tract. Folate supplementation may offset this increased risk. Concurrent ingestion of antacids and manganese may reduce manganese absorption.

H₂ Receptor Antagonists

The H_2 blocker cimetidine reacts with many drugs, including caffeine and alcohol. Cimetidine may also increase the likelihood of alcohol intoxication.

H_2 blockers decrease the body's ability to excrete caffeine; consequently, large quantities of caffeine may cause tremors, insomnia, or heart palpitations. Folate absorption or use may be impaired by H_2 blockers, which may increase risk of neural tube defects and congenital anomalies of heart, palate, and urinary tract. Folate supplementation may offset this increased risk.

H_2 blockers may impair iron absorption through effects on the pH of the digestive tract. H_2 blockers may also impair absorption of selenium. Vitamin B_{12} from food is impaired by H_2 blockers, but absorption of B_{12} supplements is not affected. Magnesium supplements can interfere with absorption of H_2 blockers. Magnesium supplements should be taken at least 2 hours before or after this medication.

Proton Pump Inhibitors

Proton pump inhibitors (PPIs) may hinder absorption of iron products, thus lessening their effectiveness. PPIs may also impair absorption of selenium. Vitamin B_{12} from food is impaired by PPIs, but absorption of B_{12} supplements is not affected. PPIs may potentiate phototoxic effects of *Hypericum* (St. John's wort).

Data from Bratman S, Girman AM: *Mosby's handbook of herbs and supplements and their therapeutic use*, St Louis, 2003, Mosby.

---

common disease. Regurgitation of acid gastric contents into the lower part of the esophagus creates constant tissue irritation because the wall of the esophagus is not protected from the acid of the stomach. During reflux, many patients feel a burning sensation behind the sternum that radiates toward the mouth, producing the most common symptom of GERD: heartburn (**pyrosis**), which is unrelated to disease of the heart (see the Diet-Medications Interactions box, "Potential Food Interactions with Drugs Used to Treat Heartburn"). Additional symptoms of GERD include acid indigestion and regurgitation, which often have a negative effect on quality of life.[2]

Other, less common symptoms include iron deficiency anemia with chronic bleeding and aspiration, which may cause cough, dyspnea, or pneumonitis. Sometimes substernal pain radiates into the neck and jaw or down the arms. Acid reflux may be worsened by a hiatal hernia, pregnancy (estrogen and progesterone have been shown to reduce LES pressure), obesity, pernicious vomiting, or nasogastric tubes. A number of drugs also lower LES pressure, causing GERD and heartburn to be a side effect of drugs used in the treatment of other conditions.

Acid and pepsin cause tissue erosion with symptoms of substernal burning, cramping, pressure sensation, or severe pain.[2] Symptoms are aggravated by lying down or any increase of abdominal pressure, such as that caused by tight clothing. The condition is related to (1) a nonfunctioning gastroesophageal sphincter, (2) frequency and duration of the acid reflux, and (3) inability of the esophagus to produce normal secondary peristaltic waves to prevent prolonged contact of the mucosa with the acid pepsin. A hiatal hernia (Fig. 20.4) may or may not be present. The most common complications of GERD are stenosis and esophageal ulcer.

Treatment of GERD is aimed at one or more aspects that cause or continue symptoms (Table 20.2). Nutrition therapy plays only a minor role in the management (Box 20.1) of GERD, and none of the dietary measures can be classified as *evidence-based treatment*.

Hiatal Hernia

The esophagus normally enters the chest cavity at the hiatus, an opening in the diaphragm membrane, and immediately joins the upper portion of the stomach. A hiatal hernia occurs when a portion of the upper part of the stomach at this entry point of the esophagus

---

KEY TERMS

Abdominal Thrust

A first aid maneuver to relieve a person who is choking from blockage of the breathing passageway by a swallowed foreign object or food particle. Standing behind the person, clasp the victim around the waist, placing one fist under the sternum (breastbone) and grasping the fist with the other hand. Then make a quick, hard, thrusting movement inward and upward.

Achalasia

Failure to relax the smooth muscle fibers of the gastrointestinal (GI) tract at any point of juncture of its parts, especially the failure of the esophagogastric sphincter to relax when swallowing, as a result of degeneration of ganglion cells in the wall of the organ. The lower esophagus also loses its normal peristaltic activity. Also called *cardiospasm*.

Pyrosis

Heartburn.

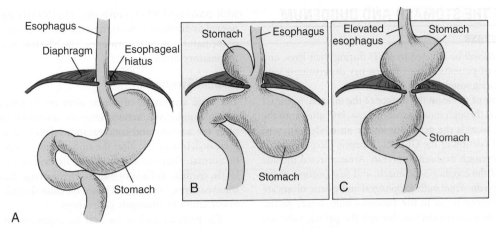

FIG. 20.4 Hiatal hernia compared with normal stomach placement. (A) Normal stomach. (B) Paraesophageal hernia (esophagus in normal position). (C) Esophageal hiatal hernia (elevated esophagus).

TABLE 20.2   Treatment of Gastroesophageal Reflux Disease Stages

Category	Recommended Treatments
Mild heartburn only (occasional bouts for >1 week)	Early low-fat dinners Elevation of head of bed H₂ antagonist >6 weeks and alkali antacids prn
Moderately severe heartburn (months of daily symptoms of heartburn/chest pressure) or poor response to H₂ receptor antagonist	PPIs single dose >6 weeks
Recurrence and persistence of moderately severe GERD symptoms (rapid recurrence of symptoms after course of PPI therapy; occasional odynophagia/dysphagia)	Gastroenterology consultation; endoscopy and biopsy of esophageal-gastric junction for Barrett metaplasia Recurrent courses of PPI therapy
Severe, persistent GERD symptoms (daily symptoms, often with odynophagia; dysphagia)	Continuous PPI therapy (often two capsules per day) Add cisapride Consider referral for laparoscopic fundoplication
Recalcitrant GERD symptoms (persistent daily/nightly symptoms with regurgitation; odynophagia, dysphagia, poor response to full drug therapy)	Maximal PPI therapy and cisapride Laparoscopic fundoplication

GERD, Gastroesophageal reflux disease; *PPIs,* proton pump inhibitors; *prn,* as needed.
Data from Gray GM: *Gastro-esophageal reflux disease (GERD): the spectrum of esophagitis, Barrett's, dysphagia, and cancer,* New York, 1996–2010, interMDnet Corporation. http://www.cyberounds.com/cmecontent/art104.html?pf=yes.

BOX 20.1   Management of Gastroesophageal Reflux Disease

Self-Care
- Over-the-counter (OTC) therapy
- Antacids
- Alginate/antacids
- H₂ receptor antagonists

Lifestyle
- Stop smoking.
- Avoid alcohol, chocolate, fatty foods, large meals at night.
- Refrain from lying down after meal.
- Elevate head of bed or use pillows.

Primary Care (Primary Care Physicians)
- Proton pump inhibitors (PPIs) or combination of alginate/antacid and acid suppressive therapy

Secondary Care (Specialists)
- Endoscopic examination
- PPIs

Data from Tytgat GN, McColl K, Tack J, et al: New algorithm for the treatment of gastro-esophageal reflux disease, *Aliment Pharmacol Ther* 27(3):249, 2008.

protrudes through the hiatus alongside the lower portion of the esophagus (see Fig. 20.4). Food is easily held in this herniated area of the stomach and mixed with acid and pepsin; then it is regurgitated back up into the lower part of the esophagus. Gastritis can occur in this herniated portion of the stomach and cause bleeding and anemia. Reflux of gastric acid contents causes symptoms similar to those described earlier.

A regular diet of choice using frequent small feedings for comfort is usually tolerated. In addition, because obesity is often associated with hiatal hernia, weight reduction is a primary goal. Avoid tight clothing, to help relieve discomfort. Patients will need to avoid leaning over or lying down immediately after meals and should sleep with the head of the bed elevated. Antacids help relieve the burning sensation. Large hiatal hernias or smaller sliding hernias may require surgical repair.

KEY TERM

Gastritis
Inflammation of the stomach.

PROBLEMS OF THE STOMACH AND DUODENUM

Peptic Ulcer Disease

One in 10 Americans will be affected by PUD during their lives, and approximately 10% of patients seen in emergency departments with abdominal pain are diagnosed with PUD.[2]

An ulcer is the loss of tissue on the surface of the mucosa. In the GI tract an ulcer extends through mucosa, submucosa, and often into the muscle layer. *Peptic ulcer* is the general term for an eroded mucosal lesion in the central portion of the GI tract. A peptic ulcer can occur in any area of the stomach exposed to pepsin. Areas affected include the lower portion of the esophagus, stomach, and first portion of the duodenum, called the *duodenal bulb.* Esophageal and gastric ulcers are less common. Most ulcers occur in the duodenal bulb, where gastric contents emptying into the duodenum through the pyloric valve are most concentrated. Gastric ulcers occur usually along the lesser curvature of the stomach. PUD itself is a benign disease, but ulcers do tend to recur. Gastric ulcers are more prone to develop into malignant disease. Weight loss is common in patients with gastric ulcers. Patients with duodenal ulcers may gain weight from frequent eating to counteract pain.

Peptic ulcer is caused by *Helicobacter pylori* in the stomach or intake of nonsteroidal antiinflammatory drugs (NSAIDs).[3] Nutrition or diet is not thought to play a significant role in the cause. *H. pylori* is a short, spiral-shaped, microaerophilic gram-negative bacillus (Fig. 20.5) that attaches itself to gastric mucosa.[3] It is able to survive the acidic environment of the stomach by secreting enzymes to neutralize the acid. This allows *H. pylori* to find its way to the protective mucous lining of the stomach, and its spiral shape facilitates burrowing through the lining.[4]

Intake of aspirin or other NSAIDs such as ibuprofen (Motrin), naproxen (Naprosyn), and etodolac (Lodine) induces ulcer formation by interfering with formation of prostaglandins, the chemicals that help the mucosal lining resist caustic acid damage.[5] They irritate gastric mucosa and cause bleeding, erosion, and ulceration, especially

FIG. 20.5 *Helicobacter pylori.* (From Kumar V, Abbas AK, Fausto N: *Robbins and Cotran pathologic basis of disease,* ed 7, Philadelphia, 2005, Saunders.)

with prolonged or excessive use. The NSAID group of drugs is so named to distinguish them from the corticosteroids, synthetic variants of the natural adrenal hormones. The NSAIDs include a dozen antiinflammatory drugs.

Clinical Symptoms

The basic symptoms of peptic ulcer are increased gastric tone and painful hunger contractions when the stomach is empty. In a duodenal ulcer the amount and concentration of hydrochloric acid (HCl) are increased. In a gastric ulcer the amount and concentration of HCl may be normal. Nutritional deficiencies are evident in low plasma protein levels, anemia, and loss of weight. Hemorrhage may be the first sign in some patients. Diagnosis is based on clinical findings, radiographs, or visualization by fiberoptic gastroscopy.

The primary goal of medical management for PUD is control of *H. pylori.* Additional supportive goals are to (1) alleviate symptoms, (2) promote healing, (3) prevent recurrences, and (4) prevent complications. In addition to general traditional measures, the rapidly expanding knowledge base and development of a number of new drugs have increased the physician's available management tools.

General Therapeutic Measures

Adequate rest, relaxation, and sleep have long been a foundation for general care of PUD to enhance the body's natural healing process. Positive stress-coping and relaxation skills, which help patients deal with personal psychosocial stressors, can be learned and practiced. Simple encouragement to talk about anxieties, anger, and frustrations helps make patients feel better, and as soon as they are able, appropriate physical activity helps work out tensions. Habits that contribute to ulcer development, such as smoking and alcohol use, should be eliminated. Common drugs such as aspirin and NSAIDs should be avoided.

Pharmacologic Management

Current pharmacologic management of PUD includes a wider choice of drugs to control underlying physiologic cause and clinical symptoms, as well as to support healing. In various ways the following five types of drugs suppress gastric acid and pepsin secretion, protect mucosal tissue, buffer acid, and eliminate infection:

1. H_2 receptor antagonists: These agents, commonly called H_2 blockers, are popular drugs for controlling gastric acid secretion. They decrease HCl production by competing with histamine for receptor sites on parietal cells. Normally, histamine attaches to its specific cellular receptors (type H_2) on acid-producing parietal cells of gastric mucosa and mediates secretion of HCl. Thus the blocking action of these agents effectively controls acid and pepsin because inactive pepsinogen requires acid for activation. The four drugs in this classification have now been reclassified for over-the-counter (OTC) purchase: (1) cimetidine (Tagamet), (2) ranitidine (Zantac), (3) famotidine (Pepcid), and (4) nizatidine (Axid).

2. *PPIs:* This newer class of drugs, more potent than H_2 blockers, also suppresses gastric acid but by a different action. For example, prostaglandin analog, misoprostol, can be used with NSAIDs to prevent ulcer. This class of medication should not be used by pregnant women. Long-term use of PPIs may lead to hypomagnesemia, and it is recommended that serum magnesium levels should be monitored. In the parietal cells, the PPIs irreversibly inhibit a key enzyme, H^+/K^+-ATPase, that actively secretes hydrogen ions needed for HCl production. Without available H_2 ions, HCl cannot be made, and without acid, ulcers can heal rapidly. The US Food and Drug Administration (FDA) has approved five drugs in this category: (1) lansoprazole (Prevacid), (2) omeprazole (Prilosec),

(3) esomeprazole (Nexium), (4) rabeprazole (Aciphex), and (5) pantoprazole (Protonix). PPIs may interfere with liver metabolism of anticoagulants, diazepam (Valium), or phenytoin (Dilantin). Serum levels of these drugs should be monitored during concurrent therapy.

3. *Mucosal protectors:* Drugs of this type act as cytoprotective agents by helping the stomach heal itself. They produce a gel-like suspension that binds to the ulcer base and covers it and surrounding normal mucosal tissue to protect involved tissue from harm while it heals. This drug also forms complexes with pepsin that inactivate pepsin. An example of this type of drug is sucralfate (Carafate). These drugs are not as effective as the other options.

4. *Antacids:* These well-known substances counteract or neutralize acidity. They are safe and inexpensive to use. Two main types are (1) magnesium-aluminum compounds (Maalox, Mylanta) and (2) aluminum hydroxide (Basaljel, Amphojel). Aluminum-based preparations may cause constipation; magnesium-based preparations may cause diarrhea.

5. *Antibiotics:* Drugs of this type are used to control the *H. pylori* infection associated with PUD. Treatment using one or two antibiotics such as amoxicillin, tetracycline (not to be used for children younger than age 12), metronidazole, or clarithromycin is recommended for 10 days to 2 weeks, in conjunction with either ranitidine bismuth citrate, bismuth subsalicylate, or a PPI. The combination of acid suppression by the H₂ blocker or PPI with antibiotics helps alleviate ulcer-related symptoms (e.g., abdominal pain, nausea) and heal inflammation and may enhance efficacy of the antibiotics.[5] Currently the FDA has approved eight *H. pylori* treatment regimens (Box 20.2), although other combinations have been used effectively. Better eradication rates have been demonstrated using triple-therapy regimens rather than dual therapy, longer length of treatment (14 days instead of 10 days), or both. Major reasons for treatment failure are antibiotic resistance and patient noncompliance.[5]

Nutritional Management

Pharmacologic therapy is the treatment of choice for PUD. No evidence indicates that diet plays a significant role in treatment when compared with pharmacologic regimens.[6] Dietary recommendations are formed from individual tolerance and should be considered supplemental to pharmacologic therapy. No conclusive evidence supports use of a traditional "bland" diet to decrease gastric acid secretion or increase the time it takes to heal ulcers.[2] In short, individuals with PUD should be encouraged to eat a healthy diet from foods they enjoy.

BOX 20.2   US Food and Drug Administration–Approved Treatment Options for Peptic Ulcer Disease

Proton Pump Inhibitor (PPI)–Based Triple Therapies
- PPI (lansoprazole or omeprazole), amoxicillin, and clarithromycin
- The above three packaged together: Prevpac (using the PPI lansoprazole)
- PPI (lansoprazole or omeprazole), metronidazole, and clarithromycin or amoxicillin

"Conventional Triple Therapy" for *Helicobacter pylori*
- Bismuth (Pepto-Bismol), metronidazole, and tetracycline or amoxicillin, combined with an H₂ blocker (cimetidine, famotidine, nizatidine, or ranitidine) or a PPI (lansoprazole or omeprazole)
- The three packaged together: Helidac combined with an H₂ blocker (cimetidine, famotidine, nizatidine, or ranitidine) or a PPI (lansoprazole or omeprazole)

Note: Dual therapy of single PPI and a single antibiotic is not recommended.
Data from Stratemeier MW, Vignogna L, Hale KL: Peptic ulcers. eMedicine. http://www.emedicinehealth.com/peptic_ulcers/article_em.htm, 2014.

General nutritional therapeutic recommendations include the following[7]:
- Emphasize a balanced, nutritious diet.
- Limit the following foods and seasonings, and encourage avoidance of lifestyle habits known to increase acid secretion, inhibit healing, or both:
  - Caffeine (including coffee, tea, or decaffeinated coffee)
  - Black pepper
  - Chocolate
  - Foods that are irritating or not well tolerated
  - Alcohol
  - Eating less than 2 hours before bedtime

Personal Focus

Sound nutritional management plays an important supportive role in total medical care of persons with PUD. The individual must be the focus of treatment. The patient is not *an ulcer;* he or she is a person *with an ulcer.* The course of the disease is conditioned by the individuality of the patient and his or her life situation. The presence of the ulcer affects the patient's life and quality of life. In the long run a wide range of foods, attractive to the eye and the taste, and regular, unhurried eating habits provide the best course of action (see the Case Study box, "The Patient With Peptic Ulcer Disease").

CASE STUDY

The Patient With Peptic Ulcer Disease

Lowell is a 40-year-old businessman who was admitted to the city hospital 3 weeks ago after vomiting bright-red blood. A medical history revealed that a dull, gnawing pain in the upper abdomen began several months ago and has increased in severity during that time. It became more severe after his most recent out-of-state trip to one of his stores. Because the pain was usually accompanied by headaches, he took aspirin to help relieve it.

Initial hospital treatment consisted of blood transfusions, intravenous fluids and electrolytes, and vitamin C. Lowell continued to feel nauseated and weak, but he stopped vomiting. However, he passed several large, tarry stools during the first 24 hours. His initial nutrition assessment results included weight 68 kg (150 lb), height 175 cm (5′ 9″), albumin 2.8 g/dL, prealbumin 14 mg/dL, transferrin 18% saturation value, hemoglobin (Hb) 11 g/dL, and hematocrit 35%. His medications included cimetidine, sucralfate, magnesium-aluminum hydroxide, and triple antibiotic therapy.

The patient began slowly to tolerate sips of clear liquids and then advanced to a regular diet as tolerated, showing continued improvement. Before he was discharged at the end of the second week, the registered dietitian (RD) discussed general nutritional needs with Lowell and his wife. He was advised to eat meals regularly in as relaxed a setting and manner as possible, eliminate his frequent between-meal snacks, and take his multivitamin supplement daily with his

Continued

meals. In addition, general guidelines and a list of a few food-related items or habits to avoid were reviewed. He was also advised to stop smoking and to rest as much as possible before returning to work. His physician had also advised him to reduce his workload and scheduled a follow-up appointment in 1 week.

Lowell's wife accompanied him to the next appointment and reported she was pleased with his ability to put aside business duties and take more time to enjoy his family. Lowell stated his two teenage sons had been surprisingly supportive in assisting him in following the prescribed regimen, and he plans to make it his general habit.

Questions for Analysis

1. The radiographic diagnosis of Lowell's illness was a gastric ulcer in the antrum lesser curvature. What does this mean? Where do most ulcers occur? Why?

2. What factors contributed to Lowell's ulcer? What effect did each of them have?

3. Evaluate the results of Lowell's initial nutrition assessment data. How would you use this information in nutrition counseling?

4. Identify Lowell's basic nutritional needs. Outline a teaching plan based on these needs that you would use to help him with his new diet plan. How would you include his wife in formulating and implementing his nutrition care plan?

5. What role does vitamin C play in Lowell's therapy?

6. Why should Lowell give up coffee, cigarettes, and alcohol? What problems do you think he may encounter in trying to change these habits?

DISORDERS OF THE SMALL INTESTINE

Diarrhea and Malabsorption

Diarrhea

Diarrhea is not a disease; it is a symptom that can be attributed to many medical conditions (see the Perspectives in Practice box, "Nutritional Aspects of Diarrhea"). *Diarrhea* is defined as an increase in frequency of bowel movements compared with the usual pattern, an excess water content of stools affecting consistency or volume, or both. Diarrhea most directly involves the large intestine but may be caused by disease of the small intestine, pancreas, or gallbladder. General diarrhea may result from basic dietary excesses. Fermentation of sugars or excess fiber stimulation of intestinal muscle function may be involved.

Chronic diarrhea may occur as a result of GI tract motility dysfunction such as irritable bowel syndrome (IBS), malabsorption, metabolic disorders, food intolerances (e.g., lactose intolerance), food poisoning,

PERSPECTIVES IN PRACTICE

Nutritional Aspects of Diarrhea

Gastrointestinal (GI) disease so often presents barriers to efficient nutrient absorption that nutritional deficiencies are planned for automatically. Unfortunately, many of these conditions also frequently lead to diarrhea, which results in further loss of fluids and electrolytes. As expected, replacement of these fluids is the initial and primary concern of therapy. However, different types of diarrhea also present other differences; control of type-specific problems requires different modes of treatment coordinated with treatment of the disease it accompanies. Before looking into possible treatment modes, three of the most common types of diarrhea should be examined: (1) watery, (2) fatty, and (3) small volume.

Watery diarrhea occurs when the amount of water and electrolytes moving into intestinal mucosa exceeds that amount absorbed into the bloodstream. This movement of water and electrolytes into the mucosa may be secretive or osmotic. If this movement of water and electrolytes into the mucosa is secretive, then it may be active or passive. Active movement occurs with excessive gastric hydrochloric acid (HCl) secretion or enterotoxin-induced infections such as cholera. Passive movement occurs with a rise in hydrostatic pressure that accompanies such infectious diseases as salmonellosis or tuberculosis, nonbacterial infections, fungal infections, renal failure, irradiation enteritis, and inflammatory bowel disease (IBD). Other conditions associated with watery diarrhea include hyperthyroidism, thyroid carcinoma, and hypermotility of the GI tract.

If this movement of water and electrolytes into the mucosa is osmotic, it will occur when nutrients are not absorbed because of intolerable levels of nonabsorbable particles present in intestinal chyme. Such particles include lactose (milk sugar) in individuals with lactase deficiency or gluten (a cereal protein found in wheat and rye and to a lesser degree in barley and oats) in persons with a reduced GI transit time caused by the removal of part of the intestinal tract.

Fatty diarrhea, or steatorrhea, occurs with maldigestion or malabsorption. Maldigestion involves a lack of enzymatic activity required to completely digest food, such as reduced pancreatic exocrine activity (release of intestinal enzymes from the pancreas) caused by pancreatic insufficiency. Malabsorption means digested materials do not make it across the intestinal mucosa to enter the bloodstream. This failure occurs in conditions in which the intestinal villi are destroyed, such as celiac disease (CD).

Small-volume diarrhea occurs mainly when the rectosigmoid area of the colon is irritated, such as in IBD (Crohn disease or ulcerative colitis [UC]). It also occurs when inflammatory conditions affect areas adjacent to the colon, as in pelvic inflammatory disease, diverticulitis, appendicitis, or hemorrhagic ovarian cysts.

Metabolic consequences of each type of diarrhea are similar. Uncontrolled, they result in syncope, hypokalemia, acid-base imbalances, and hypovolemia, with resulting renal failure. They may also be accompanied by low levels of fat-soluble vitamins, vitamin B_{12}, or folic acid, or eventually lead to protein-energy malnutrition (PEM). In addition to these conditions, each type also manifests problems associated with the disorder they accompany. Workers with the Memorial Sloan Kettering Cancer Center in New York and the Department of Medicine at Brooke Army Medical Center in Texas have developed recommendations for treating GI diseases associated with each type of diarrhea. These are summarized as follows, with the focus on the diarrheal aspects of disease:

- Watery diarrhea often accompanies inflammatory bowel conditions, such as Crohn disease, for which nutrition therapy involves (1) increased protein and kcalories, (2) low fats and lactose, and (3) avoidance of foods that stimulate peristalsis. Thus secretive diarrhea, caused by microscopic colitis, is reduced by eliminating foods that may stimulate gastric acid secretion, and all types of watery diarrhea can be avoided by reducing the motility of the GI tract. In other conditions in which osmotic diarrhea occurs, such as dumping syndrome, this problem is prevented by giving fluids between meals to avoid any extreme difference in osmotic pressures on either side of the intestinal wall. Small, frequent meals also help prevent this problem, as well as painful distention.

- Steatorrhea frequently accompanies conditions associated with maldigestion such as chronic pancreatitis or gall bladder obstruction. Nutritional management of this disease involves (1) frequent meals high in protein and carbohydrates and low in fat; (2) use of medium-chain triglycerides (MCTs), which are

Nutritional Aspects of Diarrhea—cont'd

more easily absorbed under adverse conditions; and (3) avoiding gastric stimulants, especially caffeine and alcohol. Steatorrhea also accompanies conditions of malabsorption, such as gluten-sensitive enteropathy. In addition to the nutritional management strategies listed, treating this type of diarrhea requires removal of products that damage the mucosal villi, including lactose and gluten, which is found in wheat, rye, barley, and oats, and food products and fillers such as hydrolyzed vegetable protein products. It sometimes requires restricting fat as well. In both cases the primary concern is to monitor fats that would otherwise appear in the feces. As therapy progresses, fat content of the meal can be increased as tolerated to normal levels to improve palatability.

- Small-volume diarrhea may accompany diverticulosis of the colon. A high-residue diet is recommended to increase fecal bulk, thereby preventing diarrhea. To prevent flatulence and distention, fiber should be added to the diet gradually.

All types of diarrhea can result in malnutrition, primarily because of electrolyte and fluid losses. It is important to identify the type of diarrhea occurring with each patient; only then can an effective nutritional management strategy be designed to replace those losses, as well as to eliminate or prevent other nutrition-related problems that are possible for each case.

---

infections, and human immunodeficiency virus (HIV) infection. In the case of lactose intolerance, the accumulated concentration of undigested lactose in the intestine, resulting from the lack of the enzyme lactase, creates increased osmotic pressure. This pressure effectively draws water into the gut and stimulates hypermotility, abdominal cramping, and diarrhea. Milk treated with lactase enzyme is tolerated by these persons without the difficulty encountered with regular milk. Secretory, osmotic, and inflammatory processes in the intestine result in increased losses of fluid and electrolytes from diarrhea.[8]

Malabsorption

In a normally functioning body, foods are digested and then nutrients are absorbed into the bloodstream, mostly from the small intestine. Malabsorption occurs either because a disorder interferes with how food is digested or because a disorder interferes with how nutrients are absorbed. Multiple causes of a malabsorption condition exist.[8] Symptoms of malabsorption include a change in bowel habits, apathy, fatigue, and a smooth surface on the lateral tongue. Some of these causes include the following:

- *Maldigestion problems:* pancreatic disorders, biliary disease, bacterial overgrowth, ileal disease (inflammatory bowel disease [IBD])
- *Intestinal mucosal changes:* mucosal surface alterations, intestinal surgery such as resections that shorten the bowel, lymphatic obstruction, intestinal stasis
- *Genetic disease:* cystic fibrosis (CF), with its complications of pancreatic insufficiency and lack of the pancreatic enzymes lipase, trypsin, and amylase
- *Intestinal enzyme deficiency:* lactose intolerance caused by lactase deficiency
- *Cancer and its treatment:* absorbing surface effect of radiation and chemotherapy
- *Metabolic biochemical defects:* absorbing surface effects of pernicious anemia or gluten-induced enteropathy (celiac disease [CD])

Here we briefly review four of these malabsorptive conditions: (1) CD, (2) CF, (3) IBD, and (4) short bowel syndrome (SBS).

Celiac Disease
Metabolic Defect

In 1889 a London physician named Gee observed a number of malnourished children having steatorrhea and distended abdomens. He gave the name *celiac* to the general clinical condition from the Greek word *kolia*, meaning belly or abdomen. It was not until the mid-1950s that the Dutch pediatrician Willem-Karel Dicke and his associates discovered the causative agent. Their tissue studies confirmed that the gliadin fraction of the protein gluten in wheat produced the fat malabsorption; furthermore, what had been called *celiac disease* in children and *nontropical*

sprue in adults was a single disease, which came to be called *celiac sprue.*[9] As currently used, the alternative terms *CD* and *gluten-sensitive enteropathy* are synonymous with celiac sprue. In all cases, such diseased tissues consistently show an eroded mucosal surface lacking the number and form of normal villi and having few microvilli, resulting in malabsorption of most nutrients (Fig. 20.6). (For more information regarding genetic malabsorption diseases, see the Evidence-Based Practice box, "Food Intolerances from Genetic-Metabolic Disease," and the Focus on Culture box, "Did Your Ancestors Herd Dairy Cattle?")

FIG. 20.6 Comparison of normal intestinal villi and those in an individual with celiac disease. (A) Biopsy specimen of diseased mucosa shows diffuse severe atrophy and blunting of villi. (B) Normal mucosal biopsy specimen. (From Kumar V, Abbas AK, Fausto N: *Robbins and Cotran pathologic basis of disease,* ed 7, Philadelphia, 2005, Saunders.)

EVIDENCE-BASED PRACTICE

Food Intolerances from Genetic-Metabolic Disease

Certain food intolerances may stem from underlying genetic disease that affects metabolism of one or more specific nutrients. Genetic disease results from the individual's specific gene inheritance. Genes in each cell control the metabolic functions of the cell. They regulate synthesis of approximately 1000 or more specific cell enzymes that control metabolism within the cell. A specific gene controls the synthesis of a specific enzyme. When that gene sequence is abnormal due to mutation, the cell is unable to make the enzyme. In turn, the specific metabolic reaction controlled by that specific missing enzyme cannot take place. Specific genetic disease caused by this metabolic block then manifests clinical symptoms connected with resulting abnormal metabolic products. As primary examples here, we look briefly at two such genetic diseases affecting food-nutrient intolerances: (1) phenylketonuria (PKU), which affects metabolism of amino acid and phenylalanine, leading to the need to limit certain protein foods; and (2) galactosemia, which affects carbohydrate metabolism, specifically food sources that contain lactose. Both are detected by newborn screening procedures that are mandatory by law.

Phenylketonuria

Phenylketonuria results from the missing cell enzyme phenylalanine hydroxylase, which metabolizes one of the essential amino acids, phenylalanine, to tyrosine, another nonessential amino acid. Phenylalanine then accumulates in the blood, and its alternate metabolites, the phenyl acids, are excreted in the urine. One of these urinary acids, phenylpyruvic acid, is a phenylketone, hence the name of the disease. Untreated, PKU can produce devastating effects, but current nutrition therapy can avoid these results. In past years, before current newborn screening laws and dietary treatment practices from birth, the most profound effect observed in persons with untreated PKU was severe mental retardation. The intelligence quotient (IQ) of affected persons was usually less than 50 and often less than 20. Central nervous system (CNS) damage caused irritability, hyperactivity, convulsive seizures, and bizarre behavior.

PKU can now be well controlled by special nutrition therapy. After screening at birth, a special low-phenylalanine diet effectively controls serum phenylalanine levels so that they are maintained at appropriate amounts to prevent clinical symptoms and promote normal growth and development. Because phenylalanine is an essential amino acid necessary for growth, it cannot be totally removed from the diet. Blood levels of phenylalanine need to be constantly monitored, and the metabolic team nutritionist calculates the special diet for each infant and child to allow only a limited amount of phenylalanine that can be tolerated. In addition, without phenylalanine hydroxylase, tyrosine becomes essential amino acid for individuals with PKU. Based on extensive studies, guidelines for nutritional management of PKU are currently being used effectively to build lifetime habits; research now indicates that no safe age exists at which a child may discontinue the diet. This dietary management is built on two basic components: (1) a substitute for milk (a special medical food continued past infancy and childhood into adolescence and adulthood) and (2) guidelines for adding solid foods (both regular and special low-protein products) and then building continuing food habits.

Initial education and continuing support of parents is essential, because dietary management of PKU is the only known effective method of treatment and maintaining the diet becomes more difficult as the child grows older. Parents must understand and accept the necessity of the diet, and this requires patience, understanding, and continued reinforcement. The PKU team, together with parents, provides initial and continuing care so that the child with PKU will grow and develop normally. When PKU is diagnosed at birth, as a result of widespread screening programs, a child can have a healthy and happy life, instead of the profound disease consequences experienced in the past. Current practice of long-term nutritional management is especially critical for young women with PKU who are considering pregnancy. At least 6 months before becoming pregnant, women with PKU should meet with a metabolic team to discuss treatment and follow-up. It is possible for women with PKU to have normal children. However, maternal PKU presents the possibility of a potentially high-risk pregnancy if a low-phenylalanine diet is not strictly followed.

Galactosemia

This genetic disease affects carbohydrate metabolism so that the body cannot use the monosaccharide galactose. Three enzymes are responsible for conversion of galactose to glucose, and in galactosemia at least one of the enzymes is defective or missing. Milk, infants' first food, contains a large amount of the precursor lactose (milk sugar). When infants with galactosemia are given breast milk or regular infant formula, they vomit and have diarrhea. After galactose is initially combined with phosphate to begin metabolic conversion to glucose, it cannot proceed further in the infant with galactosemia. Galactose rapidly accumulates in the blood and in various body tissues. In the past, excess tissue accumulations of galactose caused rapid damage in the untreated infant. Clinical symptoms appeared soon after birth, and the child failed to thrive. Continued liver damage brought **jaundice**, an enlarged liver with **cirrhosis**, enlarged spleen, and ascites. Without treatment, death usually resulted from liver failure. If the infant survived, then continuing tissue damage and hypoglycemia in the optic lens and the brain caused cataracts and mental retardation. However, with current newborn screening programs, infants with galactosemia are diagnosed at birth and started on special dietary management. With this vital nutrition therapy, children can grow and develop normally.

The main indirect source of dietary galactose is the lactose in milk. A galactose-free diet (free of all forms of milk and lactose) is observed, and the infant is fed a soy-based formula. Breastfeeding is not an option when this genetic condition is present. The body synthesizes the amount of galactose needed for body structures. As solid foods are added to the infant's diet at approximately 6 months of age, careful attention must be given to avoiding lactose from other food sources. Parents quickly learn to check labels carefully on all commercial products to detect any lactose or lactose-containing substances.

Websites of Interest

Galactosemia

- National Organization for Rare Disorders:
  https://www.rarediseases.org
- Parents of Galactosemic Children, Inc.:
  http://www.galactosemia.org/understanding-galactosemia/

Phenylketonuria (PKU)

- Children's PKU Network:
  http://www.pkunetwork.org/Childrens_PKU_Network/Home.html
- National Coalition for PKU and Allied Disorders:
  http://www.pku-allieddisorders.org
- National PKU News:
  https://www.pkunews.org

Data from Nelms MN, Sucher K, Long S: *Understanding nutrition therapy and pathophysiology*, Belmont, CA, 2007, Wadsworth/Thomson Learning.

🌐 FOCUS ON CULTURE

Did Your Ancestors Herd Dairy Cattle?

Do you or anyone you know experience these symptoms—cramps, bloating, gas, diarrhea, nausea—anywhere from 30 min to 2 h after consuming a food or beverage containing lactose? As you learned in Chapter 3, lactose is found in milk and some dairy products, and the enzyme lactase is necessary for us to digest lactose. Lack of this mucosal enzyme, lactase, results in a condition called *lactose intolerance.*

Humans are the only mammals that continue to drink milk past weaning. Most mammals produce lactase until they are weaned and stop drinking milk. Cessation of milk drinking and lactase production characterizes most of the world's population, especially those of Asian and African ancestry. For children older than 5 years, 90% to 95% of people of color (African Americans, Asians, Hispanics) are lactose intolerant, whereas only 20% to 25% of those of northern European descent do not tolerate dairy products. Lactose intolerance is usually referred to as a *disease* or *disorder*. Does this seem logical? Why is a trait found in 90% to 95% of the world's population abnormal? Perhaps lactose intolerance should be considered a normal adult condition.

Researchers from Cornell University believe lactose tolerance is the outcome of a genetic mutation that sustains the functionality of lactase production into adulthood, allowing consumption of milk throughout life. This mutation occurs commonly among populations from Northern Europe, where raising cattle and other ruminant animals has been practiced for centuries because the environment made it safe and economical to do so.

It appears that the ability to produce lactase and absorb lactose is nutritionally beneficial for adults only if milk is consistently available. To test this theory, data were collected on adult lactose absorption and malabsorption from 270 indigenous African and Eurasian populations. Adult lactose malabsorption was found to be associated with extreme hot or cold climates (high and low latitudes). In addition to the geographic and climatic features of these regions that preclude the raising of dairy herds, historical evidence (pre-1900) indicates that nine deadly communicable cattle diseases occurred in these regions. The researchers concluded that areas of the world where adult lactose malabsorption predominates are the same areas in which it is dangerous or impossible to sustain dairy herds. Thus the ability to digest lactose appears for the most part to be a genetic mutation.

Data from Bloom G, Sherman PW: Dairying barriers affect the distribution of lactose malabsorption, *Evol Hum Behav* 26(4):301, 2005.

Gluten molecules trigger an autoimmune and inflammatory response in the small intestine, causing the usually brushlike lining of the intestine to flatten, thereby becoming much less able to digest and absorb foods. Damage is reversed when gluten is removed from the diet. It is unclear why an immunologic response occurs when gluten is ingested by genetically predisposed persons.[10] The resulting malabsorption promotes malnutrition and severe debilitation.[8] Gluten is a protein present in some grains such as wheat, rye, and barley but not oats, rice, or corn.

CD occurs in approximately 1 in 133 persons in the United States, but only a small percentage of people with it have been diagnosed. CD, as a rule, commonly occurs in women, Caucasians and others of European ancestry, and first-degree relatives. It can occur at any age from infancy to late adulthood.[11]

Clinical Symptoms

Symptoms vary significantly from person to person. They may be intestinal or nonintestinal in nature, which makes diagnosis difficult. One person may present with diarrhea, another with constipation, and yet another with no stool elimination problems.[11] Children with CD most often display failure to thrive, with or without malabsorption. Adults most frequently present with anemia caused by iron or folate deficiency (or both).[11] A partial listing of GI symptoms is summarized in Table 20.3.

Diagnosis

Individuals in the general population may not be identified by clinical symptoms, therefore remaining underdiagnosed, but screening remains controversial. Tissue transglutaminase antibodies (tTG-IgA) have been found to be a sensitive marker for CD.[11] Intestinal biopsy is then used to confirm diagnosis in patients with positive serologic tests. Depending on the degree of intestinal involvement, a complete blood count (CBC); levels of serum iron or ferritin, red cell folate, vitamin B_{12}, serum calcium, alkaline phosphatase, albumin, and β-carotene; and prothrombin time (PT) should be obtained in patients suspected of malabsorption problems.

KEY TERMS

Jaundice
A syndrome characterized by hyperbilirubinemia and deposits of bile pigment in the skin, mucous membranes, and sclera, giving a yellow appearance to the patient.

Cirrhosis
Chronic liver disease, characterized by loss of functional cells, with fibrous and nodular regeneration.

TABLE 20.3 Gastrointestinal Symptoms Associated With Celiac Disease

Symptom	Comments
Abdominal pain	
Abdominal distention	Bloating, gas, indigestion
Constipation	
Decreased appetite	May also be increased or unchanged
Diarrhea	Chronic or occasional
Lactose intolerance	Common on diagnosis; usually resolves after treatment
Nausea and vomiting	
Steatorrhea	Stools that float, are foul smelling, bloody, or "fatty"
Weight loss	Unexplained (people can be overweight or normal weight on diagnosis)

Data from US National Library of Medicine, National Institutes of Health: *Medline Plus A.D.A.M. medical encyclopedia: celiac disease-sprue*, Atlanta, GA2005, A.D.A.M. Inc. https://www.nlm.nih.gov/medlineplus/ency/article/000233.htm.

Nutritional Management

The goal of nutritional management is to control intake of dietary gluten and prevent malnutrition. The diet is better defined as *low gluten* rather than *gluten free* because it is impossible to remove all gluten. Newer products labeled *gluten free* can contain wheat starch as a thickening agent, which cannot be recommended.[12] Wheat and rye are the main sources of glutenlike proteins; it is also present in oats and barley. Thus these four grains have always been eliminated from the diet. However, a growing body of evidence suggests that moderate amounts of oats may be safely used in diets of most adults with CD.[13] Corn and rice are usually the substitute grains used. Parents of children with CD need special instructions about food products to avoid, what constitutes a basic meal pattern, and recipes for food preparation. Careful label reading must be discussed, because many commercial products use the offending grains as thickeners or fillers and parents' knowledge of food products that contain gluten is highly variable and influences the child's attitudes toward dietary compliance. Good dietary management varies according to the child's age, pathologic conditions, and clinical status. In general, a dietary program based on the low-gluten diet should be followed (Box 20.3). In a small subgroup of patients, symptoms persist despite strict adherence to the diet. In rare instances, persons with such a refractory form of the disease respond only to parenteral nutrition (PN) support.

Cystic Fibrosis

Genetic-Metabolic Defect

CF is inherited as an autosomal recessive trait in approximately 3% of the Caucasian population. It is the most common fatal genetic disease among Caucasians, occurring in about 1 in 3300 live Caucasian births, 1 in 15,300 African-American births, and 1 in 32,000 Asian-American births.[14] Approximately one-third of CF cases in the United States involve adults. The leading characteristic of CF is hypersecretion of abnormal, thick mucus that obstructs exocrine glands and ducts.[14] Therefore it can be classified as a *respiratory disease* or *GI disorder*.

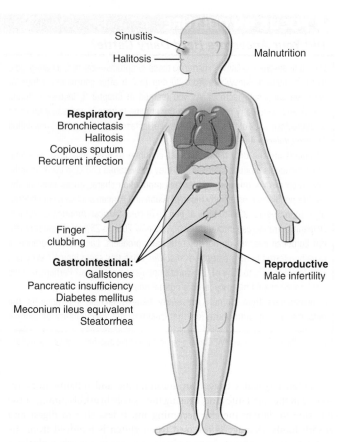

FIG. 20.7 Cystic fibrosis. (From Axford JS, O'Callaghan CA: *Medicine*, ed 2, Malden, MA, 2004, Blackwell Science.)

The CF gene (found on chromosome 7q) is very large, and more than 600 mutations that cause CF have been described.[14] The gene product is the cystic fibrosis transmembrane regulator (CFTR) protein, which regulates chloride transport and water flux across epithelial cells.[14] This results in an abnormally high concentration of sodium in perspiration and low water content in mucus.[14] CF primarily affects the pancreas, intestinal tract, sweat glands, and lungs; it causes infertility in male patients (Fig. 20.7).[14] For additional information, refer to Cystic Fibrosis Foundation at: https://www.cff.org/What-is-CF/About-Cystic-Fibrosis/.

Clinical Symptoms

Classic clinical symptoms of CF can vary widely from person to person; in general, they include the following conditions that affect the body organ systems[14]:

- Thick mucus in the lungs that accumulates and clogs air passages, damages epithelial tissue of these airways, and leads to chronic obstructive pulmonary disease (COPD) and frequent respiratory infections, both of which contribute to increased metabolism and increased energy-nutrient needs
- Pancreatic insufficiency caused by progressive clogging of pancreatic ducts and functional tissue degeneration, resulting in lack of normal pancreatic enzymes leading to bulky, foul-smelling, oily stools (steatorrhea); progressive loss of functional insulin-producing beta cells in the islets of Langerhans, resulting in type 1 diabetes mellitus
- Malabsorption of undigested food nutrients and extensive malnutrition and stunted growth

---

BOX 20.3 Sample Gluten-Free Menu

Breakfast
- Denver omelet made with low-fat natural cheddar or Monterey Jack cheese and fresh vegetables
- Rice cake (ingredient list should be checked to ascertain it is gluten free) topped with fruit jelly
- Orange juice

Lunch
- Tacos made with corn tortilla, black beans, fresh vegetables, low-fat natural cheese
- Fresh green salad with oil and vinegar dressing
- Homemade lemon/limeade

Evening Meal
- Shrimp and fresh vegetable stir-fry in oil and spices
- Brown rice or enriched white rice, plain
- Sorbet
- Cranberry juice/seltzer water spritzer

Snack
- All-natural yogurt mixed with fresh peaches (or other fruit in season)

FIG. 20.8 Clubbing of the fingers. (From Axford JS, O'Callaghan CA: *Medicine*, ed 2, Malden, MA., 2004, Blackwell Science.)

- Excessive sweating in hot weather that may lead to dehydration and circulatory failure
- Biliary cirrhosis caused by progressive clogging of bile ducts producing biliary obstruction and functional liver tissue degeneration
- Inflammatory complications that may include arthritis, finger clubbing (Fig. 20.8), or vasculitis
- Gallbladder disease, PUD, GERD, or episodes of partial intestinal obstruction
- Delayed puberty and maturity, probably the result of chronic malnutrition (men are typically infertile because the vas deferens fails to develop.)

Nutritional Management

The overall nutritional goal is to support normal nutrition and growth for all ages[15]:

- Unrestricted diet, including high-fat foods and additives
- Three meals and two to three snacks each day
- Vitamin supplementation
- Pancreatic enzymes
- Supplements and nutrient-dense nourishments may help
- Encouragement to consume whole grains, nuts, fruits, and vegetables for adequate vitamin and mineral intake
- Extra salt to replace that lost in sweat
- Adequate calcium, vitamin D, and vitamin K

Nutrition intervention is based on an initial and ongoing schedule for assessment, including anthropometrics, laboratory studies, and nutrition evaluation (Table 20.4). Related therapy is then outlined in five levels according to individual assessment results and nutrition care needs and actions (Table 20.5).

Inflammatory Bowel Diseases
Nature and Incidence

The two most common forms of IBD are Crohn disease and ulcerative colitis (UC).[16] Both conditions produce extended mucosal tissue lesions, although these lesions differ in extent and nature (Fig. 20.9). However, they have been classified medically in a single group because they are similar in their clinical symptoms and management. Their causes remain unknown, although heredity, environment, and immune functions are thought to be contributing factors.[16] Incidence of these diseases, especially Crohn disease, has increased worldwide. Crohn disease is particularly prevalent in industrialized areas of the world. It also appears among otherwise low-risk persons who move from rural to urban centers, with incidence being highest in people from 20 to 40 years of age and those of Jewish heritage.

Clinical Manifestations

Also called *regional enteritis* and *granulomatous colitis*, inflammation produced by Crohn disease extends through all layers of the intestinal wall, most commonly in the proximal portion of the colon and less often the terminal ileum.[17] UC is an inflammatory disease of mucosal

Key Assessments	Monitoring Schedule and Indications
TABLE 20.4 Basic Nutrition Assessment for Nutritional Management of Cystic Fibrosis	
Anthropometry	
Weight	Every 3 months or as needed for growth evaluation
Height (length)	
BMI (adults)	
Head circumference (until child is age 2)	
Midarm circumference	
Triceps skinfold	
Midarm muscle circumference (derived)[a]	
Biochemical Data	
CBC	Yearly routine care, interim as needed to detect deficiencies, iron status
TIBC, serum iron, ferritin	
Plasma/serum retinol, α-tocopherol	As indicated, weight loss, growth failure, clinical deterioration
Albumin, prealbumin	
Electrolytes, acid-base balance	Summer heat, prolonged fever
Random glucose	Annually to detect CFDM
Dietary Evaluation	
Dietary intake	As indicated, history and food records, full energy-nutrient analysis
Three-day fat balance study[b]	As indicated, weight loss, growth failure, clinical deterioration
Anticipatory guidance	Yearly, interim as needed according to growth or situational needs

BMI, Body mass index; *CBC,* complete blood count; *CFDM,* cystic fibrosis–related diabetes mellitus; *TIBC,* total iron-binding capacity.
[a]See Chapter 16 for equations.
[b]Three-day food records for analysis of fat intake; stool collections for analysis of fat content and degree of malabsorption.
Data from Hollander FM, De Roos NM, De Vries JH, et al: Assessment of nutritional status in adult patients with cystic fibrosis: whole-body bioimpedance vs body mass index, skinfolds, and leg-to-leg bioimpedance, *J Am Diet Assoc* 105(4):549, 2005; Ramsey BW, Farrell PM, Pencharz P: Nutritional assessment and management in cystic fibrosis: a consensus report—The Consensus Committee, *Am J Clin Nutr* 55:108, 1992; Yankaskas JR: Cystic fibrosis adult care: consensus conference report, *Chest* 125:1S, 2004.

TABLE 20.5	Levels of Nutrition Care for Management of Cystic Fibrosis	
Levels of Care	**Patient Groups**	**Nutrition Actions**
Level I—routine care	All	Diet counseling, food plans, enzyme replacement, vitamin supplements, nutrition education, exploration of problems
Level II—anticipatory guidance	Greater than 90% ideal weight-height index but at risk of energy imbalance; severe pancreatic insufficiency, frequent pulmonary infections, normal periods of rapid growth	Increased monitoring of dietary intake, complete energy-nutrient analysis, increased kcaloric density as needed; assess behavioral needs; provide counseling, nutrition education
Level III—supportive intervention	85%–90% ideal weight-height index, decreased weight-growth velocity	Reinforce all previously mentioned actions, add oral supplements (energy-nutrient dense)
Level IV—rehabilitative care	Consistently less than 85% ideal weight-height index, nutritional and growth failure	All of the previously mentioned plus EN support by nasoenteric or enterostomy tube feeding (see Chapter 19)
Level V—resuscitative or palliative care	Less than 75% ideal weight-height index, progressive nutritional failure	All of the previously mentioned plus continuous enteral tube feedings or TPN (see Chapter 19)

EN, Enteral nutrition; *TPN,* total parenteral nutrition.
Modified from Ramsey BW, Farrell PM, Pencharz P: Nutritional assessment and management in cystic fibrosis: a consensus report—The Consensus Committee, *Am J Clin Nutr* 55:108, 1992.

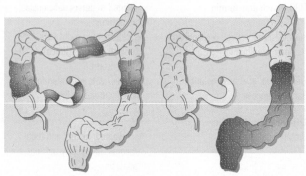

FIG. 20.9 Crohn disease *(left)* and ulcerative colitis (UC) *(right).* Crohn disease typically involves the small and large intestine in a segmental manner; UC generally starts in the rectum and progresses to involvement of varying lengths of the colon. (Modified from Cotran CS, Kumar V, Robbins SJ: *Robbins' pathologic basis of disease,* ed 4, Philadelphia, 1989, Saunders.)

layers of the rectum and colon.[18] Similarities and differences between the two diseases are summarized in Table 20.6.

Medical Management

Because the cause of IBD is unknown, treatment is focused on alleviating and reducing inflammation. Similar drug therapies are used for Crohn disease and UC: antibiotics, immunosuppressants, immunomodulators, and biologic therapies.[2,18] A small percentage of patients with UC require surgery.[18] Most common surgical procedures include total colectomy or ileostomy (Fig. 20.10). Approximately 80% of patients with Crohn disease will eventually require surgery. Fifty percent of these patients will require a second surgery within 10 years as a result of disease recurrence. Strictures often require minimal resection; colitis may require colectomy with ileorectal anastomosis or ileostomy. Abscesses are drained, and enteric fistulas are resected.[17,18]

Nutrition Therapy

Nutrition therapy centers on supporting the healing process and avoiding nutritional deficiency states and will be contingent on functional condition of the GI tract. Nutrition intervention depends on the functional status of the GI tract: extent of exacerbation, extent of diarrheal output, obstruction, surgery, and bleeding. When an oral diet cannot meet nutritional needs, enteral nutrition (EN) or PN is used[19]:
- Enteral feedings or total parenteral nutrition (TPN)

- Progression to low-fat, low-residue, high-protein, high-calorie, small, frequent meals
- Vitamin and mineral supplements: vitamin D, zinc, calcium, magnesium, folate, vitamin B_{12}, iron

Nutrition Therapy During Remission

Nutrition therapy in remission includes the following[19]:
- Tailor for the patient's current GI function
- Energy and protein at levels to maintain weight and replenish nutrient stores
- Avoid foods high in oxalate (see Appendix B)
- Increase antioxidant intake (see Chapter 6)
- Consider supplementation with omega-3 fatty acids and glutamine
- Use **probiotics** and **prebiotics**
- Diet as complete as possible

Short Bowel Syndrome
Cause

SBS is a malabsorptive condition secondary to surgical removal of parts of the small intestine with extensive dysfunction of the remaining portion of the organ. Severity of malabsorption is contingent on the amount and location of bowel resection. Removal of the distal two-thirds of ileum and ileocecal valve often results in severe malnutrition because the ileocecal valve controls the transit time of intestinal contents. Removal often promotes a transit time too rapid for sufficient absorption of nutrients. Absorption of water, electrolytes, protein, fat, carbohydrates, vitamins, and minerals is significantly reduced when large portions of the small intestine are lost.[8,20]

Typically, in an adult the small intestine is 20 feet long and the large intestine is 7 feet long. A general definition for SBS is a resection of more than 50% of the small intestine. Resections result from inherent conditions such as Crohn disease or radiation enteritis, surgical bypass, or massive abdominal injury and trauma. They may also be required for vascular problems such as blood clots that cause the death of involved tissue or for extensive fistula formation, radiation injury, congenital abnormalities, or cancer. After resection, the remaining small intestine has remarkable ability to adapt.[2] Remaining villi may enlarge and lengthen, consequently increasing absorptive surface area of the remaining intestine. Nutrients must be ingested orally for this adaptive sequence to take place, and gradual increase in oral intake after resection could promote gradual recovery in absorptive capability. PN support may be necessary for the short term or indefinitely after surgical shortening of the gut.

TABLE 20.6 Similarities and Differences Between Crohn Disease and Ulcerative Colitis

Manifestation	Crohn Disease	Ulcerative Colitis
Cause	Unknown	Unknown
Genetics	Increased prevalence in first-degree relatives; *NOD2* gene mutation on chromosome 16	Increased prevalence in first-degree relatives; susceptibility loci on chromosomes 2 and 6
Site of inflammation	Any part of the gastrointestinal (GI) tract	Rectum (and spreads proximally)
Mucosal layers affected		Epithelial
Abdominal pain	Common	Common
Diarrhea	Common	Common
Rectal bleeding	Sometimes	Common
Perforations	Common	Yes
Fibrosis, stricture, and fistulas	Common	No
Toxic megacolon	Rare	Common
Weight loss	Common	Common
Steatorrhea	Sometimes	No
Perianal disease	Common	No
Fever	Yes	No
Epidemiology	Developed countries, major age peak at ages 20–40, more common in women	Developed countries, major age peak at ages 20–40, more common in women
Relapses and remissions	Chronic	Usually no symptoms between attacks
Complications	Abscess, obstruction, fistulas, perianal disease, increased risk of colon cancer, malabsorption, kidney stones (oxalate and uric acid), gallstones	Many and varied including joint disorders, fatty liver, disorders of the eyes and skin
Prophylactic therapy	Not well established	Colonoscopy with multiple biopsies every 1–3 years
Prognosis	Recurrent morbidity throughout lives; risk of death approximately twice the general population	Mortality rate similar to general population

Data from Sartin JS: Gastrointestinal disorders. In Copstead LC, Banasik JL, editors: *Pathophysiology*, ed 4, St Louis, 2009, Saunders.

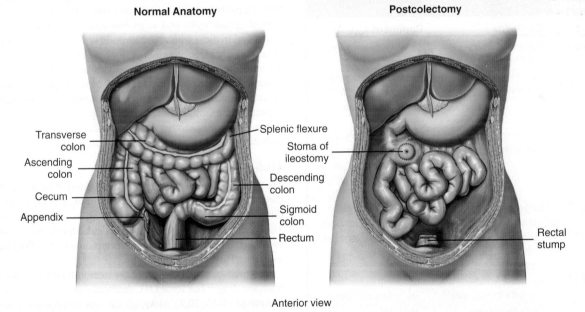

FIG. 20.10 Colectomy (colon removal) with ileostomy. (Medical Illustration Copyright 2006 Nucleus Medical Art, All rights reserved. https://www.nucleusinc.com.)

KEY TERMS

Probiotics
Microbial foods or supplements that can be used to modify or reestablish intestinal flora and improve health of the host.

Prebiotics
Nondigestible food products that promote growth of symbiotic bacterial species already present in the colon.

Nutritional Management

Degrees of surgical resection create different problems, and nutrition therapy must be tailored to individual's remaining functional capacity. Initial nutritional needs are usually supplied by early EN or PN support (see Chapter 19). Frequent monitoring of the patient's responses to nutrition support, especially fluid and electrolyte balances and malnutrition signs, is essential. The patient is weaned from nutrition support to an oral diet as tolerated, accompanied by vitamin and mineral supplementation. Nutritional status should continue to be monitored. As adaptation progresses, early restriction of fat may be liberalized somewhat with moderate use of the more easily absorbed MCT oil to obtain needed kcalories.

Bowel Transplantation

Patients with complications such as recurrent sepsis, thrombosis of access sites, metabolic disorders, cholestasis, and hepatic dysfunction resulting from TPN failure may be considered candidates for intestine transplant, which may involve the entire small intestine or just a segment of it. Most intestine transplants are whole organ transplants and are often performed in combination with a liver transplant.

Patients who undergo small-bowel transplantation can have problems transitioning to oral nutrition. Furthermore, special feeding considerations should be taken into consideration during the initial phase after transplant when the graft begins to function (Table 20.7). Large amounts of fluids lost after surgery must be replaced to prevent dehydration. Oral rehydration solutions may be used, although intravenous fluids may be required to replace not only lost fluids but also magnesium, zinc, bicarbonate, potassium, and sodium. Fiber, pectin, paregoric, and loperamide may enhance intestinal absorption by slowing transit time.

TABLE 20.7 Guidelines for Initiating Enteral Nutrition in Intestine Transplant Recipients

Nutrient	Guideline	Comment
Carbohydrates	Concentrated sweets and hyperosmolar fruit juice may cause osmotic diarrhea.	Carbohydrate malabsorption and secondary lactase deficiency may increase luminal osmolarity and increase stomal output.
Fat	MCT or intravenous lipids short term.	Lacteals and lymphatics of small intestine are severed during organ retrieval causing fat malabsorption initially.
Glutamine	Long-chain fatty acid absorption may improve within 2–6 weeks as lacteals and lymphatics are regenerated.	Glutamine is a conditionally essential amino acid and fuel for enterocytes.
Bicarbonate	An enteral formula enriched with glutamine may theoretically improve absorptive function and mucosal structure after transplantation.	Bicarbonate losses from the ostomy are often increased.
Fluid	Supplement. Rehydration solutions may be helpful.	High intestinal losses are common.

MCT, Medium-chain triglyceride.
Modified from Hasse JM: Nutrition assessment and support of organ transplant recipients, *J Parenter Enteral Nutr* 25:120, 2001. Reprinted with permission of SAGE Publications.

DISORDERS OF THE LARGE INTESTINE

Flatulence

Everyone has it. Most believe they have too much, and everyone is embarrassed if they pass gas in the wrong place at the wrong time. History views flatulence with mixed reviews. Hippocrates professed, "Passing gas is necessary to well-being." The Roman Emperor Claudius decreed, "All Roman citizens shall be allowed to pass gas whenever necessary." Regrettably for flatulent Romans, Emperor Constantine later overturned this pronouncement.

Cause

Flatulence is the condition of having excessive stomach or intestinal gas. Gas in the gut is the result of swallowed air or production in the intestines. Air swallowing (aerophagia) is a common cause of gas in the stomach. Small amounts of air are swallowed when eating and drinking. Some people swallow additional air while they eat or drink rapidly, chew gum, smoke, or wear dentures that are too loose. Most swallowed air is expelled from the stomach by burping or belching. Residual gas moves into the small intestine and is partially absorbed. A small quantity of gas travels to the large intestine and is expelled through the rectum.

Gas is produced in the intestines when normal, harmless bacteria in the large intestine break down undigested foods humans cannot because of a lack of specific digestive enzymes. Gas in the intestines is made of primarily odorless vapors such as carbon dioxide (CO_2), oxygen, nitrogen, hydrogen, and sometimes methane. The unpleasant odor of flatulence is produced by bacteria in the large intestine that release small amounts of gases that contain sulfur. These gases eventually exit the body through the rectum. Hydrogen and CO_2 are produced after ingestion of certain fruits and vegetables containing indigestible carbohydrates and in those with malabsorption syndromes (CF, CD, pancreatic insufficiency). Large amounts of disaccharides pass into the colon and are fermented to hydrogen in those with lactose deficiency. Methane is produced in approximately one-third of the population and is influenced minimally by food ingestion. The tendency to produce methane appears to be a familial trait.[21] Foods that produce gas in one person may not produce gas in another. Most foods that produce gas contain carbohydrates (Table 20.8); fats and proteins cause little gas.

Medical Management

The most common ways to reduce production of gas are to change the diet, take medications, and reduce the amount of air swallowed. The difficulty in suggesting dietary modification is individual tolerances. The quantity of gas produced by particular foods varies from person to person. Effective dietary change is typically the result of learning by way of trial and error.

Few well-controlled studies have demonstrated a clear-cut benefit from any drug,[22] but some OTC medicines are available to help reduce symptoms (Table 20.9). Although gas may be unpleasant and embarrassing, it is not life threatening. Education concerning causes, ways to reduce symptoms, and treatment help most people to find relief.[22]

Irritable Bowel Syndrome
Cause

Sometimes called *spastic colon,* IBS is a recurring functional disorder typified by abdominal pain or discomfort with alternating diarrhea and constipation for which no organic explanation is available.[8] For those with IBS, the quantity of symptoms is not as important as quality of life. Work, social life, and even sexual intercourse can be disrupted by IBS.[8] IBS is an extremely common disorder, affecting up to 20% of the US population, but most never seek medical attention.[2]

TABLE 20.8 Foods That May Cause Gas

Category	Food Sources
Sugars	
Raffinose	Beans, cabbage, Brussels sprouts, broccoli, asparagus, other vegetables, whole grains
Lactose	Milk, milk products (cheese, ice cream, processed foods)
Fructose	Onions, artichokes, peas, wheat (fructose also used as a sweetener in some soft drinks and fruit drinks)
Sorbitol	Fruits: apples, pears, peaches, prunes (sorbitol also used as an artificial sweetener in many dietetic foods and sugar-free candies and gums)
Starches	Potatoes, corn, noodles, wheat products (only starch that does not produce gas is rice)
Fiber	
Soluble	Oat bran, beans, peas, most fruits
Insoluble	Wheat bran, some vegetables

Modified from National Digestive Disease Information Clearinghouse (NDDIC), National Institute of Diabetes and Digestive and Kidney Diseases (NIDDK), National Institutes of Health (NIH): *Gas in the digestive tract*, NIH Pub No 08-883, Bethesda, MD, 2008, National Digestive Diseases Information Clearinghouse. https://www.digestive.niddk.nih.gov/ddiseases/pubs/gas/.

TABLE 20.9 Nonprescription Medications Used to Treat Flatulence

Medication	Classification	Action
Simethicone • Mylanta II • Maalox II • Di-Gel	Antacid	Foaming agent that joins gas bubbles in the stomach, making gas more easily belched away; no effect on intestinal gas
Lactase • Lactaid • Lactrase	Enzyme	Aids lactose digestion
Beano α-Galactosidase	Enzyme supplement	Contains sugar-digesting enzyme the body lacks to digest sugar in beans and many vegetables; has no effect on gas caused by lactose or fiber
Charcocaps	Activated charcoal	May produce relief from gas produced in colon

Data from National Digestive Disease Information Clearinghouse (NDDIC), National Institute of Diabetes and Digestive and Kidney Diseases (NIDDK), National Institutes of Health (NIH): *Gas in the digestive tract*, NIH Pub No 08-883, Bethesda, MD, 2008, NIH. https://www.digestive.niddk.nih.gov/ddiseases/pubs/gas/. Maslar J, Kreplick LW: *Flatulence (gas)*, Omaha, NE, 2005, eMedicine Consumer Health. https://www.emedicinehealth.com/Articles/5940-1.asp.

Clinical Symptoms

Manifestation of IBS may differ to a great extent from person to person. Some experience only diarrhea or constipation, whereas others experience an alternating pattern of both problems.[8] Some symptoms may be more marked than others. No physical findings or diagnostic tests confirm the diagnosis of IBS.[23] Diagnosis is determined by the presence of congruent symptoms and after ruling out organic diseases.[23] More than half of those diagnosed with IBS are female patients.[23]

The symptom-based Rome III diagnostic criteria for IBS emphasize a clear-cut diagnosis instead of excluding other medical conditions.[23] These criteria are based on a detailed history, physical examination, and limited diagnostic tests, as well as presentation of a particular set of symptoms (for the past 3 months, with symptom onset at least 6 months before diagnosis) as follows[24]:

- Recurrent abdominal pain or discomfort (*discomfort* means an uncomfortable sensation not described as pain) at least 3 days per month in the last 3 months associated with two or more of the following:
  - Improvement with defecation
  - Onset associated with a change in frequency of stool
  - Onset associated with a change in form (appearance) of stool
- The following other symptoms support, but are not essential, to the diagnosis of IBS:
  - More than three bowel movements per day or fewer than three bowel movements per week
  - Lumpy-hard or loose-watery stool form
  - Abnormal stool passage (straining, urgency, or feeling of incomplete evacuation)
  - Passage of mucus
  - Bloating or feeling of abdominal distention

Medical Management

Possibly the most helpful treatment intervention is to proffer assurance and a straightforward explanation of the functional nature of symptoms. Patients should be assured that their symptoms are real (i.e., not caused by stress or a psychologic or psychiatric disorder), although in some individuals stress can trigger or exacerbate symptoms of IBS.[24,25]

A chronic disorder, IBS can be treated but not cured. Therapy is directed at specific symptoms.[25] Antidiarrheal agents can decrease the motility and increase the consistency of stools for patients with diarrhea-predominant IBS. An α-adrenergic stimulating agent is sometimes used to treat diarrhea and abdominal pain by inhibiting norepinephrine activity. Other medications often used to treat IBS and assist in pain control are tricyclic antidepressants and selective serotonin reuptake inhibitors (SSRIs). Constipation-predominant IBS is often treated with bulking agents and osmotic laxatives. The newest medications for IBS are medications that work as 5-hydroxytryptamine (serotonin) ($5\text{-}HT_4$) receptor agonists and are effective in treating constipation-predominant IBS.[2]

Nutritional Management

Dietary triggers of IBS have not been established; however, dietary modification may provide symptomatic benefit. For some, a food diary in which food intake, symptoms, and activities are recorded may uncover dietary or psychosocial aspects that predispose symptoms. Malabsorption of lactose, fructose, and sorbitol can cause bloating, distention, flatulence, and diarrhea. An assortment of foods can trigger flatulence (see Table 20.8), which may cause pain and distention in some patients. To identify triggers, follow a low FODMAP (fermentable oligosaccharides, disaccharides, and monosaccharides and polyols) diet for 6 weeks and add high FODMAP food one at a time in small amounts to identify food that triggers the symptoms. Once identified, these foods can be limited to prevent "triggers." For a list of low FODMAP food choices, refer to Table 20.9. For additional information regarding low FODMAP diet, visit the Stanford Health Care website at: https://www.stanford-healthcare.org/medical-treatments/l/low-fodmap-diet.html.

For patients with constipation-predominant IBS, a high-fiber diet (20–30 g/day) may ease symptoms. Bran powder (1 tbsp, 2–3 times daily with food or in 8 oz. or more of liquid) provides the recommended amount. Some patients may report increased gas and distention from

TABLE 20.10 Low Fodmap Food Choices

Food Group	Foods to Eat	Foods to Limit
Meats, poultry, fish, eggs	Beef, chicken, canned tuna, eggs, egg whites, fish, lamb, pork, shellfish, turkey, cold cuts	Foods made with high FODMAP fruits, sauces, or with HFCS
Dairy	Lactose-free dairy, small amounts of cream cheese, half and half, hard cheese (cheddar, Colby, parmesan, Swiss), mozzarella, sherbet	Buttermilk, chocolate, cottage cheese, ice cream, creamy/cheesy sauces, milk (from cow, sheep, or goat), sweetened condensed milk, evaporated milk, soft cheeses (brie, ricotta), sour cream, whipped cream, yogurt
Meat, nondairy alternatives	Almond milk, rice milk, rice milk ice cream, nuts, nut butters, seeds	Coconut milk, coconut cream, beans, black eyed peas, hummus, lentils, pistachios, soy products
Grains	Wheat-free grains/wheat-free flours (gluten-free grains are wheat free): bagels, breads, hot/cold cereals (corn flakes, Cheerios, cream of rice, grits, oats, etc.), crackers, noodles, pastas, quinoa, pancakes, pretzels, rice, tapioca, tortillas, waffles	Chicory root, inulin, grains with HFCS or made from wheat (terms for wheat: einkorn, emmer, kamut, spelt), wheat flours (terms for wheat flour: bromated, durum, enriched, farina, graham, semolina, white flours), flour tortillas, rye
Fruits	Bananas, berries, cantaloupe, grapes, grapefruit, honeydew, kiwi, kumquat, lemon, lime, mandarin orange, passion fruit, pineapple, rhubarb, tangerine	Avocado, apples, applesauce, apricots, dates, canned fruit, cherries, dried fruits, figs, guava, lychee, mango, nectarines, pears, papaya, peaches, plums, prunes, persimmon, watermelon
Vegetables	Bamboo shoots, bell peppers, bok choy, cucumbers, carrots, celery, corn, eggplant, lettuce, leafy greens, pumpkin, potatoes, squash (butternut, winter), yams, tomatoes, zucchini	Artichokes, asparagus, beets, leeks, broccoli, Brussels sprouts, cabbage, cauliflower, fennel, green beans, mushrooms, okra, snow peas, summer squash
Desserts	Any made with allowed foods	Any with HFCS or made with foods to limit
Beverages	Low FODMAP fruit/vegetable juices (limit to 1/2 cup at a time), coffee, tea	Any with HFCS, high FODMAP fruit/vegetable juices, fortified wines (sherry, port)
Seasonings, condiments	Most spices and herbs, homemade broth, butter, chives, flaxseed, garlic flavored oil, garlic powder, olives, margarine, mayonnaise, onion powder, olive oil, pepper, salt, sugar, maple syrup without HFCS, mustard, low FODMAP salad dressings, soy sauce, marinara sauce (small amounts), vinegar, balsamic vinegar	HFCS, agave, chutneys, coconut, garlic, honey, jams, jellies, molasses, onions, pickle, relish, high FODMAP fruit/vegetable sauces, salad dressings made with high FODMAPs, artificial sweeteners: sorbitol, mannitol, isomalt, xylitol (cough drops, gums, mints)

FODMAP, Fermentable oligosaccharides, disaccharides, and monosaccharides and polyols; *HFCS*, high-fructose corn syrup.
Table from http://www.stanfordhospital.org/digestivehealth/nutrition/DH-Low-FODMAP-Diet-Handout.pdf, Stanford Hospitals and Clinics, August 2012.

fiber supplementation with bran; therefore psyllium, methylcellulose, or polycarbophil is often better tolerated. For management of flatulence, refer to Table 20.10 for nonprescription medications and supplements.

Diverticular Disease
Nature and Cause
A diverticulum is a small tubular sac that protrudes from a main canal or cavity in the body (Fig. 20.11). Formation and presence of small diverticula protruding from the intestinal lumen, usually the colon, produce the condition *diverticulosis*. More often, diverticulosis occurs in older adults. It develops at points of weakened musculature in the bowel wall, along the track of blood vessels entering the bowel from within. Direct cause is a progressive increase in pressure within the bowel from segmental circular muscle contractions that normally move the remaining food mass along and form the feces for elimination. When pressures become sufficiently high in one of these segments and dietary fiber is insufficient to maintain the necessary bulk for preventing high internal pressures within the colon, diverticula, small protrusions of the muscle layer, develop at that point. The condition causes no problem unless small diverticula become infected and inflamed from fecal irritation and colon bacteria. This diseased state is called *diverticulitis*. The commonly used collective term covering diverticulosis and diverticulitis is *diverticular disease*.

Clinical Symptoms
As the inflammatory process grows, increased hypermotility and pressures from luminal segmentation cause pain. Pain and tenderness are usually localized in the lower left side of the abdomen and are

FIG. 20.11 Diverticula. (From Lewis SM, Heitkemper M, Dirksen S: *Medical-surgical nursing: assessment and management of clinical problems*, ed 6, St Louis, 2004, Mosby.)

accompanied by nausea, vomiting, distention, diarrhea, intestinal spasm, and fever. If the process continues, then intestinal obstruction or perforation may necessitate surgical intervention.

Nutritional Management
Diverticular disease is a common GI disorder among middle-aged persons and older adults. Aggressive nutrition therapy hastens recovery from an attack, shortens hospital stay, and reduces costs. Numerous studies and extensive clinical practice have demonstrated better management of chronic diverticular disease with an increased amount of dietary

fiber than with old practices of restricting fiber. However, in acute episodes of active disease, the amount of dietary fiber should be reduced. The relationship of dietary fiber and diverticular disease has been further reinforced by studies of populations, such as those in Japan, that have recently experienced the westernization of their culture. Chapter 3 provides an extended discussion of dietary fiber and its relation to health and disease. Historically, avoidance of nuts, seeds, and hulls has been recommended, but current literature indicates this is not required.[26-29]

Constipation

A common disorder, usually of short duration, constipation is characterized by retention of feces in the colon beyond normal emptying time. Americans spend a quarter of a billion dollars each year on laxatives for this problem. However, "regularity" of elimination is highly individual, and it is not necessary to have a bowel movement every day to be healthy. Usually this common, short-term problem results from various sources of nervous tension, worry, and changes in social setting. Such situations include vacations and travel with alterations in usual routines. In addition, it may be caused by prolonged use of laxatives or cathartics, low-fiber diets, inadequate fluid intake, or lack of exercise, all of which can contribute to a decreased intestinal muscle tone. Increasing activity and improving dietary intake to include adequate fiber (with a goal of 25–35 g/day) and fluid are usually sufficient strategies to remedy the situation. However, if chronic constipation persists, then agents that increase stool bulk may be necessary. These bulking agents include bran or more soluble forms of fiber. Taking laxatives or enemas on a regular basis should be avoided. The problem of constipation occurs in all age groups but is almost epidemic in older adults. In all cases a personalized approach to management of constipation is fundamental.

DISEASES OF THE GASTROINTESTINAL ACCESSORY ORGANS

The liver, gallbladder, and pancreas (Fig. 20.12) are three major accessory organs that lie adjacent to the GI tract and produce important

digestive agents that enter the intestine and aid in processing of food substances. Specific enzymes are produced for each of the major nutrients, and bile is added to assist in enzymatic digestion of fats. Diseases of these organs can easily affect GI function and cause problems in the normal handling of specific types of food.

Viral Hepatitis
Cause

Viral hepatitis (inflammation of the liver) is a major public health problem throughout the world, affecting hundreds of millions of people. It causes considerable illness and death in human populations from acute infection or its effects, which may include chronic active hepatitis, cirrhosis, and primary liver cancer. During the past few years, knowledge of viruses that cause different types of hepatitis has grown rapidly. Currently, six unrelated human hepatitis viruses—A, B, C, D, and E—have been isolated and described. The three most common and well known are A, B, and C, which serve as examples, as follows:

- *Hepatitis A virus (HAV):* HAV is transmitted via the classic oral-fecal route through contaminated food and water. It is a prevalent infection worldwide, especially where overcrowding and poor hygiene or sanitation exists. An HAV vaccine has been developed that is far more effective than the former large and painful injection of gamma globulins, antibodies isolated from the blood. This vaccine protects travelers to developing countries, where the virus is endemic and may easily contaminate water and food.[30]

- *Hepatitis B virus (HBV):* HBV is mainly spread via parenteral contact with infected blood or blood products, including contaminated needles, and sexual contact.[26] It has now been implicated worldwide as the major cause of chronic liver disease and associated liver cancer. HBV infection is closely related to the body's immune system. Approximately 10% to 20% of those who become infected with HBV become chronic carriers. Of this number, approximately 20% acquire chronic hepatitis that

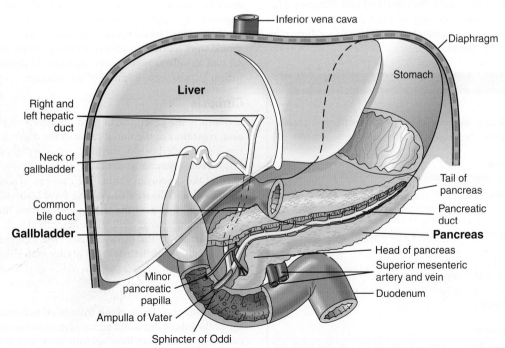

FIG. 20.12 Liver, pancreas, and gallbladder. (From Copstead LE, Banasik JL: *Pathophysiology*, ed 4, Philadelphia, 2009, Saunders.)

eventually progresses to cirrhosis and for some individuals, to liver cancer.[30] Universal immunization is recommended for persons of any age, but particularly for the following high-risk groups: male homosexuals, Alaska Natives, immigrants from highly endemic areas, illicit drug users, domestic associates of HBV carriers, hemodialysis patients, residents of institutions, medical and dental personnel, patients needing frequent transfusions, and those planning to reside in high-risk areas (e.g., Far East and sub-Saharan Africa).[30]

- *Hepatitis C virus (HCV):* HCV is mainly transmitted via blood from a person infected with HCV through infected needles syringes or blood products. According to the Center for Disease Control and Prevention, hepatitis is a leading cause of liver transplants and liver cancer. Three in four people with hepatitis C were born from 1945 – 65 and 50% of people with hepatitis C do not know they are infected. Most infected people develop chronic hepatitis C. There is no vaccine available for hepatitis C (https://www.cdc.gov/hepatitis/abc/index.htm).

Clinical Symptoms

Viral agents of hepatitis produce diffuse injury to liver cells, especially parenchymal cells. In milder cases, liver injury is largely reversible, but with increasing severity, more extensive necrosis occurs. In some cases, massive necrosis may lead to liver failure and death. A cardinal symptom of hepatitis is anorexia, which contributes to the risk of malnutrition. Varying clinical symptoms appear depending on the degree of liver injury. Jaundice, a major symptom, may or may not be obvious, depending on severity of the disease, and it can have nutritional and psychologic effects. In an outbreak of hepatitis, many infected persons may be nonicteric and thus go undiagnosed and untreated because jaundice has not developed sufficiently to be seen. Malnutrition and impaired immunocompetence contribute to spontaneous infections and continuing liver disease. General symptoms, in addition to anorexia, include malaise, weakness, nausea and vomiting, diarrhea, headache, fever, enlarged and tender liver, and enlarged spleen. When jaundice develops, it usually occurs for a preicteric period of 5 to 10 days, deepens for 1 to 2 weeks, then levels off and decreases. After this crisis point, a sufficient recovery of injured cells occurs, and a convalescence of 3 weeks to 3 months follows. Optimal care during this time is crucial to avoid relapse.

KEY TERMS

Endemic
Characterizing a disease of low morbidity that remains constantly in a human community but is clinically recognizable in only a few.

Parenchymal Cells
Functional cells of an organ, as distinguished from the cells constituting its structure or framework.

Necrosis
Cell death caused by progressive enzyme breakdown.

Icteric (Jaundice)
Alternative term for jaundice, yellowing of the sclerae of the eyes. (*Nonicteric* indicates absence of jaundice and *preicteric* indicates a state before development of icterus, or jaundice.)

Immunocompetence
The ability or capacity to develop an immune response (i.e., antibody production or cell-mediated immunity [or both]), after exposure to antigen.

General Treatment

Bed rest is essential. Physical activity and exercise increases the severity and duration of the disease. A daily intake of 3000 to 3500 mL of fluid guards against dehydration and gives a general sense of well-being and improved appetite. However, optimal nutrition is the major therapy. It provides the essential foundation for recovery of the injured liver cells and overall return of strength. Regular monitoring for signs of liver disease progression is important for patients with hepatitis infection.

Nutrition Therapy

A complete nutrition assessment and initial personal history provide the basis for planning care. Nutrition therapy principles relate to the liver's function in metabolizing each of the nutrients, as follows[31]:

- *Adequate protein:* Protein is essential for liver cell regeneration, as well as for maintaining all essential bodily functions. It also provides lipotropic agents such as methionine and choline for conversion of fats to lipoproteins and removal from the liver, thus preventing fatty infiltration. The daily diet should supply 1.0 to 1.2 g/kg of actual body weight (ABW) of high-quality protein. This amount is usually enough to achieve a positive nitrogen balance.
- *Low fat:* Less than 30% of calories should come from fat in case of steatorrhea.
- *Four to six small feedings:* To promote adequate intake and minimize loss of muscle, at least three meals and a bedtime snack are recommended.
- *Sodium:* If fluid retention is present, then limit sodium to 90 mEq/day (approximately 2000 mg).

Meals and Feedings

The problem of supplying a diet adequate to meet increased nutritional demands of a patient with an illness that makes food almost repellent calls for creativity and supportive encouragement. As the patient improves, appetizing and attractive food is needed. Because nutrition therapy is key to recovery, a major nutrition and nursing responsibility requires devising ways to encourage the increased amounts of food intake needed. The clinical dietitian and nursing staff should work together to achieve mutual goals planned for the patient. All staff attendants must observe appropriate precautions in handling patient trays to prevent spread of the infection.

Cirrhosis

Cirrhosis is the general term used for advanced stages of liver disease, regardless of the initial cause of the disease. Among all digestive diseases, cirrhosis of the liver, caused by chronic alcohol abuse, is the leading nonmalignant cause of death in the United States and most of the developed world. The majority of deaths occur among young and middle-aged adults. The French physician René Laënnec (1781–1826) first used the term *cirrhosis* (from the Greek word *kirrhos*, meaning orange-yellow) to describe the abnormal color and rough surface of the diseased liver. The cirrhotic liver is a firm, fibrous, dull-yellowish mass with orange nodules projecting from its surface (Fig. 20.13).

Cause

Some forms of cirrhosis result from biliary obstruction, with blockage of the biliary ducts and accumulation of bile in the liver.[32] Other cases may result from liver necrosis from undetermined causes or, in some cases, from previous viral hepatitis. Most common causes of cirrhosis are due to chronic hepatitis C, alcohol-related liver

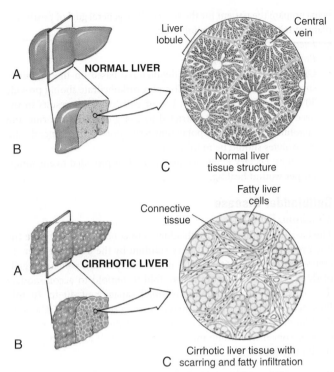

FIG. 20.13 Comparison of normal liver and liver with cirrhotic changes. (A) Anterior view of organ. (B) Cross section. (C) Tissue structure. (Medical and Scientific Illustration.)

disease, nonalcoholic fatty liver disease (NAFLD), and nonalcoholic steatohepatitis (NASH). A common problem is fatty cirrhosis, associated with the complicating factor of malnutrition. Continuing fatty infiltration causes cellular destruction and fibrotic tissue changes.

Clinical Symptoms

Early signs of cirrhosis include GI disturbances such as nausea, vomiting, loss of appetite, distention, and epigastric pain. In time, jaundice may appear, with increasing weakness, edema, ascites, and anemia from GI bleeding, iron deficiency, or hemorrhage. A specific macrocytic anemia from folic acid deficiency is also frequently observed. Steatorrhea is a common symptom. Major symptoms are caused by a basic protein deficiency and its multiple metabolic problems: (1) plasma protein levels fall, leading to failure of the capillary fluid shift mechanism (see Chapter 2), causing ascites; (2) lipotropic agents are not supplied for fat conversion to lipoproteins, and damaging fat accumulates in the liver tissue; (3) blood-clotting mechanisms are impaired because factors such as prothrombin and fibrinogen are not adequately produced; and (4) general tissue catabolism and negative nitrogen balance continue the overall degenerative process.

As the disease progresses, increasing fibrotic scar tissue impairs blood circulation through the liver, resulting in portal hypertension.[32] Contributing further to the problem is continuing ascites. Impaired portal circulation with increasing venous pressure may lead to esophageal varices, with danger of rupture and fatal massive hemorrhage.

Drug therapy includes use of broad-spectrum antibiotics to limit growth of intestinal bacteria and laxatives to speed intestinal transit time, limiting the amount of time available for bacteria to produce ammonia in the GI tract. Lactulose, a synthetic derivative of lactose

consisting of one molecule of galactose and one molecule of fructose, is a laxative that is used in the treatment of hepatic encephalopathy. Lactulose is ionized, cannot diffuse across the colon membrane, and is excreted in the stool. Lactulose can reduce blood ammonia levels by 25% to 50%. Diuretics may be given to reduce fluid retention and prevent ascites.

Nutrition Therapy

When alcoholism is an added underlying problem, treatment is difficult. Each patient requires supportive care. Therapy is usually aimed at correcting fluid and electrolyte problems and providing as much nutrition support as possible for hepatic repair. In any case, guidelines for nutrition therapy for cirrhosis of the liver should include the following principles[2,33]:

- *Energy:* 40 to 50 kcal/kg body weight. Fluid retention, if present, will affect the accuracy of estimating kcalorie needs. As muscle tissue is wasted, it is often replaced by fluid weight. An estimated dry weight (postparacentesis of ascites or well diuresed) should be used when feasible to estimate kcalorie needs.
- *Protein intake:* 1 to 1.5 g/kg body weight. Intake should be adequate to regenerate liver cells and prevent infections but not excessive to the point of aggravating ammonia buildup and inducing hepatic coma. Protein estimations should be based on dry weight whenever possible.
- *Sodium:* Intake is usually restricted to less than 2000 mg/day to help reduce fluid retention. A sodium intake level of less than 2000 mg/day is considered quite restrictive, and palatability of food is usually a problem. It may be necessary to liberalize the sodium restriction to improve intake.
- *Texture:* If esophageal varices develop, then it may be necessary to give soft foods that are smooth in texture to prevent the danger of rupture and hemorrhage.
- *Carbohydrate:* Adequate intake is needed to prevent catabolism of body protein for energy, which would further increase blood ammonia. Intestinal bacteria make ammonia from undigested proteins (proteins from shed mucosal cells, protein from GI tract bleed, and dietary proteins).
- *Fat:* Fat restriction should be less than 30% of calories (with or without MCT supplements) in patients with steatorrhea.
- *Vitamins and minerals:* The central role of the liver is to metabolize and store vitamins and minerals. Usually all people with advanced liver disease require supplementation of some vitamins, minerals, and trace elements. Nutrient supplementation is determined by monitoring serum levels and checking for clinical signs of deficiencies.
- *Alcohol:* To protect the liver from further injury, abstinence from alcohol is mandatory.
- *Personalized food plan:* Adequate intake is more likely, thus hastening recovery, if the food plan is developed based on the likes and dislikes and real-life schedule of the patient. If appetite is a problem, then several small meals per day instead of full meals may be required.
- *Fluids:* Fluids should be encouraged unless ascites or edema is present. Water is the fluid of choice. Calorie-dense beverages such as juicelike drinks and soft drinks provide excess calories with little nutrient, often taking the place of nutrient-dense foods.

Hepatic Encephalopathy

The term *encephalopathy* refers to any disease or disorder that affects the brain, especially chronic degenerative conditions such as end-stage liver disease. Accumulation of toxic substances such as ammonia in the blood as a result of liver failure impairs consciousness and contributes to memory loss, personality change, tremors, seizures, stupor, and coma.

Cause

As cirrhotic changes continue in the liver, portal blood circulation diminishes and liver functions begin to fail. The normal liver has a major function of removing ammonia from blood by converting it to urea for excretion. The failing liver can no longer inactivate, detoxify substances, metabolize, or synthesize body compounds. A key factor involved in the progressive disease process is an elevated blood level of ammonia, and ammonia is one of the compounds that accumulate in the blood due to the liver's inability to convert it to urea. The resulting hepatic encephalopathy brings changes in consciousness, behavior, and neurologic status.

Clinical Symptoms

Typical response involves disorders of consciousness and alterations in motor function. Apathy, confusion, inappropriate behavior, and drowsiness are seen, progressing to coma. Speech may be slurred or monotonous. A coarse, flapping tremor known as *asterixis* is observed in the outstretched hands, caused by a sustained contraction of a group of muscles. Breath may have a fecal odor, called *fetor hepaticus.*

Basic Treatment Objectives

Fundamental objectives of treatment are twofold: (1) removal of sources of excess ammonia and (2) provision of nutrition support. Parenteral fluid and electrolytes are used to restore normal balances. Lactulose and neomycin may be used to control ammonia levels. Neomycin is an antibiotic that reduces the population of urea-splitting organisms within the bowel that produce ammonia.

Nutrition Therapy

General nutrition support for hepatic encephalopathy is based on the following five principles of dietary management[34]:
1. *Alcohol:* Abstinence is necessary.
2. *Energy:* Moderately high energy intake (25–40 kcal/kg) is needed to prevent breakdown of body tissue. Moderate fat intake of 30% of total kcal or less is encouraged unless steatorrhea is present. In the case of steatorrhea, fat intake can be reduced. Carbohydrates provide the majority of energy intake.
3. *Protein:* In general, protein intake is limited to 1.0 to 1.5 g/kg unless encephalopathy is associated. If encephalopathy is present, then protein should be limited to 60 g/day. Protein intake can be increased gradually as the patient improves. Plant protein seems to be better tolerated than animal protein by some patients.
4. *Meals:* Small frequent meals are better tolerated than large, less frequent meals. Soft foods that are low in fiber help prevent bleeding from esophageal varices.
5. *Supplements:* Water-soluble and fat-soluble vitamin supplements are often necessary.

Liver Transplantation

Liver transplantation is the treatment of choice for patients with end-stage liver disease who have not responded to conventional treatment. Patients being considered for liver transplantation undergo extensive physiologic and psychologic evaluations to detect possible contraindications to the procedure.[2]

As with all major surgery, aggressive nutrition support reduces risks. Careful pretransplantation nutrition assessment and support helps prepare the patient for the surgery. The general goal of posttransplant nutrition therapy is as follows[2]:
- *Energy:* 35 to 45 kcal/kg.
- *Protein:* 1.0 to 1.2 g/kg.
- *Other nutrients:* These are individualized based on the immunosuppressant drug regimen. (Complex carbohydrate should provide 50%–60% of total kcalories. Use of corticosteroids results in the need for sodium to be restricted to 2–4 g/day. Cyclosporine and tacrolimus may require potassium restriction. Other minerals and electrolytes should be monitored.)
- *Vitamins:* Dietary Reference Intake (DRI) is provided to encourage proper wound healing.

Gallbladder Disease
Metabolic Function

The basic function of the gallbladder is to concentrate and store the bile produced in its initial watery solution by the liver. The liver secretes approximately 600 to 800 mL of bile per day, which the gallbladder normally concentrates fivefold to tenfold to accommodate this daily bile production in its small capacity of 40 to 70 mL. Presence of fat in the duodenum releases cholecystokinin (CCK) into the blood, which stimulates contraction of the gallbladder with release of concentrated bile into the common duct and then into the small intestine.

Cholecystitis and Cholelithiasis

The prefix *chole* of the two terms *cholecystitis* and *cholelithiasis* comes from the Greek word *chole,* which means bile. Thus cholecystitis is an inflammation of the gallbladder, and cholelithiasis is the formation of gallstones. Incidence of gallstones is associated with age, gender, and an assortment of medical factors (Box 20.4).

Inflammation of the gallbladder usually results from a low-grade chronic infection and may occur with or without gallstones. However, in 90% to 95% of patients, acute cholecystitis is associated with gallstones and is caused by the obstruction of the cystic duct by stones, resulting in acute inflammation of the organ. Gallstones can be classified into the following two main groups: (1) cholesterol stones and (2) pigment stones[35]:
1. *Cholesterol stones:* In the United States and most Western countries, more than 75% of gallstones are cholesterol stones. The infectious process produces changes in gallbladder mucosa, which affects its absorptive powers. The main ingredient of bile is cholesterol, which is insoluble in water. Normally, cholesterol is kept in solution by

---

BOX 20.4 **Risk Factors for Gallbladder Disease**

- Female gender
- Ethnicity: Native American, particularly Pima Indians of North America
- High-cholesterol diet
- Use of oral contraceptives
- Obesity (body mass index [BMI] >30)
- Ileal resection or disease
- Diabetes mellitus
- Rapid weight loss (in obese persons)
- Positive family history
- Some medications (e.g., lipid-lowering agents)
- Gallbladder hypomobility

Data from Sartin JS: Alterations in function of the gallbladder and exocrine pancreas. In Copstead LC, Banasik JL, editors: *Pathophysiology,* ed 4, St Louis, 2009, Saunders.

other ingredients in bile. However, when the absorbing mucosal tissue of the gallbladder is inflamed or infected, changes occur in the tissue. The absorptive powers of the gallbladder may be altered, affecting the solubility of the bile ingredients. Excess water or excess bile acid may be absorbed. Under these abnormal absorptive conditions, cholesterol may precipitate, forming gallstones of almost pure cholesterol.

2. *Pigment stones:* Black and brown pigment gallstones, although they differ in chemical composition and clinical features, are colored by the presence of bilirubin, the pigment in red blood cells. They are associated with chronic hemolysis in conditions such as sickle cell disease, thalassemia, cirrhosis, long-term TPN, and advancing age. Pigment stones are often found in bile ducts and may be related to a bacterial infection with *Escherichia coli.*

Clinical Symptoms

When inflammation, stones, or both are present in the gallbladder, contraction from the cholecystokinin-pancreozymin (CCK-PZ) mechanism causes pain, which is sometimes severe. Fullness, distention after eating, and particular difficulty with fatty foods are noted.

General Treatment

Surgical removal of the gallbladder, a cholecystectomy (Fig. 20.14), is usually indicated. If the patient is obese, then some weight loss before surgery is advisable if surgery can be delayed. Supportive therapy is largely nutritional. Several nonsurgical treatments for removing the stones, using chemical dissolution or mechanical stone fragmentation, have been developed. These methods provide effective alternatives to surgery in some cases.[35]

Nutrition Therapy

Basic principles of nutrition therapy for gallbladder disease include the following:
- *Fat:* Because dietary fat is the principal cause of contraction of the diseased organ and subsequent pain, it is poorly tolerated. Energy

should come primarily from carbohydrates, especially during acute phases. Control of fat will also contribute to weight control, a primary goal because obesity and excess food intake have been repeatedly associated with the development of gallstones.
- *Energy content:* If weight loss is indicated, then recommended energy intake will be reduced according to need. Principles of weight management are discussed in Chapter 6. Usually such a diet will have a relatively low percentage of calories from fat, meeting the needs of the patient for fat moderation.
- *Cholesterol and "gas formers":* Two additional modifications usually found in traditional diets for gallbladder disease concern restriction of foods containing cholesterol and foods labeled *gas formers.* Neither modification has a valid rationale. The body synthesizes more cholesterol per day than is present in an average diet. Thus restriction of dietary cholesterol has little effect in reducing gallstone formation. Total dietary fat reduction is more important. As for the use of gas formers, such as legumes, cabbage, or fiber, blanket restriction seems unwarranted because food tolerances in any circumstances are highly individual.

Diseases of the Pancreas
Pancreatitis

Acute inflammation of the pancreas (pancreatitis) is caused by digestion of the organ tissues by enzymes it produces, principally trypsin. Normally, enzymes remain in inactive form until pancreatic secretions reach the duodenum through the common duct. However, gallbladder disease may cause a gallstone to enter the common bile duct and obstruct flow from the pancreas or cause a reflux of these secretions and bile from the common duct back into the pancreatic duct. This mixing of digestive materials activates powerful pancreatic enzymes within the gland. In such activated form, they begin their damaging effects on pancreatic tissue itself, causing acute pain. Sometimes infectious pancreatitis may occur as a complication of mumps or a bacterial disease. Mild or moderate pancreatitis may

Open Cholecystectomy
Removal of gallbladder through
open incision with lysis of adhesions

Laparoscopic Cholecystectomy
Not performed due to
excessive adhesions

Laparoscopic instruments placed
through separate stab incisions

FIG. 20.14 Open and laparoscopic cholecystectomy. (Medical Illustration Copyright 2006 Nucleus Medical Art, All rights reserved. https://www.nucleusinc.com.)

subside completely, but it has a tendency to recur. Alcohol in Western societies and malnutrition worldwide are the major causes of chronic pancreatitis.

General Treatment

Initial care consists of measures recommended for acute disease involving shock. These measures include intravenous feeding at first, replacement therapy of fluid and electrolytes, blood transfusions, antibiotics and pain medications, and gastric suction.

Nutrition Therapy

In early stages (i.e., acute pancreatitis), oral feedings are withheld because entry of food into the intestines stimulates pancreatic secretions and usually causes pain. Nutritional status is maintained by intravenous fluids or jejunal enteral feeding with peptide-based or elemental EN formulas. Most patients with pancreatitis are able to resume oral feeding in 2 to 5 days.[34]

PN is generally not recommended in pancreatitis unless a patient fails an enteral feeding trial. Pseudocysts, intestinal and pancreatic fistulas, pancreatic abscesses, and pancreatic ascites may make enteral feeding impossible.

▌HEALTH PROMOTION

A single layer of cells maintains a barrier between toxins and infections in the GI tract. At the same time, this same layer of cells absorbs macronutrients, micronutrients, and water and puts them into circulation. If that is not enough, then these cells also regulate bodily functions via hormonal and immunologic mechanisms. It is plain to see why we would want to keep this remarkable organ healthy.

In 1998 Hasler[36] summarized research that identified foods that provide several physiologic benefits. Among the findings are the following:

- Individuals who consume diets high in fruits and vegetables have only one-half the cancer risk of those who consume very little of these foods.
- Intake of lycopene, the primary carotenoid found in tomatoes, is inversely associated with reduced risk of digestive tract cancer, among other cancers.
- Garlic and onions *might* offer a protective effect on cancers of the GI tract.
- Probiotics (fermented dairy products, such as yogurt) reduce risk of various cancers, particularly colon cancer.
- Prebiotics (fermentable carbohydrates such as starches, dietary fibers, other nonabsorbable sugars, sugar alcohols, and oligosaccharides) stimulate growth and activity of one or more of the "friendly" bacteria that live in the gut.

In addition to how we eat, how we live plays an important role in GI health. Strong evidence indicates that physical activity reduces risk of colon cancer by half. Physical activity might also reduce risk of cholelithiasis, constipation, diverticulosis, GI hemorrhage, and IBD.[37] Washing the hands for a minimum of 20 seconds (the amount of time it takes to sing "Happy Birthday") with hot, soapy water will reduce risk of oral-fecal contamination that could cause foodborne illnesses and certain types of hepatitis.

This information can be summed up very simply: Mom was right when she asked you to do the following:

- Eat your fruits and vegetables
- Go out and play (get plenty of physical activity)
- Wash your hands frequently and especially before eating

TO SUM UP

Nutrition therapy for GI disease is based on careful consideration of the following four major factors:

1. Secretory functions, providing chemical agents and environment necessary for digestion to occur
2. Neuromuscular functions required for motility and mechanical digestion
3. Absorptive functions, enhancing entry of nutrients into the circulatory system
4. Psychologic factors reflected by changes in GI function

Esophageal problems vary widely from simple dysphagia to serious diseases or obstruction. Nutrition therapy and mode of intake vary according to degree of dysfunction.

PUD is a common GI problem affecting millions of Americans. It is an erosion of the mucosal lining, mainly in the duodenal bulb and less commonly in the lower antrum portion of the stomach. PUD results in increased gastric tone and painful hunger contractions on an empty stomach, as well as nutrition problems such as low plasma protein levels, anemia, and weight loss. Current medical management consists of acid and infection control with a coordinated system of drugs, rest, and a regular diet (with few food and drink considerations) to supply essential nutrition support for tissue healing.

Intestinal diseases are classified as (1) *anatomic changes*, such as development of small tubular sacs branching off the main alimentary canal in diverticular disease; (2) *malabsorption*, from multiple maldigestive and malabsorptive conditions; (3) *IBD*, resulting from mucosal changes and infectious processes, as seen in UC and Crohn disease; or (4) *SBS*, resulting from surgical resection of parts of the intestine. Nutrition therapy involves fluid and electrolyte replacement, modifications in the diet's protein and energy content and food texture, and increased vitamins and minerals, with continuous adjustment of the diet according to changes in toleration for specific foods. Allergic responses to common food allergens, as well as missing cell enzymes in genetic disease, may also contribute to GI and metabolic problems from related food intolerances.

Accessory organs to the GI tract—liver, gallbladder, and pancreas—have important functions related to digestion, absorption, and metabolism, and diseases of these organs interfere with the normal functions of the GI tract. Common liver disorders include hepatitis, usually caused by viral infection, and cirrhosis, an advanced liver disease leading to hepatic encephalopathy and progressive liver failure. The requirement of nutrient and energy levels vary with each condition.

Diseases of the gallbladder include cholecystitis, inflammation that interferes with the absorption of water and bile acids, and cholelithiasis, or gallstone formation. Treatment generally involves a reduced-fat diet and surgical removal of the gallbladder. Diseases of the pancreas include acute and chronic forms of pancreatitis, in which alcohol abuse can be a primary cause. Other causes include biliary disease, malnutrition, drug reactions, abdominal injury, and genetic predisposition. In acute pancreatitis, pain is severe because of pancreatic enzyme reflux with self-digestion of pancreatic tissue by its own enzymes. PN support is used to avoid enzyme stimulus, with gradual return to small, frequent meals as the attack subsides. In chronic pancreatitis, which is caused by alcoholism in Western societies and malnutrition worldwide, maldigestion from lack of enzymes because of pancreatic insufficiency creates nutrition problems. Nutrition care focuses on a nourishing diet with enzyme replacement and vitamin-mineral supplementation.

QUESTIONS FOR REVIEW

1. What is the basic principle of diet planning for patients with esophageal problems? Outline a general nutrition care plan for a patient with GERD complicated by a hiatal hernia.

2. In current practice, what are the basic principles of diet planning for patients with PUD? How do these principles differ from former traditional therapy?

3. Outline a course of nutritional management for a person with PUD, based on the current approaches to medical management. How would you plan nutrition education for continuing self-care and avoidance of recurrence?

4. Describe the cause, clinical signs, and treatment of each of the following intestinal diseases: malabsorption and diarrhea, IBD, diverticular disease, IBS, and constipation.

5. Compare the basics of food intolerances resulting from food allergy with those resulting from a specific genetic disease such as CF.

6. How are the major metabolic functions of the liver affected in liver disease? Give some examples.

7. What is the rationale for treatment in the spectrum of liver disease: hepatitis, cirrhosis, and hepatic encephalopathy?

8. Develop a 1-day food plan for a 45-year-old man, 183 cm (6 ft 1 in) tall, weighing 90 kg (200 lb), with infectious hepatitis. Develop another plan for a similar patient with cirrhosis of the liver. What principles of diet therapy apply for each?

9. What are the principles of nutrition therapy for gallbladder disease? Write a 1-day meal plan for a 30-year-old woman, 165 cm (5 feet 6 inches) tall, weighing 81 kg (180 lb), who has an inflamed gallbladder with stones and is scheduled for a cholecystectomy.

10. Compare acute and chronic forms of pancreatitis in terms of cause, symptoms, and nutrition therapy. What role does special EN and PN support play in this therapy?

REFERENCES

1. Fisichella PM, Patti MG: *Achalasia*, Omaha, Neb., 2008, eMedicine.com, Inc. Retrieved from https://emedicine.medscape.com.

2. Nelms MN, Sucher K, Long S: *Understanding nutrition therapy and pathophysiology*, ed 3, Boston, MA, 2016, Cengage Learning.

3. Blaser MJ: The bacteria behind ulcers, *Sci Am* 274(2):104, 1996.

4. Marchetti M, Aricò B, Burroni D, et al: Development of a mouse model of *Helicobacter pylori* infection that mimics human disease, *Science* 267(5204):1655, 1995.

5. Division of Bacterial and Mycotic Disease, Centers for Disease Control and Prevention: *Helicobacter pylori and peptic ulcer disease*, Atlanta, Ga., 2005, Centers for Disease Control and Prevention. Retrieved from www.cdc.gov/ulcer/.

6. Merck & Co, Inc.: *The Merck manual of diagnosis and therapy: helicobacter pylori infection*, Whitehouse Station, N.J., 2007, Merck & Co, Inc. Retrieved from http://www.merckmanuals.com/professional.

7. American Dietetic Association: *Nutrition care manual: peptic ulcers: nutrition prescription*, Chicago, 2009, Author. Retrieved from www.nutritioncaremanual.org.

8. Sartin JS: Gastrointestinal disorders. In Copstead LC, Banasik JL, editors: *Pathophysiology*, ed 4, Philadelphia, PA, 2009, Saunders.

9. Trier JS: Celiac sprue, *N Engl J Med* 325(24):1709, 1991.

10. Beyer P: Medical nutrition therapy for lower gastrointestinal tract disorders. In Mahan LK, Escott-Stump S, editors: *Krause's food, nutrition, and diet therapy*, ed 12, Philadelphia, PA, 2007, Saunders.

11. Mariné M, Fernández-Bañares F, Alsina M, et al: Impact of mass screening for gluten-sensitive enteropathy in working population, *World J Gastroenterol* 15(11):1331, 2009.

12. US National Library of Medicine, National Institutes of Health: *Medline Plus medical encyclopedia: celiac disease-sprue*, Bethesda, MD, 2005, National Institutes of Health. Retrieved from www.nlm.nih.gov/medlineplus/ency/article/000233.htm.

13. Academy of Nutrition and Dietetics: *Nutrition care manual: celiac disease: nutrition care FAQs*, Chicago, 2009. Retrieved from www.nutritioncaremanual.org.

14. Merck & Co, Inc.: *The Merck manual of diagnosis and therapy: cystic fibrosis*, Whitehouse Station, NJ, 2008, Merck & Co, Inc. Retrieved from http://www.merckmanuals.com/professional.

15. Academy of Nutrition and Dietetics: *Nutrition care manual: cystic fibrosis: nutrition intervention*, Chicago, 2009, Retrieved from www.nutritioncaremanual.org.

16. Merck & Co, Inc.: *The Merck manual of diagnosis and therapy: inflammatory bowel disease*, Whitehouse Station, NJ, 2007, Merck & Co, Inc. Retrieved from http://www.merckmanuals.com/professional.

17. Merck & Co, Inc.: *The Merck manual of diagnosis and therapy: Crohn's disease (regional enteritis; granulomatous ileitis or ileocolitis)*, Whitehouse Station, NJ, 2008, Merck & Co, Inc. Retrieved from http://www.merckmanuals.com/professional

18. Merck & Co, Inc.: *The Merck manual of diagnosis and therapy: ulcerative colitis*, Whitehouse Station, NJ, 2008, Merck & Co, Inc. Retrieved from http://www.merckmanuals.com/professional.

19. Academy of Nutrition and Dietetics: *Nutrition care manual: Crohn's and ulcerative colitis: nutrition intervention*, Chicago, 2009. Retrieved from www.nutritioncaremanual.org.

20. Merck & Co, Inc.: *The Merck manual of diagnosis and therapy: short bowel syndrome*, Whitehouse Station, NJ, 2008, Merck & Co, Inc. Retrieved from http://www.merckmanuals.com/professional.

21. Weseman RA: Adult small bowel transplantation. In Hasse JM, Blue LS, editors: *comprehensive guide to transplant nutrition*, Chicago, 2002, American Dietetic Association.

22. Merck & Co, Inc.: *The Merck manual of diagnosis and therapy: gas-related complaints*, Whitehouse Station, NJ, 2007, Merck & Co, Inc. Retrieved from http://www.merckmanuals.com/professional.

23. Sperber, A.D., Shvartzman, P., Friger, M., et al. A Comparative reappraisal of the Rome II and Rome III diagnostic creteria: are we getting closer to the "true" prevalence of irritable bowel syndrome? *Eur J Gastroenterol Hepatol* 19(6):441–447, 2007.

24. International Foundation for Functional Gastrointestinal Disorders: *About irritable bowel syndrome (IBS)*, Milwaukee, WI, 1999-2010, International Foundation for Functional Gastrointestinal Disorders. Retrieved from www.aboutibs.org. Accessed December 14, 2017.

25. Merck & Co, Inc.: *The Merck manual of diagnosis and therapy: irritable bowel syndrome*, Whitehouse Station, NJ, 2007, Merck & Co, Inc. Retrieved from http://www.merckmanuals.com/professional.

26. Sheth AA, Longo W, Floch MH: Diverticular disease and diverticulitis, *Am J Gastroenterol* 103(6):1550, 2008.

27. Strate LL, Liu YL, Syngal S, et al: Nut, corn, and popcorn consumption and the incidence of diverticular disease, *JAMA* 300(8):907, 2008.

28. Eglash A, Lane CH, Schneider DM: What is the most beneficial diet for patients with diverticulosis? *J Fam Pract* 55(9):813, 2006.

29. Jacobs DO: Diverticulitis, *N Engl J Med* 357(20):2057, 2007.

30. Merck & Co, Inc.: *The Merck manual of diagnosis and therapy: irritable bowel syndrome*, Whitehouse Station, NJ, 2007, Merck & Co, Inc. Retrieved from http://www.merckmanuals.com/professional.

31. Academy of Nutrition and Dietetics: *Nutrition care manual: hepatitis: nutrition prescription*, Chicago, 2009, Retrieved from https://www.nutritioncaremanual.org.

32. Merck & Co, Inc.: *The Merck manual of diagnosis and therapy: cirrhosis*, Whitehouse Station, NJ, 2007, Merck & Co, Inc. Retrieved from http://www.merckmanuals.com/professional.

33. Academy of Nutrition and Dietetics: *Nutrition care manual: cirrhosis: nutrition prescription*, Chicago, 2009, Retrieved from https://www.nutritioncaremanual.org.

34. Moore MC: *Pocket guide to nutrition assessment and care*, ed 6, St Louis, 2009, Mosby.

35. Sartin JS: Alterations in function of the gallbladder and exocrine pancreas. In Copstead LC, Banasik JL, editors: *Pathophysiology*, ed 4, Philadelphia, PA, 2009, Saunders.

36. Hasler CM: Scientific status summary: functional foods—their role in disease prevention and health promotion, *Food Technol* 52(11):63, 1998.

37. Peters HPF, De Vries WR, Vanberge-Henegouwen GP, et al: Potential benefits and hazards of physical activity and exercise on the gastrointestinal tract, *Gut* 48:435, 2001.

FURTHER READINGS AND RESOURCES

Websites of Interest

Celiac Disease

- Ask the Dietitian, Gluten Intolerance and Celiac Disease: https://www.dietitian.com/gluten.html
- Celiac Disease Foundation: https://www.celiac.org
- National Celiac Association: https://www.csaceliacs.org

Cirrhosis

- American Gastroenterological Association, Cirrhosis of the liver: https://www.gastro.org
- American Liver Foundation: https://www.liverfoundation.org
- National Institute of Diabetes and Digestive and Kidney Diseases: https://www.niddk.nih.gov

Dysphagia

- American Speech-Language-Hearing Association: http://www.asha.org/PRPSpecificTopic.aspx?folderid=8589942550&section=Resources
- Dysphagia-Dietcom: https://www.dysphagia-diet.com

- Nestle Health Science management of Dysphagia: https://www.nestlehealthscience.com/health-management/gastro-intestinal/dysphagia/dysphagia-hcp

Gastroesophageal Reflux Disease

- About GERD: https://www.aboutgerd.org
- American Gastroenterological Association: https://www.gastro.org
- National Institute of Diabetes and Digestive and Kidney Diseases: https://www.niddk.nih.gov/health-information/digestive-diseases/acid-reflux-ger-gerd-adults

Celiac Disease

- Celiac Disease Foundation: https://www.celiac.org
- Medline Plus, Celiac disease: https://www.nlm.nih.gov/medlineplus/celiac-disease.html
- National Institute of Diabetes and Digestive and Kidney Diseases, Celiac disease: https://www.digestive.niddk.nih.gov/ddiseases/pubs/celiac/

Cystic Fibrosis

- Canadian Cystic Fibrosis Foundation: http://www.cysticfibrosis.ca
- Cystic Fibrosis Foundation: https://www.cff.org/home/
- CysticFibrosis.com: https://www.cysticfibrosis.com

Irritable Bowel Syndrome

- About IBS: https://www.aboutibs.org
- Irritable Bowel Syndrome Self Help and Support Group: https://www.ibsgroup.org

Pancreatitis

- eMedicine (search for pancreatitis for a number of resources): https://emedicine.medscape.com
- National Institute of Diabetes and Digestive and Kidney Diseases: https://www.niddk.nih.gov/health-information/digestive-diseases/pancreatitis
- Tummyhealth.com: https://www.tummyhealth.com

Peptic Ulcer Disease

- National Institute of Diabetes and Digestive and Kidney Diseases: https://www.niddk.nih.gov
- National Library of Medicine, *Helicobacter pylori* in Peptic Ulcer Disease: https://www.nlm.nih.gov/archive/20040830/pubs/cbm/pepulcer.html

21

Diseases of the Heart, Blood Vessels, and Lungs

Joyce Gilbert

ⓔ http://evolve.elsevier.com/Williams/essentials/

In this chapter, we consider interrelated diseases of the circulatory system—heart, blood vessels, and lungs. In recent decades, these diseases of modern civilization have become the major causes of death of men and women in the United States and most other Western societies. One out of every three deaths is caused by heart disease—more than cancer, accidents, and acquired immunodeficiency syndrome combined. The magnitude of this overall health care problem is enormous.

OUTLINE

CORONARY HEART DISEASE

Atherosclerosis

Underlying Disease Process. Atherosclerosis, the major arteriosclerosis disease and underlying pathologic process in coronary heart disease (CHD), is paramount in ongoing study in modern medicine. It is not a solitary disease entity but somewhat a pathologic progression that can involve vascular systems throughout the body, resulting in an extensive variety of clinical manifestations.[1]

An inflammatory process, the characteristic lesions involved are raised fibrous plaques (Fig. 21.1) resulting from injury on the interior surface (intima) of blood vessels.[1] After injury has occurred, plaques first appear as discrete lumps elevated above unaffected surrounding tissue and ranging in color from pearly gray to yellowish gray. Possible causes of injury are as follows[1]:

- Smoking
- Hypertension
- Diabetes
- Increased serum levels of low-density lipoprotein (LDL)-cholesterol
- Decreases serum levels of high-density lipoprotein (HDL)-cholesterol
- High levels of homocysteine
- Elevated C-reactive protein
- Increased serum fibrinogen
- Insulin resistance
- Oxidative stress
- Infection
- Periodontal disease

Additional risk factors are shown in Box 21.1 (see also the Focus on Culture box, "Is Cardiovascular Disease an Equal Opportunity Disease?").

Approximately 90% of CHD patients have elevated levels of serum cholesterol, hypertension, smoke, or have diabetes.[2] The major risk factor for plaque development is a lipoprotein (LDL-cholesterol) that carries cholesterol in the blood.[3] Oxidation of LDL-cholesterol is the principal step in this process of atherogenesis. Inflammation with oxidative stress and activation of macrophages is the principal method of this step. The oxidized LDL-cholesterol is toxic to the intima, initiates smooth muscle propagation, and triggers further immune and inflammatory responses causing formation of lesions called *fatty streaks*.[1]

This fatty degeneration and thickening narrow the vessel lumen and may allow a blood clot (or an embolus) to develop from its irritating presence. Eventually the clot may cut off blood flow in the involved artery. If the artery is a critical one, such as a major coronary vessel, then a heart attack occurs. Tissue area serviced by the involved artery is deprived of its vital oxygen and nutrient supply, a condition called ischemia, and the cells die. The localized area of dying or dead tissue is called an infarct. Because the artery involved supplies cardiac muscle, the *myocardium*, the result is called an *acute myocardial infarction (AMI)*. The two major coronary arteries, with their many branches, are so named because they lie across the brow of the heart muscle and resemble a crown (Fig. 21.2). Fig. 21.3 shows the anterior internal view of the normal human heart.

Cholesterol, Lipoproteins, and Lipids. Cholesterol is a soft, fat-like substance found in all cell membranes and blood and is a precursor of bile acids and steroid hormones. Cholesterol and triglycerides cannot dissolve in blood and must be transported to and from cells by individual components containing lipid and proteins (lipoproteins). The following five types of lipoproteins (Fig. 21.4)

Endothelium
Intima
Media
Adventitia

1. Chronic endothelial "injury":
   • Hyperlipidemia
   • Hypertension
   • Smoking
   • Homocysteine
   • Hemodynamic factors
   • Toxins
   • Viruses
   • Immune reactions

Response to injury

2. Endothelial dysfunction (e.g., increased permeability, leukocyte adhesion, monocyte adhesion) and emigration

3. Smooth muscle emigration from media to intima; macrophage activation

Fatty streak

4. Macrophages and smooth muscle cells engulf lipid

Lymphocyte

Fibrofatty atheroma

5. Smooth muscle proliferation, collagen and other extracellular matrix (ECM) deposition, extracellular lipid

Lymphocyte   Collagen

Lipid debris

FIG. 21.1 Raised fibrous plaques. (From Kumar V, Cotran R, Robbins S: *Robbins basic pathology*, ed 7, Philadelphia, 2003, Saunders.)

KEY TERMS

Atherosclerosis
Common form of arteriosclerosis, characterized by the gradual formation—beginning in childhood in genetically predisposed individuals—of yellow cheeselike streaks of cholesterol and fatty material that develop into hardened plaques in the intima or inner lining of major blood vessels, such as coronary arteries, and eventually, in adulthood, cutting off blood supply to the tissue served by the vessels; the underlying pathologic process of coronary heart disease (CHD).

Arteriosclerosis
Blood vessel disease characterized by thickening and hardening of artery walls, with loss of functional elasticity, mainly affecting the intima (inner lining) of the arteries.

Intima
General term indicating an innermost part of a structure or vessel; inner layer of the blood vessel wall.

Plaque
Thickened deposits of fatty material, largely cholesterol, within the arterial wall that eventually may fill the lumen and cut off blood supply to the tissue served by the damaged vessel.

Ischemia
Deficiency of blood to a particular tissue, resulting from functional blood vessel constriction or actual obstruction of walls in atherosclerosis.

Infarct
An area of tissue necrosis caused by local ischemia, resulting from obstruction of blood circulation to that area.

are classified according to fat content and thus their density, with those having the highest fat content possessing the lowest density[4]:

1. Chylomicrons have the highest lipid content and lowest density and are composed mostly of dietary triglycerides, with a small amount of carrier protein. They accumulate in portal blood after a meal and are efficiently cleared from the blood by the specific enzyme lipoprotein lipase.

2. Very-low-density lipoproteins (VLDLs) still carry a large lipid (triglyceride) content but include approximately 20% cholesterol. These lipoproteins are formed in the liver from endogenous fat sources.

3. Intermediate-density lipoproteins (IDLs) continue the delivery of endogenous triglycerides to cells and carry approximately 40% cholesterol.

4. LDLs carry, in addition to other lipids, approximately two-thirds or more of total plasma cholesterol formed in blood serum from catabolism of VLDL. Because LDL carries cholesterol to cells for deposit in tissues, it is considered the main agent in elevated serum cholesterol levels, or the "bad" cholesterol.

5. HDLs carry less total lipid and more carrier protein. They are formed in the liver from endogenous fat sources. Because HDL carries cholesterol from tissues to the liver for catabolism and excretion, higher serum levels of this "good" cholesterol form are considered protective against CVD. A value of 60 mg/dL or more contributes definite protection and decreased risk.

BOX 21.1 Major Risk Factors in Cardiovascular Disease

Lipid Risk Factors
- Low-density lipoprotein (LDL)-cholesterol >130 mg/dL
- High-density lipoprotein (HDL)-cholesterol <40 mg/dL
- Total cholesterol >200 mg/dL
- Triglycerides >150 mg/dL

Nonlipid Risk Factors
Modifiable
- Tobacco smoke and exposure to tobacco smoke
- Hypertension (>140/90 mm Hg)
- Physical inactivity
- Obesity (body mass index [BMI] >30 kg/m²) and overweight (BMI 25.0–29.9 kg/m²)
- Diabetes mellitus
- Atherogenic diet (high intakes of saturated fats and cholesterol)
- Thrombogenic state
- Excessive alcohol consumption (>1 drink/day for women and >2 drinks/day for men)
- Individual response to stress and coping
- Some illegal drugs (cocaine and intravenous drug abuse)

Nonmodifiable
- Male gender
- Age (men >45 years, women >55 years)
- Heredity (including race)
- Family history of premature coronary heart disease (CHD) (myocardial infarction [MI] or sudden death <55 years of age in father or other male first-degree relative, or <65 years of age in mother or other female first-degree relative)

Probable Risk Factors (Emerging)
- Lipoprotein (a)
- Small LDL particles (pattern B)
- HDL subtypes
- Apolipoprotein B
- Homocysteine
- Fibrinogen
- High-sensitivity C-reactive protein
- Impaired fasting glucose (100–125 mg/dL)

Data from National Cholesterol Education Program (NCEP): *Third report of the NCEP Expert Panel on Detection, Evaluation, and Treatment of High Blood Cholesterol in Adults (Adult Treatment Panel III), full report,* Washington, DC, 2002, National Institutes of Health, National Heart, Lung, and Blood Institute. https://www.nhlbi.nih.gov/guidelines/cholesterol/atp3_rpt.htm; Banasik JL: Alterations in cardiac function. In Copstead LC, Banasik JL, editors: *Pathophysiology,* ed 3, St Louis, 2005, Saunders.

⊕ FOCUS ON CULTURE

Is Cardiovascular Disease an Equal Opportunity Disease?

"Race and ethnicity in the United States are associated with health status."

Marian E. Gornick

The Pfizer Journal Panel[1] states the following:

The system of health care that exists in this country was developed at a time when life expectancy was short, diseases generally came on quickly and were all too frequently fatal, and patients needed lifesaving interventions at a relatively young age. The system has not changed, yet individuals who need health care now live a very long life, develop diseases that are chronic and disabling, and need prevention during a longer life span. One-hundred million Americans have at least one chronic condition, and half of them have more. Among Americans older than 65 years, 88% have one or more chronic illnesses, and one-quarter of them have at least four conditions that should be treated.

After controlling for differences in age, health insurance status, disease severity, and other health problems, the following research findings might not be surprising but nonetheless are disheartening:

- African Americans, Hispanics, and other minorities on average have more underlying risk factors for cardiovascular disease (CVD), including hypertension, obesity, smoking, physical inactivity, higher level of body mass index (BMI), and low high-density lipoprotein (HDL)-cholesterol.
- After minority patients develop CVD, they are less likely to receive higher-quality care and as a result are more likely to die.
- African Americans receive clot-reducing drugs after a heart attack less often than Caucasians.
- Approximately 18% of African-American patients have angioplasty surgery within 48 hours of a heart attack or stroke, compared with almost 30% of Caucasian patients.
- African-American women are "less familiar" with early warning signs of CVD.

- CVD deaths are highest among African Americans at all ages.
- All low-income and less-educated US residents have higher mortality rates for heart disease and stroke than other residents.

During the past 30 years, CVD mortality rates have been decreasing across all racial and ethnic groups, but decline has been much greater for Caucasian Americans. African Americans have mortality rates for CVD approximately 50% higher than those of Caucasian Americans. Hispanic Americans are substantially more likely to be uninsured than Caucasian Americans, and Hispanic Americans are far more likely to lack a usual source of health care than any other group. Research has also found some immigrant families who assimilate into the United States, many of whom are Hispanic, experience deteriorating health status in subsequent generations.

So there is more to CVD than just risk factors. It may not be enough to teach prevention to the masses. Different life experiences attributed to different ethnic groups, as well as economic, time, and residential constraints, may compete with heart-healthy behaviors to increase risk of CVD. So if you are a college student reading this information, then be thankful. You have just decreased your risk of CVD simply by being educated.

Reference

1. Pfizer Journal Panel: The quality of health care in the United States: building quality into the health care system, *Pfizer J* 9(9):1, 2005. https://www.thepfizerjournal.com/default.asp?a=journal&n=tpj41.

Bibliography

Cook NL, Ayanian JZ, Orav EJ, et al: Differences in specialist consultations for cardiovascular disease by race, ethnicity, gender, insurance status, and site of primary care, *Circulation* 119:1–8, 2009. https://www.circ.ahajournals.org.

De Lew N, Weinick RM: An overview: eliminating racial, ethnic, and SES disparities in health care, *Health Care Financ Rev* 21(4):1, 2000.

Continued

⊕ **FOCUS ON CULTURE**

Is Cardiovascular Disease an Equal Opportunity Disease?—cont'd

Gornick ME: Disparities in medicare services: potential causes, plausible explanations, and recommendations, *Health Care Financ Rev* 21(4):23, 2000.

The Henry J. Kaiser Family Foundation: *Racial/ethnic differences in cardiac care: the weight of the evidence*, 2002, USAID Highlights. http://www.kff.org/uninsured/20021009c-index.cfm.

McWilliams JM, Meara E, Zaslavsky AM, et al: Differences in control of cardiovascular disease and diabetes by race, ethnicity, and education: US trends from 1999 to 2006 and effects of Medicare coverage, *Ann Intern Med* 150:505, 2009.

Thomas AJ, Eberly LE, Smith GD, et al: Race/ethnicity, income, major risk factors, and cardiovascular disease mortality, *Am J Public Health* 95(8):1417, 2005.

Winkleby MA, Kraemer HC, Ahn DK, et al: Ethnic and socioeconomic differences in cardiovascular disease risk factors: findings for women from the Third National Health and Nutrition Examination Survey, 1988-1994, *JAMA* 280(23):1989, 1998.

FIG. 21.2 Coronary blood circulation. (From Seely RR, Stephens TD, Tate P: *Anatomy and physiology*, ed 3, St Louis, 1995, McGraw Hill.)

The characteristics of these classes of lipoproteins are summarized in Table 21.1.

Functional Classification of Lipid Disorders. Current clinical practice is based on a useful functional classification that reveals two important factors: (1) recognition of genetic factors involved and (2) focus on the role of apolipoproteins in the course of lipoprotein formation, transport, or destruction. Both factors will be encountered in readings and in clinical work with patients. Thus the outline provided in this discussion is useful in understanding clinical problems involved and in counseling patients.

Apolipoproteins. The term *apolipoprotein* refers to a major protein part of a combined metabolic product, in this case a specific protein part of a combined lipid-protein molecule. For example, apolipoprotein B is a common attachment to LDL and serves two basic functions: (1) it aids transport of lipids in a water medium (i.e., blood), and (2) it transports lipids into cells for metabolic purposes. When apolipoprotein B-100, a single large protein molecule, attaches to one pole of the LDL, it provides a recognition site for LDL receptors on the cell, causing the entire LDL to be transported by pinocytosis into the cell for use in cell metabolism.[4]

KEY TERMS

Homocysteine

An amino acid produced in the human body; high serum homocysteine levels can damage the linings of the arteries and possibly make it easier for blood to clot. Most individuals with high homocysteine levels have low dietary intakes of folic acid, vitamin B_6, or vitamin B_{12}.

C-reactive Protein

A protein found in the blood; levels rise in response to inflammation.

Apolipoproteins

Separate protein compounds that attach to specific receptor sites on particular lipoproteins and activate certain functions, such as protein synthesis of a related enzyme. For example, apolipoprotein C-II is an apolipoprotein of high-density lipoprotein (HDL) and very-low-density lipoprotein (VLDL) that functions to activate the enzyme lipoprotein lipase.

Various types of LDL have specific receptor sites for particular apolipoproteins to which the apolipoprotein is attracted and that in large measure determine function.

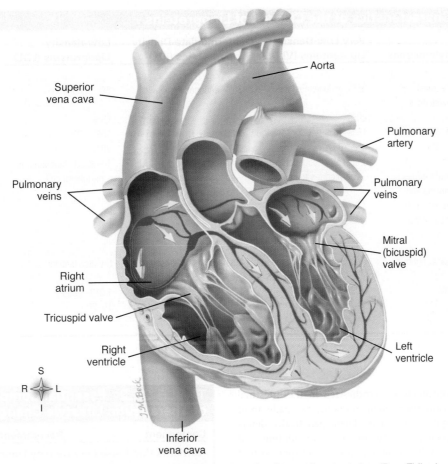

FIG. 21.3 The normal human heart. Anterior internal view showing cardiac circulation. (From Thibodeau GA, Patton KT: *Anatomy and physiology*, ed 6, St Louis, 2007, Mosby.)

FIG. 21.4 Composition of lipoproteins and transport of lipoproteins in blood. *HDL,* High-density lipoprotein; *LDL,* low-density lipoprotein. (From Gould BE: *Pathophysiology for the health professionals,* ed 3, Philadelphia, 2006, Saunders.)

TABLE 21.1 Characteristics of the Classes of Lipoproteins

Characteristic	Chylomicrons	Very Low-Density Lipoproteins (VLDL)	Intermediate-Density Lipoproteins (IDL)	Low-density Lipoproteins (LDL)	High-Density Lipoproteins (HDL)
Composition					
Triglycerides	85%, diet, exogenous	55%, endogenous	30%, endogenous	5%, endogenous	5%, endogenous
Cholesterol	5%	20%	40%	55%	20%
Phospholipid	3%–6%	15%–20%	20%	15%–22%	25%–30%
Protein	1%–2%	5%–10%	10%	20%	50%
Function	Transport dietary triglycerides to plasma and tissues, cells	Transport endogenous triglycerides to cells	Continue transport of endogenous triglycerides to cells	Transport cholesterol to peripheral cells	Transport free cholesterol from membranes to liver for catabolism
Place of Synthesis	Intestinal wall	Liver	Liver	Liver	Liver
Size and Density					
Description	Largest, lightest	Next largest, next lightest	Intermediate size, lighter	Smaller, heavier	Smaller, densest, heaviest
Density	0.095	0.095–1.006	1.00–1.03	1.019–1.063	1.063–1.210
Size in nanometers (nm)	80–1000	30–80	25–40	15–20	5–10

Function. When lipoproteins are synthesized in the intestinal wall, liver, and blood serum, the protein component is made up of varying kinds of apolipoprotein parts. These genetically determined components influence the structure, receptor binding, and metabolism of lipoproteins. It is an apolipoprotein component that helps form special spherical droplets of lipid material for transport in the bloodstream (see Chapter 4). Apolipoprotein determination is currently a useful laboratory tool for identifying persons at high risk for CHD.[3]

Defects in synthesis of apolipoproteins. The current functional approach classifies lipid disorders into four major groups based on the underlying functional problem: (1) defects in apolipoprotein synthesis, (2) enzyme deficiencies, (3) LDL receptor deficiency, and (4) other inherited hyperlipidemias.[3]

General Principles of Nutrition Therapy

Basic guidelines. The National Cholesterol Education Program (NCEP) periodically publishes revised guidelines for clinical management of high serum cholesterol. The Adult Treatment Panel I (ATP I) delineated strategy for primary prevention of CHD in persons with high levels of LDL-cholesterol (160 mg/dL) or those with borderline-high LDL-cholesterol (130–159 mg/dL) and two or more risk factors. The ATP II substantiated these strategies and made further recommendations for intensive management of LDL-cholesterol in persons with established CHD. A new lower LDL-cholesterol of 100 mg/dL was established. The ATP III report identified more intensive LDL-lowering therapy. The ATP III[3] suggests a comprehensive lifestyle approach to reducing risk for CHD called *therapeutic lifestyle changes (TLC)* and incorporates the following components[2,3]:

- Reduced intake of saturated fats and cholesterol
- Therapeutic dietary options to enhance the lowering of LDL (plant stanols and sterols and increased soluble fiber)
- Weight reduction
- Increased regular physical activity

TABLE 21.2 Essential Components of Therapeutic Lifestyle Changes

Component	Recommendation
Nutrients that Raise Low-Density Lipoprotein (LDL)	
Saturated fats	<7% of total energy intake
Dietary cholesterol	<200 mg/day
Therapeutic Options for Lowering LDL	
Plant stanols/sterols	2 g/day
Soluble fiber	10–25 g/day
Total energy (kilocalories)	Adjust total energy intake to maintain desirable body weight/prevent weight gain
Physical activity	Include enough moderate exercise to expend at least 200 kcal/day
Trans fats	Avoid
Limit sodium to 2400 mg/day	When indicated

Data from National Cholesterol Education Program (NCEP): *Third report of the NCEP Expert Panel on Detection, Evaluation, and Treatment of High Blood Cholesterol in Adults (Adult Treatment Panel III), full report,* Washington, D.C., 2002, National Institutes of Health, National Heart, Lung, and Blood Institute. https://www.nhlbi.nih.gov/guidelines/cholesterol/atp3_rpt.htm; American Dietetic Association: *Nutrition care manual,* Chicago, 2005, American Dietetic Association. https://www.nutritioncaremanual.org.

Components of TLC are outlined in Table 21.2. The ATP III also suggests ranges for other macronutrients in the TLC diet (Table 21.3). *Components of the therapeutic lifestyle changes diet.*

Saturated fat and cholesterol. In view of the fact that the major LDL-raising nutrient components are saturated fat and cholesterol, reducing saturated fat (< 7% of total energy intake) and cholesterol (less than 200 mg/day) in the diet is the foundation of the TLC diet. The strongest nutritional influence on serum LDL-cholesterol levels is

TABLE 21.3 Nutrient Composition of the Therapeutic Lifestyle Changes Diet

Component	Recommendation
Polyunsaturated fat, including omega-3 fatty acids	Up to 10% total energy intake
Monounsaturated fat	Up to 20% total energy intake
Total fat	25%–35% total energy intake[a]
Carbohydrate[b]	50%–60% total energy intake
Dietary fiber	20–30 g/day
Protein	Approximately 15% total energy intake

[a]Adult Treatment Panel III (ATP III) allows for increase of total fat to 35% total energy intake and reduction in carbohydrate to 50% for persons with the metabolic syndrome. Any increase in fat intake should be in the form of either polyunsaturated or monounsaturated fat.
[b]Carbohydrates should come primarily from foods rich in complex carbohydrates, including grains—especially whole grains—fruits, and vegetables.
Data from National Cholesterol Education Program (NCEP): *Third report of the NCEP Expert Panel on Detection, Evaluation, and Treatment of High Blood Cholesterol in Adults (Adult Treatment Panel III), full report,* Washington, DC, 2002, National Institutes of Health, National Heart, Lung, and Blood Institute. https://www.nhlbi.nih.gov/guidelines/cholesterol/atp3_rpt.htm; American Dietetic Association: *Nutrition care manual,* Chicago, 2005, American Dietetic Association. https://www.nutritioncaremanual.org.

saturated fats.[3] In fact, a "dose-response relationship" exists between saturated fats and LDL-cholesterol levels. For every 1% increase in kilocalories (kcalories or kcal) from saturated fats as a percentage of total energy, serum LDL-cholesterol increases approximately 2%. On the other hand, a 1% decrease in saturated fats will lower serum cholesterol by approximately 2%.[3] Although weight reduction by itself, even of a few pounds, will reduce LDL-cholesterol levels, weight reduction attained using a kcalorie-controlled diet low in saturated fats and cholesterol will improve and maintain LDL-cholesterol lowering. Although dietary cholesterol does not have the same influence as saturated fat on serum LDL-cholesterol levels, high cholesterol intakes raise LDL-cholesterol levels. Therefore reducing dietary cholesterol to less than 200 mg/day decreases serum LDL-cholesterol in most persons.[3]

Monounsaturated fat. The TLC diet recommends substitution of monounsaturated fat for saturated fats at an intake level of up to 20% of total energy intake, because monounsaturated fats lower LDL-cholesterol levels relative to saturated fats without decreasing HDL-cholesterol or triglyceride levels. It is recommended that plant oils and nuts be used because they are the best sources of monounsaturated fats.[3]

Polyunsaturated fats. Polyunsaturated fats, in particular linoleic acid, reduce LDL-cholesterol levels when used instead of saturated fats. However, they can also bring about small reductions in HDL-cholesterol when compared side by side with monounsaturated fats. The TLC diet recommends liquid vegetables oils, semiliquid margarines (soft, tub margarines), and other margarines low in *trans fatty acids* be used because they are the best sources of polyunsaturated fats; intakes can range up to 10% of total energy intake.[3]

***Trans* fatty acids.** Two types of *trans* fatty acids exist: (1) those appearing naturally in foods (mostly meat products) and (2) those produced by the process of hydrogenation of unsaturated fats. Trans fats from partially hydrogenated fats are more harmful than naturally occurring trans fats,[5] raising serum LDL-cholesterol and lowering serum HDL-cholesterol.

KEY TERM

Trans Fatty Acids
Fatty acids that have been hydrogenated to be used in margarine and in the food industry; have been shown to increase low-density lipoprotein (LDL)-cholesterol and lower high-density lipoprotein (HDL)-cholesterol.

Total fat. In view of the fact that only saturated fats and trans fatty acids increase LDL-cholesterol levels,[5] serum levels of LDL-cholesterol are unrelated to total fat intake per se. For that reason the ATP III suggests it is not crucial to limit total fat intake for the specific goal of reducing LDL-cholesterol levels, provided saturated fats are decreased to goal levels.[2]

Carbohydrates. When saturated fats are replaced with carbohydrates, LDL-cholesterol levels are reduced. On the other hand, very high intakes of carbohydrates (greater than 60% of total energy intake) are associated with a reduction in HDL-cholesterol and an increase in serum triglyceride. Increasing soluble fiber intake can sometimes reduce these responses. On average, increasing soluble fiber to 10–25 g/day is accompanied by an approximately 5% reduction in LDL-cholesterol.[2]

Protein. Despite the fact that dietary protein as a rule has an insignificant effect on serum LDL-cholesterol level, replacing animal protein with plant-based protein has been reported to decrease LDL-cholesterol.[2] This may be the result of plant-based foods providing good sources of proteins (legumes, dry beans, nuts, whole grains, and vegetables) containing less saturated fat than many animal proteins and no cholesterol. This is not to say animal proteins cannot be low in saturated fat and cholesterol. Fat-free and low-fat dairy products, egg whites, fish, skinless poultry, and lean cuts of beef and pork are also low in saturated fat and cholesterol. All foods of animal origin will contain cholesterol.

Further dietary options for reducing LDL-cholesterol. Adding 5–10 g of soluble fiber (oats, barley, psyllium, pectin-rich fruit, and beans) per day is associated with approximately a 5% reduction in LDL-cholesterol and is regarded as a therapeutic option to enhance reduction of LDL-cholesterol. Plant sterols present an additional therapeutic option.[2] Daily intakes of 2–3 g plant stanol and sterol esters (isolated from soybean and tall pine tree oils) have been shown to lower LDL-cholesterol by 6–15%.[2]

General Approach to Therapeutic Lifestyle Changes. The ATP III[2] suggests patients at risk for CHD or with CHD be referred to registered dietitians (RDs) or other qualified nutritionists for the duration of all stages of nutrition therapy (NT). After 6 weeks of TLC, LDL-cholesterol should be measured to evaluate response to TLC. If the LDL-cholesterol target has been realized or an improvement in LDL lowering has occurred, then NT should be uninterrupted. If the goal has not been attained, then the physician can select from a number of alternatives. First, NT can be reexplained and reinforced. Next, therapeutic dietary options can be integrated into TLC. The response to NT should be assessed in an additional 6 weeks. If the LDL-cholesterol target is achieved, then the current intensity of NT should be continued indefinitely. If downward movement is seen in LDL-cholesterol measures, then thought should be given to continuing NT before adding LDL-lowering medications. If it looks unlikely the LDL target will be realized with NT, then medications should be considered.[2] The "Guide to Therapeutic Lifestyle Changes: Healthy Lifestyle Recommendations for a Healthy Heart" is shown in Box 21.2.

BOX 21.2 Guide to Therapeutic Lifestyle Changes: Healthy Lifestyle Recommendations for a Healthy Heart

Food Items to Choose More Often
Breads and Cereals
- Six servings per day, adjusted to caloric needs.
- Breads, cereals, especially whole grains; pasta; rice; potatoes; dry beans and peas; low-fat crackers and cookies.

Vegetables
Three to five servings per day fresh, frozen, or canned, without added fat, sauce, or salt.

Fruits
Two to four servings per day fresh, frozen, canned, dried.

Dairy Products
Two to three servings per day fat-free, ½%, 1% milk, buttermilk, yogurt, cottage cheese, fat-free and low-fat cheese.

Eggs
Fewer than two egg yolks per week; egg whites or egg substitute.

Meat, Poultry, Fish
Five ounces per day.
Lean-cut beef tenderloin, ground round, extra-lean hamburger; cold cuts made with lean meat or soy protein; skinless poultry; fish.

Fats and Oils
Amount adjusted to caloric level: unsaturated oils; soft or liquid margarines and vegetable oil spreads; salad dressings, seeds, and nuts.

Therapeutic Lifestyle Changes Diet Options
Stanol/sterol-containing margarines; soluble-fiber food sources: barley, oats, psyllium, apples, bananas, berries, citrus fruits, nectarines, peaches, pears, plums, prunes, broccoli, Brussels sprouts, carrots, dry beans, soy products (tofu, miso).

Food Items to Choose Less Often
Breads and Cereals
- Many baked products, including doughnuts, biscuits, butter rolls, muffins, croissants, sweet rolls, Danish pastries, cakes, pies, coffee cakes, cookies.
- Many grain-based snacks, including chips, cheese puffs, snack mix, regular crackers, buttered popcorn.

Vegetables
Vegetables fried or prepared with butter, cheese, or cream sauce.

Fruits
Fruits fried or served with butter or cream.

Dairy Products
Whole milk, 2% milk, whole-milk yogurt, ice cream, cream, cheese.

Eggs
Egg yolk, whole eggs.

Meat, Poultry, Fish
Higher-fat meat cuts: ribs, T-bone steak, regular hamburger, bacon, sausage; cold cuts: salami, bologna, hot dogs; organ meats: liver, brains, sweetbreads; poultry with skin; fried meat; fried poultry; fried fish.

Fats and Oils
Butter, shortening, stick margarine, chocolate, coconut.

Recommendations for Weight Reduction
Weigh Regularly
Record weight, body mass index (BMI), and waist circumferences.

Lose Weight Gradually
Goal: lose 10% of body weight in 6 months; lose ½–1 lb per week.

Develop Healthy Eating Patterns
- Choose healthy foods (see "Food Items to Choose More Often").
- Reduce your intake of foods in "Food Items to Choose Less Often."
- Limit the number of eating occasions.
- Avoid second helpings.
- Identify and reduce hidden fat by reading food labels to choose products lower in saturated fat and calories, and ask about ingredients in ready-to-eat foods prepared away from home.
- Identify and reduce sources of excess carbohydrates such as fat-free and regular crackers, cookies and other desserts, snacks, and beverages that contain sugar.

Recommendations for Increased Physical Activity
Make Physical Activity Part of Daily Routines
- Reduce sedentary time.
- Walk or bike ride more and drive less.
- Take the stairs instead of an elevator.
- Get off the bus a few stops early and walk the remaining distance.
- Mow the lawn with a push mower, rake leaves, and work in a garden.
- Push a stroller.
- Clean your house.
- Do exercises or pedal a stationary bike while watching television.
- Play actively with your children.
- Take a brisk 10-minute walk or bike ride before work, during your work break, and after dinner.

Make Physical Activity Part of Exercise or Recreational Activities
- Walk or jog.
- Ride a bicycle or use an arm pedal bicycle.
- Swim or do water aerobics.
- Play basketball.
- Join a sports team.
- Play wheelchair sports.
- Play golf, pulling or carrying clubs.
- Go canoeing, cross-country skiing, or dancing.
- Take part in an exercise program at work, at home, at school, or at the gym.

Data from US Department of Health and Human Services, Public Health Service, National Institutes of Health, National Heart, Lung, and Blood Institute: *Your guide to lowering your blood pressure with DASH,* NIH Pub No 06-4082, Bethesda, MD, 2006, US Government Printing Office. https://www.nhlbi.nih.gov.

Metabolic syndrome is the name for a group of metabolic risk factors that increase risk for heart disease, type 2 diabetes, peripheral vascular disease (PVD), and stroke. Any one of these risk factors may develop, but they tend to occur together. Although no well-accepted criteria exist for diagnosis of metabolic syndrome, it is identified by the presence of at least three of the following:

- Abdominal obesity
  - Men: ≥40 inches (102 cm)
  - Women: ≥35 inches (88 cm)
- Elevated triglycerides (≥150 mg/dL)
- Reduced HDL-cholesterol
  - Men: <40 mg/dL
  - Women: <50 mg/dL
- Elevated blood pressure (≥130/85 mm Hg)
- Elevated fasting blood glucose (≥100 mg/dL)

Data from American Heart Association: *Metabolic syndrome: information for professionals*, Dallas, Texas, 2009, American Heart Association. https://www.americanheart.org/presenter.jhtml?identifier=534; National Institutes of Health, National Heart, Lung, and Blood Institute: *Diseases and conditions index: metabolic syndrome*, Washington, DC, 2010, National Institutes of Health, National Heart, Lung, and Blood Institute. https://www.nhlbi.nih.gov/health/dci/Diseases/ms/ms_whatis.html.

Drug Therapy. Although use of TLC will help many individuals attain their LDL-cholesterol target goal, a segment of the population will need LDL-lowering medications to achieve the prescribed goal for LDL-cholesterol. If treatment with TLC alone is unsuccessful after 3 months, then the ATP III recommends initiation of drug treatment. However, when drugs are used, TLC also should continue to be used concomitantly. NT affords further CHD risk reduction beyond drug efficacy.[2] The combined use of TLC and LDL-cholesterol–lowering medications may include the following actions[5]:

- Intensive LDL lowering with TLC, including therapeutic dietary options
- May prevent need for drugs
- Can augment LDL-lowering medications
- May allow for lower doses of medications
- Weight control plus increased physical activity
- Reduces risk beyond LDL-cholesterol lowering

- Constitutes principal management of metabolic syndrome (see margin box)
- Raises HDL-cholesterol
- Initiating TLC before medication consideration
- For most people a trial of NT of approximately 3 months is advised before initiating drug therapy
- Ineffective trials of NT exclusive of medications should not be protracted for indefinite period if the goals of therapy are not approached in reasonable time (medication should not be withheld if it is needed to reach targets in persons with high short-term or long-term CHD risk)
- Initiating drug therapy simultaneously with TLC
- For severe hypercholesterolemia in which NT alone cannot attain LDL-cholesterol targets
- For those with CHD or CHD risk equivalents in whom NT alone will not attain LDL-cholesterol targets

The general strategy for initiation and progression of drug therapy is outlined in Fig. 21.5. (For information about particular herbs and supplements that affect the cardiovascular system, see the Complementary and Alternative Medicine [CAM] box, "It Does a Heart Good . . . or Does It?" and the Diet-Medications Interactions box, "Possible Interactions Between Cardiovascular Diseases and Natural Therapies.")

Acute Cardiovascular Disease: Myocardial Infarction

Medical Management. Initial medical treatment of myocardial infarction (MI), or heart attack, usually includes strong analgesics (usually morphine sulfate) for severe unremitting pain, oxygen therapy, intravenous nitroglycerin for ischemic discomfort, control of hypertension or management of pulmonary congestion, and aspirin to produce a rapid antithrombotic effect.[4] This protocol is sometimes referred to as *MONA* (morphine, oxygen, nitroglycerin, and aspirin).

Nutritional Management. In the initial acute phase of CVD, an MI requires close attention to dietary modifications. The basic clinical objective is cardiac rest to allow the healing process to begin. All care is directed toward this basic need for cardiac rest so that the damaged heart can be restored to normal functioning. In addition to TLC (see Table 21.3), sodium may be restricted to 2 to 4 g for hypertension or to control edema (see the Case Study box, "The Patient with Myocardial Infarction").[2]

FIG. 21.5 Progression of drug therapy. *LDL*, Low-density lipoprotein. (From the National Cholesterol Education Program [NCEP]: *Third report of the NCEP Expert Panel on Detection, Evaluation, and Treatment of High Blood Cholesterol in Adults [Adult Treatment Panel III], full report*, Washington, DC, 2001, National Institutes of Health, National Heart, Lung, and Blood Institute.)

COMPLEMENTARY AND ALTERNATIVE MEDICINE (CAM)

It Does a Heart Good . . . or Does It?

Herbs are used by many to treat "what ails them." Although research is constantly being undertaken to test the efficacy of herbs, available information remains limited. The following table reviews the efficacy of herbal medicines that affect the cardiovascular system. In an effort to simplify the information, herbs are classified under the primary diseases they treat. However, please keep in mind most herbal medicines have multiple, overlapping cardiovascular effects. It is also important to remember that herbs sold in the United States are not standardized doses or preparations; therefore no regulation exists regarding the safety of herbal products.

Cardiovascular Disorder	Commonly Used Herb/ Supplement	Efficacy of Herb/Supplement
Congestive heart failure (CHF)	Coenzyme Q$_{10}$ (CoQ$_{10}$) (mitoquinone, ubidecarenone, ubiquinone)	Reasonably good evidence supports use of CoQ$_{10}$ as adjunct therapy; thought to work by improving efficiency of cardiac muscle
	Hawthorn (*Crataegus laevigata, C. monogyna, C. oxyacantha, C. pentagyna*)	No evidence hawthorn reduces CHF morbidity or mortality
	Carnitine	Improves myocardial contractility and relaxation and cardiac pump function in patients with ventricular dysfunction
	Taurine	Might be useful in adjuvant therapy in class II, III, and IV CHF
	Arginine	Might improve some CHF symptoms
	Creatine	Might improve skeletal muscle exercise tolerance in patients with CHF
	Vitamin B$_1$ (thiamin)	Slight evidence that intravenous thiamin followed by oral supplementation could improve heart function in patients with CHF
	Vitamin E (α-tocopherol)	Ineffective for treatment of CHF
High blood pressure	Garlic (*Allium* spp., including *A. sativum*)	Might mildly reduce blood pressure (approximately 10 mm Hg systolic and 5 mm Hg diastolic)
	CoQ$_{10}$	Adjunctive treatment with 120 mg CoQ$_{10}$ daily has been shown to reduce average blood pressure by about 9%; might prolong hypotensive effects of enalapril and nitrendipine without changing their maximal effect
	Fish oils (alternative names/supplement forms: docosahexaenoic acid [DHA], eicosapentaenoic acid [EPA], omega-3 fatty acids, omega-3 oils)	Might have slight antihypertensive effect
	Hawthorn	Might increase exercise tolerance
	Carnitine	Might increase exercise tolerance; decrease number of premature ventricular contractions (PVCs); might decrease need for some medications such as nitroglycerides, β-blockers, antihypertensives, diuretics, anticoagulants, antiarrhythmics, and hypolipidemics
	Inositol hexaniacinate (a form of niacin)	Might improve walking distance
	L-carnitine	Improves muscle energy use
	Mesoglycans	Might improve walking distance
	Policosanol	Improves walking distance
	Oxerutins	In combination with compression stockings, effective in reducing leg edema
	Diosmin/hesperidin (citrus bioflavonoids)	Significantly improves symptoms
	Butcher's broom (*Ruscus aculeatus*)	Improves symptoms of venous insufficiency
	Grape leaf	Dose-dependent improvements in symptoms
	Oligomeric proanthocyanidin complexes (OPCs)	Provide significant benefit in chronic venous insufficiency
	Gotu kola (*Centella asiatica*)	Dose-dependent improvements in symptoms
Angina pectoris	N-acetylcysteine (NAC) (modified form of the dietary amino acid cysteine)	Given in combination with nitroglycerin is more effective than either drug alone in preventing death, myocardial infarction (MI), or need for revascularization; unfortunately, combined treatment also associated with high rate of severe headache
Hypertension	Stevia	Might possess antihypertensive effects; considered safe when used at recommended doses
Peripheral vascular disease (PVD) (intermittent claudication)	Ginkgo (*Ginkgo biloba*)	Modest improvement in pain-free walking
Venous insufficiency	Horse chestnut (*Aesculus hippocastanum*)	Used in combination with compression stockings, useful treatment for pain, itching, leg fatigue, and feelings of tension in the legs

Bibliography

Bratman S, Girman AM: *Mosby's handbook of herbs and supplements and their therapeutic uses*, St Louis, 2003, Mosby.

Kuhn MA, Winston D: *Herbal therapy and supplements: a scientific and traditional approach*, Philadelphia, 2001, Lippincott Williams & Wilkins.

Springhouse Corporation: *Professional guide to complementary and alternative therapies*, Baltimore, MD, 2001, Springhouse.

⬥ DIET-MEDICATIONS INTERACTIONS

Possible Interactions Between Cardiovascular Diseases and Natural Therapies

Pharmaceutical Class	Natural Therapy	Interaction
Warfarin	Coenzyme Q10 (CoQ10)	Concurrent use could reduce effectiveness of drug; might increase excretion or metabolism of warfarin
ACE inhibitors	Arginine, potassium	Possible hyperkalemia
	Dong quai (Angelica polymorpha sinensis), St. John's wort (Hypericum perforatum)	Possible increased risk of photosensitivity
	Iron	Mutual absorption interference; possible reduction of ACE inhibitor–induced cough
	Licorice (natural)	Antagonism of drug action
	Zinc	Correction of possible drug-induced depletion
Digitoxin, digoxin	Eleutherococcus (Siberian ginseng)	Interference with laboratory measurement of digoxin levels
	Hawthorn (Crataegus laevigata, C. monogyna, C. oxyacantha, C. pentagyna)	Might interfere with effects of digoxin or serum monitoring
	Horsetail, licorice (natural)	Possible hypokalemia leading to increased drug toxicity
	Magnesium	Absorption interference
	St. John's wort	Decreased serum levels of drug with possible rebound toxicity if herb is stopped
Loop diuretics	Dong quai, St. John's wort	Possible increased risk of photosensitivity
	Licorice (natural)	Potentiation of hypokalemic action of drug
Potassium-sparing diuretics	Arginine	Possible increased risk of hyperkalemia
	Licorice (natural)	Antagonism of drug action
	Magnesium	Risk of hypermagnesemia
	White willow (Salix alba)	Possible interference of salicylate content with spironolactone action
	Zinc	Excessive zinc levels with spironolactone
Thiazide diuretics	Calcium	Potential risk of hypercalcemia
	Dong quai, St. John's wort	Possible increased risk of photosensitivity
	Licorice (natural)	Potentiation of hypokalemic action of drug
Fluoroquinolones, tetracyclines	Calcium	Mutual absorption interference
Levothyroxine	Calcium	Possible absorption interference
Calcium channel blockers (CCBs)	Combined high-dose calcium and vitamin D, grapefruit juice	Possible antagonism of drug action
Anticoagulant and antiplatelet agents	Fish oil	Possible increased risk of bleeding complications
	Vitamin C	Possible antagonism of drug action
	Garlic, ginkgo, high-dose vitamin E, policosanol	Possible increased risk of bleeding complications
	Horse chestnut, oligomeric proanthocyanidin complexes (OPCs)	Possible increased risk of bleeding complications
Amiloride	Magnesium	Possible hypermagnesemia
β-blockers	Calcium	Absorption interference
	Chromium	Increased high-density lipoprotein (HDL) levels
Nitrates	N-acetylcysteine (NAC)	Increase of headache side effects

Bibliography

Bratman S, Girman AM: *Mosby's handbook of herbs and supplements and their therapeutic uses,* St Louis, 2003, Mosby.

Kuhn MA, Winston D: *Herbal therapy and supplements: a scientific and traditional approach,* Philadelphia, 2001, Lippincott Williams & Wilkins.

Springhouse Corporation: *Professional guide to complementary and alternative therapies,* Baltimore, MD, 2001, Springhouse.

CASE STUDY

The Patient With Myocardial Infarction

Edward is a 37-year-old sedentary executive who was seen for an annual physical examination 6 months ago. He had no complaints other than feeling the "everyday pressures" of his job as a corporate attorney and head of the legal division. He admitted smoking two packs of cigarettes a day as a means of relieving stress.

Edward is 175 cm (5′ 9″). At the time of his examination, he weighed 83 kg (185 lb). His blood pressure was 148/90 mm Hg, and his serum cholesterol level

was 285 mg/dL. He was advised to quit smoking, exercise daily at a moderate pace, and lose 9 kg (20 lb).

Edward arrived in the hospital emergency department 3 months later complaining of severe chest pains and difficulty breathing. His wife reported that he had appeared pale that evening, had broken out into a cold sweat, and had vomited shortly after arriving home from work. Once regular breathing was restored by the emergency medical team and his pain subsided, a number of

Continued

The Patient With Myocardial Infarction—cont'd

laboratory tests were ordered. These tests included serum glutamic-oxaloacetic transaminase (SGOT), lactate dehydrogenase (LDH), prothrombin time (PT), lipid panel plus high-density lipoprotein (HDL)-cholesterol, sedimentation rate, coagulation times, fasting plasma glucose (FPG), blood urea nitrogen (BUN), and complete blood count (CBC). An electrocardiogram (ECG) was also ordered. The patient was then transferred to the coronary care unit for closer monitoring.

The following test results were elevated: SGOT, LDH, LDL, as well as total cholesterol, triglycerides, glucose, PT, white blood cell count, and sedimentation rate. HDL level was low. The ECG revealed an infarction of the posterior wall of the myocardium. The diagnosis was myocardial infarction (MI), with underlying familial hypercholesterolemia.

In consultation with the hospital's registered dietitian (RD), the cardiologist ordered a liquid diet, increasing it to a soft diet with low saturated fats 2 days later. The RD noted continued improvement in the patient's appetite accompanying recovery and recommended changing the diet order to the therapeutic lifestyle changes (TLC) diet.

One week later, Edward was discharged. During his convalescence, the RD and nurse met with him and his wife several times to discuss his continuing care at home. At each follow-up clinic visit with the physician and nutritionist, Edward showed good general recovery and enjoyment of his new modified fat and cholesterol food habits.

Questions for Analysis
1. What predisposing factors in Edward's lifestyle place him in the high-risk category for coronary heart disease (CHD)?
2. Why was moderate, consistent exercise originally recommended?
3. Explain the causes for Edward's initial symptoms.
4. How does each laboratory test ordered in the emergency department relate to cell metabolism? Why were the results elevated?
5. Explain the association between the final diet order and his lipid disorder.
6. What nondietary needs might Edward have while convalescing at home? What community agencies might be of assistance?

Metabolic Syndrome. If the patient has metabolic syndrome, further attention must be given to the following[4]:
- Weight management
- Gradual increase in physical activity under physician's supervision
- Limiting alcohol intake

Chronic Coronary Heart Disease

Congestive Heart Failure. In chronic CHD a condition of congestive heart failure (CHF) may develop over time. Each year more than 550,000 new cases are diagnosed.[1] The progressively weakened heart muscle, the myocardium, is unable to maintain an adequate cardiac output to sustain normal blood circulation. Resulting fluid imbalances cause edema, especially pulmonary edema, to develop. This condition brings added problems in breathing called *respiratory distress* or *dyspnea*, which places added stress on the laboring heart. The most common cause of CHF is myocardial ischemia from coronary artery disease, hypertension, and cardiomyopathy. Approximately half of CHF patients suffer diastolic dysfunction, whereas systolic function is preserved. This is more likely to develop in older adults, women, and those without history of MI.[1]

Etiology: Relationship to Sodium and Water. Fluid congestion of chronic heart disease relates to imbalances in the body's capillary fluid shift mechanism and its resulting hormonal effects, as follows:
- *Imbalance in capillary fluid shift mechanism:* As the heart fails to pump out returning blood fast enough, venous return is delayed. This causes a disproportionate amount of blood to accumulate in the vascular system working with the right side of the heart. Venous pressure rises, a sort of "backup" pressure effect, and overcomes the balance of filtration pressures necessary to maintain the normal capillary fluid shift mechanism (see Chapter 7). Fluid that would normally flow between interstitial

spaces and blood vessels is held in the tissue spaces rather than recirculated.
- *Hormonal mechanisms:* Two hormonal mechanisms are involved in fluid balance in normal circulation. In this instance, both of the following contribute to cardiac edema:
  1. *Aldosterone mechanism:* This mechanism, described more completely by its full name, the *renin-angiotensin-aldosterone mechanism,* is normally a lifesaving sodium- and water-conserving mechanism that ensures essential fluid balances. However, in this case, it only compounds the edema problem. As the heart fails to propel blood circulation forward, deficient cardiac output effectively reduces blood flow through kidney nephrons. Decreased renal blood pressure triggers the renin-angiotensin system. Renin is an enzyme from the renal cortex that combines in blood with its substrate, angiotensinogen, which is produced in the liver, to produce in turn angiotensin I and II. Angiotensin II acts as a stimulant to the adrenal glands to produce aldosterone. This hormone in turn effects a reabsorption of sodium in an ion exchange with potassium in the distal tubules of the nephrons, and water reabsorption follows. Ordinarily this is a lifesaving mechanism to protect the body's vital water supply. However, in CHF, it only adds to the edema problem. The mechanism reacts as if the body's total fluid volume is reduced, when in truth the fluid is excessive; it is just that it is not in normal circulation but is being retained in the body's tissues.
  2. *Antidiuretic hormone (ADH) mechanism:* This water-conserving hormonal mechanism also adds to edema. Cardiac stress and reduced renal flow cause the release of ADH, also known as *vasopressin,* from the pituitary gland. ADH then stimulates still more water reabsorption in nephrons of the kidney, further increasing the problem of edema.

Increased Cellular Free Potassium. As reduced blood circulation depresses cell metabolism, cell protein is broken down and releases its bound potassium in the cell. As a result the amount of free potassium inside the cell is increased, which increases intracellular osmotic pressure. Sodium ions in fluid surrounding the cell then also increase in number to balance increased osmotic pressure within the cell and to prevent cell dehydration. In time, the increased sodium outside the cell causes still more water retention.[6]

KEY TERM

Pulmonary Edema
Accumulation of fluid in tissues of the lung.

Antidiuretic Hormone (ADH)
Water-conserving hormone from the posterior lobe of pituitary gland; causes resorption of water by kidney nephrons according to body need.

Vasopressin
Alternative name of antidiuretic hormone.

Nutritional Management. The basis for all care of the person with CHF is improving cardiac output while reducing the workload of the heart and minimizing congestive symptoms. Medical treatment involves oxygen therapy, decreased physical activity, and drug therapy with (1) diuretic and vasodilator agents to control fluid congestion in the lungs; (2) digitalis drugs to strengthen contractions of the heart muscle; and (3) sympathetic antagonists, angiotensin-converting enzyme (ACE) inhibitors, nitrate, and vasodilators to decrease workload of the heart.[7] Nutrition support involves the following[8]:

- *Sodium* is usually restricted to 2 g/day and may be adjusted upward to 3 g/day if necessary to promote food and nutrient intake.
- *Fluids* may be restricted to 1500 mL/day, if necessary.
- *Texture* may be modified to soft foods so that little physical effort is needed.
- *Meals* may be divided into smaller feedings to also decrease effort necessary for eating.
- *Alcohol* is generally limited to one drink per day. If alcohol is thought to be a causative factor in the heart disease, then abstinence is mandatory.

Cardiac Cachexia

Etiology. Sometimes with prolonged myocardial insufficiency and heart failure, an extreme clinical condition of cardiac cachexia develops. Progressive, profound malnutrition results from an insufficient oxygen supply that cannot meet demands of red blood cell formation by bone marrow or energy needs for basic breathing. The enlarged, laboring heart is unable to maintain a sufficient blood supply to the body tissues, and nutrient delivery to cells is impaired. Edema, unpalatable sodium-restricted diets, drug reactions, and postoperative complications of cardiac surgery all worsen the anorexia and reduce food intake. In addition, the individual has probably become hypermetabolic and hypercatabolic. It should be no surprise that the incidence of nosocomial (hospital-induced) cardiac cachexia is a common occurrence.

Nutrition Therapy. The goal is to help restore heart-lung function as much as possible and rebuild body tissue. Team care involving the physician, clinical dietitian, nurse, patient, and family is essential. Nutrition support focuses on energy, nutrients, supplements, and feeding plan, as follows[4]:

- *Energy:* Sufficient kcalories are needed to cover basal energy needs, as well as energy for minimal activity and the hypermetabolism of severe CHF; more kcalories may be needed if major surgery is planned. Depending on the extent of malnutrition indicated by nutrition assessment, an increase of 30–50% of basal needs may be indicated.
- *Fluids:* Sufficient but not excessive fluid intake is needed, at a rate of approximately 0.5 mL/kcal/day or 1000–1500 mL/day.
- *Protein:* Approximately 1.0–1.5 g/kg body weight is needed to replace tissue losses and cover malabsorption.

- *Sodium:* Sodium restriction varies with individual status, usually in a range of 1–2 g/day, with attention to multiple alternate seasonings to enhance palatability of food.
- *Mineral-vitamin supplementation:* May need to supplement intake with folate, magnesium, thiamin, zinc, and iron depending on serum levels. Increasing vitamins E, B_6, B_{12}, and thiamin may be beneficial.
- *Feeding plan:* Small, frequent feedings are better tolerated. Large meals add to the risk of carbon dioxide (CO_2) accumulation and respiratory failure.
- *Enteral nutrition (EN) and parenteral nutrition (PN) support:* Tube feedings or PN may be appropriate. Several EN feeding formulas are available that have a low volume with a high density of kcalories. These are suitable for patients who require fluid restriction.

ESSENTIAL HYPERTENSION AND VASCULAR DISEASE

Hypertension

High blood pressure is one of the most prevalent vascular diseases worldwide. As the population ages, the prevalence of hypertension will increase. It is a major factor in the development of stroke, heart attack, heart failure, and kidney disease.[8] At least 95% of these individuals have essential hypertension, meaning its cause is unknown, although a strong familial predisposition exists, with its onset in young teenage years. It has often been called the *silent disease* because it carries no overt signs, but it can have serious implications if not treated and controlled.[9] The large United States study—Dietary Approaches to Stop Hypertension (DASH)—has clearly indicated that a diet rich in fruits, vegetables, and low-fat dairy foods and with reduced saturated and total fat can substantially lower blood pressure.[10] Individual treatment uses current antihypertensive drugs as needed.

Blood Pressure Controls.

Arterial pressure. As commonly measured, blood pressure is an indication of arterial pressure in vessels of the upper arm. This measure is obtained by an instrument for determining force of the pulse (Fig. 21.6). This instrument is called a *sphygmomanometer,* from the

Essential Hypertension
An inherent form of hypertension with no specific discoverable cause and considered to be familial; also called *primary hypertension.*

FIG. 21.6 Monitoring blood pressure. (From Potter PA, Perry AG: *Basic nursing: essentials for practice,* ed 5, St Louis, 2003, Mosby.)

Greek words *sphygmos* (meaning pulse), *manos* (meaning thin), and *metron* (meaning measure). Pulse pressure is measured in millimeters of mercury (mm Hg) rise or in equivalent values read on gauges or digital indicators. The higher, or upper, value recorded is systolic pressure from contraction of the heart muscle. The lower value recorded is diastolic pressure, produced during the relaxation phase of the cardiac cycle.

Several factors contribute to maintaining fluid dynamics of normal blood pressure: (1) increased pressure on forward blood flow; (2) increased resistance from blood vessels through which the blood is flowing; and (3) increased viscosity of blood itself, making movement through vessels more difficult. Of these factors, increased viscosity is a rare event. Thus, in discussing high blood pressure in general terms, we are dealing with the first two factors: (1) the pumping pressure of the heart muscle propelling blood forward and (2) resistance to this forward flow presented by blood vessel walls normally or by any abnormal added constriction or thickening.

Muscle tone of blood vessel walls. In hypertension, the body's finely tuned mechanisms designed to maintain fluid dynamics are not operating effectively. Normally these systems include several agents that act to variously dilate and constrict blood vessels to meet whatever need is present at a given time. However, in a person with hypertension, dilation or constriction of blood vessels does not occur in the normal manner. If not effectively treated, then uncontrolled elevated blood pressure results. Body systems that operate to help maintain normal blood pressure include: (1) neuroendocrine functions of the sympathetic nervous system, mainly mediated by chemical neurotransmitters such as norepinephrine; (2) hormonal systems such as the renin-angiotensin-aldosterone mechanism and its vasopressor effect; and (3) enzyme systems such as the kallikrein-kinin mechanism (sometimes operating with prostaglandins), which controls substances that act to dilate or constrict smooth muscle as needed.

Classifications of Blood Pressure. Hypertension is defined as systolic blood pressure of 140 mm Hg or higher, diastolic blood pressure of 90 mm Hg or higher or taking antihypertensive medication. The objective of identifying and treating hypertension is to reduce morbidity and

mortality. For that reason, classification of adult (older than 18 years of age) blood pressure (Table 21.4) provides a mechanism for identifying high-risk individuals and provides guidelines for follow-up and treatment.[7]

Prevention and Treatment. The goal of prevention and management of hypertension is to reduce morbidity and mortality by the least intrusive means possible.[7] Lifestyle modifications (Table 21.5) offer the potential for preventing hypertension. They have been shown capable of lowering blood pressure and can reduce cardiovascular risk factors at minimal cost and risk.[7]

Nutritional Management of Hypertension. Taste for a given amount of salt with food is an acquired one, not a physiologic necessity. Sufficient sodium for the body's need is provided as a natural mineral in foods consumed. Some persons salt their foods heavily and thus form high salt taste levels. Others form lighter tastes by using smaller amounts. Common daily adult intakes of sodium range widely from approximately 2–4 g with lighter tastes to as high as 10–12 g with heavier use. Salt (sodium chloride [NaCl]) intakes are approximately twice these amounts, because sodium makes up approximately 40% of the NaCl molecule. The large amount of salt in the American diet, estimated to be approximately 6–15 g of sodium per day (260–656 mEq), is largely a result of the increased use of many processed food products. The main source of dietary sodium is food processing (approximately 75%). Approximately 10–11% occurs naturally in foods, approximately 15% is discretionary (half of which is contributed by table salt and half by cooking), and less than 1% comes from water.

Other nutrients that affect blood pressure are potassium and calcium. High potassium intake from food sources (see the Perspectives in Practice box, "Dietary Approaches to Stop Hypertension [DASH] Diet Pattern") such as fresh fruits and vegetables may protect against the development of hypertension and improve blood pressure control in those who do have hypertension.[7] Calcium in the form of low-fat dairy products (which are also low in saturated and total fat) is also recommended to reduce blood pressure. Moderate consumption of alcohol (equivalent to two drinks per day for men and one drink per day for women) is also known to reduce blood pressure.[7]

TABLE 21.4   Classification of Blood Pressure for Adults

Blood Pressure Classification	Systolic (in mm Hg)[a]	Diastolic (in mm Hg)	Lifestyle Modification	INITIAL DRUG THERAPY Without Compelling Indication	INITIAL DRUG THERAPY With Compelling Indication[b]
Normal[c]	<120	and <80	Encourage	No antihypertensive drug indicated	None
Prehypertension	120–139	or 80–89	Yes	No antihypertensive drug indicated	Drug(s) for compelling indications[d]
Stage 1 hypertension[e]	140–159	or 90–99	Yes	Thiazide-type diuretics for most; consider ACEI, ARB, BB, CCB, or combinations	Drug(s) for the compelling indications[d] Other antihypertensive drugs (diuretics, ACEI, ARB, BB, CCB) as needed
Stage 2 hypertension[e]	>160	or >100	Yes	Two-drug combination for most[d]	

[a]Treatment determined by highest blood pressure category.
[b]Heart failure, post-MI, high coronary disease risk, chronic kidney disease, recurrent stroke prevention.
[c]Optimal blood pressure with respect to cardiovascular risk is less than 120/80 mm Hg. However, unusually low readings should be evaluated for clinical significance.
[d]Initial combined therapy should be used cautiously in those at risk for orthostatic hypotension.
[e]Based on the average of two or more readings taken at each of two or more visits after initial screening.
ACEI, Angiotensin-converting enzyme inhibitor; *ARB,* aldosterone receptor blocker; *BB,* β-blocker; *CCB,* calcium channel blocker.
Data from National High Blood Pressure Program: *The seventh report of the Joint National Committee on Prevention, Detection, Evaluation, and Treatment of High Blood Pressure (JNC 7), National Institutes of Health, National Heart, Lung, and Blood Institutes,* NIH Pub No 04-5230, Washington, DC, 2004, US Government Printing Office. http://www.nhlbi.nih.gov/guidelines/hypertension/jnc7full.htm.

TABLE 21.5   Lifestyle Modifications to Manage Hypertension[a]

SYSTOLIC BLOOD PRESSURE

Modification (Range)	Recommendations	Approximate SBP Reduction (Range)
Weight reduction	Maintain normal body weight (BMI, 18.5–24.9 kg/m^2).	5–20 mm Hg per 10-kg weight loss
Adapt DASH eating plan	Consume a diet rich in fruits and vegetables and low in fat.	8–14 mm Hg
Dietary sodium reduction	Reduce dietary sodium intake to no more than 2.4 g sodium or 6 g sodium chloride (NaCl).	2–8 mm Hg
Physical activity	Engage in regular aerobic physical activity such as brisk walking (at least 30 min/day, most days of the week).	4–9 mm Hg
Moderation of alcohol consumption	Limit consumption to no more than two drinks (1 oz or 30 mL ethanol [e.g., 24 oz beer, 10 oz wine, or 3 oz 80-proof whiskey]) per day in most men and to no more than one drink per day in women and lighter-weight persons.	2–4 mm Hg

[a]For overall cardiovascular risk reduction, stop smoking. The effects of implementing these modifications are dose and time dependent and could be increased for some individuals.

BMI, Body mass index; *DASH*, Dietary Approaches to Stop Hypertension; *SBP*, systolic blood pressure.

Data from National High Blood Pressure Program: *The seventh report of the Joint National Committee on Prevention, Detection, Evaluation, and Treatment of High Blood Pressure, National Institutes of Health, National Heart, Lung, and Blood Institutes,* NIH Pub No 04-5230, Washington, DC, 2004, US Government Printing Office.

PERSPECTIVES IN PRACTICE

Dietary Approaches to Stop Hypertension Diet Pattern

The following list indicates the number of recommended daily servings from each food group, with examples of food choices (based on the 2000-kcal reference diet). The number of servings may increase or decrease, depending on individual calorie needs, and can be found on the Dietary Approaches to Stop Hypertension (DASH) website: https://www.nhlbi.nih.gov/health/public/heart/hbp/dash/.

Food Group	Daily Serving (Except Where Noted)	Serving Sizes	Examples and Notes	Significance to the DASH Diet Pattern
Grains and grain products	7–8	1 slice of bread 1 oz of dry cereal[a] ½ cup of cooked rice, pasta, or cereal	Whole wheat bread, English muffin, pita bread, bagel; cereals; grits; oatmeal	Major source of energy and fiber
Vegetables	4–5	1 cup of raw, leafy vegetables ½ cup of cooked vegetables 6 oz of vegetable juice	Tomatoes, potatoes, carrots, peas, squash, broccoli, turnip greens, collard greens, kale, spinach, artichokes, beans, sweet potatoes	Rich sources of potassium, magnesium, and fiber
Fruits	4–5	6 oz of fruit juice 1 medium fruit ¼ cup of dried fruit ½ cup of fresh, frozen, or canned fruit	Apricots, bananas, dates, grapes, oranges, orange juice, tangerines, strawberries, mangoes, melons, peaches, pineapple, prunes, raisins	Important sources of potassium, magnesium, and fiber
Low-fat or nonfat dairy foods	2–3	8 oz of milk 1 cup of yogurt 1½ oz of cheese	Fat-free or 1% milk, fat-free or low-fat buttermilk; nonfat or low-fat yogurt; part-nonfat mozzarella cheese, nonfat cheese	Major sources of calcium and protein
Meat, poultry, and fish	<2	3 oz of cooked meats, poultry, or fish	Select only lean meats; trim away visible fats; broil, roast, or boil, instead of frying; remove skin from chicken	Rich sources of protein and magnesium
Nuts, seeds, and legumes	4–5/week	1½ oz or ½ cup of nuts ½ oz or 2 tbsp of seeds ½ cup of cooked legumes	Almonds, filberts, mixed nuts, peanuts, walnuts, sunflower seeds, kidney beans, lentils	Rich sources of energy, magnesium, potassium, protein, and fiber

Continued

Dietary Approaches to Stop Hypertension Diet Pattern—cont'd

Food Group	Daily Serving (Except Where Noted)	Serving Sizes	Examples and Notes	Significance to the DASH Diet Pattern
Fats and oils[b]	2–3	1 tsp of soft margarine 1 tbsp of low-fat mayonnaise or salad dressing 2 tbsp of light salad dressing 1 tsp of vegetable oil	Soft margarine, low-fat mayonnaise, light salad dressing, vegetable oil (e.g., olive, corn, canola, safflower)	DASH has 27% of calories as fat, including that in or added to foods
Sweets	5/week	1 tbsp of sugar 1 tbsp of jelly or jam ½ oz of jelly beans 8 oz of lemonade	Maple syrup, sugar, jelly, jam; fruit-flavored gelatin, jelly beans, fruit punch, sorbet, ices, hard candy	Sweets should be low in fat

[a]Equals ½–¼ cup, depending on cereal type. Check the product's nutrition label.
[b]Fat content changes serving counts for fats and oils. For example, 1 tbsp of regular salad dressing equals 1 serving; 1 tbsp of low-fat dressing equals ½ serving; 1 tbsp of fat-free dressing equals 0 servings.

Strategies for Adopting DASH

Dietary changes are best achieved through small changes in food selections. Use this list of tips as a way to initiate discussion and dietary compliance to reduce hypertension among your clients.

Tips on Eating the DASH Way

- Change gradually.
- If you now eat one or two vegetables a day, then add a serving at lunch and another at dinner.
- If you do not eat fruit now or have only juice at breakfast, then add a serving to your meals or have it as a snack.
- Gradually increase your use of fat-free and low-fat dairy products to three servings a day. For example, drink milk with lunch or dinner instead of soda, sugar-sweetened tea, or alcohol. Choose low-fat (1%) or fat-free (skim) dairy products to reduce your intake of saturated fat, total fat, cholesterol, and kcalories.
- Read food labels on margarines and salad dressings, and choose those lowest in unsaturated fat. Some margarines are now trans-fat free.
- Treat meat as one part of the whole meal instead of the focus.
- Limit meat to 6 oz a day (two servings), which is all that is needed (3–4 oz is approximately the size of a deck of cards).
- If you now eat large portions of meat, cut them back gradually, by one-half or one-third at each meal.
- Include two or more vegetarian-style (meatless) meals each week.

- Increase servings of vegetables, rice, pasta, and dry beans at meals. Try casseroles, pasta, and stir-fry dishes that have less meat and more vegetables, grains, and dry beans.
- Use fruit or other foods low in saturated fat, cholesterol, and kcalories as desserts and snacks.
- Fruits and other low-fat foods offer great taste and variety. Use fruits canned in their own juices. Fresh fruits require little or no preparation. Dried fruits are a good choice to carry with you or to have ready in the car.
- Try these snacks ideas: unsalted pretzels or nuts mixed with raisins, graham crackers, low-fat and fat-free yogurt and frozen yogurt, popcorn with no salt or butter added, and raw vegetables.
Try these additional tips:
- Choose whole grain foods to get added nutrients such as minerals and fiber. For example, choose whole wheat bread and whole grain cereals.
- If you have trouble digesting dairy products, then try taking lactase enzyme pills or drops (available at drugs and grocery stores) with the dairy foods or buy lactose-free milk or milk with lactase enzyme added to it.
- Use fresh, frozen, or no-salt-added canned vegetables.

Bibliography

US Department of Health and Human Services, Public Health Service, National Institutes of Health, National Heart, Lung, and Blood Institute: *Your guide to lowering your blood pressure with DASH*, NIH Pub No 06-4082. Bethesda, MD, 2006, US Government Printing Office. https://www.nhlbi.nih.gov.

Cerebrovascular Accident

Arteriosclerotic vascular injury and hypertension may also affect blood vessels in the brain. A cerebrovascular accident (CVA), or stroke, occurs when a blood vessel carrying oxygen and nutrients to the brain ruptures (hemorrhagic stroke) or is clogged by a blood clot (ischemic stroke), interrupting blood flow to an area of the brain. When any part of the brain does not receive blood and oxygen, nerve cells in the affected area die, resulting in loss of control of the abilities that area of the brain once controlled. During the past 20 years, with the declining US early death rate from heart disease, stroke stands in third place as a leading cause of death of adults ages 25–65 years.[11] Nearly 170,000 Americans die annually of stroke, meaning someone in the United States experiences a stroke every 45 seconds.[2] Among all US population groups, the incident rate for

first stroke among African Americans is almost double that of European Americans.[12]

Four main types of stroke exist: two are caused by blood clots, and two are caused by ruptured blood vessels. Cerebral thrombosis and cerebral embolism account for approximately 70–80% of all strokes. Cerebral thrombosis, the most common stroke, occurs when a thrombus forms and blocks blood flow in an artery bringing blood to part of the brain. They usually occur at night or first thing in the morning when blood pressure is low. They are often preceded by a transient ischemic attack (TIA), or "ministroke." Cerebral embolism occurs when an embolus forms away from the brain, usually in the heart. The clot is carried in the bloodstream until it lodges in an artery leading to or in the brain and blocks the flow of blood.[2] A subarachnoid hemorrhage occurs when a blood vessel on the brain's surface ruptures and bleeds into the space between the brain and skull. A cerebral hemorrhage occurs when a defective artery in the brain bursts, flooding the surrounding tissue with blood.[2]

Nutrition Therapy. Paralysis and other problems may occur, depending on the site and extent of brain damage resulting from a stroke. Patients who experience left-sided CVA most commonly experience sight and hearing losses, including the ability to see where food is on plates or trays. Right-hemisphere, bilateral, or brainstem CVA causes significant problems with feeding and swallowing, in addition to speech problems.[7]

Dysphagia often occurs, and foods that cause choking or that are hard to manage should be avoided (dry or crisp foods, peanut butter, thinly pureed foods, raw vegetables, to mention a few). If the patient has problems with saliva production, then foods can be moistened with small amounts of liquid (au jus or gravy). Because thin liquids are often difficult to swallow, thickeners are used to make semisolid foods from soups, beverages, and juices.[7]

Peripheral Vascular Disease

Peripheral vascular disease (PVD) is characterized by narrowing of blood vessels in the legs and sometimes the arms. Blood flow is restricted and causes pain in affected area. Contributory risk factors include hypertension and diabetes mellitus. However, the greatest risk factor is cigarette smoking, which constricts blood vessels. More than 90% of patients with PVD are or were moderate to heavy smokers.

Symptoms and Complications. As arteries gradually narrow because of atherosclerosis (the most common cause), an aching, tired feeling occurs in leg muscles when walking. Resting the leg for a few minutes relieves pain, but it recurs shortly when walking is resumed. For this reason the symptom is called *intermittent claudication.* Sometimes a sudden arterial blockage occurs when a blood clot develops on the top of a plaque or a clot formed in the heart is carried to a peripheral artery and blocks it. The blockage causes sudden severe pain in the affected area, which becomes cold and either pale or blue and has no pulse. Movement and sensation are lost.

Treatment. By far the most important treatment for the patient is to stop smoking. As with coronary vessels, surgery on diseased vessels is sometimes required: (1) arterial reconstructive surgery to bypass them, (2) endarterectomy to remove obstructing fatty deposits on inner linings, or (3) balloon angioplasty to widen vessels. Drug therapy may include antiplatelet or anticoagulant agents to prevent blood clotting. NT consists of regular fat and cholesterol modifications described for CHD. Exercise is also important. The person should walk every day with medical clearance, gradually increasing

to approximately 1 hour, stopping whenever intermittent pain occurs and resuming when it stops. Regular inspection of feet, daily washing and stocking change, good-fitting shoes to avoid pressure, and scrupulous foot care (ideally by a podiatrist) are essential to prevent infection.

PULMONARY DISEASES

Chronic Obstructive Pulmonary Disease

Clinical Characteristics. Progressive CHF contributes to lung disease and risk of respiratory failure. Malnutrition is common with the debilitating condition of chronic obstructive pulmonary disease (COPD). This term describes a group of disorders in which airflow in the lungs is limited and respiratory failure develops. Chronic bronchitis and emphysema are two main interrelated COPD conditions. Malnutrition usually accompanies COPD, and its presence increases illness and death rates associated with the disease process. Anorexia and significant weight loss reflect a growing inability to maintain adequate nutritional status, which in turn severely compromises pulmonary function. Progression of the disease process, with its increasing shortness of breath, prevents the person from living a normal life, and prognosis is poor. Eventually, in progressive respiratory failure, the patient becomes dependent on a mechanical respirator and controlled oxygen supply. A poor prognosis is associated with a compromised nutritional status in these patients.

Nutritional Management. Respiratory failure is actually a failure of pulmonary exchange of oxygen and CO_2. Thus its common manifestations are hypoxemia, deficient oxygenation of blood, and hypercapnia, excess CO_2 in the blood. Patients with COPD have increased energy requirements, which will vary for each individual. Requirements for carbohydrate, protein, and fat will be determined by the underlying lung disease, oxygen therapy, medications, weight status, and any acute fluid fluctuations.[4] A balanced proportion of protein (15–20% total kcalories) with fat (30–45% total kcalories) and carbohydrate (40–55% total kcalories) is necessary to maintain appropriate respiratory quotient (RQ) from substrate use.[4] Although it is important not to overfeed patients with COPD (especially too much carbohydrate), these patients often have difficulty taking in sufficient amounts of food because of fatigue (food preparation, shortness of breath, the act of eating) and lose weight. Commonly, other coexisting diseases (CVD, diabetes mellitus, renal disease, or cancer) may be present, thereby influencing total amount and kind of carbohydrate, protein, and fat prescribed.[4]

Pneumonia

The term *pneumonia* comes from the Greek word *pneuma,* meaning breath. It is an acute inflammation of the lung caused by an infectious agent and can stem from three sources: (1) aspiration of normal bacterial flora, gastric contents, or both in oropharyngeal secretions; (2) inhalation of contaminants (e.g., virus); or (3) contamination from systemic circulation. A common disorder, community-acquired pneumonia is the most lethal infectious disease in the United States and the sixth leading cause of death.[13]

Symptoms. In general, the immune response—cough with or without sputum production, sneezing, and mucociliary clearance (pulmonary defense mechanisms)—guards against pneumonia.[13] Community-acquired pneumonia is usually bacterial in origin and produces exudate that is hard to expectorate. Viral pneumonia does not produce exudate.[13] Hospital-acquired, or nosocomial, pneumonia develops in up to 5% of hospitalized patients.[13] Nosocomial pneumonia and community-based pneumonia are caused by different pathogens. Aspiration of infected pharyngeal or gastric secretions delivers bacteria straight to the lungs. This is promoted by exogenous factors such as contamination by dirty hands and equipment, treatment with broad-spectrum antibiotics that promote emergence of drug-resistant organisms, and patient factors such as malnutrition, smoking, preexisting lung disease, advanced age, swallowing disorders, and chest or upper abdominal surgery. Signs and symptoms are nonspecific; however, fever, purulent sputum, and leukocytosis are present in most patients.[13]

Treatment. Sputum and blood specimens are cultured before antibiotic treatment. The usual treatment is with a broad-spectrum penicillin antibiotic. Erythromycin may be added if the presence of an atypical organism is suspected. Oxygen therapy is often used, and in severe cases the patient may be ventilated. Nosocomial pneumonia is treated more aggressively with broad-spectrum antibiotics and tailored to a specific clinical setting because of the high mortality rate.[13]

Nutritional Management. Sufficient fluids (3–3.5 L) should be given daily if not contraindicated. Frequent small meals may be better tolerated. A multivitamin and mineral supplement may be beneficial, and fiber should be encouraged to avoid constipation. Adequate fruit and fruit juice intake will supply necessary potassium.[7]

Tuberculosis

Tuberculosis (TB), caused by *Mycobacterium tuberculosis,* is one of the world's more widespread and deadly diseases. It occurs disproportionately among disadvantaged populations such as the malnourished, the homeless, and those living in overcrowded and substandard housing. *M. tuberculosis* is an airborne disease, and strains resistant to one or more first-line antituberculosis drugs are increasing.[13]

Symptoms. Typical symptoms of TB are malaise, anorexia, weight loss, fever, and night sweats. Chronic cough is the most universal pulmonary symptom. It may be dry at first but becomes productive of purulent sputum as the disease progresses. More often than not, the sputum is blood streaked. Patients appear chronically ill and malnourished.[3,11]

Treatment. The basic goals of TB treatment are as follows[13]:
- Administer multiple drugs to which organisms are susceptible.
- Add at least two new antitubercular agents to a regimen when treatment failure is suspected.
- Provide the safest, most effective therapy in the shortest period of time.
- Ensure adherence to therapy.

Nonadherence (because of adverse drug reaction) to treatment is a major cause of treatment failure, continued transmission of TB, and development of drug resistance. Hospitalization for initial therapy of TB is not necessary for most patients,[13] but hospitalization has

increased because of increasing resistance of the organism to treatment and an increasing number of cases.[4]

Nutritional Management. The objective of nutritional management is to maintain weight or prevent weight loss. If febrile, then patients will be hypermetabolic. A well-balanced diet with liberal amounts of protein and adequate kcalories is usually necessary. Ensure the patient is consuming adequate amounts of calcium, iron, vitamin C, and B-complex vitamins.[4]

HEALTH PROMOTION

ADDED FOOD FACTORS IN CORONARY HEART DISEASE THERAPY

The primary focus of NT for CHD is on control of lipid factors, including cholesterol and saturated fats. However, two other food factors play a different role. In varying ways they help protect us from the development of CHD.[3]

Dietary Fiber

Studies indicate water-soluble types of dietary fiber have significant cholesterol-lowering effect. Soluble fiber includes gums, pectin, certain hemicelluloses, and the body's storage polysaccharide, glycogen. Foods rich in soluble fiber include oat bran and dried beans, with additional amounts in barley and fruits. Oat bran, for example, contains a primary water-soluble gum, β-glucan, which is a lipid-lowering agent. Soluble dietary fiber has the following properties:
- Delays gastric emptying
- Slows intestinal transit time
- Slows glucose absorption
- Is fermented in the colon into short-chain fatty acids that may inhibit liver cholesterol synthesis and help clear LDL-cholesterol

On the other hand, insoluble dietary fiber—cellulose, lignin, and many hemicelluloses—found in vegetables, wheat, and most other grains does not have these lipid-lowering effects. Thus an increased use of soluble fiber food sources, especially oat bran and legumes, would have beneficial effects.

Omega-3 Fatty Acids

Studies indicate omega-3 fatty acids, eicosapentaenoic acid (EPA) and docosahexaenoic acid (DHA) (see Chapter 4), found mostly in seafood and marine oils, also have protective functions. They can do the following:
- Change pattern of plasma fatty acids to alter platelet activity and reduce platelet aggregation that causes blood clotting, thus lowering the risk of coronary thrombosis
- Decrease the synthesis of VLDL
- Increase antiinflammatory effects

It would seem, then, that factors in foods such as oats, dried beans, and fatty fish would provide valuable lipid-lowering additions to our diets.

TO SUM UP

CHD remains the leading cause of death in the United States. Atherosclerosis, its underlying pathologic process, involves the formation of plaque, a fatty substance that builds up along the interior surfaces of blood vessels, interfering with blood flow and damaging blood vessels. If this buildup becomes severe, then it cuts off blood supplies of oxygen and nutrients to tissue cells, which in turn begin to die. When this occurs in a coronary artery, the result is an MI, or heart attack. When it occurs in a brain vessel, the result is a CVA, or stroke.

Risk for atherosclerosis increases with the amount and type of blood lipids (lipoproteins) available. The apolipoprotein portion of lipoproteins is an important genetically determined part of the disease process. Elevated serum LDL-cholesterol level is a primary factor in atherosclerosis development.

Initial dietary recommendations for acute CVD (heart attack) include caloric restriction, soft-textured foods, and small, frequent meals to reduce the metabolic demands of digestion, absorption, and metabolism of foods and their nutrients. Maintenance of a lean body weight is important. Persons with chronic CHD (e.g., CHF) and those with essential hypertension benefit from weight management, exercise, and sodium restriction to overcome cardiac edema and to help control elevated blood pressure.

Current dietary recommendations to help prevent CHD involve maintaining a healthy weight; limiting fats to 25–30% of all kcalories, with the majority being unsaturated food forms; limiting sodium intake to 2–3 g/day; and increasing exercise.

Concerted efforts are needed to combat development of cardiac cachexia in progressive heart failure. In addition, atherosclerotic plaques may occur in the extremities, usually the legs, causing PVD and the pain of intermittent claudication when walking. Progressive respiratory failure interferes with normal exchange of blood gases, oxygen and CO_2, and results in COPD, for which changed ratios of the fuel macronutrients are sometimes indicated.

KEY TERM

Hyperlipoproteinemia
Elevated level of lipoproteins in the blood.

QUESTIONS FOR REVIEW

1. Which types of hyperlipoproteinemia occur most often? Identify lipids that are elevated in each case, as well as predisposing factors. Describe the types of diet recommended for each.
2. Identify four dietary recommendations that should be made for the person with a heart attack. Describe how each recommendation helps recovery.
3. What dietary changes can the average American make to reduce saturated fats and to substitute polyunsaturated fats?
4. What does the term *essential hypertension* mean? Why would weight management and sodium restriction contribute to its control?
5. Outline NT for cardiac cachexia and discuss the rationale for each aspect of the feeding plan.
6. Discuss the cause and treatment of PVD.
7. Outline NT for COPD, and discuss the rationale for the fuel macronutrient adjustments.

REFERENCES

1. Brashers VL: Alterations of cardiovascular function. In McCance KL, Huether SE, editors: *Pathophysiology: the biologic basis for disease in adults and children*, ed 3, St Louis, 2006, Mosby.
2. American Heart Association: *Heart disease and stroke statistics*, Dallas, TX, 2009, American Heart Association. Retrieved from www.americanheart.org.
3. National Cholesterol Education Program (NCEP): *Third report of the NCEP Expert Panel on Detection, Evaluation, and Treatment of High Blood Cholesterol in Adults (Adult Treatment Panel III), full report*, Washington, DC, 2002, National Institutes of Health, National Heart, Lung, and Blood Institute. Retrieved from www.nhlbi.nih.gov/guidelines/cholesterol/atp3_rpt.htm.
4. Mahan LK, Escott-Stump S, editors: *Krause's food & nutrition therapy*, ed 12, St Louis, 2008, Saunders.
5. Mozaffarian D, Katan MB, Ascherio A, et al: Trans fatty acids and cardiovascular disease, *N Engl J Med* 354(15):1601, 2006.
6. Banasik JL: Alterations in cardiac function. In Copstead LC, Banasik JL, editors: *Pathophysiology*, ed 3, St Louis, 2005, Saunders.
7. Banasik JL: Heart failure and dysrhythmias: common sequelae of cardiac diseases. In Copstead LC, Banasik JL, editors: *Pathophysiology*, ed 3, St Louis, 2005, Saunders.
8. Antman EM, Anbe DT, Armstrong PW, et al: ACC/AHA guidelines for the management of patients with ST-elevation myocardial infarction—executive summary: a report of the ACC/AHA Task Force on Practice Guidelines (Committee to Revise the 1999 Guidelines on the Management of Patients With Acute Myocardial Infarction), *Circulation* 110:588, 2004.
9. National High Blood Pressure Program: *The seventh report of the Joint National Committee on Prevention, Detection, Evaluation, and Treatment of High Blood Pressure, National Institutes of Health, National Heart, Lung, and Blood Institutes*, Washington, DC, 2004, US Government Printing Office. NIH Pub No 04-5230.
10. Sacks FM, Svetkey LP, Vollmer WM, et al: Effects on blood pressure of reduced dietary sodium and the Dietary Approaches to Stop Hypertension (DASH), *N Engl J Med* 344:3, 2001.
11. National Center for Health Statistics, Centers for Disease Control and Prevention: *Stroke/cerebrovascular disease*, Hyattsville, MD, 2009, Centers for Disease Control and Prevention. Retrieved from www.cdc.gov/nchs/fastats/stroke.htm.
12. American Heart Association: *Stroke statistics*, Dallas, TX, 2005, American Heart Association. Retrieved from www.americanheart.org.
13. Schumann L: Restrictive pulmonary disorders. In Copstead LC, Banasik JL, editors: *Pathophysiology*, ed 3, St Louis, 2005, Saunders.

FURTHER READINGS AND RESOURCES

Websites of Interest

- American Heart Association. Information for health professionals and consumers regarding cardiovascular diseases and stroke. https://www.americanheart.org
- Centers for Disease Control and Prevention: Health Topic: Heart Disease. This website provides credible and reliable health information for consumers, health professionals, policy makers, and the media. http://www.cdc.gov/heartdisease/index.htm.
- MedlinePlus, Heart Diseases. This is the National Institutes of Health website for consumers. It is produced by the National Library of Medicine to provide reliable, up-to-date health information about diseases, conditions, and wellness issues. https://www.nlm.nih.gov/medlineplus/heartdiseases.html.
- Womenshealth.gov: Heart Health and Stroke. http://www.womenshealth.gov/heart-disease-and-stroke. The Office of Women's Health is housed in the US Department of Health and Human Services to promote health equity for women and girls through sex/gender-specific approaches. http://www.womenshealth.gov/heart-stroke/heart-disease-stroke-prevention/index.cfm.
- World Health Organization (WHO): Cardiovascular Diseases. Part of the United Nations, WHO is responsible for providing leadership on global health matters. https://www.who.int/cardiovascular_diseases/en/.

22

Diabetes Mellitus

Joyce Gilbert

ⓔ http://evolve.elsevier.com/Williams/essentials/

In this chapter of our continuing clinical nutrition series, we look at the problem of diabetes. We seek to understand its nature and how it can be managed to maintain good health and avoid complications. Diabetes is a serious, costly, and increasingly common chronic disease. In the United States, 25.86 million people (8.3% of the population) have diabetes. An estimated 18.8 million Americans have diagnosed diabetes, and an additional 7 million have undiagnosed diabetes. Approximately 1.9 million new cases of diabetes are diagnosed each year.[1] Diabetes can be diagnosed on the basis of two fasting glucose readings of 126 mg/dL or higher or a random glucose level of 200 mg/dL or higher and symptoms such as polyuria, polydipsia, and unexplained weight loss.[2] Although elevation of blood glucose level is the hallmark characteristic of diabetes, it is a group of metabolic disorders resulting from a defect in insulin secretion, insulin action, or both. These defects interfere with normal cellular uptake of glucose and use of glucose within cells. Restoring normal metabolic function is the goal in the early diagnosis and treatment of diabetes. Restoration of normal metabolism can prevent many of the short-term complications such as hyperglycemia and hypoglycemia and the longer-term microvascular, macrovascular, and neurologic complications that affect multiple body systems. Direct and indirect health costs of diabetes were estimated to be $245 billion in 2012 in the United States (or more than 1 out of every 5 health care dollars).[3] The death rate among middle-aged people with diabetes is double the death rate of those who do not have diabetes. Diabetes causes preventable complications that can be life threatening, including heart disease. Lifestyle changes can delay the progression of diabetes, as can controlling blood glucose, lipids, and blood pressure.

OUTLINE

Nature of Diabetes
General Management of Diabetes
Rationale for Diabetes Nutrition Therapy
Implementing Nutrition Therapy

Issues Related to Medical Therapy
Management of Diabetes Nutrition Therapy
Diabetes Education Program
Health Promotion

NATURE OF DIABETES

History

The metabolic disease we know currently as *diabetes mellitus* has been with us for a long time. Ancient records describe its devastating effects as observed by early healers. In the first century AD, the Greek physician Aretaeus wrote of a malady in which the body "ate its own flesh" and gave off large quantities of urine. He gave it the name *diabetes*, from the Greek word meaning *siphon* or *to pass through*. Much later, in the 17th century, the word *mellitus*, from the Latin word for *honey*, was added because of the sweet nature of the urine. This addition also distinguished it from diabetes insipidus (*insipid*, meaning tasteless, or not sweet), another disorder, although uncommon, in which the passage of copious amounts of urine had been observed. Currently, use of the single name diabetes always means diabetes mellitus.

As medical knowledge began to grow, early clinicians—such as Rollo in England and Bouchardat in France—observed that diabetes became

less severe in overweight patients who lost weight. Later, another French physician, Lancereaux, and his students described two kinds of diabetes: (1) *diabète gras* ("fat diabetes") and (2) *diabète maigre* ("thin diabetes").[4] All of these observations preceded any knowledge about insulin or any relation to the pancreas. During these times, which have aptly been called the *diabetic dark ages*, individuals with diabetes had short lives and were maintained on a variety of semistarvation diets.[5]

Later, evidence began to point to the pancreas as a primary organ involved in the disease process. Paul Langerhans (1847–88), a young German medical student, found special clusters—or islets—of cells scattered throughout the human pancreas that were different from the rest of the tissue. Although their function was still unknown, these special islet cells were named for their young discoverer: the islets of Langerhans. Research at that time focused on the pancreas. Finally, in 1921 and 1922 a University of Toronto team discovered and successfully used the controlling agent from the "island cells," naming it *insulin* for its source.[6]

KEY TERMS

Diabetes Insipidus

A condition of the pituitary gland and insufficiency of one of its hormones, vasopressin (antidiuretic hormone); characterized by a copious output of a nonsweet urine, great thirst, and sometimes a large appetite. However, in diabetes insipidus these symptoms result from a specific injury to the pituitary gland, not a collection of metabolic disorders as in diabetes mellitus. The injured pituitary gland produces less vasopressin, a hormone that normally helps the kidneys reabsorb adequate water.

Insulin

Hormone formed in the beta cells of the islets of Langerhans in the pancreas. It is secreted when blood glucose and amino acid levels rise and assists their entry into body cells. It also promotes glycogenesis and conversion of glucose into fat and inhibits lipolysis and gluconeogenesis (protein breakdown). Commercial insulin is manufactured from pigs and cows; new "artificial" human insulin products have recently been made available.

Classification

The American Diabetes Association classifies diabetes into the four categories[2]:

1. Type 1 diabetes mellitus (T1DM), formerly called insulin-dependent diabetes mellitus
2. Type 2 diabetes mellitus (T2DM), formerly called non–insulin-dependent diabetes mellitus
3. Gestational diabetes mellitus (GDM)
4. Other specific types

The terms *insulin-dependent diabetes mellitus* (IDDM) and *non–insulin-dependent diabetes mellitus* (NIDDM) should no longer be used because they are confusing and have often resulted in classifying patients based on treatment rather than cause of their diabetes.[2]

T1DM is characterized by sudden, severe insulin deficiency requiring insulin therapy to prevent ketoacidosis, coma, and death. T1DM generally appears during childhood or adolescence and accounts for 5%–10% of the cases of diabetes. However, T1DM can occur at any age, and almost half of new cases are diagnosed after 20 years of age. Two forms of T1DM exist: (1) immune-mediated diabetes and (2) idiopathic diabetes. Immune-mediated diabetes results from a cellular-mediated autoimmune destruction of the beta cells of the pancreas.[7] Idiopathic diabetes has no known cause.

The onset of T1DM is often rapid, accompanied by classic symptoms of weight loss and increased urination and thirst, especially if a viral infection or other stress increases the need for insulin. Onset may be less acute, or a "honeymoon period" of 6–12 months may occur in which the diabetes may appear to be "cured" after an initial acute onset and initiation of insulin therapy. Destruction of the beta cells in the pancreas and loss of insulin production are usually gradual, accounting for the honeymoon period after insulin therapy restores normal glucose and metabolic stress is resolved.

T2DM is associated with insulin resistance and obesity combined with inadequate insulin produced in the pancreatic beta cells to compensate for the insulin resistance or an insulin secretory defect with insulin resistance.[2] T2DM accounts for 90%–95% of all cases of diabetes, and symptoms may include poor wound healing, blurred vision, or recurrent gum or bladder infections. Many individuals are not symptomatic, and the diabetes may be detected as the result of a routine blood test. Obesity and physical inactivity are strong risk factors for T2DM.[8-10] A large waist circumference is considered to be a biomarker for insulin resistance and the metabolic syndrome associated with diabetes, hypertension, and dyslipidemia (typically low high-density cholesterol and elevated triglyceride

levels).[11] Although T2DM is associated with insulin resistance and is typically diagnosed after 40 years of age, it is occurring in epidemic proportions in younger populations, including children and adolescents. Most children diagnosed with T2DM have a family history of T2DM, are overweight or obese, are insulin resistant, or have physical signs of insulin resistance such as acanthosis nigricans.[10] Undiagnosed, these young people may be at early risk for cardiovascular disease (CVD).[10] Current testing criteria and diabetes risk factors to help identify T2DM before the onset of complications has been developed by the American Academy of Pediatrics and the American Dietetic Association (ADA).[11]

GDM is defined as carbohydrate intolerance of variable severity with onset or first recognition during pregnancy. GDM develops in 2%–5% of all pregnancies, and 30%–40% of women with GDM are likely to develop T2DM.[12] In T2DM and GDM a relative insulin deficiency exists because the pancreas fails to produce the level of insulin needed to compensate for insulin resistance.

Other specific types of diabetes include genetic defects of the beta cell, genetic defects in insulin action, disease of the exocrine pancreas, endocrinopathies, and other uncommon forms of immune-mediated diabetes.[2]

The American Diabetes Association identified an intermediate classification of individuals whose glucose levels do not meet the criteria but are still considered high risk for developing diabetes.[2] This category consists of individuals diagnosed with *prediabetes*. If cross-sectional data were applied to the 2007 US population, approximately 57 million adults (20 years or older) in the United States are estimated to have had prediabetes in 2007.[1] People are considered to have prediabetes if they have impaired fasting glucose (IFG) or impaired glucose tolerance (IGT); some people have both conditions.[1] IFG is identified through fasting blood glucose, and IGT is identified by an oral glucose tolerance test (OGTT).[11] Formerly called *borderline diabetes,* IFG, IGT, and prediabetes are associated with metabolic syndrome that includes abdominal obesity, dyslipidemia (high triglycerides, low high-density lipoprotein [HDL]-cholesterol, or both), and hypertension.[1] Research has shown lifestyle interventions can reduce the rate of progression to T2DM.[13,14] Table 22.1 outlines criteria used to diagnose diabetes.

Contributing Causes

Genetics. For some time, early insulin assay tests developed to measure the level of insulin activity in blood found insulin-like activity in diabetes to be 2 or 3 times normal insulin levels. It is now evident that diabetes is a syndrome with multiple forms, resulting from (1) lack of insulin or (2) insulin resistance (or from both).[2]

Diabetes has long been associated with body weight, since the early observations of differences in "fat diabetes" and "thin diabetes."[4] Current research has reinforced the relation of overweight state to development of T2DM. Obesity can increase circulating insulin levels, which will ultimately lead to increased insulin resistance. In addition, individuals with a family history may have mutations on genes that control insulin production or may inherit insulin resistance not directly related to obesity. Thus multiple genetic mutations may interact to increase the risk of T2DM.

Environmental Role: "Thrifty Gene". Environmental factors apparently play a role in unmasking the underlying genetic susceptibility—a "thrifty" diabetic genotype that probably developed during primitive times. This theory indicates diabetes may be associated with past genetic modifications for survival during varying periods of food availability. Gene mutations and the thrifty trait associated with T2DM facilitated more efficient use of limited food during times of difficult survival conditions. As food supplies became more plentiful, negative

TABLE 22.1 Criteria for Diagnosing Diabetes

Diabetes Type	Former Terms	Etiology	Criteria
Type 1 diabetes mellitus (T1DM)[a]: immune-mediated or idiopathic	Insulin-dependent diabetes mellitus (IDDM), type I diabetes, juvenile-onset diabetes, ketosis-prone diabetes, brittle diabetes	Beta cell destruction, usually leading to absolute insulin deficiency	Symptoms[b] of diabetes mellitus and casual plasma glucose $\leq$200 mg/dL (*casual* is defined as any time of day without regard to last meal) *or*
Type 2 diabetes mellitus (T2DM) (adults)	Non-insulin-dependent diabetes mellitus (NIDDM), T2DM, adult-onset diabetes, maturity-onset diabetes, ketosis-resistant diabetes, stable diabetes	Insulin resistance with insulin secretory defect	Fasting plasma glucose (FPG) $\leq$126 mg/dL (*fasting* is defined as no kcalorie intake for at least 8 h) *or* 2-h postprandial plasma glucose (PPG) $\leq$200 mg/dL during oral glucose tolerance test (OGTT) (performed as described by the World Health Organization [WHO] using glucose load containing the equivalent of 75 g anhydrous glucose dissolved in water)
T2DM (children)			Overweight (body mass index [BMI] >85th percentile for age and gender, weight for height >85th percentile, or weight >120% of ideal for height) *Plus* Any two of the following: • Family history of T2DM in first- or second-degree relative • Native American, African American, Latino, Asian American, Pacific Islander • Signs of insulin resistance or conditions associated with insulin resistance (acanthosis nigricans, hypertension, dyslipidemia, or polycystic ovary syndrome [PCOS])
Gestational diabetes (GDM)			One-step approach: diagnostic OGTT Two-step approach: initial screening to measure plasma or serum glucose concentration 1 h after 50 g oral glucose load (glucose challenge test [GCT]) and perform diagnostic OGTT on those women exceeding glucose threshold value on GCT (glucose threshold >140 mg/dL identifies >80% of women with GDM)
Impaired glucose tolerance (IGT)	Borderline diabetes, chemical diabetes		2-h PPG >140 mg/dL and <200 mg/dL

[a]Patients with any form of diabetes may require insulin treatment at some stage of their disease. Such use of insulin does not classify the patient as having T1DM.
[b]Symptoms include polyuria, polydipsia, and unexplained weight loss.
Data from American Diabetes Association: Standards of medical care in diabetes—2008, *Diabetes Care* 31(Suppl 1):S12, 2008, with permission from The American Diabetes Association.

aspects of the thrifty trait began to appear. Such is indeed the case with the experience of Pima Indians in Arizona, as earlier studies and recent archeological excavations have indicated.[15] In earlier times, this group ate a limited diet mainly of carbohydrate foods harvested through heavy physical labor in a primitive agricultural climate. Now, however, with the "progress" of civilization, the Pimas have become obese, and half of the adults have T2DM (the highest reported rate of this type of diabetes in the world). Native Americans develop diabetes at almost 3 times the rate of Caucasians. This same pattern is seen among populations of now-urbanized Pacific Islanders, South Asians, Asian Indians, and Creoles, although less is known about the exact numbers.[8,9]

Other at-risk populations include Hispanic and Latino Americans, who are 1.5 times as likely to develop diabetes as Caucasians, and African Americans, who develop diabetes at 1.6 times the rate of Caucasians.[1] Thus evidence suggests that these groups have a genetic susceptibility to T2DM (diabetic genotype) and that the disease is triggered by environmental factors, including obesity (see the Focus on Culture box, "Type 2 Diabetes: An Equal Opportunity Disease?"). Several specific genes involved in energy metabolism are thought to increase the risk for developing obesity, T2DM, or both. As we commonly observe, lifestyle (dietary and physical activity habits) can interact with genetics in the development of T2DM.

FOCUS ON CULTURE

Type 2 Diabetes: An Equal Opportunity Disease?

Type 2 diabetes mellitus (T2DM) occurs disproportionately in minorities throughout the United States. Rates of T2DM are 2–6 times higher in Native Americans, Alaska Natives, African Americans, and Hispanic Americans than in the non-Hispanic Caucasian population. In addition, people within these ethnicities experience onset at an earlier age, and their complications are harsher. Although the cause for these ethnic disparities has not been identified, it is hypothesized that the differences may lie in the interaction of inherent susceptibility and modifiable risk factors such as physical inactivity and poor diet.

Ethnic Group	Prevalence (Ages 20+)	Additional Information
Non-Hispanic Caucasians	6.6%	
Native Americans	16.5% of the population: 6.0% among Alaska Natives, 29.3% among Native Americans	Diagnosis 2.2 times more likely than Caucasians Pima tribe has highest rate of diabetes in the world: 50% Complications of diabetes are major causes of death and health problems in most Native American populations
African Americans	11.8%	Diagnosis 1.6 times more likely; 25% between ages 65 and 74 have diabetes; 1 in 4 women older than age 55 has diabetes
Latinos/Hispanics	10.4%	Diagnosis 1.5 times more likely Approximately 11.9% of Mexican Americans have diabetes Approximately 12.6% of Puerto Rican Americans have diabetes Approximately 8.2% of Cuban Americans have diabetes

Bibliography

Brown TL: Ethnic populations. In Ross TA, Boucher JL, O'Connell BS, editors: *American Dietetic Association guide to diabetes medical nutrition therapy and education*, Chicago, 2005, American Dietetic Association.

Centers for Disease Control and Prevention: *National diabetes fact sheet: general information and national estimates on diabetes in the United States*, 2007, Atlanta, GA, 2008, US Department of Health and Human Services, Centers for Disease Control and Prevention. https://www.cdc.gov/diabetes/pubs/pdf/ndfs_2007.pdf.

Symptoms

Symptoms of T1DM in its uncontrolled state include the following:

- Increased thirst (polydipsia)
- Increased urination (polyuria)
- Increased hunger (polyphagia)
- Weight loss (more common with T1DM)
- Fruity smell to breath (symptom of ketoacidosis)
- Fatigue or weakness

These symptoms occur because, in an insulin-deficient state, blood glucose levels and renal filtration of glucose are increased beyond the kidney's threshold for reabsorption; as the level of glucose excreted increases, urine volume increases. Without adequate glucose use, fat mobilization increases, and an increased breakdown of fat leads to excess ketone formation.

T2DM may be asymptomatic, or symptoms may be more subtle and may include the following:

- Poor wound healing or recurrent infections
- Blurred vision (result of effects of hyperglycemia on shape of the cornea, which is returned to normal after glucose levels are stabilized)
- Skin irritation or infection
- Recurrent gum or bladder infections

Classic symptoms of diabetes are the result of short-term effects of hyperglycemia. These symptoms are reversible if blood glucose levels are returned to a normal or near-normal level.

Metabolic Pattern of Diabetes

Overall Energy Balance and Energy Nutrients.
Because initial symptoms of glycosuria and hyperglycemia are related to excess glucose, historically diabetes was called a *disease of carbohydrate metabolism*. However, as more becomes known about the intimate interrelationships of carbohydrate, fat, and protein metabolism, we view it in more general terms. It is a metabolic disorder resulting from lack of insulin (absolute, partial, or unavailable) affecting more or less each basic energy nutrient. It is especially related to metabolism of the two fuels in the body's overall energy system: (1) carbohydrate and (2) fat.

Normal Blood Glucose Control. Control of blood glucose level within its normal range of 70–120 mg/dL (3.9–6.7 mmol/L) is vital to normal overall fuel metabolism and other metabolic functions. A knowledge of factors involved in maintaining a normal blood glucose level is essential to understanding the impairment of these factors (see Chapters 3 and 5). An overview of these normal balancing controls is illustrated in Fig. 22.1.

Sources of Blood Glucose. Two sources of blood glucose ensure a constant supply of this primary body fuel: (1) diet, energy nutrients in our food (i.e., dietary carbohydrate, protein, fat); and (2) glycogen, the backup source from constant turnover of "stored" liver glycogen by a process called glycogenolysis.

Uses of Blood Glucose. To prevent continued rise of blood glucose above the normal range, excess glucose is converted to other substances based on need. These include the following: (1) glycogenesis, conversion of glucose to glycogen for storage in liver and muscle; (2) lipogenesis, conversion of glucose to fat and storage in adipose tissue; and (3) glycolysis, cell oxidation of glucose for energy.

Pancreatic Hormonal Controls. The following three types of islet cells scattered in clusters throughout the pancreas (islets of Langerhans) provide hormones closely integrated in the regulation of blood glucose levels.

1. *Alpha cells:* Arranged around the outer rim of the islets are alpha cells, one to two cells thick, making up approximately 30% of the total cells. These cells synthesize glucagon.
2. *Beta cells:* The largest portion of islets is occupied by beta cells filling the central zone or approximately 60% of the gland. These primary cells synthesize insulin.

FIG. 22.1 Sources of blood glucose (food and stored glycogen) and normal routes of control.

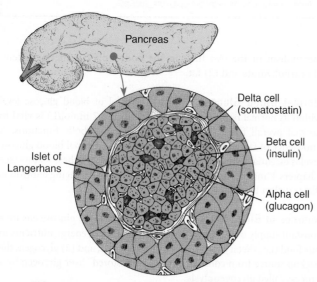

FIG. 22.2 Islets of Langerhans, located in the pancreas.

3. *Delta cells:* Interspersed between alpha and beta cells, or occasionally between alpha cells alone, are delta cells, the remaining 10% of total cells. These cells synthesize somatostatin.

This specific arrangement of human islet cells is illustrated in Fig. 22.2.

Interrelated Hormone Functions. Juncture points of the three types of islet cells act as sensors of blood glucose concentration and its rate of change. They constantly adjust and balance the rate of secretion of insulin, glucagon, and somatostatin to match whatever conditions prevail at any time. Each of the following three hormones has specific interbalanced functions:

1. *Insulin:* Although the precise mechanisms are not entirely clear in every case, insulin has a profound effect on glucose control. It functions extensively in the metabolism of all three energy nutrients, as follows:
   - Insulin facilitates transport of glucose through cell membranes by way of special insulin receptors. These receptors are located on the membrane of insulin-sensitive cells, including those in adipose tissue, muscle tissue, and monocytes. These insulin receptors mediate all metabolic effects of insulin. Research has shown that cells of obese persons with diabetes have fewer than the normal number of insulin receptors. Weight loss in obese individuals and physical exercise increase the number of these receptors. The insulin receptor also appears to control several metabolic steps within the cell.
   - Insulin enhances conversion of glucose to glycogen and its consequent storage in the liver (glycogenesis). Insulin also, then, inhibits the breakdown of glycogen to glucose and its release into the body.
   - Insulin stimulates conversion of glucose to fat (lipogenesis) for storage as adipose tissue.
   - Insulin inhibits fat breakdown (lipolysis) and the breakdown of protein.
   - Insulin promotes uptake of amino acids by skeletal muscles, thus increasing protein synthesis.
   - Insulin influences glucose oxidation through the main glycolytic pathway.

2. *Glucagon:* The hormone glucagon functions as a balancing antagonist to insulin. It rapidly causes breakdown of liver glycogen and, to a lesser extent, fatty acids from adipose tissue to serve as body fuel. This action raises blood glucose levels to protect the brain and other body tissues. It helps maintain normal blood glucose levels during fasting hours of sleep. A lowering of the blood glucose concentration, increased amino acid concentrations, or sympathetic nervous system stimulation triggers glucagon secretion.

3. *Somatostatin:* Although pancreatic islet delta cells are the major source of somatostatin, this hormone is also synthesized and secreted in different regions of the body, including the hypothalamus. It acts

Glycogenolysis
Production of blood glucose from liver glycogen.

Glycogenesis
Synthesis of glycogen from blood glucose.

Lipogenesis
Synthesis of fat from blood glucose.

Glycolysis
Cell oxidation of glucose for energy.

Glucagon
A polypeptide hormone secreted by the alpha cells of the pancreatic islets of Langerhans in response to hypoglycemia; has an opposite balancing effect to that of insulin, raising the blood sugar, and thus is used as a quick-acting antidote for the hypoglycemic reaction of insulin. It stimulates the breakdown of glycogen (glycogenolysis) in the liver by activating the liver enzyme phosphorylase and thus raises blood sugar levels during fasting states to ensure adequate levels for normal nerve and brain function.

Somatostatin
A hormone formed in the delta cells of the pancreatic islets of Langerhans and the hypothalamus. It is a balancing factor in the maintenance of normal blood glucose levels by inhibiting insulin and glucagon production in the pancreas as needed.

in balance with insulin and glucose to inhibit their interactions as needed to maintain normal blood glucose levels. It also helps regulate blood glucose levels by inhibiting the release of a number of other hormones as needed.

Metabolic Changes in Diabetes

In uncontrolled diabetes, insulin is lacking to facilitate operation of normal blood glucose controls; abnormal metabolic changes occur, as follows, that affect glucose, fat, and protein and account for symptoms of diabetes:

- *Glucose:* Blood glucose cannot be oxidized properly through the main glycolytic pathway in the cell to furnish energy (see Chapter 8), and a lack of insulin allows the breakdown of hepatic glycogen and the release of glucose; therefore glucose builds up in the blood (hyperglycemia).
- *Fat:* Formation of fat (lipogenesis) is curtailed, and fat breakdown (lipolysis) increases. This leads to excess formation and accumulation of ketones (ketoacidosis). Appearance of the major ketone, acetone, in urine indicates development of ketoacidosis.
- *Protein:* Tissue protein is also broken down in an effort to secure energy. This causes weight loss and nitrogen excretion in the urine.

GENERAL MANAGEMENT OF DIABETES

Treatment Goals: Basic Objectives

The diabetes care team—the physician, dietitian, nurse, and person with diabetes—are guided by the following three basic objectives:

1. *Maintain optimal nutrition:* The first objective is to fulfill the basic nutritional requirement for health, growth and development, and a desirable body weight.
2. *Prevent hypoglycemia or hyperglycemia:* This second objective is designed to keep the person relatively free of hypoglycemia or insulin

reaction, which requires immediate countermeasures, and hyperglycemia, which, if untreated, contributes to more serious ketoacidosis or diabetic coma.

3. *Prevent complications:* The third objective recognizes the increased risk a person with diabetes faces for developing complications that reflect the damaging effects of chronic diabetes on the tissues of small and large blood vessels and peripheral nerves. These damages may occur in tissues such as eyes (**retinopathy**), nerves (**neuropathy**), and kidneys (**nephropathy**). In addition, coronary artery disease occurs in persons with diabetes approximately 4 times as often as in the general population. Peripheral vascular disease (PVD) occurs approximately 40 times as often.

In all of these areas, evidence indicates that consistent, well-planned food habits and exercise, balanced as needed with early aggressive insulin therapy, can significantly help normalize metabolism and thereby reduce risks of these potentially serious complications.[16]

This aggressive insulin therapy consists of multiple daily injections or continuous subcutaneous infusion by an insulin pump (Fig. 22.3). Self-monitoring of blood glucose (SMBG) levels is used to guide decisions to improve glycemic control. The added cardiovascular risk associated with diabetes is reflected in having blood pressure and lipid goals for diabetes management that are similar to those used in treating individuals who have diagnosed CVD (Table 22.2).

Self-Care Role of the Person with Diabetes

To effectively control diabetes, the person with diabetes must play a central role. Daily self-discipline and informed self-care, supported by a skilled and sensitive health care team, are required for sound diabetes management. Ultimately, all persons with diabetes must treat themselves. This is especially true with the stricter normal blood glucose control currently being used, with frequent SMBG and multiple insulin injections or an insulin infusion pump. Thus even greater need currently exists for comprehensive diabetes education programs that encourage self-monitoring and self-care responsibility. Diabetes-related issues also need to be addressed as an integral component of primary care. Weight, activity, variety, and excess are themes that are relevant for assessing basic needs and providing basic recommendations.

Retinopathy
Noninflammatory disease of the retina—the visual tissue of the eye—characterized by microaneurysms, intraretinal hemorrhages, waxy yellow exudates, "cotton wool" patches, and macular edema; a complication of diabetes that may lead to proliferation of fibrous tissue, retinal detachment, and blindness.

Neuropathy
General term for functional and pathologic changes in the peripheral nervous system; in diabetes, a chronic sensory condition affecting mainly the nerves of the legs, marked by numbness from sensory impairment, loss of tendon reflexes, severe pain, weakness, and wasting of muscles involved.

Nephropathy
Disease of the kidneys; in diabetes, renal damage associated with functional and pathologic changes in the nephrons, which can lead to glomerulosclerosis and chronic renal failure.

FIG. 22.3 Insulin injecting using an insulin pump. (From Peckenpaugh NJ: *Nutrition essentials and diet therapy*, ed 11, St. Louis, 2010, Saunders.)

TABLE 22.2   Metabolic Goals in Diabetes Management

Indicator	Normal Value	Goal	Additional Action Suggested[a]
Plasma Values (mg/dL)			
Average preprandial glucose	<110	90–130	>90/<150
Average bedtime glucose	<120	110–150	>110/<180
Whole Blood Values[b] (mg/dL)			
Average preprandial glucose	<100	80–120	>80/<140
Average bedtime glucose	<110	100–140	>100/<160
Hemoglobin A₁c (HbA₁c) (%)	<6	<7	<8
Low-density lipoprotein (LDL)-cholesterol		<100 mg/dL	
High-density lipoprotein (HDL)-cholesterol		Men: >55 mg/dL	
		Women: >55 mg/dL	
Triglycerides		<150 mg/dL	
Blood pressure		<130/80 mm Hg	

[a]Depends on individual patient circumstances.
[b]Measurement of capillary blood glucose.
Data from American Diabetes Association: Standards of medical care in diabetes—2008, *Diabetes Care* 31(Suppl 1):S12, 2008, with permission from The American Diabetes Association.

RATIONALE FOR DIABETES NUTRITION THERAPY

Nutrition therapy (NT) for diabetes is multifaceted. Physicians and nurses can no longer rely on preprinted diet sheets to assume they are providing nutrition care for patients.[17] No standard American Diabetes Association or diabetic diet exists. The American Diabetes Association does not sanction any single meal plan or specific percentages of nutrients.[18] It is essential that persons with diabetes are assessed by a registered dietitian (RD) to determine an appropriate nutrition prescription and plan for self-management education.[11] In addition, diet orders such as *no sugar added, no concentrated sweets, low sugar,* and *liberal diabetic* are not considered suitable because they do not reflect diabetes nutritional recommendations and pointlessly restrict sucrose. Such meal plans support the erroneous concept that simply limiting sucrose-sweetened foods will enhance blood glucose control.[18]

NT should be individualized, taking usual eating habits and other lifestyle factors into consideration.[19] Consistency within an eating pattern will result in better glycemic control than abiding by an arbitrary eating style. Nutrition recommendations are the same for individuals with diabetes as for the general population in regard to total fat, saturated fat, cholesterol, fiber, vitamins, and minerals. Recommendations for protein, carbohydrates, sucrose, and alcohol are modified, depending on the nature of diabetes in relation to carbohydrate metabolism or effects of complications.[17]

Type 1 Diabetes Mellitus

Recognizing the need for a more comprehensive program of care of diabetes, based on the individual metabolic balance concept and designed to help delay or avoid life-threatening complications of this chronic disease, a national US clinical research study supported by the National Institutes of Health was organized. The Diabetes Control and Complications Trial (DCCT)[16] involved 1441 subjects in 29 clinical centers across the country for approximately 10 years. The study was designed to compare the effects of intensive insulin therapy aimed at achieving blood glucose levels as close as possible to the normal non-diabetic range with effects of conventional therapy on early microvascular complications of T1DM. The DCCT demonstrated that lowering hemoglobin A₁c (HbA₁c) from 9% to 7% in the intensively treated group reduced the risk of the development or progression of eye, kidney, and neurologic complications by 50%–75%.[11,20] Dietary strategies played an important role in achieving control in the intensively treated group.[21] Reduction in complications was linearly related to improvement in glycemic control, indicating risk reduction can be achieved even if intensification of treatment fails to achieve a near-normal HbA₁c.[17,22] The adverse effects of intensive therapy included a twofold to threefold increase in severe hypoglycemia and a weight gain of 10 lb (4.5 kg).[16] Initial weight was considerably higher, but providing consultation about overeating to prevent or treat hypoglycemia appears to attenuate the weight gain.

Type 2 Diabetes Mellitus

The United Kingdom Prospective Diabetes Study (UKPDS) evaluated the effects of treatments to improve glycemic control and cardiovascular risk factors in individuals with newly diagnosed diabetes. Glycemic control and cardiovascular risk reduction therapies reduced rates of macrovascular and microvascular complications. The UKPDS confirmed DCCT findings with respect to preventing microvascular complications of diabetes and provided evidence that a comprehensive risk reduction approach could also reduce macrovascular complications.[23-26] The major cause of morbidity and mortality in persons with diabetes is CVD. T2DM and its common coexisting conditions (e.g., hypertension, dyslipidemia) are considered to be independent risk factors for macrovascular disease.[11]

Gestational Diabetes Mellitus

For women with preexisting diabetes or GDM, risks of fetal abnormalities and mortality are increased in the presence of hyperglycemia. Maternal insulin does not cross the placenta, but glucose does, causing the fetus's pancreas to increase insulin production if the mother becomes hyperglycemic. This increased production of insulin causes macrosomia, which is the most typical characteristic of babies born to women with diabetes. Other problems such as hyperinsulinemia and hyperglycemia may occur.[27] Therefore every effort should be made to control blood glucose levels.[11] All women with GDM should receive counseling by an RD when possible.[28] Individualized medical nutrition therapy (MNT), contingent on maternal weight and height, should include provision of adequate kilocalories (kcalories or kcal) and nutrients to meet the needs of the pregnancy and be consistent with established maternal blood glucose goals.[28] At the start, SMBG should be planned 4 times a day (fasting and 1 or 2 hours postprandial). Frequency can be decreased after glycemic control is established. Blood glucose goals during pregnancy are as follows[28]:

- *Fasting:* ≤105 mg/dL
- *1 hour postprandial:* ≤155 mg/dL
- *2 hours postprandial:* ≤130 mg/dL

IMPLEMENTING NUTRITION THERAPY

Nutrition intervention is governed by consideration of treatment goals and lifestyle changes the person with diabetes is ready to make, preferably to predetermined energy levels and percentages of carbohydrates, protein, and fat. The objective of NT is to support and facilitate individual lifestyle and behavior changes that will lead to improved glycemic control. Cultural and ethnic preferences should be taken into consideration, and individuals with diabetes should be included in the decision-making process.[17]

Current nutrition principles and recommendations focus on lifestyle goals and strategies for treatment of diabetes. For the first time the 2002 evidence-based nutrition recommendations purposely address lifestyle approaches to diabetes prevention, because MNT for treating and managing diabetes may not necessarily be the same for preventing or delaying onset of diabetes.[17] Goals of NT that apply to all persons with diabetes are as follows[17]:

- Attain and maintain optimal metabolic outcomes.
- Blood glucose levels in the normal (or near-normal) range
- Lipid and lipoprotein profiles that reduce risk for macrovascular diseases
- Blood pressure levels that reduce risk for vascular disease
- Prevent and treat chronic complications.
- Improve health through healthy food choices and physical activity.
- Address individual nutritional needs, taking into consideration personal and cultural preferences and lifestyle while respecting individuals' wishes and willingness to change.

Additional, more specific medical nutrition goals include the following[17]:

- *Youth with T1DM:* NT goals for children and adolescents with T1DM should ensure provision of sufficient energy for normal growth and development. Insulin regimens should be integrated into usual eating and physical activity habits.
- *T2DM in children and adolescents:* Goals for NT for children and adolescents with T2DM should facilitate changes in eating and physical activity habits to decrease insulin resistance and enhance metabolic status.
- *Pregnant and lactating women:* NT goals for pregnant and lactating women should provide adequate energy and nutrients necessary for optimal pregnancy outcomes.
- *Older adults:* Nutritional and psychosocial needs of an aging individual should be provided in NT goals.
- *Individuals treated with insulin or insulin secretagogues:* Self-management education for treatment and prevention of hypoglycemia, acute illness, and exercise-related blood glucose problems should be included in MNT goals for individuals treated with insulin or insulin secretagogues.
- *Individuals at risk for diabetes:* For those at risk for developing diabetes, physical activity should be encouraged and food choices that facilitate moderate weight loss (or at least prevent weight gain) should be promoted.

In addition, any medications a person has been prescribed should be considered as well; certain foods and drinks may interfere with them (see the Diet-Medications Interactions box, "Interactions with Diabetes Drugs").

DIET-MEDICATIONS INTERACTIONS

Interactions with Diabetes Drugs

Drug Class	Drug Names	Interactions/Instructions
α-Glucosidase inhibitor agents	Acarbose: Precose	Take with first bite of main meal
	Miglitol: Glyset	Limit alcohol
Biguanide agents	Metformin: Glucophage	Take with meals to decrease GI distress
	Metformin and glibenclamide: Glucovance, Glucophage, glyburide	May cause anorexia
DPP-4 inhibitors	Sitagliptin: Januvia	Does not cause hypoglycemia when used as a single agent
	Saxagliptin: Onglyza	Increases insulin release after meals; lowers glucagon release
Insulin and related agents	Insulin mixtures, intermediate acting, long acting, rapid acting, short acting	May increase weight
		Should use alcohol with caution and under advice from physician (alcohol increases hypoglycemic effect of insulin)
		Large weight gain increases insulin needs

Continued

🔶 DIET-MEDICATIONS INTERACTIONS

Interactions With Diabetes Drugs—cont'd

Drug Class	Drug Names	Interactions/Instructions
Meglitinide agents (nonsulfonylurea insulin releasers)	Nateglinide: Starlix Repaglinide: Prandin	Take 15–30 min before meals May increase weight Tooth disorders Nausea/vomiting Diarrhea/constipation Limit alcohol May increase risk of hypoglycemia in malnutrition
Sulfonylurea agents	Acetohexamide: Dymelor Tolazamide: Tolinase Tolbutamide: Orinase Chlorpropamide: Diabinese	Take with first meal of the day Nausea Avoid alcohol Increased risk of hypoglycemia in geriatric or malnourished patients
Sulfonylurea agents—second generation	Glimepiride: Amaryl Glyburide: DiaBeta, Micronase, Glynase PresTabs	Take 30 min before first meal of the day Hyperglycemia with high doses of nicotinic acid May increase or decrease appetite Increased weight Dyspepsia, nausea Constipation/diarrhea Avoid alcohol Possible hypoglycemia in geriatric or malnourished patients
Thiazolidinedione agents	Pioglitazone: Actos Rosiglitazone: Avandia	Take once a day without regard to food Increased weight
Pramlintide agent	Symlin	Used with insulin, an increased risk of insulin-induced severe hypoglycemia, particularly in patients with T1DM; seen usually within 3 h of injection
Exenatide	Byetta	Hypoglycemia can occur when combined with sulfonylureas, or Byetta combined with metformin and a sulfonylurea

GI, Gastrointestinal; *DPP-4*, dipeptidyl peptidase-4; *T1DM*, type 1 diabetes.

Bibliography

American Diabetes Association: *Living with diabetes: what are my options?* Alexandria, VA, 2010, American Diabetes Association. http://www.diabetes.org/living-with-diabetes/treatment-and-care/medication/oral-medications/what-are-my-options.html.

Drugs A-Z. Rancho Santa Fe, CA, 2005, RxList. https://www.rxlist.com.

Pronsky ZM: *Food medication interactions*, ed 16, Birchrunville, PA, 2010, Food-Medication Interactions.

ISSUES RELATED TO MEDICAL THERAPY

Blood Glucose Control

Insulin Therapy. The management goal for persons with T1DM is to maintain a normal blood glucose level as closely as possible. Strong evidence from the DCCT, as well as accumulating practice experience, indicates that maintaining such a "normoglycemic" state helps prevent the chronic complications of long-term uncontrolled hyperglycemia.[29] To achieve this goal, more intensive insulin therapy with the different types of insulin now available is being used. Insulin is increasingly being used as adjunctive therapy in T2DM.

Types of insulin. A number of insulin preparations are available for therapeutic use, and new ones are constantly being developed to meet medical care needs for individual patients and market changes. Individual responses to insulin types is highly variable. According to time of action, they are as follows:

1. *Rapid-acting insulins:* These insulins have various names (e.g., Humulin R, Semilente, Velosulin R), depending on the manufacturer. Rapid-acting insulins have their onset of action within approximately ½ hour after injection and stay in the body for less than 5 hours. This type of insulin peaks approximately 2 hours after injection. Human insulin analog Humalog (generic name, insulin lispro) has the shortest time-action curve of any insulin currently available. Short-acting insulins have their onset of action in ½–1 hour and have a 6- to 8-hour duration. Short-acting insulins peak at approximately 3 hours. A number of variables influence absorption rate, such as site of injection, physical activity, skin temperature, and any circulating antiinsulin antibodies. The effect on blood glucose can be detected in approximately 1 hour, peaks at 4–6 hours, and lasts approximately 12–16 hours.

2. *Intermediate-acting insulins:* These insulins include Humulin L, Lente, NPH, Insulatard N, and Insulatard. Effect is detected in approximately 2 hours, peaks at approximately 11 hours, and lasts approximately 20–29 hours.

3. *Long-acting insulins:* These insulins include Humulin U. Its duration is somewhat longer than that of intermediate-acting insulins. It can be difficult to use because basal insulin is difficult to predict or control when the insulin peaks. Insulin glargine recombinant deoxyribonucleic acid (rDNA), which was first released in 2001, is a rDNA insulin analog specifically formulated to provide a long, flat response. However, insulin glargine rDNA (trade name, Lantus) cannot be mixed with other insulins, and two injections are needed to combine the action with a short-acting insulin. It is a long-acting

insulin that works slowly over 24 hours and may not be used in combination with another type of insulin or an oral hypoglycemic medication to keep blood glucose regulated. Treatment algorithms are developed to adjust insulin on the basis of lifestyle and SMBG.

The process of intensifying T1DM management occurs in several stages. The initial dose of insulin is usually calculated based on current body weight with 0.5–0.6 units of insulin/kg/day, with approximately half being for basal needs and half being as boluses for meals. During this initial phase a consistent carbohydrate intake is needed to identify a blood glucose pattern. Next, the client can move on to more complex planning using monitoring results to achieve better glycemic control and a more flexible lifestyle. Bolus requirement varies widely, but the initial dose is often estimated to provide 1 unit of short-acting insulin per 15 g of carbohydrate. Gradually the client learns to adjust insulin for changes in food or activity using a ratio of carbohydrate intake to insulin dose. A similar approach is used for insulin therapy in other forms of diabetes. In the treatment of T2DM, insulin may be used alone or in conjunction with an oral agent.

Insulin and exercise balance. Exercise benefits all persons with diabetes through its action in increasing the number of insulin receptors on muscle cells, thus increasing insulin efficiency. However, physical activity must be regular to be effective. A detailed history of personal activity and exercise habits provides information that is needed to help a client plan a wise program of regular moderate exercise. Guidelines for extra food to cover periods of heavier exercise, athletic practice, or competition can be included (Table 22.3).

Insulin delivery systems. Intensive insulin therapy for maintaining more normal blood glucose control requires multiple injections of rapid-acting insulin, alone or in combination with basal intermediate-acting insulin. This is accomplished either by regular injection with disposal syringes or with an insulin pump. The pump is not for everyone, but for many, using an insulin pump to achieve a basal insulin infusion and bolus insulin for meals has made life easier. It is a small device that is easily worn on the belt, with a subcutaneous needle in the abdomen and buttons the wearer pushes to obtain a fixed programmed flow of insulin in balance with food intake. Frequent monitoring is needed to adjust insulin dose with either multiple injections or the insulin pump.

Oral Antidiabetic Drugs. Five classes of oral antidiabetic drugs are used to treat hyperglycemia in T2DM: (1) sulfonylurea, (2) biguanide, (3) thiazolidinedione, (4) meglitinide, and (5) α-glucosidase inhibitor. When lifestyle changes alone cannot normalize metabolism, MNT should help optimize metabolic control and reduce potential medication side effects. Table 22.4 provides a brief review of insulin and oral antidiabetic drugs (see the Complementary and Alternative Medicine [CAM] box, "Herbs and Supplements Commonly Used in Diabetes Mellitus").

COMPLEMENTARY AND ALTERNATIVE MEDICINE (CAM)

Herbs and Supplements Commonly Used in Diabetes Mellitus

Herb/ Supplement	Common Uses	Efficacy	Safety	Drug-Herb Interactions	Interaction
Chromium	Glycemic control	Improved glycemic control	No adverse effects reported	Hyperglycemic agents and any other agent used for glycemic control	Possible risk of hypoglycemia
Cinnamon (Cinnamomum verum)	Glycemic control	Increases use of endogenous insulin	Large amounts increase heart rate and intestinal motility, followed by sleepiness and depression. As a spice, long-term use safe	None known	
Ginseng (Panax ginseng)	Glycemic control	Improved glycemic control	Possible overstimulation and insomnia	Hyperglycemic agents and any other agent used for glycemic control	Possible risk of hypoglycemia
				May enhance effect of stimulants, antibiotics, MAOIs	Estrogenic effects of ginseng may cause vaginal bleeding and breast nodules
				Antagonism of warfarin; might falsely elevate digoxin levels	
				Increases alcohol clearance; might decrease diuretic effect of furosemide	
				Might potentiate effects of hormones and anabolic steroid therapies	
Evening primrose oil (Oenothera biennis)	Peripheral neuropathy	May be helpful	No adverse effects reported	Phenothiazines	Might increase risk of seizures

Continued

❧ COMPLEMENTARY AND ALTERNATIVE MEDICINE (CAM)

Herbs and Supplements Commonly Used in Diabetes Mellitus—cont'd

Herb/ Supplement	Common Uses	Efficacy	Safety	Drug-Herb Interactions	Interaction
Lipoic acid	Neuropathy	Slight evidence intravenous lipoic acid can reduce symptoms of peripheral neuropathy in the short term. Evidence for oral lipoic acid inadequate	No adverse reactions documented	Some concern that lipoic acid potentiates the effects of insulin, but this has not been documented in formal studies	None noted
Vanadium	Glycemic control	May improve glycemic control	Usually well tolerated, but GI disturbances can occur. Studies suggest excess is toxic (hepatotoxicity, nephrotoxicity, teratogenicity, and developmental/reproductive toxicity)	Might cause hypoglycemia if used in conjunction with an effective antidiabetic regimen	None noted

GI, Gastrointestinal; *MAOIs,* monoamine oxidase inhibitors.

Bibliography

Bratman S, Girman AM: *Mosby's handbook of herbs and supplements and their therapeutic uses,* St. Louis, 2003, Mosby.

Contributors and Consultants: *Professional guide to complementary and alternative therapies,* Springhouse, PA, 2001, Springhouse.

Kuhn MA, Winston D: *Herbal therapy and supplements: a scientific and traditional approach,* Philadelphia, 2001, Lippincott Williams & Wilkins.

TABLE 22.3   Meal-Planning Guide for Active People With Type 1 Diabetes Mellitus

Exchange Needs	Sample Menus
Moderate Activity	
30 Minutes	
1 bread *or*	1 bran muffin *or*
1 fruit	1 small orange
1 Hour	
2 bread + 1 meat *or*	Tuna sandwich *or*
2 fruit + 1 milk	½ cup fruit salad + 1 cup milk
Strenuous Activity	
30 Minutes	
2 fruit *or*	1 small banana *or*
1 bread + 1 fat	½ bagel + 1 tsp cream cheese
1 Hour	
2 bread + 1 meat + 1 milk *or*	Meat and cheese sandwich + 1 cup milk *or*
2 bread + 2 meat + 2 fruit	Hamburger + 1 cup orange juice

Insulin is often used in T2DM as adjunctive therapy when oral agents are not achieving glycemic control. A nighttime dose of insulin is commonly used to help reduce fasting glucose levels, especially if fasting levels are 13.9 mmol/L (250 mg/dL) or higher. Insulin therapy is also commonly used as adjunctive therapy when glycemic control is not achieved with oral agent monotherapy or combination therapy.

Adjunctive Therapies. Two new injectable drugs have been approved by the US Food and Drug Administration (FDA). Exenatide (Byetta) is first in its class of drugs for treatment of T2DM for patients taking metformin, a sulfonylurea, or a combination of metformin and a sulfonylurea. This class of drugs is referred to as *incretin mimetics.*

Isolated from the saliva of Gila monsters, exenatide works to lower blood glucose levels by increasing insulin secretion. It has this effect only in the presence of elevated blood glucose levels; therefore it does not tend to increase risk of hypoglycemia on its own.

Pramlintide (Symlin) is a synthetic form of the hormone amylin. Amylin and insulin are produced by the beta cells in the pancreas. Amylin, insulin, and glucagon work together to maintain normal blood glucose levels. Pramlintide injections taken with meals modestly improve HbA$_{1c}$ levels by slowing gastric emptying rate without altering overall absorption of nutrients. In addition, pramlintide suppresses glucagon secretion from the liver and regulates food intake because of centrally mediated modulation of appetite.

Testing Methods for Monitoring Results. Frequent testing of blood glucose levels is necessary for successful **tight control** of T1DM and to reduce risk of complications.

Self-monitoring of blood glucose. For insulin doses to be administered in sufficient time intervals and amounts to maintain normal blood glucose, close monitoring of immediate blood glucose levels is mandatory. Small, lightweight, easy-to-use, hand-sized meters, easily carried in pockets and handbags, are available for convenient use. A reagent test strip is inserted into the blood glucose meter, a drop of capillary blood from the finger obtained with an automatic lancet is placed on the reagent test strip, and a digital reading of the blood glucose level appears on the meter. The frequency of monitoring varies according to need for control and goal of care. More frequent self-monitoring is indicated for unstable forms of diabetes, persons using insulin pumps, and those who want close control and freedom of movement. Usually two to eight before- and after-meal tests are

KEY TERM

Tight Control
Keeping blood glucose levels as close to normal as possible.

TABLE 22.4   Medications Used to Treat Diabetes

Drug Class	Drug Names	Action	Target Organs	Side Effects	How Taken
α-Glucosidase inhibitor agents	Acarbose: Precose Miglitol: Glyset	Delays absorption of glucose from GI tract	Small intestine	Excess flatulence, diarrhea (particularly after high-carbohydrate meal), abdominal pain; may interfere with iron absorption	Must be taken with meals three times/day
Biguanide agents	Metformin: Glucophage	Decreases hepatic glucose production and intestinal glucose absorption; improves insulin sensitivity	Liver, small intestine, and peripheral tissues	Less likely to gain weight; may lose weight; anorexia, nausea, diarrhea, metallic taste; may reduce absorption of vitamin B_{12} and folic acid; rarely suitable for adults <80 years old	Take with first main meal
Insulin and related agents	Insulin mixtures: Humulin 50/50, Humulin 70/30, Novolin 70/30	Exogenous insulin preparations	Cells	Hypoglycemia, fatigue, hunger, nausea, muscular weakness or trembling, headache, sweating, blurred vision, fainting, weight gain, skin irritation	Subcutaneous injection
	Intermediate acting: Humulin L, Humulin N, Iletin II Lente, Iletin II NPH, Novolin L, Novolin N	Exogenous insulin preparations		Hypoglycemia, fatigue, hunger, nausea, muscular weakness or trembling, headache, sweating, blurred vision, fainting, weight gain, skin irritation	Subcutaneous injection
	Long acting: Humulin U, Lantus (insulin glargine)	Exogenous insulin preparations		Hypoglycemia, fatigue, hunger, nausea, muscular weakness or trembling, headache, sweating, blurred vision, fainting, weight gain, skin irritation	Subcutaneous injection
	Rapid acting: Humalog, insulin lispro, insulin aspart	Exogenous insulin preparations		Hypoglycemia, fatigue, hunger, nausea, muscular weakness or trembling, headache, sweating, blurred vision, fainting, weight gain, skin irritation	Subcutaneous injection, intramuscular or intravenous in special situations
	Short acting: Humulin R, Iletin II Regular, Novolin R, Novolin BR	Exogenous insulin preparations		Hypoglycemia, fatigue, hunger, nausea, muscular weakness or trembling, headache, sweating, blurred vision, fainting, weight gain, skin irritation	Subcutaneous injection, intramuscular or intravenous in special situations
Meglitinide agents (nonsulfonylurea insulin releasers)	Nateglinide: Starlix Repaglinide: Prandin	Stimulates secretion of insulin	Pancreatic beta cells	Hypoglycemia and weight gain; repaglinide (Prandin) has a slightly increased risk for cardiac events	Take with meals
Sulfonylurea agents—first generation	Acetohexamide: Dymelor Tolazamide: Tolinase Tolbutamide: Orinase Chlorpropamide: Diabinese	Stimulates secretion of insulin	Pancreatic beta cells	Hypoglycemia and weight gain; tolbutamide may be associated with cardiovascular complications; chlorpropamide (Diabinese) can cause hyponatremia and should not be used by women who are pregnant, who are nursing, or those individuals allergic to sulfa drugs; sulfonylurea interacts with many other drugs (prescription, OTC, and alternative); Diabinese: avoid alcohol	Take before or with meals
Sulfonylurea agents—second generation	Glimepiride: Amaryl Glyburide: DiaBeta, Micronase, Glynase PresTabs				
Thiazolidinedione agents	Pioglitazone: Actos Rosiglitazone: Avandia	Improves insulin sensitivity	Activates genes involved with fat synthesis and carbohydrate metabolism	Possible liver damage, weight gain, mild anemia	Once or twice daily

GI, Gastrointestinal; *OTC,* over the counter.

Data from Nelms MN, Sucher K, Lacey L, Long S: *Nutrition therapy and pathophysiology,* ed 2, Belmont, CA, 2010, Thomson Cengage; Mahan LK, Escott-Stump S, editors: *Krause's food & nutrition therapy,* ed 12, St. Louis, 2008, Saunders.

performed daily. During pregnancy, postprandial monitoring is performed at 1 hour after meals. Glucose goals are lower during pregnancy because of the dilution effect of having increased blood volume.

Glycated hemoglobin. The most common glycated hemoglobin (Hb) test is the HbA_{1c}. Glycated Hb molecules are relatively stable within the red blood cell. During the 120-day life of the red blood cell, glucose molecules attach themselves to Hb. This irreversible glycosylation of Hb depends on the concentration of blood glucose. The glycosylation of proteins in various body systems appears to play a role in the development of diabetic complications. The greater the level of circulating glucose is during the life of the red blood cells, the greater is the concentration of glycohemoglobin. Thus measurement of HbA_{1c} relates to the level of blood glucose during a longer period. It provides an effective tool for evaluating the long-term management of diabetes and degree of control.[11] Because glucose attaches to Hb during the life of the red blood cell, the test gives an accumulated history of glucose levels across time, providing an effective management tool for evaluating progress and making decisions about treatment changes. Obtaining an HbA_{1c} level every 6–8 weeks can be used to monitor the overall glucose control.

Physical Activity Habits

In counseling clients with diabetes, a detailed history of personal activity and physical exercise habits should be discussed. This information is then used as a basis for planning a wise program of regular moderate exercise. Guidelines for extra food to cover periods of heavier exercise or athletic practice and competition are included (see Table 22.3). Self-monitoring is a regular procedure now used by most persons with T1DM and T2DM. It is a helpful means of determining the balance needed at any point in time between exercise, insulin, and food.

Gestational Diabetes

Occasionally the stress of pregnancy may bring about GDM, which is a form of glucose intolerance that has onset during pregnancy and is resolved on parturition.[30] Risk of fetal abnormalities and mortality are increased in the presence of hyperglycemia; therefore every effort should be made to control blood glucose levels. All women with GDM should receive nutrition counseling by an RD when possible.[28]

Changes that take place during pregnancy greatly affect insulin use. Some hormones and enzymes produced by the placenta are antagonistic to insulin, thus reducing its effectiveness. Maternal insulin does not cross the placenta, but glucose does, causing the fetal pancreas to increase insulin production if maternal blood glucose levels get too high. Increased production of insulin causes the most predictable characteristic of infants born to women with diabetes, macrosomia, in addition to other problems such as respiratory difficulties, hypocalcemia, hypoglycemia, hypokalemia, and jaundice.[27]

Individualization of NT based on maternal weight and height is recommended.[28] MNT should include the provision of adequate kcalories and nutrients to meet pregnancy needs and should be consistent with accepted maternal blood glucose goals.[28] SMBG provides important information about the effect of food on blood glucose levels. At the beginning of the pregnancy, minimal daily SMBG should be planned 4 times a day (fasting, and 1 or 2 hours after each meal). Blood glucose goals during pregnancy are fasting, less than 105 mg/dL; 1 hour postprandial, 155 mg/dL; and 2 hour postprandial, less than 130 mg/dL.[28] The frequency of SMBG may be decreased after blood glucose control is established. However, some monitoring should continue throughout pregnancy.

Recommended weight gains and nutrient requirements are the same as for established pregnancy guidelines, as follows[27]:

- Underweight (body mass index [BMI] less than 18.5): 28–40 lb
- Normal/healthy weight (BMI 18.5–24.9): 25–35 lb
- Overweight (BMI 25–29.9): 15–25 lb
- Obesity (class 1) (BMI 30–34.9): less than 15 lb
- Obesity (class 2) (BMI 35–39.9): not available
- Obesity (class 3) (BMI greater than 40): not available

No kcalorie modifications are needed for the first trimester.[17] During the second and third trimesters, increased energy intake of approximately 180 kcal/day is suggested.[27] High-quality protein should be increased by 25 g/day. As with any pregnancy, 600 mcg/day of folic acid is recommended for prevention of neural tube defects (NTDs) and other congenital abnormalities.[27] Alcohol consumption is not recommended in any amount.

Kcaloric restriction must be considered with care. A minimum of 1700–1800 kcal/day of carefully selected foods has been shown to prevent ketosis. Intakes less than this level are not advised.[28] Weight gain goals are established using prepregnancy BMI. Weight gain should still occur even if patients have gained substantial weight before the onset of GDM. Each patient with GDM should be evaluated individually by an RD, their care plans should be fine-tuned, and patient education should be provided as required to realize weight goals.

Impaired Fasting Glucose and Impaired Glucose Tolerance

The terms *IFG* and *IGT* refer to a metabolic stage somewhere between normal glucose homeostasis and overt diabetes. Although not clinical entities in their own right, these conditions are risk factors for future diabetes and CVD.[2,11] Lifestyle interventions should be consistent with current guidelines for overweight and obesity and address cardiovascular risk factors and common concomitant conditions. The Da Qing IGT and Diabetes Study provided preliminary evidence that diet and exercise intervention can lower the conversion to overt diabetes during the 6-year period.[14] The Finnish Diabetes Prevention Study demonstrated that a lifestyle change program could reduce the risk for developing T2DM by 58% during a 3-year period.[13] In the United States the Diabetes Prevention Program (DPP) has confirmed the findings of the Finnish trial in a highly diverse US population with IGT. The DPP addressed how an intensive diet and exercise intervention compares with metformin in a three-arm randomized clinical trial that uses placebo as the third arm.

MANAGEMENT OF DIABETES NUTRITION THERAPY

Counseling Process in Nutrition Therapy for Diabetes

NT for diabetes is highly individualized. The American Diabetes Association recommendations clearly state that no single diabetic or American Diabetes Association diet exists. Currently the recommended diet is a dietary prescription based on individual nutrition assessment and treatment goals.[19] This model emphasizes actions of the diabetes team clinical dietitian in an individualized, integrated four-point approach: (1) assessment, (2) goal setting, (3) nutrition intervention, and (4) evaluation, as follows[31]:

1. *Assessment:* The first step involves a comprehensive assessment of the client's background. It includes clinical information, medical and lifestyle data such as personal SMBG, and dietary history. Interview follow-up tools such as questionnaires and food records assess general food patterns and nutrient intake.
2. *Nutrition diagnosis:* The second step identifies and labels problems the client may have.

3. *Nutrition intervention:* The third step guides the client in selecting and using the most appropriate meal-planning guide from the number that are now available, based on individual needs for knowledge and skills to change or maintain eating habits and daily living practices.

4. *Monitoring and evaluation:* Together the client and dietitian evaluate goals and nutrition intervention, as well as ongoing clinical data, to help the client succeed at the established individual program. They then make any desired adjustments, and the dietitian provides continuing counseling and education as needed.

Diabetes Meal-Planning Tools

Since the DCCT, growing emphasis has been placed on selecting a planning approach that meets the needs of each client from a wide array of meal-planning guides. Regardless of the diabetes NT management tool, the first vital principle in working with persons who have diabetes is to begin where they are physically, mentally, and emotionally. Any food-planning process must focus first on the unique individual rather than on the case or disease. Numerous planning approaches are used by skilled and sensitive clinical dietitians who tailor their actions to the person's learning needs and abilities, as well as his or her nutritional needs, personal needs, and lifestyle issues. The use of the exchange lists as a dietary management tool is widespread; they are outlined on the Evolve website.

Carbohydrate Counting.

Carbohydrate counting is one of the most commonly used methods of meal planning. Research shows carbohydrate is the primary nutrient affecting postprandial blood glucose level and consequently insulin requirements.[21,22] Carbohydrate quantity and distribution can affect metabolic control.[22] Carbohydrate counting can help people with diabetes become more aware of carbohydrate content of the foods they eat and consistency of food consumption at meals and when snacking.[19]

At an advanced level, carbohydrate counting is a tool that allows the person with diabetes to focus on adjustment of foods, medication, and activity based on patterns from daily food intake records and blood glucose records.[19] To use carbohydrate counting effectively, the dietetic professional and person with diabetes must have a good understanding of intensive insulin therapy.[22]

Carbohydrate content can be measured in grams of carbohydrate or servings: one carbohydrate serving equals 15 g carbohydrate. Most people find it easier to count the number of carbohydrate servings consumed rather than keeping track of grams of carbohydrate consumed.[22] Box 22.1 provides a brief outline of carbohydrate content of foods to equal one serving of carbohydrate.

Planning for Special Needs

Sick days. When general illness occurs, food and insulin amounts must be adjusted accordingly. Texture may be modified as needed to use easily digested and absorbed liquid foods while still maintaining as many as possible glucose equivalents of the usual food plan.

Physical activity. For any strenuous physical activity, the client with T1DM must make special advanced plans. This is particularly true of a young person with diabetes who is engaging in athletic practice or competition. Energy demands of exercise are discussed in Chapter 14.

Travel. When a trip is planned, the clinical dietitian must confer with the client to guide food choices according to what will be available. SMBG levels, insulin therapy equipment, and making food plans are just as important on a trip as they are at home. The traveler always needs to plan ahead with the health care team (see

---

> ### BOX 22.1   Equivalents to One 15-g Carbohydrate Serving[a]
>
> **Grains, Breads, Cereals, Starches**
> - 1 slice bread
> - ¾ cup dry cereal
> - ½ cup cooked cereal
> - ⅓ cup cooked rice or pasta
>
> **Milk and Yogurt**
> - 1 cup milk
> - ⅓ cup (6 oz) unsweetened or sugar-free yogurt
>
> **Fruits**
> - 1 small fresh fruit
> - ½ cup canned fruit (canned in juice)
> - 1 cup melon or berries
> - ¼ cup dried fruit
> - ½ cup unsweetened fruit juice
>
> **Vegetables**
> - ½ cup cooked potatoes, peas, or corn
> - 3 cups raw vegetables
> - 1½ cups cooked vegetables
> - Small portions (½ cup) of nonstarchy vegetables are free
>
> **Sweets and Snack Foods**
> - ½ cup or ¾ oz snack food (pretzels, chips)
> - 4–6 snack crackers
> - 1 oz sweet snack (two small cookies)
> - ½ cup regular ice cream
> - 1 tbsp sugar

[a]Reproduction of the Exchange Lists in whole or part without permission of the American Dietetic Association or the American Diabetes Association, Inc., is a violation of federal law. This material has been modified from *Choose Your Foods: Exchange Lists for Diabetes*, which is the basis of a meal planning system designed by a committee of the American Diabetes Association and the American Dietetic Association. Although designed primarily for people with diabetes and others who must follow special diets, the Exchange Lists are based on principles of good nutrition that apply to everyone.

Data from American Diabetes Association, American Dietetic Association: *Choose your foods: exchange lists for diabetes,* ed 6, Alexandra, VA/Chicago, 2008, American Diabetes Association, American Dietetic Association. Copyright 2008 by the American Diabetes Association.

---

the Perspectives in Practice box, "Travel and Illness: 'Real-Life' Situations").

Dining out. Provide similar guidelines and suggestions for various situations when the client eats meals away from home. As a general rule, the plan must be made ahead of time; therefore accommodations for what is eaten at home before and after the restaurant meal will reflect the continuing balance needs of the day. Have the client get the menu ahead of time. Many restaurants are willing to fax their menus, or they may be available on websites.

Stress. Any form of emotional stress is reflected in variations of diabetes control.[22] These variations are caused by hormonal responses that act as antagonists to insulin. The clinical dietitian must help the client learn and practice a variety of useful stress reduction activities.

PERSPECTIVES IN PRACTICE

Travel and Illness: "Real-Life" Situations

People do not stop living their lives just because they have diabetes. They still travel, and they still catch colds, influenza, and other common illnesses. Special considerations to all areas of diabetes management will enhance safe traveling, as well as the traveler's health. What kind of information does the person with diabetes need to know when traveling or if he or she becomes too ill to eat? The following are a few helpful hints you may want to offer clients for these situations.

Traveling Safely With Diabetes
General Tips

1. Ensure that you have sufficient medication (insulin or oral glucose-lowering medication) for the entire trip.
2. Carry some form of medical identification that includes the type of diabetes you have, name, address, telephone number, emergency contact information, medications taken, physician's name and phone number, and additional relevant medical conditions. Preferably, this information should be worn on a necklace or bracelet (rather than carrying it in a wallet or purse).
3. Take extra snacks such as cereal bars, vanilla wafers, peanut butter crackers, or glucose tablets or gel.
4. Always keep insulin cool, especially when vacationing in warm climates.
5. Keep some money available for food purchases if necessary. Change for vending machines may not always be available.
6. Always carry blood glucose monitoring equipment. Blood glucose levels should be checked before beginning a trip, as well as every 2 hours. An extra check should be done whenever symptoms of hypoglycemia occur, even if recent blood glucose checks were acceptable.
7. Walking around and stretching every 2–4 hours helps stimulate circulation.
8. Whenever possible, travel with a companion.
9. Wear comfortable shoes.
10. Plan for time zone changes. Meal schedules may need to be revised to balance with insulin activity pattern.
11. If traveling abroad, learn to say the following in the local language: "I have diabetes. Please give me something sweet to drink."
12. If travel is frequent, contact a registered dietitian (RD) or diabetes educator for ideas for healthful, portable meals and snacks.

Driving Tips

1. If diabetes medications have the potential to cause hypoglycemia, medications and meals will need to be scheduled during a long trip.
2. If diabetes medications have the potential to cause hypoglycemia, food should be eaten before leaving home or snacks should be taken in the automobile. Traffic may not be conducive to stopping at a favorite store or restaurant for a quick meal or snack.
3. Keep nonperishable, carbohydrate-containing foods in the automobile in case flat tires, traffic jams, or breakdowns occur. Handy, premeasured carbohydrate amounts may be beneficial to avoid overeating or undereating. Replenish the food supply as needed to avoid running out at inopportune times.
4. Always carry blood glucose monitoring equipment when driving. Blood glucose levels should be checked before the trip begins, as well as every 2 hours while driving. An extra check should be done if symptoms of hypoglycemia occur (even if recent blood glucose checks have been acceptable).
5. An extra glucose meter should not be kept in an automobile. Internal automobile temperatures can get very hot and very cold. Strips and meters exposed to extreme temperatures may not be accurate or function properly.

6. High blood glucose levels may cause the following symptoms that can affect driving:
   - Fatigue related to the body's inability to use glucose for energy
   - Increased urination, causing preoccupation, repeated stops, and a delay in arriving at destination
   - Blurry vision, which may impair ability to see road signs clearly; blurry vision may be especially problematic at night or while driving in rain or snow
   - Numbness or tingling in hands or feet, which may impair ability to steer, accelerate, and stop the vehicle
7. Prompt attention to hypoglycemia and treatment is necessary to prevent mental confusion and even losing consciousness. When blood glucose is low, the first organ affected is the brain. Keep appropriate sources of carbohydrates available in the automobile.
8. If driving hours at a time, it is important to stop the automobile, get out and stretch, and walk around every 2–4 hours.
9. Wear medical identification. Law enforcement officers may not be familiar with diabetes or symptoms of hypoglycemia or hyperglycemia. They can mistake impaired awareness and judgment for drunkenness.
10. Whenever possible, drive with a friend.
11. If driving for several hours, set an alarm as a reminder for blood glucose checks, meals, and even times to stretch and walk.
12. Visual disturbances can occur with either hyperglycemia or hypoglycemia.
13. If driving long distances, take twice as many diabetes supplies as thought to be needed. Be aware of all medicines taken (prescription and over-the-counter [OTC] medications).
14. Always carry money for toll booths, parking fees, and telephone calls. Consider keeping a cell phone to call for assistance.

Flying Tips

1. Call ahead to airlines to advise them that you have diabetes and supplies you may need.
2. Carry a copy of your physician's prescription for insulin and other medications.
3. Carry a letter from the physician explaining the need to carry syringes/injection devices and insulin.
4. If problems are encountered, request to speak to a manager or supervisor.
5. Carry insulin onto the aircraft. Insulin should not be packed in luggage that will be stored in the hold of an airplane. Low temperatures can damage the insulin.
6. Notify the Transportation Security Administration (TSA) representative that you have diabetes and are carrying your supplies with you. The following are allowed through the checkpoint once screened:
   - Insulin and insulin-loaded dispensing products clearly marked and labeled
   - Unlimited number of unused syringes when accompanied by insulin or other injectable medication
   - Lancets, blood glucose meters, blood glucose meter test strips, alcohol swabs, meter-testing solutions
   - Insulin pump and supplies
   - Glucagon emergency kit clearly identified and labeled
   - Urine ketone test strips
   - Unlimited number of used syringes when transported in sharps disposal container or other similar hard-surfaced container

Sick Day Survival

1. Keep taking diabetes medications even if solid foods cannot be eaten.
2. For insulin users the physician may prescribe extra doses or increased amounts of insulin during an illness.
3. Blood glucose should be tested and recorded every 4 hours.

4. Test for ketones in urine if blood glucose level stays at or greater than 240 mg/dL for at least 4 hours.
5. Try to use regular meal plan and diet, but if that is not possible, soft foods or liquids can be consumed to take the place of carbohydrates usually eaten. Some easily digested foods to replace one serving (15 g) of carbohydrate include the following:
   - ⅓ – ½ cup fruit juice
   - ½ cup regular soft drink
   - ½ cup regular gelatin
   - ½ cup hot cereal
   - ½ cup vanilla ice cream
   - 1 cup broth-based soup
6. To prevent dehydration, sip 3–6 oz of noncaffeinated, sugar-free beverages or water every hour. Sugar-free fluids may be alternated with liquids containing sugar to help control blood glucose levels.
7. Keep a thermometer on hand to determine body temperature.
8. When buying OTC medicines, choose one that is sugar free. In addition to the word *sugar* on labels, *dextrose, fructose, lactose, sorbitol, mannitol, xylitol,* and *honey* indicate that a product contains sugar.
9. OTC cold medications containing epinephrine-like compounds (including ephedrine, pseudoephedrine, phenylpropanolamine, phenylephrine, and epinephrine) can raise blood glucose levels and should only be used with a physician's approval.
10. *Planning ahead:* Keep the following items on hand in case of colds, influenza, or other kinds of illnesses:
    - Thermometer
    - Urine test strips for ketones (check expiration date periodically)
    - Approved OTC cold and influenza medicines
    - Syringes or prescription for them (if insulin is not usually taken but is part of a sick day plan)
    - Short-acting insulin (keep refrigerated)
    - Extra prescriptions for all medications usually taken (or have on file at pharmacy)
    - Nonperishable foods such as noncaffeinated soft drinks (regular and diet), regular gelatin, Popsicles, sport drinks, saltines, and canned fruit juices

11. Call the physician if any of the following occurs:
    - Vomiting for several hours
    - Diarrhea recurring within 6 hours
    - Difficulty breathing
    - Blood glucose levels greater than 240 mg/dL for 24 hours if using oral medications; blood glucose levels greater than 240 mg/dL for two consecutive tests (4 hours apart) after taking supplemental insulin
    - Blood glucose levels less than 60 mg/dL
    - Moderate to large amounts of ketones in urine and no improvement after at least 12 hours
    - Signs of dehydration such as dry skin or mouth, sunken eyes, or weight loss
    - Sickness that continues from 12 to 48 hours without improvement
    - Increased fatigue
    - Stomach or chest pain
    - Temperature that stays at higher than 101°F
    - Acute loss of vision
12. When calling your physician, he or she will want to know your blood glucose levels and urine ketone levels, how long the illness has lasted, what medicines have been taken, temperature, how much you have had to eat or drink, and other symptoms that have been experienced.
13. If it is necessary to go to the emergency department, the staff should be informed that you have diabetes.

In summary, in all cases the client must be advised to (1) maintain a steady intake of food every day, (2) replace the carbohydrate value of solid foods with that of liquid or soft foods as needed, (3) monitor blood and urine frequently for sugar and ketone levels, and (4) contact the physician if the illness lasts more than a day or so.

Bibliography

American Diabetes Association: *Traveling with diabetes supplies,* Alexandria, VA, 2006, American Diabetes Association. https://www.diabetes.org/advocacy-and-legalresources/discrimination/public_accommodation/travel.jsp.
Diabetes Mall: FAA regulations for diabetes supplies. *Diabetes News,* 2001. https://www.diabetesnet.com/news/news100701.php.
National Diabetes Information Clearinghouse: *What I need to know about eating and diabetes.* Bethesda, MD, 2003, National Institute of Diabetes and Digestive and Kidney Diseases, National Institutes of Health. NIH Pub No 03-5043.

DIABETES EDUCATION PROGRAM

Goal: Person-Centered Self-Care

In past years the traditional medical model has guided diabetes education in its methods, language, and the respective roles assumed. Professionals have viewed themselves as having major authoritative roles and have assigned to the person with diabetes the more passive role of patient. With notable exceptions in certain places, this model has been followed in most cases. However, with the increasing movement toward changing roles of practitioners and consumers in the health care system, persons with diabetes are assuming a more active voice in planning and conducting their own care. Several barriers in our traditional system stem from three sources: (1) our culture, (2) our health care delivery system, and (3) our professional training habits. Essentially, much of the core problem focuses on communication. For example, a list of words we use too commonly that may be objectionable to persons with diabetes, along with the preferred language, includes the following:

- Diabetic used as a noun: The word *diabetic* is an adjective and should not be used alone as a noun. Instead, use the phrase *person with diabetes.*
- Compliance: The word *compliance* raises red flags in minds of persons with diabetes. It is a purely medical term and connotes an authoritative physician position. Instead, the word *adherence* should be used, which has been adopted by national committees and associations working in the field of diabetes. The word *adherence* indicates placement of more decision-making responsibility on the person with diabetes to determine courses of action in varying situations, which is, of course, the necessity.
- Patient: Instead of *patient,* the phrase *person with diabetes* should be used. Persons with diabetes are patients only when they are in the hospital or seeing a physician for an illness.
- Cheating: A particularly abusive word in the minds of many persons with diabetes, especially parents of children and young people with diabetes, is the word *cheating* because it suggests dishonesty or failure to live up to an external code. By and large, persons with diabetes do not cheat. They may kid themselves, or they may be inaccurate in their reporting, but they do not cheat. Instead, phrases such as *having difficulty* or *having a problem with* should be used.

Contents: Tools for Self-Care

A plan for diabetes education must recognize the need for building self-sufficiency and responsibility within persons with diabetes and their families. It should provide practical guidelines that build on

The Woman With Type 2 Diabetes Mellitus

Angela is a 35-year-old woman diagnosed 2 years ago with type 2 diabetes mellitus (T2DM). She has three children whose birth weights were in the range of 4.5–5 kg (10–11 lb). The children, now teenagers, show no signs of diabetes, and their weights are reported to be within normal limits despite their mother's fondness for cooking. Her husband, an underpaid construction worker, is slightly overweight.

Approximately 6 months ago, Angela was seen with a complaint of a series of infections that lasted longer than usual during the past 2 months. At that time she was measured as 165 cm (5'5") and 71 kg (156 lb). Her glucose tolerance test was positive. She was seen for follow-up twice during the next month, each time showing hyperglycemia and glycosuria. At the second follow-up, an oral antidiabetic medication was prescribed, and she was referred for medical nutrition therapy (MNT).

Angela did not keep this appointment or her subsequent medical appointment. She was not seen again until 1 month ago, when she arrived at the emergency department with ketoacidosis. She responded well to treatment and was placed on a 1200-kcal diet and a mixture of intermediate- and rapid-acting insulin given in two injections a day. Her discharge plan included a referral for an MNT consultation session and diabetes education classes.

Questions for Analysis
1. What factors do you think contributed to the ketoacidosis?
2. What relation do these factors have to diabetes control?
3. Why did Angela first appear to have T2DM?
4. Assume that Angela administers insulin before breakfast and before the evening meal. What additional information is necessary to develop an individualized meal plan?
5. Identify any personal factors that may affect Angela's adherence to her treatment plan. Do you anticipate any problems?
6. If so, then how would you attempt to help her solve them?
7. Outline a diabetes education plan for Angela.

necessary skills that a person with diabetes must have for the best possible control, as well as additional surrounding factors related to life situations and psychosocial needs. Content areas include needs in relation to the nature of diabetes, nutrition and basic meal planning, insulin (or oral medication) effects and how to regulate them, monitoring of blood glucose, how to deal with illness, and, if relevant, urine ketones (see the Case Study box, "The Woman with Type 2 Diabetes Mellitus").

Educational Materials: Person-Centered Standards

A broad, confusing array of diabetes education materials are available. Some are excellent, and some should be discarded. Whatever is used should measure up to several basic person-centered requirements by doing the following:

- Give the intended receiver credit for having some intelligence and wanting new information.
- Inform persons fully and completely, giving both sides when experts disagree (as they surely do on occasion).
- Appeal to various levels of audience, ranging from basic to sophisticated.
- Never be patronizing, dehumanizing, or childish.

HEALTH PROMOTION

Nutrition Questions From Persons With Diabetes

Persons with diabetes have many questions about their diets, especially when they are newly diagnosed and anxieties are high. They do not want just a yes-or-no answer. For any diet item of concern, they want

to know if it can be used. If use of the diet item should be limited, then they want to know why this is so and exactly how often they can use it.

Alcohol and Diabetes: Do They Mix?

Questions about alcohol and various sweeteners are common. People with diabetes should follow the same sensible drinking guidelines as people without diabetes, as follows[17,32,33]:

- Use alcohol only in moderation (one drink/day for women, two drinks/day for men).
- One drink = 12 oz regular beer, 5 oz wine, or 1½ oz of 80-proof distilled spirits (whiskey, scotch, rye, vodka, brandy, cognac, rum).
- Never drink alcohol on an empty stomach.
- Some medications may not mix with alcohol; check with physician or pharmacist.
- Never drink and drive.
- Never drink if pregnant or trying to become pregnant.
- Above all, use common sense.

Having diabetes should not prevent consumption of alcohol; however, some considerations must be made. Alcoholic beverages, depending on amount and type, can cause hyperglycemia and hypoglycemia. Alcohol moves very quickly from the stomach into the bloodstream; it does not require digestion or metabolism. Approximately 30–90 minutes after an alcoholic drink is consumed, alcohol in the bloodstream is at its highest concentration. Because the liver plays the biggest role in removing alcohol from the blood, it stops making glucose while cleansing alcohol from the body. If blood glucose levels are falling during the same time, then hypoglycemia can occur very quickly. Those who take insulin or oral hypoglycemic agents should also be aware that these can lower blood glucose levels. This is why two shots of whiskey on an empty stomach lower blood sugar dramatically.

Alcoholic beverages can be high in kcalories (and low in food value) and can raise blood glucose, especially if mixed with sweet mixers, fruit juices, or ice cream. Two ounces of 90-proof alcohol contain almost 200 kcal. Wine coolers, liqueurs, and port wines are also high in sugar and kcalories. This can interfere with weight loss goals and practicing tight control. Alcohol also increases serum cholesterol levels, although this effect is transient. In addition, it can lead to hyperlipoproteinemia, with high triglyceride levels in susceptible individuals, including persons with diabetes, when it is excessive. Alcohol can also make neuropathy and retinopathy worse.

For clients who choose to use alcohol, they should ask themselves the following three basic questions:
1. Is my diabetes under control?
2. Does my health care provider agree that I am free from any health problems that alcohol can make worse (e.g., high blood pressure, neuropathy)?
3. Do I know how alcohol can affect me and my diabetes?

If the answer to all three questions is *yes,* then the client can have an occasional drink. In addition to the sensible drinking guidelines listed earlier, the following recommendations should also be considered:

- Discuss the use of alcohol with your physician or dietitian.
- Drink with caution, and carry identification.
- Choose drinking buddies wisely. (Make sure at least one friend or trusted companion knows that you have diabetes and is aware of what should be done in case of hypoglycemia.)
- Have a snack before going to bed to prevent hypoglycemia during sleep.
- Do not drink if you are practicing tight control (because alcohol impairs judgment); have neuropathy, hypertriglyceridemia, or hypertension; or are taking Diabinese (which causes nausea, flushing, headache, or dizziness when mixed with alcohol); or Glucophage (which can cause lactic acidosis).
- Always sip alcoholic drinks slowly.

- If you are a man and taking insulin, you can include two alcoholic beverages in addition to your regular meal plan. If you are a woman taking insulin, then you can include one alcoholic beverage. Do not omit food in exchange for an alcoholic drink.
- If you are not taking insulin (and watching your weight), you can substitute alcohol for fat choices and in some cases extra starch choices (sweet wines, sweet vermouth, and wine coolers).

Can I Use Fructose in My Diabetic Diet?

How would you answer this question from your diabetic client? Fructose has been touted as a sweetener for persons with diabetes because it is a naturally occurring sugar that is as much as 1.5 times as sweet as sucrose. However, can the person with diabetes use it safely?

Although fructose as a sweetener is not for all persons with diabetes, generally you can reply, "Yes, but with qualifications." The following should be considered:

- Advertising claims promoting fructose are sometimes so misleading that many consumers mistakenly believe that it can be used as a "free" food. However, fructose has the same nutritive value as other sugars—4 kcal/g. Persons with T1DM should especially be instructed to use fructose as carefully as they use any other food with a caloric and carbohydrate value.
- The quantity must be limited. If used, then the maximum amount is 75 g/day.
- Consumption of fructose in large amounts may have adverse effects on plasma lipids. It may also cause loose stools and gas when consumed in amounts greater than approximately 25 g/serving.
- The sweetness of fructose varies with temperature, acidity, and dilution. It has been used satisfactorily in some cooked desserts. However, with high temperatures, a rise in pH, and increased concentration of solution, its sweetness is reduced.

TO SUM UP

Whatever methods or materials we use, one central fact remains: The person who has diabetes is the most important and a fully equal member of the diabetes care team. Interdisciplinary approaches and strategies that involve this recognition can be developed.

Diabetes mellitus is a syndrome composed of many metabolic disorders collectively characterized by hyperglycemia and other symptoms. Treatment relies heavily on a basic type of therapy—a carefully controlled diet. Diabetes is classified in four categories: (1) *T1DM*, (2) *T2DM*, (3) *GDM*, and (4) *prediabetes*.

Blood glucose levels are controlled primarily by hormones of pancreatic islet cells: insulin, which facilitates passage of glucose through cell membranes via special membrane receptors; glucagon, which ensures adequate levels of glucose to prevent hypoglycemia; and somatostatin, which controls the actions of insulin and glucagon to maintain normal blood glucose levels. Diabetes results from inadequate insulin secretion or insulin resistance from too few receptor sites. Symptoms range from polydipsia, polyuria, polyphagia, and signs of abnormal energy metabolism to fluid and electrolyte imbalances, acidosis, and coma in seriously uncontrolled conditions.

Approximately 5%–10% of all persons with diabetes have T1DM, which often develops during childhood or adolescence. Treatment involves blood glucose self-monitoring, insulin administration, and regular meals and exercise to balance insulin activity. T2DM occurs mostly in adults, particularly those who are overweight. Acidosis is rare. Treatment consists of weight management and exercise. The food plan for both types of diabetes should be low in saturated fats and cholesterol to reduce cardiovascular risk. Moderate regular exercise increases efficiency of insulin and aids in weight management. GDM occurs in 2%–5% of all pregnancies.

QUESTIONS FOR REVIEW

1. Describe the major characteristics of T1DM and T2DM. Explain how these characteristics influence differences in NT. List and describe medications used to control these conditions.
2. Identify and explain symptoms of uncontrolled diabetes mellitus.
3. Describe three major complications of uncontrolled diabetes. What therapy is used in the DCCT designed to achieve and maintain normal blood glucose levels and help avoid these complications?
4. Glenn just found out that he has diabetes mellitus. He is a sedentary, 45-year-old man who is 170 cm (5'8") tall and weighs 94 kg (210 lb). No medications were prescribed for him. What is his BMI? If he decides to drink, then how much alcohol could be allowed and how should he fit it into his diet? Defend your answer. Glenn wants to help his children reduce their chances of developing diabetes. What advice would you offer?

REFERENCES

1. Centers for Disease Control and Prevention: *National diabetes fact sheet: general information and national estimates on diabetes in the Unit*, 2011, US Department of Health and Human Services, Centers for Disease Control and Prevention. from: http://www.cdc.gov/DIABETES/pubs/pdf/ndfs_2011.pdf.
2. American Diabetes Association: Diagnosis and classification of diabetes mellitus. Diabetes Care 33(Suppl 1):S62, 2010.
3. American Diabetes Association: The cost of diabetes, Alexandria, VA, 2012, American Diabetes Association. from: http://www.diabetes.org/advocate/resources/cost-of-diabetes.html.
4. Whitehouse FW: Classification and pathogenesis of the diabetes syndrome: a historical perspective. *J Am Diet Assoc* 81(3):243, 1982.
5. Nestle M: A case of diabetes mellitus. *N Engl J Med* 81:127, 1982.
6. Bliss M: The discovery of insulin. Chicago, 1982, University of Chicago Press.
7. Atkinson MA, Eisenbarth GS: Type 1 diabetes: new perspectives on disease pathogenesis and treatment. *Lancet* 358(9277):221, 2001.
8. McKeigue PM, Shah B, Marmot MG: Relation of central obesity and insulin resistance with high diabetes prevalence and cardiovascular risk in South Asians. *Lancet* 337:382, 1991.
9. Dowse GK, Zimmet PZ, Gareeboo H, et al: Abdominal obesity and physical inactivity as risk factors for NIDDM and impaired glucose tolerance in Indian, Creole, and Chinese Mauritians. *Diabetes Care* 14(4):271, 1991.
10. National Diabetes Education Program: Overview of diabetes in children and adolescents, Washington, DC, June 2011, US Department of Health and Human Services. from: <www.ndep.nih.gov/diabetes/youth/youth_FS.htm#IdentifyingType2>.
11. American Diabetes Association: Standards of medical care in diabetes—2011. *Diabetes Care* 34(Suppl 1):S11, 2011.
12. Dabelea D, Snell-Bergeon JK, Heartsfield CL, et al: Increasing prevalence of gestational diabetes mellitus (GDM) over time and by birth cohort. *Diabetes Care* 28:579, 2005.
13. Tuomilehto J, Lindstrom J, Eriksson JG, et al: Prevention of type 2 diabetes mellitus by changes in lifestyle among subjects with impaired glucose tolerance. *N Engl J Med* 344:1343–1350, 2001.

14. Pan XR, Li GW, Hu YH, et al: Effects of diet and exercise in preventing NIDDM in people with impaired glucose tolerance: the Da Qing IGT and Diabetes Study. *Diabetes Care* 20:537, 1997.

15. Wendorf M, Goldfine ID: Archeology of NIDDM—excavation of the thrifty genotype. *Diabetes* 40:161, 1991.

16. Diabetes Control and Complications Trial Research Group: The effect of intensive treatment of diabetes on the development and progression of long-term complications in insulin-dependent diabetes mellitus. *N Engl J Med* 329:977, 1993.

17. Franz MJ, Bantle JP, Beebe CA, et al: Evidence-based nutrition principles and recommendations for the treatment and prevention of diabetes and related complications. *Diabetes Care* 25:148, 2002.

18. American Diabetes Association: Translation of the diabetes nutrition recommendations for health care institutions. *Diabetes Care* 25(Suppl): S61, 2002.

19. American Diabetes Association: Nutrition recommendations and interventions for diabetes. *Diabetes Care* 31(Suppl):S61, 2008.

20. American Diabetes Association: Implications of the Diabetes Control and Complications Trial (position statement). *Diabetes Care* 25:S25, 2002.

21. Delahanty LM, Halford BN: The role of diet behaviors in achieving improved glycemic control in intensively treated patients in the Diabetes Control and Complications Trial. *Diabetes Care* 16:1453, 1993.

22. Harris MI, Eastman RC: Is there a glycemic threshold for mortality risk? *Diabetes Care* 21:331, 1998.

23. The Oxford Center for Diabetes, Endocrinology and Metabolism Diabetes Trials Unit: UK prospective diabetes study, Oxford, England, 1998, Oxford Center for Diabetes, Endocrinology and Metabolism. from: http://www.dtu.ox.ac.uk/ukpds_trial/index.php.

24. Murray P, Chune GW, Raghavan VA: Legacy effects from DCCT and UKPDS: what they mean and implications for future diabetes trials. *Curr Atheroscler Rep* 12(6):432, 2010.

25. Ousman Y, Sharma M: The irrefutable importance of glycemic control. *Clin Diabetes* 19:71, 2001.

26. American Diabetes Association: Implications of the United Kingdom Prospective Diabetes Study (position statement). *Diabetes Care* 25:S28, 2002.

27. Thomas AM, Gutierrez YM: American Dietetic Association guide to gestational diabetes mellitus. Chicago, 2005, American Dietetic Association.

28. American Diabetes Association: Gestational diabetes mellitus (position statement). *Diabetes Care* 27(Suppl):88S, 2004.

29. Anderson EJ, Richardson M, Castle G, et al: The DCCT Research Group: nutrition interventions for the intensive therapy in the Diabetes Control and Complications Trial. *J Am Diet Assoc* 93(7):768, 1993.

30. Buchanan TA, Xiang A, Kjos SL, et al: What is gestational diabetes? *Diabetes Care* 30(Suppl 2):S105, 2007.

31. Ross TA, Boucher JL, O'Connell BS: American Dietetic Association guide to diabetes medical nutrition therapy and education. Chicago, 2005, American Dietetic Association.

32. American Diabetes Association: Alcohol, Alexandria, Va., 2010, American Diabetes Association. from: http://www.diabetes.org/food-and-fitness/food/what-can-i-eat/alcohol.html.

33. Joslin Diabetes Center: Managing diabetes: Fitting alcohol into your meal plan. Boston, 2006, Joslin Diabetes Center. from: http://www.joslin.org/info/Fitting_Alcohol_Into_Your_Meal_Plan.html.

FURTHER READINGS AND RESOURCES

Websites of Interest

American Association of Diabetes Educators (AADE): As a multidisciplinary organization of health professionals who teach about diabetes, the AADE and its website provide information about the scope of practice and standards related to diabetes education; the website also has information and AADE publications: https://www.aadenet.org.

American Diabetes Association: The American Diabetes Association publishes many health professional and client materials in addition to its scientific journals; in an annual supplement to *Diabetes Care*, the American Diabetes Association reissues its practice guidelines that address a wide array of clinical issues, including nutrition; these guidelines can be downloaded from the American Diabetes Association website free of charge; local information about American Diabetes Association activities can be obtained from either the website or toll-free telephone number; diabetes self-management educational programs that are reviewed and receive American Diabetes Association "recognition" are covered by Medicare and other third-party payers: http://www.diabetes.org; 1-800-DIABETES.

Centers for Disease Control and Prevention, National Center for Chronic Disease Prevention and Health Promotion, Diabetes Public Health Resource: This site has information about the Diabetes Control Program in each state and diabetes-related statistics such as the rise in the prevalence and incidence of diabetes; the National Diabetes Fact Sheet *CDC Information* is available as a downloadable file: https://www.cdc.gov/diabetes; 1-877-CDC-DIAB.

Diabetes Care and Education (DCE) Practice Group of the Academy of Nutrition and Dietetics: The DCE publishes *On the Cutting Edge*, a theme-centered newsletter on timely topics related to nutrition and diabetes; educational materials developed by the DCE are available for purchase from the Academy of Nutrition and Dietetics; the DCE website provides information about the Medicare MNT benefits for persons with diabetes, Health Care Financing Administration (HFCA) rules for American Diabetes Association Education Recognition Programs reimbursement, and Current Procedural Terminology (CPT) codes for MNT; the website also provides information about the DCE publications and e-mail listserv: https://www.dce.org; http://www.eatright.org.

National Diabetes Education Program (NDEP): The NDEP is a federally sponsored initiative that involves public and private partnerships to improve the treatment and outcomes for people with diabetes through a variety of activities; the NDEP publications include a newsletter, materials for people with diabetes (in several languages), materials for health care providers, materials for organizations, and media kits; single copies of most materials are available free of charge or can be downloaded from the NDEP website: https://www.ndep.nih.gov; 1-800-860-8747.

National Institutes of Diabetes and Digestive and Kidney Diseases (NIDDK), National Diabetes Information Clearinghouse (NDIC): The NIDDK website provides information about its diabetes-related clinical trials and other research programs, a directory of diabetes organizations, health education programs, and diabetes-related topics; downloadable files include *Diabetes Dateline*, an NIDDK newsletter; client education materials; and information for health professionals; the NIDDK website also includes the National Diabetes Information Clearinghouse, which disseminates information about online and print materials and provides access to database searches for diabetes-related references: https://www.niddk.nih.gov.

23

Renal Disease

Joyce Gilbert

ⓔ http://evolve.elsevier.com/Williams/essentials/

This chapter reviews basic kidney function and pathophysiology of kidney diseases. Nutrition assessment methodology and nutritional recommendations for chronic kidney disease (CKD), maintenance dialysis therapy, postrenal transplantation, acute renal failure (ARF), renal stones, and urinary tract infection (UTI) are discussed.

OUTLINE

Basic Kidney Function
Chronic Kidney Disease
  Pathophysiology of Glomerular Disease
  Treatment of Chronic Kidney Disease
  Nutrition Assessment of Patients With Chronic Kidney Disease
  Altered Nutrient Requirements With Chronic Kidney Disease
  Medical Nutrition Therapy

Acute Renal Failure
Urolithiasis (Calculi or Kidney Stones)
Urinary Tract Infection
Resources
Health Promotion
  Omega-3 Fatty Acids and Renal Disease

BASIC KIDNEY FUNCTION

The main functions of the kidney are excretory, regulatory, and endocrine. The excretory function serves to remove potentially toxic metabolic waste products such as urea, the major end product of protein metabolism, from the blood. The regulatory function controls electrolyte, acid-base, and fluid balance. The result is maintenance of proper serum concentrations of sodium, potassium, calcium, phosphorus, chloride, bicarbonate, and hydrogen ions. The endocrine functions include conversion of the biologically inactive form of vitamin D (25-hydroxycholecaliciferol) to the biologically active vitamin D (1,25-dihydroxycholecalciferol), synthesis of erythropoietin (needed for red blood cell production in the bone marrow), and synthesis and release of renin, which regulates systemic blood pressure.[1]

These functions are accomplished by the unique architecture of the nephron, the basic functioning unit of the kidney. Each human adult kidney consists of approximately 1 million nephrons (Fig. 23.1). The key structures of the nephron are the glomerulus and the tubules.

Glomerulus

At the head of each nephron, blood enters in a single capillary and then branches into a group of collateral capillaries. This tuft of collateral capillaries is held closely together in a cup-shaped membrane. This cup-shaped capsule is named *Bowman capsule* for the young English physician Sir William Bowman. In 1843 Bowman established the basis of plasma filtration and consequent urine secretion from the interrelationship of blood-filled glomeruli and enveloping membrane. The filtrate formed here is cell free and virtually protein free.

Tubules

Continuous with the base of Bowman capsule, nephron tubules wind in a series of convolutions toward their terminal in the renal pelvis. The following list details specific reabsorption functions performed by the four sections of the tubule:

1. *Proximal tubule:* In the first section nearest the glomerulus, major nutrient reabsorption occurs. Essentially, 100% of the glucose and

---

> ### KEY TERM
>
> **Nephron**
> Microscopic anatomic and functional unit of the kidney that selectively filters and resorbs essential blood factors, secretes hydrogen ions as needed for maintaining acid-base balance, and then resorbs water to protect body fluids and forms and excretes a concentrated urine for elimination of wastes. The nephron includes the renal corpuscle (glomerulus), proximal convoluted tubule, loop of Henle, distal convoluted tubule, and collecting tubule, which empties the urine into the renal medulla. The urine passes into the papilla and then to the pelvis of the kidney. Urine is formed by filtration of blood in the glomerulus and by the selective reabsorption and secretion of solutes by cells that constitute the walls of the renal tubes. Approximately 1 million nephrons exist in each kidney.

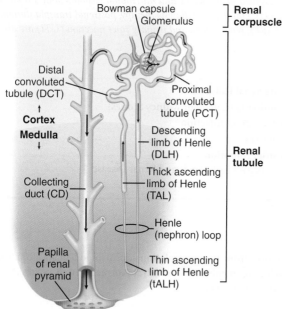

FIG. 23.1 (A) Kidney structure. **(B)** Components of nephron. (From Thibodeau GA, Patton KT: *Anatomy & physiology*, ed 7, St Louis, 2010, Mosby.)

amino acids and 80%–85% of the water, sodium, potassium, chloride, and most other substances are reabsorbed. Only 15%–30% of the filtrate remains to enter the next section.

2. *Loop of Henle:* This narrowed midsection of the renal tubule is named for the German anatomist Friedrich Henle, who in 1845 first demonstrated its unique structure and function in creating the necessary fluid pressures for ultimately forming concentrated urine. At this narrowed midsection, the thin loop of the tubule dips into the central renal **medulla**. Here, through a balanced system of water and sodium exchange through sodium pumps in the limbs of the loop (the countercurrent system), important fluid density is created surrounding the loop. This area of increased density in the central part of the kidney is important to concentrate urine through osmotic pressure, because the lower collecting tubule later passes through this same area of the kidney.

3. *Distal tubule:* This latter portion of tubule functions primarily in providing acid-base balance through secretion of ionized hydrogen. It also conserves sodium by reabsorbing it under the influence of the hormones aldosterone and vasopressin (also called *antidiuretic hormone* [ADH]).

4. *Collecting tubule:* In this final widened section of the tubule, filtrate is concentrated to save water and form urine for excretion. Water is absorbed under the influence of pituitary hormone vasopressin (ADH) and osmotic pressure of the denser surrounding fluid in this central part of the kidney. The resulting volume of urine, now concentrated and excreted, is only 0.5%–1% of the original water and solutes filtered at the beginning in Bowman capsule.

It is through these specialized anatomic components that the kidney serves to maintain homeostasis of the body's internal environment.[1]

KEY TERM

Medulla
Inner tissue substance of the kidney.

CHRONIC KIDNEY DISEASE

Chronic kidney disease (CKD) is a syndrome in which progressive, irreversible losses of excretory, endocrine, and metabolic capacities of the kidney occur as a result of kidney damage (Table 23.1). Determination of renal function requires evaluation of glomerular filtration rate (GFR), which is accomplished through clearance tests. Clearance tests measure the rate at which substances are cleared from the plasma by the glomerulus. In clinical practice, GFR is best approximated by using prediction equations and factoring in serum creatinine concentration, age, gender, race, and body size. Recommended prediction equations for adults are the Modification of Diet in Renal Disease (MDRD) study and Cockcroft-Gault equations.[2] A normal GFR is 125 mL/min/1.73 m². As kidney disease progresses, the GFR falls. Chronic renal failure progresses slowly over time and may include periods during which kidney function remains stable. However, once the disease progresses to stage 5 kidney failure, continuance of life requires initiation of maintenance **dialysis** therapy or subsequent kidney transplantation[3] (see the Case Study box, "The Patient with Chronic Renal Failure").

CKD is a public health problem. The incidence and prevalence of end-stage renal disease (ESRD) have increased 20% to 25% in the United States during the past decade.[4] Of the group being treated by dialysis, 97 per million were older than age 70, compared with 2.1 per million who were children[3] (see the Focus on Culture box, "Kidney Failure: Another Equal Opportunity Disease?"). The total cost for the CKD problem continues to increase.

TABLE 23.1   Stages of Chronic Kidney Disease[a]

Stage	Description	GFR Range (mL/min/1.73 m²)
1	Kidney damage with normal or ↑ GFR	≥90
2	Kidney damage with mild ↓ GRF	60–89
3	Moderate ↓ GFR	30–59
4	Severe ↓ GFR	15–29
5	Kidney failure	<15 (or dialysis)

[a]CKD is defined as either kidney damage or GFR <60 mL/min/ 1.73 m² for ≥3 months. Kidney damage is defined as pathologic abnormalities or markers of damage, including abnormalities in blood or urine tests or imaging studies.

CKD, Chronic kidney disease; *GFR,* glomerular filtration rate.
Modified from National Kidney Foundation: K/DOQI clinical practice guidelines for chronic kidney disease: evaluation, classification and stratification, *Am J Kidney Dis* 39(Suppl 1):S1, 2002.

CASE STUDY

The Patient With Chronic Renal Failure

Mr. Steinberg is 45 years old, married, and works as a city planner for a large municipal government. He cited a recent history of nausea, anorexia, **hematuria**, and swollen ankles during a physical examination. His wife reported that he had been tiring more easily than usual during the past year. A history of prior illnesses proved negative, except for a severe case of influenza with sore throat 10 years before during an epidemic when he was stationed with the Army overseas. Tests were ordered, and the patient was advised to return in 1 week for review of the test results (and sooner if any changes in his symptoms were noted).

Mr. Steinberg did return, with additional symptoms of headaches and occasionally blurred vision. At that time his blood pressure was 160/98 mm Hg, his temperature was 37.5°C (99.6°F), and he had lost 4 kg (8¾ lb). Laboratory tests showed albumin and red and white blood cells in the urine, with an elevated **blood urea nitrogen (BUN)**; a phenolsulfonphthalein (PSP) test indicated a reduced filtration rate. The diagnosis was chronic renal failure.

The physician discussed the diagnosis and its serious prognosis with Mr. and Mrs. Steinberg, giving them the benefits and disadvantages of **hemodialysis** and kidney transplantation. Antihypertensive medication was prescribed along with other drugs to minimize discomfort.

During the following weeks, Mr. Steinberg continued to lose weight, had increasing joint pain, and became anemic. He found it increasingly difficult to maintain his hectic schedule of frequent meetings, conferences, and public speeches because of gastrointestinal (GI) bleeding, increasing nausea, and occasional muscle spasms. Small mouth sores made eating very difficult.

Finally, the Steinbergs informed the physician of their decision to accept the kidney transplant as a means of controlling the disease process. They were referred to the registered dietitian (RD) for renal diet counseling to control protein, sodium, potassium, phosphate, and fluids, as well as to ensure adequate kilocalorie (kcalories or kcal) intake. After discussing these needs for nutritional maintenance before surgery, the RD helped them develop a meal plan based on Mr. Steinberg's food preferences. Food selection and preparation were discussed in detail, with many ideas for building in as much variety and taste appeal as possible.

The Steinbergs' follow-up with the food plan was excellent. One month later the laboratory values were almost normal, blood pressures averaged 140/88 mm Hg, the headaches and blurred vision had virtually disappeared, and Mr. Steinberg had gained 3.2 kg (7 lb) of his lost weight. The nutrient supplements, including the amino acid analogs, were taken each day as instructed.

Fortunately a kidney donor was soon found, and with the aid of drug control of immune responses the transplant surgery was apparently a success. Mr. Steinberg convalesced well at home, kept all follow-up visits with the health care team, and has continued to be asymptomatic 1 year after surgery.

Questions for Analysis

1. Identify a metabolic imbalance caused by chronic renal failure that may account for each symptom presented by Mr. Steinberg.
2. What factors affect the amount of protein needed by persons with chronic renal failure? What amounts are usually used? Why? What are the amino acid analogs used with the low-protein diet, and why are they used?
3. What factors affect the amount of sodium needed by persons with chronic renal failure? How much is usually recommended?
4. Why is it important to control potassium levels? How much is recommended? What clinical signs presented by Mr. Steinberg may indicate that he had not been getting enough potassium?
5. Why is control of phosphate important in the diet for chronic renal failure? What additional means may be used to control it?
6. What factors affect fluid balance in chronic renal failure? How much is usually allowed?
7. Outline a general teaching plan you would use to instruct the Steinbergs about the presurgical and postsurgical dietary needs.

KEY TERMS

Dialysis
Process of separating crystalloids and colloids in solution by the difference in their rates of diffusion through a semipermeable membrane; crystalloids pass through readily, and colloids pass through only very slowly or not at all.

Hematuria
The abnormal presence of blood in the urine.

Blood Urea Nitrogen (BUN)
The nitrogen component of urea in the blood; a measure of kidney function; elevated levels of BUN indicate a disorder of kidney function.

Hemodialysis
Removal of certain elements from the blood according to their rates of diffusion through a semipermeable membrane (e.g., by a hemodialysis machine).

KEY TERMS

Glomerulonephritis
A form of nephritis affecting the capillary loops in an acute short-term infection. It may progress to a more serious chronic condition leading to irreversible renal failure.

PATHOPHYSIOLOGY OF GLOMERULAR DISEASE

The majority of nondiabetic glomerular diseases are the result of immune-mediated mechanisms. Although renal injury induced by antibody alone is known to occur, the mechanisms involved in renal injury that results from antigen-antibody complex formation are better understood. Antigen-antibody complex formation occurs as a result of antibody reacting either to circulating antigens or to native kidney antigens expressed on renal cell membranes. Immune complex deposition may occur within the glomerular basement membrane (GBM), between the GBM and epithelial cell (subepithelial), between the GBM and endothelial cell (subendothelial), or within the mesangial matrix. The pattern of immune complex deposition within the glomerulus is helpful diagnostically because different diseases have characteristic patterns.[4,5] For example, membranous nephropathy is characterized in part by subepithelial immune complex deposition (Figs. 23.2 and 23.3).

The most common causes of CKD are diabetic nephropathy and hypertension. Other common causes of kidney failure include glomerulonephritis, cystic kidney disease, and urologic disease.[4] Table 23.1 outlines the stages of chronic kidney disease.

FOCUS ON CULTURE

Kidney Failure: Another Equal Opportunity Disease?

Of the millions of Americans currently living with kidney disease, a disproportionate number are African American. This reflects an incidence rate fourfold greater than that of European-Americans and is most commonly attributed to increased prevalence of high blood pressure, diabetes, and a familial history of the disease. However, not only are African Americans at an increased risk for developing kidney disease, but they also seem to acquire it earlier in life, with almost half not knowing they have the condition until dialysis is required.

This is a startling realization, considering early interventions can limit damage done to the kidneys. Later diagnosis of kidney disease can result in increased rates of chronic problems, dialysis dependency, and need for transplantation. The difficulty is that relatively few African Americans receive screening or intervention. Adding to the problem, with diabetes being the primary risk factor for kidney disease, one-third of the cases of diabetes among African Americans go undiagnosed, demonstrating the need for further screening.

According to the National Kidney Foundation, African Americans represent 13% of the American population but make up 35% of those on kidney transplant waiting lists. Consequently, although an increased kidney transplant demand exists for African Americans, a moderately low donorship rate is seen from this group, compounding the problem.

Whether the increased rate of kidney disease in African Americans stems from lack of awareness, lack of health care, or genetic factors, the fact remains that African Americans possess many risk factors affecting renal health. Screenings and education about blood glucose and blood pressure control at a younger age, along with lifestyle and medication interventions, have been shown to have dramatic results in kidney health. Unfortunately, only a small percentage actually receives these screenings or treatment. This problem is a major one that is made all the more disheartening by the unnecessary suffering involved. It is hoped that with increased attention brought to kidney disease, the incidence rate in the African-American population will decline.

Bibliography

Freedman BI, Spray BJ, Tuttle AB, et al: The familial risk of end-stage renal disease in African Americans, *Am J Kidney Dis* 21(4):387, 1993.

National Kidney Foundation: *Diabetes, chronic kidney disease and special populations*, New York. http://www.kidney.org/professionals/tools/diabetesandckd.cfm.

National Kidney and Urologic Diseases Information Clearinghouse, National Institute of Diabetes and Digestive and Kidney Diseases, National Institutes of Health: *Strategic plan on minority health disparities*, Bethesda, MD. http://www2.niddk.nih.gov/AboutNIDDK/ReportsAndStrategicPlanning/Strategic_Plan_Minority_Health_Disparities.htm.

Reif M, Hall P: *Kidney failure among African Americans*, Cincinnati, OH, 2001, Net Wellness. http://www.netwellness.org/healthtopics/kidney/faq2.cfm.

Tarver-Carr M, Powe NR, Eberhardt MS, et al: Excess risk of chronic kidney disease among African-American versus white subjects in the United States: a population-based study of potential explanatory factors, *J Am Soc Nephrol* 13:2363, 2002.

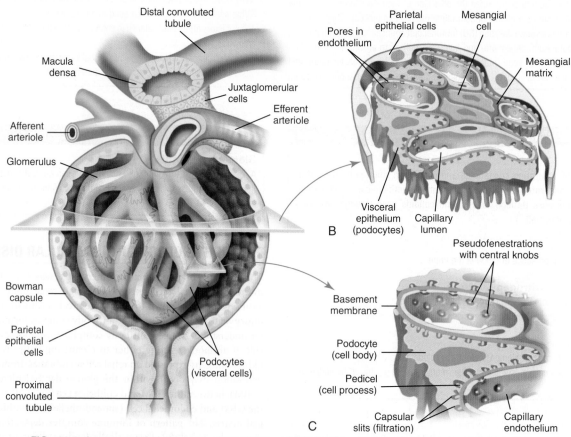

FIG. 23.2 Anatomy of the glomerulus and juxtaglomerular apparatus. **(A)** Longitudinal cross-section of glomerulus and juxtaglomerular apparatus. **(B)** Horizontal cross-section of glomerulus. **(C)** Enlargement of glomerular capillary filtration membrane. (From McCance K, Huether S: *Pathophysiology: the biologic basis for disease in adults and children*, ed 5, St Louis, 2006, Mosby.)

FIG. 23.3 Glomerular capillary. (A) Scanning electron micrograph of normal glomerular capillary (C) enclosed by podocytes (P) with primary processes and interdigitating foot processes. (B) Glomerular capillary wall showing foot processes of endothelial podocytes (F), filtration slit membrane (arrow), basement membrane (M), and fenestrated endothelium (E) (magnification, ×40,000). (From Kissane JM, editor: *Anderson's pathology*, ed 9, St Louis, 1990, Mosby.)

KEY TERMS

Complement
A complex series of enzymatic proteins occurring in normal serum that interact to combine with and augment (fill out, complete) the antigen-antibody complex of the body's immune system, producing lysis when the antigen is an intact cell; composed of 11 discrete proteins or functioning components, activated by the immunoglobulin factors IgG and IgM.

Deposition of immune complexes leads to activation of the complement system, which mediates injury through inflammatory or noninflammatory mechanisms. Chemotactic complement components formed as products of the activated complement cascade result in the migration of inflammatory cells into glomeruli. These cells, which include platelets, macrophages, and polymorphonuclear neutrophils (leukocytes), all produce products that are either directly cytotoxic or serve as mediators for further cell or matrix injury (e.g., proteases, reactive oxygen species, lipid mediators, cytokines). When subepithelial immune complexes activate complement, a noninflammatory mechanism is responsible for glomerular injury.[6]

TREATMENT OF CHRONIC KIDNEY DISEASE

The approach to treatment of CKD has shifted focus from diagnosis and treatment of established kidney diseases to detection and treatment at much earlier stages.[3] The clinical course of this disease can be significantly improved if specific interventions are instituted early in development of the disease. These include annual screening for microalbuminuria (greater than 30 mg/day or 20 mcg/min of albumin in the urine); improving glycemic control; aggressive antihypertensive therapy with angiotensin-converting enzymes or angiotensin receptor blockers; and lifestyle modifications that include weight loss, reduction in salt and alcohol intake, and exercise.[7]

Less traditional interventions that have been explored for their beneficial effects on renal disease include nutrients such as amino acids and carbohydrates. A class of nutrients that continues to be investigated for

potential benefits on progression of renal disease is omega-3 fatty acids (see section "Health Promotion" later in this chapter).

Through its initiative, *K/DOQI: Kidney Disease Outcomes Quality Initiative*, the National Kidney Foundation recently published clinical practice guidelines for evaluation, classification, and stratification of CKD.[3] A main rationale for development of these clinical guidelines was the accumulation of evidence that adverse effects of CKD, including kidney failure, cardiovascular disease (CVD), and premature death can be prevented or delayed by earlier testing and treatment of CKD.[3]

K/DOQI guidelines for CKD recommend that during health evaluations all individuals be evaluated as to whether they are at increased risk of having or developing renal disease. Individuals are to be considered at risk if they have diabetes, hypertension, autoimmune diseases, systemic infections, exposure to drugs or procedures associated with acute decline in kidney function, recovery from acute kidney failure, are older than 60 years, have a family history of kidney disease, or reduced kidney mass.[3] Table 23.1 identifies the stages of disease and associates each stage with a level of GFR. As the GFR falls below 60 mL/min/1.73 m², nutrition intervention becomes an important component of medical care.

NUTRITION ASSESSMENT OF PATIENTS WITH CHRONIC KIDNEY DISEASE

Malnutrition is a significant comorbidity of CKD, including patients on hemodialysis or peritoneal dialysis therapy.[5] Life-threatening malnutrition is present in 5%–10% of patients, and moderate malnutrition is present in an additional 20%–40%.[8] Factors contributing to malnutrition in patients with renal failure are listed in Box 23.1.

Evaluating and monitoring nutritional status are vital components of nutrition care of patients with kidney disease. The high prevalence of malnutrition, large number of aberrations in normal metabolism, and complications including anorexia and catabolism all indicate the need for consistent monitoring. Nutrition assessment is best completed by a registered dietitian (RD) who has received special training in renal nutrition care.

When completing a nutrition assessment, an array of indexes, each representing a specific data category, are measured independently and then evaluated collectively to ascertain the nutritional status of the renal patient. Table 23.2 lists the data categories that encompass the nutrition assessment of the renal patient. Specific indexes used to evaluate biochemical values are listed in Table 23.3. Following is a review of indexes most commonly measured from each data category.[9]

History and Physical Examination

Medical History. The medical record should include information concerning comorbid conditions, medications, past hospitalizations,

---

BOX 23.1 Factors Contributing to the Presence of Malnutrition in Patients With Chronic Renal Failure

1. Anorexia as a result of the following:
   - Nausea, emesis, medications
   - Uremia/uremic state of metabolism
   - Underdialysis
   - Accumulation of uremic toxins not completely removed by dialysis
2. Metabolic acidosis
3. Endocrine disorders (insulin resistance, **hyperparathyroidism**, impaired response to insulin-like growth factor I)
4. Comorbidity (infections, intercurrent illnesses)
5. Reduced nutrient intake

6. Dialysis related to the following:
   - Inadequate dose of dialysate
   - Catabolism (bioincompatible membrane)
   - Loss of amino acids and protein to the dialysate
   - Dialysate reused with bleach
7. Psychosocial
   - Depression
   - Inability to purchase or prepare food adequately
   - Loss of or poorly fitting dentures

Data from Wolfson M: Causes, manifestations, and assessment of malnutrition in chronic renal failure. In Kopple JD, Massry SG, editors: *Nutrition management of renal disease*, ed 2, Philadelphia, 2004, Lippincott Williams & Wilkins.

TABLE 23.2 Nutrition Assessment Parameters in Chronic Kidney Disease

Parameter	What It Measures	Components
History and physical examination	Past and present nutritional status; areas that should be addressed when developing a plan of care	Review of medical record
		Patient, family, and/or caregiver interview
		Psychosocial history
		Ability to obtain, prepare, ingest, and enjoy food
		Mental status
		Educational level
		Functional status
		Person responsible for shopping/preparing food
		Patient's functional status (activities of daily living)
		Diet histories: usual food intake, food intake patterns, and factors affecting intake
		Religious/cultural beliefs
		Use of supplements and alternative or complementary therapies
		Past diet restrictions (and education)
		Patient's ability to chew, swallow, taste, and smell foods
		Changes in appetite and eating pattern
		Food preferences, allergies, and intolerances
		Use of alcohol
		Practice of pica
Anthropometric assessment	Weight status; nutritional status; distribution of body fat, lean muscle mass, and bone	Body weight (can be difficult to determine because of fluid retention)
		Estimated dry weight or edema-free body weight
		Hemodialysis: weight post dialysis
		Peritoneal dialysis: weight after drainage of dialysate with peritoneum empty
		Interdialytic weight gains
		Fluid gains between hemodialysis treatments
		Height
		Initial measurement essential
		Recumbent bed height, arm span, or knee height may be used if patient cannot stand
		Estimation of frame size
		Body mass index
		Estimate of body composition
		Skinfold thicknesses

TABLE 23.2 Nutrition Assessment Parameters in Chronic Kidney Disease—cont'd

Parameter	What It Measures	Components
Energy and nutrient requirements	Must be individually assessed based on type of dialysis, cause of kidney disease, and other comorbidities	Kcalories per kg formulas
Subjective global assessment	Useful measure of protein-energy nutritional status in maintenance dialysis patients	4-item, 7-point scale Medical history Weight change during previous 6 months Dietary intake Gastrointestinal symptoms Physical examination Visual assessment of subcutaneous tissue and muscle mass
Biochemical parameters	Monitored on ongoing basis to assess nutritional status	See Table 23.3

Data from Barbá PD, Goode JL: Nutrition assessment in chronic kidney disease. In Byham-Gray L, Wiesen K, editors: *A clinical guide to nutrition care in kidney disease*, Chicago, 2004, American Dietetic Association.

TABLE 23.3 Biochemical Parameters for Assessing Nutritional Status

Parameter	Substance	Normal Range	CKD Range
Visceral protein stores	Albumin	3.5–5.0 g/dL	WNL for laboratory or >4.0 g/dL
	Prealbumin (transthyretin)	15–36 mg/dL	>30 mg/dL
	Transferrin	Female subjects: 15%–50% Male subjects: 20%–50%	WNL
	CRP	0.8 mg/dL	2–15 mg/dL
Static (somatic) protein reserves	Serum creatinine	Female subjects: 0.5–1.1 mg/dL Male subjects: 0.6–1.2 mg/dL	2–15 mg/dL
Other estimates of protein reserves	Nitrogen balance		
Fluid, electrolyte, and acid-base status	Sodium	135–145 mEq/L	WNL
	Potassium	3.5–5.0 mEq/L	3.5–6.0 mEq/L
	Calcium	WNL for laboratory	Normal: 8.4–10.2 mg/dL; preferably at low end of normal (8.4–9.5 mg/dL)
	Phosphorus	3.0–4.5 mg/dL	3.5–5.5 mg/dL
	CO_2	23–29 mEq/L	22–25 mEq/L
	Glucose	70–105 mg/dL	WNL <200 nonfasting before dialysis; intake has influence
Indirect indices of renal function and dialysis adequacy	Serum creatinine	Female subjects: 0.5–1.1 mg/dL Male subjects: 0.6–1.2 mg/dL	2–15 mg/dL
	BUN	10–20 mg/dL	60–80 mg/dL in anuric; well dialyzed and eating adequate protein
	Kt/V (hemodialysis)	N/A	1.2
	Kt/V (peritoneal dialysis)	N/A	2.0–2.2
Anemia	Hb	Female subjects: 12–16 g/dL Male subjects: 14–18 g/dL	Variable: 11–12 g/dL
	Ferritin	Female subjects: 10–150 mg/mL Male subjects: 12–300 mg/mL	≥100 mg/mL, but no known benefit >800 mg/mL
	Serum iron	Female subjects: 50–170 mcg/dL Male subjects: 60–175 mcg/dL	WNL
Hyperlipidemia	Serum cholesterol	<200 mg	WNL <150 mg; evaluate for nutrient deficit
	Triglycerides	Female subjects: 35–135 mg/dL Male subjects: 40–160 mg/dL	WNL <200 mg/dL
Renal osteodystrophy	Calcium	WNL for laboratory	Normal: 8.4–10.2 mg/dL; preferably at low end of normal (8.4–9.5 mg/dL)
	Alkaline phosphatase	30–85 U/mL	WNL for laboratory
	PHT (i) intact	10–65 pg/mL	150–300 pg/mL
	Biointact (third generation)	60–140 pg/mL	80–160 pg/mL

BUN, blood urea nitrogen; *CKD*, chronic kidney disease; *CRP*, C-reactive protein; *Hb*, hemoglobin; *Kt/V*, K-dialyzer clearance of urea; t-dialysis time; V-volume of distribution of urea; *N/A*, not applicable; *PHT*, parathyroid hormone; *WNL*, within normal limits.

Data from Barbá PD, Goode JL: Nutrition assessment in chronic kidney disease. In Byham-Gray L, Wiesen K, editors: *A clinical guide to nutrition care in kidney disease*, Chicago, 2004, American Dietetic Association; Wilkens KG: Medical nutrition therapy for renal disorders. In Mahan LK, Escott-Stump S, editors: *Krause's food & nutrition therapy*, ed 12, St. Louis, 2008, Saunders.

weight history, socioeconomic status, and functional status, as well as information from the physical examination. Any major organ or gastrointestinal (GI) diseases, surgeries, or previous symptoms of malabsorption or other digestive problems, including nausea, vomiting, and diarrhea, should be noted. Impairment in fluid and electrolyte balance, hypertension and hypotension, proteinuria, and any previous symptoms of uremia that affect appetite, food intake, digestion, or nutritional status should also be noted.

Psychosocial History. A psychosocial history evaluates a patient's mental status, as well as factors regarding economics, education level, physical home environment, food shopping and preparation capabilities, and available support systems. The goal is to create an individualized intervention the patient or patient's support system can understand and apply. Factors that might compromise nutritional status include depression or improper food preparation and storage equipment. This component of the assessment process helps identify patients requiring social services to assist with economic needs or special services to provide regular access to food and medications.

Demographics. Information on age, marital status, gender, and ethnicity is needed to assess nutritional status. Many reference standards used to classify clinical indexes adjust for gender and age. Knowledge of ethnicity affects the ability to individualize nutrition therapy; marital status helps identify support systems.

Physical Activity. Assessment of the patient's physical capabilities is needed to maintain activities of daily living (ADLs) and proper level of physical exercise for psychologic and physical therapeutics. The following questionnaires have been validated for the purpose of measuring physical activity and physical functioning in the ESRD patient population: the Stanford 7-Day Physical Activity Recall, Physical Activity Scale for the Elderly, Human Activity Profile, and Medical Outcomes Study Short-Form 36-Item Questionnaire.

Current Medical and Surgical Issues. Identification of nutritional implications of medical and surgical problems is imperative for the nutrition assessment procedure. For the patient with chronic, progressive disease, this requires acknowledgment of any newly diagnosed medical and surgical illnesses.

Diet and Food Intake

This category relies on subjective patient reporting to evaluate qualitative and quantitative aspects of food intake. One of the most useful outputs from this category is calculation of nutrient intake. Other outputs include information related to past and current food intake (qualitative and quantitative), eating patterns, and specific food preferences. This information allows an approximation of the diet's adequacy. It also helps identify nutrient factors that may be contributing to medical problems. Qualitative data are essential for formulation of individual diet therapy, including meal plans and menus.

Diet History. Nutrition history is usually obtained at the initial meeting. It is an all-inclusive collection of some objective, but primarily subjective, information concerning the patient's food consumption, such as aversions, allergies, preferences, and intake. Information on previous and current diet intake assists in devising interventions to improve diet or devising an acceptable therapeutic meal plan. The most commonly used tools to obtain food intake information differ in approach to data collection, retrospective versus prospective, and whether the information is a qualitative description of intake versus a quantitative one.

Food record. A food record provides qualitative and approximate quantitative food intake information that is best collected prospectively. The minimal time recommended for data collection is 3 days; a reasonable maximum is 5 days. The patient should provide intake information for weekends and weekdays so that variability can be determined. For the dialysis patient, it is strongly recommended the food record include intake for days on which dialysis takes place, as well as those on which it does not, in addition to a weekend versus weekday pattern. A difference in food intake between dialysis and nondialysis days has been noted in the type and amount of food selected.

The patient should be provided with instructions on how to approximate food portion sizes and servings of fluid to ensure accurate reporting. Use of food models is very helpful. The food record should include time of day of any intake (meals and snacks), names of foods eaten, approximate amount of food ingested, method of preparation, and special recipes or steps taken in the food preparation. The same instructions apply to fluid intake. Brand names are requested when available.

Some patients find it is more convenient to record food intake at the end of the day. This is an inferior method because the data collection becomes retrospective and more subject to error. Calculation of intake of total protein, protein quality, carbohydrate, fat, fatty acid classes, and other selected nutrients is best completed by a computerized nutrient analysis program.

24-Hour food recall. The 24-hour food recall is an interactive tool in which the clinician assists the patient in remembering qualitative and quantitative food intake via prompting. The clinician can sit with a patient during dialysis and slowly help the patient recall the previous day's intake of food and fluid. Food models or drawings can be used to help the patient identify portion size. However, one 24-hour recall does not provide sufficient information to ascertain total food intake.

A variation of the 24-hour recall for a dialysis patient is to meet with the patient during three consecutive treatments, or at least four sessions within a 2-week period, and obtain one 24-hour recall at each visit. Effort should be made to obtain a recall for a weekend day, a dialysis day, and a nondialysis day. To obtain a total food intake on a dialysis day, the practitioner can ask the patient what he or she had to eat so far that day and record it. The patient or family member can finish recording for the rest of the day, or the clinician can meet with the patient at the next session to help him or her recall what was eaten for the rest of that day. Calling the patient's home on a daily basis to obtain the needed information is an option but is not practical.

Food frequency questionnaires. Food frequency questionnaires (FFQs) approximate nutrient intake by identifying periodicity of intake of specific foods within food groups that are significant sources of a particular nutrient or nutrients (e.g., dairy products are a good source of calcium, vitamin D, and protein). A food frequency consists of listing foods according to group, such as vegetables, fruits, dairy, protein, and so forth. The patient is questioned as to how often he or she eats this food per day, per week, and per month. An approximation of adequacy of intake of specific nutrients can be calculated from the results.

Biochemical Values

Serum biochemical values are used to assess and monitor nutritional status over time. Selected serum values pertain to visceral protein stores, static protein reserves, overall protein nutriture, immune competence, and iron stores, as well as vitamin, mineral, and trace element status. In addition to

---

KEY TERM

Proteinuria
The presence of an excess of serum proteins, such as albumin, in the urine.

these components, nutrition assessment involves evaluating fluid, electrolyte, and acid-base status; renal function; dialysis adequacy for the patient receiving replacement therapy; serum lipid levels; and bone health.

Visceral Protein Stores

Serum albumin. Albumin, the most abundant plasma protein, functions to maintain plasma oncotic pressure and serves as a major carrier protein for drugs, hormones, enzymes, and trace elements. Clinically significant hypoalbuminemia occurs with different types of malnutrition besides kidney disease (e.g., protein-energy kwashiorkor, uncomplicated) in children and adults. In these conditions, hypoalbuminemia usually indicates other metabolic derangements, as well as a poor prognosis. From these observations, serum albumin became a part of routine nutrition assessment of the hospitalized patient and subsequently the renal patient.

Although serum albumin levels have been used extensively in clinical practice, research studies, and nutritional surveys to assess nutritional status of the CKD population, reliability and sensitivity of this parameter have been questioned. Concerns are independent of conditions that change serum albumin as a marker of visceral protein stores. Use of albumin for assessment purposes has been criticized because of its long half-life, averaging 14–20 days, and large body pool, 4–5 mg/kg, making albumin slow to respond to changes in visceral protein stores. It is therefore a late marker of malnutrition.

Prealbumin (thyroxine-binding prealbumin, transthyretin). Prealbumin is a carrier protein for retinol-binding protein (RBP) and thus has a major role in transport of thyroxine. Its short half-life of 2–3 days and its small body pool make it more sensitive than albumin to changes in protein status. This was the first visceral protein found to be low in healthy children who were eating marginal amounts of protein. In primates, prealbumin reflects overall nitrogen balance during starvation and refeeding. Decreases in serum levels occur independently of nutritional status when acute metabolic stress is seen, including trauma, minor stress, and inflammation. Serum concentration has also been observed to decrease in liver disease and with iron supplementation. Prealbumin can be useful as a nutritional marker after acute metabolic stress.

The low molecular weight of prealbumin (approximately 54,980 daltons) precludes its use as a marker of nutritional status in patients with CKD who have a decreased GFR. Prealbumin levels have been reported to be elevated in the euvolemic patient with chronic renal failure. In hemodialysis patients, high levels have been observed and are attributed to decreased renal catabolism. A decline in the proportion of circulating free

prealbumin versus that complexed with RBP may explain the diminished catabolism and therefore the elevated levels. A concentration of less than 30 mg/dL (normal range, 10–40 mg/dL) may indicate malnutrition in the hemodialysis patient and has recently been associated with an increased risk of death. These studies indicate prealbumin level may serve as a better nutrition assessment tool and predictor of patient outcome than the traditionally used serum albumin in the dialysis population.

Transferrin (siderophilin). The main function of transferrin is to bind ferrous iron and to transport iron to the bone marrow. Its half-life of 8–10 days and small body pool enable it to respond more rapidly to short-term changes in protein status, compared with albumin. Its value is influenced by iron pool status and needs to be assessed in conjunction with this value.

C-reactive protein. C-reactive protein (CRP) mirrors the acute-phase response to inflammation. Increases are regulated by the rise in circulating cytokines and tumor necrosis factor-α (TNF-α), very powerful determinants of albumin levels in CKD patients.

Body Weight

Initial assessment of body weight and monitoring of weight change over time represent critical components of the nutrition assessment process. Weight loss in excess of 5%–10%, depending on the patient's overall nutritional status, or substandard weight for height should be considered a risk factor for malnutrition. Interrelationships between weight loss over time and outcome in the renal patient population have not yet been reported.

Body mass index (BMI), current weight, usual weight, ideal body weight (IBW), percentage usual weight, percentage IBW, and, particularly, percentage weight change over a defined time period are important parameters of body weight. A database or sheet in the patient's chart committed to record body weight is recommended for every patient.

ALTERED NUTRIENT REQUIREMENTS WITH CHRONIC KIDNEY DISEASE

Nutrition intervention for patients with CKD includes modifications for sodium, fluid, potassium, phosphorus, calcium, vitamin D, iron, calories, and protein. Although global recommendations are available, nutrition care must be individualized based on serum chemistry levels, fluid balance, and nutritional status. These concerns are addressed in the following discussion (see the Diet-Medications Interactions box, "Common Drugs Used for Renal Disorders and Potential Food-Drug Interactions").

DIET-MEDICATIONS INTERACTIONS

Common Drugs Used for Renal Disorders and Potential Food-Drug Interactions

Drugs	Potential Food-Drug Interactions, Side Effects, and Recommendations
Pyelonephritis and Urinary Tract Infections	
Ceftriaxone and gentamicin	Sufficient water and fluids should be consumed
	Monitor glucose changes in persons with diabetes mellitus
	Avoid use with alcohol
Sulfisoxazole (Gantrisin)	Can deplete folacin and vitamin K
Trimethoprim (Trimpex), trimethoprim/sulfamethoxazole (Bactrim, Septra, Cotrim)	May cause diarrhea, gastrointestinal (GI) distress, stomatitis
Nitrofurantoin (Furadantin, Macrodantin)	Sufficient fluid intake necessary
Quinolones: ofloxacin (Floxin), norfloxacin (Noroxin), ciprofloxacin (Cipro), trovafloxacin (Trovan)	Should be taken with food or milk
	Adequate dietary protein is necessary
	Nausea, vomiting, anorexia are common
	Milk, yogurt, and calcium supplements should be avoided when taking Cipro; caffeine intake should be limited
	Floxin should be taken separately from vitamin supplements; nausea is one side effect

Continued

◆ DIET-MEDICATIONS INTERACTIONS

Common Drugs Used for Renal Disorders and Potential Food-Drug Interactions—cont'd

Drugs	Potential Food-Drug Interactions, Side Effects, and Recommendations
Urolithiasis/Nephrolithiasis (Kidney Stones)	
Allopurinol (Zyloprim) and probenecid (usually used instead of or in conjunction with purine-restricted diet)	Drink 10–12 glasses of fluid daily
	Avoid concomitant intake of vitamin C supplements
	Patient should maintain alkaline urine
	Side effects include nausea, vomiting, diarrhea, abdominal pain
Thiazide diuretics	Increase intake of high-potassium foods
	Control sodium intake
	Increase magnesium intake
	Dry mouth or GI distress may occur
d-Penicillamine	Requires vitamin B_6 and zinc supplementation
	Increase fluid intake with cystinuria
	Take 1–2 hours before/after meals
	Stomatitis, diarrhea, nausea, vomiting, abdominal pain may occur
Demerol and similar medications	Dry mouth, constipation, nausea, vomiting can occur
Acute Renal Failure	
Exchange resins (Kayexalate)	Take separately from calcium and antacids by several hours
Sorbitol	Bloating, flatulence, diarrhea may occur
Chronic Kidney Disease	
Phosphate binders: calcium acetate or calcium carbonate	Nausea/vomiting may occur
Ergocalciferol (vitamin D analog)	Additional water necessary to prevent constipation
	Monitor fluids carefully if urine output decreased
	Avoid long-term use
Recombinant human erythropoietin (r-HuEPO)	Iron supplements necessary
	Do not take iron supplement at same time as calcium
Hemodialysis	
Kayexalate	Take separately from calcium supplements or antacids
Transplantation (patients are usually on three to four of the five drugs listed following)	
Corticosteroids (prednisone, Solu-Cortef)	Increased catabolism of proteins
	Negative nitrogen balance
	Hyperphagia
	Ulcers
	Decreased glucose tolerance
	Sodium and fluid retention
	Impaired calcium absorption and osteoporosis
	Cushing syndrome
	Obesity
	Muscle wasting
	Increased gastric secretion
Cyclosporine	Nausea, vomiting, diarrhea
	Hyperlipidemia and hyperkalemia may occur
	Elevated glucose and lipids
Immunosuppressants (Muromonab, Orthoclone [OKT3], antithymocyte globulin [ATG])	Nausea, anorexia, diarrhea, vomiting
Azathioprine (Imuran)	Fever
	Stomatitis
	Leukopenia, thrombocytopenia
	Oral and esophageal sores
	Macrocytic anemia
	Pancreatitis
	Vomiting, diarrhea
	Folate supplementation may be needed
	Dietary modifications (liquid or soft diet, use of oral supplements) may be needed
Tacrolimus (Prograf, FK506)	GI distress, nausea, vomiting, diarrhea
	Hyperglycemia

Data from Escott-Stump S: *Nutrition and diagnosis-related care*, ed 6, Philadelphia, 2007, Lippincott Williams & Wilkins.

TABLE 23.4 Recommended Dietary Nutrient Intake for Patients With Chronic Kidney Disease

Nutrient	Stages 1 and 2	Stage 3	Stage 4	Stage 5
Protein (g/kg/day)	0.75	0.75	0.6	0.6–0.75
Energy (kcal/kg/day)	Based on energy expenditure	Based on energy expenditure	30–35 kcal/kg/day	30–35 kcal/kg/day
Sodium (mg/day)	1–4 g/day, depending on comorbidities	1–4 g/day, depending on comorbidities	1–4 g/day, depending on comorbidities	1–4 g/day, depending on comorbidities
Potassium (mEq/day)	Usually no restriction unless serum level high	Usually no restriction unless serum level high	Usually no restriction unless serum level high	Usually no restriction unless serum level high
Phosphorus (mg/kg/day)	Monitor and restrict if serum levels >4.6	8–12 mg/g protein or 800–1000 mg/day	8–12 mg/g protein or 800–1000 mg/day	8–12 mg/g protein or 800–1000 mg/day
Calcium (mg/day)	1.2–1.5 mg/day; serum calcium should be maintained on lower end	1.2–1.5 mg/day; serum calcium should be maintained on lower end	Same as stages 1–3, but not to exceed 2000 mg/day	Same as stages 1–3, but not to exceed 2000 mg/day
Vitamins and minerals	Dietary Reference Intakes (DRIs) for all	DRIs for B complex and C vitamins; individualize vitamin D, zinc, and iron	DRIs for B complex and C vitamins; individualize vitamin D, zinc, and iron	DRIs for B complex and C vitamins; individualize vitamin D, zinc, and iron

Modified from Fedje L, Karalis M: Nutrition management in early stages of chronic kidney failure. In Byham-Gray L, Stover J, Wiesen K, editors: *A clinical guide to nutrition care in kidney disease, ed 2*, Chicago, 2013, Academy of Nutrition and Dietetics. Copyright Academy of Nutrition and Dietetics. Reprinted with permission.

Sodium and Potassium

As kidney function declines, the ability of the nephrons to maintain sodium balance through sodium excretion diminishes. However, an adaptive mechanism results in undamaged nephrons being able to excrete an increased percentage of filtered sodium, with the effect being a decrease in the fractional reabsorption and an increase in fractional excretion of sodium by renal tubules. As GFR falls to 10 mL/min, a sodium restriction of 2–3 g may be required to maintain sodium and fluid balance. Clinical symptoms of excessive sodium intake include shortness of breath, hypertension, congestive heart failure (CHF), and edema.

Kidney regulation of potassium balance is obtained by renal excretion of potassium in an amount equal to that absorbed by the GI tract. Potassium balance is dependent on the ability of the tubules to continue to secrete potassium into the ultrafiltrate. This ability will decrease as kidney failure progresses. As serum potassium levels increase to more than 5.0 mg/dL, dietary potassium restriction to approximately 3–4 g/day may be needed.[10]

Phosphorus, Calcium, and Vitamin D

The consequence of abnormalities of calcium, phosphorus, and vitamin D metabolism seen in CKD is development of bone diseases, which are referred to as *renal osteodystrophy*. Diagnoses include osteoporosis, osteosclerosis, osteomalacia, and osteitis fibrosa. The healthy kidney filters approximately 7 g of phosphorus per day, of which 80%–90% is reabsorbed by the renal tubules and the remaining 10% is excreted into urine. Phosphorus balance can be maintained until the GFR falls below 20 mL/min. At that point, phosphorus accumulation occurs in the serum. In addition, conversion of vitamin D to the active form 1,25-dihydrocholecalciferol is diminished, resulting in low serum calcium levels and elevated parathyroid hormone (PTH) levels. Dietary intervention for bone disease management is dietary phosphorus restriction to 8–12 mg of phosphorus per kilogram of body weight per day. In addition to dietary phosphate restriction, most patients require oral calcium, oral or intravenous vitamin D, or vitamin D analogs (or a combination of these therapies). Serum PTH, calcium, and phosphorus levels must be monitored closely to avoid excesses and deficiencies that can exacerbate the bone disease.[10]

Iron

Because of the diminished ability of the failing kidney to synthesize adequate amounts of erythropoietin, most patients with chronic renal failure develop anemia if left untreated. Recommended levels for hematocrit are 33%–36%; for hemoglobin (Hb), 11–12 g/dL. These target levels are accomplished through administration of recombinant human erythropoietin (r-HuEPO) and 10–18 mg oral iron. Doses are individualized. If left untreated, then adverse clinical events can occur, including increased mortality rates, malnutrition, angina, cardiac enlargement, and impaired immunologic response.

Calories and Protein

K/DOQI guidelines for CKD recommend 0.6 g protein/kg of body weight per day when GFR is less than 25 mL/min and the patient is not on dialysis. For individuals who do not want to observe this diet or are unable to maintain adequate caloric intake, a diet providing protein in the amount of 0.75 g/kg/day should be considered. At this same level of GFR, caloric intake for patients younger than 60 years is recommended to be 35 kcal/kg/day; for those 60 years or older, 30–35 kcal/kg/day.[11] Other diet recommendations that integrate current data concerning protein, calories, fatty acids, vitamins, and minerals until additional data are available are listed in Table 23.4.

MEDICAL NUTRITION THERAPY

Chronic Kidney Disease Stages 1–4

Nutrition goals for CKD stages 1–4 should center on comorbid states (diabetes, hypertension, and hyperlipidemia) and slowing development of potential CVD[3,11]:

- Protein: 0.60–0.75 g/kg of body weight, 50% or greater high biologic value (HBV) protein
- Energy: 35 kcal/kg of body weight for younger than 60 years; 30–35 kcal/kg of body weight for older than 60 years
- Sodium: 1–3 g/day
- Potassium: usually unrestricted unless serum level is high
- Phosphorus: 800–1000 mg/day when serum phosphorus is greater than 4.6 mg/dL or PTH is elevated
- Calcium 1.0–1.5 g/day, not to exceed 2 g/day with binder load
- Fluid: no restriction
- Vitamins/minerals: Daily Reference Intakes (DRIs) for B complex and vitamin C; individualize vitamin D, iron, and zinc

KEY TERMS

Osteodystrophy
Defective bone formation.

Chronic Kidney Disease Stage 5

A patient requiring maintenance hemodialysis usually requires two or three treatments per week, with each treatment lasting 2½ to 5 hours. During treatment the patient's blood circulates through the dialysis solution in an artificial kidney (the dialyzer), maintaining normal blood levels of life-sustaining substances the patient's own kidneys can no longer accomplish. An alternative form of peritoneal dialysis is practical for long-term ambulatory therapy at home.

The diet of a patient on kidney dialysis is a vital aspect of maintaining biochemical control. Several basic objectives govern each individually tailored diet, designed to (1) maintain adequate protein and calorie intake, (2) prevent dehydration or fluid overload, (3) maintain normal serum potassium and sodium blood levels, and (4) maintain acceptable phosphate and calcium levels[3,11]:

- Protein: 1.2 g/kg or more of body weight, 50% or greater HBV protein (at least 50% of dietary protein should come from HBV protein [meats, poultry, game, fish, eggs, soy, and dairy])
- Energy: 35 kcal/kg of body weight for patients younger than 60 years; 30–35 kcal/kg of body weight for patients older than 60 years
- Sodium: 1–3 g/day
- Potassium: 2–3 g/day; adjust based on serum levels
- Phosphorus: 800–1000 mg/day when serum phosphorus is greater than 5.5 mg/dL or PTH is elevated
- Calcium: 2 g/day or less; include binder load
- Fluid: urine output +1000 mL

- Vitamins/minerals:
  - Vitamin C: 60–100 mg/day
  - Vitamin B_6: 2 mg/day
  - Folate: 1 mg/day
  - Vitamin B_{12}: 3 mcg/day
  - DRIs for all other water-soluble vitamins
  - Vitamin E: 15 IU/day
  - Zinc: 15 mg/day
  - Iron and vitamin D: individualize

Stage 5: Peritoneal Dialysis. An alternative form of dialysis, peritoneal dialysis, allows dialysate solutions to flow directly through a catheter port established through the abdominal wall into the abdominal cavity. The solution is typically a dextrose-salt solution. High osmolality of the solution causes waste materials to diffuse across the saclike **peritoneum** lining the abdominal cavity (see the Perspectives in Practice box, "Peritoneal Dialysis"). Then this dialysate collection of waste materials flows back into the dialysate bag for disposal. The peritoneal membrane serves as the filtering mechanism.[12]

KEY TERM

Peritoneum

A strong smooth surface—a serous membrane—lining the abdominal and pelvic walls and the undersurface of the diaphragm, forming a sac that encloses the body's vital visceral organs within the peritoneal cavity.

 PERSPECTIVES IN PRACTICE

Peritoneal Dialysis

A variety of types of peritoneal dialysis exist; the two main types are continuous ambulatory peritoneal dialysis (CAPD) and continuous cyclic peritoneal dialysis (CCPD). The choice of which type of peritoneal dialysis to perform depends on lifestyle and clinical considerations, much the same way the decision to choose hemodialysis or peritoneal dialysis is made. CAPD is an ambulatory dialysis procedure that introduces dialysate directly into the peritoneal cavity. Solutes and water flow across the peritoneal membrane into dialysate fluid. This is accomplished by attaching a disposable bag containing dialysate to a catheter permanently inserted into the peritoneal cavity, waiting an individually prescribed amount of time (i.e., "dwell time") for solution exchange, and then lowering the bag to allow the force of gravity to cause the waste-containing fluid to drain into it. When the bag is empty, it can be folded around the waist or tucked into a pocket, allowing the user mobility.

The exchange takes place via osmosis and diffusion, with the rate being determined in part by the amount of dextrose in the solution. The most common dialysate solutions are 1.5%, 2.5%, or 4.25% dextrose in 1.5–2 L of solution. The actual rate of solute transport, type and number of peritoneal dialysis exchanges, and solution dwell times vary among patients. Each patient is prescribed an individualized dialysis prescription that includes the number and type of dialysate solutions to use each day and the length of dwell times. A method to determine membrane function and the optimal peritoneal dialysis method for each patient is the peritoneal equilibration test. Peritoneal solute and solvent movement rates vary among patients and over time can vary even within the same patient. Therefore clinical monitoring of dialysis adequacy is important. Patients using CAPD as a renal replacement therapy have better mobility than those on hemodialysis. In addition, they typically have a more liberal diet in regard to dietary potassium, phosphorus, and total fluid intake due in large part to the more continuous nature of the therapy. Protein requirement is increased and can be a challenge for some patients.

Table 23.5 lists the nutritional recommendations for patients on peritoneal dialysis. Special nutrient considerations are as follows:

- *Protein and amino acid* losses average 5–15 g/24 hours; amino acid losses average 3 g/day (see Table 23.5 for protein requirements).
- *Potassium* requirements depend on the number of solution exchanges, whether the patient has any residual renal function, and the individual clearance characteristics of the patient's peritoneal membrane. On average, potassium recommendation is 3–4 g/day. Some patients will require potassium supplementation.
- *Phosphorus-binding antacids* are not as needed because of improved control of phosphorus blood levels with CAPD use.
- *Dietary sodium* is usually restricted to 2–4 g/day. The recommendation must be individualized in accordance to the patient's fluid status, blood pressure, and thirst.
- *Fluid* requirements depend on weight, blood pressure, and residual renal function.

CAPD poses nutrition-related problems related to weight gain from the dialysate and, on the other end of the spectrum, anorexia because of glucose absorption from the dialysate.

One method available to calculate glucose absorption in an individualized manner is the D/D_0 formula: grams of glucose absorbed.

$$\text{Glucose (g)} = (1 - D/D_0)x_i$$

where D_0 is initial dextrose in the dialysate at zero hours (g); D is remaining dextrose in the dialysate after an appropriate dwell time (g); D/D_0 is the fraction of glucose remaining in the dialysate; and x_i is initial glucose instilled:

- 13 g/L for 1.5% dextrose
- 22 g/L for 2.5% dextrose
- 38 g/L for 4.25% dextrose

Peritoneal Dialysis—cont'd

In addition to posing possible weight management problems, extra dextrose can lead to elevated triglycerides and low-density lipoprotein (LDL) levels and depressed levels of protective high-density lipoproteins (HDLs), thus increasing risk of coronary heart disease in long-term users.

Nutritionists and nurses who counsel patients being transferred from hemodialysis to a CAPD regimen may find that patients need guidance in adjusting to their new diet. The following guidelines may be helpful:

- Increase potassium intake by eating a wide variety of fruits and vegetables each day.
- Encourage liberal fluid intake to prevent dehydration.
- Encourage complex carbohydrates while avoiding overindulging in concentrated sweets to help control triglyceride and HDL levels.
- Maintain lean body weight by incorporating the kcalories provided by the dialysate into the total meal plan (to be calculated and explained to the patient by the renal dietitian).

Bibliography

National Kidney Foundation: K/DOQI clinical practice guidelines for nutrition in chronic renal failure, *Am J Kidney Dis* 35(Suppl 2):S9, 2000.

National Kidney Foundation: Kidney disease outcomes quality initiative (K/DOQI): practice guidelines for peritoneal dialysis adequacy, *Am J Kidney Dis* 37(Suppl 1):S55, 2001.

Passadakis P, Vargemezis V, Oreopoulos DG, et al: Peritoneal dialysis: better than, equal to, or worse than hemodialysis? Data worth knowing before choosing a dialysis modality, *Perit Dial Int* 21:25, 2001.

Theofilou P: Quality of life in patients undergoing hemodialysis or peritoneal dialysis treatment, *J Clin Med Res* 3(3):132–138, 2011.

Valderrábano F1, Jofre R, López-Gómez JM: Quality of life in end-stage renal disease patients, *Am J Kidney Dis* 38(3):443, 2001.

Wiggins K: *Guidelines for nutrition care of renal patients*, ed 3, Chicago, 2002, American Dietetic Association.

Two main types of peritoneal dialysis exist:
1. Continuous ambulatory peritoneal dialysis (CAPD), in which a dialysis solution in a plastic pouch is infused and drained via gravity each day (24 hours), 5 times at 4-hour intervals
2. Continuous cyclic peritoneal dialysis (CCPD), in which three or four machine-delivered exchanges are given at night, approximately 3 hours each, leaving about 2 L of dialysate solution in the peritoneal cavity for 12–15 hours during the day

Nutritional concerns specific to peritoneal dialysis involve calories contributed by the dialysate, which are usually 1.5%, 2.5%, or 4.25% dextrose in 1.5–2 L of solution, and the concern that fluid and potassium intake can be liberalized compared with hemodialysis because of the enhanced clearance of potassium.
- Protein: 1.2–1.3 g/kg or more of body weight, 50% or greater HBV
- Energy: 35 kcal/kg of body weight for patients younger than 60 years; 30–35 kcal/kg of body weight for patients older than 60 years, including dialysate calories
- Sodium: 2–4 g/day; monitor fluid balance

- Potassium: 3–4 g/day; adjust to serum levels
- Phosphorus: 800–1000 mg/day when serum phosphorus is more than 5.5 mg/dL or PTH is elevated
- Calcium: 2 g/day or less; include binder load
- Fluid: maintain balance
- Vitamins/minerals:
  - Vitamin C: 60–100 mg/day
  - Vitamin B_6: 2 mg/day
  - Folate: 1 mg/day
  - Vitamin B_{12}: 3 mcg/day
  - Vitamin B_{12}: may need 1.5–2 mg/day because of dialysis losses
  - DRIs for all other B vitamins
  - Vitamin E: 15 IU/day
  - Zinc: 15 mg/day
  - Iron and vitamin D: individualize

Table 23.5 summarizes dietary recommendations for patients receiving hemodialysis and peritoneal dialysis.

TABLE 23.5 Nutritional Recommendations for Patients on Hemodialysis and Peritoneal Dialysis Therapy

Nutrient	Hemodialysis	Peritoneal Dialysis
Protein (g/kg)[a]	1.2 average weight (50% HBV)	1.2–1.3 SBW or adjusted BW (>50% HBV)
Energy (kcal/kg)[a]	30 kcal/kg if <60 years of age and 30–35 kcal/kg if >60 years of age or obese	30–35 if >60 years of age and 35 if <60 years of age
If patient <90% or >115% of median standard weight, use aBW$_{ef}$		
Phosphorus	800–1000 mg/day or <17 mg/kg IBW or SBW	800–1000 mg or 10–15 mg phosphorus/g protein
Sodium	2–4 g if fluid output ≥1 L	2–4 g
	2 g if fluid output ≤1 L	
	2 g if anuria	
Potassium	40 mg/kg IBW or SBW	2–4 g (considered consistent with unrestricted diet)
Fluid	2 L if fluid output ≥1 L	1–3 L/day
	1–1.5 L if fluid output ≤1 L	
	1 L if anuria	
Calcium	Individualized	<2000 mg including diet and binders

[a]For continuous ambulatory peritoneal dialysis (CAPD) and automated peritoneal dialysis (APD) include dialysate calories.
BW, Body weight; *aBW$_{ef}$,* edema-free adjusted body weight; *HBV,* high biologic value; *IBW,* ideal body weight; *SBW,* standard body weight.
Data from Biesecker R, Stuart N: Nutrition management of the adult hemodialysis patient. In Byham-Gray L, Wiesen K, editors: *A clinical guide to nutrition care in kidney disease,* Chicago, 2004, American Dietetic Association; McCann L: Nutrition management of the adult peritoneal dialysis patient. In Byham-Gray L, Wiesen K, editors: *A clinical guide to nutrition care in kidney disease,* Chicago, 2004, American Dietetic Association.

TABLE 23.6 Nutritional Guidelines for Adult Kidney Transplant Recipients

Nutrient	Acute Period	Chronic Period
Protein	1.3–2 g/kg[a]	0.8–1 g/kg; limit with chronic graft dysfunction
Energy	30–35 kcal/kg[a] or BEE × 1.3 (may increase with postoperative complications)	Adjust calories to maintain desirable body weight
Carbohydrates	Limit simple carbohydrate intake with elevated blood glucose levels and/or unwanted weight gain	Emphasize complex carbohydrate intake and distribution
Fat	Remainder of calories	Emphasize PUFA and MUFA
Potassium	2–4 g if hyperkalemic	Unrestricted unless hyperkalemic
Sodium	Restrict if blood pressure/fluid status dictates	2–4 g with hypertension and/or edema
Calcium	1200–1500 mg	1200–1500 mg
Phosphorus	DRIs; may need supplementation to normalize serum levels	DRIs[b]
Fluids	Limited only by graft function (generally unrestricted)	Limited only by graft function (generally unrestricted)

[a]Based on standard or adjusted body weight.
[b]Due to lack of research, no specific recommendations are available for this population. Currently the DRI is used as guideline.
BEE, Basal energy expenditure; *DRIs,* Dietary Reference Intakes; *MUFA,* monounsaturated fatty acids; *PUFA,* polyunsaturated fatty acids.
From Cochran CC, Kent PS: Nutrition management of the renal transplant patient. In Byham-Gray L, Stover J, Wiesen K, editors: *A clinical guide to nutrition care in kidney disease,* ed 2, Chicago, 2013, Academy of Nutrition and Dietetics. Copyright Academy of Nutrition and Dietetics. Reprinted with permission.

Kidney Transplantation

Nutritional care of kidney transplant recipients is divided into three phases: (1) pretransplantation, (2) acute posttransplantation, and (3) chronic posttransplantation. Pretransplant nutrition concerns are based on current renal replacement therapy, if any, along with assessment of nutritional status.[13]

The nutritional challenges of the acute posttransplant period are most often related to posttransplantation medications (see the Evidence-Based Practice box, "Kidney Transplantation"). Hyperlipidemia, weight gain, and abnormal blood glucose levels can result, often because of side effects of the antirejection medications such as corticosteroids and cyclosporine A.[14] Foodborne infections can be life-threatening for transplant patients receiving immunosuppressive medications; therefore food safety education should be routinely included.

During the chronic posttransplant period, overnutrition may lead to complications such as obesity, dyslipidemias, diabetes mellitus, and hypertension. Nutritional goals are to provide adequate nutrition, prevent infection, and manage long-term nutritional complications.[13] A summation of nutritional guidelines for this patient group is provided in Table 23.6.

EVIDENCE-BASED PRACTICE

Kidney Transplantation

Thousands of patients await transplantation every year. Others cannot consider a transplant because of medical or psychosocial issues (or because of both). Overall, kidney transplantation remains the treatment of choice for the majority of patients with chronic kidney disease (CKD). Advances in solid organ transplantation and immunosuppressive therapy have resulted in improved patient survival and improved viability of transplanted kidneys.

Nearly 50% of all kidney transplant recipients will be alive with a successful functioning transplant 10 years after transplantation. One-year cadaver kidney success rates are 89%, and 5-year success rates are 65%. In comparison, success rates for recipients of living donor kidneys are 97% at 1 year and 78% at 5 years. A patient who is trouble free for the first 3 months after the transplantation has an excellent prognosis. Most common causes of death after the first year are cardiovascular disease (CVD), infection, and cancer.

The patient who receives a kidney transplant has a challenging first year. Visits to the transplant team occur an average of 2 or 3 times per week during the first month and once per week for up to 3 months after the surgery. Visits then drop to once monthly during the first year if no problems occur. After the first year, it is recommended that patients have their laboratory parameters monitored every 1–2 months.

Medication regimens are challenging for the transplant recipient. Immunosuppressive agents, lipid-lowering drugs, antihypertensives, and hypoglycemic agents are needed for quite some time. Significant side effects can occur from these medicines, and adherence to the rigid medication schedule is critical for successful allograft survival. Medical problems that can develop during the first year include infections such as cytomegalovirus, hyperlipidemia, bone disease,

diabetes, CVD, hypertension, and dental problems. Weight gain as a side effect of medications can also become a problem (Table 23.6 for nutritional recommendations for the kidney transplant recipient).

Morbidity and mortality rates for kidney transplantation are clinically significant. These statistics should improve as advances in the technology of the surgery and pharmacologic management occur over time. Not every patient will medically qualify for transplantation, and every candidate must be assessed for his or her ability to meet the demands of the posttransplantation period. In addition, evidence suggests that living kidney donors have survival similar to nondonors, and their risk of CKD is not increased.

In the future, perhaps the availability of organs for transplantation will be increased by improvements in living-related surgeries, development of artificial organs, and most optimistically, finding a cure for progressive kidney disease.

Bibliography

2001 Annual report: End Stage Renal Disease Clinical Performance Measures Project, *Am J Kidney Dis* 39(Suppl 2):S1, 2002.

Baiardi F, Degli Esposti E, Cocchi R, et al: Effects of clinical and individual variables on quality of life in chronic renal failure patients, *J Nephrol* 15(1):61, 2002.

Braun WE: Update on kidney transplantation: increasing clinical success, expanding waiting lists, *Cleve Clin J Med* 69(6):501, 2002.

Ibrahim HN, Foley R, Tan L, et al: Long-term consequences of kidney donation, *N Engl J Med* 360(5):459, 2009.

Matas AJ, Halbert RJ, Barr ML, et al: Life satisfaction and adverse effects in renal transplant recipients: a longitudinal analysis, *Clin Transplant* 16(2):113, 2002.

ACUTE RENAL FAILURE

The catabolic acute renal failure (ARF) patient, most frequently encountered in the intensive care setting, presents a management challenge to the entire team of physicians, nurses, dietitians, respiratory therapists, dialysis staff, pharmacists, and other technicians. These patients are in negative nitrogen balance and generate much urea resulting from the catabolic process. Infection is a major threat, and it aggravates the existing malnutrition.

Disease Process

Renal failure may occur acutely with sudden shutdown of renal function after some metabolic insult or traumatic injury to normal kidneys. It is typically characterized by retention of nitrogenous waste products, fluid overload, acid-base disturbances, electrolyte imbalance, and hemodynamic instability. ARF is linked with major in-hospital morbidity and mortality.[15] Immediate and continuing nutrition support is essential.

ARF may have various causes: (1) severe injury such as extensive burns or crushing injuries that cause widespread tissue destruction; (2) infectious diseases such as peritonitis; (3) traumatic shock after surgery on the abdominal aorta; (4) toxic agents in the environment such as carbon tetrachloride or poisonous mushrooms; or (5) immunologic drug reactions such as penicillin reaction in allergic or sensitive persons.[15]

Clinical Symptoms

The major sign of ARF is oliguria (diminished urine output) often accompanied by proteinuria or hematuria. This diminished urine output is brought on by underlying tissue problems that characterize ARF. Usually blockage of tubules is seen, caused by cellular debris from tissue trauma or urinary failure with backup retention of filtrate materials.[15]

Oliguria. Diminished urinary output is a cardinal symptom of oliguria, often with proteinuria or hematuria accompanying the small output. Water balance becomes a crucial factor. The course of the disease is usually divided into an oliguric phase followed by a diuretic phase. The urinary output during the oliguric phase varies from as little as 20–200 mL/day.

Anorexia, Nausea, and Lethargy. During this initial phase of ARF, the patient may be lethargic and anorectic and experience nausea and vomiting. Blood pressure elevation and signs of uremia may be present. Oral intake is usually difficult in this catabolic period.[15]

Increasing Serum Urea Nitrogen and Creatinine Levels. During the initial catabolic period after injury, surgery, or some other metabolic dysfunction, the serum urea nitrogen level increases along with the creatinine level. These increases result from tissue breakdown of muscle mass. Blood potassium, phosphate, and sulfate levels also increase, and sodium, calcium, and bicarbonate levels decrease.[15]

Basic Treatment Goals

Treatment must be individualized, adjusted according to the progression of the illness, the type of treatment being used, and the patient's response. In general, however, basic therapy objectives are as follows[15]:

- Reduce and minimize protein breakdown
- Prevent protein catabolism, and minimize uremic toxicity

KEY TERM

Oliguria
Secretion of a very small amount of urine in relation to fluid intake.

- Prevent dehydration or overhydration
- Correct acidosis carefully
- Correct electrolyte depletions, and avoid excesses
- Control fluid and electrolyte losses from vomiting and diarrhea
- Maintain optimal nutritional status
- Maintain appetite, general morale, and sense of well-being
- Control complications—hypertension, bone pain, nervous system problems

Nutritional Requirements for Patients With Acute Renal Failure

The nutrition requirements for the ARF patient are directly influenced by the type of renal replacement therapy (if any), nutritional and metabolic status, and degree of hypercatabolism. Current recommendations for protein and calories for this patient population are defined in the following discussion.

When energy requirements cannot be measured directly, calorie requirements can usually be met by providing 25–35 kcal/kg IBW, reserving the upper limit of the range for patients who are severely catabolic and whose nitrogen balance does not improve at lower intakes.[15] Protein sources containing essential and nonessential amino acids should be provided. For patients whose ARF is expected to resolve in a few days and who are not catabolic and will not need dialysis, 0.8–1.2 g/kg body weight of protein is recommended. The patient's nutritional and metabolic status and renal diagnosis determine the exact dose. For patients who are catabolic, receiving acute hemodialysis, or both, the recommendation is 1.2–1.5 g/kg body weight of protein.[15]

Total fluid intake for any patient depends on the amount of residual renal function (i.e., if the patient is oliguric or anuric) and fluid and sodium status. In general, fluid intake can be calculated by adding 500 mL (for insensible losses) to the 24-hour urine output. During diuresis, fluids should be increased to prevent dehydration.[15]

Although the diet should be as liberal as possible to support sufficient intake, nutrient needs should be frequently reevaluated, because requirements may change as a consequence of resumption of kidney function, use of dialysis, and anabolism. Sodium needs may increase to restore losses from diuresis, but the general recommendation is 2–3 g per day. Potassium requirements depend on lab values and the degree of hyperkalemia. In general, 2–3 g/day is suggested, but requirements may possibly increase with dialysis, restoration of kidney function, and anabolism. Phosphate binders may be necessary, along with a restriction of 8–15 mg/kg body weight per day. Requirements may increase with daily dialysis, return of kidney function, and anabolism.[15]

UROLITHIASIS (CALCULI OR KIDNEY STONES)

Disease Process

Kidney stone disease is an ancient medical problem. Records of its incidence have appeared in medical documents since the days of Hippocrates. It continues to be a prevalent health problem. Multiple stone attacks affect 12% of American men and 5% of women during their lifetimes.[16]

Kidney stone disease appears to be chronic and recurrent. Calculi form when excessive amounts of reasonably insoluble salts are found in the urine or when inadequate fluid intake creates highly concentrated urine. When any solid substance forms, sediment continues to build up. The salts that form crystals can grow to form stones.[16] Immobility can also cause calculi because of stasis of urine and ensuing chemical alterations.[16,17] The existence of stones typically becomes evident only when they obstruct the flow of urine.[17]

Although the basic cause of kidney stones remains unknown, many factors contribute directly or indirectly to their formation. These

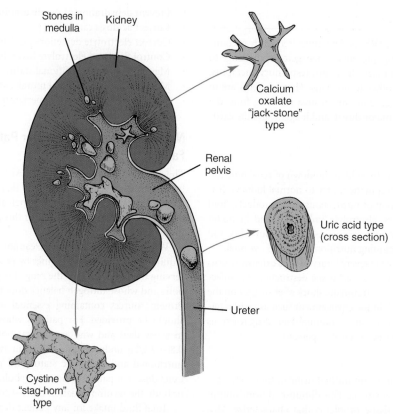

FIG. 23.4 Renal stones in kidney, pelvis, and ureter.

factors relate to the nature of the urine itself or to conditions of the urinary tract environment. The risk for urinary calculi development is affected by a number of factors, including age, gender, race, geographic location, seasonal factors, fluid intake, diet, and occupation. Geographic locations affect stone formation as the result of indirect factors such as average temperature, humidity, and rainfall, and their influence on fluid and dietary patterns.[16] According to the concentration of urinary constituents, approximately 75% of major stones formed are calcium stones. The rest consist chiefly of uric acid, struvite, or cystine (Fig. 23.4).[17]

Major Types of Stones

Calcium Stones. Calcium stones are composed of calcium compounds, usually calcium oxalate, calcium carbonate, or calcium phosphate. Calcium stones form as a result of hypercalciuria that can result from alkaline urine, inadequate fluid intake, high levels of dietary oxalate (see Appendix B), prolonged immobilization, or parathyroid tumor.[16,17] Oxalates occur naturally only in a few food sources, and individual absorption and excretion rates influence availability. Only eight foods cause a significant increase in urinary oxalate excretion: (1) spinach, (2) rhubarb, (3) beets, (4) nuts, (5) chocolate, (6) tea, (7) wheat bran, and (8) strawberries. Nutrition therapy for individuals prone to stone formation may be limited to restriction of these eight foods, with results monitored by laboratory analysis of urine composition.

- *Animal protein:* A diet high in animal protein, such as the typical American diet, has been linked to increased excretions of calcium, oxalate, and urate. A vegetarian type of diet has been recommended by some investigators as a wise choice for persons prone to stone formation.
- *Dietary fiber:* Added dietary fiber has been found to reduce risk factors for stone formation, especially calcium stones.

Struvite Stones. Next to calcium stones in frequency are struvite stones, composed of a single compound—magnesium ammonium phosphate ($MgNH_4PO_4$). These are often called *infection stones* because they are associated with urinary tract infections (UTIs). The offending organism in the infection is *Proteus mirabilis.* This is a urea-splitting bacterium that contains urease, an enzyme that hydrolyzes urea to ammonia. Thus urinary pH becomes alkaline. In the ammonia-rich environment, struvite precipitates and forms large, "staghorn" stones.[16] Surgical removal is usually indicated.

Uric Acid Stones. Excess uric acid excretion may be caused by an impairment in intermediary metabolism of purine, as occurs in gout. Cancer chemotherapy may also cause urine to be acidic, which aids in hyperuricemia.

Cystine Stones. A hereditary metabolic defect in renal tubular reabsorption of the amino acid cystine causes this substance to accumulate in urine. This condition is called *cystinuria.* Because this is a genetic disorder, it is characterized by early onset and a positive family history. This is one of the most common metabolic disorders associated with kidney stones in children before puberty.

Clinical Symptoms

Severe pain and numerous urinary symptoms may result, with general weakness and sometimes fever. Laboratory examination of urine and chemical analysis of any stone passed help determine treatment.

General Treatment

Fluid Intake. Large fluid intake produces a more dilute urine and is a foundation of therapy. Dilute urine helps prevent concentration of stone constituents.

Urinary pH. An attempt to control solubility factor is made by changing urinary pH to an increased acidity or alkalinity, depending on the chemical composition of the stone formed. An exception is calcium oxalate stones, because solubility of calcium oxalate in urine is not pH dependent. Conversely, calcium phosphate is soluble in an acid urine.

Stone Composition. When possible, dietary constituents of the stone are controlled to reduce the amount of the substance available for precipitation.

Binding Agents. Materials that bind stone elements and prevent their absorption in the intestine cause fecal excretion. For example, sodium phytate is used to bind calcium, and aluminum gels are used to bind phosphate. Glycine and calcium have a similar effect on oxalates.

Alternative Remedies. A number of herbs are also used to help prevent the development of kidney stones (see the Complementary and Alternative Medicine [CAM] box, "Common Herbal Treatments for Kidney Stones").

Nutrition Therapy

Manipulation of single nutritional components is usually not effective. General nutrition recommendations for kidney stones entail the following[18]:

- Protein: not to exceed the DRI of 0.8–1.0 g/kg body weight/day
- Calcium: should not be restricted; intake should be balanced throughout the day
- Fluids: 12–16 cups to produce urine volume to more than 2.5 L/day
- Oxalate: less than 40–50 mg/day

COMPLEMENTARY AND ALTERNATIVE MEDICINE (CAM)

Common Herbal Treatments for Kidney Stones

Patients interested in complementary and alternative medicine may also be interested in knowing low fluid intake greatly increases risk of developing all types of kidney stones.

Herb	Efficacy	Side Effects and/or Risks	Drug Interaction
Citrate	Might help prevent oxalate and acid stones by binding with calcium in urine, reducing the amount of calcium available to form calcium oxalate stones. It also alkalizes urine, inhibiting development of calcium oxalate and uric acid stones.		Increases serum levels of ephedra, flecainide, mecamylamine, and methamphetamine. Decreases serum levels of lithium, methotrexate, salicylates, sulfonylureas, and tetracyclines. Hyperkalemia can occur when taking ACE inhibitors and potassium-sparing diuretics.
Calcium	Calcium supplements might slightly increase kidney stone risk, whereas dietary calcium reduces risk of kidney stones.	Increased intakes are associated with increased risk of prostate cancer.	Concurrent use of calcium with pheasant's eye (Adonis vernalis) increases risk of cardiac toxicity. CCBs can be affected by combinations of calcium supplements and high doses of vitamin D. Might decrease blood level of atenolol (β-blocker) and possibly other β-blockers. Interferes with absorption of tetracyclines and levothyroxine. Excess intake can interfere with absorption of iron, zinc, magnesium, iodine, manganese, and copper.
Magnesium (magnesium oxide or magnesium hydroxide)	No strong evidence that magnesium prevents calcium oxalate stones.	Should not be taken by those with severe heart or kidney disease without consultation with a health care provider.	Might decrease absorption of psyllium.
Vitamin B$_6$ (pyridoxamine)	Weak evidence indicates that vitamin B$_6$ might help prevent calcium oxalate stones.	Vitamin B$_6$ deficiency increases the amount of oxalate in urine. Large doses may cause nausea, vomiting, and potential risk of neurotoxicity.	None were found.
GLA (omega-6 oils, omega-6 fatty acids, evening primrose oil, black currant oil, borage oil)	No evidence is available.	No adverse effects have been noted.	Increases bleeding time when used with anticoagulant therapy. GLA is synergistic with paclitaxel.

Bibliography

Bratman S, Girman AM: *Mosby's handbook of herbs and supplements and their therapeutic uses*, St Louis, 2003, Mosby.

Herr SM: *Herb-drug interaction handbook*, ed 2, Nassau, NY, 2002, Church Street Books.

ACE, Angiotensin-converting enzyme; *CCBs*, calcium channel blockers; *GLA*, γ-linolenic acid.

- Sodium: decrease intake to 2300 (100 mEq) to 3450 (250 mEq) mg/day
- Energy: level to maintain healthy weight
- Vitamin and mineral supplements: vitamin C should be restricted to DRI; B vitamins have not been shown to be harmful

URINARY TRACT INFECTION

Disease Process

The term *UTI* refers to a wide variety of clinical infections in which a significant number of microorganisms are present in any portion of the urinary tract. A common form is cystitis, an inflammation of the bladder that is very prevalent in young women. At least 20% of women experience a UTI during their lifetime, of which the vast majority are cases of uncomplicated cystitis.[16,17] The condition is called *recurrent UTI* if three or more bouts are experienced in 1 year.

The majority of cases are caused by aerobic members of the fecal flora, especially *Escherichia coli*. The presence of these organisms in urine is termed *bacteriuria*. Urine produced by the normal kidney is sterile and remains so as it travels to the bladder. However, in UTIs the normal urethra has microbial flora; therefore any voided urine generally contains many bacteria. Bacteriuria is present when the quantity of organisms is more than 100,000/mL of urine. The female anatomy is more conducive to entry of these bacteria into the urinary tract. Recurrent cystitis occurs mostly in young and otherwise healthy women who have infections that usually correspond with sexual activity and continued diaphragm use. In most cases, simply changing to another birth control method will solve the problem. Cystitis is characterized by frequent voiding and burning on urination.

Treatment

Although regular consumption of cranberry juice can help prevent UTIs, it is not effective for treatment. Intake of adequate fluids helps produce a dilute urine. It is important to control a UTI, because UTIs are a risk factor in stone formation.

RESOURCES

The renal diet is complex and presents a challenge to practitioners and even more so to patients. A basic resource, the National Renal Diet educational series, provides valuable guides. These standardized guidelines for nutrition intervention and patient education in renal disease have been developed by the collaborative work of renal dietitians from the Academy of Nutrition and Dietetics Renal Dietitians Dietetic Practice Group and the National Kidney Foundation Council on Renal Nutrition. The *Professional Guide* can be used in conjunction with other guides from the Academy of Nutrition and Dietetics for the care of renal disease patients. Because dietary management must be tailored to the stage of the disease and method of treatment, the series of materials contains a professional guide and six client booklets, each designed with special food lists to meet specific needs of the various renal disease requirements. These Academy of Nutrition and Dietetics resources give the practitioner a comprehensive basis for individualizing dietary instructions and provide the patient and family with a practical guide for everyday decisions and plans for food choices.

The Council on Renal Nutrition of the National Kidney Foundation is an expert resource for information. Membership includes a subscription to the *Journal of Renal Nutrition,* a quarterly publication geared toward nutritionists, scientists, and physicians interested and working in the fields of nephrology and renal nutrition. (For contact information, see the Websites of Interest section at the end of this chapter.)

Nutritional status and care have been documented to have important roles in patient outcomes; therefore interest in renal nutrition and the number of online resources have substantially increased. (See the Websites of Interest section for a listing of websites that provide excellent information and links to other sites pertaining to renal nutrition and nephrology.)

HEALTH PROMOTION

OMEGA-3 FATTY ACIDS AND RENAL DISEASE

Despite countless research efforts, the mechanisms responsible for the progressive nature of renal disease remain elusive. Historically, nutrition science has been an inherent component of research directed toward identifying nutrient manipulations that ameliorate kidney disease, metabolic abnormalities associated with chronic renal insufficiency, and mechanisms by which nutrients modulate factors involved in promoting exacerbation of existing disease. In all of these research areas, dietary protein, phosphorus, and caloric deprivation have been more widely studied than other nutrients. However, more recently, research interest has become directed toward dietary essential fatty acids (EFAs). This shift is in response to a growing body of evidence indicating that fatty acid substitution of cell membrane phospholipids modulates biochemical pathways implicated in the pathophysiology of progressive kidney disease and CVD, which are so prominent in the renal patient population.

It has been demonstrated that altering the availability of EFAs can influence the natural course of several important diseases in the mammalian organism. For example, epidemiologic studies of the Dutch, Japanese, and native Greenland Eskimo populations attribute their low incidence of heart disease to a fish diet high in omega-3 fatty acids. Beneficial observations have included an improved lipid profile, prolonged survival, and improved renal function.

Dietary EFAs are direct precursors to the biologically diverse and potent class of compounds called *eicosanoids*. EFAs can also modulate cellular production of interleukins (ILs). Several chronic inflammatory and renal diseases are characterized in part by an overproduction of eicosanoids and ILs. These facts suggest manipulation of dietary fatty acids might contribute a therapeutic influence by altering proinflammatory and other activated pathways in disease processes.

TO SUM UP

Through its unique functional units, the nephrons, the kidneys act as a filtration system, reabsorbing substances the body needs, secreting additional hydrogen ions to maintain a proper pH balance in the blood, and excreting unnecessary materials in a concentrated urine.

Renal function may be impaired by a variety of conditions. These include inflammatory and degenerative diseases, infection and obstruction, chronic diseases such as hypertension and diabetes, environmental agents such as insecticides and solvents and other toxic substances, and some medications and trauma. Some clinical conditions that affect structure and function include glomerulonephritis, ARF and chronic renal failure, renal calculi, and UTIs.

Stage 5 of CKD is treated by dialysis—hemodialysis or peritoneal dialysis—and kidney transplantation. The diet for CKD needs to include ample calories and protein, with restrictions for GFR of less than 25 mL/min per 1.73 m^2 only if the patient is able to maintain adequate caloric intake. Dialysis patients must be monitored closely for calories, protein, fluid, and electrolyte balance. All of the diets need to be individualized to ensure overall nutritional adequacy and adherence. Monitoring of nutritional status is important for all patients.

QUESTIONS FOR REVIEW

1. For each of the following conditions, outline nutritional components of therapy, explaining effect of each on kidney function: glomerulonephritis, ARF (renal insufficiency), and chronic renal failure.
2. Identify four clinical conditions that impair renal function. Give an example of each, describing its effect on various structures in the kidney.
3. List nutritional factors that must be monitored in individuals undergoing renal dialysis.
4. Summarize the rationale and nutrient recommendations for patients who have received a renal transplant.
5. Outline nutrition therapy used for patients with various types of kidney stones. Describe each type of stone and explain the rationale for each aspect of therapy.
6. For what condition is a UTI a predisposing factor? What general nutrition principles are recommended in the treatment of such infections?

REFERENCES

1. Huether SE: Structure and function of the renal and urologic systems. In Huether SE, McCance KL, editors: *Understanding pathophysiology*, ed 4, St Louis, 2008, Mosby.
2. National Kidney Foundation: K/DOQI clinical practice guidelines and clinical practice recommendations for diabetes and chronic kidney disease, *Am J Kidney Dis* 49(Suppl 2):S12, 2007.
3. National Kidney Foundation: K/DOQI clinical practice guidelines for chronic kidney disease: evaluation, classification and stratification, *Am J Kidney Dis* 39(Suppl 1):S1, 2002.
4. UUS Renal Data System: *USRDS 2008 Annual Report: Atlas of chronic kidney disease and end-stage renal disease in the United States*, Bethesda, MD, 2008, National Institutes of Health, National Institute of Diabetes and Digestive and Kidney Diseases.
5. Beekley MD: Update on nutrition and chronic kidney disease. In *Medscape Nephrology*, Chronic Kidney Disease Expert Column, 2007. From http://www.medscape.com.
6. Gray M, Huether SE, Forshee BA: Alterations of renal and urinary tract function. In McCance KL, Huether SE, editors: *Pathophysiology. The biologic basis for disease in adults and children*, ed 5, St Louis, 2006, Saunders.
7. American Diabetes Association: Diabetic nephropathy, *Diabetes Care* 25(Suppl 1):S85, 2002.
8. Kalantar-Zadeh K, Kopple J: Malnutrition as a risk factor for morbidity and mortality in maintenance patients. In Kopple J, Massry S, editors: *Nutritional management of renal disease*, Philadelphia, 2004, Lippincott Williams & Wilkins.
9. Barbá PD, Goode JL: Nutrition assessment in chronic kidney disease. In Byham-Gray L, Wiesen K, editors: *A clinical guide to nutrition care in kidney disease*, Chicago, 2004, American Dietetic Association.
10. Fedje L, Karalis M: Nutrition management in early stages of chronic kidney failure. In Byham-Gray L, Wiesen K, editors: *A clinical guide to nutrition care in kidney disease*, Chicago, 2004, American Dietetic Association.
11. National Kidney Foundation: K/DOQI clinical practice guidelines for nutrition in chronic renal failure, *Am J Kidney Dis* 35(Suppl 2):S9, 2000.
12. Biesecker R, Stuart N: Nutrition management of the adult hemodialysis patient. In Byham-Gray L, Wiesen K, editors: *A clinical guide to nutrition care in kidney disease*, Chicago, 2004, American Dietetic Association.
13. Cochran CC, Kent PS: Nutrition management of the renal transplant patient. In Byham-Gray L, Wiesen K, editors: *A clinical guide to nutrition care in kidney disease*, Chicago, 2004, American Dietetic Association.
14. Weil SE: Nutrition in the kidney transplant recipient. In Danovitch GM, editor: *Handbook of kidney transplantation*, ed 5, Philadelphia, 2010, Lippincott, Williams & Wilkins.
15. Bickford A, Schatz SR: Nutrition management in acute renal failure. In Byham-Gray L, Wiesen K, editors: *A clinical guide to nutrition care in kidney disease*, Chicago, 2004, American Dietetic Association.
16. Huether SE, Gray M: Alterations of renal and urinary tract functions. In Huether SE, McCance KL, editors: *Understanding pathophysiology*, ed 4, St Louis, 2008, Mosby.
17. Gould BE: *Pathophysiology for the health professions*, ed 3, St Louis, 2006, Mosby.
18. American Dietetic Association: *Nutrition care manual. Celiac disease: nutrition care FAQs*, Chicago, 2009, Author. from http://www.nutritioncaremanual.org.

FURTHER READINGS AND RESOURCES

Websites of Interest

- Academy of Nutrition and Dietetics: The website of the world's largest food and nutrition professionals organization provides information regarding nutrition and health through research, education, and advocacy: http://www.eatright.org.
- American Journal of Kidney Diseases: This is the website of the official journal of the National Kidney Foundation: http://www.ajkd.org.
- Da Vita: Provider of dialysis services and education for patients with CKD: http://www.davita.com.
- Hypertension, Dialysis and Clinical Nephrology (HDCN): Provides up-to-date, selected information on renal disorders and their treatment: http://www.hdcn.com.
- *Journal of the American Society of Nephrology:* http://www.jasn.org.
- *Journal of Renal Nutrition.* This site also provides links to the homepage of the National Kidney Foundation and the Council on Renal Nutrition: http://www.jrnjournal.org.
- National Kidney Foundation: http://www.kidney.org
- Nephrology News and Issues Online (NephrOnline): http://www.nephron-line.com.

24

Acquired Immunodeficiency Syndrome

Adriana Campa

ⓔ http://evolve.elsevier.com/Williams/essentials/

The human immunodeficiency virus (HIV) and its end stage, acquired immunodeficiency syndrome (AIDS), are nutrition-related conditions.1 Nutrition status and nutrition interventions are critical in the care of people living with HIV. Several international studies have shown that mild to moderate malnutrition impairs the immune response and increases the severity and mortality of infections.[2-4] Although the advent of potent combined antiretroviral therapy (cART) has not provided a permanent cure, it has transformed HIV into a manageable, chronic disease. As a consequence, nutrition interventions in those living with HIV are rapidly evolving to tailor nutrition support to the special needs created by the stages of the infection and its treatment.

OUTLINE

Evolution of Human Immunodeficiency Virus and the Acquired Immunodeficiency Syndrome Epidemic
Medical Management

Nutrition Therapy
Goals of Nutrition Therapy
To Sum Up

EVOLUTION OF HIV AND THE AIDS EPIDEMIC

HIV/AIDS is a pandemic that has claimed more than 25 million lives globally since the first case was reported in June 1981, including more than 619,000 in the United States.[5] There are 33.4 million people living with HIV/AIDS worldwide, and approximately 1.2 million in this country. The incidence of new cases in the United States is approximately 50,000 annually. Homosexual men (61% of new cases in 2010), drug users, and minorities account for most US new cases.[5] Approximately 97% of the cases of HIV/AIDS are found in low- and middle-income countries, especially in sub-Saharan Africa, with the number of new cases increasing in Asia.[6]

On June 30, 2013, the World Health Organization (WHO) revised their HIV treatment guidelines by recommending starting ART at a CD4 cell count of 500 cells/μL or less. Simultaneously, the treatment progress update issued by the WHO, the *Joint United Nations Programme on HIV/AIDS* (UNAIDS), and the United Nations Children's Fund (UNICEF) identified challenges in providing access to treatment for all eligible persons, because many of the most affected countries have limited resources to attain this standard.[7,8]

In addition to causing disease and death, the pandemic impacts families, communities, and the economic development of countries. Many of the regions hardest hit by HIV are limited-resource countries with high prevalence of other infectious diseases, food insecurity, and social and political problems. The most common method of transmission in the rest of the world is by heterosexual contact. HIV is a bloodborne virus transmitted by direct contact with infected body fluids via

unprotected heterosexual and homosexual intercourse, through intravenous needle sharing, and from mother to child during pregnancy, delivery, and breast-feeding. Worldwide, approximately half of all persons living with HIV/AIDS are women who acquire HIV mainly via heterosexual contact.[6]

The epidemic of HIV/AIDS has transformed our perception of public health, research, cultural attitudes, and social behaviors.[9] The incidence of new cases has decreased, and prevention has helped reduce HIV prevalence rates in several countries. In addition, the number of people with HIV receiving treatment in resource-poor countries has increased since 2002.[5]

Disease Progression

As shown in Fig. 24.1, HIV infection has several phases.[10] The Centers for Disease Control and Prevention (CDC) and the WHO have developed several classification systems that define four clinical stages using CD4 cell counts and clinical conditions for stages 2, 3, and 4.[11] For easier understanding, we have defined disease progression in three major phases: (1) acute infection, (2) asymptomatic and latency, and (3) AIDS. The acute stage occurs when the virus is transmitted and enters the bloodstream. From that moment on, the infection becomes a progressive disease, with the condition worsening over time. Without proper treatment, infected persons are likely to advance to AIDS, the final stage of the disease. The rate of progression is different depending on the characteristics of the host (exposure to infection, nutritional status, access to care, etc.) and the virus (HIV subtypes, superinfections, resistance to treatment, etc.).

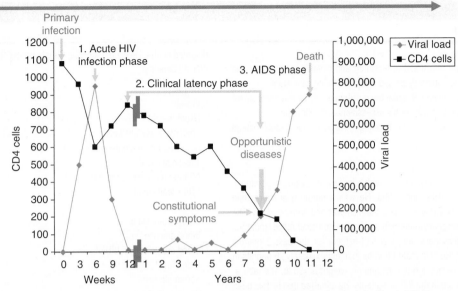

FIG. 24.1 Phases of HIV disease progression. (Adapted from Pantaleo G, Graziosi C, Fauci AS: New concepts in the immunopathogenesis of human immunodeficiency virus infection. *New Engl J Med* 328[5]:327-335, 1993.)

Acute Infection Stage

The genetic information of HIV, a retrovirus, is in the form of ribonucleic acid (RNA). HIV uses a reverse transcriptase enzyme to change RNA into double-stranded deoxyribonucleic acid (DNA) (Fig. 24.2). The new DNA is inserted by integrase, another viral enzyme, into the infected cell's genetic material. When the new DNA is activated, the viral information is translated, causing a sequence of cellular events that end with cell death, and the dead cell sheds infectious HIV particles called virions. If the cell remains dormant, then the viral genetic material may remain dormant for years, which makes HIV difficult to cure.[12] Although the acute stage of HIV infection may vary, typically it lasts for 3–6 weeks after the primary infection. Most individuals experience varying nonspecific symptoms of fatigue, sore throat, muscle pain, fever, night sweats, and enlarged lymph nodes.[12,13] The process of developing antibodies to HIV is called *seroconversion*, and it may last days or weeks. Subsequent HIV testing by enzyme-linked immunosorbent assay (ELISA) becomes positive.

Asymptomatic Stage (Latency)

Following the acute stage, HIV enters a period of inactivity or latency. An extended asymptomatic period usually continues for the next 10–12 years. However, this seemingly inactive period of relative wellness

can be deceiving. Antibodies typically appear within 4–7 weeks after infection through blood products but may remain seronegative for 6–14 months after sexual transmission. This phase between infection and manifestation of antibody is referred to as the *window period*.[12] During the asymptomatic stage of infection, viral replication continues and cellular destruction takes place in many tissues and organs of the body. The virus continues to proliferate during this phase.[13] During this protracted phase, many individuals will still not exhibit clinical signs of the infection, whereas others have generalized enlarged lymph nodes[14] and may present clinical manifestations of CDC clinical stages 2 and 3.[11] Viral replication appears to be reduced during this time. CD4 cell count decreases slowly, resulting in a weaker immune response.[13]

Final Stage (AIDS)

This is the last stage of the HIV infection, which is characterized by severe damage to the immune system and immune failure. CD4 cell count is 200 cells/μL or less. Opportunistic infections and AIDS-defining conditions manifest in this stage with numerous serious complications such as gastrointestinal (GI) effects and neurologic effects such as AIDS dementia (see the Case Study box "HIV in an Adult").

Diagnosis of hIV Infection
Testing Procedures[15]

HIV infection is diagnosed by detection of the virus or by the detection of specific antibodies, as is done in the routine screening of blood and blood products for transfusion and in most epidemiologic studies. The recommended procedure for virus detection is a two-step process. The first step is ELISA screening. Second, suspected positive samples from the ELISA screening are followed with Western blot testing for confirmation. Both tests are highly sensitive and specific, and both are used to confirm the results before informing the individual. Because a positive test is such a personal and life-changing event, most experienced physicians caring for HIV-infected patients repeat all positive tests again, even when they have been confirmed by Western blotting, before informing the individual.

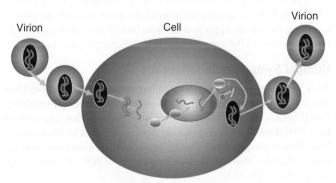

FIG. 24.2 HIV life cycle.

CASE STUDY

HIV in an Adult

Nutritional Assessment:

- Please do a complete nutritional assessment and develop a treatment and follow-up plan for the patient described in the following case study.
- You also need to identify and describe the nutritional indices and assessment tools that you are going to use for his assessment and follow-up.
- Please justify and discuss why you are using these assessment tools instead of others.

Case Study

Paul is a 58-year-old male Army veteran, with a history of cocaine dependence and a medical history of HIV since 1993. He was a heroin user more than 10 years ago, while in the Army. Paul is a chain smoker and drinks socially. The patient came to the emergency room (ER), reporting depressed mood, thoughts of worthlessness, helplessness, and low self-esteem for the past 2 months previous to the ER visit. He also stated that he lost approximately 25 pounds in the past 3 months. His height is 6 ft 2 in., and his weight is 155 lb. The laboratory values for this visit are in the following table. He admitted that he has been neglecting his care, not taking his antiretroviral medication, which consists of one tablet of Atripla daily. He also reports to be unable to sleep for more than 3 h per night. He admitted that he felt so "down" that last night he binged on crack cocaine. The patient also described severe difficulties with his family and friends. He left his wife 2 months ago after an argument. He described insomnia and nightmares for 3–4 weeks, describing that he witnessed his friend being murdered in a drug-related affair. He also described multiple losses, including the death of his older daughter (the oldest of four daughters) to AIDS in 2006. He was arrested in 2008 for assault. He has a history of multiple suicide attempts by hanging and overdose of psychiatric medications while in jail. He missed his last health care appointment 3 months ago. The patient finished high school and has been working on and off as a security officer. He is currently unemployed. Paul is presently on Supplemental Security Income benefits for disabled adults. He is not receiving Supplemental Nutrition Assistance Program (SNAP) benefits.

Height	188 cm
Weight	70.4 kg
Usual weight	81.9 kg
Percentage weight loss	14%
Body weight (percentage of usual)	86%
Triceps skinfold	<25th percentile
Midarm muscle circumference	<25th percentile
CD4+ cell count	118 cells/μL
Viral load	3.2 log copies/mL
Serum potassium	3.1 mEq/dL
Blood glucose	70 mg/dL
Blood urea nitrogen (BUN)	32 mg/dL
Creatinine	0.4 mg/dL
Serum albumin	2.8 mg/dL
Serum osmolality	325 mOsm/kg
Calculated basal energy expenditure (BEE)	2450 kcal/day

Questions for Analysis

1. Is Paul's HIV infection under control? Is his adherence to medication adequate?
2. Is he involved in risky behaviors for transmitting the disease?
3. Based on laboratory and anthropometric data, does Paul appear to be malnourished? Please support your response with evidence.
4. Assess Paul's food security and access to food. What type of assessment could help you determine this?
5. What are the acute or immediate nutrition goals? What about long-term goals?
6. What nutritional information will Paul need based on his ART regimen?
7. What type of referrals or follow-up is Paul going to need to prevent further nutritional depletion?

There are enzyme immunoassay (EIA) tests that use other body fluids to look for antibodies to HIV. These tests work in a similar manner to the standard blood ELISA tests and require a confirmatory Western blot in the same fluid. These new tests include the oral fluid (not saliva) test that is collected from the mouth using a special collection device and the urine tests. The sensitivity and specificity (accuracy) of the urine tests are somewhat less than that of the blood and oral fluid tests.[15]

Rapid HIV Testing

Rapid tests have also been developed. The CDC has published guidelines for their use, training, and counseling. These tests use blood from venipuncture, finger-stick, or oral fluids, producing results in 20 minutes. As with the previously described tests, they need a confirmatory Western blot test.[16]

Home Testing Kits

This type of test was first licensed in 1997. Currently only the Home Access HIV-1 Test SystemExternal Link is approved by the US Food and Drug Administration. This is not a true home test, but a home collection kit, which can be found in most drug stores. The collection procedure involves pricking a finger with a device, depositing blood drops from the pricked finger on a special card, and then mailing the card in to be tested at a licensed laboratory. The kit provides an identification number to use when contacting the laboratory for the results. Callers may speak to a counselor before taking the test, while waiting for the test result, and when the results are given. All individuals who receive a positive test result are provided referrals for a follow-up confirmatory test, as well as information and resources on treatment and support services.[15,17]

RNA Viral Assays

Viral load assays are used to assess prognosis, determine the need for and type of cART to use, and monitor the effectiveness of the treatment. RNA tests look for genetic material of the virus and can be used in screening the blood supply and for detection of very early cases of the infection when ELISA tests are unable to detect antibodies to HIV.[15]

Clinical Symptoms and Illnesses

Early clinical symptoms that may follow initial exposure to the virus add further confirmation to the HIV-seropositive testing procedures. Initial symptoms and possible associated diseases that characterize later HIV stages have been generally described earlier in discussion of basic disease progression. Some examples of these common opportunistic infections that manifest depending on CD4+ cell count range are listed in Table 24.1.

TABLE 24.1 Common Infectious Complications of AIDS

Microorganism	Nutritional Implications
Parasites	
Pneumocystis carinii	Dyspnea, fever, weight loss
Toxoplasma gondii	Fever
Cryptosporidium	Malabsorption, diarrhea
Isospora belli	Diarrhea
Microspora	Malabsorption, diarrhea
Entamoeba histolytica	Diarrhea
Giardia lamblia	Diarrhea
Acanthamoeba	Meningoencephalitis
Bacteria	
Campylobacter	Abdominal pain, cramping, bloody diarrhea, fever
Legionella	Fever
Listeria monocytogenes	Fever
Mycobacterium avium-intracellulare	Fever, weight loss, diarrhea, malabsorption
Salmonella	Diarrhea, bacteremia
Shigella	Abdominal pain, bloody diarrhea, fever
Fungi	
Aspergillus	Fungemia, fevers, weight loss
Candida albicans	Thrush, stomatitis, esophagitis, nausea
Cryptococcus neoformans	Fever, nausea, vomiting
Histoplasma capsulatum	Fever, weight loss, dysphagia
Viruses	
Cytomegalovirus	Esophagitis, colitis, diarrhea
Herpes simplex virus	Ulcerative mucocutaneous lesions, stomatitis, esophagitis, pneumonia
Epstein-Barr virus	Oral hairy leukoplakia
Hepatitis B	Nausea, vomiting, fever
Herpes zoster	Mucocutaneous lesions

Data from the Academy of Nutrition and Dietetics: *Manual of clinical dietetics*, ed 6, Chicago, 2000, Academy of Nutrition and Dietetics; Gold JWM: HIV-1 infection: diagnosis and management. *Med Clin North Am* 76(1):1, 1992; Bernard EM, Sepkowitz KA, Telzak EE, et al: Pneumocystosis. *Med Clin North Am* 76(1):107, 1992; and Ralten DJ: Nutrition and HIV infection: a review and evaluation of the extent of knowledge of the relationship between nutrition and HIV infection. *Nutr Clin Pract* 6(3):1S, 1991.

MEDICAL MANAGEMENT

With the advent of antiretroviral treatments in 1996, HIV became a chronic disease. The treatment regimen for HIV is cART. The standard combination includes nucleoside reverse transcriptase inhibitors (NRTIs), protease inhibitors (PIs), and non-nucleoside reverse transcriptase inhibitors (NNRTIs). New families of ART are now being used, such as fusion inhibitors and the HIV integrase strand transfer inhibitors that are to be used when the first lines of ART fail to control the viral load.[18] Although resistant viral strains to these medications have been recognized, the death rate from AIDS-related diseases has been significantly decreased with ART.[19]

Combination ART is used to achieve long-term viral suppression (measured by HIV viral load) and immunologic restoration (measured by CD4+ T-cell count) as a means to decrease HIV-related morbidity and mortality and improve quality of life. This is frequently complicated because retroviruses incorporate into the genetic material of the host and may not be removed by ART. Therefore medications to manage HIV are typically prescribed for the lifetime of the infected individual. Furthermore, HIV may hide in "sanctuaries," which are body regions where the cART may not be active, such as the central nervous system (CNS).[19]

Indications for starting ART were updated in February 2013, with recommendations to start ART at CD4+ T-cell count less than 500 cells/mm^3 to reduce risk of disease progression and to prevent transmission of HIV.[20] ART is recommended for pregnant women, those with HIV-associated nephropathy, and individuals coinfected with hepatitis B virus (HBV) regardless of CD4+ T-cell count.[19] Adherence to this drug regimen can be demanding for the HIV-infected individual and health care providers. It is critical to assess the patient's commitment to ART adherence because of its importance for successful therapy, and the patient's understanding of the benefits and risks of treatment. Furthermore, dosing convenience, drug safety profiles, viral genetic testing, and drug-drug interactions ought to be considered for the selection of treatment for each individual. On the whole, ART toxicities can be common and should be evaluated and compared with the benefits of favorable virologic and immunologic responses.[20]

Classes of Drugs

More than 26 antiretroviral agents are now available, with many combinations provided in one to two capsules daily from six classes of drugs (Table 24.2):

- Nucleoside reverse transcriptase inhibitors (NRTIs)
- Non-nucleoside reverse transcriptase inhibitors (NNRTIs)

TABLE 24.2   **Classes of Antiretroviral Drugs**

Drug Class	Generic Name (Other Names and Acronyms)	Brand Name	FDA Approval Date
Nucleoside Reverse Transcriptase Inhibitors (NRTIs)			
NRTIs block reverse transcriptase, an enzyme HIV needs to make copies of itself.	abacavir (abacavir sulfate, ABC)	Ziagen	December 17, 1998
	didanosine (delayed-release didanosine, dideoxyinosine, enteric-coated didanosine, ddl, ddl EC)	Videx / Videx EC (enteric-coated)	October 9, 1991 / October 31, 2000
	emtricitabine (FTC)	Emtriva	July 2, 2003
	lamivudine (3TC)	Epivir	November 17, 1995
	stavudine (d4T)	Zerit	June 24, 1994
	tenofovir disoproxil fumarate (tenofovir DF, TDF)	Viread	October 26, 2001
	zidovudine (azidothymidine, AZT, ZDV)	Retrovir	March 19, 1987
Non-Nucleoside Reverse Transcriptase Inhibitors (NNRTIs)			
NNRTIs bind to and later alter reverse transcriptase, an enzyme HIV needs to make copies of itself.	efavirenz (EFV)	Sustiva	September 17, 1998
	etravirine (ETR)	Intelence	January 18, 2008
	nevirapine (extended-release nevirapine, NVP)	Viramune / Viramune XR (extended release)	June 21, 1996 / March 25, 2011
	rilpivirine (rilpivirine hydrochloride, RPV)	Edurant	May 20, 2011
Protease Inhibitors (PIs)			
PIs block HIV protease, an enzyme HIV needs to make copies of itself	atazanavir (atazanavir sulfate, ATV)	Reyataz	June 20, 2003
	darunavir (darunavir ethanolate, DRV)	Prezista	June 23, 2006
	fosamprenavir (fosamprenavir calcium, FOS-APV, FPV)	Lexiva	October 20, 2003
	indinavir (indinavir sulfate, IDV)	Crixivan	March 13, 1996
	nelfinavir (nelfinavir mesylate, NFV)	Viracept	March 14, 1997
	ritonavir (RTV)[a]	Norvir	March 1, 1996
	saquinavir (saquinavir mesylate, SQV)	Invirase	December 6, 1995
	tipranavir (TPV)	Aptivus	June 22, 2005
Fusion Inhibitors			
Fusion inhibitors block HIV from entering the CD4 cells of the immune system.	enfuvirtide (T-20)	Fuzeon	March 13, 2003
Entry Inhibitors			
Entry inhibitors block proteins on the CD4 cells that HIV needs to enter the cells.	maraviroc (MVC)	Selzentry	August 6, 2007

TABLE 24.2　Classes of Antiretroviral Drugs—cont'd

Drug Class	Generic Name (Other Names and Acronyms)	Brand Name	FDA Approval Date
Integrase Inhibitors Integrase inhibitors block HIV integrase, an enzyme HIV needs to make copies of itself.	dolutegravir (DTG, dolutegravir sodium)	Tivicay	August 13, 2013
	elvitegravir (EVG)	Vitekta	September 24, 2014
	raltegravir (raltegravir potassium, RAL)	Isentress Isentress HD	October 12, 2007 May 26, 2017
Pharmacokinetic Enhancers Pharmacokinetic enhancers are used in HIV treatment to increase the effectiveness of an HIV medicine included in an HIV regimen.	cobicistat (COBI)	Tybost	September 24, 2014
Combination HIV Medicines Combination HIV medicines contain two or more HIV medicines from one or more drug classes.	abacavir and lamivudine (abacavir sulfate/lamivudine, ABC/3TC)	Epzicom	August 2, 2004
	abacavir, dolutegravir, and lamivudine (abacavir sulfate/dolutegravir sodium/lamivudine, ABC/DTG/3TC)	Triumeq	August 22, 2014
	abacavir, lamivudine, and zidovudine (abacavir sulfate/lamivudine/zidovudine, ABC/3TC/ZDV)	Trizivir	November 14, 2000
	atazanavir and cobicistat (atazanavir sulfate/cobicistat, ATV/COBI)	Evotaz	January 29, 2015
	darunavir and cobicistat (darunavir ethanolate/cobicistat, DRV/COBI)	Prezcobix	January 29, 2015
	efavirenz, emtricitabine, and tenofovir disoproxil fumarate (efavirenz/emtricitabine/tenofovir DF, EFV/FTC/TDF)	Atripla	July 12, 2006
	elvitegravir, cobicistat, emtricitabine, and tenofovir alafenamide fumarate (elvitegravir/cobicistat/emtricitabine/tenofovir alafenamide, EVG/COBI/FTC/TAF)	Genvoya	November 5, 2015
	elvitegravir, cobicistat, emtricitabine, and tenofovir disoproxil fumarate (QUAD, EVG/COBI/FTC/TDF)	Stribild	August 27, 2012
	emtricitabine, rilpivirine, and tenofovir alafenamide (emtricitabine/rilpivirine/tenofovir AF, emtricitabine/rilpivirine/tenofovir alafenamide fumarate, emtricitabine/rilpivirine hydrochloride/tenofovir AF, emtricitabine/rilpivirine hydrochloride/tenofovir alafenamide, emtricitabine/rilpivirine hydrochloride/tenofovir alafenamide fumarate, FTC/RPV/TAF)	Odefsey	March 1, 2016
	emtricitabine, rilpivirine, and tenofovir disoproxil fumarate (emtricitabine/rilpivirine hydrochloride/tenofovir disoproxil fumarate, emtricitabine/rilpivirine/tenofovir, FTC/RPV/TDF)	Complera	August 10, 2011
	emtricitabine and tenofovir alafenamide (emtricitabine/tenofovir AF, emtricitabine/tenofovir alafenamide fumarate, FTC/TAF)	Descovy	April 4, 2016
	emtricitabine and tenofovir disoproxil fumarate (emtricitabine/tenofovir DF, FTC/TDF)	Truvada	August 2, 2004
	lamivudine and zidovudine (3TC/ZDV)	Combivir	September 27, 1997
	lopinavir and ritonavir (ritonavir-boosted lopinavir, LPV/r, LPV/RTV)	Kaletra	September 15, 2000

[a]Although ritonavir is a protease inhibitor (PI), it is generally used as a pharmacokinetic enhancer as recommended in the *Guidelines for the Use of Antiretroviral Agents in HIV-1-Infected Adults and Adolescents* and the *Guidelines for the Use of Antiretroviral Agents in Pediatric HIV Infection*.
From FDA: Antiretroviral Drugs Used in the Treatment of HIV Infection; National Institute of Allergy and Infectious Diseases: Drugs That Fight HIV-1; National Library of Medicine: Drug information from the DailyMed website; US Department of Health and Human Services: Drugs. From https://aidsinfo.nih.gov/drugs; https://aidsinfo.nih.gov/understanding-hiv-aids/fact-sheets/21/58/fda-approved-hiv-medicines.

- Protease inhibitors (PIs)
- Fusion inhibitors (block HIV from entering the CD4 cells of the immune system.)
- Entry inhibitors (block proteins on the CD4 cells that HIV needs to enter the cells.
- Integrase inhibitors (block HIV integrase, an enzyme HIV needs to make copies of itself.)

In addition, there are new pharmacokinetic enhancers, which are used in HIV treatment to increase the effectiveness of antiretroviral; there are also combination HIV medicines that contain two or more HIV medicines from one or more drug classes. This makes treatment regimens easier, lessens pill burden, and optimistically increases patient medication compliance (see Table 24.2). The wide variety of medicines to choose from has made the HIV viral control more effective, to the point where nutrition interventions need to focus more on the treatment of the disease of aging, and the potential side effects of the drugs.

Many side effects occur from these drugs, which may contribute to noncompliance with drug regimens, as listed in the *Diet-Medications Interactions* box, "Protease Inhibitor Drug-Nutrient Side Effects and Interactions." Side effects such as nausea and diarrhea may require diet modifications (Table 24.3).

TABLE 24.3 Antiretroviral Drugs Used to Treat HIV/AIDS and Potential Adverse Nutritional Consequences

BRAND NAME	Generic Name	Manufacturer Name	Potential Adverse Nutritional Consequences
Multi-Class Combination Products			
Atripla	Efavirenz, emtricitabine and tenofovir disoproxil fumarate	Bristol-Myers Squibb and Gilead Sciences	It should be taken on an empty stomach, long-term intake associated with reduced bone density. Common gastrointestinal (GI) reactions to tenofovir are diarrhea, nausea.
Complera	Emtricitabine, rilpivirine, and tenofovir disoproxil fumarate	Gilead Sciences	Take with meal. Although uncommon, it has been associated with abdominal fullness, flatulence, indigestion, lack of appetite, diarrhea, nausea, and vomiting. Potential redistribution of body fat. It contains tenofovir, and its long-term intake has been associated with reduced bone density.
Stribild	Elvitegravir, cobicistat, emtricitabine, tenofovir disoproxil fumarate	Gilead Sciences	Nausea and diarrhea.
Nucleoside Reverse Transcriptase Inhibitors (NRTIs)[a]			
Combivir	Lamivudine and zidovudine	GlaxoSmithKline	Take without regard to meals; constipation, taste alterations possible; macrocytic anemia or neutropenia possible. Uncommon side effects are abdominal pain, nausea, vomiting.
Emtriva	Emtricitabine, FTC	Gilead Sciences	Take without regard to meals; snacks may reduce GI upset.
Epivir	Lamivudine, 3TC	GlaxoSmithKline	Take without regard to meals; snacks may reduce GI upset.
Epzicom	Abacavir and lamivudine	GlaxoSmithKline	Take without regard to meals; snacks may reduce GI upset; alcohol can increase drug levels; nausea, vomiting, diarrhea, and loss of appetite possible.
Hivid	Zalcitabine, dideoxycytidine, ddC (no longer marketed)	Hoffmann-La Roche	Take without regard to meals; vomiting, stomach/abdominal pain, oral lesions, constipation, or persistent nausea may occur; rare chance of pancreatitis.
Retrovir	Zidovudine, azidothymidine, AZT, ZDV	GlaxoSmithKline	Take without regard to meals; constipation, taste alterations possible; macrocytic anemia or neutropenia possible.
Trizivir	Abacavir, zidovudine, and lamivudine	GlaxoSmithKline	Take without regard to meals; snacks may reduce GI upset; alcohol can increase drug levels; nausea, vomiting, diarrhea, and loss of appetite possible.
Truvada	Tenofovir disoproxil fumarate and emtricitabine	Gilead Sciences	Take without regard to meals; diarrhea, nausea, vomiting, and flatulence possible.
Videx EC	Enteric-coated didanosine, ddI EC	Bristol Myers-Squibb	Take 30 min before or 2 h after meal; do not mix with acidic liquid (e.g., grapefruit juice, oranges, other citrus; tomatoes or tomato juice); do not take antacids with magnesium or aluminum within 2 h; nausea possible.
Videx	Didanosine, dideoxyinosine, ddI	Bristol Myers-Squibb	
Viread	Tenofovir disoproxil fumarate, TDF	Gilead Sciences	Take without regard to meals; diarrhea, nausea, vomiting, and flatulence possible.
Zerit	Stavudine, d4T	Bristol Myers-Squibb	Take without regard to meals; snacks may limit GI upset; mouth/esophageal ulcers possible.
Ziagen	Abacavir sulfate, ABC	GlaxoSmithKline	Take without regard to meals; snacks may reduce GI upset; alcohol can increase drug levels; nausea, vomiting, diarrhea, and loss of appetite possible.

TABLE 24.3   Antiretroviral Drugs Used to Treat HIV/AIDS and Potential Adverse Nutritional Consequences—cont'd

BRAND NAME	Generic Name	Manufacturer Name	Potential Adverse Nutritional Consequences
Non-Nucleoside Reverse Transcriptase Inhibitors (NNRTIs)[a]			
Edurant	Rilpivirine	Tibotec Therapeutics	Take with meal, a protein drink alone does not replace a meal. Although uncommon, it has been associated with abdominal fullness, flatulence, indigestion, lack of appetite, nausea and vomiting.
Intelence	Etravirine	Tibotec Therapeutics	Take after a meal; nausea possible.
Rescriptor	Delavirdine, DLV	Pfizer	Take without regard to meals; avoid St. John's wort; constipation, diarrhea, dry mouth, and flatulence possible; decreased appetite possible.
Sustiva	Efavirenz, EFV	Bristol Myers-Squibb	High-fat/high-calorie meals increase peak plasma concentrations; take on empty stomach; take at bedtime to decrease adverse effects; taste alterations, potential loss of appetite, and flatulence possible.
Viramune (Immediate Release)	Nevirapine, NVP	Boehringer Ingelheim	Take without regard to meals; snacks may limit GI upset; nausea and loss of appetite possible
Viramune XR (Extended Release)	Nevirapine, NVP	Boehringer Ingelheim	
Protease Inhibitors (PIs)[b]			
Agenerase	Amprenavir, APV (no longer marketed)	GlaxoSmithKline	Take on empty stomach; low fat limits GI upset (avoid high fat meals); avoid grapefruit juice; increase fluid intake; avoid taking antacids within 2 h; nausea, vomiting, gas, and diarrhea possible.
Aptivus	Tipranavir, TPV	Boehringer Ingelheim	Take with a fatty meal.
Crixivan	Indinavir, IDV	Merck	Avoid grapefruit juice; avoid St. John's wort; (unboosted) take 2 h before or 2 h after meals; take on empty stomach, but if not tolerated may take with nonfat milk; eat low-fat meals and light snacks; (ritonavir [RTV] boosted) timing of food intake not a consideration; loss of appetite, nausea, and metallic taste possible.
Invirase	Saquinavir mesylate, SQV	Hoffmann-La Roche	Take within 2 h of a meal; GI intolerance, nausea, and diarrhea possible.
Kaletra	Lopinavir and ritonavir, LPV/RTV	Abbott Laboratories	Time of food not a consideration; nausea, vomiting, and diarrhea possible.
Lexiva	Fosamprenavir calcium, FOS-APV	GlaxoSmithKline	Take without regard to meals; diarrhea, nausea, and vomiting possible.
Norvir	Ritonavir, RTV	Abbott Laboratories	Take with food if possible (may improve tolerability); nausea, vomiting, diarrhea, and taste changes possible.
Prezista	Darunavir	Tibotec, Inc.	Take with food; diarrhea and nausea are possible.
Reyataz	Atazanavir sulfate, ATV	Bristol-Myers Squibb	Take with food; avoid taking simultaneously with antacids or H_2 blockers.
Viracept	Nelfinavir mesylate, NFV	Agouron Pharmaceuticals	Diarrhea is possible.
Fusion Inhibitors[c]			
Fuzeon	Enfuvirtide, T-20	Hoffmann-La Roche & Trimeris	Not applicable. It is a subcutaneous application.
Entry Inhibitors: CCR5 Co-Receptor Antagonist[d]			
Selzentry	Maraviroc	Pfizer	No food effect; take with or without food; abdominal pain possible.
HIV Integrase Strand Transfer Inhibitors[e]			
Isentress	Raltegravir	Merck & Co., Inc.	Take with or without food; nausea and diarrhea possible.
Tivicay	Dolutegravir	GlaxoSmithKline	Take 2 h before or 6 h after taking cation-containing antacids or laxatives, sucralfate, oral iron supplements, oral calcium supplements, or buffered medications. Body fat redistribution is possible.

[a]Nucleoside/nucleotide reverse transcriptase inhibitors (NRTIs) and non-nucleoside reverse transcriptase inhibitors (NNRTIs) prevent reverse transcriptase from making more copies of the human immunodeficiency virus (HIV) genome.

[b]Protease inhibitors (PIs) prevent protease from breaking apart long strands of viral proteins to make the smaller, active proteins HIV needs to reproduce.

[c]Fusion inhibitors are specific types of entry inhibitors that prevent fusion between HIV's outer envelope and the cell's outer membrane.

[d]Entry Inhibitors—CCR5 co-receptor antagonists are chemokine receptor antagonists; they are the first antiretrovirals to bind a cellular protein of the host.

[e]Integrase inhibitors prevent integrase from inserting HIV's genetic material into an infected cell's genetic material.

Data from Dong KR, Mangili A: Highly active antiretroviral therapy (HAART). In Hendricks KM, Dong KR, Gerrior JL, editors: *Nutrition management of HIV and AIDS*, Chicago, 2009, Academy of Nutrition and Dietetics; Panel on Antiretroviral Guidelines for Adults and Adolescents: *Guidelines for the use of antiretroviral agents in HIV-1-infected adults and adolescents*, Washington, DC, 2008, Department of Health and Human Services; Keithley JK, Swanson B: *Nursing guidelines: HIV and nutrition*, ANAC, Ohio. From http//www.nursesinaidscare.org.

NUTRITION THERAPY

Basic Role of Nutrition in the HIV Disease Process

Infections generally create an environment that leads to reduction in nutrient intake and absorption, as well as an increase in the use and requirement for nutrients.[21,22] HIV infection is associated with the destruction of the immune system. As a result, it is critical to maintain adequate nutritional status in HIV-infected individuals. The disease, in combination with underlying or consequent malnutrition, creates a vicious cycle that aggravates disease progression and affects chances of survival.[23] Poor nutritional status may accelerate disease progression and lead to poor outcomes. In addition, HIV infection impairs nutrient intake, digestion, absorption, and use, leading to weight loss, nutrient deficiencies, and compromised immune function and competence, as well as susceptibility to infections.[22,23]

In people living with HIV, clinical symptoms and treatment side effects such as loss of appetite, and nausea and vomiting may lead to reduction in food and nutrient intake.[24-26] This contributes to weight loss and nutrient deficiency even in asymptomatic patients.[24,27] Weight loss has been persistent among people who are infected with HIV even in the era of ART.[27] In addition to inadequate intake, diarrhea and malabsorption of macronutrients and micronutrients are also common during HIV infection. These conditions are exacerbated by infections from pathogens such as *Cryptosporidium* and *Cytomegalovirus*. When fat malabsorption is present, it may cause decreased bioavailability or deficiency of fat-soluble vitamins.[23] Even among asymptomatic patients, HIV infection can lead to intestinal defects like permeability and epithelial damage.[23,28,29] The infection can also alter the body's ability to metabolize and store nutrients such as carbohydrates,[24] proteins, and fats by altering the effect of enzymes and hormones needed for their metabolism. HIV infection may impair the production of enzymes and transport proteins in the GI tract that are needed for nutrient digestion and absorption.[22]

Poor nutritional status impairs immune function either directly or indirectly. Directly, nutritional deficiency can interfere with the primary activity of the lymphoid system such as during immune cell triggering, interaction, and differentiation. Indirectly, it can affect other metabolic and cellular processes needed for immune regulation.[30] Several micronutrients are necessary for proper immune function. Vitamin A is important for the growth and function of T and B cells, antibody responses, as well as for the maintenance of the epithelial integrity of the respiratory and GI tract.[23] Vitamin E is essential for the function of T, B, and phagocytic cells.[31] It also acts as an antioxidant protecting vitamin A and fats from oxidation.[22] Zinc and selenium are important nutrients for the immune system, acting as antioxidants, with involvement in the development of cell-mediated and nonspecific immunity, as well as vitamin A transport.[22] Several other vitamins and minerals play a role in immune function, either at the physical barrier (skin/mucosal) level, cellular immunity level, or antibody production level.[32] Vitamins B_6, B_{12}, C, D, folic acid, iron, and copper all work to enhance the protective activities of immune cells. With the exception of vitamin C and iron, the rest of the nutrients work to support antibody production.[32] Nutritional deficiency during HIV infection could result in increased levels of prooxidants, leading to oxidative stress, which may hasten HIV replication through nuclear factor κB (NF-κB), a transcriptional promoter of proteins involved in HIV transcription.[23] It can also result in immunosuppression, which may affect viral expression and replication and ultimately disease progression and death. Factors that could contribute to poor nutrition include inadequate nutrient intake and absorption, poor appetite, metabolic problems, chronic infection, and limited food availability, among others.[22]

HIV-infected individuals are more susceptible to infections because of compromised immunity. Chronic HIV infection also increases the nutritional requirements of those infected above those who are uninfected.[23,33,34] ART medications can also affect energy expenditure, contributing to higher caloric needs.[34] HIV-infected individuals who are asymptomatic require on average 10% more energy intake than what is recommended for noninfected healthy individuals for the same age and sex.[33] This requirement increases to 20%–30% during the symptomatic phase. Increased energy requirement, among other nutrient needs, has made optimal nutrition critical for managing the HIV infection.[35]

Nutritional Status During HIV Infection

Nutritional status, defined by *Mosby's Medical Dictionary* as the "extent to which nutrients are available to meet metabolic needs,"[36] is a good predictor of morbidity and mortality in the course of HIV infection.[37,38] There are several indicators used in measuring nutritional status, such as anthropometric measures (weight, height, body mass index [BMI], and body composition), biochemical measures (such as serum levels of nutrients), clinical measures (such as hemoglobin, hematocrit, and serum albumin), and dietary intake of nutrients. The impact that an infection has on nutritional status is dependent on the baseline nutritional status, as well as the nature and severity level of the infection.[39] During HIV infection, higher mortality rates are predicted by poor nutritional status, even when treatment is initiated.[40,41] When compared with noninfected individuals, HIV-infected patients have lower serum concentration of nutrients and were more susceptible to nutritional deficiencies.[42-45]

Early HIV studies reported a severe impact of the disease on nutritional status before the era of ART. Malnutrition, often associated with low serum levels of micronutrients, was common regardless of the socioeconomic status of the population infected, and serum nutrient deficiencies were associated with disease progression.[23,44,46] Review articles that examined the prevalence and impact of micronutrient deficiency in HIV patients in the pre-ART era reported deficiencies in vitamins A, C, E, B_{12}, zinc, and selenium.[23,47,48] Vitamin B_6 and vitamin D deficiencies were also reported in HIV patients prior to ART use.[44,49] Since the advent of ART use, morbidity and mortality in HIV-infected individuals has declined; however, poor nutritional status is still being reported among some populations.[41,50]

Studies conducted in developed countries among HIV patients receiving ART report conflicting results on micronutrient status, even when supplementation was sometimes provided.[51-58] Some studies found significant differences in serum concentrations of α-tocopherol, α- and β-carotene, vitamin B_{12}, and folate between those receiving ART and controls.[53,55,58] Other cross-sectional and longitudinal studies found no differences in vitamins A and E,[54,55] B_6 and folate,[52] selenium, zinc, iron, and copper between those receiving ART and controls.[51,54] One study found those who received ART to have lower plasma concentration of vitamin A compared with controls.[56] A recent study reported 77% of HIV-infected study participants to be malnourished. However, it is unclear whether these individuals were receiving ART treatment or not.[59]

Most studies investigating micronutrient status in HIV-infected individuals used serum or plasma measures.[23,46] These measures have some limitation because they may not be sensitive indicators of micronutrient status,[23] and most of these micronutrients are acute-phase reactants and will vary in body compartments during an infection.[46] HIV-infected individuals are susceptible to opportunistic infections; hence, unless other infections were accounted and controlled for in these studies, the results might have limitations. A consistent body of literature exists that supports a strong relationship between HIV infection and poor nutritional status.[46] Most evidence supports that this relationship is a reciprocal, vicious, and deadly cycle, in which malnutrition and HIV infection advance each other.[22,23]

Weight loss is another indicator of nutritional status, and it has been linked to adverse outcomes during HIV infection.[60] Although ART treatment improved survival rates, weight loss (even as low as 5%) continued to be an independent predictor of morbidity and mortality in this population up until the early years of the millennium, when ART was available and reports of increased overweight/obesity started to emerge among the population.[27,61] In 2000 the Nutrition for Healthy Living (NFHL) found 13% of its 633 participants to have wasting at the time of enrollment to the study.[38] At follow-up visits, 18% and 21% had, respectively, lost more than 10% and more than 5% of their body weight, with 8% having a BMI of less than 20.38 kg/m². The weight loss observed in this group occurred in patients successfully treated with ART, in those for whom ART treatment failed, and also in ART-naïve patients.[50] The weight loss was also found to be a combination of fat and lean body mass loss, depending on initial body weight and etiology of weight loss (i.e., whether it was a result of abnormalities in intake or altered metabolism).[27,62]

The NFHL also reported overweight in its cohort to be between 33% and 40% in men and 27% and 34% in women. Among this same cohort, obesity rates were 6–13% in men and 21–29% in women.[63,64] Other studies have also reported increasing overweight and obesity rates among HIV-infected individuals, with several studies reporting higher prevalence of overweight and obesity compared with wasting in the study populations.[65-68] It appears that overweight/obesity is being reported at diagnosis, with continued weight gain during HIV infection. One author suggests this to be a reflection of improved health status in this population, even as the trend mirrors what is being observed in the general public.[67] With between 46% and 60% overweight/obesity rates being reported in certain HIV-infected populations, obesity, and not weight loss or wasting, seems to be the new nutritional concern for this population, especially when coronary heart disease is on the rise in the ART-treated individuals.[67,68] Lack of access to nutritious foods, metabolic abnormalities, and illicit drug use, all of which can aggravate weight loss and the catabolic nature of the HIV disease, are still common; hence it is important not to completely rule out weight loss as a nutrition concern in this population.[69-78] The new epidemic of overweight and obesity may be attributed to unhealthy eating habits, excessive caloric and fat intake, and treatment-related metabolic alterations, especially with lipid metabolism.[64,79-83]

Several studies have reported on issues of dietary and nutrient intake of HIV-infected individuals.[84-90] Caloric and fat overconsumption seems to be a consistent theme in developed areas.[84,85,87-89] In low-income settings the opposite problem exists, with numerous studies reporting inadequate nutrient intake to be common among HIV-infected people, especially in those regions where ART is still not widely available.[24,91,92] In resource-adequate areas, low intakes have been reported in HIV-infected sociodemographic groups such as women, drug abusers, and minorities at risk for health care disparities and adverse clinical outcomes.[25,91,93] On the other hand, adequate nutrient consumption is found in HIV-infected men who are educated, high-income earners, and users of supplements.[86,87] Two studies found nutrient intake among these economically advantaged HIV-infected individuals to be higher than that reported by HIV-noninfected populations.[86,93] Some studies that have investigated biochemical markers such as hemoglobin, hematocrit, and albumin among HIV-infected people have consistently reported these parameters as low in this population.[59,84,89,90,94-96] However, most of the studies have been conducted in low-resource areas. A multicenter study, conducted among women in North America, reported low albumin levels in those infected with HIV and concluded that baseline albumin level independently predicted mortality in this group, with a 48% mortality rate in the lowest serum albumin category compared with 11% in the highest category.[97]

In summary, the impact that an infection has on nutritional status is dependent on the nutritional status at the onset of the infection, as well as the nature and severity of the infection. In HIV infection the literature is consistent in demonstrating a strong relationship between HIV infection and poor nutritional status. Most evidence supports that this relationship is a reciprocal, vicious, and deadly cycle, in which malnutrition and HIV infection advance each other. In the United States, where ART is available and HIV has become a manageable disease, the nutritional care has shifted its emphasis from preventing wasting toward preventing obesity, hyperlipidemias, and other long-term complications of treatment, as described in Box 24.1.

BOX 24.1   Nutrition-Related Complications of AIDS and Nutritional Care

Nutrition-Related Complications of AIDS	Nutrition Care and Recommendations
Wasting/Rapid Weight Loss due to: • Reduced intake • Excessive nutrient losses due to vomit, diarrhea, or malabsorption • Hypermetabolism • Adverse gastrointestinal (GI) reactions to treatment	• Recommend a high calorie (35 kcal/kg), high protein (1.5–2 g/kg) diet with snacks between meals • Oral high calorie or protein supplement if extra calories/protein needed • The physician may prescribe appetite stimulants if needed (Megace, Marinol, etc.)
Nutritional Anemias: • Microcytic anemia/iron deficiency • Macrocytic anemia/folate or vitamin B_{12} deficiency	**Iron deficiency anemia**: • Daily oral iron supplements and recommend iron-rich foods, such as meat, fish, poultry, beans, dried fruits and fortified grains, cereals, and energy bars. Also good sources of vitamin C (orange juice, cantaloupe slices) at every meal • Avoid iron-binding foods such as tea, coffee, or milk with meals or supplements. **Folate or vitamin B_{12} deficiency anemia:** • Oral folate supplements • Intermuscular (IM) or subcutaneous (SQ) injections of vitamin B_{12} • A high-protein diet (1.5 g/kg); meats, eggs, and milk products are rich in vitamin B_{12} • Fresh fruits, and vegetables and their juices

Continued

BOX 24.1 Nutrition-Related Complications of AIDS and Nutritional Care—cont'd

Nutrition-Related Complications of AIDS	Nutrition Care and Recommendations
Insulin Resistance	• Monitor insulin resistance by measuring blood sugar, triglycerides, and Hgb$_{A1c}$ if fasting glucose levels are consistently elevated, and adjust the diet accordingly • Diabetic diet if needed
Lipodystrophy/Lipoatrophy: Loss of peripheral fat, in the face, arms, legs and/or buttocks, and an accumulation of central fat in the intraabdominal area, upper back (buffalo hump), and/or breasts	• A healthy diet using the MyPlate recommendations and an exercise regimen similar to those recommended for uninfected individuals • Caloric intake should be adjusted to achieve and maintain a healthy body weight
Hyperlipidemias: • Triglyceridemias • Total and low-density lipoprotein cholesterolemia	• The National Cholesterol Education Program (NCEP) Therapeutic Lifestyle Changes (TLC) diet • For a complete description of this diet, please access the National Heart, Lung, and Blood Institute website at http://www.nhlbi.nih.gov/guidelines/cholesterol/index.htm
Sore Mouth/Throat, Stomatitis	• Eat cold foods such as ice creams, Popsicles, and Italian ices • Moisten foods by adding gravies or sauces or soaking in liquids; prefer soft foods • Avoid hard foods, and acidic, spicy, hot foods or beverages
Diarrhea	• Avoid beverages that irritate or stimulate motility such as drinks that contain alcohol, and carbonated or caffeinated beverages • Eat easy-to-digest foods, such as canned peaches, cooked carrots, baked chicken, turkey, or fish • Avoid lactose-containing products such as milk and its products • Avoid gassy foods • Eat binding foods such as bananas, rice, applesauce, tea, toast, and gummy bears • Replace fluid and electrolytes with electrolyte-containing foods and fluids • Use safety strategies for food handling, storage, and preparation, as well as strategies for eating safely in restaurants and traveling abroad
HIV Dementia	• The care of a caregiver, who actively supports the nutritional care of the patient, is essential to maintain adequate nutritional status, adherence to medication, and prevent HIV disease progression

Data from Keithley JK, Swanson B: *Nursing guidelines: HIV and nutrition*, ANAC, Ohio. From http//www. nursesinaidscare.org.; US Food and Drug Administration: *Protecting and promoting your health. Antiretroviral drugs used in the treatment of HIV infection.* From http://www.fda.gov/ForConsumers/byAudience/ForPatientAdvocates/HIVandAIDSActivities/ucm118915.htm.

Food Insecurity Among HIV–Infected Persons

In 2011 more than 50 million individuals lived in households that experienced food insecurity.[98] According to the US Department of Agriculture (USDA), these included 17.9 million households, 11 million of which experienced low food security and 5.7% of which experienced very low food security.[98] Several studies have evaluated the prevalence of food insecurity among people infected with HIV, and their reports suggest that the prevalence is higher than those recorded at the national level, especially in resource-adequate settings. One study[61] found that 81% of HIV-infected adults surveyed in Miami who experienced wasting were food insecure, whereas another study conducted in Miami and Atlanta among a similar population reported 34% food insufficiency.[99] In British Columbia, 48% of HIV-positive study participants were reported to be food insecure,[72] and another study conducted in the same province, but among HIV-infected intravenous drug users, had a food insecurity prevalence of 64%.[100] Among homeless and marginally housed HIV-infected individuals in San Francisco,[75] it was estimated that 49% had food insecurity. Another study involving HIV-infected patients from eight veterans' clinics, in the Veteran Aging Cohort Study, reported that 24% of participants receiving ART treatment were food insecure.[101]

Food insecurity needs to be addressed because it has been found to contribute to HIV transmission, especially among food-insecure women responsible for their households.[102,103] Food insecurity also impacts HIV transmission by compromising nutritional status, and consequently, immunologic status.[104] Inadequate nutrient intake may affect the mucosal integrity of the genitalia and GI tract, leading to increased risk of HIV transmission. Compromised nutritional status has been associated with mother-to-child transmissions in resource-constrained settings.[105,106]

Food insecurity interferes with HIV-related care and services.[106-110] A recent study found food insecurity to be associated with missed clinic visits, with 17% of study participants having to give up ART treatment, and 30% and 32% did not access outpatient and inpatient treatment, respectively, because of competing demands for food.[77] HIV-infected persons who are food insecure, especially those with low socioeconomic status and limited resources, frequently need to choose between receiving HIV-related services or food procurement.[106,108]

ART for HIV infection is most effective when adherence to treatment is greater than 95%.[111] Studies conducted in developed countries and resource-limited settings have identified that food-insecure HIV-infected individuals are less likely to adhere to treatment, compared with their food-secure counterparts.[75,112] However, adherence to treatment increased among those who received food assistance, stressing the importance of food assistance among low-income HIV-infected patients.[113-115]

During the nutritional assessment and care of the HIV patient, it is important to ask questions on food insecurity and refer the patient to the community and government programs, such as SNAP and food pantries, that provide a food security net for these patients who are at very high nutritional risk.

Nutrition Assessment

A thorough initial nutrition assessment for people living with HIV is important for the continuing nutrition care that follows.

A registered dietitian (RD) should perform an assessment that provides the necessary information for planning and individualizing the nutritional support for the HIV-infected person. The nutritional assessment should establish rapport between the patient and the provider, creating a human context within which this continuum of nutritional care and support is provided. The basic nutrition assessment will provide a practical guide for HIV-infected patients, using the framework of the Nutrition Care Process[116] and these four steps: (1) nutrition assessment and reassessment, (2) nutrition diagnosis, (3) nutrition intervention, and (4) nutrition monitoring and evaluation.

Components of the Nutrition, Clinical, and Biochemical Assessments

Components of Nutritional Assessment

- Diet Intake Assessment
  - Usual intake, current intake, restrictions, modifications (use 24-hour recall and food diaries)
  - Ethnic and cultural food practices
  - Limitations in food access, food preparation, or both
  - Food intolerances, allergies, or both
  - Use of macronutrient or micronutrient supplements (or use of both)
  - Alcohol intake
  - Patient's goals for improving his or her intake
  - Use of fraudulent nutrition products or fads
- Psychosocial issues and comorbidities related to nutrition
  - Living situation, personal support
  - Food environment, types of meals, eating assistance needed
  - History of eating disorders or body image concerns
  - Housing status
- Food insecurities
  - Access to safe food and water
  - Comorbidities related to the disease and treatment
  - Other related comorbidities
- Medications related to the disease and/or comorbidities

Components of Clinical Assessment[116]

- Medical history
- Physical parameters related to nutrition care
- Physical activity level
- Existing nutrition-related issues:
  - Hepatitis
  - Diabetes
  - Oral health issues
  - Bone disorders
- Family history of nutrition-related issues
- Weight history
- Usual level of physical activity
- GI complications
- Medications:
  - Potential food and drug interactions
  - Nutrition-related adverse effects
- Use of any complementary therapies (see the Complementary and Alternative Medicine [CAM] box, "Are Persons with HIV and AIDS Vulnerable to Nutritional Quackery?")
- Presence of opportunistic infections that may affect intake or metabolism
- Anthropometric measurements
  - Weight
  - BMI
  - Subcutaneous fat stores

COMPLEMENTARY AND ALTERNATIVE MEDICINE(CAM):

Are Persons With HIV and AIDS Vulnerable to Nutritional Quackery?[116]

People with chronic diseases, such as AIDS, who lack curative therapy and have poor prognoses are susceptible to claims of unproved therapies and nutrition quackery. The following questionable practices are some of the nutritional quackery being touted as treatments for HIV infection.

Megadoses of Nutrients

Large doses of vitamins A and C, selenium, and zinc have been recommended to restore cell-mediated immunity by increasing T-cell number and activity. The value of such large doses has not been established in controlled clinical studies. In fact, the opposite is true; megadoses of these nutrients can be dangerous. Chronic intakes of vitamin A in excess of 25,000 IU/day can be toxic, especially to the liver. Doses of vitamin C greater than 2000 mg can cause diarrhea, nausea, and GI upset; increase the risk of kidney stones; and cause a urine test to test falsely positive for diabetes. Chronic intakes of excess zinc, as little as 25 mg/day, can cause GI distress, nausea, and impaired immune function. Selenium is also toxic in high (>400 µg daily) chronic doses. In a review of the literature on HIV and micronutrients, Campa and Baum found evidence that micronutrient supplementation at nutritional doses is beneficial in people living with HIV.[117]

Components of the Biochemical Assessment

- Albumin
- Complete blood count
- Glucose
- Serum iron
- Electrolytes
- Vitamin levels
- Blood lipids
- Renal function
- Liver enzyme levels

GOALS OF NUTRITION THERAPY

Adequate nutritional status is associated with survival in individuals with HIV.[118] Nutrition interventions have been shown to reduce morbidity, improve health outcomes, reduce cost, and shorten hospital stays. Goals of nutrition intervention include the following:

- Early assessment and treatment of conditions leading to malnutrition
- Maintenance of nutrition status
  - Weight
  - Protein stores
- Management of comorbid conditions
  - Obesity
  - Diabetes
  - Hyperlipidemia
- Management of nutrition-related side effects from HIV or disease treatment

Nutrient Requirements

Adequate intake of nutrients is critical in restoring and maintaining health. The benefits of providing adequate amounts of energy, protein, fat, and micronutrients for people living with HIV are well described in the literature[1]; however, the optimal amounts of each nutrient to improve disease outcomes need more research.[117]

Energy

Individuals' energy needs will vary depending on numerous factors, including nutrient malabsorption, altered metabolism, nutrient depletion, severity of disease, and opportunistic infections. Adequate energy intake is important to prevent weight loss and loss of lean body mass. Care should be taken to estimate recommendations for daily energy intake, although no standard level of energy intake has been established.[1]

Protein

A diet that offers a protein intake ranging from 1.2–2.0 g protein/kg body weight may be beneficial for people living with HIV who have suffered wasting due to HIV progression, secondary opportunistic infections, and/or severe socioeconomic conditions. For those patients early in the disease who are asymptomatic, the Dietary Reference Intakes (DRIs) or 0.8 g protein/kg body weight may be adequate. Although high biologic value protein is desirable, a balanced combination of animal and vegetarian sources of protein may be used. Strict vegetarians should eat an extensive variety of foods to achieve sufficient intake of essential amino acids. In general, vegetarians will benefit from additional protein (1 g protein/kg/day), calorie, iron, and vitamin B_{12} supplementation.

Fat

Fat requirements of individuals with HIV do not seem to be different from the general population. Some medications, therapies for HIV, symptoms of infections (i.e., diarrhea), and malabsorption syndromes will possibly necessitate modification in the timing, quality, and type of fat intake for some persons. It is crucial to work with each individual closely to determine his or her needs.

Micronutrients

Currently, the complete function of micronutrients in treatment of HIV is not completely known. However, individuals are sure to benefit from a varied diet rich in micronutrients.

Food and Water Safety

The compromised immune system of individuals with AIDS puts them at great risk for foodborne or waterborne (Box 24.2) illnesses. Fortunately, nearly all cases of foodborne and waterborne illnesses can be reduced or prevented with appropriate safety measures, including safe food handling and use of safe water sources (see Box 24.1). It is essential for the RD to stress food and water safety in nutrition counseling for individuals living with HIV, their significant others, and their caretakers.

According to the CDC, boiling municipal tap water and use of bottled water are not essential unless a local public health department has issued notice that public drinking water is not safe for individuals living with HIV. Ice and fountain drinks in restaurants are often made from municipal water and should be avoided if safety of the water is unknown. Food and water sanitation may not be adequate when traveling abroad. Guidelines for choosing safer beverages are outlined in Box 24.3.

Antiretroviral Therapy–Associated Metabolic and Body Composition Changes

Although ART has revolutionized medical treatment of HIV and AIDS and reduced incidence of malnutrition and infections, its adverse effects continue to be a major obstacle to patient compliance and a limiting factor that drives the cost-benefit ratio for pharmacologic therapy. Lipodystrophy and its related fat distribution complications have become the major nutrition issues in patients being treated with PIs. Lipodystrophy syndrome consists of changes in body shape that

---

BOX 24.2 Extra Precautions to Ensure Safe Water

Persons living with HIV should avoid drinking water straight from lakes, rivers, streams, springs, or the ocean. Current recommendations from the Centers for Disease Control and Prevention (CDC) state the following:

- Because it might not be possible to be sure if tap water is safe, it is advisable to avoid tap water, including water or ice from a refrigerator ice maker, which is made with tap water.
- Always check with the local health department and water utility to see if they have issued any special notices for people with HIV about tap water.
- You may also wish to boil or filter your water, or drink bottled water.
- Drinks made at a fountain might not be safe because they are made with tap water.
- If you choose to boil or filter your water or drink only bottled water, do this all the time, not just at home.
- Boiling is the best way to kill germs in your water. Heat your water at a rolling boil for 1 minute. After the boiled water cools, put it in a clean bottle or pitcher with a lid and store it in the refrigerator. Use the water for drinking, cooking, or making ice.
- Water bottles and ice trays should be cleaned with soap and water before use. Don't touch the inside of them after cleaning. If you can, clean your water bottles and ice trays yourself.

BOX 24.3 Choosing Safer Beverages

Safer Beverages
- Carbonated beverages ("sodas") that come in cans or bottles (check seal to ensure safety)
- Fruit drinks that come in cans or bottles (check seal to ensure safety)
- Steaming hot tea or coffee
- Pasteurized milk and other dairy products
- Pasteurized juices

Beverages That May Not Be Safe
- Fountain drinks or drinks served over ice
- Drinks made by mixing frozen concentrate with water
- Iced tea or coffee
- Unpasteurized milk and other dairy products
- Fresh fruit juices (e.g., unpasteurized cider, fresh-squeezed orange juice)

Reprinted with permission from Vining L: General nutrition issues for healthy living with HIV infection. In Hendricks KM, Dong KR, Gerrior JL, editors: *Nutrition management of HIV and AIDS*, Chicago, 2009, Academy of Nutrition and Dietetics. Data from Centers for Disease Control and Prevention: *Safe food and water*. From http://www.cdc.gov/hiv/resources/brochures/food.htm; Keithley JK, Swanson B: *Nursing guidelines: HIV and nutrition*, ANAC, Ohio. From http//www.nursesinaidscare.org.

---

are caused by abnormal redistribution of fat. Fat accumulates in the abdominal area (truncal and visceral obesity), in the axillary pads, and in the dorsocervical pads ("buffalo hump") but decreases in the legs, arms, and nasolabial and cheek pads.[118,119] Lipodystrophy, although not life threatening, can cause varying degrees of depression, anxiety, social withdrawal, and low self-esteem, which can ultimately lead to poor medication compliance.[1] Many patients discontinue therapy, risking progression of HIV infection. ART can also cause hyperlipidemia (especially hypertriglyceridemia and hypercholesterolemia) and insulin resistance, which can significantly increase the risk of developing cardiovascular disease (CVD). This is a major concern and potentially a major deterrent to early or continuous therapy. Overall, the risk of myocardial infarction (MI) in HIV-infected patients taking PIs appears to be twofold to threefold greater than in the general population.[120] Persons on ART are also at increased risk of developing diabetes, hypertension, and osteoporosis.

Obtaining baseline anthropometrics (waist-hip ratio, bioelectric impedance analysis, skinfold measurements) and serial measurements (i.e., at each clinic visit) is important for monitoring changes in body composition. In addition, baseline measurements of triglycerides, total cholesterol and lipoproteins (high-density lipoprotein [HDL], low-density lipoprotein [LDL], very-low-density lipoprotein [VLDL]), blood glucose, and blood pressure should be obtained (also at each clinic visit to monitor for changes). Diet, exercise, and pharmacologic agents are useful in the treatment of lipodystrophy syndrome. Patients with abnormal LDL, HDL, and total cholesterol levels may benefit from observing the therapeutic lifestyle changes (TLC) diet, which emphasizes grains, cereals, legumes, fruits, vegetables, lean meats, poultry, fish, and low-fat dairy products. Diet-resistant hyperlipidemia may need to be controlled with lipid-lowering agents. Currently researchers are trying to determine which drugs can be used safely and effectively in persons on anti-HIV drugs. Individuals with insulin resistance and hyperglycemia will need counseling for carbohydrate counting and may benefit from a tailored diabetic diet. An individual with hypertriglyceridemia will need to limit intake of simple carbohydrates and alcohol. Exercise, especially weight training, may help prevent muscle wasting in the arms, legs, and buttocks, whereas aerobic exercise may help control abdominal visceral fat accumulation. Clinical trials are ongoing to determine actual benefits (see Box 24.1).

Use of Anabolic Agents in HIV and AIDS

The use of anabolic agents has been recommended as an effective way of improving gains in lean body mass. Anabolic agents such as oxandrolone and nandrolone decanoate are known to promote protein anabolism and are generally safe when taken as prescribed.[121] Recombinant human growth hormone (rhGH) (trade name Serostim) is the most extensively studied anabolic agent; it has also been shown to significantly improve lean body mass and nitrogen balance in treatment of HIV/AIDS wasting.[122] Human growth hormone therapy may help control some of the body composition changes seen in some individuals with lipodystrophy. However, many potential side effects exist for anabolic agents, including gynecomastia, testicular atrophy and decreased fertility, salt retention, lipid and carbohydrate abnormalities, and acne. Resistance or weight training have shown benefits in people living with HIV, and they have been found safe and effective for maintaining and improving lean body mass in infected people who are physically able to exercise.[123]

Nutrition Counseling, Education, and Supportive Strategies

Professionals and patients must be involved throughout the progressive course of the disease, because the patient's wishes and needs are ultimately paramount in various treatments and decisions about care. The goal of nutrition counseling is to make the fewest possible changes in the person's lifestyle and food patterns to promote optimal nutritional status while providing comfort and quality of life. In this person-centered care process, several counseling principles are particularly pertinent:

- *Motivation:* Changed behavior in any area requires motivation, desire, and ability to achieve one's goals. Until the patient perceives food patterns and behaviors as appropriate goals, it is best to wait for a better time and begin with establishing a general supportive climate in which to continue working together. Any specific obstacle raised by the patient, such as time, physical limitations, money,

or increased anxiety, can be met with related suggestions for the patient to consider. Priorities among needs should be recognized in the care plan, and items should be introduced according to order of importance and immediacy of the patient's nutrition problems.
- *Justification:* Any diet or food behavior change, with possible benefits and risks, must be clearly explained to the patient. The reason *why* something is being done is important to everyone. Understanding may increase compliance.
- *Provider-patient agreement:* In the best interests of all concerned, the patient and health care provider must agree to changes. Any change should be structured around daily routines and include caregivers. The nutrition counselor should provide any needed information and encouragement throughout the process.
- *Manageable steps:* All information given and actions agreed on should proceed in manageable steps, as small as necessary, in order of complexity and difficulty. Information overload can discourage anyone, and the particular stress load at any point can be intolerable for the patient. At such points of stress, patients are more vulnerable to the lure of unproved HIV/AIDS therapies.

Special Considerations for Children With AIDS[1]

Malnutrition, particularly inadequate calories and protein, and dehydration are serious issues in children with AIDS. In adults, the disease affects nutritional status. In children, not only is nutritional status affected but also growth and development can be significantly impaired, resulting in growth failure. A strong relationship exists between early nutritional status—poor growth, cachexia, poor oral intake, taste changes, decreased absorption of nutrients, and increased energy expenditure—and mortality risk; poor nutritional status increases mortality.

Nutrition assessments should be performed routinely in all children with AIDS so that any problems can be identified and treated as they occur and nutritional deficits can be minimized. As with adults, assessments should include evaluation of anthropometrics, visceral protein stores, red blood cell indexes, and electrolytes. In addition, growth assessment should be performed as frequently as needed, or following the standard pediatric schedule to monitor growth curves. Appetite, intake, and feeding ability should also be assessed. Developmental delays related to the disease can also increase the risk for developing failure to thrive.

Providing adequate calories to maintain linear growth and support weight gain can be difficult as a result of chronic infections, fever, and medications. The CDC revised the criteria for pregnant women, infants, and children in July 2012 and issued the following recommendation for the postnatal management of the HIV-exposed neonate[124]:

- A complete blood count and differential should be performed on newborns as a baseline evaluation.
- Decisions about the timing of subsequent monitoring of hematologic parameters in infants depend on baseline hematologic values, gestational age at birth, clinical condition of the infants, the zidovudine dose being administered, receipt of other antiretroviral drugs and concomitant medications, and maternal antepartum ART.
- If hematologic abnormalities are identified in infants receiving prophylaxis, decisions on whether to continue infant antiretroviral prophylaxis need to be individualized. Consultation with an expert in pediatric HIV infection is advised if early discontinuation of prophylaxis is considered.
- Some experts recommend more intensive monitoring of hematologic and serum chemistry and liver function assays at birth and when diagnostic HIV polymerase chain reaction tests are obtained in infants exposed to combination antiretroviral (ARV) drug regimens in utero or during the neonatal period.

- A recheck of hemoglobin and neutrophil counts is recommended 4 weeks after initiation of prophylaxis for infants who receive combination zidovudine/lamivudine-containing ARV prophylaxis regimens.

- Routine measurement of serum lactate is not recommended. However, measurement can be considered if an infant develops severe clinical symptoms of unknown etiology (particularly neurologic symptoms).

- Virologic tests are required to diagnose HIV infection in infants younger than 18 months of age and should be performed within the first 14–21 days of life, at 1–2 months, and at 4–6 months of age.

- To prevent *Pneumocystis jiroveci* pneumonia (PJP), all infants born to women with HIV infection should begin PJP prophylaxis at ages 4–6 weeks, after completing their ARV prophylaxis regimen, unless there is adequate test information to presumptively exclude HIV infection (see USPHS/IDSA Guidelines for the Prevention and Treatment of Opportunistic Infections in HIV-Exposed and Infected Children at http://aidsinfo.nih.gov/guidelines).

- Health care providers should routinely inquire about premastication of foods fed to infants, instruct HIV-infected caregivers to avoid this practice, and should advise on safer feeding options.

Diarrhea and malabsorption in the infected child can result in dehydration, which can be very serious in infants and young children, and the onset may occur suddenly.[1] To prevent dehydration, offer Popsicles, Jell-O, juices, and other beverages frequently. Oral rehydration fluids, such as Pedialyte, will also help replace electrolytes lost with acute or chronic diarrhea.

The following list contains suggestions to provide supplemental calories and nutrient intake[1]:

- Use a calorie-dense formula (24–27 kcal/oz) for infants. Add glucose polymers or medium-chain triglycerides (MCTs) to formulas, or reduce the amount of water added to powdered formulas to boost calories.

- Try liquid medical nutritional supplements, such as PediaSure, to provide supplemental calories.

- Add fats such as butter, margarine, or mayonnaise to foods to boost calories.

- Encourage nutrient-dense snacks such as raisins and peanuts or peanut butter.

- For the older, lactose-tolerant child, add skim milk powder to whole milk to boost calories and proteins.

- Make adjustments in diet consistency and temperatures to overcome eating difficulties associated with disease complications and any other eating problems.

- For lactose-intolerant children with AIDS, use soy-based infant formulas instead of milk.

- Add Lactaid (the enzyme lactase) to milk for better tolerance and digestion.

- Use low-lactose dairy foods such as yogurt and mild cheddar cheese, if tolerated.

Vitamin and mineral supplements in amounts one or two times the Recommended Dietary Allowance (RDA) may ensure adequate intake of these nutrients and contribute to meeting increased requirements that occur during hypermetabolic states. Attention should also be given to drug-nutrient interactions and other effects of these drugs on nutritional status.

Caregivers need to be particularly careful about food safety and sanitation. Safe food preparation is as important for children as it is for adults with HIV/AIDS, and the same food safety guidelines also apply.

Proper procedures and sanitary formula preparation must be followed for infants being bottle-fed. Infants should not be put to bed with a bottle of milk or juice, because these are easily contaminated. Unpasteurized milk and milk products should never be given because they may be a source of *Salmonella* and other microorganisms that can cause intestinal infections.

Children should never be fed any food directly from a jar, to avoid possible bacterial contamination of the remaining food from the child's mouth. Fruits and vegetables should be peeled or cooked, and meat, chicken, and fish should be well cooked. All utensils and dishes should be washed in a dishwasher or in hot, soapy water.

TO SUM UP

The viral evolution and current worldwide spread of HIV infection have reached epidemic proportions and are still growing. Disease progression follows three distinct stages (1) HIV acute infection; (2) asymptomatic (latency) stage, and (3) final full-blown AIDS, with complicating diseases leading to death. This overall disease progression from initial infection to death lasts approximately 10–12 years or in some cases even longer. The Public Health Service and the CDC are responsible for monitoring the disease and providing leadership in research and treatment development, based on collaborative information exchange with scientists worldwide.

During the initial decade of the epidemic in the 1980s, scientists learned the nature and life cycle of the new mutation of HIV, as well as its transmission modes and population groups at risk. Development of diagnostic-testing procedures has enabled population surveillance, individual detection of disease, and personal care to proceed. The important role of nutrition support in the personal care of HIV-infected individuals has become evident.

Medical management of HIV infection, which is without a vaccine or cure, involves supportive treatment of associated illnesses and complicating diseases coupled with administration of ART. In the terminal HIV stage, the virus eventually gains sufficient strength to destroy white blood cells of the host's immune system and death follows.

Nutritional management focuses on providing personal individual nutrition support to address the nutrition-related diseases associated with HIV itself, its complications, and its long-term treatment, as well as the aging of people living with HIV. The process of nutrition care involves performing a comprehensive nutrition, clinical, and biochemical assessment, which includes evaluation of personal needs, planning care with each patient and his or her caregivers, and meeting practical food needs. Throughout the nutrition care process, nutrition counseling, education, and strategic services, it is also important to provide or refer the patient and caregivers to psychosocial support. Although HIV/AIDS cannot be cured with nutrition, appropriate individualized nutritional support can prolong life.

QUESTIONS FOR REVIEW

1. Describe the evolutionary history of HIV and its current worldwide epidemic spread. How is it transmitted, and why do you think it has spread so rapidly? Identify major population groups at risk.

2. Describe the nature of HIV and its action in the human body. What is a retrovirus?

3. Describe the progression of HIV infection in terms of its stages of development from initial infection to death.

4. Identify the drugs currently used in the medical management of HIV/AIDS, and describe any associated actions, side effects, or toxicities that may relate to dietary management.
5. Discuss the causes of HIV wasting and its medical and nutrition therapies.
6. Outline the basic parts of a comprehensive initial nutrition assessment of a patient with HIV/AIDS.

7. Describe the general process of planning nutrition care based on patient assessment information and the main types of nutrition problems in patients with HIV/AIDS. Devise a related plan of action for each type of problem. Can you give an example of how you might follow up to determine which parts of your plan worked and which parts did not work? List any adjustments that should be made to your original nutrition care plan based on that follow-up.

REFERENCES

1. Fields-Gardner C, Campa A, American Dietetic Association: Position of the American Dietetic Association: nutrition intervention and human immunodeficiency virus infection, *J Am Diet Assoc* 110(7):1105–1119, 2010.
2. Tomkins A: Malnutrition, morbidity and mortality in children and their mothers, *Proc Nutr Soc* 59(1):135–146, 2000.
3. Caulfield LE, de Onis M, Blössner M, et al: Undernutrition as an underlying cause of child deaths associated with diarrhea, pneumonia, malaria, and measles, *Am J Clin Nutr* 80(1):193–198, 2004.
4. Blössner M, de Onis M: *Malnutrition: quantifying the impact at national and local levels*, Geneva, 2005, WHO.
5. AIDS.gov: *HIV/AIDS Basics.* http://aids.gov/hiv-aids-basics/hiv-aids-101/statistics/index.html. Reviewed June 6, 2012. Accessed May 17, 2013.
6. World Health Organization: *Data and Statistics.* Annex 8. HIV and AIDS statistics by WHO and UNICEF regions, 2010. http://www.who.int/hiv/data/en/. Accessed July 5, 2013.
7. Piot P, Quinn TC: Response to the AIDS pandemic—a global health model, *N Engl J Med* 368(23):2210–2218, 2013.
8. World Health Organization: *WHO issues new HIV recommendations calling for earlier treatment*, 2013. http://www.who.int/mediacentre/news/releases/2013/new_hiv_recommendations_20130630/en/index.html. Accessed July 3, 2013.
9. Brandt AM: How AIDS invented global health, *N Engl J Med* 368(23):2149–2152, 2013.
10. Pantaleo G, Graziosi C, Fauci AS: New concepts in the immunopathogenesis of human immunodeficiency virus infection, *N Engl J Med* 328(5):327–335, 1993.
11. HIV Classification: *CDC and WHO Staging Systems.* http://hab.hrsa.gov/deliverhivaidscare/clinicalguide11/cg-205_hiv_classification.html. Accessed July 9, 2013.
12. Rote NS: Hypersensitivities, infection, and immune efficiencies. In Huether SE, McCance KL, editors: *Understanding pathophysiology*, ed 4, St Louis, 2008, Mosby.
13. Rote NS: Alterations in immunity and inflammation. In McCance KL, Huether SE, editors: *Pathophysiology: the biologic basis for disease in adults and children*, ed 5, St Louis, 2006, Mosby.
14. Gould BE: *Pathophysiology for the health professions*, ed 3, St Louis, 2006, Mosby.
15. Centers for Disease Control and Prevention: *National HIV and STD Testing Resources, HIV Testing.* http://hivtest.cdc.gov/faq.aspx#tested. Accessed July 11, 2013.
16. Centers for Disease Control and Prevention: *Division of HIV/AIDS Prevention. National Center for HIV/AIDS, Viral Hepatitis, STD, and TB Prevention, Rapid HIV testing.* Last modified July 27, 2012. http://www.cdc.gov/hiv/topics/testing/rapid/index.htm. Accessed July 11, 2013.
17. US Department of Health and Human Services, US Food and Drug Administration: http://www.fda.gov/BiologicsBloodVaccines/BloodBloodProducts/ApprovedProducts/LicensedProductsBLAs/BloodDonorScreening/InfectiousDisease/UCM080466. Accessed July 15, 2013.
18. HIV and AIDS Activities: Antiretroviral drugs used in the treatment of HIV infection.
19. Dong KR, Mangili A: Highly active antiretroviral therapy (HAART). In Hendricks KM, Dong KR, Gerrior JL, editors: *Nutrition management of HIV and AIDS*, Chicago, 2009, American Dietetic Association.
20. *Guidelines for the use of antiretroviral agents in HIV-1 in adults and adolescents.* aidsinfo.nih.gov/contentfiles/lvguidelines/adultandadolescentgl.pdf. Accessed July 15, 2013.
21. Katona P, Katona-Apte J: The interaction between nutrition and infection, *Clin Infect Dis* 46(10):1582–1588, 2008.
22. Piwoz E, Preble E: *HIV/AIDS and nutrition: a review of the literature and recommendations for nutritional care and support in sub-Saharan Africa*, Washington, DC, 2000, Academy for Educational Development [AED], Support for Analysis and Research in Africa Project [SARA].
23. Semba RD, Tang AM: Micronutrients and the pathogenesis of human immunodeficiency virus infection, *Br J Nutr* 81(3):181–189, 1999.
24. McCorkindale C, Dybevik K, Coulston AM, et al: Nutritional status of HIV-infected patients during the early disease stages, *J Am Diet Assoc* 90(9):1236–1241, 1990.
25. Kim JH, Spiegelman D, Rimm E, et al: The correlates of dietary intake among HIV-positive adults, *Am J Clin Nutr* 74(6):852–861, 2001.
26. Baum M, Cassetti L, Bonvehi P, et al: Inadequate dietary intake and altered nutrition status in early HIV-1 infection, *Nutrition* 10(1):16–20, 1994.
27. Mangili A, Murman DH, Zampini AM, et al: Nutrition and HIV infection: review of weight loss and wasting in the era of highly active antiretroviral therapy from the nutrition for healthy living cohort, *Clin Infect Dis* 42(6):836–842, 2006.
28. Babameto G, Kotler DP: Malnutrition in HIV infection, *Gastroenterol Clin North Am* 26(2):393–415, 1997.
29. Keating J, Bjarnason I, Somasundaram S, et al: Intestinal absorptive capacity, intestinal permeability and jejunal histology in HIV and their relation to diarrhoea, *Gut* 37(5):623–629, 1995.
30. Cunningham-Rundles S: Effects of nutritional status on immunological function, *Am J Clin Nutr* 35(Suppl 5):1202–1210, 1982.
31. Meydani SN, Beharka AA: Recent developments in vitamin E and immune response, *Nutr Rev* 56(1 Pt 2):S49–S58, 1998.
32. Maggini S, Wintergerst ES, Beveridge S, et al: Selected vitamins and trace elements support immune function by strengthening epithelial barriers and cellular and humoral immune responses, *Br J Nutr* 98(1):S29–S35, 2007.
33. WHO: *Nutrient requirements for people living with HIV/. AIDS: report of a technical consultation*, Geneva, 2003, WHO.
34. Shevitz AH, Knox TA, Spiegelman D, et al: Elevated resting energy expenditure among HIV-seropositive persons receiving highly active antiretroviral therapy, *AIDS* 13(11):1351–1357, 1999.
35. FANTA: *Food assistance programming in the context of HIV. Food and Nutrition Technical Assistance (FANTA) Project and World Food Programme (WFP)*, Washington, DC, 2007, FANTA Project, Academy for Educational Development.
36. *Mosby's medical dictionary*, ed 8, St Louis, 2009, Elsevier.
37. Melchior JC, Niyongabo T, Henzel D, et al: Malnutrition and wasting, immunodepression, and chronic inflammation as independent predictors of survival in HIV-infected patients, *Nutr* 15(11–12):865–869, 1999.
38. Chlebowski RT, Grosvenor MB, Bernhard NH, et al: Nutritional status, gastrointestinal dysfunction, and survival in patients with AIDS, *Am J Gastroenterol* 84(10):1288–1293, 1989.
39. Scrimshaw NS: Effect of infection on nutritional status, *Proc Natl Sci Counc Repub China B* 16(1):46–64, 1992.
40. Liu E, Spiegelman D, Semu H, et al: Nutritional status and mortality among HIV-infected patients receiving antiretroviral therapy in Tanzania, *J Infect Dis* 204(2):282–290, 2011.

41. Koethe JR, Heimburger DC: Nutritional aspects of HIV-associated wasting in sub-Saharan Africa, *Am J Clin Nutr* 91(4):S1138–S1142, 2010.

42. Semba RD, Shah N, Strathdee SA, et al: High prevalence of iron deficiency and anemia among female injection drug users with and without HIV infection, *J Acquir Immune Defic Syndr* 29(2):142–144, 2002.

43. Periquet BA, Jammes NM, Lambert WE, et al: Micronutrient levels in HIV-1-infected children, *AIDS* 9(8):887–893, 1995.

44. Beach RS, Mantero-Atienza E, Shor-Posner G, et al: Specific nutrient abnormalities in asymptomatic HIV-1 infection, *AIDS* 6(7):701–708, 1992.

45. Lacey CJ, Murphy ME, Sanderson MJ, et al: Antioxidant-micronutrients and HIV infection, *Int J STD AIDS* 7(7):485–489, 1996.

46. Tang AM, Lanzillotti J, Hendricks K, et al: Micronutrients: current issues for HIV care providers, *AIDS* 19(9):847–861, 2005.

47. Tang AM, Smit E: Selected vitamins in HIV infection: a review, *AIDS Patient Care STDS* 12(4):263–273, 1998.

48. Baum MK: Role of micronutrients in HIV-infected intravenous drug users, *J Acquir Immune Defic Syndr* 25:S49–S52, 2000.

49. Haug CJ, Aukrust P, Haug E, et al: Severe deficiency of 1,25-dihydroxyvitamin D3 in human immunodeficiency virus infection: association with immunological hyperactivity and only minor changes in calcium homeostasis, *J Clin Endocrinol Metab* 83(11):3832–3838, 1998.

50. Wanke CA, Silva M, Knox TA, et al: Weight loss and wasting remain common complications in individuals infected with human immunodeficiency virus in the era of highly active antiretroviral therapy, *Clin Infect Dis* 31(3):803–805, 2000.

51. Batterham M, Gold J, Naidoo D, et al: A preliminary open label dose comparison using an antioxidant regimen to determine the effect on viral load and oxidative stress in men with HIV/AIDS, *Eur J Clin Nutr* 55(2):107–114, 2001.

52. Look MP, Riezler R, Berthold HK, et al: Decrease of elevated N, N-dimethylglycine and N-methylglycine in human immunodeficiency virus infection during short-term highly active antiretroviral therapy, *Metabolism* 50(11):1275–1281, 2001.

53. Remacha AF, Cadafalch J, Sardà P, et al: Vitamin B-12 metabolism in HIV-infected patients in the age of highly active antiretroviral therapy: role of homocysteine in assessing vitamin B-12 status, *Am J Clin Nutr* 77(2):420–424, 2003.

54. Rousseau MC, Molines C, Moreau J, et al: Influence of highly active antiretroviral therapy on micronutrient profiles in HIV-infected patients, *Ann Nutr Metab* 44(5–6):212–216, 2000.

55. Tang AM, Smit E, Semba RD, et al: Improved antioxidant status among HIV-infected injecting drug users on potent antiretroviral therapy, *J Acquir Immune Defic Syndr* 23(4):321–326, 2000.

56. Toma E, Devost D, Chow Lan N, et al: HIV-protease inhibitors alter retinoic acid synthesis, *AIDS* 15(15):1979–1984, 2001.

57. Wellinghausen N, Kern WV, Jöchle W, et al: Zinc serum level in human immunodeficiency virus-infected patients in relation to immunological status, *Biol Trace Elem Res* 73(2):139–149, 2000.

58. Woods MN, Tang AM, Forrester J, et al: Effect of dietary intake and protease inhibitors on serum vitamin B12 levels in a cohort of human immunodeficiency virus—positive patients, *Clin Infect Dis* 37(Suppl 2):S124–S131, 2003.

59. Khalili H, Soudbakhsh A, Hajiabdolbaghi M, et al: Nutritional status and serum zinc and selenium levels in Iranian HIV infected individuals, *BMC Infect Dis* 8:165, 2008.

60. Wheeler DA, Gibert CL, Launer CA, et al: Weight loss as a predictor of survival and disease progression in HIV infection, *J Acquir Immune Defic Syndr Hum Retrovirol* 18(1):80–85, 1998.

61. Campa A, Yang Z, Lai S, et al: HIV-related wasting in HIV-infected drug users in the era of highly active antiretroviral therapy, *Clin Infect Dis* 41(8):1179–1185, 2005.

62. Tang AM, Forrester J, Spiegelman D, et al: Weight loss and survival in HIV-positive patients in the era of highly active antiretroviral therapy, *J Acquir Immune Defic Syndr* 31(2):230–236, 2002.

63. Hendricks KM, Willis K, Houser R, et al: Obesity in HIV-infection: dietary correlates, *J Am Col. Nutr* 25(4):321–331, 2006.

64. Shevitz AH, Knox TA: Nutrition in the era of highly active antiretroviral therapy, *Clin Infect Dis* 32(12):1769–1775, 2001.

65. Amorosa V, Synnestvedt M, Gross R, et al: A tale of 2 epidemics: the intersection between obesity and HIV infection in Philadelphia, *J Acquir Immune Defic Syndr* 39(5):557–561, 2005.

66. Crum-Cianflone N, Roediger MP, Eberly L, et al: Increasing rates of obesity among HIV-infected persons during the HIV epidemic, *PLoS One* 5(4):e10106, 2010.

67. Crum-Cianflone N, Tejidor R, Medina S, et al: Obesity among patients with HIV: the latest epidemic, *AIDS Patient Care STDS* 22(12):925–930, 2008.

68. Hodgson LM, Ghattas H, Pritchitt H, et al: Wasting and obesity in HIV outpatients, *AIDS* 15(17):2341–2342, 2001.

69. Campa A, Yang Z, Sales S, et al: Inadequate food and micronutrient intake in HIV+ drug users. International conference on AIDS, Barcelona, Spain, 2002.

70. Anema A, Weiser SD, Fernandes KA, et al: High prevalence of food insecurity among HIV-infected individuals receiving HAART in a resource-rich setting, *AIDS Care* 23(2):221–230, 2011.

71. Quach LA, Wanke CA, Schmid CH, et al: Drug use and other risk factors related to lower body mass index among HIV-infected individuals, *Drug Alcohol Depend* 95(1–2):30–36, 2008.

72. Normén L, Chan K, Braitstein P, et al: Food insecurity and hunger are prevalent among HIV-positive individuals in British Columbia, Canada, *J Nutr* 135(4):820–825, 2005.

73. Vogenthaler N, Hadley C, Rodriguez AE, et al: Depressive symptoms and food insufficiency among HIV-infected crack users in Atlanta and Miami, *AIDS Behav* 15(7):1520–1526, 2011.

74. Weiser SD, Bangsberg DR, Kegeles S, et al: Food insecurity among homeless and marginally housed individuals living with HIV/AIDS in San Francisco, *AIDS Behav* 13(5):841–848, 2009.

75. Weiser SD, Frongillo EA, Ragland K, et al: Food insecurity is associated with incomplete HIV RNA suppression among homeless and marginally housed HIV-infected individuals in San Francisco, *J Gen Intern Med* 24(1):14–20, 2009.

76. Weiser SD, Fernandes KA, Brandson EK, et al: The association between food insecurity and mortality among HIV-infected individuals on HAART, *J Acquir Immune Defic Syndr* 52(3):342–349, 2009.

77. Weiser SD, Tsai AC, Gupta R, et al: Food insecurity is associated with morbidity and patterns of healthcare utilization among HIV-infected individuals in a resource-poor setting, *AIDS* 26(1):67–75, 2012.

78. Baum MK, Jayaweera DT, Duan R, et al: Quality of life, symptomatology and healthcare utilization in HIV/HCV co-infected drug users in Miami, *J Addict Dis* 27(2):37–48, 2008.

79. Dorey-Stein Z, Amorosa VK, Kostman JR, et al: Severe weight gain, lipodystrophy, dyslipidemia, and obstructive sleep apnea in a human immunodeficiency virus-infected patient following highly active antiretroviral therapy, *J Cardiometab Syndr* 3(2):111–114, 2008.

80. Grinspoon S: Insulin resistance in the HIV-lipodystrophy syndrome, *Trends Endocrinol Metab* 12(9):413–419, 2001.

81. Batterham MJ, Garsia R, Greenop PA: Dietary intake, serum lipids, insulin resistance and body composition in the era of highly active antiretroviral therapy. Diet FRS Study, *AIDS* 14(12):1839–1843, 2000.

82. Jaime PC, Florindo AA, Latorre Mdo R, et al: Central obesity and dietary intake in HIV/AIDS patients, *Rev Saude Publica* 40(4):634–640, 2006.

83. Joy T, Keogh HM, Hadigan C, et al: Dietary fat intake and relationship to serum lipid levels in HIV-infected patients with metabolic abnormalities in the HAART era, *AIDS* 21(12):1591–1600, 2007.

84. Chlebowski RT, Grosvenor M, Lillington L, et al: Dietary intake and counseling, weight maintenance, and the course of HIV infection, *J Am Diet Assoc* 95(4):428–435, 1995.

85. Hendricks KM, Dong KR, Tang AM, et al: High-fiber diet in HIV-positive men is associated with lower risk of developing fat deposition, *Am J Clin Nutr* 78(4):790–795, 2003.

86. Hendricks KM, Mwamburi DM, Newby PK, et al: Dietary patterns and health and nutrition outcomes in men living with HIV infection, *Am J Clin Nutr* 88(6):1584–1592, 2008.

87. Hendricks KM, Sansavero M, Houser RF, et al: Dietary supplement use and nutrient intake in HIV-infected persons, *AIDS Read* 17(4):211–216, 2007.

88. Smit E, Graham NMH, Tang A, et al: Dietary intake of community-based HIV-1 seropositive and seronegative injecting drug users, *Nutrition* 12 (7–8):496–501, 1996.

89. Swaminathan S, Padmapriyadarsini C, Sukumar B, et al: Nutritional status of persons with HIV infection, persons with HIV infection and tuberculosis, and HIV-negative individuals from Southern India, *Clin Infect Dis* 46(6):946–949, 2008.

90. Vorster HH, Kruger A, Margetts BM, et al: The nutritional status of asymptomatic HIV-infected Africans: directions for dietary intervention, *Public Health Nutr* 7(8):1055–1064, 2004.

91. Luder E, Godfrey E, Godbold J, et al: Assessment of nutritional, clinical, and immunologic status of HIV-infected, inner-city patients with multiple risk factors, *J Am Diet Assoc* 95(6):655–660, 1995.

92. Chlebowski RT, Grosvenor M, Kruger S, et al: Dietary intake in HIV infection: relative caloric deficiency in patients with AIDS, *Int Conf AIDS* 5:467, 1989.

93. Woods MN, Spiegelman D, Knox TA, et al: Nutrient intake and body weight in a large HIV cohort that includes women and minorities, *J Am Diet Assoc* 102(2):203–211, 2002.

94. Steenkamp L, Dannhauser A, Walsh D, et al: Nutritional, immune, micronutrient and health status of HIV-infected children in care centres in Mangaung, South Africa, *J Clin Nutr* 22(3):131–136, 2009.

95. Dusingize JC, Hoover DR, Shi Q, et al: Association of serum albumin with markers of nutritional status among HIV-infected and uninfected Rwandan women, *PLoS One* 7(4):e35079, 2012.

96. Graham SM, Baeten JM, Richardson BA, et al: A decrease in albumin in early HIV type 1 infection predicts subsequent disease progression, *AIDS Res Hum Retroviruses* 23(10):1197–1200, 2007.

97. Feldman JG, Burns DN, Gange SJ, et al: Serum albumin as a predictor of survival in HIV-infected women in the Women's Interagency HIV Study, *AIDS* 14(7):863–870, 2000.

98. Food Security in the US: Economic Research Service. USDA. http://www.ers.usda.gov/topics/food-nutrition-assistance/food-security-in-the-us.aspx. 2012. Accessed on July 12, 2013.

99. Vogenthaler NS, Hadley C, Lewis SJ, et al: Food insufficiency among HIV-infected crack-cocaine users in Atlanta and Miami, *Public Health Nutr* 13(9):1478–1484, 2010.

100. Anema A, Kerr T, Weiser SD, et al: *Prevalence and correlates of self-reported hunger among HIV+ and HIV− injection drug users in Canada*, 5th International AIDS Society Conference on HIV Pathogenesis and Treatment, Cape Town, South Africa, 2009.

101. Wang EA, McGinnis KA, Fiellin DA, et al: Food insecurity is associated with poor virologic response among HIV-infected patients receiving antiretroviral medications, *J Gen Intern Med* 26(9):1012–1018, 2011.

102. Dunkle KL, Jewkes RK, Brown HC, et al: Transactional sex among women in Soweto, South Africa: prevalence, risk factors and association with HIV infection, *Soc Sci Med* 59(8):1581–1592, 2004.

103. Oyefara JL: Food insecurity, HIV/AIDS pandemic and sexual behaviour of female commercial sex workers in Lagos metropolis, Nigeria, *Sahara J* 4(2):626–635, 2007.

104. Gillespie S, Kadiyala S, Greener R: Is poverty or wealth driving HIV transmission? *AIDS* 21(7):S5–S16, 2007.

105. Gillespie S, Kadiyala S, International Food Policy Research I: *HIV/AIDS and food and nutrition security: from evidence to action*, Washington, DC, 2005, IFPRI.

106. Anema A, Vogenthaler N, Frongillo EA, et al: Food insecurity and HIV/AIDS: current knowledge, gaps, and research priorities, *Curr HIV/AIDS Rep* 6:224–231, 2009.

107. Mshana GH, Wamoyi J, Busza J, et al: Barriers to accessing antiretroviral therapy in Kisesa, Tanzania: a qualitative study of early rural referrals to the national program, *AIDS Patient Care STDS* 20(9):649–657, 2006.

108. Tuller DM, Bangsberg DR, Senkungu J, et al: Transportation costs impede sustained adherence and access to HAART in a clinic population in southwestern Uganda: a qualitative study, *AIDS Behav* 14(4):778–784, 2010.

109. Unge C, Johansson A, Zachariah R, et al: Reasons for unsatisfactory acceptance of antiretroviral treatment in the urban Kibera slum, Kenya, *AIDS Care* 20(2):146–149, 2008.

110. Wig N, Bhatt SP, Sakhuja A, et al: Dietary adequacy in Asian Indians with HIV, *AIDS Care* 20(3):370–375, 2008.

111. Ramírez García P, Côté JK: Factors affecting adherence to antiretroviral therapy in people living with HIV/AIDS, *J Assoc Nurses AIDS Care* 14(4):37–45, 2003.

112. Olupot-Olupot P, Katawera A, Cooper C, et al: Adherence to antiretroviral therapy among a conflict-affected population in Northeastern Uganda: a qualitative study, *AIDS* 22(14):1882–1884, 2008.

113. Cantrell RA, Sinkala M, Megazinni K, et al: A pilot study of food supplementation to improve adherence to antiretroviral therapy among food-insecure adults in Lusaka, Zambia, *J Acquir Immune Def Syndr* 49(2):190–195, 2008.

114. Byron E, Gillespie S, Nangami M: Integrating nutrition security with treatment of people living with HIV: lessons from Kenya, *Food Nutr Bull* 29(2):87–97, 2008.

115. Tirivayi N, Koethe JR, Groot W: Clinic-based food assistance is associated with increased medication adherence among HIV-infected adults on long-term antiretroviral therapy in Zambia, *J AIDS Clin Res* 3(7):171, 2012.

116. Academy of Nutrition and Dietetics: *Resources for Health Practitioners*. http://www.eatright.org/HealthProfessionals/content.aspx?id=7077. Accessed July 15, 2013.

117. Campa A, Baum MK: Micronutrients and HIV-infection, *HIV Therapy* 4(4):437–469, 2010.

118. Kotler DP: *Lipodystrophy—it just gets more complicated*. Paper presented at the Eighth Annual Conference on Retroviruses and Opportunistic Infections, Chicago, February 6, 1991.

119. Scevola D, Di Matteo A, Uberti F, et al: Reversal of cachexia in patient treated with potent antiviral therapy, *AIDS Read* 10(6):365, 2000.

120. Loss JC: The use of anabolic agents in HIV disease, *Support Line* 3:1999.

121. Schambelan M, Mulligan K, Grunfeld C: Recombinant human growth hormone in patients with HIV-associated wasting: a randomized, placebo-controlled trial, *Ann Intern Med* 125:873, 1996.

122. FDC Reports: *Serono Serostim required on state Medicaid formularies, HCFA says*. FDC Reports, vol 66, Chevy Chase, MD, 1999.

123. Fillipas S, Cherry CL, Cicuttini F, et al: The effects of exercise training on metabolic and morphological outcomes for people living with HIV: a systematic review of randomised controlled trials, *HIV Clin Trials* 11(5):270–282, 2010.

124. Panel on Antiretroviral Therapy and Medical Management of HIV-Infected Children: *Guidelines for the Use of Antiretroviral Agents in Pediatric HIV Infection*. Available from http://aidsinfo.nih.gov/contentfiles/lvguidelines/pediatricguidelines.pdf. Accessed July 15, 2013.

FURTHER READING AND RESOURCE

Eatright.Store: Food safety precautions for individuals living with HIV. http://www.eatrightstore.org/search?keyword=HIV+AIDS.

25

Cancer

Joyce Gilbert

ⓔ http://evolve.elsevier.com/Williams/essentials/

This chapter focuses on cancers, which, as a group of diseases, are among the prevalent diseases in the world. We examine the nature of the cancer process, associated risk factors, and treatments, with a focus on the role of nutrition. Here we look at nutrition and cancer in two basic areas: (1) the role of nutrition in cancer development and risk reduction and (2) the role of nutrition in cancer therapy and rehabilitation. Cancer development and its prevention are discussed in relation to the interplay of environment, the body's defense system, and nutritional factors that govern each. Nutrition support has a significant role in medical therapy during both the treatment and posttreatment phases of cancer management in the effectiveness of therapy and quality of life. To understand these nutritional relationships, we must understand the nature of cancer as a growth process.

OUTLINE

PROCESS OF CANCER DEVELOPMENT

According to the National Cancer Institute (NCI) of the National Institutes of Health, the term *cancer* refers to a category of diseases in which abnormal cells divide without control and are able to invade other tissues. Cancer cells can spread to other parts of the body through the blood and **lymph** systems.

Cancer is thus a generic term encompassing more than 100 different types of conditions. Most cancers are named for the organ or type of cell in which they start; for example, cancer that begins in the colon is called *colon cancer*; cancer that begins in **melanocytes** of the skin is called *melanoma*.

Cancer types can be categorized as follows:

- Carcinoma—cancer that begins in the skin or in tissues that line or cover internal organs. There are a number of subtypes of carcinoma, including **adenocarcinoma, basal cell carcinoma, squamous cell carcinoma**, and **transitional cell carcinoma**.
- Sarcoma—**cancer** that begins in bone, cartilage, fat, muscle, blood vessels, or other connective or supportive tissue.
- Leukemia—cancer that starts in blood-forming tissue such as the bone marrow and causes large numbers of abnormal blood cells to be produced and enter the blood.
- Lymphoma and myeloma—cancers that begin in the cells of the **immune system**.
- Central nervous system cancers—cancers that begin in the tissues of the brain and spinal cord.[1]

Cancer Cell

Almost every time a cell divides, the DNA is replicated without error; this allows living organisms to grow and sustain themselves throughout their normal life span. However, there are occasional mutations that occur during DNA replication that either may be of no physiologic significance or may produce aberrations in the synthesis of various proteins and/or in phases of the cell cycle. These disruptions can have a host of implications for the organism, including the transformation of a normal cell into a cell with the capacity for the abnormal growth that results in cancers. Defining and categorizing these disruptions in the cell cycle is an area of intense scientific inquiry that has yielded significant insights over the past 3 or 4 decades.

It was once thought that cancer resulted from a single mutation or group of mutations that allowed for unregulated cell growth. In fact, it is now generally understood that cancers develop through a series of four distinct steps: (1) initiation, (2) promotion, (3) development, and (4) progression.[2]

Most errors in DNA replication are repaired by "DNA repair genes" prior to cell division and thus have minimal physiologic significance. In other instances, after cell division, some mutations trigger synthesis of various **tumor suppression genes** such as p53, which lead to cellular suicide or **apoptosis** of the mutated cell. These types of mutations may also have minimal physiologic significance. However, in certain heritable cancers, such as heritable colon cancers and melanomas, there is an inherited mutation that suppresses expression of one or more of the

Lymph

The clear fluid that travels through the lymphatic system and carries cells that help fight infections and other diseases. Also called *lymphatic fluid*.

Melanocyte

A cell in the skin and eyes that produces and contains the pigment called melanin.

Adenocarcinoma

Cancer that begins in glandular (secretory) cells. Glandular cells are found in tissue that lines certain internal organs and makes and releases substances in the body, such as mucus, digestive juices, or other fluids. Most cancers of the breast, pancreas, lung, prostate, and colon are adenocarcinomas.

Basal Cell Carcinoma

Cancer that begins in the lower part of the epidermis (the outer layer of the skin). It may appear as a small white or flesh-colored bump that grows slowly and may bleed. Basal cell carcinomas are usually found on areas of the body exposed to the sun. Basal cell carcinomas rarely metastasize (spread) to other parts of the body. They are the most common form of skin cancer. Also called basal cell cancer.

Squamous Cell Carcinoma

Cancer that begins in squamous cells. Squamous cells are thin, flat cells that look like fish scales and are found in the tissue that forms the surface of the skin, the lining of the hollow organs of the body, and the lining of the respiratory and digestive tracts. Most cancers of the anus, cervix, head and neck, and vagina are squamous cell carcinomas. Also called *epidermoid carcinoma*.

Transitional Cell Carcinoma

Cancer that begins in the transitional cells. Transitional cells are cells that vary in shape depending on whether the tissue is being stretched. Transitional cells may be stretched without breaking apart. They line hollow organs such as the bladder.

Cancer

A malignant cellular tumor with properties of tissue invasion and spreading to other parts of the body.

Immune System

A complex network of cells, tissues, organs, and the substances they make that helps the body fight infections and other diseases. The immune system includes white blood cells and organs and tissues of the lymph system, such as the thymus, spleen, tonsils, lymph nodes, lymph vessels, and bone marrow.

Thus these mutations result in a deregulation of some facet of cellular function. For example, some mutations disrupt cell signaling pathways by leading to overproduction of growth factors, cytokines, and proteases. The resulting cells produce larger volumes of these compounds and therefore affect normal neighboring cells through a variety of impacts on the cellular microenvironment. These impacts may be termed the *invasion metastasis cascade* and consist of the following critical steps: (1) local invasion, (2) the invasion of blood vessels, (3) transport of the cancer cell through the blood to a distant site, (4) escape of the cancer cell from the blood to tissue, and (5) adaptation of the relocated cancer cell to the new local environment that allows for its continued growth. The tumor microenvironment is critical in achieving these cascading steps.[5]

Regardless of the mechanism by which cells are mutated, their abnormal growth may result in neoplasms (literally new growth). These neoplasms are categorized as either benign, which lack the ability to spread to other tissues, or malignant, which possess the ability to spread to other tissues. Malignant neoplasms can spread to other tissues by direct or indirect invasion. In direct invasion, the neoplasms grow so large that they enter adjacent tissues or crowd the tissue so as to render it less effective. The indirect spread of neoplasms occurs when neoplastic cells enter the blood or lymphatic system and invade other tissues. These neoplastic cells retain the original mutation as they reproduce in their new host tissue. Therefore they retain the name of the original tissue. For example, a bone sarcoma (osteosarcoma) that has spread to the liver is termed a *hepatic osteosarcoma*, whereas a carcinoma that originated in the liver (hepatic carcinoma) and has spread to the bone is termed a *hepatic carcinoma of the bone*.

Tumor Suppression Gene

A type of gene that makes a protein called a *tumor suppressor protein* that helps control cell growth. Mutations (changes in DNA) in tumor suppressor genes may lead to cancer. Also called *antioncogene*.

Apoptosis

A type of cell death in which a series of molecular steps in a cell lead to its death. This is one method the body uses to get rid of unneeded or abnormal cells. The process of apoptosis may be blocked in cancer cells. Also called *programmed cell death*.

Chromatin

The combination of DNA and proteins that makes up the contents of the nucleus of a cell. The primary functions of chromatin are to (1) package DNA into a smaller volume to fit in the cell, (2) strengthen the DNA to allow mitosis, (3) prevent DNA damage, and (4) control gene expression and DNA replication. The primary protein components of chromatin are histones that compact the DNA.

Histone

A type of protein found in chromosomes. Histones bind to DNA, help give chromosomes their shape, and help control the activity of genes.

Epigenetics

The study of how age and exposure to environmental factors, such as diet, exercise, drugs, and chemicals, may cause changes in the way genes are switched on and off without changing the actual DNA sequence. These changes can affect a person's risk of disease and may be passed from parents to their children.

Oncogene

A gene that is a mutated (changed) form of a gene involved in normal cell growth. Oncogenes may cause the growth of cancer cells. Mutations in genes that become oncogenes can be inherited or caused by being exposed to substances in the environment that cause cancer.

tumor suppressor genes. This mutation increases the probability of developing cancers resulting from an event that would normally result in apoptosis of the mutated cell.

In other instances that may result in the development of cancer cells, there is no change in DNA sequence, but posttranscriptional and/or posttranslational modifications in DNA do not occur normally. These modifications typically involve DNA methylation or in formation of chromatin or histones. Many of these types of modifications are under environmental control, and, hence, potentially reversible. The emerging science of epigenetics focuses on the environmental control of these posttranscriptional and/or posttranslational modifications in gene expression and in DNA modification and chromatin structure.[3,4]

In still other instances, regions of mutated DNA, or oncogenes, code for the expression of proteins that leads to abnormal cell growth or division. These mutations may involve genes that (1) activate/deactivate carcinogens, (2) govern normal cell cycle, (3) govern cell senescence, (4) govern cell signaling, and (5) govern cell differentiation.

CARCINOGENS AND CANCER PREVENTION

Diet and Epigenetics

Understanding the fundamental biochemical and physiologic processes that underlie development of cancers is key to designing preventive and treatment strategies. Developments and refinements in the sciences of genetics, epigenetics, proteomics, metabolomics, and other related sciences are elucidating specific cellular alterations that may lead to neoplastic growth in some instances and not in others. Although still in their developmental phases, these areas of science hold great promise for improving evidence-based diagnostic and treatment protocols and refinement of public health recommendations. In particular, the results of epigenetic research are to allow greater understanding of the role of environmental factors, such as radiation, naturally occurring and synthetic chemicals, diet, infections, and occupation on the etiology of different forms of cancers.[6]

Researchers in epigenetics have identified several dietary constituents that may function as natural chemopreventive agents by influencing the activity or expression of DNA methyltransferases and histone-modifying enzymes. Some of these chemopreventive agents include the following:

- Micronutrients (folate, retinoic acid, and selenium compounds)
- Butyrate
- Polyphenols from green tea, apples, coffee, black raspberries, and other dietary sources
- Genistein and soy isoflavones
- Curcumin
- Resveratrol
- Dihydrocoumarin
- Nordihydroguaiaretic acid (NDGA)
- Lycopene
- Anacardic acid
- Garcinol
- Constituents of *Allium* species and cruciferous vegetables, including indol-3-carbinol (I3C), diindolylmethane (DIM), sulforaphane, phenylethyl isothiocyanate (PEITC), phenylhexyl isothiocyanate (PHI), diallyldisulfide (DADS) and its metabolite allyl mercaptan (AM)
- Cambinol
- Relatively unexplored modulators of histone lysine methylation (chaetocin, polyamine analogs)

So far, data on humans are limited, but advances in technology will allow exploration of nutriepigenomics at a genome-wide level to better understand the importance of epigenetic mechanisms for gene regulation in cancer chemoprevention.[7]

An example of the potential for understanding the role of nutrition in epigenetics is illustrated by a series of studies conducted using experimental animals. In these studies, rodents were fed diets deficient in methionine, choline, folate, and/or vitamin B_{12}, which are the micronutrients involved in methyl group metabolism. Deficiencies in these nutrients resulted in hypomethylation of DNA and an increased incidence of hepatocarcinoma in rodents. Assays revealed lower levels of S-adenosyl methionine, aberrant levels of DNA-methyltransferases, methyl CpG binding proteins, histone methyltransferase protein expression, and histone posttranslational modification.[8]

Radiation

Exposure to radiation may lead to DNA alterations through a variety of mechanisms that are not yet fully understood. Such radiation damage may be ionizing, such as from x-rays, radioactive materials, and atomic exhausts or wastes, or it may be nonionizing, such as from sunlight. Ultraviolet radiation in sunlight is one of the most prominent sources of environmental carcinogens. It is highly genotoxic but does not penetrate the skin. The common forms of skin cancers—basal cell carcinoma and squamous cell carcinoma—are easily cured by surgical removal. However, a far more lethal form of skin cancer, malignant melanoma, occurs in skin cells that produce the pigment melanin.

Viruses

Viruses may be thought of as a major risk factor for cancer development. A virus contains a small chromosome, DNA or RNA, with a relatively small number of genes, usually fewer than five and never more than several hundred. In general, when viruses produce disease, they act as parasites, taking over the cell to replicate themselves. Numerous oncogenic viruses have been identified that are capable of producing tumors only in hosts in which the virus can replicate. They transform cells by integrating a DNA copy of the virus (termed a *provirus*) into the host cell genome. Recognized examples of viral-associated cancers include the following:

- Human papillomavirus (HPV) and cervical cancer[9]
- Retroviruses and certain breast and skin cancers[10]
- Epstein-Barr virus and certain lymphomas
- Hepatitis B and C and hepatocellular carcinoma
- Human immunodeficiency virus (HIV) and Kaposi sarcoma[11]

PUBLIC HEALTH GUIDELINES FOR CANCER RISK REDUCTION

The American Cancer Society (ACS) has published guidelines for nutrition and physical activity to reduce the risk of developing cancers (Table 25.1). These guidelines emphasize individual choices that may reduce the risk of developing cancers, and include maintaining an appropriate weight and eating a diet rich in fruits and vegetables. These guidelines provide general guidance for population-based strategies for reducing the risk of developing cancers based on the available science. As advances in genetic research continue, some of these strategies may be modified to address risks for specific population groups.

In addition to the individual choice guidelines, the ACS also recommends that public, private, and community organizations work together at national, state, and local levels to apply policy and environmental changes that (1) increase access to affordable, healthful foods in communities, places of work, and schools and decrease access to and marketing of foods and drinks of low nutritional value, particularly to youth, and (2) provide safe, enjoyable, and accessible environments for physical activity in schools and workplaces and for transportation and recreation in communities.

Another set of public health guidelines for reducing cancer risk, morbidity, and mortality are provided through the Healthy People 2020 program. Healthy People 2020 provides science-based, 10-year national objectives designed to improve health of Americans. One topic area within those objectives addresses cancers. Table 25.2 lists the 20 objectives related to cancer and the target set to be achieved by 2020. The Healthy People 2020 objectives focus on reducing the incidence of common forms of cancers and improving rates of screening and not specifically on lifestyle alterations that may reduce risk; however, public health interventions to reduce risk aid in achieving these objectives. In the *2011/2012 Cancer Trends Progress Report,* the NCI, one of the National Institutes of Health, cited progress toward the major cancer-related Healthy People targets. Their conclusions are as follows:

- The rate of cancer incidence has declined since 1998.
- Death rates for the four most common cancers (prostate, female breast, lung, and colorectal), as well as for all cancers combined, have continued to decline.
- Death rates are increasing for cancer of the pancreas, liver, intrahepatic bile duct, and corpus uteri and unspecified uterus.

TABLE 25.1   American Cancer Society Guidelines for Individual Choices on Nutrition and Physical Activity

Guideline	Targets
Achieve and maintain a healthy weight throughout life	• Be as lean as possible throughout life without being underweight. • Avoid excess weight gain at all ages. For those who are overweight or obese, losing even a small amount of weight has health benefits and is a good place to start. • Get regular physical activity and limit intake of high-calorie foods and drinks as keys to help maintain a healthy weight.
Be physically active	• Adults: Get at least 150 min of moderate intensity or 75 min of vigorous intensity activity each week (or a combination of these), preferably spread throughout the week. • Children and teens: Get at least 1 h of moderate or vigorous intensity activity each day, with vigorous activity on at least 3 days each week. • Limit sedentary behavior such as sitting, lying down, watching TV, and other forms of screen-based entertainment. • Doing some physical activity above usual activities, no matter what one's level of activity, can have many health benefits.
Eat a healthy diet, with an emphasis on plant foods	• Choose foods and drinks in amounts that help you get to and maintain a healthy weight. • Limit how much processed meat and red meat you eat. • Eat at least 2½ cups of vegetables and fruits each day. • Choose whole grains instead of refined grain products.
If you drink alcohol, limit your intake	• Drink no more than 1 drink/day for women or 2/day for men.

From American Cancer Society: *Guidelines for nutrition and physical activity for cancer prevention.* http://www.cancer.org/healthy/eathealthygetactive/acsguidelinesonnutritionphysicalactivityforcancerprevention/acs-guidelines-on-nutrition-and-physical-activity-for-cancer-prevention-intro.

TABLE 25.2   Healthy People 2020 Cancer Objectives and Progress

Goal	Target
Reduce overall cancer death rate	10% improvement
Reduce lung cancer death rate	10% improvement
Reduce female breast cancer death rate	10% improvement
Reduce the death rate from cancer of the uterine cervix	10% improvement
Reduce colorectal cancer death rate	15% improvement
Reduce oropharyngeal cancer death rate	10% improvement
Reduce prostate cancer death rate	10% improvement
Reduce melanoma cancer death rate	10% improvement
Reduce invasive colorectal cancer	15% improvement
Reduce invasive uterine cervical cancer	10% improvement
Reduce late stage female breast cancer	5% improvement
Increase the number of central, population-based registries from the 50 states and the District of Columbia that capture case information on at least 95% of the expected number of reportable cancers	Total coverage
Increase the proportion of cancer survivors who are living 5 years or longer after diagnosis	10% improvement
Increase mental and physical health-related quality of life among cancer survivors	10% improvement
Increase the proportion of women who receive a cervical cancer screening based on the most recent guidelines	10% improvement
Increase the proportion of adults who receive a colorectal cancer screening based on the most recent guidelines	26% improvement
Increase the proportion of women who receive breast cancer screening based on the most recent guidelines	10% improvement
Increase the proportion of adults who were counseled about cancer screening consistent with the most recent guidelines	10% improvement
Increase the proportion of men who have discussed the advantages and disadvantages of the PSA test to screen for prostate cancer with their health care provider	10% improvement
Increase the proportion of persons who participate in behaviors that reduce their exposure to harmful UV irradiation and avoid sunburn	10% improvement

PSA, Prostate-specific antigen; *UV,* ultraviolet.
From US Department of Health and Human Services: *Healthy people 2020, goals and objectives for cancer.* http://www.healthypeople.gov/2020/topicsobjectives2020/objectiveslist.aspx?topicId=5.

• Length of cancer survival has increased for all cancers combined. For all sites, the proportion of people surviving 5 years from diagnosis in 2003 (most recent year with 5-year follow-up) was 66.7 percent.
• Incidence rates of some cancers are rising, including melanoma of the skin, non-Hodgkin lymphoma, leukemia, childhood cancer, cancers of the kidney and renal pelvis, thyroid, pancreas, liver and intrahepatic bile duct, testis, myeloma, and esophagus.
• Lung cancer incidence rates in women continue to rise but less rapidly.
• Cancer treatment spending continues to rise, along with total health care spending.

- Unexplained cancer-related health disparities remain among population subgroups. For example, African Americans have elevated rates of both new cancers and cancer deaths.
- Pap test use has declined from 81% in 2000 to 74% in 2010. Mammography rates have decreased from 69% in 2000 to 67% in 2010. Screening rates for colorectal cancer have increased from 52% in 2008 to 59% in 2010.[12]

CANCER-RELATED HEALTH DISPARITIES

Despite overall reductions in incidence of many of the most prevalent types of cancers and increased rates of survival, improvements do not affect all population groups equally. The decreased incidences are probably associated with early detection of precancerous tissue. That is, there are disparities. The NCI defines "cancer health disparities" as "differences in the incidence, prevalence, mortality, and burden of cancer and related adverse health conditions that exist among specific population groups in the United States" (http://www.crchd.cancer.gov/disparities/defined.html).

These disparities are highlighted in the *2011/2012 Cancer Trends Progress Report*.[12] African-American populations have a higher incidence of both new cancers and deaths from cancer than Caucasians. Other minority populations, such as Latinos, Native Americans, and Asian/Pacific Islanders experience disproportionately higher rates of specific forms of cancers. For example, African Americans have a higher incidence and death rate from colorectal cancer than any other racial or ethnic group. Asian/Pacific Islanders have the highest incidence of stomach cancer of any of the racial or ethnic groups in the United States and are more than twice as likely to die from stomach cancer as Caucasians.

Higher rates of incidence of specific cancers within certain racial and ethnic groups may suggest a genetic association; however, there are many complex and interrelated factors that contribute to these disparities in cancer incidence and death among these groups. The most obvious factors are associated with health care coverage and socioeconomic status.

Socioeconomic status is most often based on a person's income, education level, occupation, and other factors, such as social status in the community. It is the major predictor of access to education and health insurance, employment in certain occupations, and living conditions that are associated with the risks of developing and surviving cancer. These predictors may be positive or negative. For example, lower socioeconomic status is associated with living conditions and employment in occupations where exposure to environmental toxins is more common. Socioeconomic status also appears to play a major role in influencing the prevalence of behavioral risk factors for cancer, such as tobacco smoking, physical inactivity, obesity, and excessive alcohol intake, as well as in following cancer screening recommendations. In addition to socioeconomic status, financial, physical, and cultural beliefs may be barriers that prevent individuals or groups from obtaining effective health care.

In addition to the interactions among race, ethnicity, and socioeconomic status on the incidence of cancers, people from medically underserved populations are more likely to be diagnosed with late-stage diseases, in part because of lack of access to or knowledge of early screening tests. These late-stage cancers might have been treated more effectively or cured if diagnosed earlier.[13] An example of the effects of combinations of all these factors on morbidity and mortality from cancers among people in developing countries is discussed in the Focus on Culture box, "Cancers in Developing Countries."

🌐 FOCUS ON CULTURE

Cancers in Developing Countries

Although cancers are widely thought to be diseases of affluence among developed countries, there is increasing recognition of the prevalence of cancers in developing countries. According to 2008 World Health Organization (WHO) statistics, cancer causes approximately 7.9 million deaths worldwide each year. Approximately 70% of these deaths, or 5.5 million, occur in the developing world. This number is projected to increase to 6.7 million in 2015 and 8.9 million in 2030. In contrast, cancer deaths in wealthy countries are expected to remain fairly stable over the next 20 years.

There are many global trends that contribute to this increased incidence in cancers in the developing world, including population aging, rapid unplanned urbanization, and globalization of unhealthy lifestyles. It is estimated that 40% of all cancers worldwide, including those in developing countries, are preventable. For example, increased urbanization and globalization of unhealthful lifestyles contribute to the development of preventable cancers associated with increased exposure to carcinogens through tobacco use, unhealthful diets, and environmental pollutants.

Public health programs have been very successful in addressing deaths from communicable diseases, according to reports from the United Nations Millennium Development Goals (MDGs) project. Infant and childhood mortality has declined from 90 deaths per 1000 live births in 1990 to 48 in 2012; deaths from malaria have declined by 26% since 2001; and deaths from tuberculosis have declined by 41% since 1991. Rates of infections with HIV have decreased by 21% since 2001. These successes contribute to a rise in the proportion of populations who are adults and at an increased risk of developing cancers.

The disease burden that results from cancers is significant in developing countries. In some African countries, only 20% of patients survive cancers, such as cervical cancer, that are highly curable in developed countries. On average, 70%

of cancer patients in developing countries are diagnosed at a late stage of illness, when treatment is no longer effective and the only possible intervention is palliative care. Even basic palliative care, such as pain management, fails to reach more than 5 million terminally ill cancer patients every year.

Throughout the developing world, most health systems are designed to cope with episodes of communicable diseases. They have demonstrated an increasing capacity for effectiveness in this area as measured by achievement in meeting the MDGs. Most developing countries do not have the capacity—measured as financial resources, facilities, equipment, technology, infrastructure, staff, or training—to address care for cancers. In large parts of Africa, treatments such as surgery, radiotherapy, and chemotherapy are largely unavailable. For example, according to the director-general of the WHO, in 2010, 30 countries did not have a single radiation therapy machine.

In most developing countries the capacity for the basic components of cancer control could be built on the evidence base and technology from developed countries. Basic components of cancer control—public education, prevention, early detection, diagnosis and treatment, and palliative care—could be incorporated into other disease prevention programs using some of the strategies that have been effective in meeting the MDG targets.

Bibliography

Chan M: *Cancer in developing countries: facing the challenge.* http://www.who.int/dg/speeches/2010/iaea_forum_20100921/en/index.html.

United Nations Millennium Development Goals. http://www.un.org/millenniumgoals/.

WHO Guide for Effective Programmes: *Cancer control: knowledge into action: diagnosis and treatment,* 2008. http://www.who.int/cancer/modules/9789241547406/en/index.html.

POPULATION-BASED SCREENING RECOMMENDATIONS FOR CANCERS

Among the reasons for the decreased incidence of cancer, particularly late-stage cancers, is widespread use of screening tests for several of the most commonly diagnosed cancers. Early detection of cancer increases the probability of successful treatment. Detection and treatment of precancerous lesions before becoming malignant may also be achieved through effective implementation of screening tests. Among the most commonly used screening tests are:

- Mammography (for breast cancer)
- Pap test (for cervical cancer)
- Fecal occult blood test (for colorectal cancer)
- Colorectal endoscopy or colonoscopy (for colorectal cancer)
- Prostate specific antigen (PSA) (for prostate cancer)

The US Preventive Services Task Force (USPSTF) issues evidence-based guidelines for screening for cervical, colorectal, and breast cancers. These guidelines are regularly updated and provide resources for administration of these screening tools among population groups based on age, family history, race, and presence of risk factors. The most current recommendations may be accessed at the USPSTF website: http://www.uspreventiveservicestaskforce.org

POSTDIAGNOSTIC STAGING OF CANCERS

Cancers can be diagnosed at several points in their development as a result of screening tests or other types of physical or clinical examinations. Many malignancies are confirmed microscopically, because malignant cells have a distinctive microscopic appearance. These include abnormalities in cell shape and size, variation in nuclear size and shape, incomplete cellular differentiation, loss of normal tissue organization, and a poorly defined tumor boundary.

After cancer has been diagnosed, physicians conduct a series of tests to determine the progression of the disease. These tests may be clinical or pathologic. Clinical tests include physical examinations; imaging tests, such as computed tomography (CT) or positron emission tomography (PET) scans and magnetic resonance imaging (MRI) scans; blood tests; and biopsies. Pathologic tests are primarily conducted on tissues removed during surgery to remove the tumor and associated tissues, such as lymph nodes. The results of both clinical and pathologic tests are used to answer questions about size of the tumor, its spread to nearby lymph nodes, and the extent to which it may have metastasized to other tissues.

Based on results of these tests, the cancer is assigned a "stage." The most commonly used staging system is the TNM system, in which *T* refers to tumor size, *N* refers to lymph node involvement, and *M* refers to metastasis. Each section also includes levels; for example, a T4, N0, M0 tumor would be large (T4) but with no lymph node involvement (N0) or metastasis (M0).

Other staging systems are used for some specific types of cancers. Stages can be as a number (0, I, II, III, or IV), in which lower numbers reflect more localized growth. Stages may also be identified with terms, such as *carcinoma in situ, localized, regional,* or *distant.* In this system, carcinoma in situ refers to a highly localized area of dysplasia for which there is no evidence of spreading, whereas distant refers to cancers that have metastasized to areas of the body distant from their original location.

PRACTICE GUIDELINES FOR TREATMENT OF CANCERS

The health care team for patients with cancer includes oncologists, nurses, dietetics professionals, and other support personnel. Because there are more than 300 different forms of cancers, each with different treatment options depending on the stage of the cancer, it is difficult to generalize about treatments. Over the past decade, with the increased emphasis on evidence-based practice, professional organizations have established practice guidelines. Practice guidelines are developed through a process that includes a systematic literature review on the effectiveness of specific outcomes of specific interventions. After this systematic review, guidelines are developed based on the strength of the evidence for that particular intervention.

Professional organizations that have developed practice guidelines for treatment of various types of cancer include the National Comprehensive Cancer Network (http://www.nccn.org/professionals/physician_gls/f_guidelines.asp) and the American Society of Clinical Oncology (http://www.asco.org/institute-quality/guidelines). The Academy of Nutrition and Dietetics (AND) has practice guidelines for various aspects of oncology nutrition, such as appropriate methods to estimate resting energy expenditure (REE) and use of parenteral nutrition (http://www.andevidencelibrary.com). These guidelines are updated regularly and should be reviewed by health care professionals as part of designing treatment protocols for all patients.

TREATMENT OF CANCER

Just as knowledge of the epigenetics of cancer is changing rapidly, so too are treatments. However, most current cancer therapy takes four major forms: (1) surgery, (2) radiation, (3) chemotherapy, and (4) biologic therapy. Each of these treatment modalities entail physiologic and psychological stresses, including damage to cell DNA structure, changes in normal body function, and alterations in quality of life. Nutrition support seeks to alleviate these problems and to enhance the potential success of cancer therapy.

Surgery

Diagnosis of certain cancers in early stages of development allows for surgical removal of operable tumors as a major treatment of a large number of patients with cancer. Surgical treatment may also be used with other forms of therapy for removal of single metastases or for prevention and alleviation of symptoms.

Radiation Therapy

Radiation therapy damages DNA; therefore cell division and growth are impaired. Its effectiveness in treatments of cancer is predicated on its ability to limit neoplastic cell growth. Radiotherapy may be used alone or in conjunction with other therapies for curative and palliative care. Radiation used in cancer therapy may employ either external radiation beams or internal isotopes (brachytherapy).

- In external beam radiation therapy, radiation emitted from a linear accelerator is directed at a highly specific treatment site. This type of radiation frequently causes nutrition-related side effects and changes in quality of life.
- In brachytherapy, highly radioactive isotopes, such as cobalt 60, are placed directly into or next to the tumor to deliver a localized dose. Nutritional side effects do not generally occur from this type of radiotherapy.[14]

Chemotherapy

Chemotherapy refers to the use of chemical agents as a treatment for cancer. It may be used as the only form of treatment but is typically used in conjunction with surgery, radiation therapy, or biologic therapy. Chemotherapy can be administered as follows:

- To decrease size of a tumor before surgery or radiation therapy. This is called *neoadjuvant chemotherapy.*
- To destroy cancer cells that may remain after surgery or radiation therapy. This is called *adjuvant chemotherapy.*
- To work synergistically with radiation therapy and biologic therapy.

In general, the effectiveness of chemotherapeutic agents is greater when tumor burden is less. Tumor burden may be less because of early detection or initial treatment by surgery or radiation. Selection and dosage of chemotherapeutic agents is based on the type of cancer and the evidence-based practice guidelines that have been developed for use by physicians. The agents may be administered singly or in combination and are frequently given serially in dosages designed to halt growth of the neoplastic cells. These repeated series of chemotherapy treatments are known as "rounds," and side effects of the treatments may increase in intensity with sequential rounds of treatments.

Mode of Action. Chemotherapeutic agents are effective because they disrupt normal cellular processes responsible for cell growth and reproduction. Some agents interfere with DNA synthesis. Others disrupt DNA structure and RNA replication. Others prevent mitosis, cause hormonal imbalances, or disrupt protein synthesis by limiting the availability of specific amino acids. This diversity in mode of action provides a basis for classifying chemotherapeutic agents, as follows:

- Alkaloid agents—inhibit microtubule function
- Alkylating agents—chemically alter cellular DNA
- Antibiotic agents—prevent normal DNA functions
- Antimetabolite agents—block cell division by imitating purines or pyrimidines
- Enzymal agents—prevent normal functions of DNA
- Hormonal agents—damage cell division[15]

Chemotherapy Administration. Chemotherapy may be administered in several ways, as follows:

- *Injection*—chemotherapeutic agent is given intramuscularly or subcutaneously
- *Intraarterial (IA)*—chemotherapeutic agent is given directly into the artery that is feeding the cancer
- *Intraperitoneal (IP)*—chemotherapeutic agent is given directly into the peritoneal cavity
- *Intravenous (IV)*—chemotherapeutic agent is given directly into a vein
- *Topically*—chemotherapeutic is rubbed directly onto the skin
- *Orally*—chemotherapeutic agent is given as pills, capsules, or liquids

Biologic Therapy

Advances in cell biology and physiology, as well as epigenetics, have led to development of specific biologic, or targeted, therapies for treatment of cancers. Targeted therapies are transforming cancer treatments by facilitating discovery of therapeutic targets within cancer cells and designing treatments that selectively interfere with them.

Forms of biologic therapies include antibodies, vaccines, and small molecules that traverse the cell membrane. These treatments are often used in combination with chemotherapy or as adjuvant therapy with surgery or radiation. These therapies affect primarily or exclusively the neoplastic cell and thus limit the collateral damage to other rapidly dividing cells associated with chemotherapeutic agents.

An excellent tutorial on targeted therapies is available through the NCI at http://www.cancer.gov/cancertopics

MEDICAL NUTRITION THERAPY FOR PATIENTS WITH CANCER

Nutrition care for persons with cancer should follow the Nutrition Care Process (NCP) as outlined by the AND.[16] The NCP has four basic sequential, but interrelated, steps:

1. *Nutrition assessment* is a systematic approach to collect, record, and interpret relevant data from patients, clients, family members, caregivers, and other individuals and groups. Nutrition assessment is an ongoing, dynamic process that involves initial data collection, as well as continual reassessment and analysis of the patient's or client's status, compared with specified criteria.

2. *Nutrition diagnosis* is a food and nutrition professional's identification and labeling of an existing nutrition problem that the food and nutrition professional is responsible for treating independently.

3. *Nutrition intervention* is a purposefully planned action(s) designed with the intent of changing a nutrition-related behavior, risk factor, environmental condition, or aspect of health status. Nutrition intervention consists of two interrelated components: planning and intervention. The nutrition intervention is typically directed toward resolving the nutrition diagnosis or the nutrition etiology. Less often, it is directed at relieving signs and symptoms.

4. *Nutrition monitoring and evaluation* identify the amount of progress made and whether goals or expected outcomes are being met. Nutrition monitoring and evaluation identify outcomes relevant to the nutrition diagnosis and intervention plans and goals.

For each of these steps, the plan should include specific, measurable outcomes.

Development of an effective nutrition care plan for persons with cancer will necessarily require collaboration with other members of the health care team and caregivers, periodic monitoring, and a holistic approach to patient management. Many of the common signs and symptoms associated with cancer care are related to quality of life and activities of daily living and therefore impact food behaviors and nutrient intake (see the Case Study box, "Patient With Cancer").

CASE STUDY

Patient With Cancer

As a dietitian working with a medical oncology practice, you received a referral for Yolande, a 45-year-old mother of four who has been diagnosed with stage 1 triple negative breast cancer. She has had a lumpectomy, and the sentinel lymph node biopsy was negative. She weighs 125 lb and is 62 inches tall; results of her lab tests are unremarkable. Her recommended course of treatment includes six rounds of chemotherapy conducted over the next 3 months followed by 4 weeks of radiation therapy.

Yolande is originally from Haiti and works full time as a fulfillment clerk for an online shopping business. Her husband works 50 hours a week in construction. The two older children are in elementary school and the two younger children are in full-time day care.

Questions for Analysis

1. Outline components of the initial nutrition assessment of this client. What additional information might you need to conduct a thorough nutrition assessment?
2. Develop a nutrition diagnostic statement that follows the pattern of the Nutrition Care Process.
3. Describe the appropriate nutrition intervention, including planning and implementation steps.
4. Develop a plan for monitoring and evaluation.

After three rounds of chemotherapy, Yolande has maintained her weight and does not report significant issues with nausea. However, she reports increasing fatigue and an intolerance to intense smells during food preparation. Develop an appropriate modification to her nutrition care plan.

Nutritional Needs of Cancer Patients

Patients with cancer typically have increased needs for energy, protein, vitamins and minerals, and fluid, based on the disease itself and its treatment. Individual needs and food tolerances vary, but general guidelines are the same.

Energy. Increased energy needs of cancer patients may result from either a disease-induced hypermetabolic state or tissue-healing requirements or both. Calculation of energy needs follows determination of the REE and additional needs for activity and tissue healing, in accordance with practice guidelines for the type of cancer. Macronutrient composition should be apportioned to allow sufficient protein for tissue healing and maintenance. In general, carbohydrates comprise the majority of the calorie intake, with fat providing approximately 30% of the total calories. Overfeeding must be avoided to minimize the risk of "refeeding syndrome."

Protein. Tissue protein synthesis, a necessary component of healing and rehabilitation, requires essential amino acids and nitrogen. Efficient protein use, which depends on an optimum protein-to-calorie ratio, promotes wound repair and tissue maintenance and prevents tissue catabolism. A protein intake of approximately 0.8–1.2 g/kg/day is adequate for most patients with cancer. In some instances, such as cachexia, protein supplementation may be necessary.

Vitamins and Minerals. Adequate intakes of vitamins and minerals are important for normal tissue function and healing and for maintenance of immune function. However, there is insufficient evidence to suggest efficacy of use of vitamin or mineral supplements (see the discussion on complementary and alternative medicine [CAM]). Key vitamins and minerals control protein and energy metabolism through their roles in cell enzyme systems. Increased dietary consumption of vegetables and fruits is the best way to obtain these vitamins and minerals.

Fluids. Most adults require approximately 35 mL/kg, or between 1500 and 2000 mL, of water each day. Adequate fluid intake is important to replace gastrointestinal (GI) losses or losses caused by infection and fever and to aid in renal excretion of metabolic breakdown products from destroyed cancer cells and medications.

Medical Nutrition Therapy of the Surgery Oncology Patient

One factor in successful surgical outcomes is adequate nutritional status of the patient; this is especially true of patients with cancer because their general condition may be weakened. Working with the patient to obtain optimal nutritional status preoperatively and providing appropriate nutrition support postoperatively are fundamental to the healing process.

Development of nutrition interventions that include provision of adequate nutrient intake to facilitate healing, including energy, protein, and micronutrients, is important both preoperatively and postoperatively. In addition, postoperative care may involve diet modification, particularly for those patients whose treatment involves surgery on some component of the GI system. For these patients, there may be specific challenges with normal eating, digestion, and absorption of nutrients that necessitate modifications in nutrient content, texture, and/or timing of eating. These challenges are characteristic of the portion of the GI tract involved rather than to the cancer itself, as seen in the following:

- *Head and neck surgery*, or resections in the oropharyngeal area, will affect ability to consume foods. During the healing process, individuals may require diets with texture modifications or, in some instances, modifications in the feeding modality such as placement

of feeding tubes. Depending on the nature of the surgery, long-term adjustments in texture and/or feeding modality may be necessary.
- *Gastric or intestinal resections* may result in numerous problems related to digestion and absorption of nutrients. During the healing process, modifications in macronutrient composition of the diet and in timing of feedings may be necessary. Depending on the nature of the surgery, long-term adjustments in macronutrient composition of the diet and in timing of feeding may be necessary. Particular attention should be paid to nutritional status for fat-soluble nutrients, fluid, and electrolytes.
- *Pancreatectomy* causes loss of digestive enzymes with ensuing malabsorption and weight loss; it also induces insulin-dependent diabetes mellitus.

Medical Nutrition Therapy of the Radiation Oncology Patient

Not all patients who receive radiation therapy will experience nutrition-related side effects (Table 25.3). Those who receive radiation treatments to the head and neck region, to parts of the GI tract, or to other organs within the abdominal cavity are most likely to experience nutrition-related signs and symptoms. Current practice guidelines from the AND include strong evidence for both pretreatment evaluation and ongoing medical nutrition therapy (MNT) for patients with head and neck cancers undergoing radiation therapy.[17] MNT has been demonstrated to improve calorie and protein intake, maintain anthropometric measures, and improve quality of life for these patients.

- *Head and neck* radiation therapy typically affects oral mucosa and salivary secretions, as well as the esophagus, influencing taste sensations and sensitivity to food temperature and texture. Common side effects include mucositis, xerostomia, hypogeusia, and dysnomia (alteration in or loss of smell). MNT may include modification in texture and temperature of the diet. In addition, modifications in appearance and aroma of foods may assist with management of anorexia and hypogeusia. For treatments that impact salivary secretions, treatments to stimulate saliva production include medications and inclusion of foods such as chewing gums and hard candies that stimulate saliva production. These treatments may mitigate impact on oral mucosa and dentition.
- *Abdominal cavity* radiation therapy may produce denuded bowel mucosa and loss of villi with tissue edema and congestion; vascular changes occur as a result of intimal thickening, thrombosis, ulcer formation, or inflammation. In the intestinal wall, fibrosis, stenosis, necrosis, or ulceration may occur. Modifications in macronutrient composition and timing of feedings may be necessary. Particular attention should be given to nutritional status for fat-soluble nutrients, fluids, and electrolytes.

In addition to these specific impacts on nutritional status, fatigue is very common among radiation oncology patients. This general fatigue may impact the patient's appetite or ability to prepare and consume food. The level of fatigue typically increases with duration of the radiation treatments and may significantly impact the patient's quality of life. Fortunately, the fatigue typically resolves following treatment.

Medical Nutrition Therapy of the Chemotherapy Patient

The impact of chemotherapeutic agents on rapidly reproducing normal cells is most apparent in cells of the bone marrow, GI tract, and hair follicles and accounts for many of the side effects of chemotherapy with implications for MNT.

- *Bone marrow effects* include interference with production of red and white blood cells and platelets. Although there are medications that stimulate production of these cell types, patients may benefit from modifications in diet to increase intake of vitamins and minerals

TABLE 25.3	**Dietary Modifications for Nutrition-Related Side Effects of Cancer**
Side Effect	**Suggested Dietary Modifications**
Anorexia	Provide small, frequent meals.
	Offer high-calorie, high-protein, nutrient-dense foods.
	Encourage consumption of the highest-calorie, highest-protein foods first.
	Avoid foods with offensive odors.
	Encourage favorite foods.
Altered perception of taste and odor	Maximize use of herbs and seasonings to enhance flavor of foods.
	If the flavor and aroma of red meats are offensive, avoid these foods and use alternative protein-rich foods such as chicken, fish, cheese, eggs, and milk.
	Serve cold foods and beverages more often than hot foods and beverages.
	Vary appearance (i.e., color, texture) of foods.
	Prepare and serve food in glass or porcelain rather than metal pans or dishes.
Stomatitis and mucositis	Provide foods in liquid, semisolid, or pureed form.
	Avoid tart, citric, or acidic foods and beverages.
	Avoid extremes in temperature.
	Avoid excessively seasoned and spicy foods.
	Avoid dry, coarse foods; serve foods with sauces or gravies.
	Encourage foods that melt or are liquid or soft textured at room temperature.
	Avoid carbonated beverages.
Xerostomia	Moisten foods with sauces, gravies, liquid, melted butter, mayonnaise, or yogurt.
	Encourage naturally soft, moist foods.
	Encourage sipping of liquids throughout the day.
	Avoid alcohol.
Dysphagia	Provide foods in liquid, semisolid, or pureed form.
	Maximize calorie and protein density of food as much as possible.
	Use commercially available liquid nutritional supplements.
Nausea and vomiting	Give small, frequent meals.
	Give dry foods without added fats or sauces, such as dry toast.
	Give liquids only between meals.
	Avoid greasy, fried, high-fat foods.
	Avoid foods with strong odors.
Diarrhea	Provide small, frequent meals.
	Encourage plenty of liquids to prevent dehydration.
	Avoid greasy, fried, high-fat foods.
	Consider limiting dietary lactose if these foods exacerbate symptoms.
	Avoid high-fiber foods.
	Avoid gassy, cruciferous vegetables, such as broccoli and cauliflower.
	Avoid caffeine.

From Dobbin M, Harmuller VW: Suggested management of nutrition-related symptoms. In MacCallum PD, Polisena CG, editors: *The clinical guide to oncology nutrition*, Chicago, 2000, American Dietetic Association.

involved in blood cell and platelet formation. Additional concerns associated with leukopenia include increased risk of foodborne infections. MNT for these patients might include the use of a neutropenic diet, in which foods identified by the FDA in the US Food Code as "potentially hazardous"[18] and other foods likely to have a high microbial count, such as raw fruits and vegetables, are restricted.

- *GI effects* include nausea and vomiting, stomatitis, anorexia, ulcers, and diarrhea. Nausea and vomiting are common side effects of chemotherapy, affecting more than 50% of patients at some point in their treatment. Chemotherapy-induced emesis (CIE) is managed with increasing effectiveness by following practice guidelines on use of antiemetic medications tailored for the emetogenic potential of chemotherapeutic agents.[19] Malabsorption and fluid and electrolyte imbalances may result from inadequate control of CIE and should be monitored by the registered dietitian (RD). In addition to the direct physical effects of CIE, it also significantly impacts quality of life.

Other GI effects may include postgastrectomy "dumping" syndrome, general diarrhea, constipation, flatulence, or specific lactose intolerance or surgery responses, such as those that occur with intestinal resections and various ostomies. Helpful guidance for patients with colostomies, ileostomies, or ileoanal reservoirs is necessary.

In addition to MNT approaches to managing symptoms associated with GI distress, such as alterations in macronutrient composition and timing of feeding, nutrition professionals should also recognize the impact of these symptoms on quality of life.

ALTERATIONS IN NUTRITIONAL STATUS ASSOCIATED WITH NEOPLASTIC DISEASE PROCESS

Malnutrition is the most common secondary diagnosis in patients with cancer and is a prognostic indicator for poor response to cancer therapy and shortened survival time. The disease process itself may be associated with three basic systemic effects—(1) anorexia, (2) altered metabolic state, and (3) negative nitrogen balance—which are often accompanied by a continuing weight loss. These effects may vary widely with individual patients, according to type and stage of the disease, from mild, scarcely discernible responses to the extreme forms of debilitating cachexia seen in advanced disease, and they are estimated to cause more than 50% of the cancer deaths.[20]

Anorexia associated with cancers is frequently accompanied by depression or discomfort during normal eating. This contributes to a limited nutrient intake at a time when the disease process causes an increased metabolic rate and nutrient demand. The weight loss associated with anorexia may contribute to development of cachexia, a severe wasting process.

Cachexia is not a local effect but rather arises from systemic metabolic effects, the etiology of which is not clearly understood. This extreme weight loss and weakness are associated with abnormalities in fat, muscle, and glucose metabolism, mediated in part by natural body defense substances such as tumor necrosis factor and cytokines.[20] Not all patients who develop cachexia will respond to MNT.

COMPLEMENTARY AND ALTERNATIVE MEDICINE

Patients who face treatments for cancers may choose to incorporate some form of complementary medicine as a component of their treatment. The National Center for Complementary and Alternative Medicine (NCCAM) of the NCI defines complementary and alternative medicine (CAM) as treatments that are not currently considered to be part of conventional medicine. In general, complementary medicine refers to treatments that are used in conjunction with conventional medicine, and alternative medicine refers to treatments that are used as an alternative to conventional medicine. Another term, which is

sometimes used interchangeably with CAM, is integrative medicine. NCCAM defines integrative medicine as treatment that combines conventional medicine with CAM therapies that have been reported to be safe and effective after being studied in patients. It is important that CAM therapies that are incorporated into care processes be those for which safety and effectiveness have been studied or those which are very unlikely to cause any harm, such as relaxation and various spiritual practices.

Four of 10 adults who participated in the 2007 National Health Interview Survey reported using CAM therapy in the past 12 months, with the most commonly used treatments being natural products and deep breathing exercises.[21] Similarly, approximately 4 in 10 cancer survivors reported using complementary therapies such as prayer, faith and spiritual practice, relaxation, and nutritional supplements, including vitamins.[22] There is limited evidence to suggest benefits from use of various botanical supplements, vitamin supplements, mineral supplements, or antioxidants as a component of cancer treatment. Similarly, there is concern, but limited evidence, that use of these supplements may interfere with the efficacy of various cancer treatments, particularly chemotherapeutic agents.[23]

The Society for Integrative Oncology has developed practice guidelines designed to assist health care professionals to make evidence-based decisions on various aspects with integrative oncology. These guidelines, presented in Table 25.4, have recommendations for the

TABLE 25.4	Practice Guidelines for Integrative Oncology			
Category	**Recommendation**	**Benefits and Risks**	**Implications**
The clinical encounter	Inquire about the use of complementary and alternative therapies as a routine part of initial evaluations of cancer patients.	Benefits clearly outweigh risks or burdens	Strong recommendation; may change when higher-quality evidence is available
The clinical encounter	All patients with cancer should receive guidance about the advantages and limitations of complementary therapies in an open, evidence-based, and patient-centered manner by a qualified professional. Patients should be fully informed of the treatment approach, the nature of the specific therapies, potential risks/benefits, and realistic expectations.	Benefits clearly outweigh risks or burdens	Strong recommendation; may change when higher-quality evidence is available
Mind-body medicine	Mind-body modalities are recommended as part of a multidisciplinary approach to reduce anxiety, mood disturbance, and chronic pain and improve quality of life.	Benefits clearly outweigh risks or burdens	Strong recommendation; can apply to most patients in most circumstances without reservation
Mind-body medicine	Support groups, supportive/expressive therapy, cognitive-behavioral therapy, and cognitive-behavioral stress management are recommended as part of a multidisciplinary approach to reduce anxiety, mood disturbance, chronic pain, and improve quality of life.	Benefits clearly outweigh risks or burdens	Strong recommendation; can apply to most patients in most circumstances without reservation

Continued

TABLE 25.4   Practice Guidelines for Integrative Oncology—cont'd

Category	Recommendation	Benefits and Risks	Implications
Touch therapy	For cancer patients experiencing anxiety or pain, massage therapy delivered by an oncology-trained massage therapist is recommended as part of multimodality treatment.	Benefits clearly outweigh risks or burdens	Strong recommendation; may change when higher-quality evidence is available
Touch therapy	The application of deep or intense pressure is not recommended near cancer lesions or enlarged lymph nodes, radiation field sites, medical devices (such as indwelling intravenous catheters), or anatomic distortions such as postoperative changes or in patients with a bleeding tendency.	Benefits closely balanced with risks and burden	Weak recommendation; best action may differ depending on circumstances or patients' or societal values
Physical therapy	Regular physical activities can play many positive roles in cancer care. Patients should be referred to a qualified exercise specialist for guidelines on physical activity to promote basic health.	Benefits clearly outweigh risks or burdens	Strong recommendation; can apply to most patients in most circumstances without reservation
Energy therapy	Therapies based on a philosophy of bioenergy fields are safe and may provide some benefit for reducing stress and enhancing quality of life. There is limited evidence as to their efficacy for symptom management, including reducing pain and fatigue.	Benefits clearly outweigh risks or burdens	Strong recommendation; can apply to most patients in most circumstances without reservation
Acupuncture	Acupuncture is recommended as a complementary therapy when pain is poorly controlled, when nausea and vomiting associated with chemotherapy or surgical anesthesia are poorly controlled, or when the side effects from other modalities are clinically significant.	Benefits clearly outweigh risks or burdens	Strong recommendation; can apply to most patients in most circumstances without reservation
Acupuncture	Acupuncture is recommended as a complementary therapy for radiation-induced xerostomia.	Benefits clearly outweigh risks or burdens	Strong recommendation; can apply to most patients in most circumstances without reservation
Acupuncture	Acupuncture does not appear to be more effective than sham acupuncture for treatment of vasomotor symptoms (hot flashes) in postmenopausal women in general. However, in patients experiencing severe symptoms not amenable to pharmacologic treatment, a trial of acupuncture treatment can be considered.	Benefits clearly outweigh risks or burdens	Strong recommendation; can apply to most patients in most circumstances without reservation
Acupuncture	For patients who do not stop smoking despite use of other options or those suffering from symptoms such as cancer-related dyspnea, cancer-related fatigue, chemotherapy-induced neuropathy, or postthoracotomy pain, a trial of acupuncture may be helpful, but more clinical studies of acupuncture are warranted.	Uncertainty in estimates of benefits, risks, and burden; may be closely balanced	Very weak recommendations; other alternatives may be equally reasonable
Acupuncture	Acupuncture should be performed only by qualified practitioners and used cautiously in patients with bleeding tendencies.	Benefits clearly outweigh risks or burdens	Strong recommendation; may change when higher-quality evidence is available
Diet and nutritional supplements	Research in diet and cancer prevention is based mainly on studies of populations consuming dietary components in whole-food form, with secure food supplies and access to a variety of food and drinks. Therefore nutritional adequacy should be met by selecting a wide variety of foods; dietary supplements are usually unnecessary.	Benefits clearly outweigh risks or burdens	Strong recommendation; can apply to most patients in most circumstances without reservation
Diet and nutritional supplements	It is recommended that patients be advised regarding proper nutrition to promote basic health.	Benefits clearly outweigh risks or burdens	Strong recommendation; can apply to most patients in most circumstances without reservation
Diet and nutritional supplements	Based on a current review of the literature, specific dietary supplements are not recommended for cancer prevention.	Benefits clearly outweigh risks or burdens	Strong recommendation; can apply to most patients in most circumstances without reservation

TABLE 25.4 Practice Guidelines for Integrative Oncology—cont'd

Category	Recommendation	Benefits and Risks	Implications
Diet and nutritional supplements	Evaluation of patients' use of dietary supplements prior to the start of cancer treatment is recommended. Also recommended are referral of cancer patients to trained professionals for guidelines on diets, nutritional supplementation, promotion of optimum nutritional status, management of tumor- and treatment-related symptoms, satisfaction of increased nutritional needs, and correction of any nutritional deficits while on active treatment.	Benefits clearly outweigh risks or burdens	Strong recommendation; can apply to most patients in most circumstances without reservation
Diet and nutritional supplements	It is recommended that dietary supplements, including botanicals and megadoses of vitamins and minerals, be evaluated for possible side effects and potential interaction with other drugs. Those that are likely to interact adversely with other drugs, including chemotherapeutic agents, should not be used concurrently with immunotherapy, chemotherapy, or radiation or prior to surgery.	Benefits clearly outweigh risks or burdens	Strong recommendation; can apply to most patients in most circumstances without reservation
Diet and nutritional supplements	For cancer patients who wish to use nutritional supplements, including botanicals for purported antitumor effects, it is recommended that they consult a trained professional. During the consultation, the professional should provide support, discuss realistic expectations, and explore potential benefits and risks. It is recommended that use of those agents occur only in the context of clinical trials, recognized nutritional guidelines, clinical evaluation of the risk/benefit ratio based on available evidence, and close monitoring of adverse effects.	Benefits clearly outweigh risks or burdens	Strong recommendation; may change when higher-quality evidence is available
Diet and nutritional supplements	As with nutritional supplementation during treatment, survivors should be evaluated for supplement use and referred to a trained professional for evaluation to meet specific nutritional needs and to correct nutritional deficits as indicated. For older cancer survivors, nutritional supplementation may reduce nutrient inadequacies, although survivors who use supplements are usually the least likely to need them.	Benefits closely balanced with risks and burden	Weak recommendation; best action may differ depending on circumstances or patients' or societal values

From Deng GE, Frenkel M, Cohen L, et al: Evidence-based clinical practice guidelines for integrative oncology: complementary therapies and botanicals, *J Soc Integr Oncol* 7(3):85, 2009.

clinical encounter and for various treatment modalities. The recommendations are also evaluated based on benefits versus risks/burdens and the strength of the recommendation. These guidelines, like those of other professional organizations, are reviewed on a regular basis and updated to reflect changes in the evidence base. These recommendations support the limited evidence available for effectiveness of nutritional supplements in cancer prevention, treatment, or survivorship.

TO SUM UP

Cancer is a term applied to abnormal, malignant growths in various body tissue sites. The cancerous cell is derived from a normal cell that loses control over cell reproduction through a variety of mechanisms, including mutation, carcinogens, radiation, and oncogenic viruses. It is also influenced by many epidemiologic factors such as diet, alcohol use, and smoking, as well as physical and psychologic stress factors.

Cancer therapy consists primarily of surgery, radiation, and chemotherapy. MNT for the patient with cancer should be highly individualized and depends on the response of each body system to the disease and to the treatment itself. It should carefully follow the NCP and be based on current practice guidelines. Because the course of treatment for cancers spans several months, regular monitoring and evaluation may be needed to ensure optimal nutrition care.

■ QUESTIONS FOR REVIEW

1. What is cancer? What may be roles of DNA methylation and apoptosis in development of cancers?
2. List and describe the rationale and mode of action of the types of therapies used to treat cancer.
3. Outline the general procedure for the nutritional management of a patient with cancer.

REFERENCES

1. National Cancer Institute: What Is Cancer? Available from http://www.cancer.gov/cancertopics/cancerlibrary/what-is-cancer.
2. Reif AE, Heeren T: Consensus on synergism between cigarette smoke and other environmental carcinogens in the causation of lung cancer, *Adv Cancer Res* 76:161, 1999.
3. Bollati V, Baccarelli A: Environmental epigenetics, *Heredity (Edinb)* 105:105, 2010.
4. Shen H, Laird PW: Interplay between the cancer genome and epigenome, *Cell* 153:38, 2013.
5. Mbeunkui F, Johann DJ Jr: Cancer and the tumor microenvironment: a review of an essential relationship, *Cancer Chemother Pharmacol* 63:571, 2009.
6. Wild CP: Environmental exposure in cancer epidemiology, *Mutagenesis* 24:117, 2009.
7. Gerhauser C: Cancer chemoprevention and nutriepigenetics: state of the art and future challenges, *Top Curr Chem* 329:73, 2013.
8. Jang H, Shin H: Current trends in the development and application of molecular technologies for cancer epigenetics, *World J Gastroenterol* 19:1030, 2013.
9. Franco EL, Duarte-Franco E, Ferenczy A: Cervical cancer: epidemiology, prevention and the role of human papillomavirus infection, *CMAJ* 164:1017, 2001.
10. Sourvinos G, Tsatsanis C, Spandidos DA: Mechanisms of retrovirus-induced oncogenesis, *Folia Biol(Praha)*. 46:226, 2000.
11. Shih WL, Fang CT, Chen PJ: Anti-viral treatment and cancer control, *Recent Results Cancer Res* 193:269, 2014.
12. National Cancer Institute: Cancer Trends Progress Report—2011/2012 Update, Bethesda, MD, 2012, NIH, DHHS. Available from http://progressreport.cancer.gov.
13. National Cancer Institute Fact Sheet: Cancer Health Disparities, 2013. Available from http://www.cancer.gov/cancertopics/factsheet/disparities/cancer-health-disparities.
14. National Cancer Institute Fact Sheet: Radiation Therapy and Cancer, 2010. Available from http://www.cancer.gov/cancertopics/factsheet/Therapy/radiation.
15. MedIndia Network for Health: Chemotherapy Drugs. Available from http://www.medindia.net/Patients/PatientInfo/chemotherapy-drugs-classification.htm.
16. Writing Group of the Nutrition Care Process/Standardized Language Committee: Nutrition Care Process and Model Part I: The 2008 Update, *J Am Diet Assoc* 108:1113, 2008.
17. Academy of Nutrition and Dietetics: Oncology Evidence Based Nutrition Practice Guidelines. Available from http://andevidencelibrary.com/topic.cfm?cat=3250.
18. Food and Drug Administration: US Food Code, 2009. Available from http://www.fda.gov/Food/GuidanceRegulation/RetailFoodProtection/FoodCode/ucm186464.htm.
19. Basch E, Prestrud AA, Hesketh PJ, et al: Antiemetics: ASCO Clinical Practice Guideline Update, *J Clin Oncol* 29:4189, 2012.
20. National Cancer Institute: Nutrition in Cancer Care PDQ. Available from http://www.cancer.gov/cancertopics/pdq/supportivecare/nutrition/HealthProfessional.
21. Barnes PM, Bloom B, Nahin RL: Complementary and alternative medicine use among adults and children: United States, 2007, *Natl Health Stat Report* 12:1, 2009.
22. Gansler T, Kaw C, Crammer C, et al: A population-based study of prevalence of complementary methods use by cancer survivors: a report from the American Cancer Society's studies of cancer survivors, *Cancer* 113:1048, 2008.
23. National Cancer Institute: Cancer and CAM: What the Science Says. Available from http://nccam.nih.gov/health/providers/digest/cancer-science.htm?nav=gsa.

FURTHER READINGS AND RESOURCES

Websites of Interest

- American Cancer Society. Excellent resource for the public and medical personnel. https://www.cancer.org/.
- Breastcancer.org. This nonprofit organization's website provides reliable, complete, and up-to-date information about breast cancer. https://www.breastcancer.org/.
- MD Anderson Cancer Center (University of Texas). One of the world's most-respected medical centers devoted entirely to care of cancer patients, research, and cancer prevention. https://www.mdanderson.org/.
- National Cancer Institute. Part of the National Institutes of Health (NIH), this is the principal government agency for cancer research and training. https://www.cancer.gov/.
- OncoLink (University of Pennsylvania). Founded by Penn cancer specialists to help cancer patients, families, health care professionals, and the general public. https://www.oncolink.com/.
- WebMD. Part of the WebMD medical information network, Cancer Health Center provided information regarding cancer. https://www.webmd.com/diseases_and_conditions/cancer.htm.

APPENDICES

Body Mass Index: (Second of Two BMI Tables)

BMI	36[a]	37	38	39	40	41	42	43	44	45	46	47	48	49	50	51	52	53	54
Height	Body Weight (pounds)																		
4 ft 10 in	172	177	181	186	191	196	201	205	210	215	220	224	229	234	239	244	248	253	258
4 ft 11 in	178	183	188	193	198	203	208	212	217	222	227	232	237	242	247	252	257	262	267
5 ft	184	189	194	199	204	209	215	220	225	230	235	240	245	250	255	261	266	271	276
5 ft 1 in	190	195	201	206	211	217	222	227	232	238	243	248	254	259	264	269	275	280	285
5 ft 2 in	196	202	207	213	218	224	229	235	240	246	251	256	262	267	273	278	284	289	295
5 ft 3 in	203	208	214	220	225	231	237	242	248	254	259	265	270	278	282	287	293	299	304
5 ft 4 in	209	215	221	227	232	238	244	250	256	262	267	273	279	285	291	296	302	308	314
5 ft 5 in	216	222	228	234	240	246	252	258	264	270	276	282	288	294	300	306	312	318	324
5 ft 6 in	223	229	235	241	247	253	260	266	272	278	284	291	297	303	309	315	322	328	334
5 ft 7 in	230	236	242	249	255	261	268	274	280	287	293	299	306	312	319	325	331	338	344
5 ft 8 in	236	243	249	256	262	269	276	282	289	295	302	308	315	322	328	335	341	348	354
5 ft 9 in	243	250	257	263	270	277	284	291	297	304	311	318	324	331	338	345	351	358	365
5 ft 10 in	250	257	264	271	278	285	292	299	306	313	320	327	334	341	348	355	362	369	376
5 ft 11 in	257	265	272	279	286	293	301	308	315	322	329	338	343	351	358	365	372	379	386
6 ft	265	272	279	287	294	302	309	316	324	331	338	346	353	361	368	375	383	390	397
6 ft 1 in	272	280	288	295	302	310	318	325	333	340	348	355	363	371	378	386	393	401	408
6 ft 2 in	280	287	295	303	311	319	326	334	342	350	358	365	373	381	389	396	404	412	420
6 ft 3 in	287	295	303	311	319	327	335	343	351	359	367	375	383	391	399	407	415	423	431
6 ft 4 in	295	304	312	320	328	336	344	353	361	369	377	385	394	402	410	418	426	435	443

[a]For lower body mass index (BMI) values, see Table 8.5.

To use the table, find the appropriate height in the left-hand column. Move across to a given weight. The number at the top of the column is the BMI of that height and weight. Pounds have been rounded off.

A BMI of 18.5 to 24.9 is the range of healthy weight; a BMI of 25 to 29.9 is the range of overweight; a BMI of 30 to 39.9 is the range of obese, and a BMI of 40 or over is classified as extreme obesity.

Modified from Clinical Guidelines on the Identification, Evaluation, and Treatment of Overweight and Obesity in Adults: The Evidence Report. National Heart, Lung, and Blood Institute, Bethesda, MD. https://www.nhlbi.nih.gov/health/educational/lose_wt/BMI/bmi_tbl2.htm.

Food Sources of Oxalates

VEGETABLES

- Baked beans
- Beans, green and wax
- Beet greens
- Beets
- Celery
- Chard, Swiss
- Chives
- Collards
- Eggplant
- Endive
- Kale
- Leeks
- Mustard greens
- Okra
- Peppers, green
- Rutabagas
- Spinach
- Squash, summer
- Sweet potatoes
- Tomato soup
- Tomatoes
- Vegetable soup

FRUITS

- Berries, all
- Concord grapes
- Currants
- Figs
- Fruit cocktail
- Plums
- Rhubarb
- Tangerines

NUTS

- Almonds
- Cashews
- Peanut butter
- Peanuts

BEVERAGES

- Chocolate
- Cocoa
- Draft beer
- Tea

OTHER

- Grits
- Soy products
- Tofu
- Wheat germ

Calculation Aids and Conversion Tables[a]

In 1799 a group of French scientists set up the metric system of weights and measures that, with refinements over the years, is still in use today. It is referred to as the *Système International d'Unités* (SI) and is used in most countries throughout the world. The United States continues to follow the British/American system of weights and measures. Given here are various conversion factors to help you make these transitions in your necessary calculations.

METRIC SYSTEM OF MEASUREMENT

Similar to our monetary system, this is a simple decimal system based on units of 10. It is uniform and used internationally.

Weight Units

1 kilogram (kg) = 1000 grams (gm or g)
1 g = 1000 milligrams (mg)
1 mg = 1000 micrograms (mcg or µg)

Length Units

1 meter (m) = 100 centimeters (cm)
1000 m = 1 kilometer (km)

Volume Units

1 liter (L) = 1000 milliliters (mL)
1 mL = 1 cubic centimeter (cc)

Temperature Units

The Celsius (C) scale is based on 100 equal units between 0°C (freezing point of water) and 100°C (boiling point of water). This scale is used entirely in all scientific work.

Energy Units

Kilocalorie (kcal) = Amount of energy required to raise 1 kg water 1°C
Kilojoule (kJ) = Amount of energy required to move a 1 kg mass 1 m by a force of 1 newton
1 kcal = 4.184 kJ

BRITISH/AMERICAN SYSTEM OF MEASUREMENT

Our customary system is made up of units having no uniform relationships. It is not a decimal system, but rather a collection of different units brought together in usage and language over time. It is predominantly used in the United States.

Weight Units

1 pound (lb) = 16 ounces (oz)

Length Units

1 foot (ft) = 12 inches (in)
1 yard (yd) = 3 ft

Volume Units

3 teaspoons (tsp) = 1 tablespoon (tbsp)
16 tbsp = 1 cup
1 cup = 8 fluid ounces (fl oz)
4 cups = 1 quart (qt)
5 cups = 1 imperial quart (qt) (Canada)

Temperature Units

The Fahrenheit (F) scale is based on 180 equal units between 32°F (freezing point of water) and 212°F (boiling point of water) at standard atmospheric pressure.

CONVERSIONS BETWEEN MEASUREMENT SYSTEMS

Weight

1 oz = 28.35 g (To change oz to g multiply by 28)
2.2 lb = 1 kg (To change lb to kg multiply by 0.45)

Length

1 in = 2.54 cm (To change in to cm multiply by 2.54)
1 ft = 30.48 cm (To change ft (12 in) to cm multiply by 30.48)
39.37 in = 1 m (To change in to m multiply by 39.37)

Volume

1 tsp = 5 ml
1 tbsp = 15 ml
1.06 qt = 1 L
0.85 imperial qt = 1 L (Canada)

Temperature

Boiling point of water: 100°C; 212°F
Body temperature: 37°C; 98.6°F
Freezing point of water: 0°C; 32°F

Interconversion Formulas

Fahrenheit temperature (°F) = 9/5 (°C) + 32
Celsius temperature (°C) = 5/9 (°F − 32)

---

[a]Differences in Canadian measurements are indicated where needed.

Federal Food Assistance Programs

Programs described here are funded by the US government with state allocations based on population, numbers of eligible participants, and other factors. States may be required to provide some degree of match in support of the statewide program.

Supplemental Nutrition Assistance Program (formerly the food stamp program)

Type of Program: Entitlement program.

Supervising Agency: US Department of Agriculture.

Population Served: Individuals and families with incomes falling within 130% of the federal poverty line and assets not exceeding federal guidelines. Supplemental Nutrition Assistance Program (SNAP) eligibility and benefits take into consideration household income, household size, housing costs, total assets, and work registration requirements. Eligibility requirements and benefits are adjusted annually.

Benefits Provided/Nutrition Standards: SNAP benefits increase the amount of money participants have available to spend for food. Recipients receive electronic debit cards (also known as EBT or electronic benefit transfer cards). At the time of purchase, funds are transferred from the client's account to the retailer's account. SNAP benefits can be used to buy most foods, as well as seeds and plants for raising food for the household, although there are exceptions.

The average monthly SNAP benefit is approximately $133 per person and approximately $275 per household.

The following items cannot be purchased using SNAP benefits:

- Hot, ready-to-eat foods
- Foods that will be eaten in the store
- Vitamin or mineral supplements, or medicines
- Pet foods
- Nonfood items such as soap, cleaning supplies, paper products, toothpaste, or cosmetics
- Tobacco items
- Alcoholic beverages

Number Served: More than 47 million people are served by SNAP benefits. Nearly half (45%) are children under the age of 18, and about 9% are age 60 or older. Fifty-six percent of SNAP households with children are single-adult households.

Availability of Nutrition Education: Most states offer nutrition education in conjunction with their SNAP program, but not all families are reached, and participation is voluntary. See discussion of the Supplemental Nutrition Assistance Program-Education Program (SNAP-Ed) later.

The Emergency Food Assistance Program (TEFAP)

Type of Program: States are required to set and enforce income eligibility requirements for distribution of food for home use; persons receiving meals are considered to be low income.

Supervising Agency: US Department of Agriculture with state oversight on the local level.

Population Served: Individuals and families must meet income guidelines (usually falling at or below the federal poverty line). Food is distributed to individuals and families through local food pantries and may be made available to school meal programs, meal programs for older adults, soup kitchens and emergency feeding locations, or child care facilities.

Benefits Provided/Nutrition Standards: Specific foods available for distribution are subject to market conditions but may include meat, poultry, or fish; canned fruits and vegetables; fruit juice; dried eggs; dried beans; pasta; milk; cheese; cereals; and soups.

Number Served: More than 840 million pounds of food can be distributed annually.

Availability of Nutrition Education: No formal mandate; may be provided at facilities or locations serving meals or distributing food.

CHILD NUTRITION PROGRAMS

National School Lunch Program

Type of Program: Serves all children of school age who choose to participate. Free lunches are provided to children whose family income falls at or below 130% of the federal poverty level, and lunches are available at a reduced cost of no more than 40 cents to children whose family incomes fall between 130% and 185% of the federal poverty level. Programs can choose to receive either commodity foods or cash reimbursement, based on the number of students served.

Supervising Agency: US Department of Agriculture.

Population Served: Children in public schools, nonprofit private schools, and residential child care programs.

Benefits Provided/Nutrition Regulations: Nutritionally balanced lunches provide one-third of the Dietary Reference Intakes (DRIs) for protein, vitamin A, vitamin C, iron, and calcium. New standards limit the number of kcalories served, in an effort to combat child obesity, and mandate increased servings of vegetables and fruits and the use of whole grains to comply with recommendations of the *Dietary Guidelines for Americans*. (For details, see the table "Nutrition Standards for School Meal Programs".)

Nutrition Standards for School Meal Programs

Grades	BREAKFAST MEAL PATTERN			LUNCH MEAL PATTERN		
	K–5	6–8	9–12	K–5	6–8	9–12
Meal Pattern: Amount of Food Per Week (Minimum Per Day)						
Fruits (cups)[a]	5 (1)	5 (1)	5 (1)	2½ (½)	2½ (½)	5 (1)
Total vegetables (cups)[a]	0	0	0	3¾ (¾)	3¾ (¾)	5 (1)
Dark Green	0	0	0	½	½	½
Red/Orange	0	0	0	¾	¾	1¼
Beans/Peas (Legumes)	0	0	0	½	½	½
Starchy	0	0	0	½	½	½
Other[b]	0	0	0	½	½	¾
Additional vegetable to reach total	0	0	0	1	1	1½
Grains (oz eq)[a,c]	7–10 (1)	8–10 (1)	9–10 (1)	8–9 (1)	8–10 (1)	10–12 (2)
Meat/Meat alternates (oz eq)[a]	0	0	0	8–10 (1)	9–10 (1)	10–12 (2)
Fluid milk (cups)[d]	5 (1)	5 (1)	5 (1)	5 (1)	5 (1)	5 (1)
Other Specifications: Daily Amount Based on the Average for the Week						
Minimum/Maximum kcal[e]	350–500	400–550	450–600	550–650	600–700	750–850
Saturated fat (% of total kcal)	<10	<10	<10	<10	<10	<10
Sodium (mg)	≤430	≤470	≤500	≤640	≤710	≤740
Trans fat	Nutrition label must indicate zero grams of trans fat per serving					

[a]See Table 1.2 for specific foods included in each of these groups and their nutritional contribution.
[b]Can be met with additional amounts from the dark green, red/orange, or legumes groups.
[c]At least half of the grains offered must be whole grains.
[d]Fluid milk must be low fat (1% milk fat or less) or fat free; can be flavored or unflavored.
[e]Foods of minimal nutritional value are not allowed.

Number Served: More than 100,000 schools and child care institutions offer a school lunch program, and meals are served to 31 million children every school day. Since the program's inception in 1946, it has served more than 224 billion meals.

Availability of Nutrition Education: Team Nutrition, a comprehensive nutrition education program developed to support the National School Lunch Program, contains integrated activities for the school classroom, lunchroom, and after-school setting that promote healthy food choices, portion control, and physical activity.

National School Breakfast Program

Type of Program: Serves all children of school age who choose to participate. Free breakfasts are provided to children whose family income falls at or below 130% of the poverty level, and breakfasts are available at a reduced cost to children whose family income falls between 130% and 185% of the poverty level. Children receiving the reduced price pay no more than 30 cents.

Supervising Agency: US Department of Agriculture.

Population Served: Children in public schools, nonprofit private schools, and residential child care programs.

Benefits Provided/Nutrition Regulations: Breakfast must provide one-fourth of the DRIs for protein, calcium, iron, vitamin A, and vitamin C. New standards control kcalories and promote healthful eating according to the *Dietary Guidelines for Americans.* (For details, see the table "Nutrition Standards for School Meal Programs.")

Number Served: More than 89,000 schools offer a breakfast program, and approximately 13 million children receive a daily breakfast; more than 10 million children obtain their breakfast at a free or reduced price.

Availability of Nutrition Education: See National School Lunch Program earlier.

Summer Food Service Program

Type of Program: Entitlement program where available.

Supervising Agency: US Department of Agriculture.

Population Served: Children meeting income eligibility guidelines.

Benefits Provided/Nutrition Regulations: Provides breakfast and/or a noon meal during summer vacation periods for children who depend on school meal programs for a significant portion of their nutrient intake. Meals must meet the same nutrition standards in place for the school breakfast and lunch programs. Summer meals are usually offered as part of a summer school or camp experience sponsored by a local school district, recreation department, or other government or nonprofit community agency.

Number Served: Nearly 2.5 million children participate daily.

Availability of Nutrition Education: May be offered as part of the educational or recreational program.

School Milk Program

Type of Program: Available to all children in participating schools or child care facilities.

Supervising Agency: US Department of Agriculture.

Population Served: Children in schools or child care facilities or summer camps that do not offer a breakfast or lunch program.

Benefits Provided/Nutrition Regulations: Participating schools or programs are reimbursed for the milk provided free to children meeting income guidelines or sold to children at a nominal cost. Milk must be pasteurized, fortified with vitamins A and D according to FDA standards, and be fat free or lowfat (1% fat).

Number Served: More than 4100 schools and child care facilities participate, serving 61 million half-pints of milk annually.

Availability of Nutrition Education: Unknown.

Child and Adult Care Food Program (CACFP)

Type of Program: Available to all children and adults in participating programs and facilities.

Supervising Agency: US Department of Agriculture.

Population Served: Child care programs serving children up to 12 years of age, adult day care programs serving persons age 60 and older, or day programs caring for individuals who are chronically impaired or disabled. Such settings include Head Start, other child care and adult day care centers, after-school programs, recreation centers, and emergency shelters caring for children.

Benefits Provided/Nutrition Regulations: Cash reimbursements to the program or facility providing meals are based on the recipients' eligibility for free or reduced-price meals. Children and adults are eligible to receive two meals and one snack each day, with an additional meal or snack if care exceeds 8 hours.

Number Served: 3.3 million children and 120,000 adults.

Availability of Nutrition Education: May be offered as part of a recreational or educational program.

Special Supplemental Nutrition Program for Women, Infants, and Children (WIC)

Type of Program: Participation is based on both income and medical or nutritional risk. Income eligibility (at or below 185% of the federal poverty line) does not ensure benefits: only those judged to be at medical or nutritional risk may participate to the extent that resources are available.

Supervising Agency: US Department of Agriculture; local programs are administered through state health departments.

Population Served: Women falling within income guidelines who are pregnant, postpartum, or breast-feeding, and infants and children up to 5 years of age, who are found to be at nutritional risk. Postpartum mothers can receive supplementary food for 6 months, and breast-feeding mothers can receive supplementary food for 12 months.

Eligibility must be determined by a health professional using the following criteria:

1. *Medically based risk:* anemia; underweight; overweight; poor prior pregnancy outcome; or history of pregnancy complications.
2. *Dietary risk:* mothers, infants, or children with nutrient deficiencies or nutrition-related medical conditions; inappropriate nutrition/feeding practices; or diets that fail to meet the *Dietary Guidelines for Americans.*

Benefits Provided/Nutrition Regulations: Participants receive vouchers or electronic debit cards to purchase designated foods that are rich sources of protein, calcium, iron, vitamin A, and vitamin C. The specific types and amounts of food provided in the food packages are based on the recipient's age or condition. Vouchers or debit cards may be used to purchase fresh fruits and vegetables at local farmers' markets. Food packages have been adjusted to comply more closely with the *Dietary Guidelines for Americans.*

Approved WIC Foods:

Infants
- Iron-fortified infant formula
- Iron-fortified infant cereal
- Baby food fruits and vegetables
- Baby food meat

Women and Children
- Vitamin C–rich fruit juice (unsweetened; fruit drinks not allowed)
- Vitamin C–rich vegetable juice (unsweetened)
- Eggs
- Milk (soy beverages, cheese, and tofu are also available)

- Cheese
- Iron-fortified breakfast cereal (may not contain more than 6 gm sucrose/sugar per 1 oz of dry cereal; whole grain preferred)
- Whole wheat bread (brown rice, oatmeal, and soft corn or whole wheat tortillas, and whole grain barley are also available)
- Peanut butter
- Dried or canned legumes
- Canned fish (light tuna, salmon, sardines, and mackerel)
- Fruits and vegetables (fresh, frozen, canned, dried; no added sugar, fats, or oils)

(The regulatory requirements for WIC food packages and the alternative choices available can be found at http://www.fns.usda.gov/wic/benefitsandservices/foodpkg.htm.)

Number Served: Of the 8.9 million individuals who receive monthly benefits, 4.7 million are children, 2.1 million are infants, and 2.1 million are women.

Availability of Nutrition Education: Public health nutritionists provide nutrition counseling at every WIC visit, and nutrition education is offered to individuals and groups. WIC also provides health screening and referrals to other indicated medical or social services.

WIC has been shown to be cost-effective in (1) reducing the number of premature and very-low-birth-weight infants, (2) reducing health care expenditures within the first 60 days after birth, and (3) lowering the number of preschool children with iron-deficiency anemia.

NUTRITION PROGRAM FOR THE ELDERLY/NUTRITION SERVICES INCENTIVE PROGRAM

Type of Program: Available to all persons 60 years of age or older regardless of income, although the program targets those with greatest social or economic needs, including low-income older adults, minority older adults, those residing in rural areas with limited access to services, and those at high risk of institutionalization. Participants are encouraged to make a donation to help meet the cost of the meals provided. Growing transportation needs are putting a strain on nutrition program budgets. The Nutrition Services Incentive Program was developed to provide additional funding to be used for food only.

Supervising Agency: Administration for Community Living/Administration on Aging, US Department of Health and Human Services.

Population Served: Congregate meals are offered at noon in community centers, churches, senior housing, or similar locations with familiarity and easy access for the aging population. Meals are home delivered for those who cannot leave their homes as a result of illness, disability, or a dependent family member; certification for home-delivered meals must be renewed every 6 months by a health or social services professional.

Benefits Provided/Nutrition Regulations: A hot meal is served on weekdays at noon at congregate meal sites; delivered meals may include a cold lunch for the evening meal or cold breakfast for the following day. As the costs of daily home delivery continue to rise, programs have experimented with weekly delivery of several frozen meals that can be defrosted and reheated as needed. Unfortunately, occasional delivery of several frozen meals takes away the social aspect of a daily visitor, important to a homebound or isolated senior. Meals should provide at least one-third of the DRIs for all nutrients as defined for persons older than 50 years and conform to the *Dietary Guidelines for Americans* in total fat, percent saturated fat, and sodium.

Number Served: More than 3 million older adults receive meals regularly.

Availability of Nutrition Education: May be offered as part of the educational or recreational program at congregate sites.

EXPANDED FOOD AND NUTRITION EDUCATION PROGRAM(EFNEP)/SUPPLEMENTAL NUTRITION ASSISTANCE PROGRAM-EDUCATION (SNAP-ED)

Type of Program: Services are directed toward individuals and families falling within the federal poverty guidelines and/or receiving SNAP benefits, but SNAP recipients are not required to participate.

Supervising Agency: US Department of Agriculture.

Population Served: Families with children, older adults, and youth. Individuals are recruited through neighborhood contacts, local welfare agencies, and the Special Supplemental Nutrition Program for Women, Infants, and Children.

Benefits Provided: The Expanded Food and Nutrition Education Program (EFNEP) and SNAP-Ed do not provide actual food but support limited-resource families through education, thereby helping them obtain the knowledge and skills necessary for making healthy food choices and using their food dollars wisely. Programs are delivered to both youth and adults by Cooperative Extension agents, paraprofessionals, and volunteers. Paraprofessionals are indigenous to the communities and populations they serve.

Number Served: More than 480,000 youth and 130,000 adults are reached by EFNEP each year, with an indirect effect on an additional 400,000 family members.

Availability of Nutrition Education: An experiential series of lessons offers hands-on opportunities to develop skills in food preparation, food safety, food budgeting and management, and wise shopping. Group classes, media methods, one-on-one instruction, and educational mailings are used to reach various audiences. The EFNEP reporting system indicates that 85% of adults improve their food management practices (e.g., planning meals and shopping more wisely), and 95% increase their daily fruit and vegetable intakes by 1 cup; nearly 60% of youth improve their food preparation and food safety skills.

Further Information

Further information on all US Department of Agriculture food assistance programs can be accessed at https://www.usda.gov/topics/food-and-nutrition. An overview of nutrition programs for older adults supervised by the Administration for Community Living/Administration on Aging can be found at https://www.acl.gov/programs.